Treatment Planning Steps in
Oral Implantology
A Color Atlas

Treatment Planning Steps in
Oral Implantology
A Color Atlas

Editors

Lanka Mahesh BDS MBA DHA DHHM
Visiting Professor, Universidad Católica San Antonio de Murcia (UCAM)
Murcia, Spain
Honorary Professor, ITS College of Dentistry
Ghaziabad, Uttar Pradesh, India
Specialized Implant Practice
New Delhi, India

Praful Bali BDS MDS Cert. Implantology, UCLA (USA)
Director, Center of Advanced Dental Education (CADE)
Director, International Center of Excellence in Dentistry (ICED)
Founder Treasurer, Academy of Oral Implantology (AOI)
Fellow of International College of Oral Implantologists (ICOI), USA
Assistant Editor, International Journal of Oral Implantology and Clinical Research
New Delhi, India

Craig M Misch DDS MDS
Clinical Associate Professor
Departments of Periodontics and Prosthodontics
University of Florida
Guinesville, Florida, USA
University of Alabama
Tuscaloosa, Alabama, USA

David Morales Schwarz MDS
Specialist in Clinical Dental M & M
Valladolid, Spain

Forewords

Maurice A Salama
RK Bali

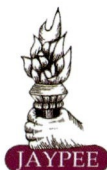

JAYPEE *The Health Sciences Publisher*
New Delhi | London | Panama

Jaypee Brothers Medical Publishers (P) Ltd

Headquarters

Jaypee Brothers Medical Publishers (P) Ltd.
4838/24, Ansari Road, Daryaganj
New Delhi 110 002, India
Phone: +91-11-43574357
Fax: +91-11-43574314
E-mail: jaypee@jaypeebrothers.com

Overseas Offices

J.P. Medical Ltd.
83, Victoria Street, London
SW1H 0HW (UK)
Phone: +44-20 3170 8910
Fax: +44(0)20 3008 6180
E-mail: info@jpmedpub.com

Jaypee Brothers Medical Publishers (P) Ltd.
17/1-B, Babar Road, Block-B, Shaymali
Mohammadpur, Dhaka-1207
Bangladesh
Mobile: +08801912003485
E-mail: jaypeedhaka@gmail.com

Jaypee-Highlights Medical Publishers Inc.
City of Knowledge, Bld. 235, 2nd Floor, Clayton
Panama City, Panama
Phone: +1 507-301-0496
Fax: +1 507-301-0499
E-mail: cservice@jphmedical.com

Jaypee Brothers Medical Publishers (P) Ltd.
Bhotahity, Kathmandu, Nepal
Phone: +977-9741283608
E-mail: kathmandu@jaypeebrothers.com

Website: www.jaypeebrothers.com
Website: www.jaypeedigital.com

Inquiries for bulk sales may be solicited at: jaypee@jaypeebrothers.com

Treatment Planning Steps in Oral Implantology: A Color Atlas

First Edition: **2018**

ISBN: **978-93-5270-059-2**

Printed at : Replika Press Pvt. Ltd.

Dedicated to

Dad and Mom wherever they maybe.

Lanka Mahesh

Contributors

Sujit Bopardikar MDS
Prosthodontist
Private Practice
Mumbai, Maharashtra, India

Cary Bopiah
BDS MFDS (RCPS Glasg) MJDF (RCS Eng)
MDS (OMFS)
Fellow ICOI, Diplomate ICOI
Director, Sensura (UK) Limited
Hornsey, London, UK

Douglas F Dompkowski
Private Practice
Maryland, USA

Stutee Grewal BDS MDS DNB
Orthodontist
Professor
Santosh Dental College and Hospital
Ghaziabad, Uttar Pradesh, India
Private Practice: Gurugram, Haryana, India

José Luis Calvo Guirado DDS PhD Eu PhD MS
Full Professor in Oral Surgery and Implant Dentistry
Universidad Católica San Antonio de Murcia (UCAM)
Murcia, Spain
Bidoctor in Dentistry and Bioengineering in Biomaterials
Chairman of International Dentistry Research Cathedra
Director of Murcia Biomaterials and Implants Research
Group (MBIRG)
Research Professor
Department of Prosthodontics and Digital Technologies
School of Dental Medicine
State University of New York
Stony Brook, New York, USA
Visiting Professor of Faculty of Medicine and Dentistry
University of Belgrade
Studentski trg 1, Belgrade, Serbia

Amit Gulati MDS
Periodontist and Implantologist
Private Practice
Mumbai, Maharashtra, India

Shweta Gupta BDS PGDHHM
Certificate Implantology
University of California,
Los Angeles, California, USA
Dental Surgeon and Implantologist
Director: Dental Solutions
Ex. Resident: Ram Manohar Lohia Hospital, New Delhi, India
Ex. Dental Surgeon: Sir Ganga Ram Hospital, New Delhi, India
Ex. Dental Surgeon: Maharaja Agrasen Hospital
New Delhi, India

Vishal Gupta
Private Practice
New Delhi and
Agra, Uttar Pradesh, India

Robert A Horowitz DDS
Clinical Assistant Professor
New York University College of Dentistry
Departments of Periodontology,
Implant Dentistry and Oral Surgery
New York, New York, USA

Saj Jivraj BDS MSED
Clinical Associate Professor
Herman Ostrow USC School of Dentistry
Los Angeles, California, USA
Honorary Clinical Teacher
Eastman Dental Institute
England, London
Private Practice Limited to
Prosthodontics and Implant Dentistry
Oxnard, California, USA

Vani Kalra BDS MDS
Prosthodontist and Implantologist
Member: German Society of Oral Implantologist
Member: International Congress of Oral Implantologist
Member: Academy of Oral Implantology
Ex-Assistant Professor: Shree Bankey Bihari Dental College
Private Practice: New Delhi, India

Jin Y Kim DDS MPH MS FACD
Diplomate, American Board of Periodontology
Diplomate, American Board of Oral Implantology/
Implant Dentistry
Diplomate, Internatonal Congress of Oral Implantologists
Fellow, American College of Dentists
Fellow, American Academy of Implant Dentistry
Fellow and Board Member, World Academy of Ultrasonic
Piezoelectric Bone Surgery
Lecturer, UCLA School of Dentistry
Los Angeles, California, USA

Sudhindra Kulkarni MDS (Perio.) DICOI
Faculty Professor and Head
Department of Implantology and Periodontics
Chief Consultant
Faculty Practice, SDM College of
Dental Sciences and Hospital
Dharwad, Karnataka, India
Private Practice
Oris Dental, Center for Oral Rehabilitation
Hubli, Karnataka, India

Tarun Kumar MDS
Professor and Head, Bapuji Implant Center
Associate Dean (Academics)
Bapuji Dental College and Hospital
Davangere, Karnataka, India

Gregori M Kurtzman
DDS MAGD FPFA FACD FADI DICOI DADIA
General Practitioner
Silver Spring, Maryland, USA

Bach Le DDS MD FICD FACD
Clinical Associate Professor
Department of Oral and Maxillofacial Surgery
The Herman Ostrow School of Dentistry of USC
Los Angeles County/USC Medical Center
Los Angeles, California, USA

Glenn Mascarenhas BDS MSC
Prosthodontist, Private Practice
Mumbai, Maharashtra, India

Ziv Mazor DMD
Periodontist, Associate Professor
Titu Majorescu University
Bucharest, Romania
Private practice: Ra'anana, Israel

Sourabh Nagpal BDS MDS
Prosthodontist and Implantologist
Director: Matrix Dental and Skin Lounge
Private Practice: New Delhi, India

Sushil Nijhawan BDS MDS MBA COI (Germany)
Prosthodontist and Implantologist
Professor and Head
Department of Dental Surgery
Muzaffarnagar Medical College, Uttar Pradesh, India
Private Practice: New Delhi, India

Jesus Gomez Perez
Private Practice
Madrid, Spain

Nitika Poonia MDS
Periodontist and Implantologist
New Delhi, India

Bassam F Rabie
Fellow American Academy of Implant Prosthodontics
Diplomat, International Congress of Oral Implantologists
Prosthodontist
Pittsburgh, Pennsylvania, USA

Monica Restrepo
Private Practice
Bogota, Columbia

Alejandro Vivas Rojo DDS MS
Oral and Maxillofacial Surgeon
DDS–Universidad Central de Venezuela, Caracas
DMD–Universidad De Granada, Spain
Residency Oral Surgery
Hospital Gregorio Marañon
Madrid, Spain

Maurice A Salama DMD
Periodontist and Orthodontist
Managing General Partner
Goldstein Garber and Salama
Founder, Dental XP
Atlanta, Georgia, USA

Dong Seok Sohn DDS PhD
Professor
Department of Oral and Maxillofacial Surgery
Catholic University Medical Center
Daegu, Republic of Korea

Narayan TV MDS
Oral Pathologist and Implantologist
Bengaluru, Karnataka, India

Associate Contributors

Dildeep Bali BDS MDS
Endodontist and Esthetic Dentist
Professor and Head
Department of Conservative Dentistry and Endodontics
Santosh Dental College and Hospital
Ghaziabad, Uttar Pradesh, India
Private Practice: New Delhi, India

Shweta Bali BDS MDS
Periodontist
Professor and Head
Santosh Dental College and Hospital
Ghaziabad, Uttar Pradesh, India
Private Practice: New Delhi, India

Ashish Chowdhary BDS MDS
Prosthodontist and Implantologist
Professor, School of Dental Sciences
Sharda University, Greater Noida
Uttar Pradesh, India
Private Practice: New Delhi, India

Sumit Datta BDS MDS
Orthodontist and Implantologist
Private Practice: New Delhi, India

Sunil Datta BDS MDS
Prosthodontist and Implantologist
Senior Consultant
Sir Ganga Ram Hospital, New Delhi, India
Private Practice: New Delhi, India

Mandeep Grewal BDS MDS
Conservative Dentistry and Endodontics
Professor and Head
PDM Dental College and Hospital
Bahadurgarh, Haryana, India
Private Practice: Gurugram, Haryana, India

Priyank Jayna BDS MDS
Orthodontist
Fellow, International College of Dentists
Member, Indian Orthodontic Society
Member, Indian Society of Cleft Lip,
Palate and Craniofacial Anomalies
Ex-Assistant Professor
Shree Bankey Bihari College
Masuri, Uttar Pradesh, India
Private Practice: New Delhi, India

Hilde Morales
Degree in Dentistry (University of Alfonso X el Sabio)
Master of Orthodontics (University of Lleida)
Master in Implantology and Oral Surgery
(University of Lleida)
Master in Methodology of Research in Health
Management
(University of Alfonso X el Sabio)
Functional occlusion course (Dawson Academy)
Private Practice
Valladolid, Spain

Foreword

Since the term osseointegration was first coined over 50 years ago by Professor Branemark, Implant Dentistry has advanced by leaps and bounds and even more so in the past two decades.

We have seen a vast increase in scientific knowledge about biological and biomechanical factors relating to the success or failure of implant therapies.

Over the years, significant advances in the evolution of Bone Grafting, Guided Bone Regeneration (GBR) and Sinus Augmentation techniques have changed the face of contemporary tooth replacement dentistry.

This book nicely demonstrates this journey through the eyes of many regarded clinicians featuring most aspects of implant therapeutics with clear illustrations of various clinical situations showcasing the most modern biomaterials, instruments, and implant systems used in implant dentistry today.

It is my pleasure to have participated in this journey with my dear friend, Dr Lanka Mahesh. I have known him to be one of the finest gentlemen and most dedicated clinicians and implantologists I have had the pleasure to interact with. I wish him and all the contributing clinicians good luck with this effort in bringing out this well designed Color Atlas of Oral Implantology which should be enjoyed by all clinicians interested in modern implant dentistry.

Maurice A Salama DMD
Periodontist and Orthodontist
Managing General Partner
Goldstein Garber and Salama
Founder, Dental XP
Atlanta, Georgia, USA

Foreword

I have had the privilege to write forewords for many books on different subjects but this one is special to me, as it is for my son. It gives me immense pleasure in writing this foreword on the Color Atlas of Oral Implantology, authored by Dr Lanka Mahesh, Dr Praful Bali, Dr Craig M Misch and Dr David Morales Schwarz. This publication covers almost all aspects of advanced Implantology, beautifully photographed and illustrated with each and every procedure simplified. I congratulate the authors and all the contributors, who have looked into each and every minor details of each case presented.

I am confident that this Atlas will be of immense help, for both budding and practicing implantologists, as they can appreciate specialized cases of different genre compiled in one time.

The photographs of this Color Atlas show that the authors are thorough clinicians and have put in a lot of hardwork, skill, experience of many many years and time to achieve such good clinical results. I congratulate them for bringing out this unique collection of their clinical work which is surely an educational resource and valuable publication.

RK Bali
Padmashree Awardee
Dr BC Roy National Awardee

Preface

"If the doors of perception were cleansed, everything would appear to man as it is, infinite."
—William Blake, The marriage of Heaven and Hell, 1793.

The information technology boom has seen the coming of age of Dentistry in general and Implant Dentistry in particular. While the burgeoning growth of social media has meant that a new type of learning, known as crowd learning has emerged, it has also meant that the control over the information transfer has been lost, and along with the good information, there is a whole lot of misinformation, anecdotal information which is contrary to the principles of evidence based dentistry as practiced today. It was this that led us, a group of conscientious clinicians from around the globe, to come together and collectively publish this *Treatment Planning Steps in Oral Implantology: A Color Atlas* with the aim of showcasing the spectrum of procedures which have shown predictable outcomes in the hands of innumerable clinicians. This is a book aimed at clinicians who are already in the practice of Implant Dentistry, to enable them to stay abreast with the latest in surgical and restorative protocols, as well as a must read for the students of Implant Dentistry, to understand the scope of the science, from procedures for developing optimal aesthetics, to managing deficient bone in the posterior maxilla and mandible, to various fixed and removable prosthetic options for full arch reconstructions and bone regeneration techniques and finally, a section on complications and their management.

Here's wishing you an enjoyable and informative reading.

Lanka Mahesh
Praful Bali

Acknowledgments

Sana and Saisha my little girls for keeping me going in this chaotic world and making life worth living.

The toughest part in writing a book is probably the acknowledgment, apart from getting a great publisher and recruiting some of the world's best known clinicians and researchers.

When there are so many people to thank one is sure to forget a name. Therefore, I would like to acknowledge the thousands of patients who reposed their faith in me, all my contributing authors, team of Jaypee Brothers Medical Publishers, New Delhi, India especially Ms Chetna Malhotra Vohra (Associate Director–Content Strategy) and Ms Nedup Bhutia (Development Editor) for their untiring effort and tolerating me when I kept breathing down their neck at all given times, thank you for tolerating me.

To my father who made me what I am and taught me life more than medicine and who taught me it is better to have a helping hand than a praying hand. I hope I have lived upto his expectations.

My teachers, colleagues and all the good human beings I interact with daily who help me keep the faith.

My special thanks to Mr Nayak for giving me most of his waking hours over the last twenty years and having helped me in hundreds of surgeries all over the country, I can never thank you enough. Mr Suresh Kumar for all his help with the photography and everything else he does for me.

To the Almighty for His constant blessings.

And to "someone somewhere" who's watching over me.

Lanka Mahesh

Acknowledgments

I share my happiness and excitement in making of this Color Atlas of Oral Implantology. This book had been a challenging job and an eye-opener for me. I bow down to all the previous authors who have taken out books, which we as budding implantologists read through. Each page, every picture, every thought that has gone into the book has taken shape very well and I am overjoyed and satisfied with the end result.

Words cannot express my love and gratitude for my parents because of whom I am what I am today. They have been the source of encouragement and support throughout my career by helping me at each stage. My father, Dr RK Bali being one of the eminent dental surgeons in the country has been one of the earliest dentists to start implantology in India and he has shared and taught me implantology at many stages during my initial days. I cannot thank enough my wife, Dr Dildeep Bali, who stood by me in tough times and had been a source of encouragement to complete this book.

My respect and gratitude to my mentor and guide, Prof Dr N Sridhar Shetty, who awakened the interest for implants during my postgraduation period.

The Basic Implantology training that I did in Manipal has been a stepping stone and has gone a long way in my overall grooming as a successful Implantologist and Dr Rudd Hertel was instrumental in the whole process.

I express my sincere thanks Dr Shahvir Nooryezdan for constant support and encouragement.

I also express my gratitude to Dr Sascha Jovanovic, Dr Egon Ewue and Dr Istvan Urban. The Masters Clinical Program, conducted by them has helped me improve my skills as an esthetic implant specialist tremendously and I consider their work a bench mark, a true inspiration for me.

I thank Dr Ruhani Cheema, Dr Radhika Chawla and Ms Jaspreet Oberoi for helping me with the book.

Lastly, my sincere thanks to Dr Lanka Mahesh to have made me do this, he pushed me to complete the book.

Love to my sister, Dr Stutee Grewal and my children Ahan and Amaiyra.

Praful Bali

Contents

SECTION 2: IMMEDIATE IMPLANTATION INTO EXTRACTED SOCKET

SECTION 3: MANAGEMENT OF POSTERIOR MAXILLA INCLUDING SINUS GRAFTING

SECTION 4: MANAGEMENT OF POSTERIOR MANDIBLE

SECTION 5: GUIDED BONE REGENERATION (GBR)

SECTION 6: SOFT TISSUE GRAFTING

SECTION 7: PROSTHETIC OPTIONS: SINGLE TOOTH TO FULL ARCH

SECTION 8: COMPLICATIONS AND FAILURES

SECTION 1

Anterior Esthetics

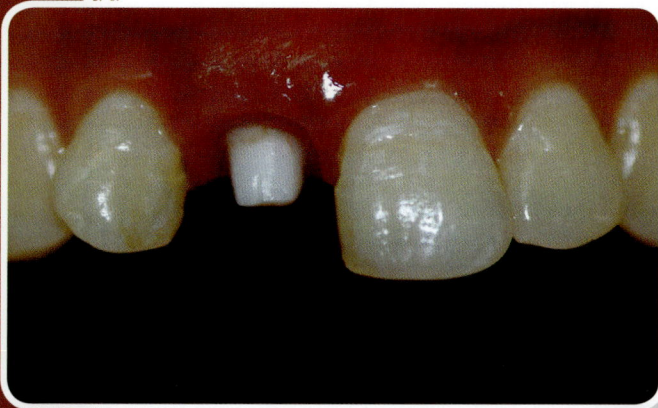

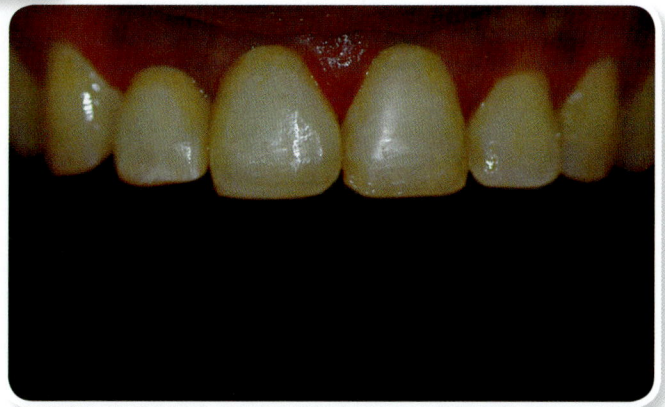

Praful Bali

HARD AND SOFT TISSUE AUGMENTATION TO ACHIEVE OPTIMAL ANTERIOR ESTHETICS. TISSUE ENGINEERING AND FINE TUNING DONE WITH SET OF PROTOTYPES

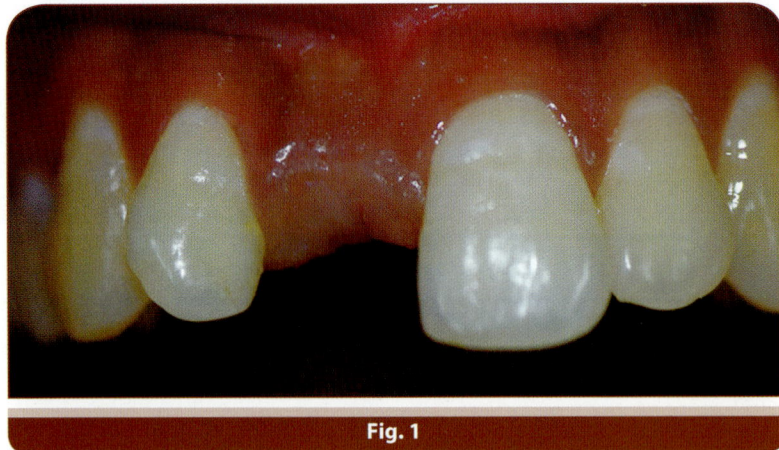

Fig. 1

Preoperative—facial view—missing tooth no #11 (right upper central incisor) **(Fig. 1)**.

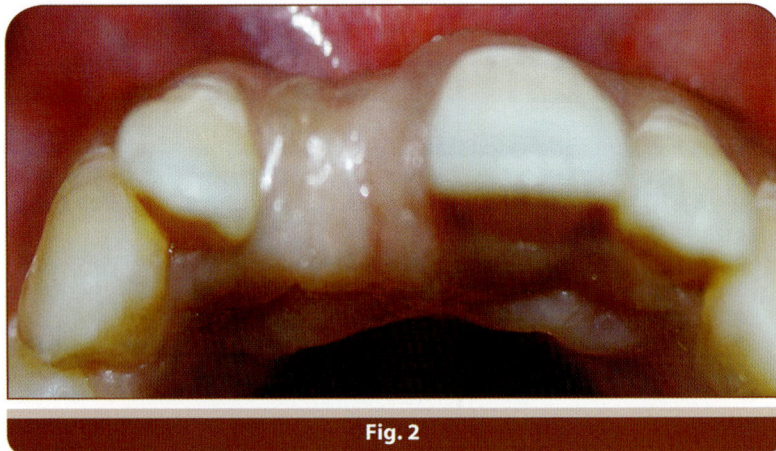

Fig. 2

Preoperative—occlusal view, note the facial dip indicating the deficiency of buccal bone. Still, there seems to be adequate bone to place a good size implant and do grafting in the same surgical visit **(Fig. 2)**.

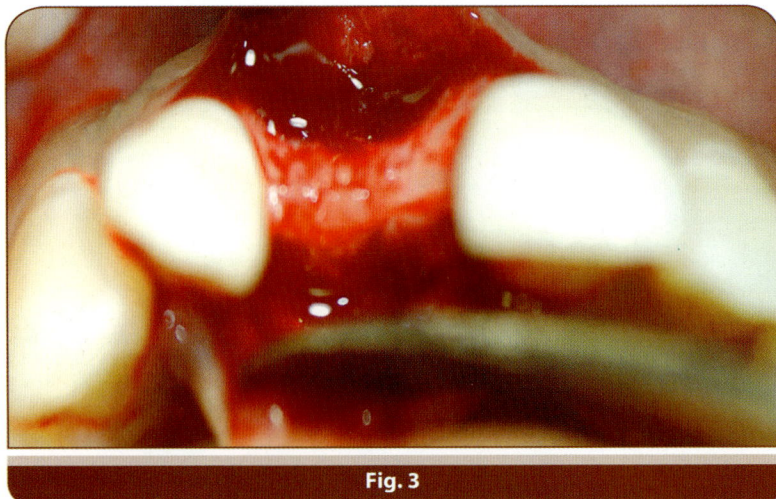

Fig. 3

Full thickness flap reflection done exposing the site of osteotomy. Note the buccal plate deficiency **(Fig. 3)**.

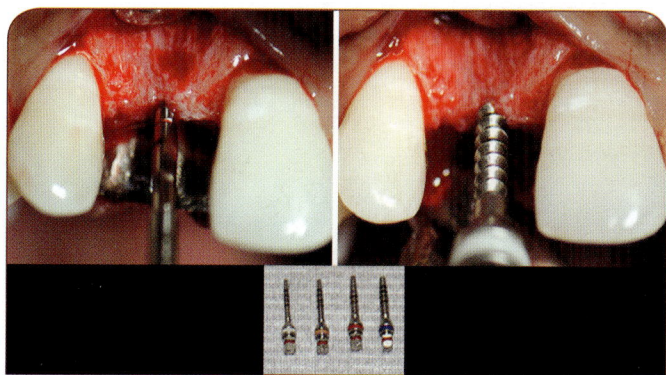

Fig. 4

Use of expanders to expand the bone and also preserving the bone at the crucial buccal area **(Fig. 4)**.

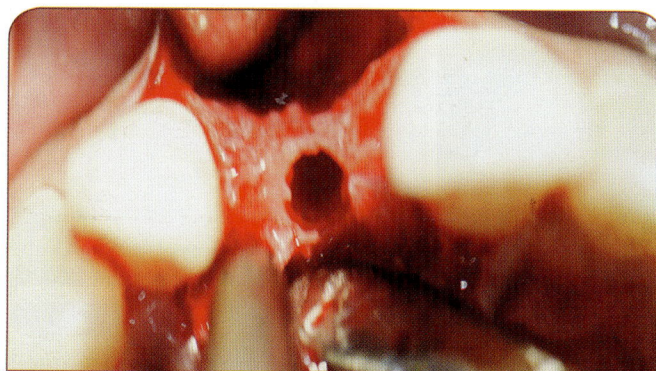

Fig. 5

Final osteotomy in 3D position **(Fig. 5)**

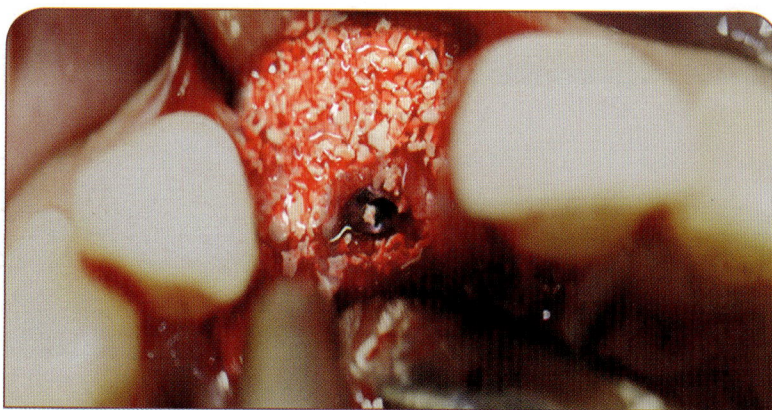

Fig. 6

GBR—Zenograft—Bio-Oss placed to create proper bone esthetics and also provide extra bulk of hard tissue around the implant **(Fig. 6)**.

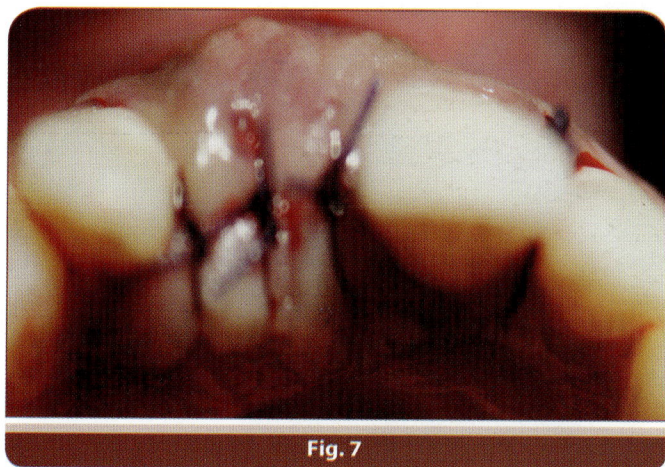

Fig. 7

Collagen membrane placed over the graft to complete the GBR and suturing done **(Fig. 7)**.

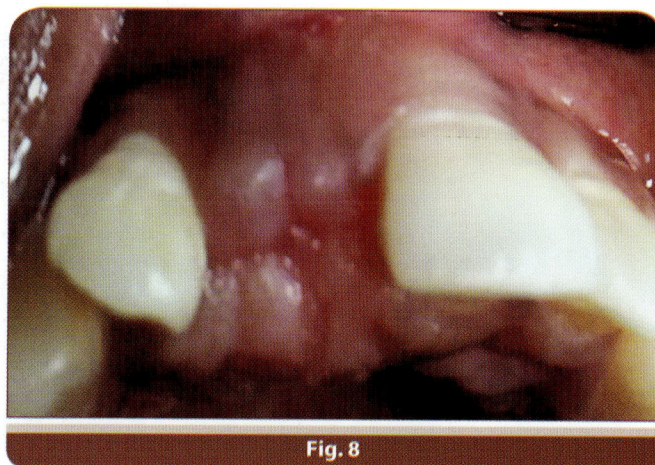

Fig. 8

4 months post healing **(Fig. 8)**.

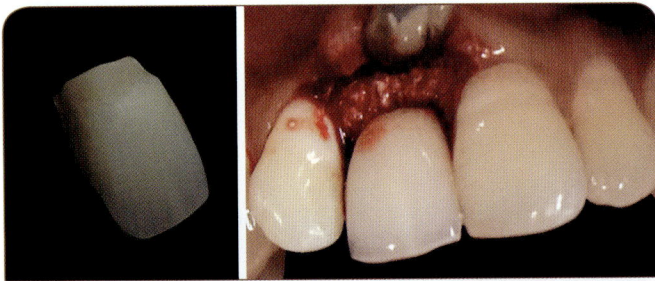

Fig. 9

A stock Zirconia abutment is shaped extraorally and torqued to 35 Ncm—One Abutment One Time Concept. A Protemp crown is cemented with temporary cement as the 1st Prototype **(Fig. 9)**.

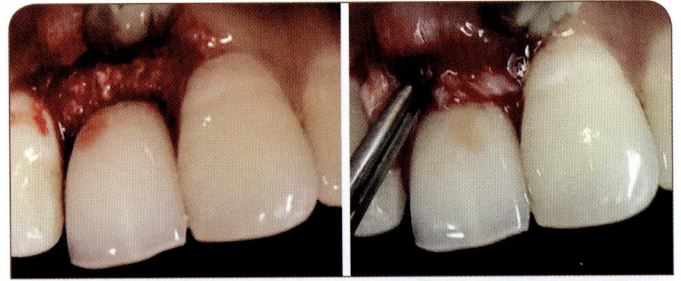

Fig. 10

Connective tissue graft done **(Fig. 10)**.

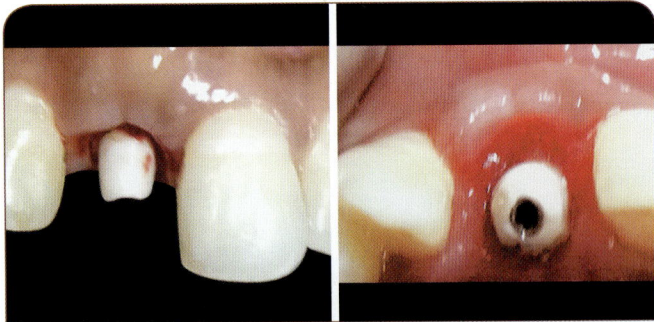

Fig. 11

Sufficient soft and hard tissue formation after GBR and connective tissue graft and a healing period of 2 months **(Fig. 11)**.

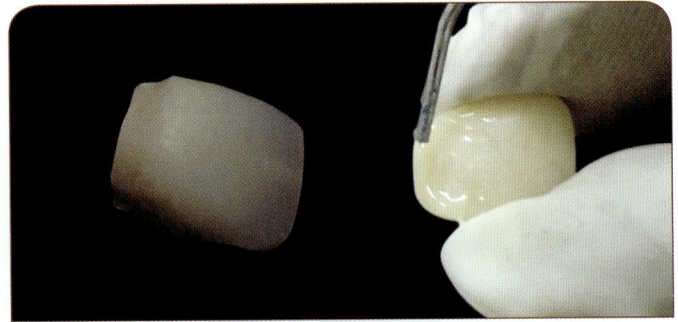

Fig. 12

A series of temporary prototypes are modified by adding composite till satisfactory gingival maturation and esthetics are achieved **(Fig. 12)**.

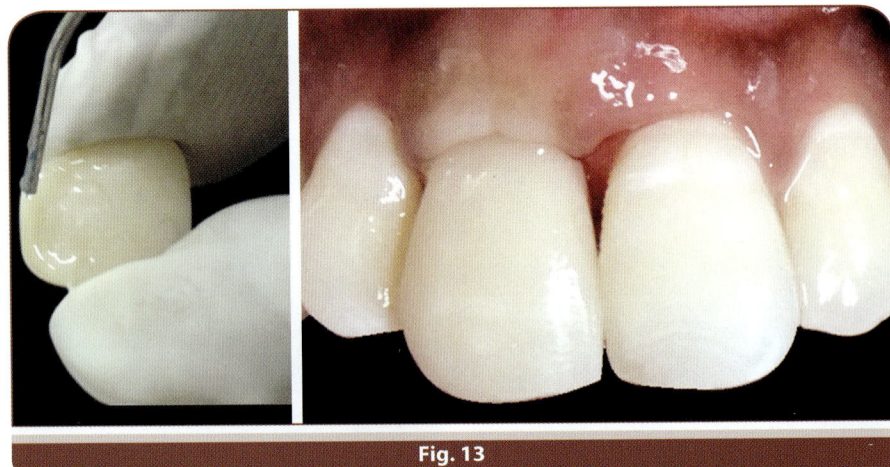

Fig. 13

Final prototype—to mimic the adjacent central incisor **(Fig. 13)**.

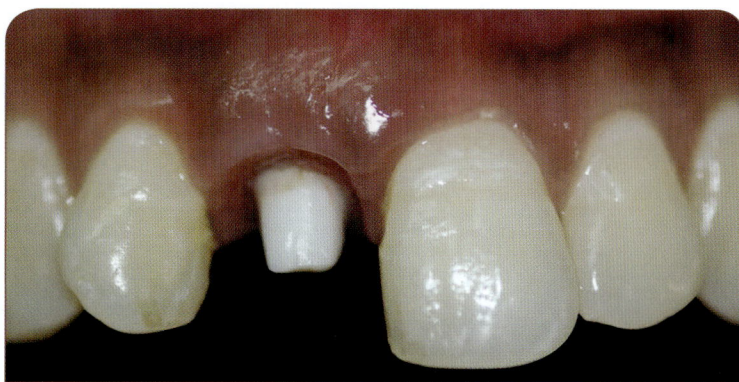

Fig. 14

Soft tissue integration around the Procera abutment. Impression made for final crown **(Fig. 14)**.

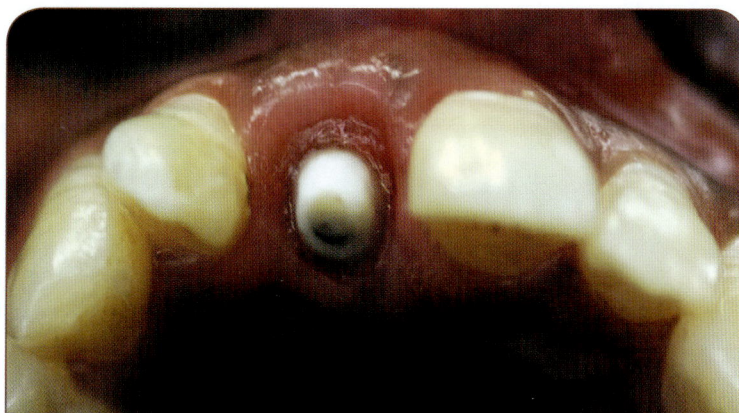

Fig. 15

Hard and soft tissue integration **(Fig. 15)**.

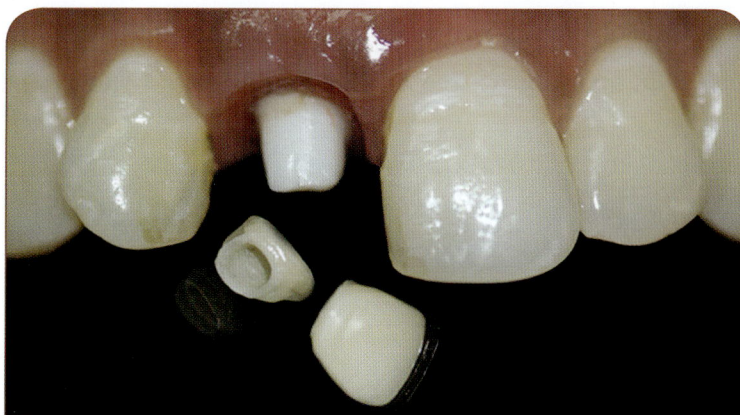

Fig. 16

Final Procera crown **(Fig. 16)**.

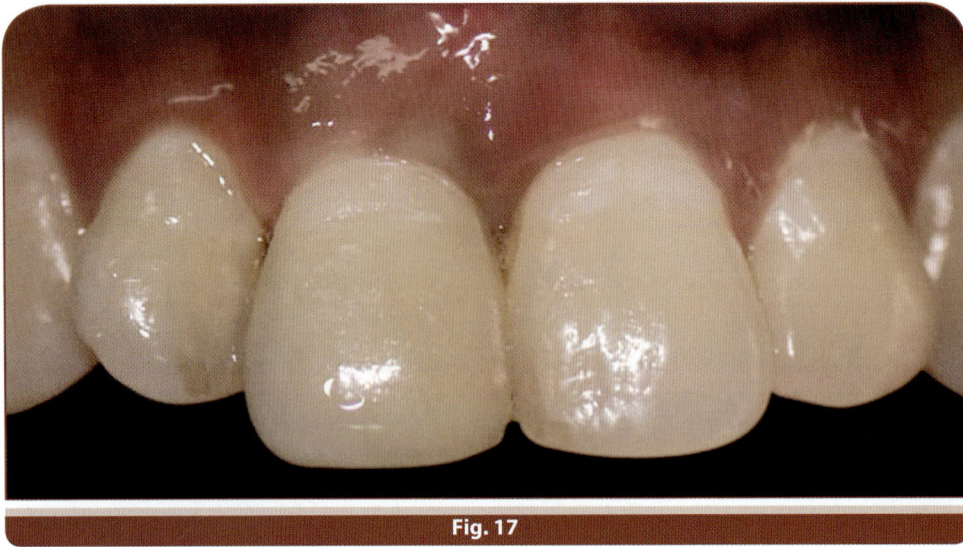

Fig. 17

Permanant Procera crown cemented in position. Tissue engineering and fine tuning of gingiva results in a near perfect result **(Fig. 17)**.

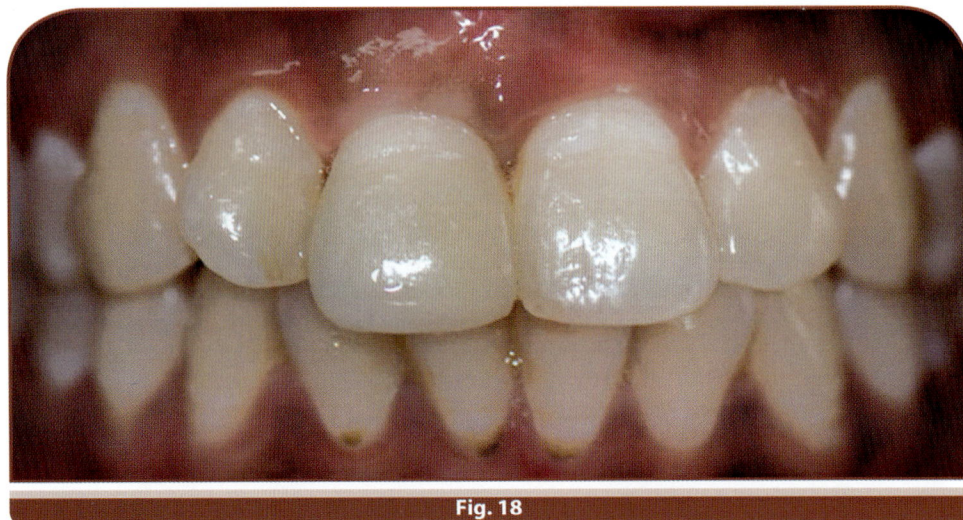

Fig. 18

Frontal view of the final prosthesis. Note the natural esthetics achieved **(Fig. 18)**.

Lanka Mahesh

SINGLE TOOTH REPLACEMENT WITH SOFT TISSUE GRAFTING IN THE ESTHETIC ZONE

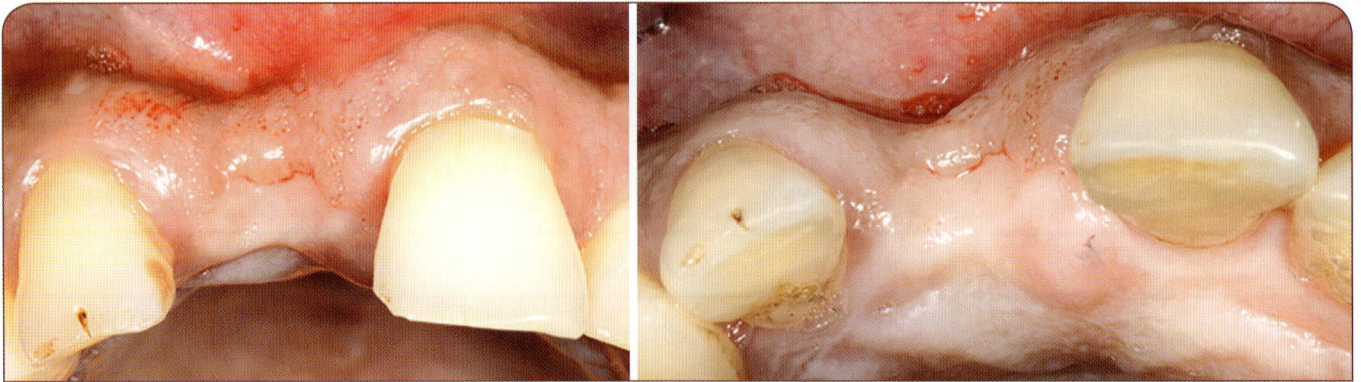

Fig. 1

Preoperative clinical situation of a missing tooth # 11. Thick gingival biotype is seen. The occlusal view shows a large soft tissue defect **(Fig. 1)**.

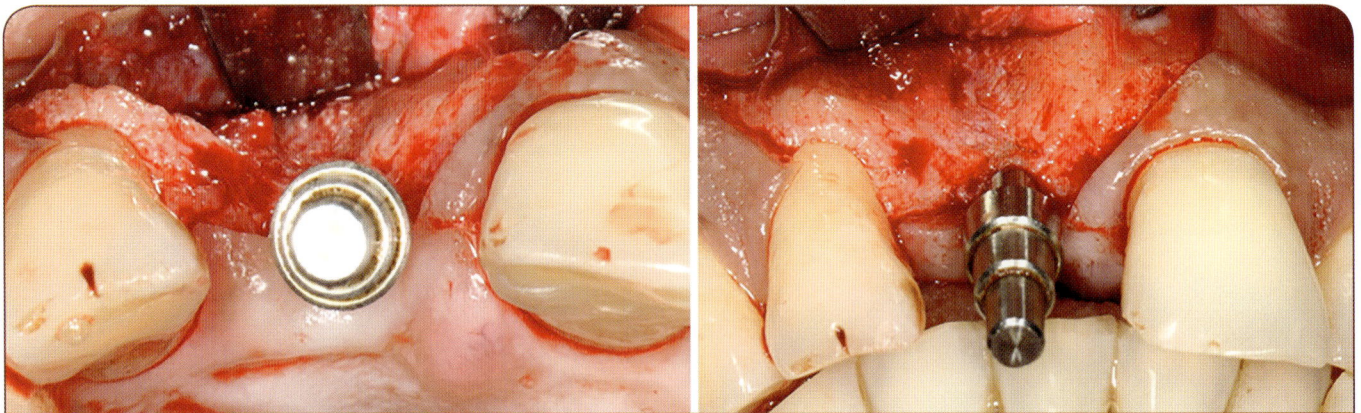

Fig. 2

After flap reflection adequate bone width is visible and the osteotomy is initiated. A parallel pin is used to verify the final implant position. An occlusal check at this stage is mandatory to verify final prosthesis and crown height space (CHS) **(Fig. 2)**.

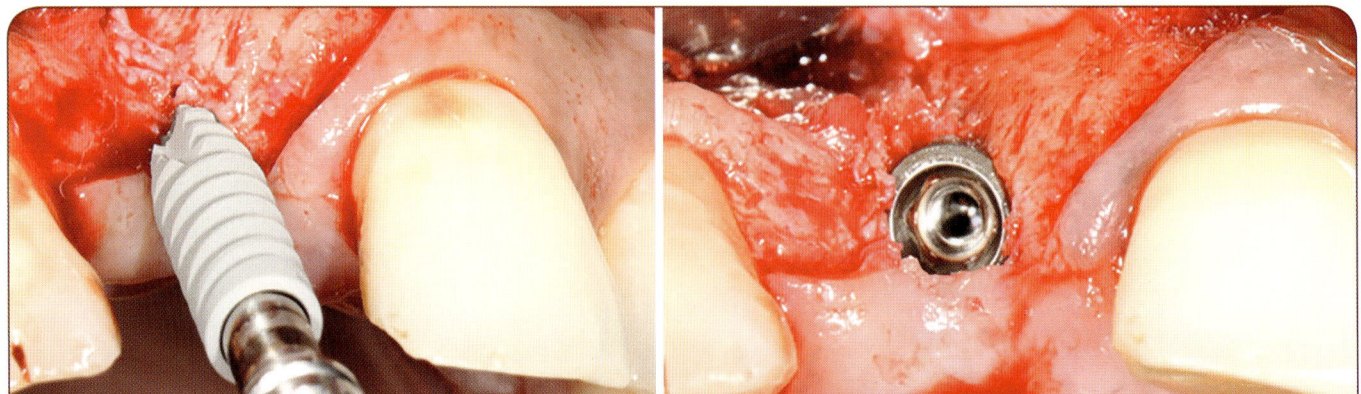

Fig. 3

A 4/11.5 mm TOP DM implant (Bioner) is inserted at 50 Ncm torque. After final seating of the implant, good bony housing was clearly seen around the implant. Therefore, a GBR procedure was ruled out **(Fig. 3)**.

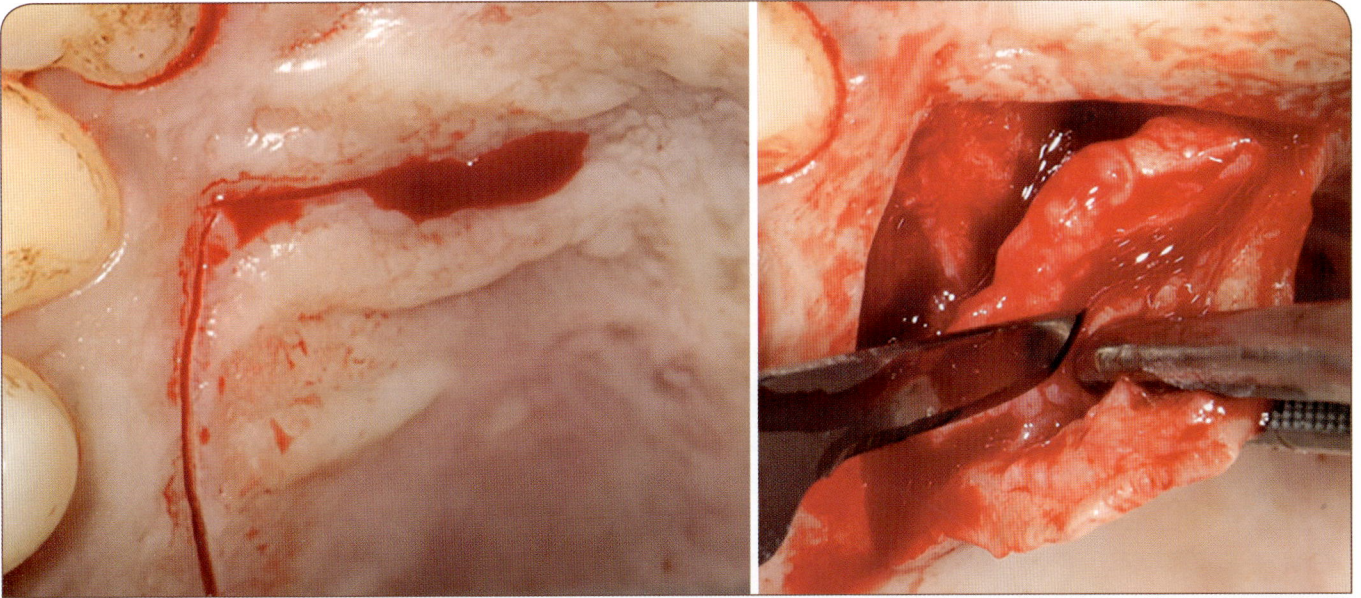

Fig. 4

A free connective tissue graft is harvested from the palate in a "L" shaped incision. A 15C blade is used to harvest the tissue **(Fig. 4)**.

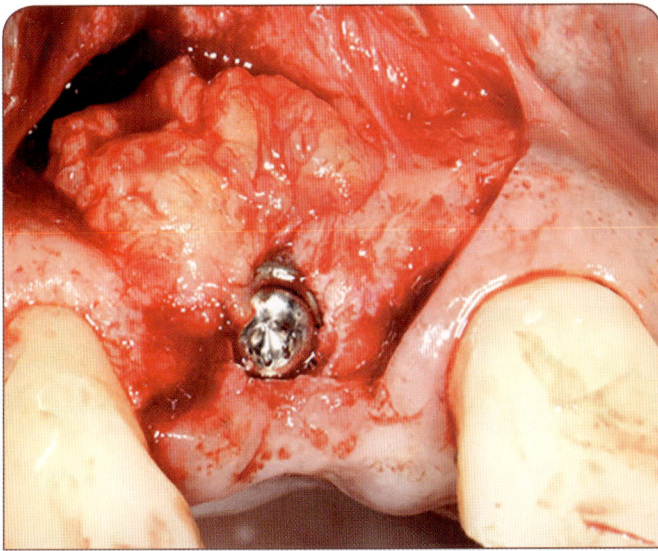

Fig. 5

The CT graft is layered on the facial wall of the implant to bulk soft tissue around the implant **(Fig. 5)**.

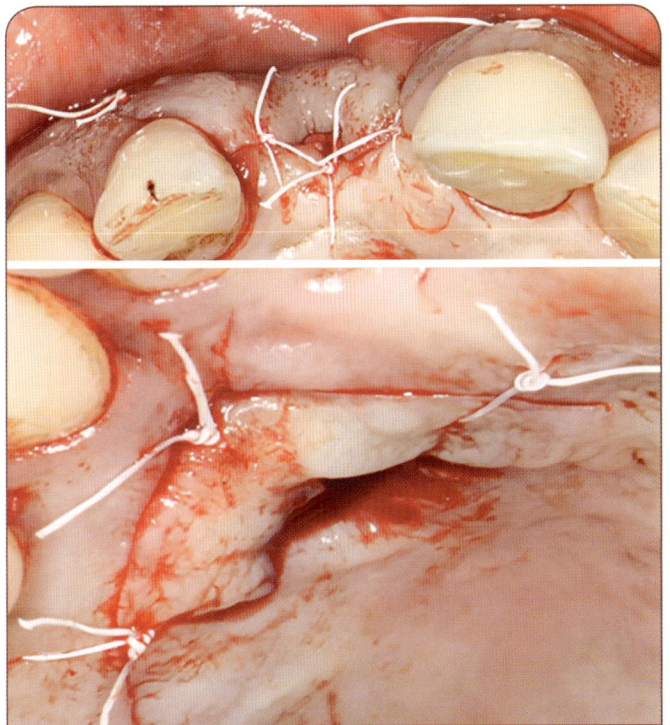

Fig. 6

The tissue at the host and donor area is closed with 3-0 cytoplast sutures (Osteogenics). The bulk of soft tissue on the facial side is immediately evident **(Fig. 6)**.

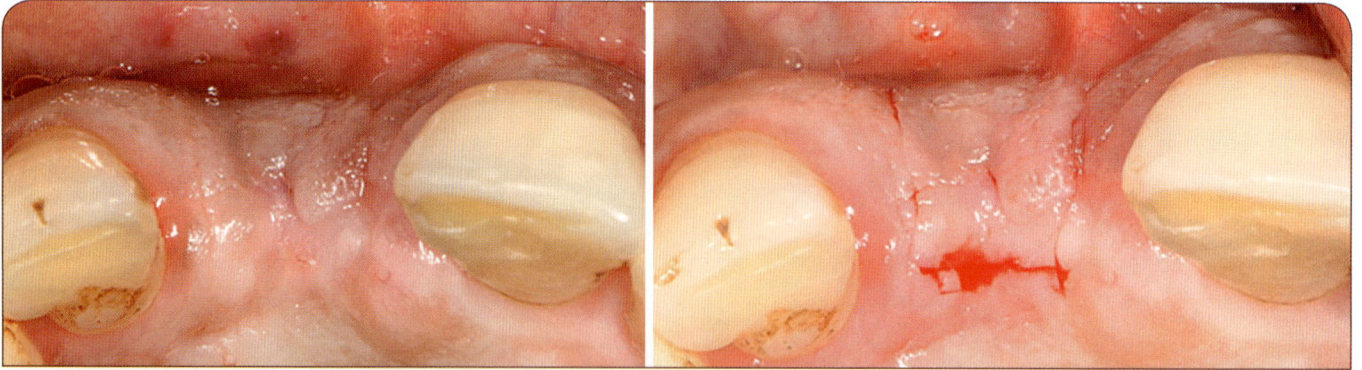

Fig. 7

At 4 months postoperative recall appointment, there is some amount of tissue shrinkage. A palatal roll flap is planned to bulk facial soft tissue, the incision borders are marked with the incision extending para-crestally **(Fig. 7)**.

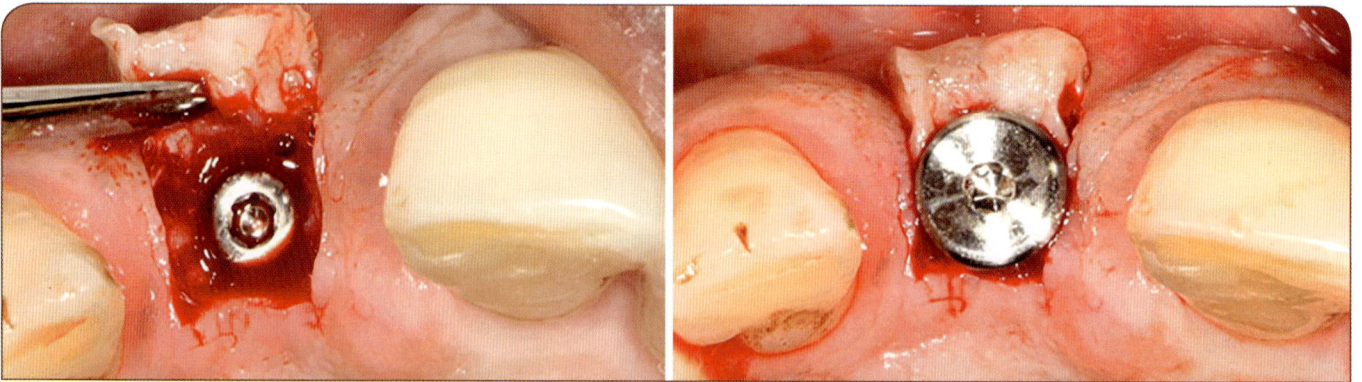

Fig. 8

The flap is elevated and rolled on the facial side providing adequate bulk. A healing collar of appropriate width is chosen to support the soft tissue from "collapsing" **(Fig. 8)**.

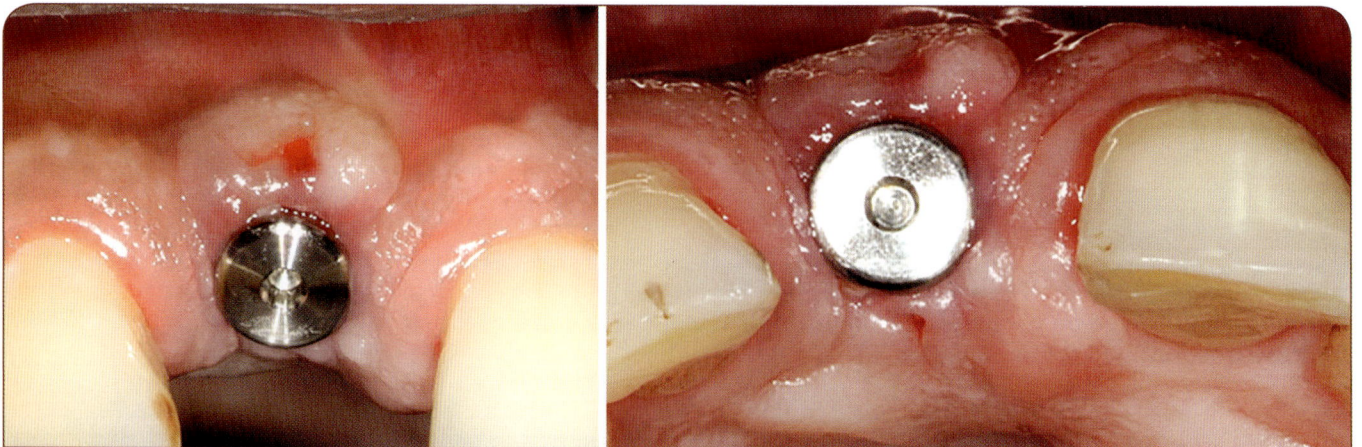

Fig. 9

At suture removal, the tissue bulk is maturing and healthy. The occlusal view is ample proof of tissue matching up to the neighboring central incisor **(Fig. 9)**.

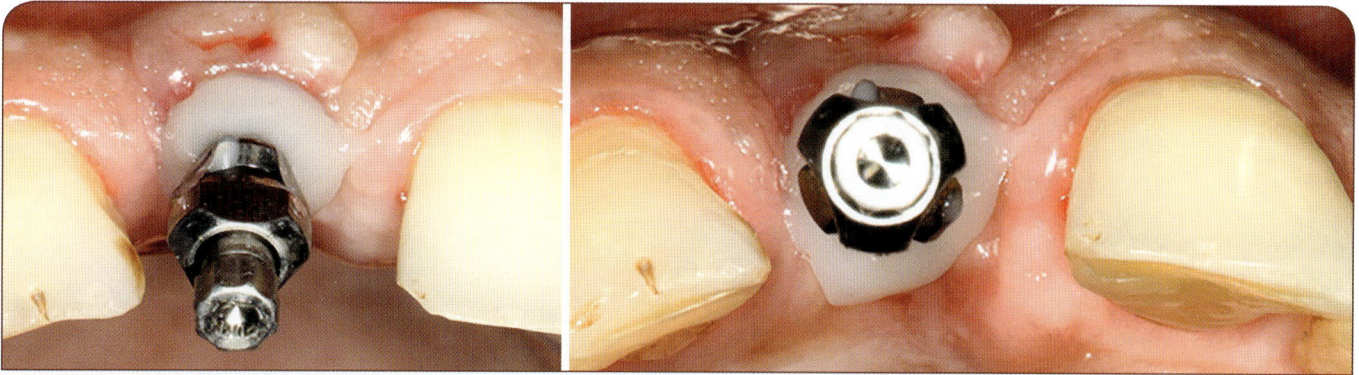

Fig. 10

A customized impression with flowable light cure composite around the sulcus area is used to capture the margins of the soft tissue. The occlusal view shows the implant in correct 3D position to the surrounding area **(Fig. 10)**.

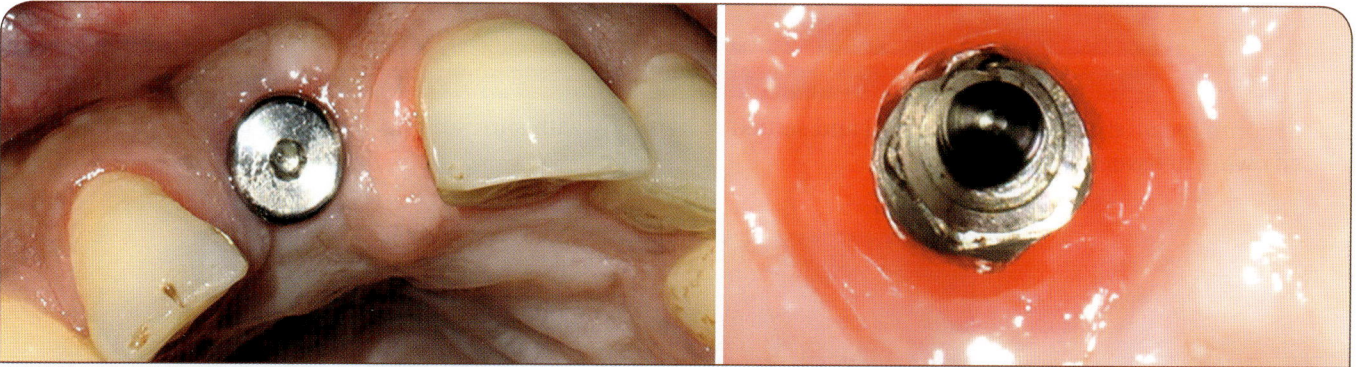

Fig. 11

Two weeks following, the impression, the tissue has healed adequately with sufficient bulk. After removal of the healing collar a very well-healed tissue surrounding the implant is visible **(Fig. 11)**.

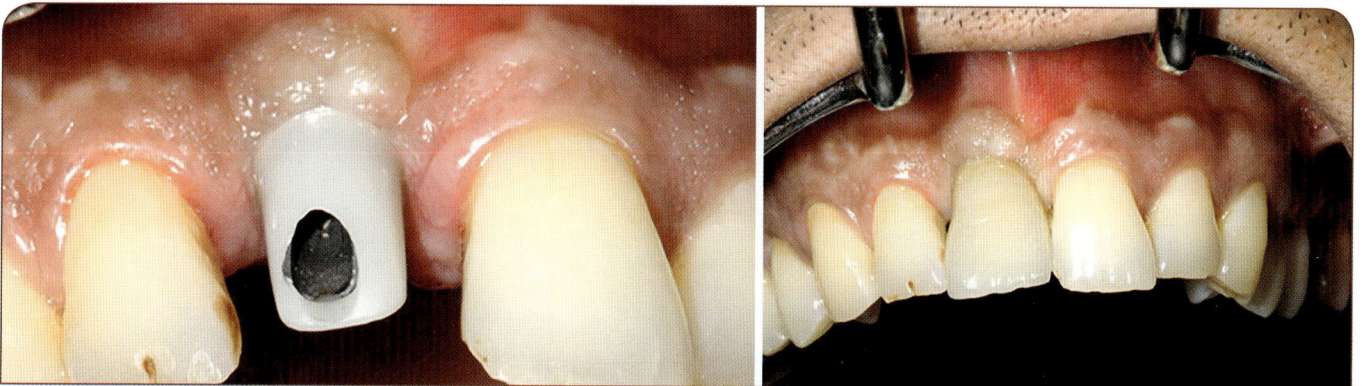

Fig. 12

A zirconia abutment (layered zirconia over a stock abutment) is torqued to 30 Ncm, tissue blanching at this stage signifies a good marginal fit. (should the blanching persist beyond ten minutes? The abutment should be removed and the tissue surface trimmed). The final zirconia prosthesis in place with good tissue stability evident. A black triangle is visible at the distal of the prosthesis **(Fig. 12)**.

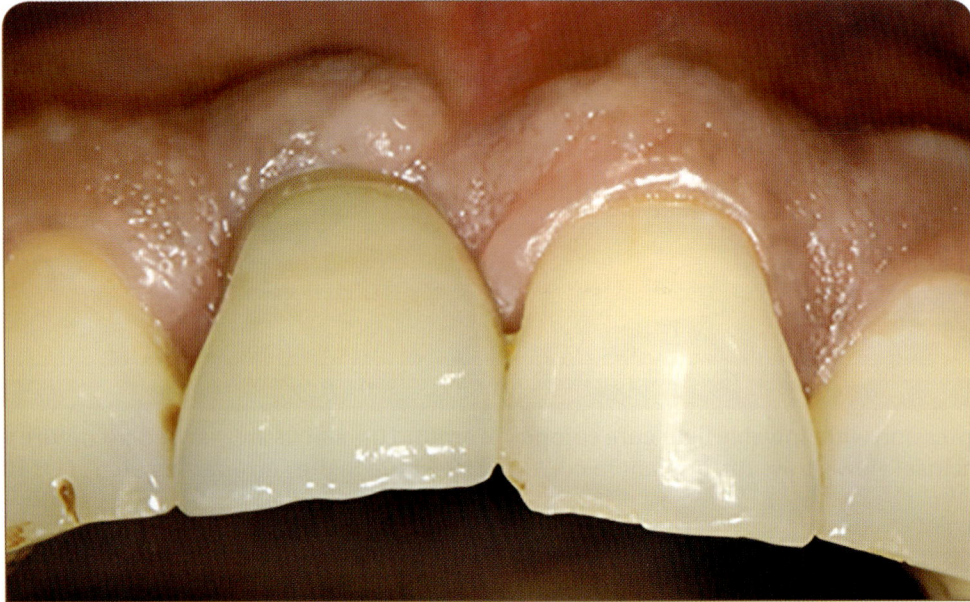

Fig. 13

At 18 month recall, the tissue has matured and settled in harmony with surrounding tissue, the black triangle has also closed owing to tissue creep **(Fig. 13)**.

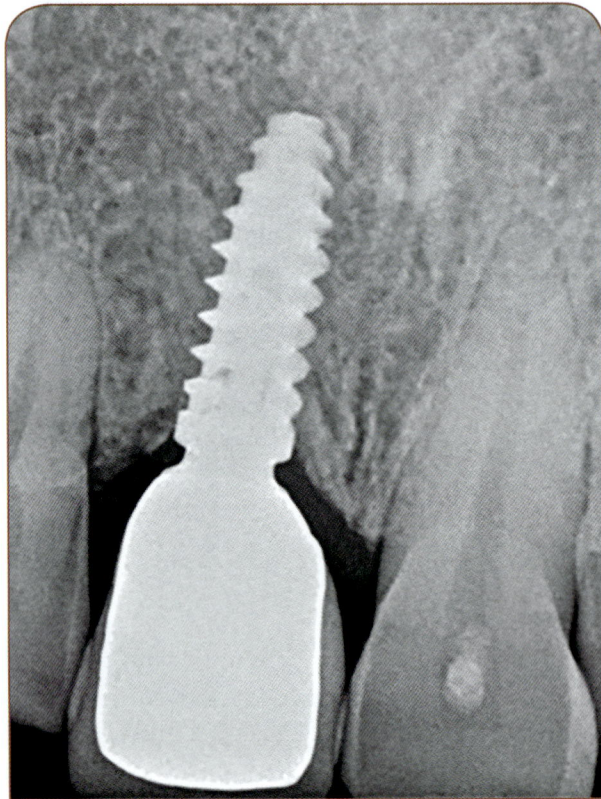

Fig. 14

The radiograph shows a good bony support around the implant **(Fig. 14)**.

Praful Bali

HARD TISSUE AUGMENTATION FOR DEFICIENT HORIZONTAL BONE AND SOFT TISSUE AUGMENTATION TO BOOST THE THIN GINGIVAL BIOTYPE FOR A MISSING RIGHT UPPER LATERAL INCISOR

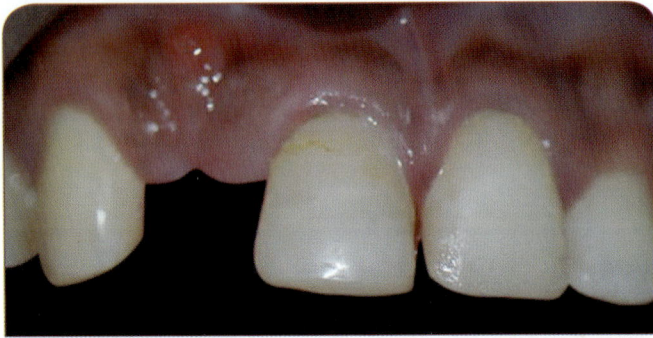

Fig. 1

Preoperative—facial view—missing tooth no #12 (right upper lateral incisor). There is a draining fistula also on the edentulous area which needs attention **(Fig. 1)**.

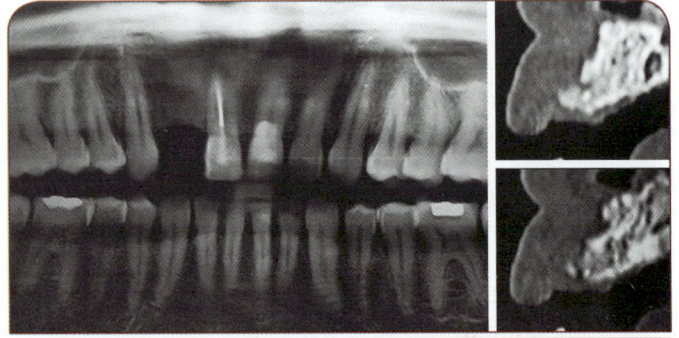

Fig. 2

Preoperative X-ray and CT scan **(Fig. 2)**.

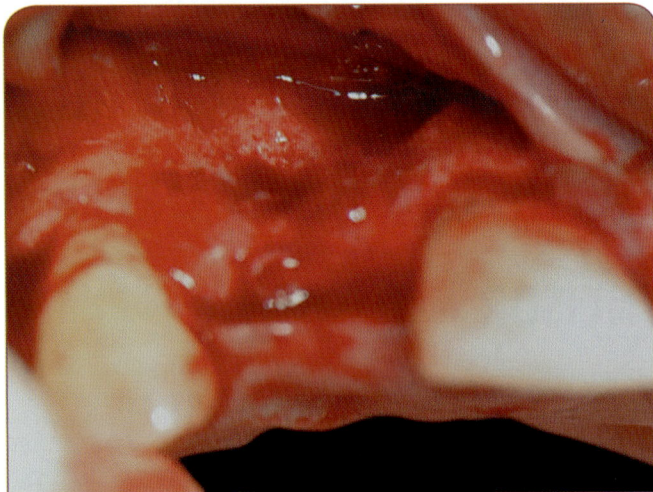

Fig. 3

Full thickness flap reflection done exposing the site of osteotomy. Note the buccal plate deficiency **(Fig. 3)**.

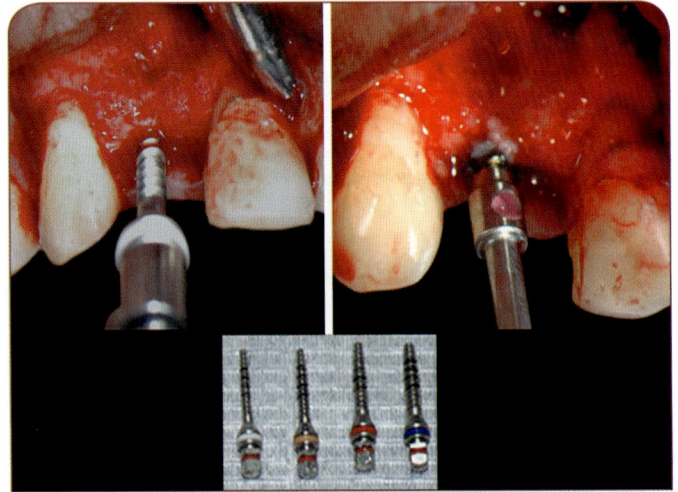

Fig. 4

Use of expanders to expand the bone and also preserving the bone at the crucial buccal area **(Fig. 4)**.

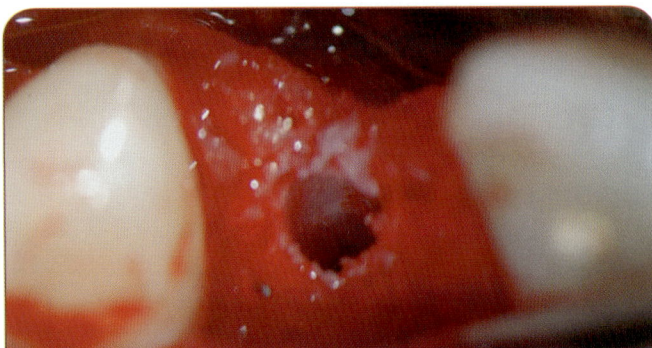

Fig. 5

Final osteotomy preparation **(Fig. 5)**.

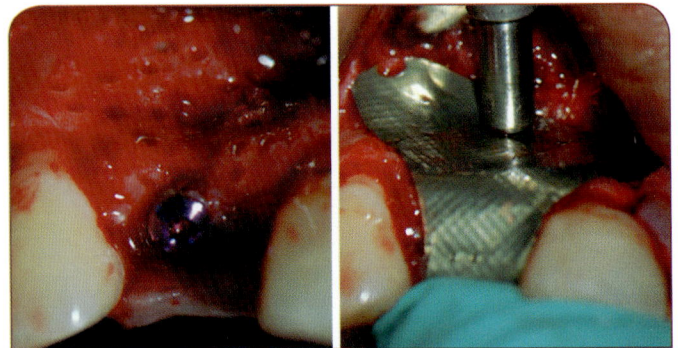

Fig. 6

3.5/13 implant placed (Nobel Biocare). Buccal bone prepared for augmentation **(Fig. 6)**.

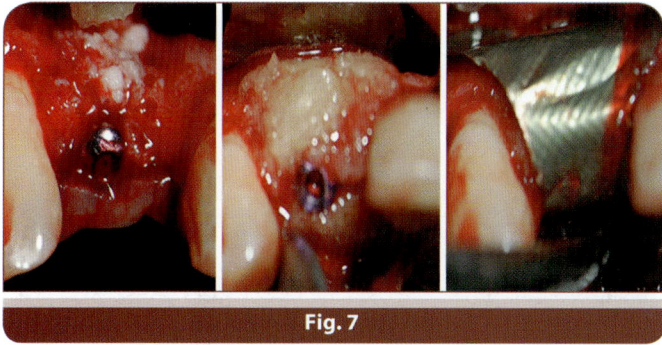

Fig. 7

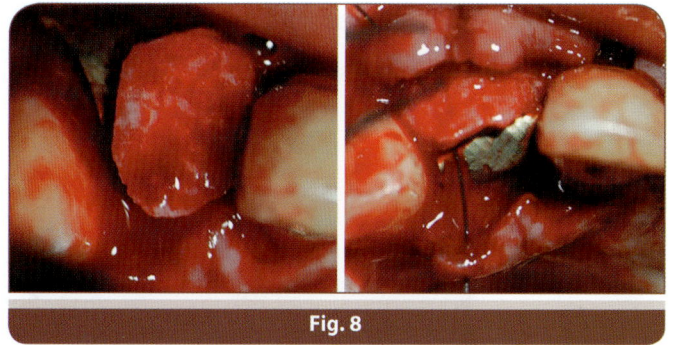

Fig. 8

Cortical bone scrapings placed as 1st layer as part of GBR procedure. Synthetic bone graft (NovaBone) placed to create proper bone esthetics and also provide extra bulk of hard tissue around the implant. Nonresorbable titanium membrane placed as a barrier **(Fig. 7)**.

Pedicle connective tissue graft taken from the palate to enhance the soft tissue **(Fig. 8)**.

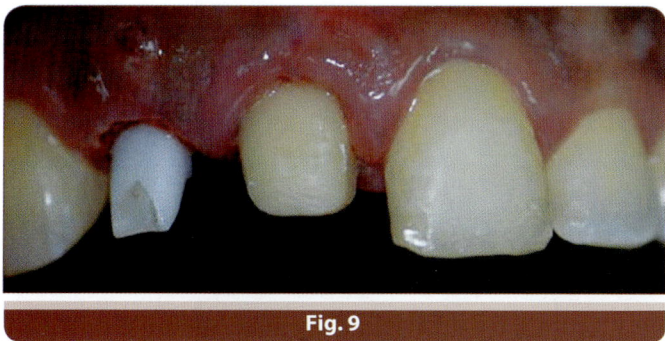

Fig. 9

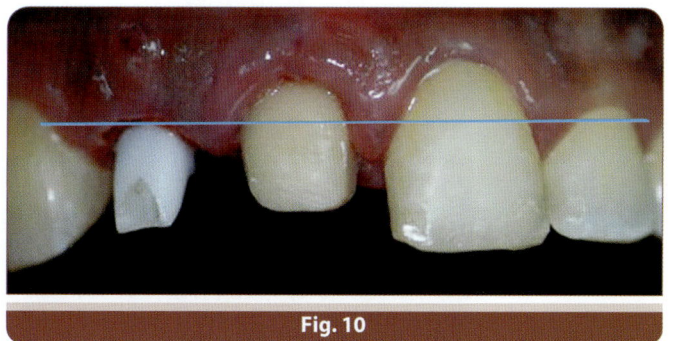

Fig. 10

A stock Procera abutment is shaped extraorally and torqued to 35 Ncm—One Abutment One Time Concept **(Fig. 9)**.

Note the emergence of the implant abutment is more positive than the contralateral side **(Fig. 10)**.

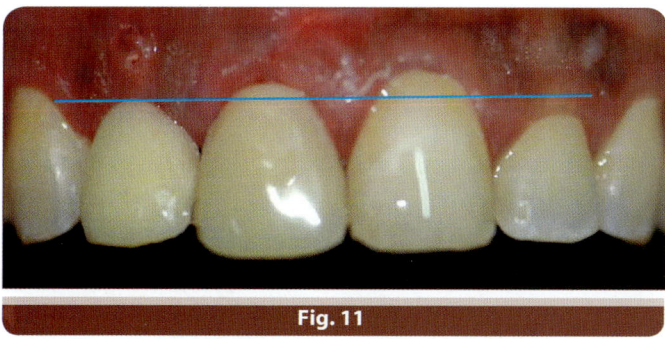

Fig. 11

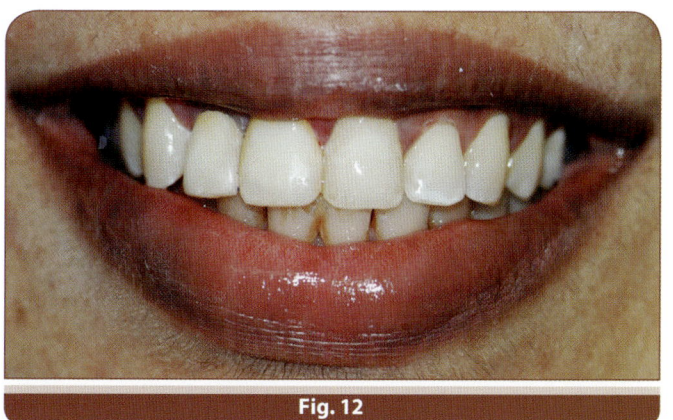

Fig. 12

This is reshaped to achieve a better result with regard to golden proportion and smile designing concept. A prototype crown is cemented with temporary cement. A temporary crown also for the right central incisor **(Fig. 11)**.

Also, the contralateral side lateral incisor is reshaped with gingivectomy to achieve optimal esthetics **(Fig. 12)**.

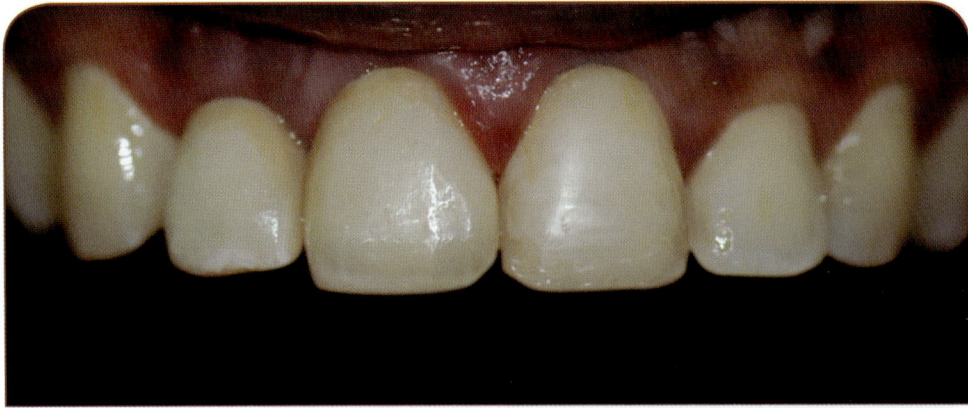

Fig. 13

Permanant E-max crown cemented in position **(Fig. 13)**.

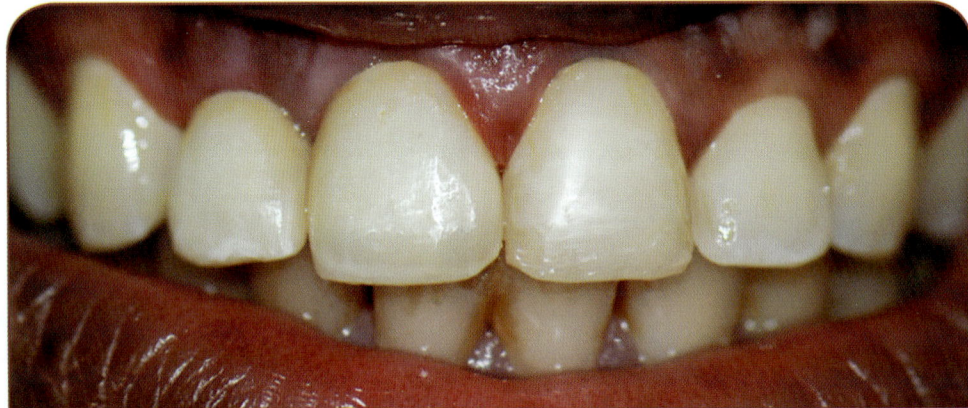

Fig. 14

One year follow-up: Excellent emergence profile of the implant restoration combined with equally good shade selection and matching **(Fig. 14)**.

Praful Bali, Stutee Grewal

A Multidisciplinary Approach to Achieve Optimal Esthetics in Compromised Bone Situation: An 8-year Follow-up

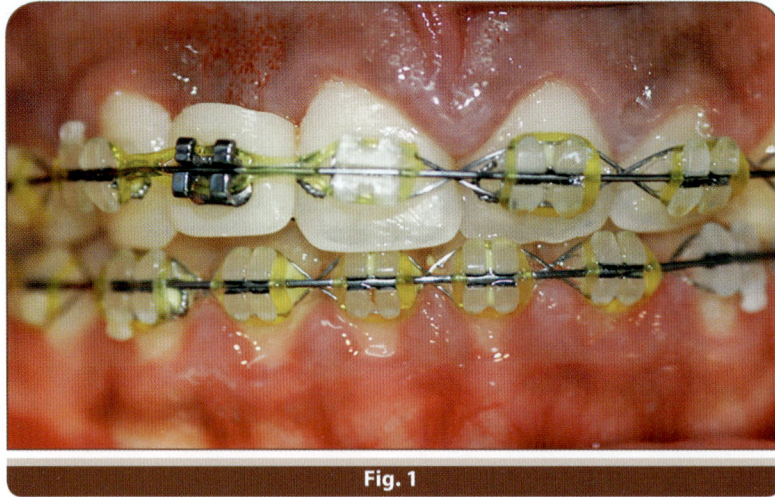

Fig. 1

Patient presents with an acrylic tooth fixed with orthodontic bands in the area of tooth # 12 as a compromised fixed temporary restoration **(Fig. 1)**.

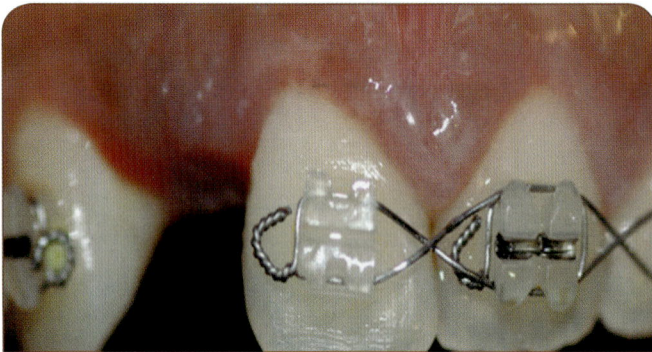

Fig. 2

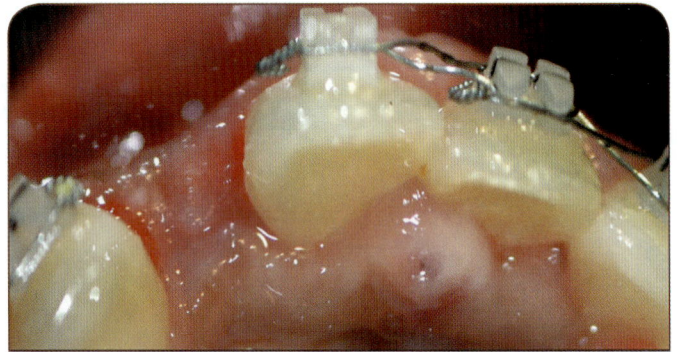

Fig. 3

Preoperative facial view—absence of interdental papillae and slight inflammation due to possible pressure from the temporary restoration **(Fig. 2)**.

Preoperative occlusal view, note the slight facial dip indicating the deficiency of buccal bone **(Fig. 3)**.

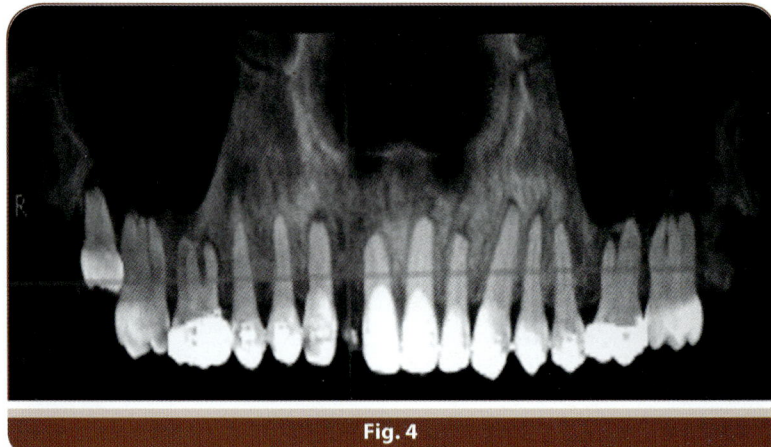

Fig. 4

Preoperative X-ray showing the absence of bone in vertical dimension **(Fig. 4)**.

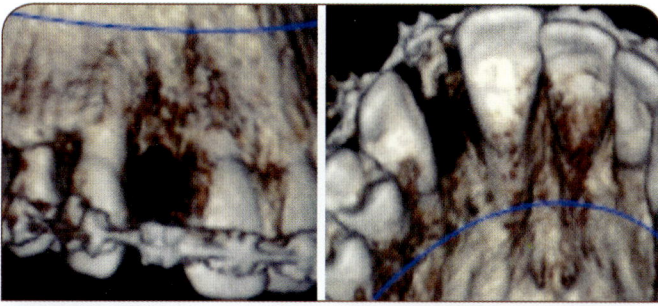

Fig. 5

Preoperative CT scan reconfirming the almost absence of bone in the verticle dimension in the area of missing lateral incisor **(Fig. 5)**.

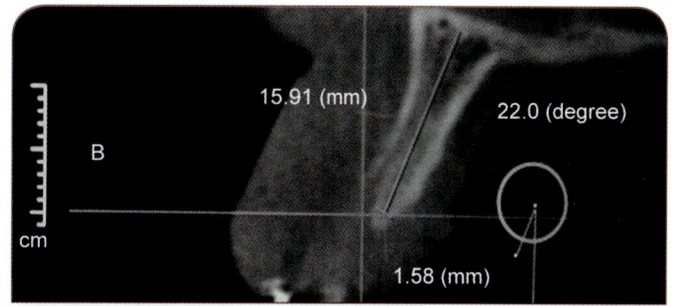

Fig. 6

Preoperative CT scan showing the absence of bone in horizontal dimension also **(Fig. 6)**.

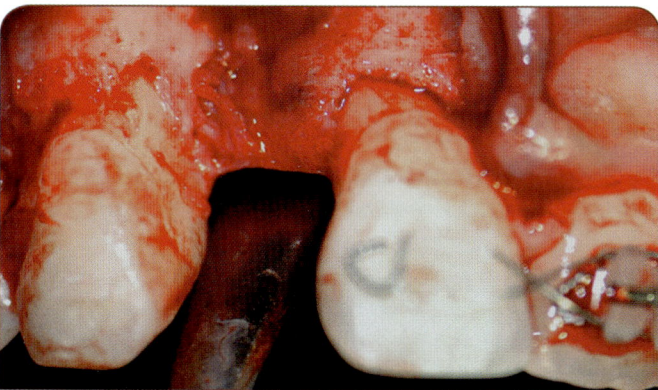

Fig. 7

Full thickness flap reflection done and the site, cleaned and prepared for grafting **(Fig. 7)**.

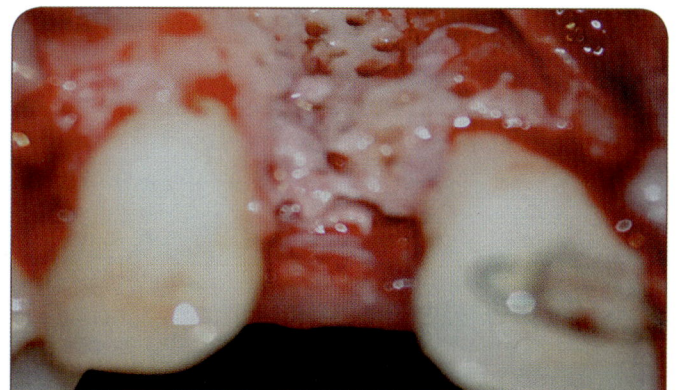

Fig. 8

De-corticisation of recipient bone to initiate bleeding in the recipient site. The amount of deficient bone cannot be rebuilt only by artificial bone substitutes so a decision is made to use autogenous bone in form of cortical bone chips taken from ramus of the mandible **(Fig. 8)**.

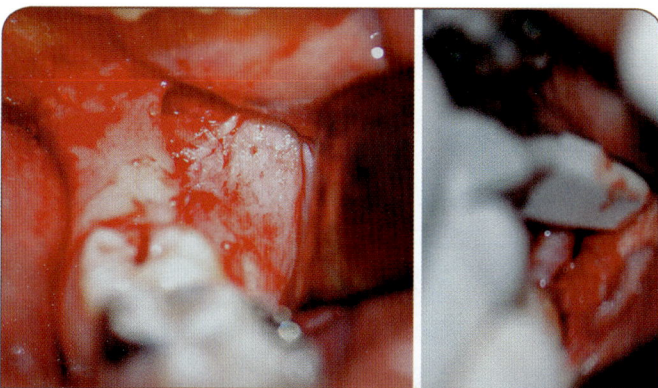

Fig. 9

Exposure of the pre-ramus area to scrape autogenous bone **(Fig. 9)**.

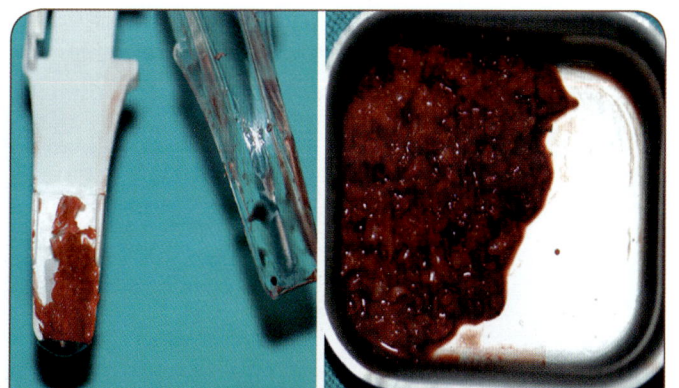

Fig. 10

Cortical bone scrapings using a disposable bone scraper (meta scraper) **(Fig. 10)**.

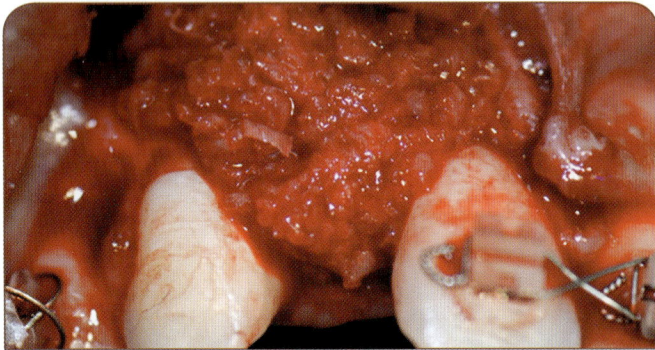

Fig. 11

Autogenous bone grafted onto the recipient bone **(Fig. 11)**.

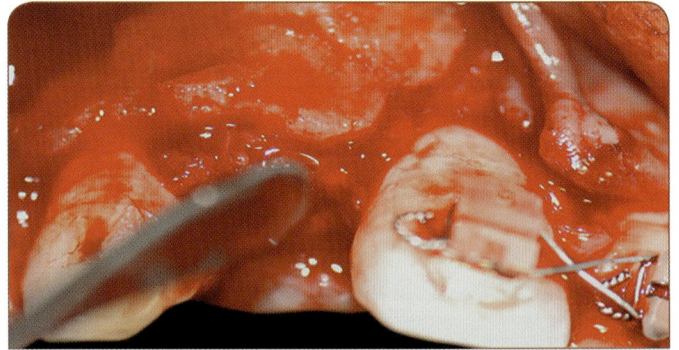

Fig. 12

Calcium phosphosilicate bone substitute (NovaBone putty) as part of the sandwitch technique used on top of the cortical bone scrappings **(Fig. 12)**.

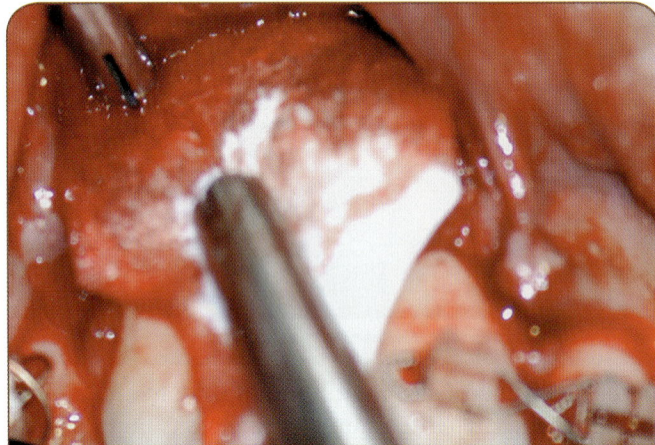

Fig. 13

GBR completed by using a Bio-Guide collagen membrane to secure the graft **(Fig. 13)**.

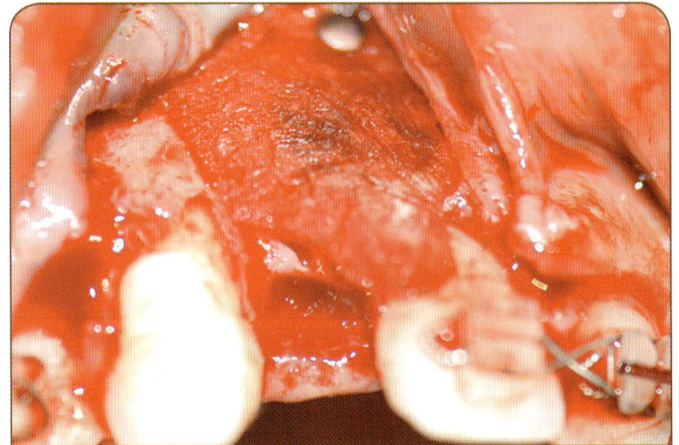

Fig. 14

Intakt (equinox) bone tags used to secure the membrane **(Fig. 14)**.

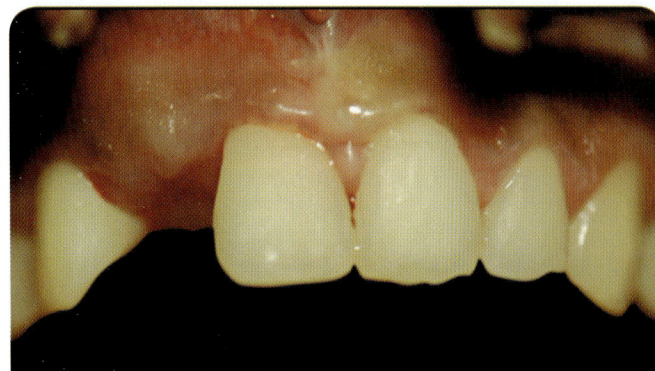

Fig. 15

Four months postoperative—Facial view **(Fig. 15)**.

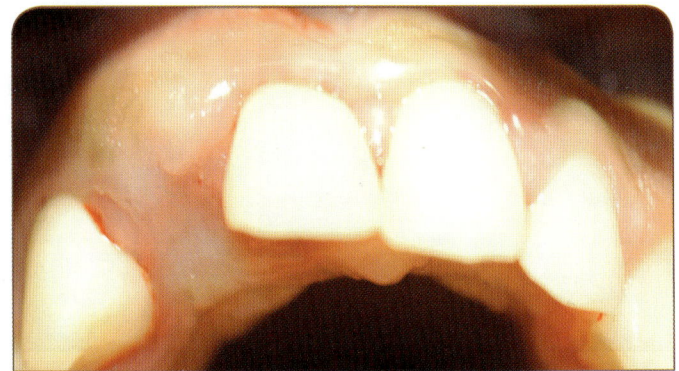

Fig. 16

Four months postoperative—Occlusal view **(Fig. 16)**.

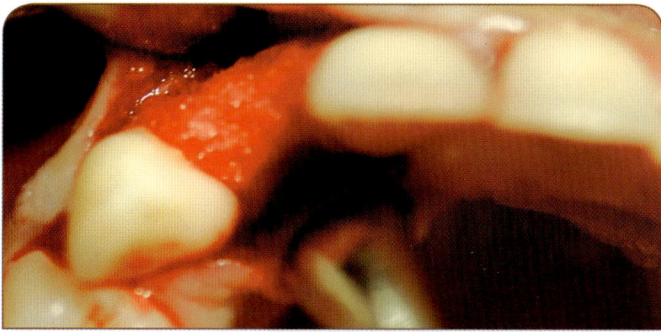

Fig. 17

9 mm bone regeneration horizontally **(Fig. 17)**.

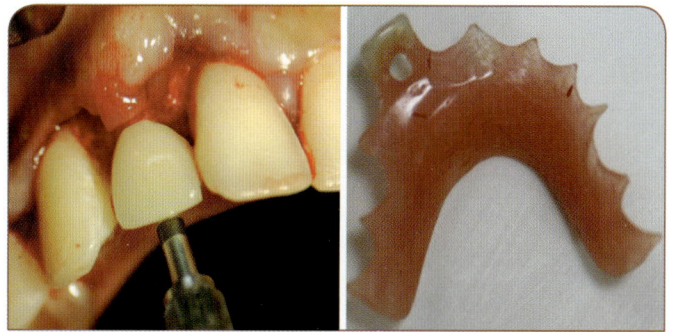

Fig. 18

Using the existing treatment partial denture of the patient as a Surgical Stent, correct implant placement is guided **(Fig. 18)**.

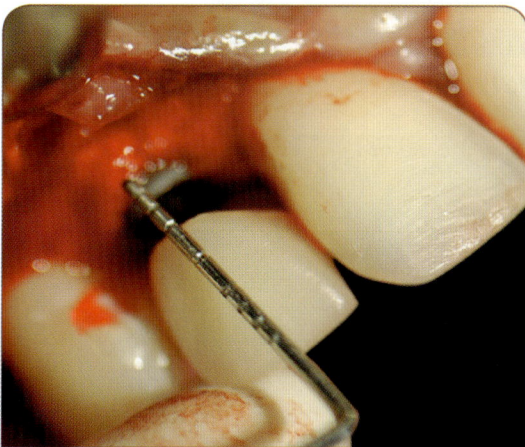

Fig. 19

3D implant placement (vertical—2–3 mm) **(Fig. 19)**.

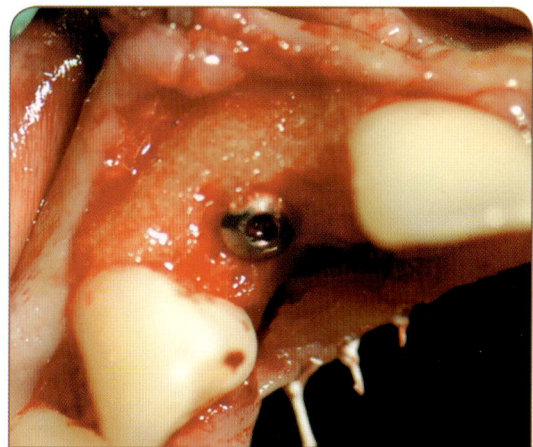

Fig. 20

NovaBone putty is augmented again to establish the buccal contour **(Fig. 20)**.

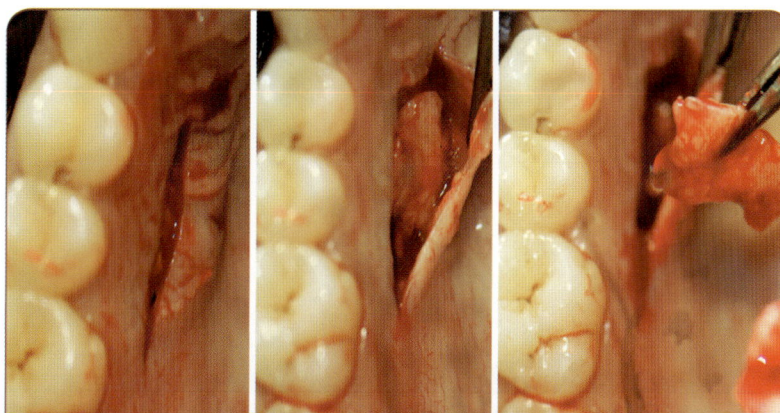

Fig. 21

Connective tissue graft secured from the palate **(Fig. 21)**.

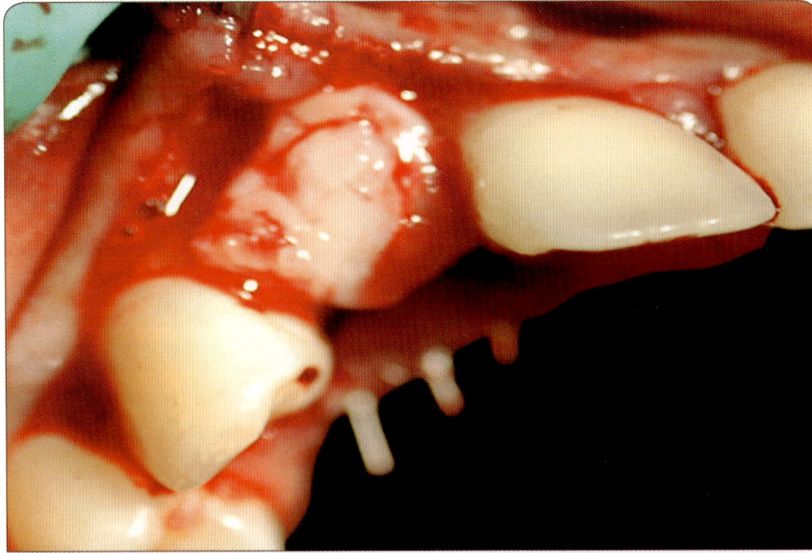

Fig. 22

Connective tissue graft done **(Fig. 22)**.

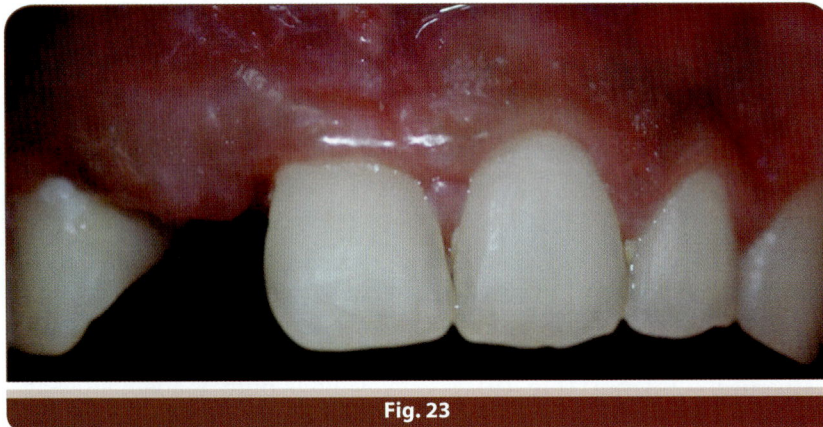

Fig. 23

Sufficient soft and hard tissue formation after GBR and connective tissue graft and a healing period of 3 months **(Fig. 23)**.

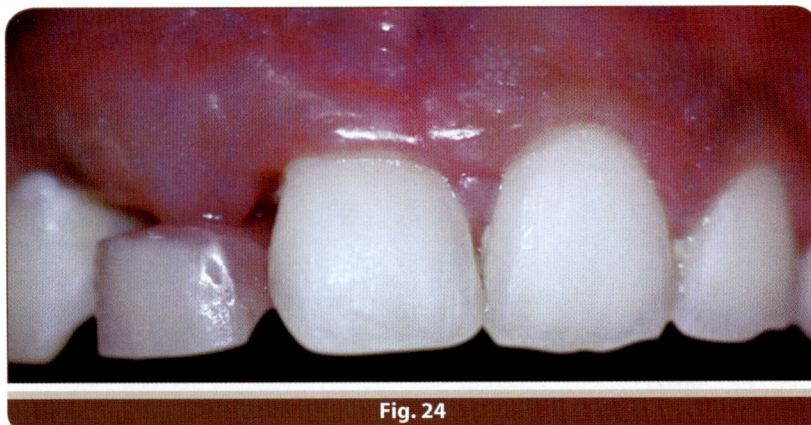

Fig. 24

Picture shows the amount of hard and soft tissue gained after the augmentation procedure. The existing partial denture of the patient was adjusted a few times to accommodate the bulk of tissue **(Fig. 24)**.

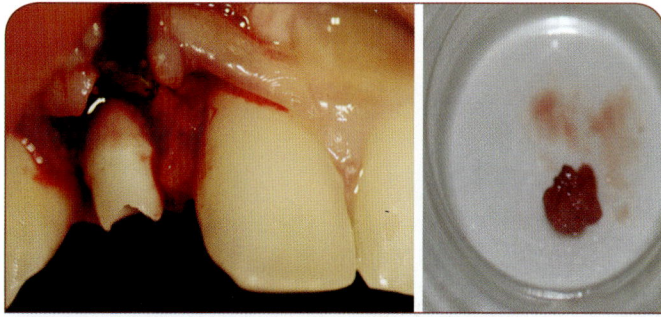

Fig. 25

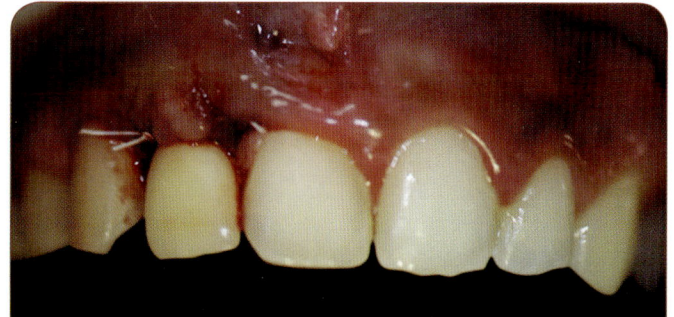

Fig. 26

A stock Zirconia abutment is customised extraorally and torqued to 35 N/cm^2—One-Abutment One Time concept. A small CT graft is also done again to build up the deficient Implant Papilla for optimal esthetics **(Fig. 25)**.

A Protemp crown is cemented with temporary cement as the 1st Prototype. 3–0 sutures are done around the crown **(Fig. 26)**.

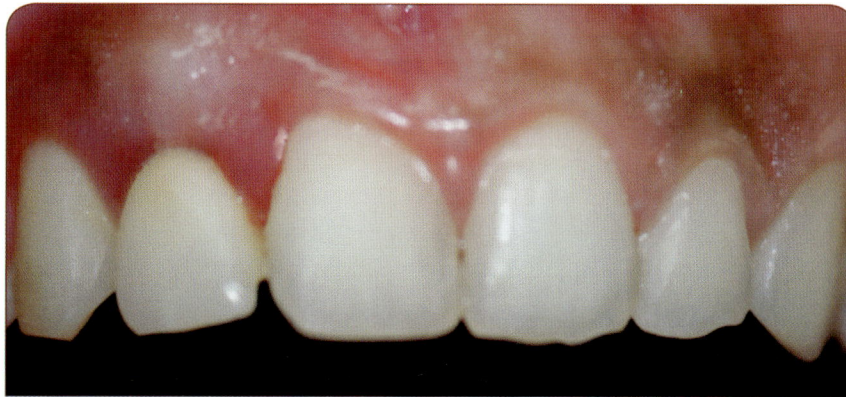

Fig. 27

A series of temporary prototypes are changed till satisfactory gingival maturation and esthetics are achieved **(Fig. 27)**.

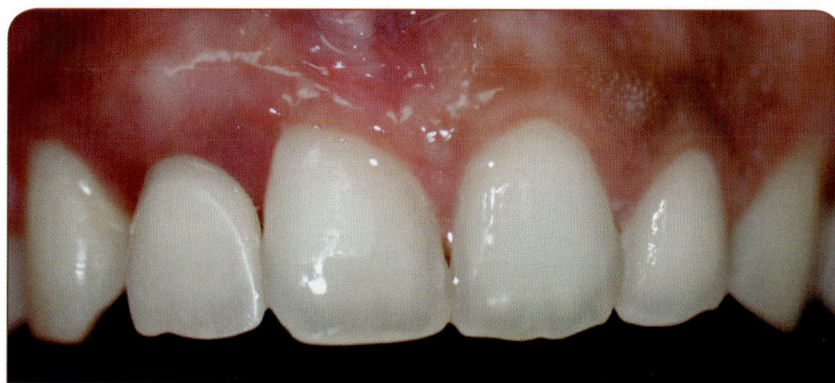

Fig. 28

E-Max full ceramic implant crown cemented. Note the soft and hard tissue esthetics achieved **(Fig. 28)**.

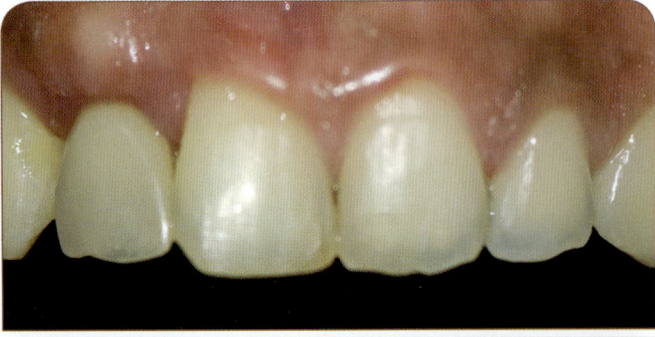

Fig. 29

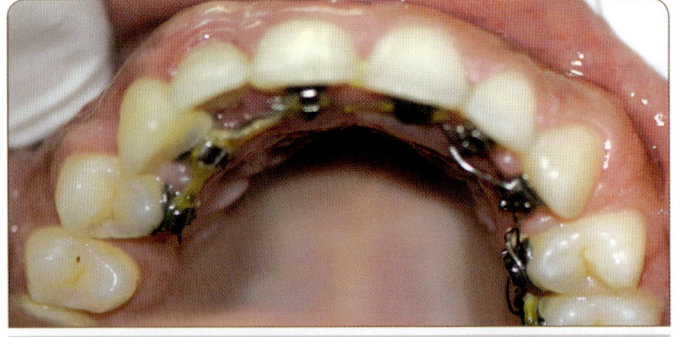

Fig. 30

18 months postoperative— remodeling of the soft tissue is evident but overall an acceptable result. The patient feels her implant crown is wider than the contra-angle side and looks for some solution **(Fig. 29)**.

Lingual orthodontics is undertaken, the canine and premolar are drifted mesially to constrict the gap. A temporary crown is given and altered during the 9 months of treatment **(Fig. 30)**.

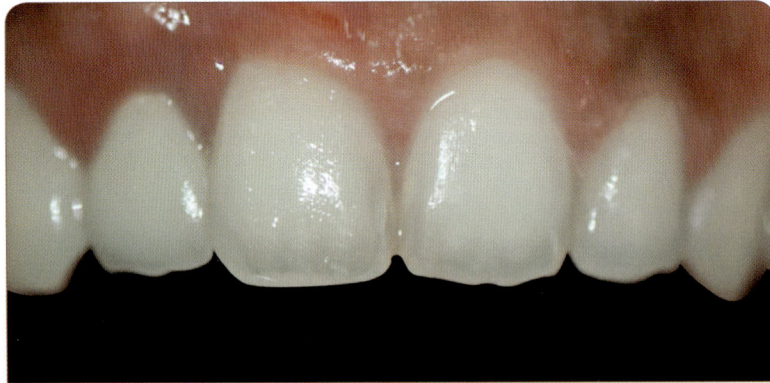

Fig. 31

A new final E-Max crown done after ortho treatment is finished. Optimum implant esthetics achieved. Note the papilla fill and optimal esthetics due to multidisciplinary approach **(Fig. 31)**.

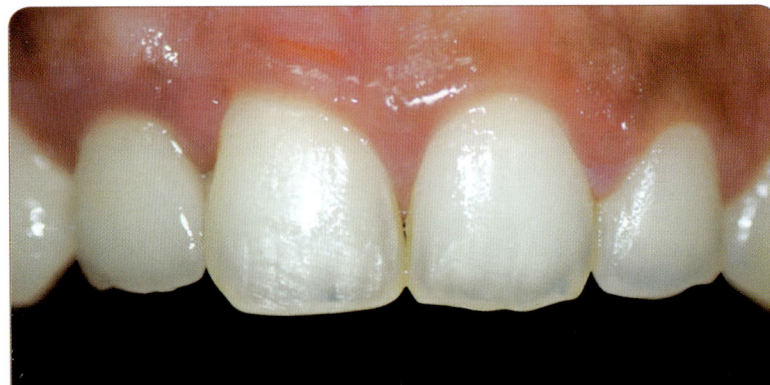

Fig. 32

An 8-year follow-up **(Fig. 32)**.

CASE STUDY 5

Praful Bali, Dildeep Bali

Hard and Soft Tissue Grafting to Achieve a Near Natural Result for a Missing Upper Central Incisor: A 4-year Follow-up

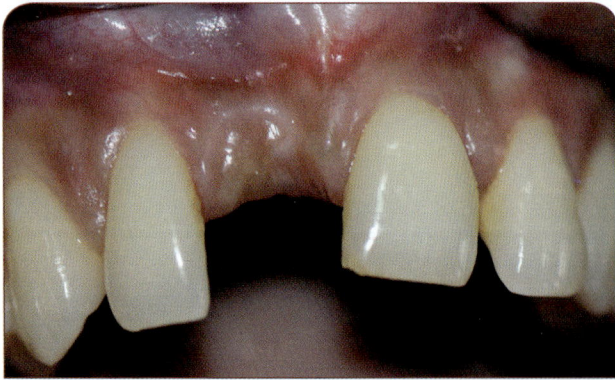

Fig. 1

A 31-year-old female patient with missing tooth # 11, tooth lost due to a road accident. Preoperative—facial view—missing tooth no #11 (right upper central incisor) **(Fig. 1)**.

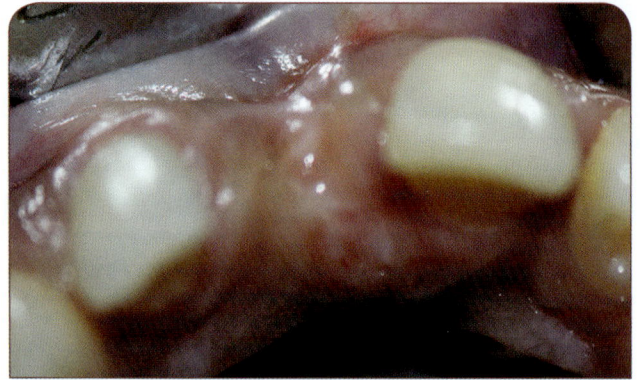

Fig. 2

Preoperative—occlusal view, note the facial dip indicating the deficiency of buccal bone. Still, there seems to be adequate bone to place a good size implant and do grafting in the same surgical visit **(Fig. 2)**.

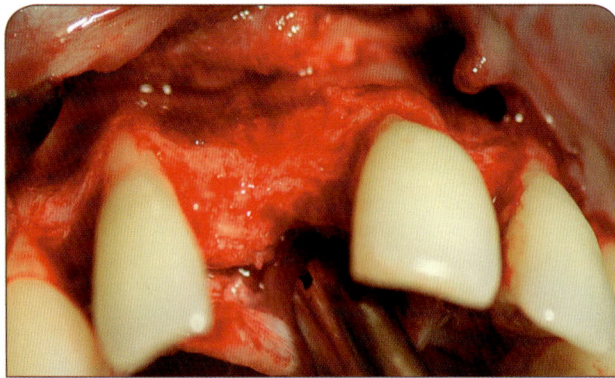

Fig. 3

Full thickness flap reflection done exposing the site of osteotomy. Note the buccal plate deficiency **(Fig. 3)**.

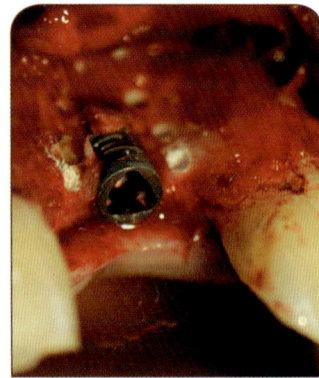

Fig. 4

There are threads of the implants exposed and it requires bone augmentation with autogenous bone—GBR to buildup the area **(Fig. 4)**.

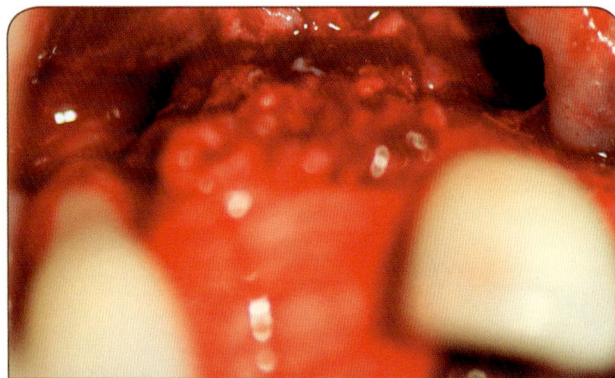

Fig. 5

Cortical scrapings placed as 1st layer as part of GBR procedure **(Fig. 5)**.

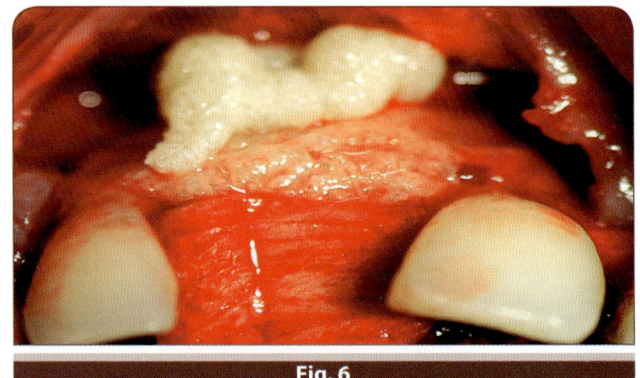

Fig. 6

GBR—Alloplastic bone graft—NovaBone placed to create proper bone esthetics and also provide extra bulk of hard tissue around the implant **(Fig. 6)**.

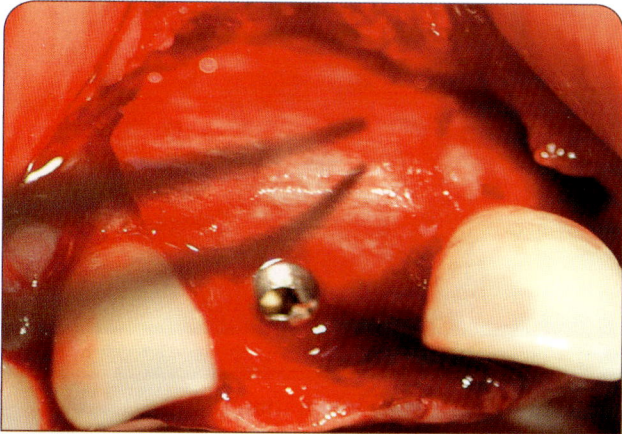

Fig. 7

Resorbable membrane placed as a barrier (**Fig. 7**).

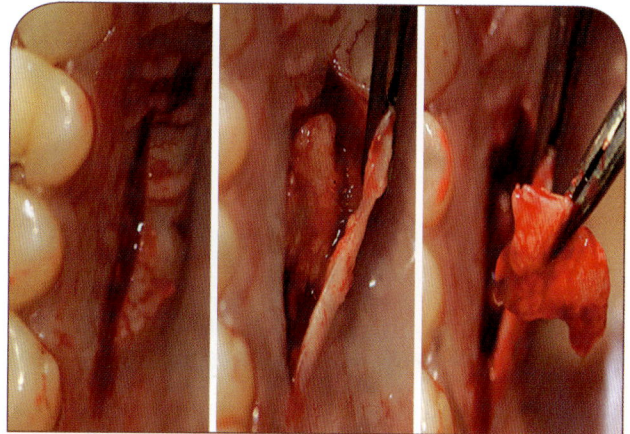

Fig. 8

Pedicle connective tissue graft taken from the palate (**Fig. 8**).

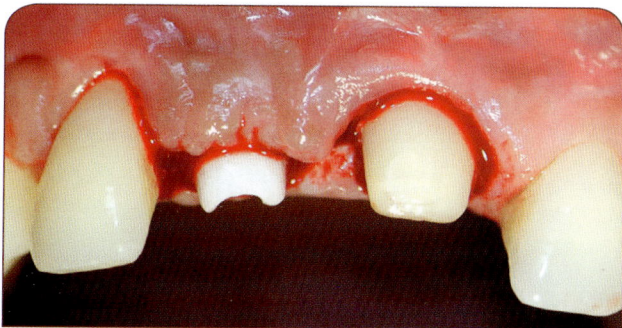

Fig. 9

A stock Zirconia abutment is shaped extraorally and torqued to 35 N/cmsq—One Abutment One Time Concept (**Fig. 9**).

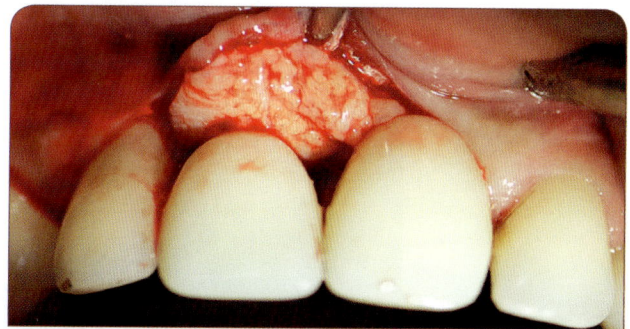

Fig. 10

A Protemp crown is cemented with temporary cement as the 1st Prototype. A temporary crown also for the left central incisor (**Fig. 10**).

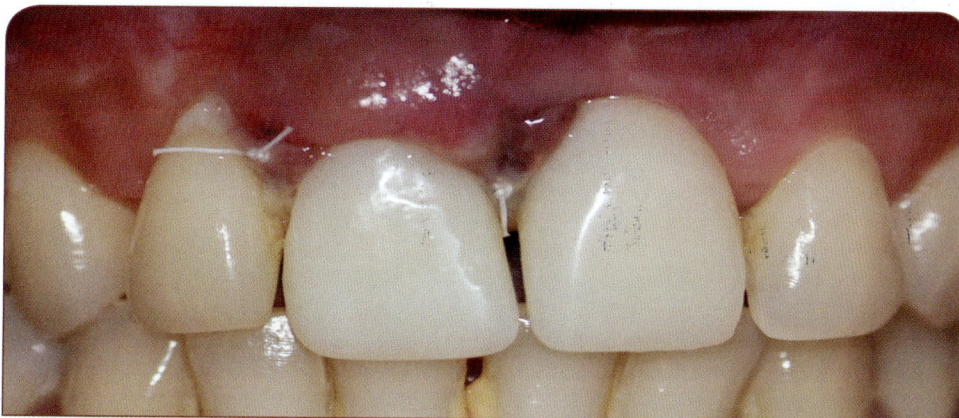

Fig. 11

One week postoperative picture after soft tissue augmentation (**Fig. 11**).

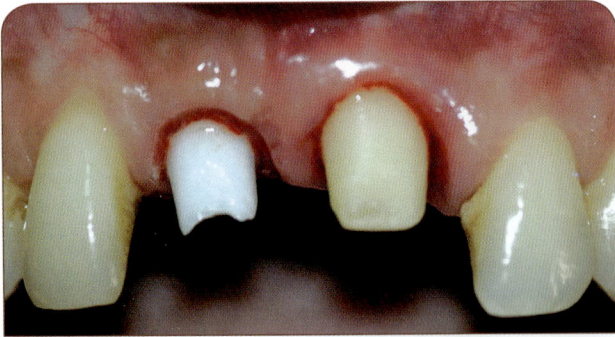

Fig. 12

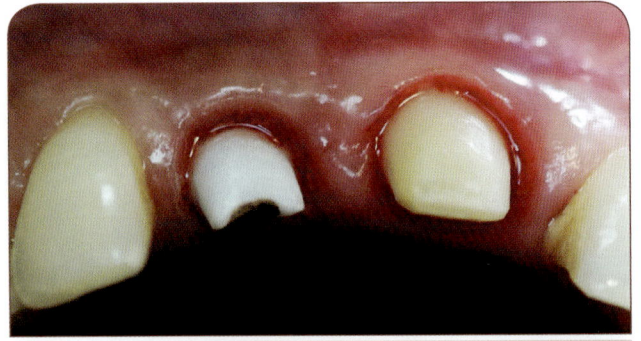

Fig. 13

Sufficient soft and hard tissue formation after GBR and connective tissue graft and a healing period of 3 months. Impressions made after gingival cord retraction (**Fig. 12**).

Soft tissue integration (**Fig. 13**).

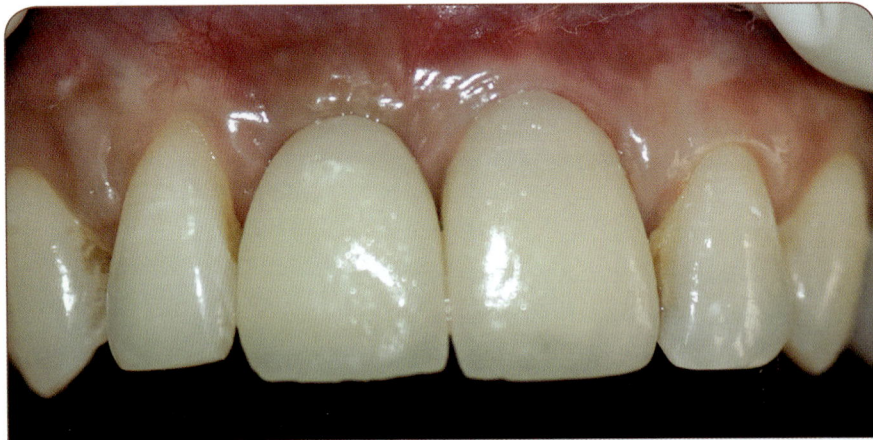

Fig. 14

Permanent Procera crown cemented in position (**Fig. 14**).

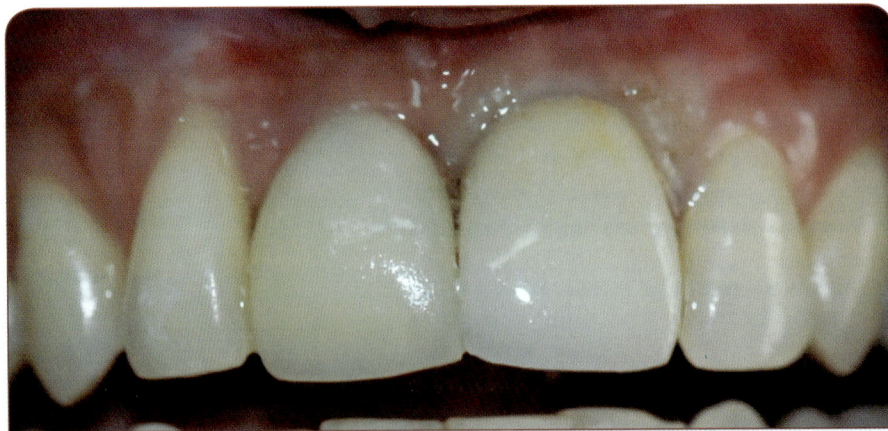

Fig. 15

Four year follow up—Optimum soft and hard tissue esthetics. The crown on left upper central incisor chipped off which was replaced by a new all ceramic prosthesis (**Fig. 15**).

MAXILLARY AUGMENTATION WITH A RAMUS BLOCK BONE GRAFT FOLLOWING REMOVAL OF AN IMPACTED CUSPID

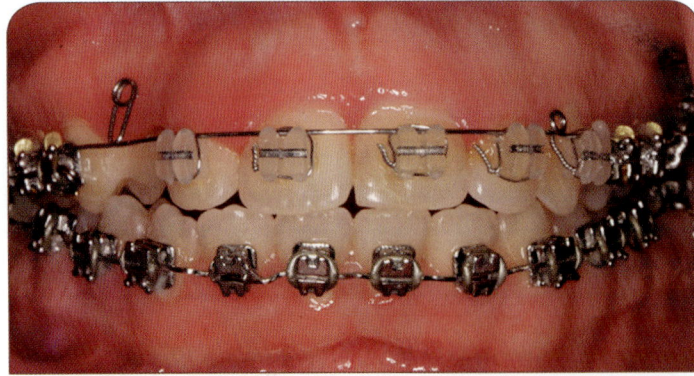

Fig. 1

A 22-year-old female patient with a history of an impacted maxillary right cuspid that could not be orthodontically erupted. No relevant medical history. Clinical exam found a significant horizontal ridge deficiency in the right anterior maxilla. Treatment plan included a block bone graft harvested from the ramus to reconstruct the site for implant replacement **(Fig. 1)**.

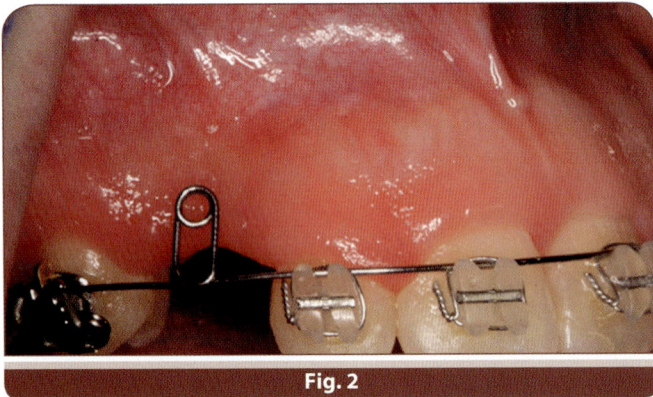

Fig. 2

The patient underwent orthodontic therapy to develop space for prosthetic replacement of the missing cuspid **(Fig. 2)**.

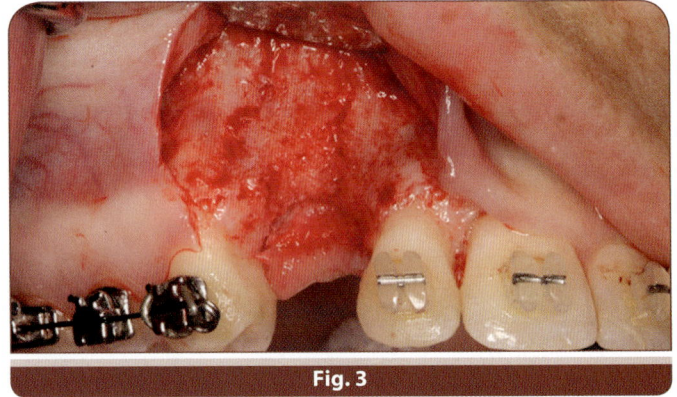

Fig. 3

Surgical exposure of the maxillary defect found significant horizontal deficiency with localized vertical loss of bone as well **(Fig. 3)**.

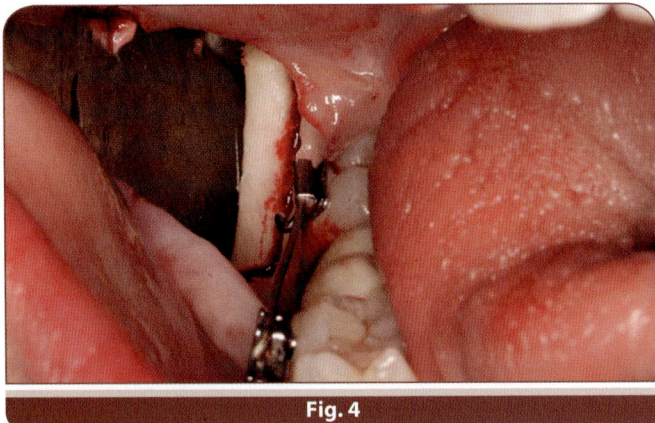

Fig. 4

A cortical block bone graft was harvested from the mandibular right ramus **(Fig. 4)**.

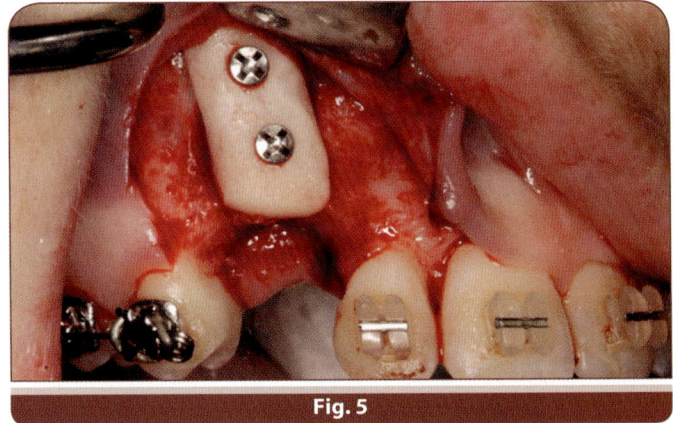

Fig. 5

The block bone graft was shaped to fit over the defect and secured with two titanium fixation screws **(Fig. 5)**.

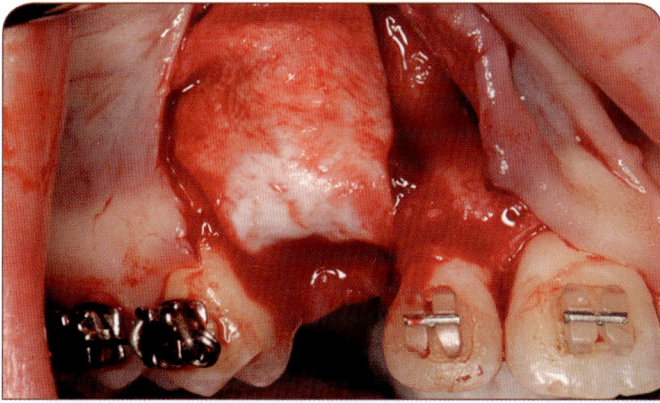

Fig. 6

The block bone graft was covered with a collagen membrane **(Fig. 6)**.

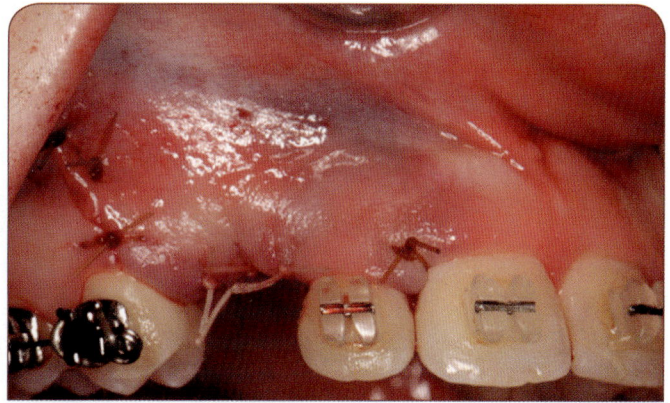

Fig. 7

An incision was made through the periosteum along the base of the buccal flap to allow advancement and tension free primary closure with 4-0 vicryl sutures **(Fig. 7)**.

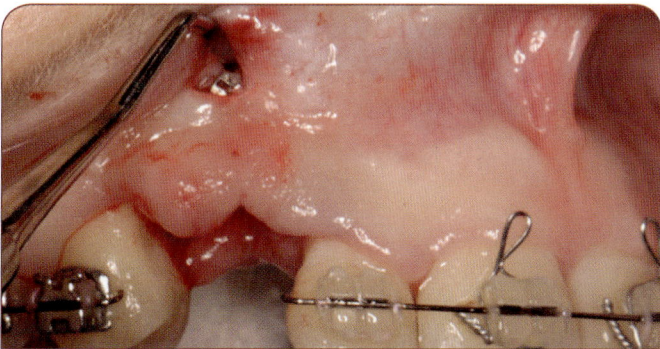

Fig. 8

The graft was allowed to heal for four months. Rather than elevating a flap and disturbing the vascular supply, the fixation screw was removed through a small remote incision **(Fig. 8)**.

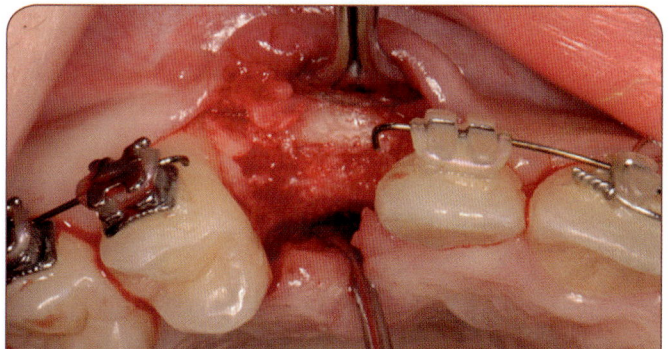

Fig. 9

Exposure of the grafted ridge found excellent incorporation of the bone graft and favorable ridge dimensions for implant placement **(Fig. 9)**.

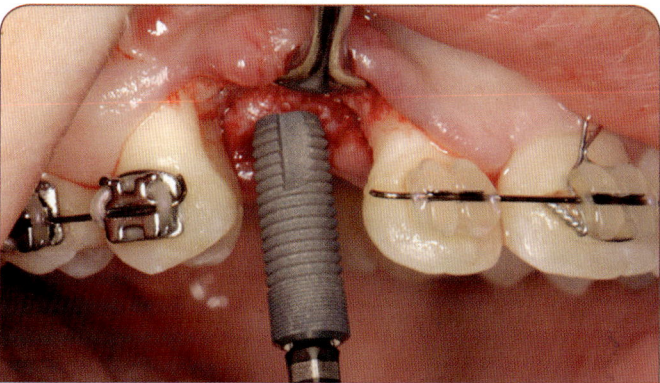

Fig. 10

A 4.0 × 13.0 mm implant was placed into the reconstructed site **(Fig. 10)**.

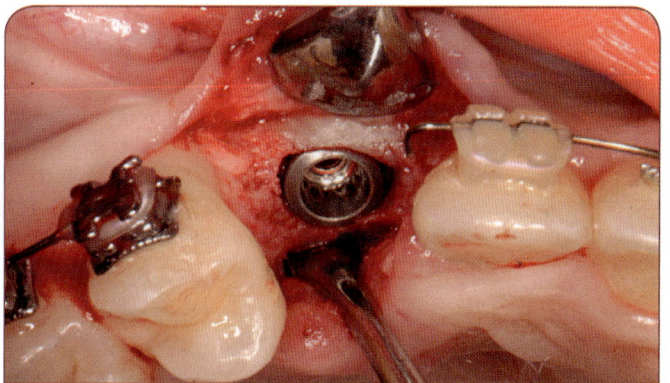

Fig. 11

The implant was positioned palatally along the ridge to leave the thick buccal cortex intact **(Fig. 11)**.

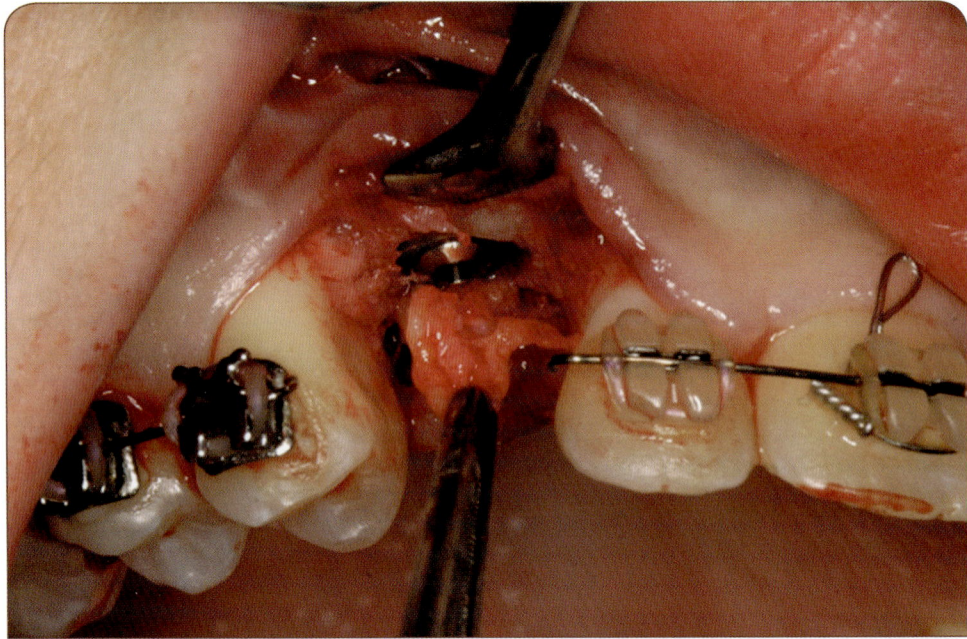

Fig. 12

A connective tissue graft was harvested from the palate to augment the soft tissue over the implant site **(Fig. 12)**.

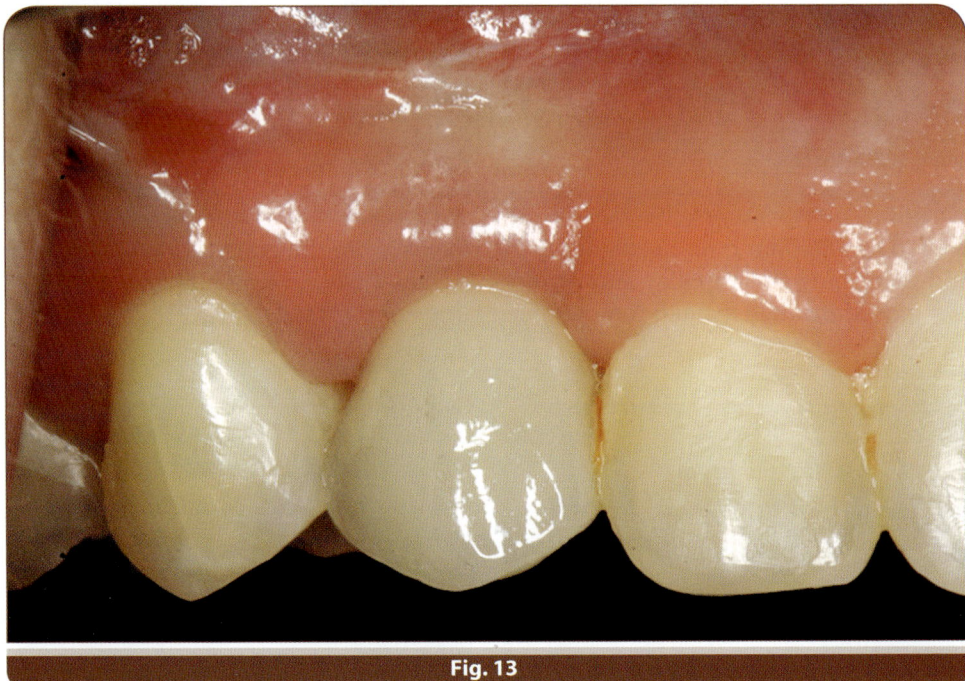

Fig. 13

The implant was restored with a custom titanium CAD/CAM abutment and a porcelain to metal cement retained crown **(Fig. 13)**.

CASE STUDY 7

Lanka Mahesh

FLAPLESS IMPLANT PLACEMENT FOR SINGLE TOOTH REPLACEMENT IN THE ESTHETIC ZONE

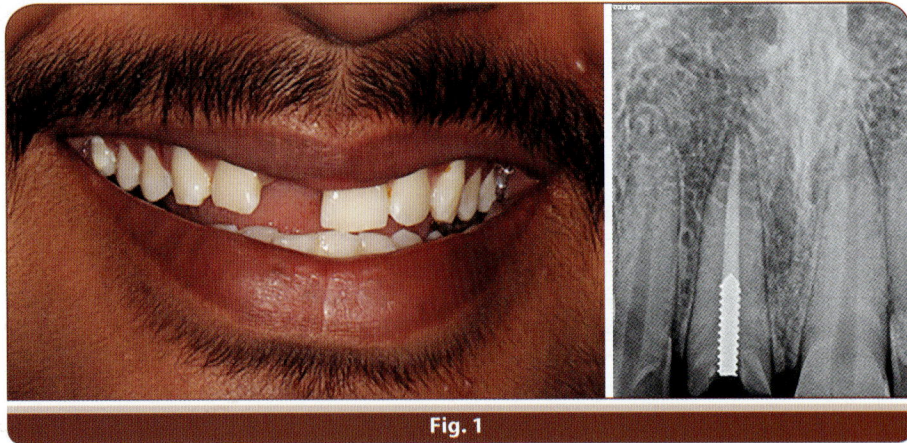

Fig. 1

A 19-year-old male, fractured tooth # 11. Medium smile line is evident. Periodontally in good overall health. IOPA X-ray reveals fracture of the crown segment previous endodontic treatment and a retention screw. Treatment plan included immediate flapless placement, an interim prostheis and a submerged healing protocol **(Fig. 1)**.

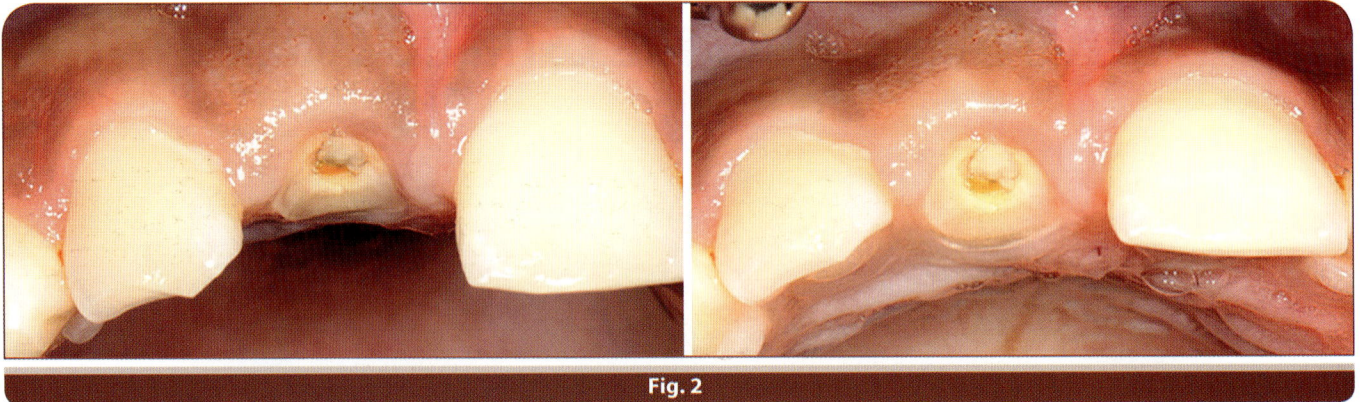

Fig. 2

Frontal and occlusal views show a thick gingival biotype and good soft tissue and adequate alveolus thickness, which are two main requisites of flapless implant placement **(Fig. 2)**.

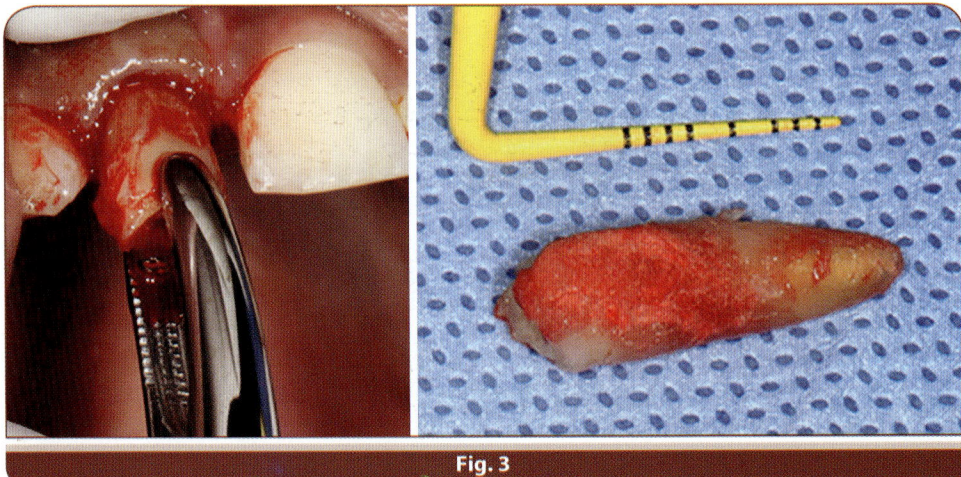

Fig. 3

The root is gently luxated with flexible luxators (Dowell) and extracted with a narrow beak serrated forceps (Medsey). It is imperative to measure the extracted fragment to know the fixture length that has to be placed ideally 3 to 4 mm of the implant should extend beyond the root apex and anchor in fresh bone **(Fig. 3)**.

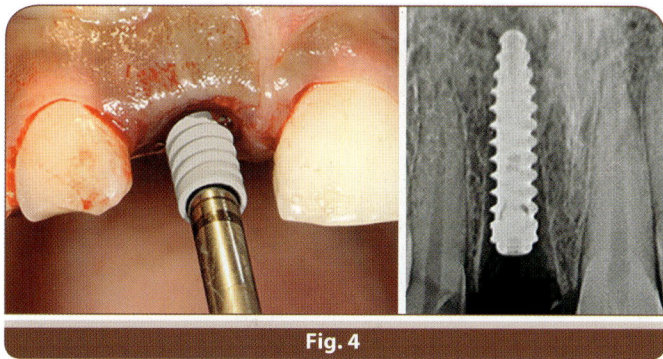

Fig. 4

A 4/15 mm Bioner DM (Bioner) implant is placed at 50 Ncm following conventional drilling protocols. Immediate postoperative X-ray shows a correct mesiodistal placement and the implant taking anchorage past the natural tooth apex (extending to the inferior nasal floor) **(Fig. 4)**.

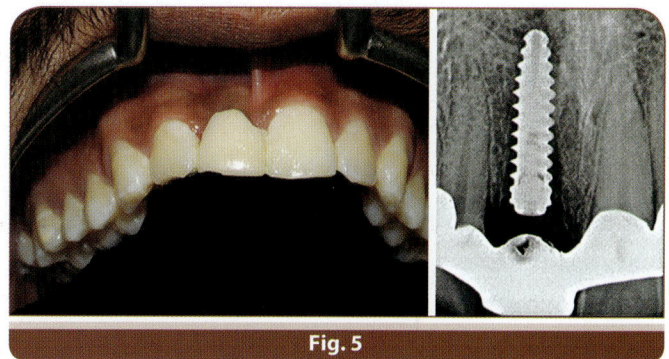

Fig. 5

A bonded metal acrylic Maryland bridge is placed on the day of surgery. At three week follow-up some collapse of soft tissue is evident. An X-ray at this stage might exhibit a slight radiolucent appearance along the length of the fixture due to on going osteoclastic activity **(Fig. 5)**.

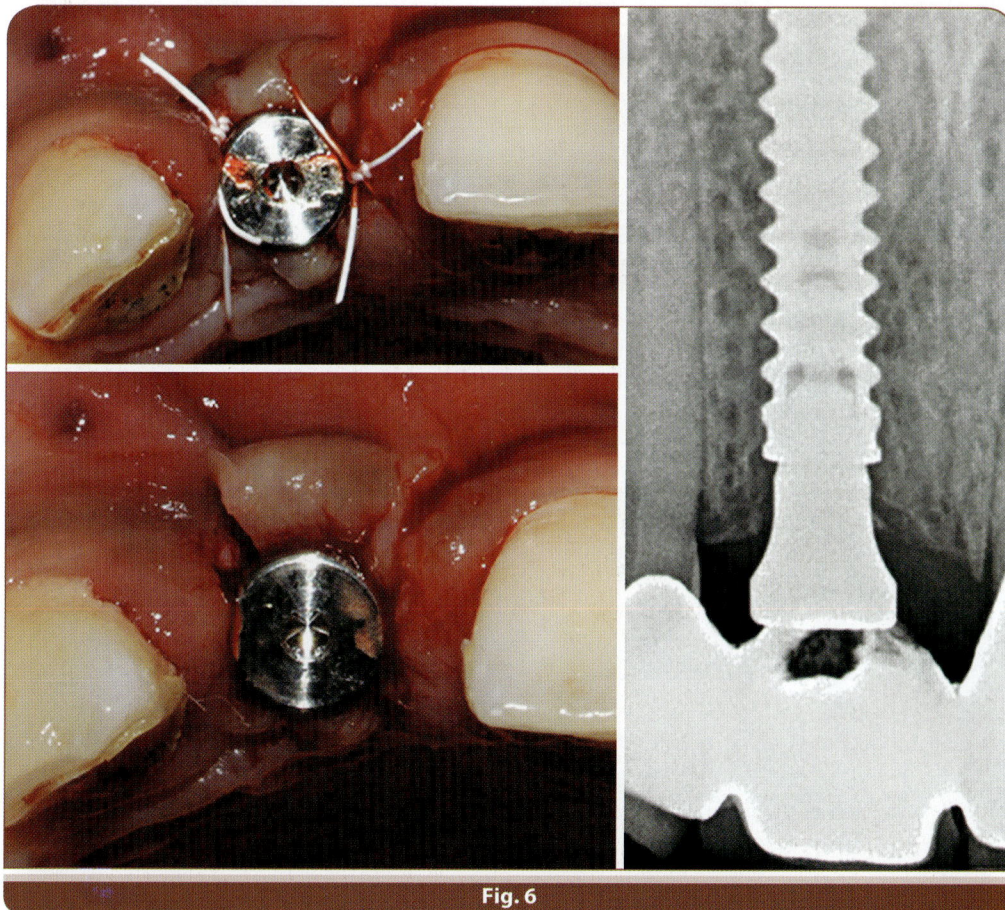

Fig. 6

At 4 months healing a palatal soft tissue roll procedure is performed to increase the thickness of tissue on the labial side. Simple interrupted sutures with 4-0 cytoplast (Osteogenics) are placed to stabilize. The tissue the X-ray with the healing collar exhibits successful osseointegration **(Fig. 6)**.

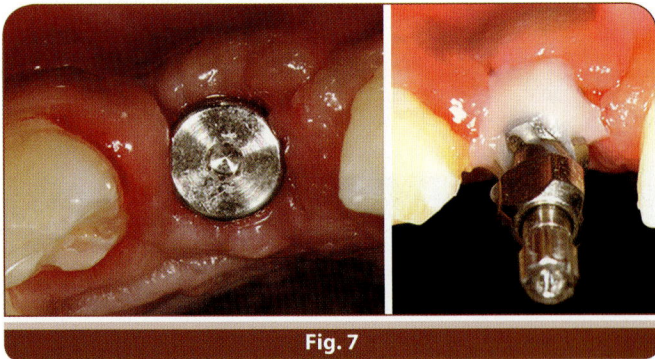

Fig. 7

At two weeks the tissue thickening is evident. An open tray impression is recorded at this stage, flowable composite is bonded to the impression post to mimic the peri-implant sulcus portion **(Fig. 7)**.

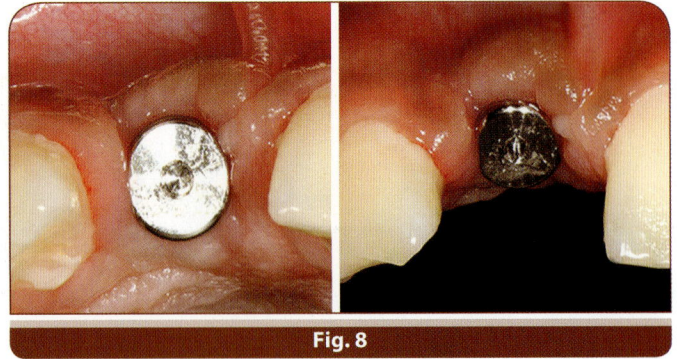

Fig. 8

At 4 weeks occlusal and frontal views clearly demonstrate a thick band of keratinized tissue around the healing collar **(Fig. 8)**.

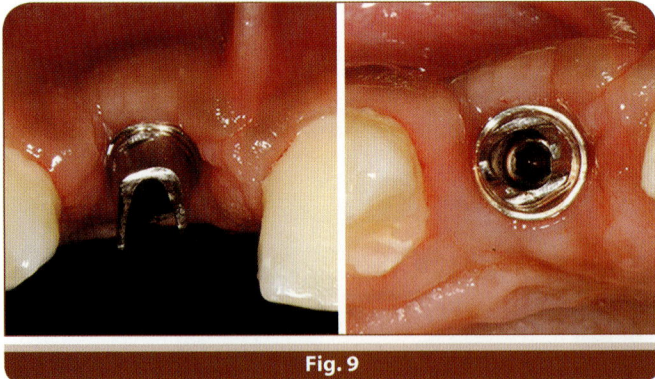

Fig. 9

Frontal and occlusal views of the final stock abutment illustrating excellent tissue health around the fixture. The abutment is torqued to 30 Ncm with a preset torque device **(Fig. 9)**.

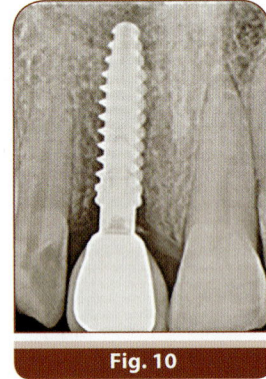

Fig. 10

Radiographic view the stable bony housing around the implant is evident with minor remodeling at the crestal region **(Fig. 10)**.

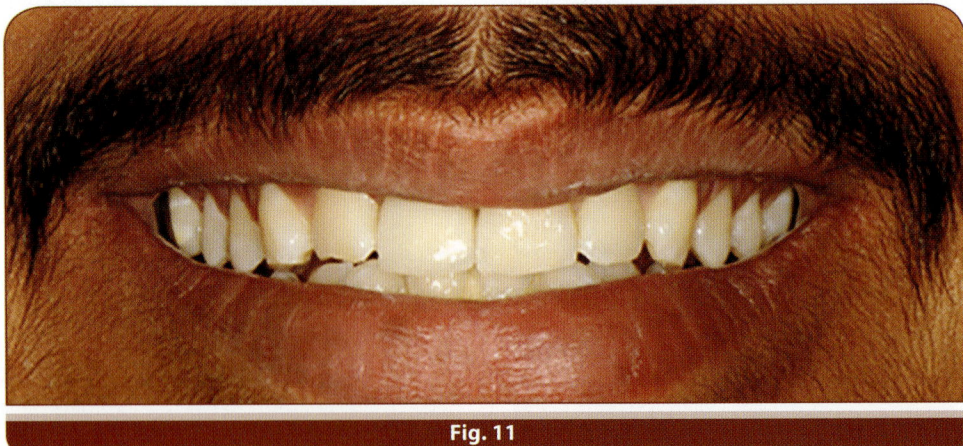

Fig. 11

One year recall clinical view of the zirconia prosthesis and smile line **(Fig. 11)**.

Lanka Mahesh, Nitika Poonia

SINGLE TOOTH REPLACEMENT IN A DEFICIENT MAXILLARY ANTERIOR ZONE WITH GBR AND SIMULTANEOUS IMPLANT

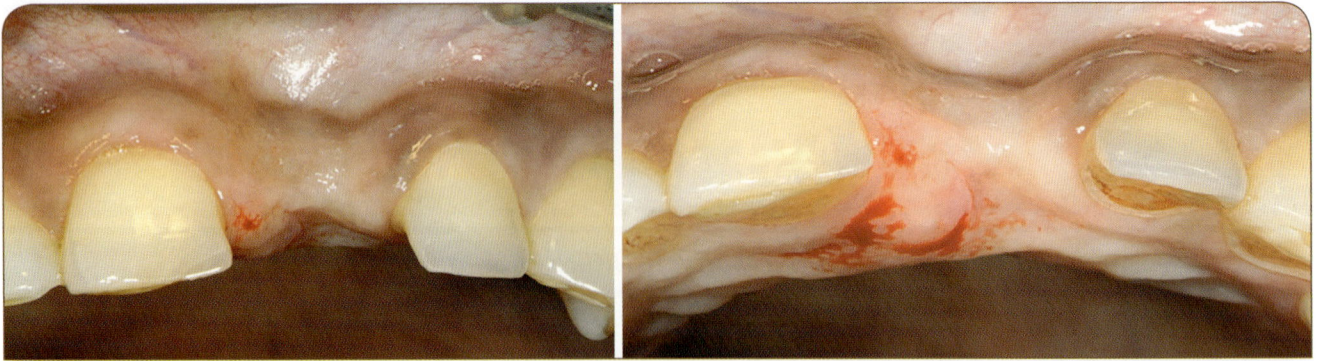

Fig. 1

Clinical frontal and occlusal view of a young male patient desiring an implant supported tooth for missing tooth #21. Other centers had advised him a block graft with delayed implant placement seeing his CBCT. A deficient ridge is evident, also soft tissue collapse is evident. Treatment plan included a simultaneous implant placement with GBR and a zirconia prosthesis **(Fig. 1)**.

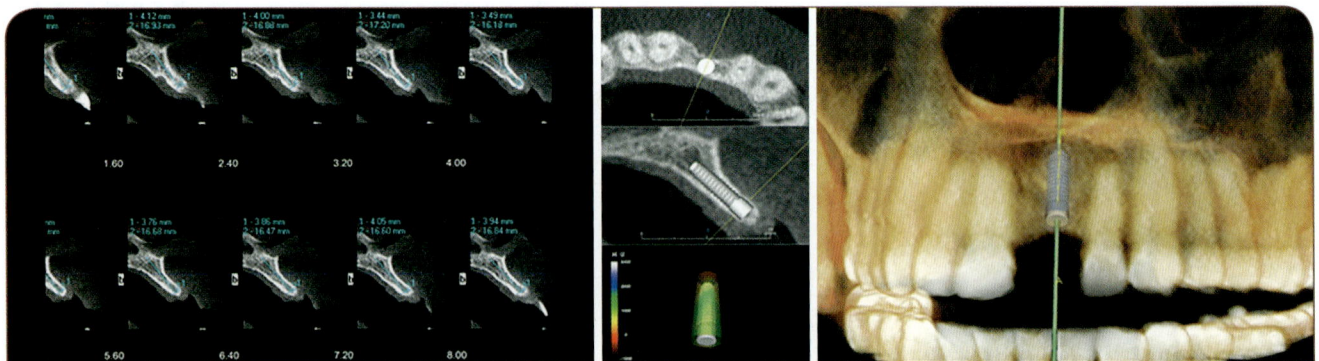

Fig. 2

The CBCT views show marked resorption. Implant simulation suggested the placement of a 3.5 mm implant with a bone graft due to narrow ridge **(Fig. 2)**.

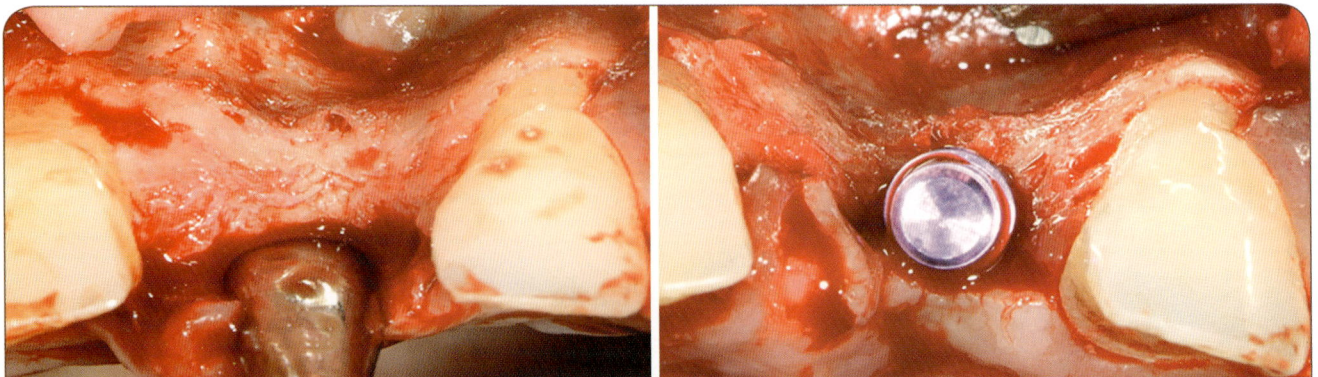

Fig. 3

Upon flap reflection the defect is clearly evident. A paralleling pin corresponding to 3.5 mm is placed to check angulation, it clearly demonstrates the facial defect although it suggests increasing the implant diameter without fracture of the facial plate **(Fig. 3)**.

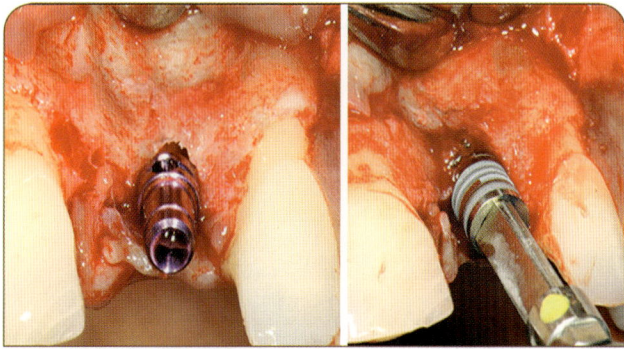

Fig. 4

Frontal view of the 3.5 mm pin showing minor cracks on the crestal area. The osteotomy is continued till the next implant size and a 4.3/11.5 nobel replace (Nobel Biocare) is placed at 45 Ncm torque **(Fig. 4)**.

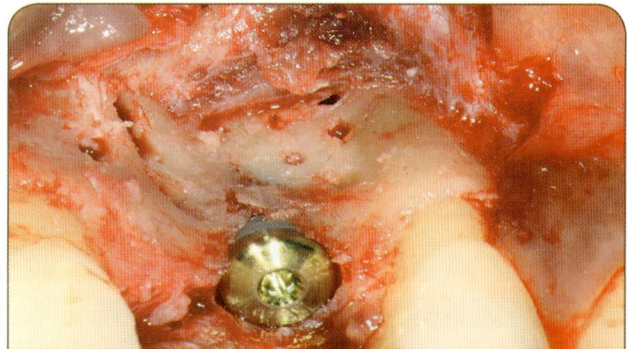

Fig. 5

Intramarrow preparation is done to accelerate the regional accelatory phenomenon, with a round bur or a lancet drill that is part of the implant surgical kit. The extremely thin facial plate and a minor fracture of the crestal area is now clearly evident **(Fig. 5)**.

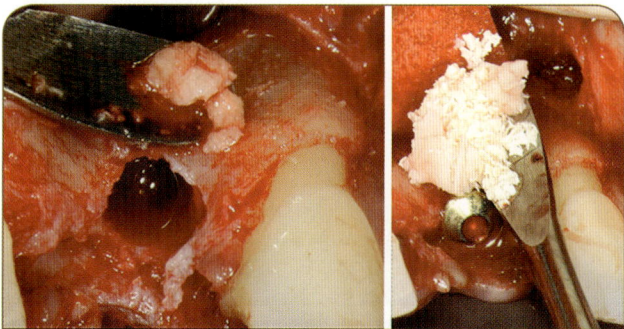

Fig. 6

Autogenous bone from the drills is collected and mixed with a bovine DBBM (cerabone, botiss). The autogenous bone should ideally contact the host bed before the bone substitute material **(Fig. 6)**.

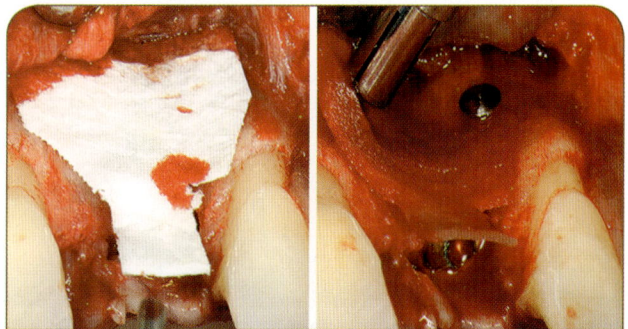

Fig. 7

A collagen membrane (RCM) is adapted over the operative site after trimming to appropriate proportion. The membrane is fixated with two tacks (Bioner) **(Fig. 7)**.

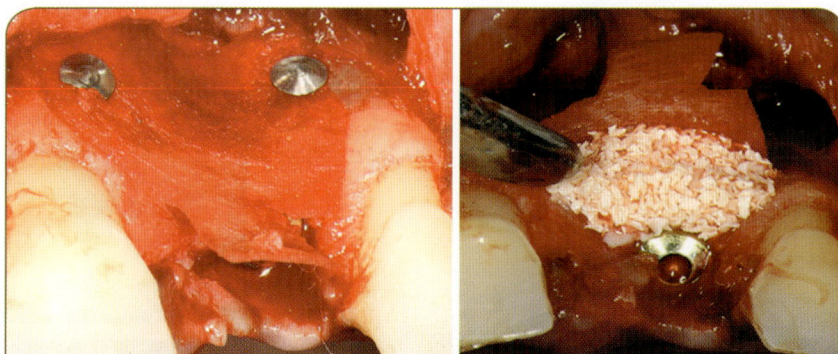

Fig. 8

The membrane is adapted with tacks and the graft is gently placed in incremental layers, it is advised that the surgical nurse hold the membrane down with an instrument of choice during this step to prevent the tacks from getting loose and the membrane getting dislodged **(Fig. 8)**.

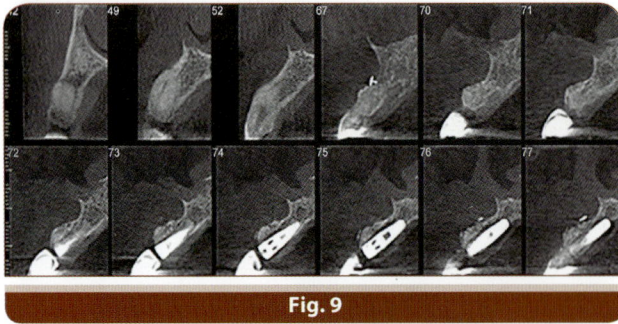

Fig. 9

This 6 month postoperative scan clearly demonstrates adequate bone graft maturation on the facial side of the implant **(Fig. 9)**.

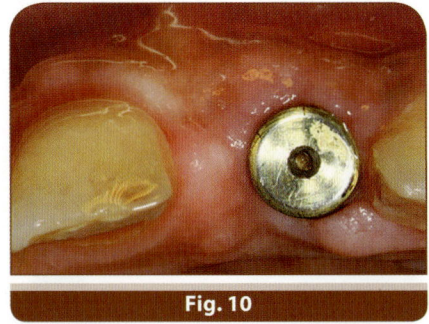

Fig. 10

A wide healing collar is used at second stage to create an adequate emergence profile **(Fig. 10)**.

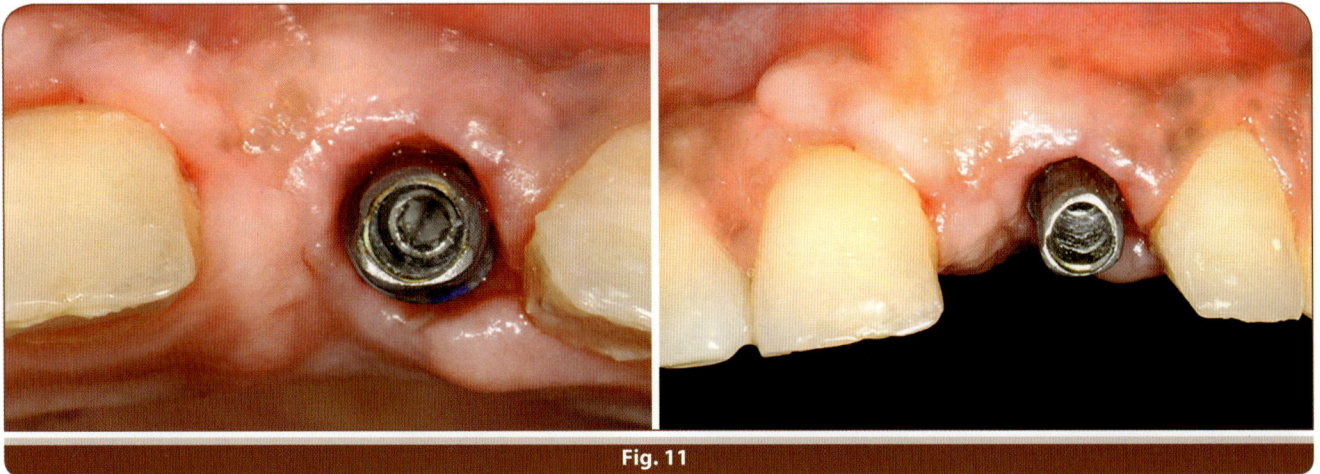

Fig. 11

Occlusal and facial views with the final abutment demonstrate adequate soft tissue bulk and contour around the implant **(Fig. 11)**.

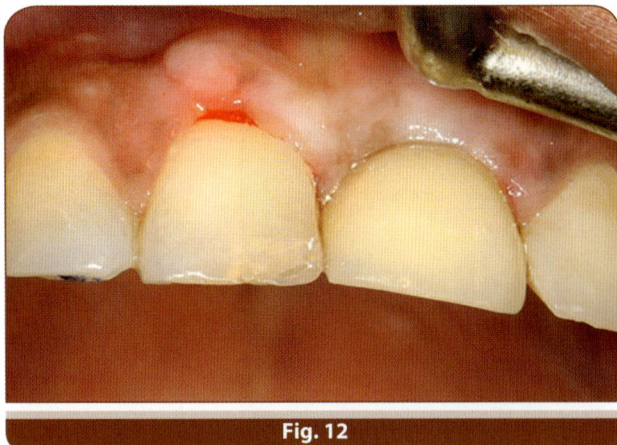

Fig. 12

Final outcome (A diastema was advised but the patient was against it and he was also against composite bonding of the adjacent tooth **(Fig. 12)**.

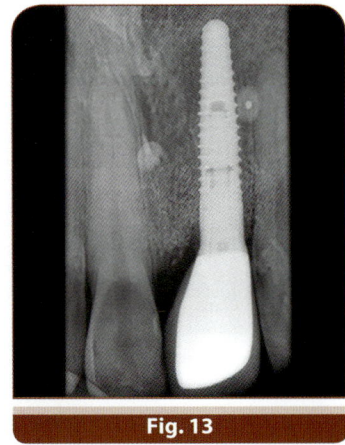

Fig. 13

Control X-ray at 1 year shows a stable crestal level (the membrane tacks can also be seen on the X-ray) **(Fig. 13)**.

Praful Bali

TISSUE ENGINEERING AND PROSTHETIC FINE TUNING TO GIVE A NEAR NATURAL OUTCOME TO AN ANTERIOR CASE DONE ON 2 IMPLANTS

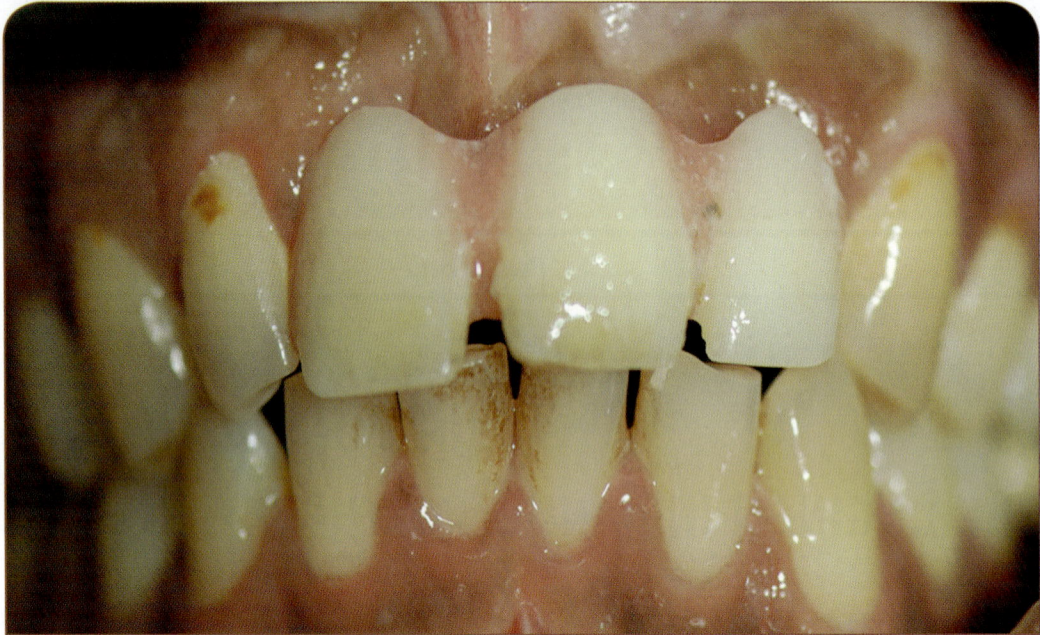

Fig. 1

Patient presents with a hopeless acrylic temporary restoration. History of failed endodontic Rx and bridge collapse leading to extraction of teeth #11, 21, 22 **(Fig. 1)**.

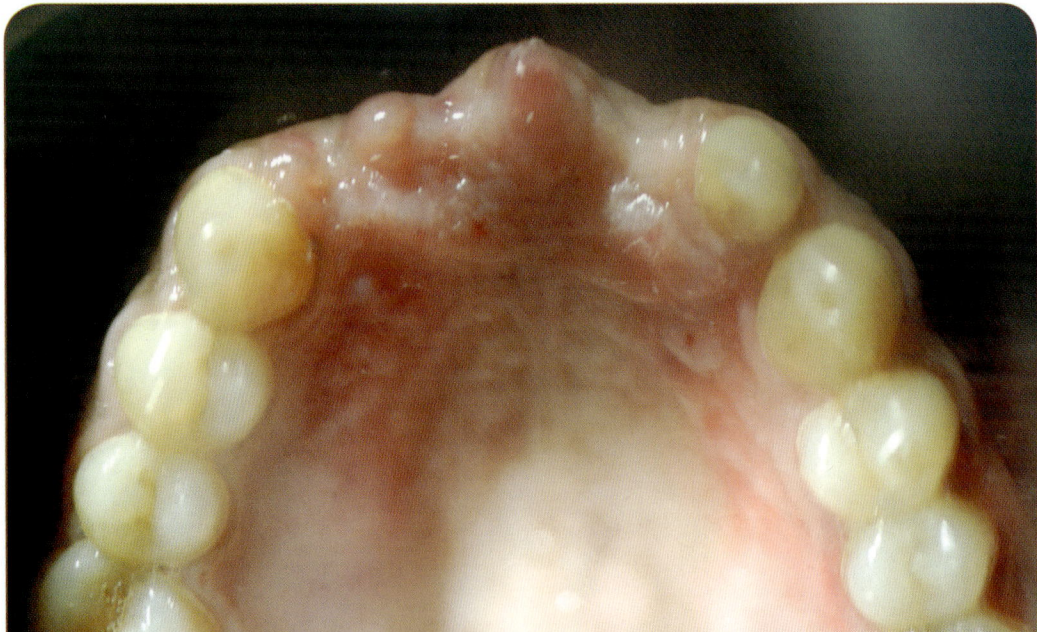

Fig. 2

A 35-year-old patient came with missing upper central incisors and upper left lateral incisor. On clinical examination and radiographic evaluation, there was deficient horizontal bone in that site and required both hard and soft tissue augmentation. Preoperative—occlusal view, note the slight facial dip in #21 area indicating the deficiency of buccal bone **(Fig. 2)**.

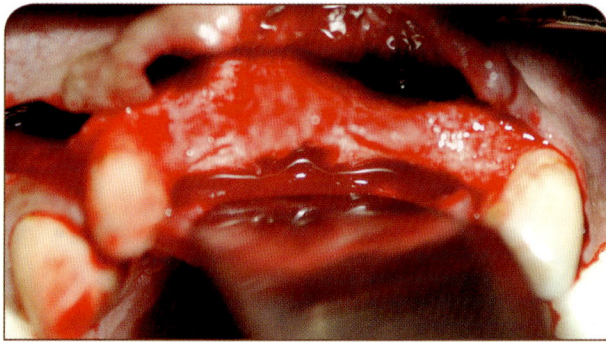

Fig. 3

Full thickness flap reflection done, note the deficient buccal bone **(Fig. 3)**.

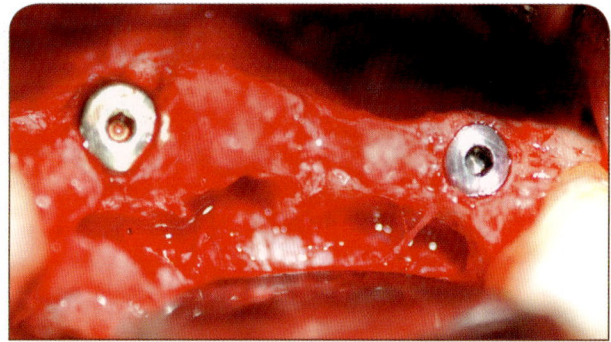

Fig. 4

Implants placed 4.3/13 and 3.5/13 (Nobel biocare). Soft tissue grafting was done to take care of the visible dip **(Fig. 4)**.

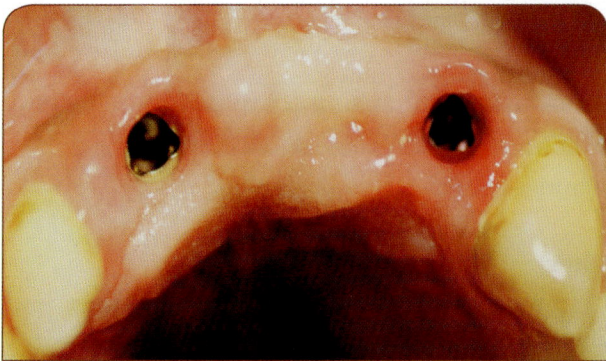

Fig. 5

Four month postoperative— occlusal view. Procera (zirconia) abutments are customized and torqued at 30 N/cm^2 **(Fig. 5)**.

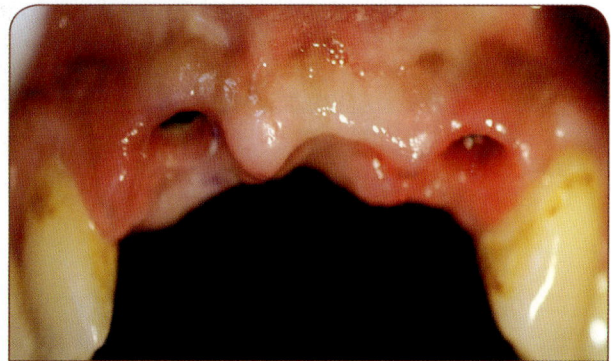

Fig. 6

Facial view: Soft tissue engineering—repeated pressure is applied on the pontic region to train the soft tissue. Repeated prototypes are made to achieve the final result **(Fig. 6)**.

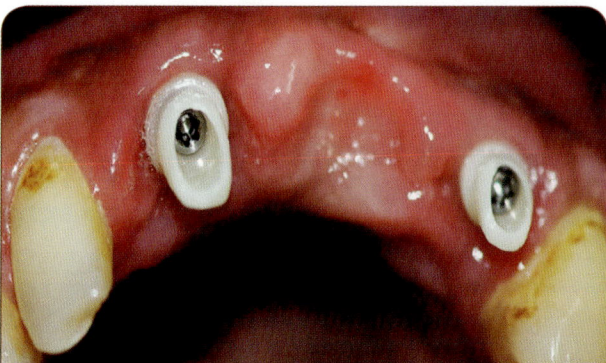

Fig. 7

Occlusal view: Soft tissue engineering—repeated pressure is applied on the pontic region to train the soft tissue **(Fig. 7)**.

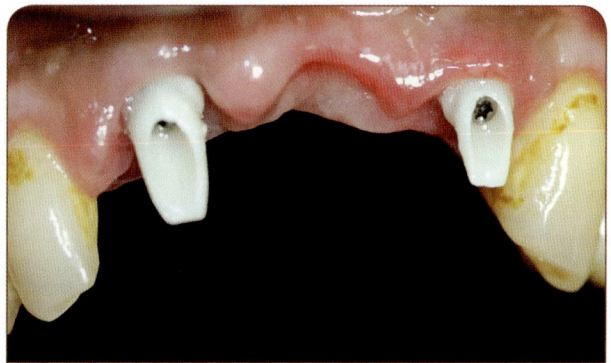

Fig. 8

Procera permanent abutment— and final soft tissue esthetics after changing prototype a number of times. (6 month after Stage II) **(Fig. 8)**.

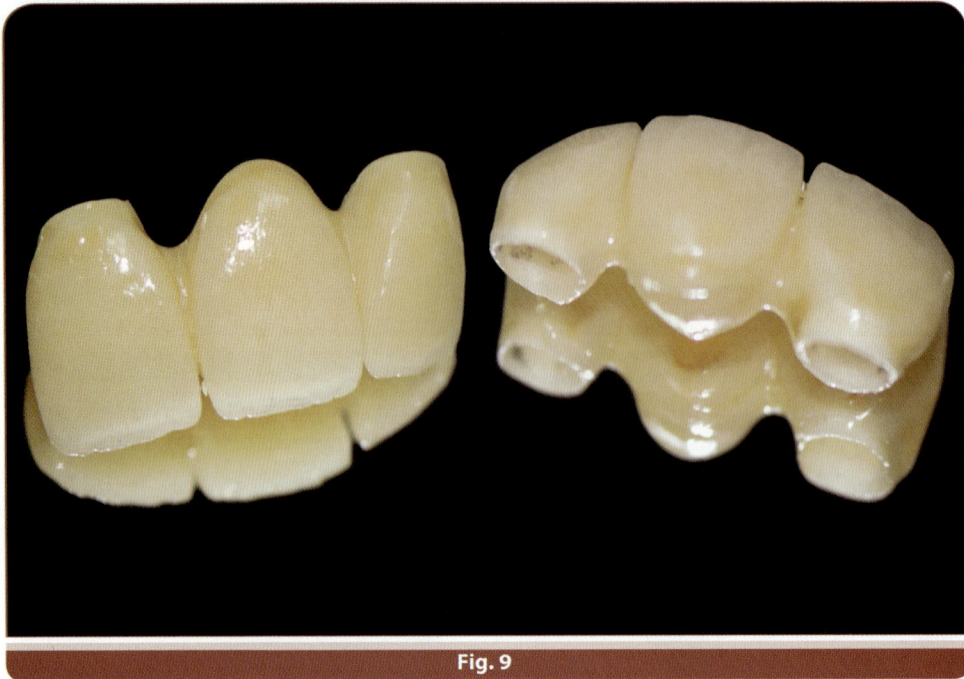

Fig. 9

Procera permanent 3 unit bridge **(Fig. 9)**.

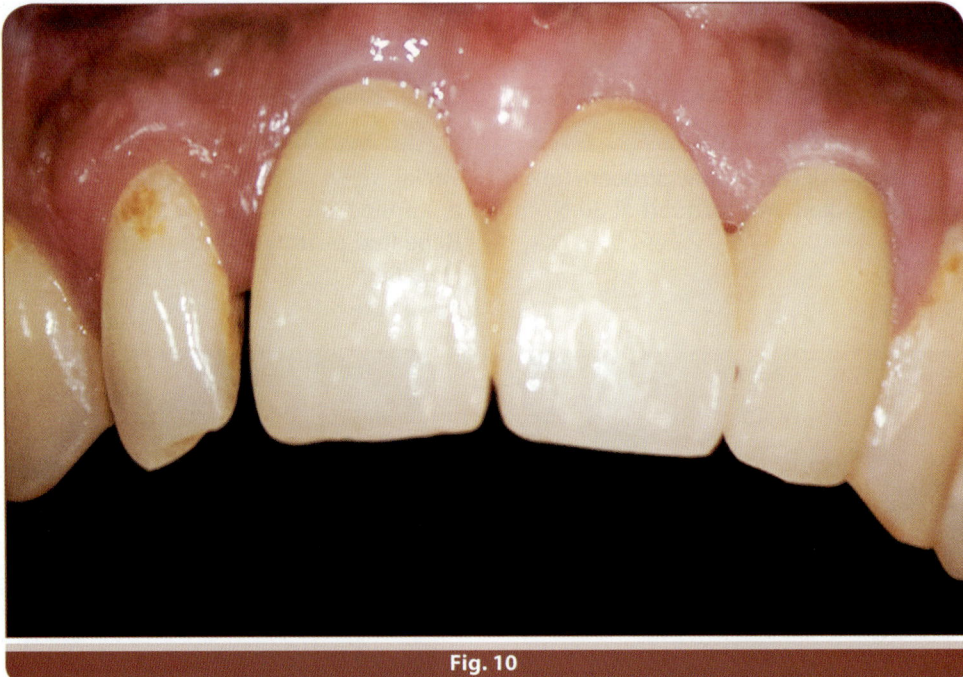

Fig. 10

Final restoration on implants, note the excellent soft tissue esthetics and pseudopapilla at the pontic area. The pontic is ovate in design to enable esthetics, hygiene and function **(Fig. 10)**.

SIMULTANEOUS GBR, SOFT TISSUE AUGMENTATION AND IMMEDIATE PROVISIONALIZATION FOR ENHANCED ESTHETIC IN AN ANTERIOR CASE

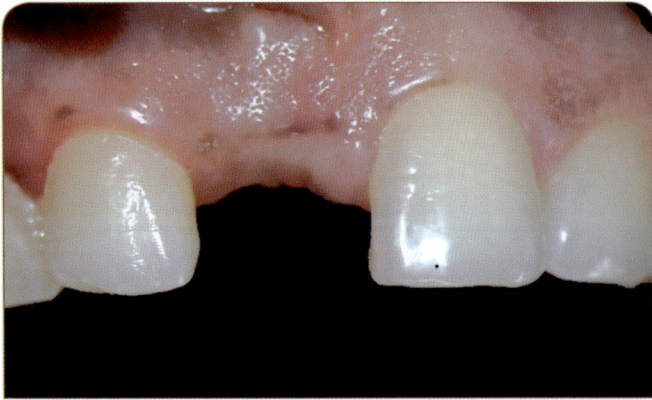

Fig. 1

Preoperative facial view of a young male patient with a missing tooth # 11 **(Fig. 1)**.

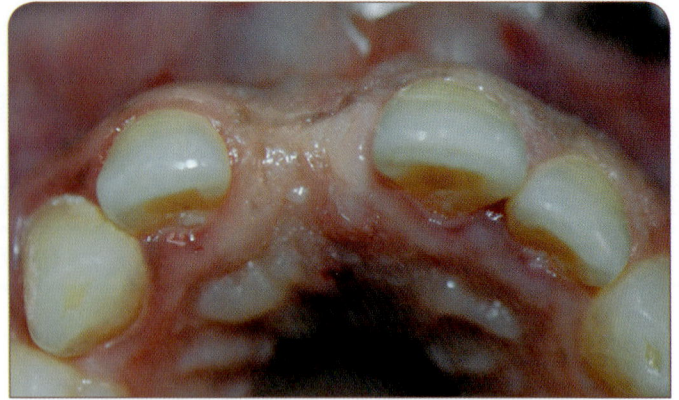

Fig. 2

Preoperative occlusal view: Note the slight buccal bone dip **(Fig. 2)**.

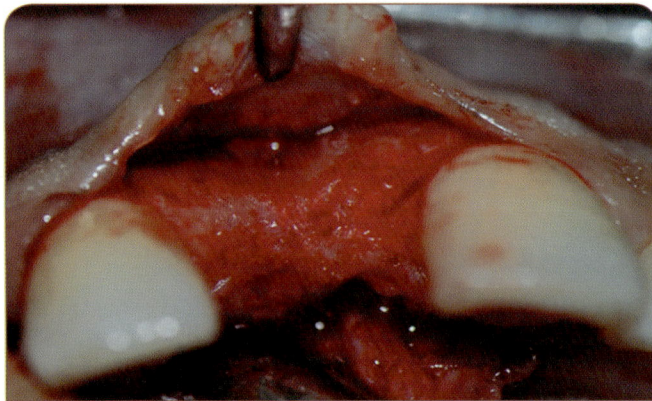

Fig. 3

A full thickness flap reflected to expose the underlying bone. Good bone width to place a decent diameter implant **(Fig. 3)**.

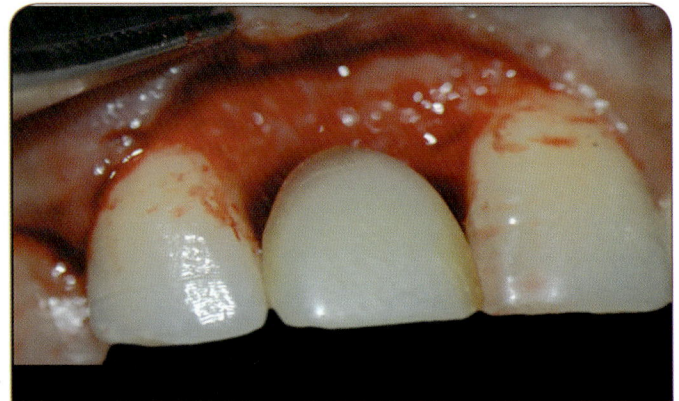

Fig. 4

Patients existing removable partial denture customized to use it as a surgical stent for a 3D implant placement **(Fig. 4)**.

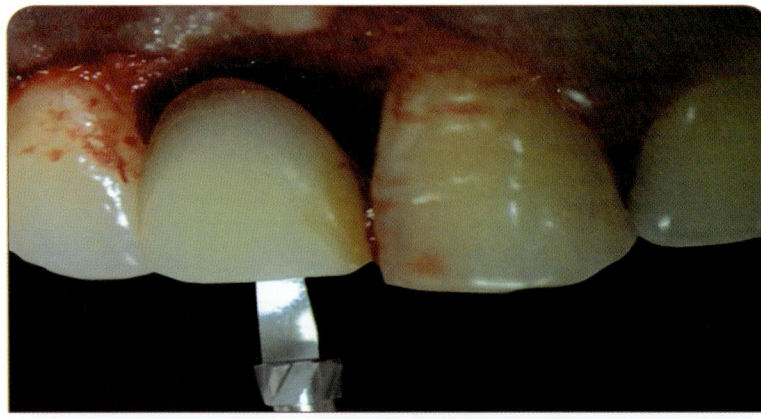

Fig. 5

The pilot drilling is done through the palatal aspect of the surgical stent so as to make sure that the position of the implant buccolingually is perfect **(Fig. 5)**.

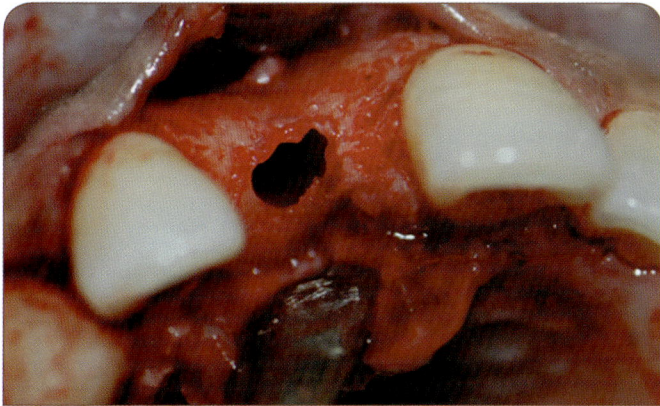
Fig. 6

The osteotomy preparation: There is adequate amount of buccal bone around the osteotomy but the evident buccal dip needs to be attended (**Fig. 6**).

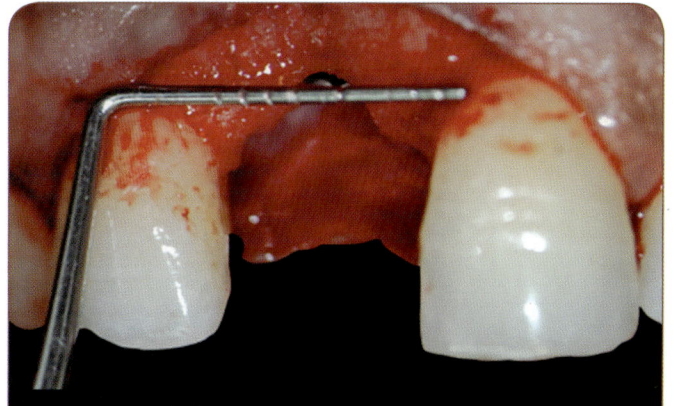
Fig. 7

3D implant placement—vertically 2–3 mm below the CE junction of the adjacent central incisor (**Fig. 7**).

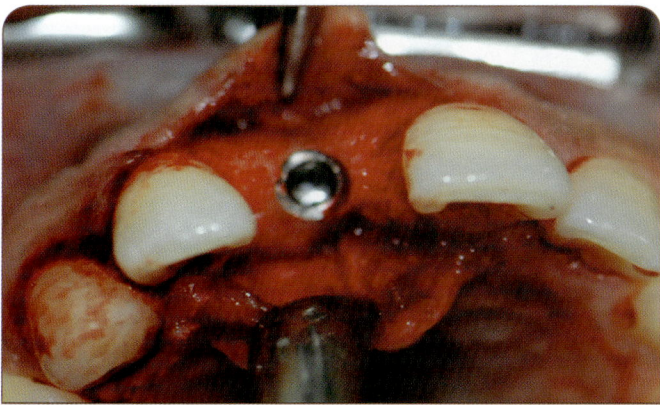
Fig. 8

Occlusal view of 4/12 blue sky implant (Bredent) in place. Implant has attained more than 50 Ncm torque fulfilling the criteria for immediate fixed temporization (**Fig. 8**).

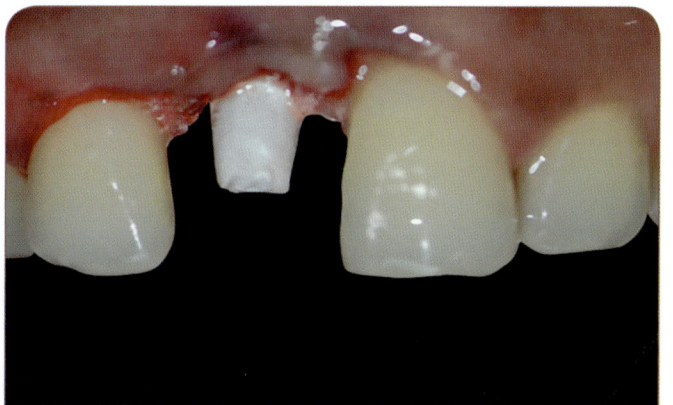
Fig. 9

A Bio-HPP permamant abutment is torqued to the implant at 35 Ncm. This is the One abutment- One time concept (**Fig. 9**).

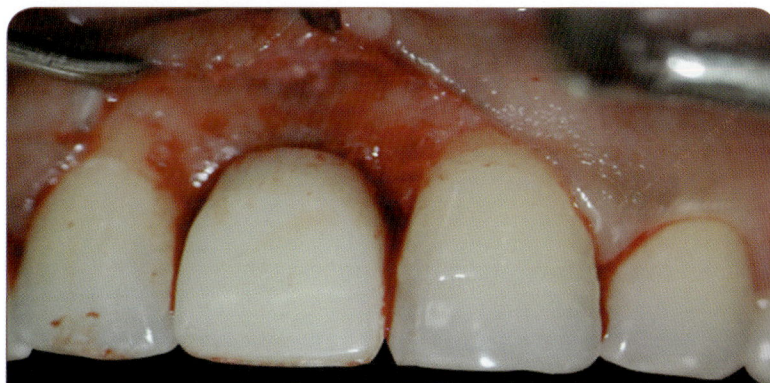
Fig. 10

An acrylic temporary crown is cemented to the Bio-HPP abutment and care is taken to remove every bit of cement after cementation (**Fig. 10**).

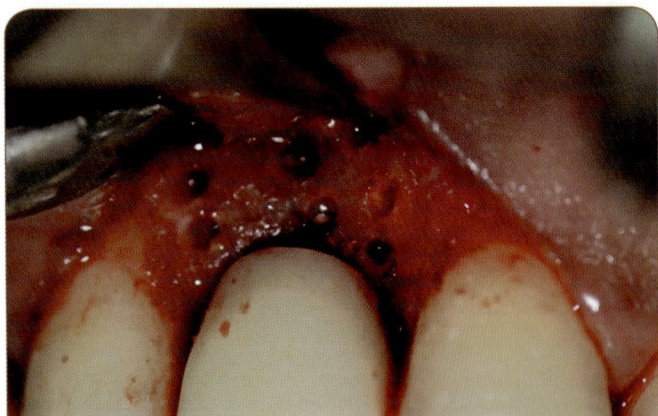
Fig. 11

The buccal bone bed is prepared for GBR procedure (Fig. 11).

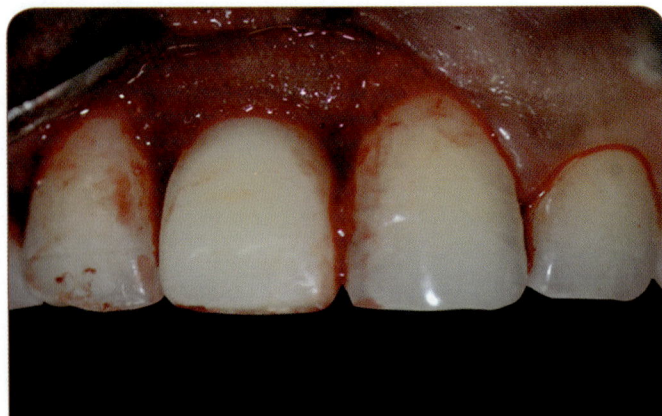
Fig. 12

Novabone Putty is augmented to add bulk to the existing dip (Fig. 12).

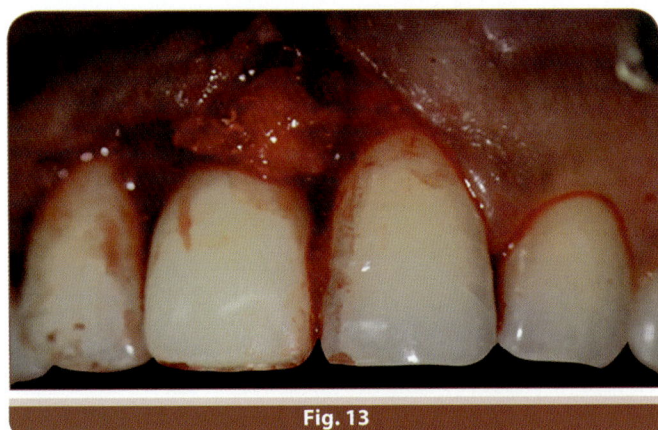
Fig. 13

A connective tissue pedicle graft is placed over the augmentation to increase the soft tissue profile (Fig. 13).

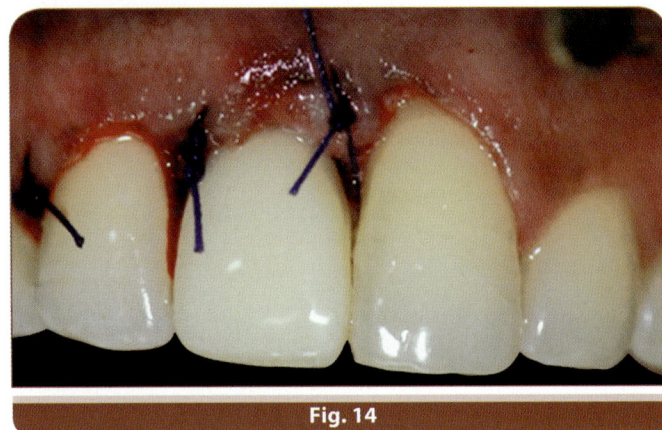
Fig. 14

Suturing done around the fixed temporary crown (Fig. 14).

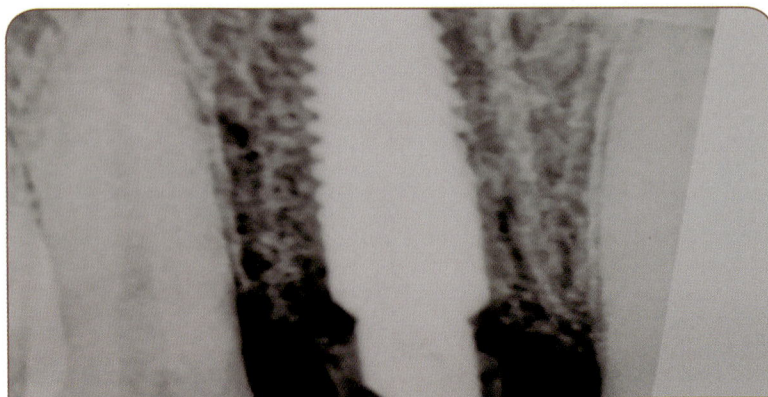
Fig. 15

Immediate postoperative IOPA X-ray (Fig. 15).

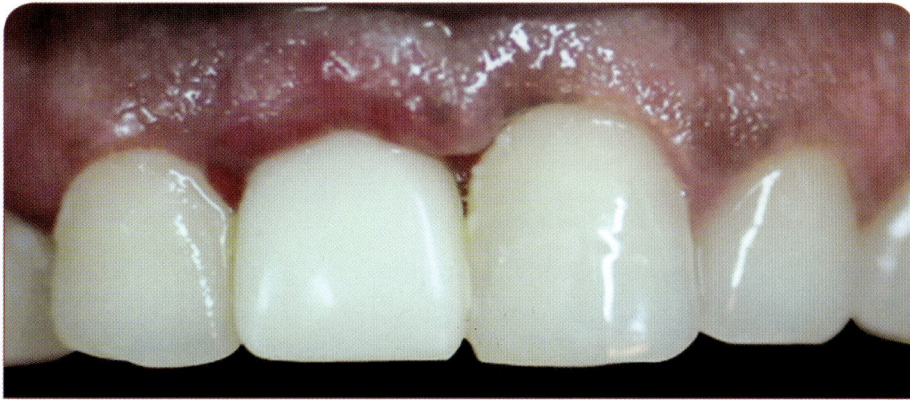

Fig. 16

Healthy tissue 2 weeks postoperative **(Fig. 16)**.

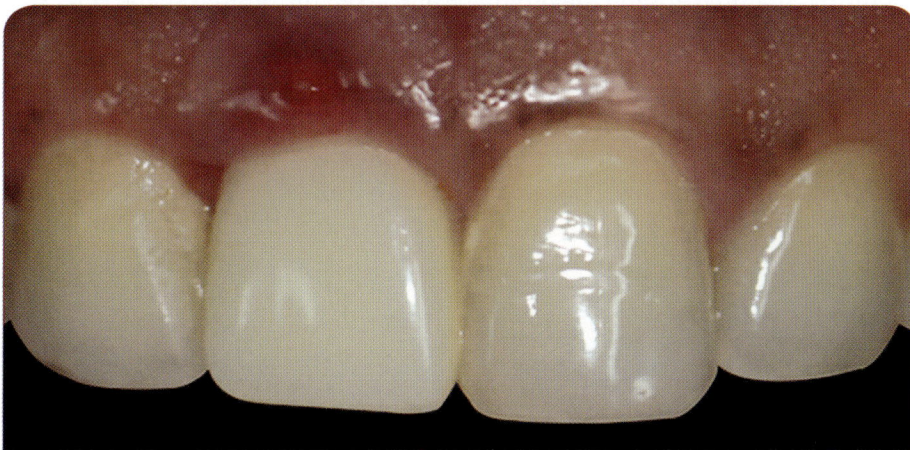

Fig. 17

3 months postoperative: excellent healing and tissue growth around the implant tooth **(Fig. 17)**.

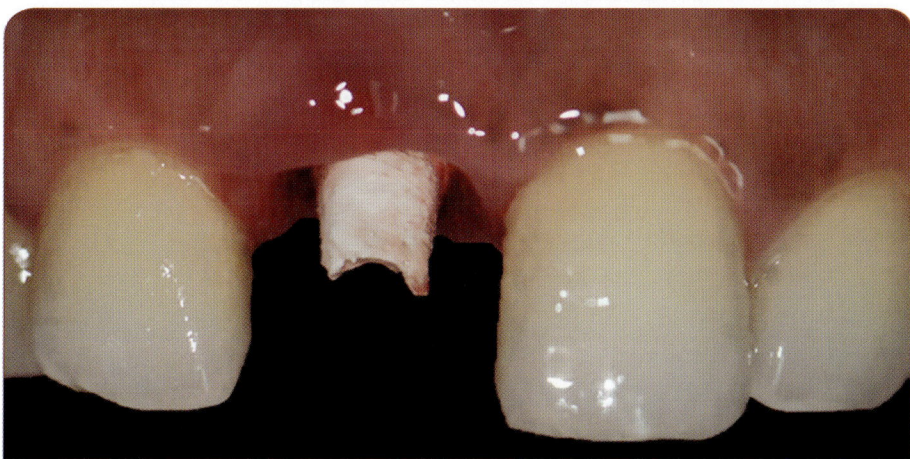

Fig. 18

3 months postoperative: excellent tissue maturation, ready for impressions **(Fig. 18)**.

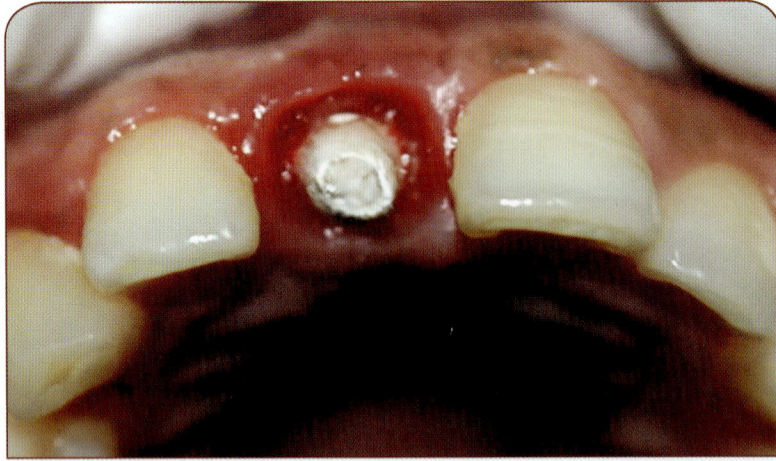
Fig. 19

Tissue has matured around the prototype and taken the desired shape **(Fig. 19)**.

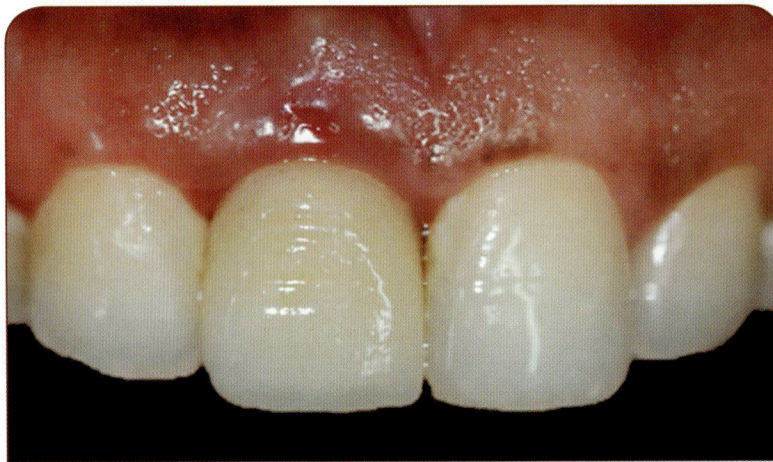
Fig. 20

Final crown over the implant tooth, excellent hard and soft tissue integration and high esthetic result **(Fig. 20)**.

Praful Bali, Stutee Grewal, Shweta Bali

ORTHO-PERIO-PROSTHO-COMBO TO ACHIEVE UTMOST ESTHETICS IN THE ANTERIOR ZONE

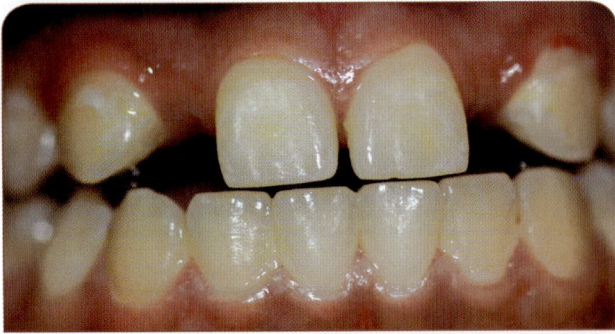

Fig. 1

Patient presents with congenitally missing upper lateral incisors. Clinical and radiographic evaluation is done and it is decided to do orthodontic correction to eliminate the central diastema and also create proper space for implants in the lateral incisor areas **(Fig. 1)**.

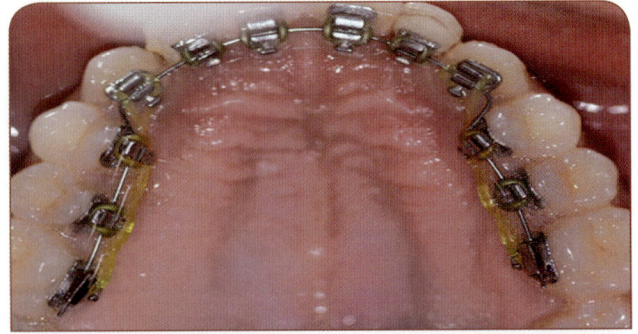

Fig. 2

Lingual orthodontics done **(Fig. 2)**.

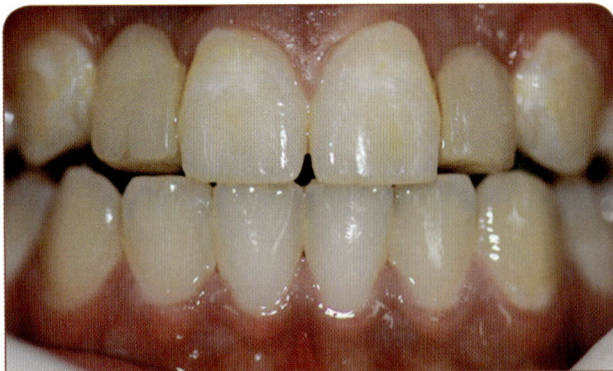

Fig. 3

Temporary acrylic teeth are bonded attached along with the lingual brackets to give a fixed temporary solution during the orthodontic treatment and also during osseointegration period. Note that the diastema between the central incisors has closed **(Fig. 3)**.

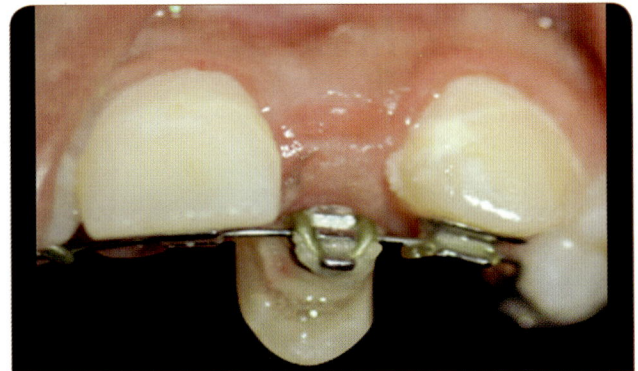

Fig. 4

Preoperative view **(Fig. 4)**.

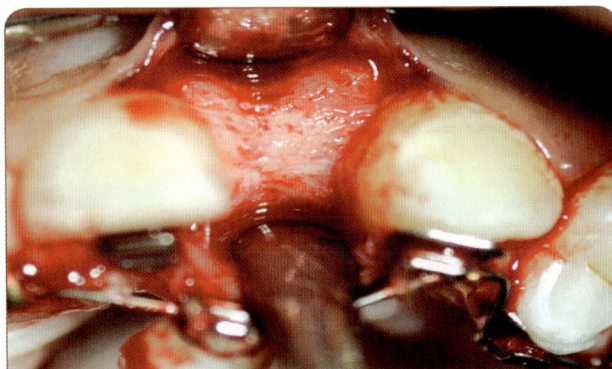

Fig. 5

A full thickness flap reflected and underlying bone exposed **(Fig. 5)**.

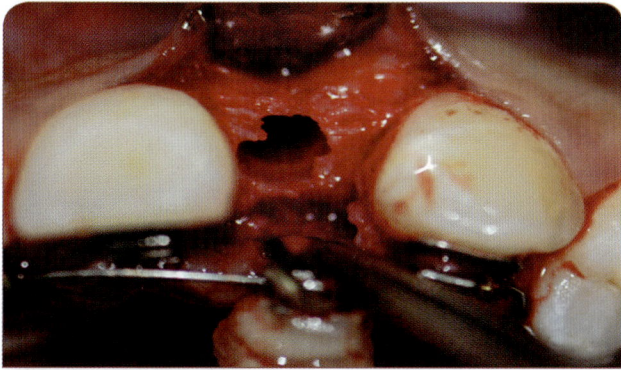

Fig. 6

Osteotomy preparation done. The remaining facial bone looks thin and a GBR procedure is planned after the placement of implants **(Fig. 6)**.

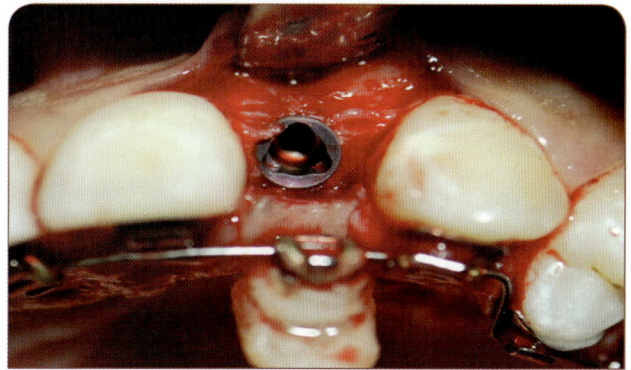

Fig. 7

A 3.5/13 Nobel groovy implant (Nobel Biocare) is placed in a 3D position **(Fig. 7)**.

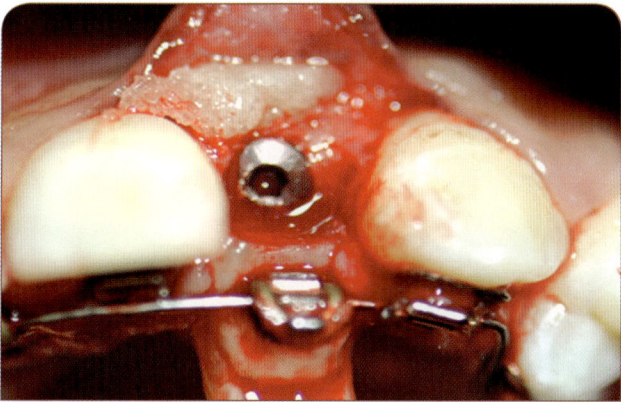

Fig. 8

Novabone putty as part of the GBR **(Fig. 8)**.

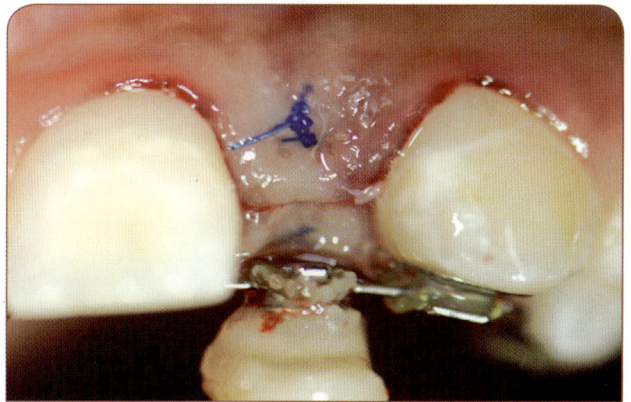

Fig. 9

Suturing done and the site left to heal up. The fixed provisional placed back **(Fig. 9)**.

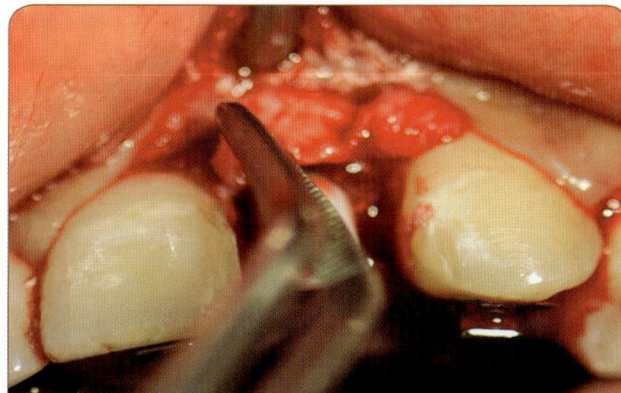

Fig. 10

A connective tissue graft taken from the palate to enhance the soft tissue architecture **(Fig. 10)**.

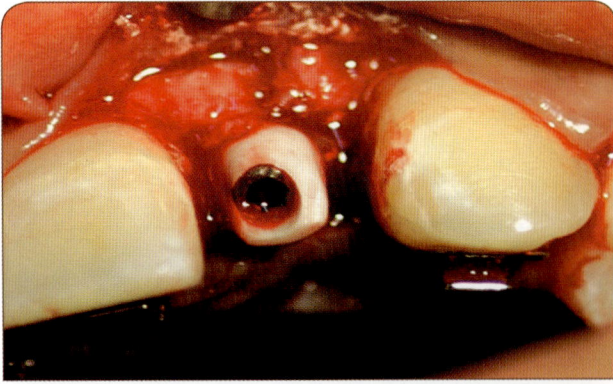

Fig. 11

The pedicle CT graft placed and a temporary made **(Fig. 11)**.

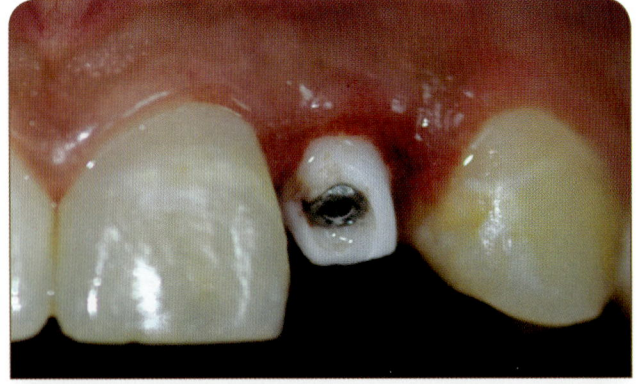

Fig. 12

Healed tissue 3 months post CT graft **(Fig. 12)**.

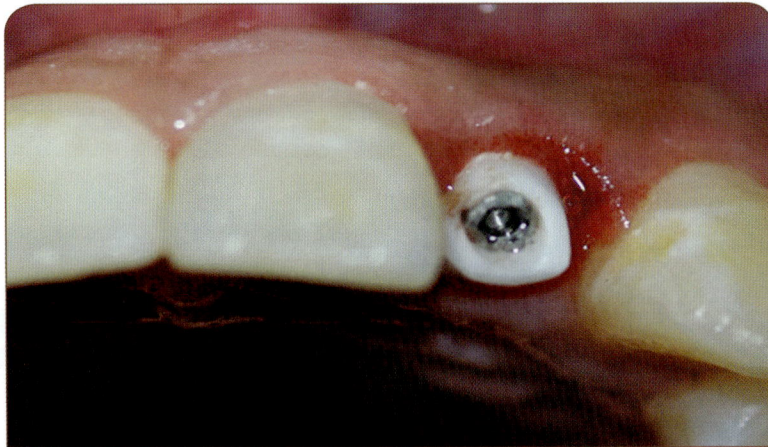

Fig. 13

Occlussal view showing good soft tissue integration **(Fig. 13)**.

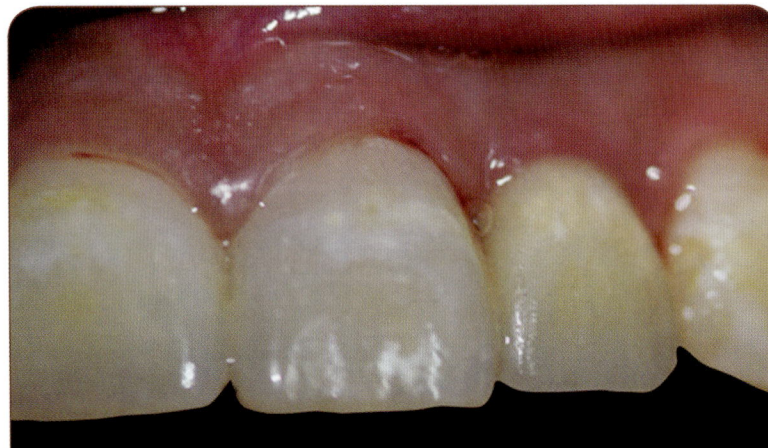

Fig. 14

Final E-Max crown over the procera abutment **(Fig. 14)**.

CASE STUDY 12

Glenn Mascarenhas

Congenitally Missing Upper Lateral Incisors Restored with Orthodontic Treatment and One-Piece Dental Implants

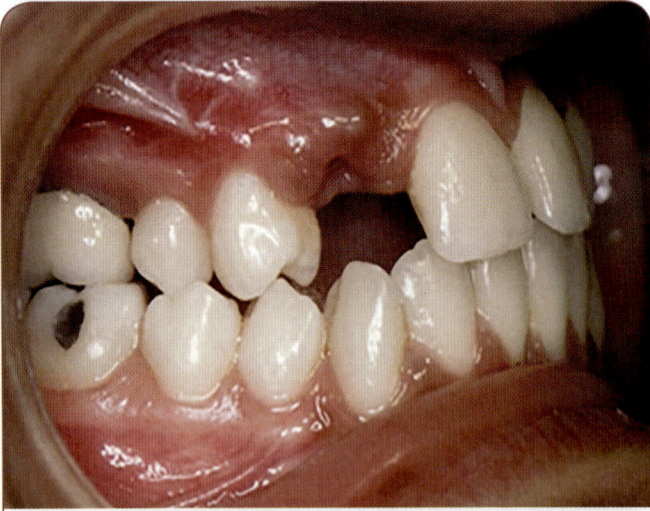

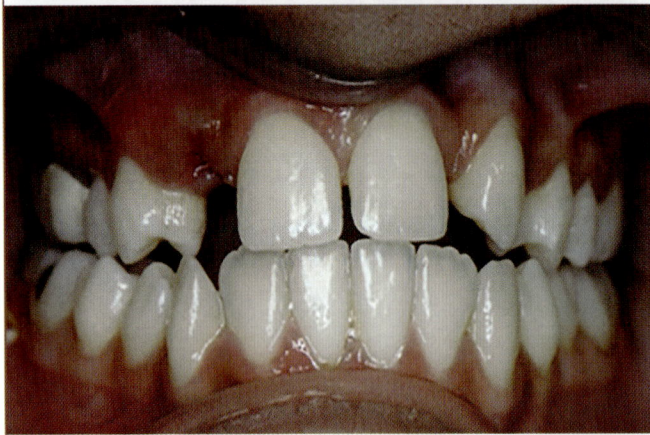

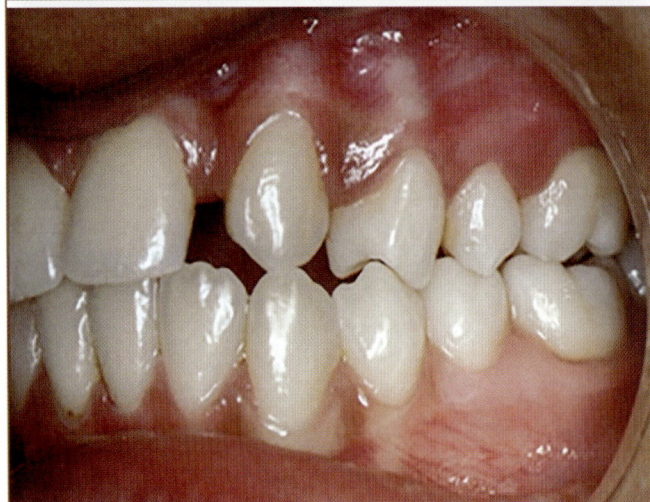

Fig. 1

Fig. 2

Right lateral view showing congenitally missing upper right lateral incisor and canine. Retracted frontal view showing congenitally missing upper right lateral incisor, canine and upper left lateral incisor. Left lateral view showing congenitally missing upper left lateral incisor **(Fig. 1)**.

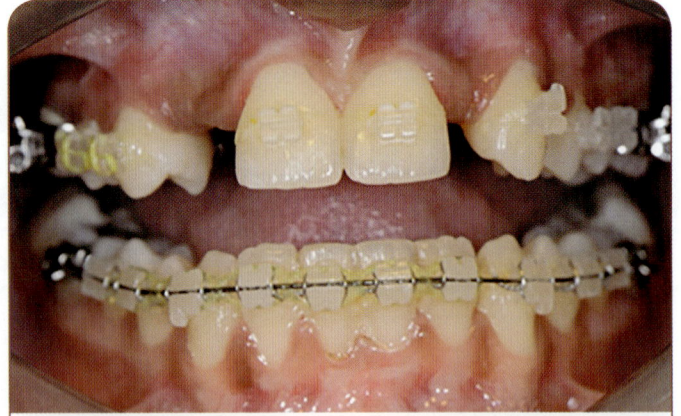

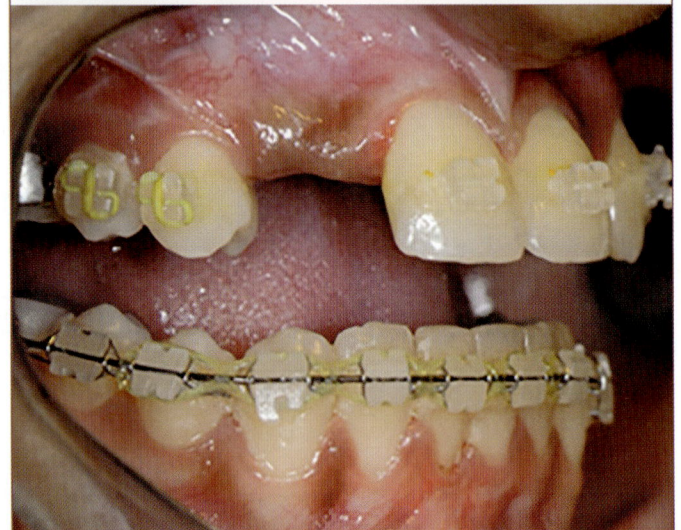

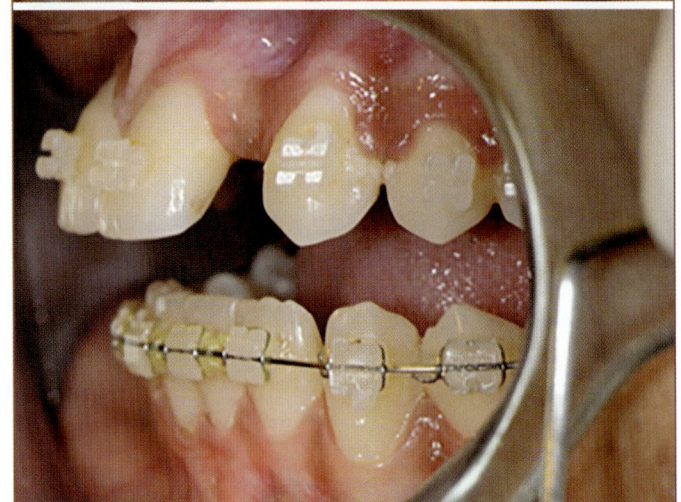

Retracted frontal view showing orthodontic treatment in progress to distribute the available space proportionately. Upper right space closure to accommodate a lateral incisor only. Upper left space being opened to accommodate a lateral incisor **(Fig. 2)**.

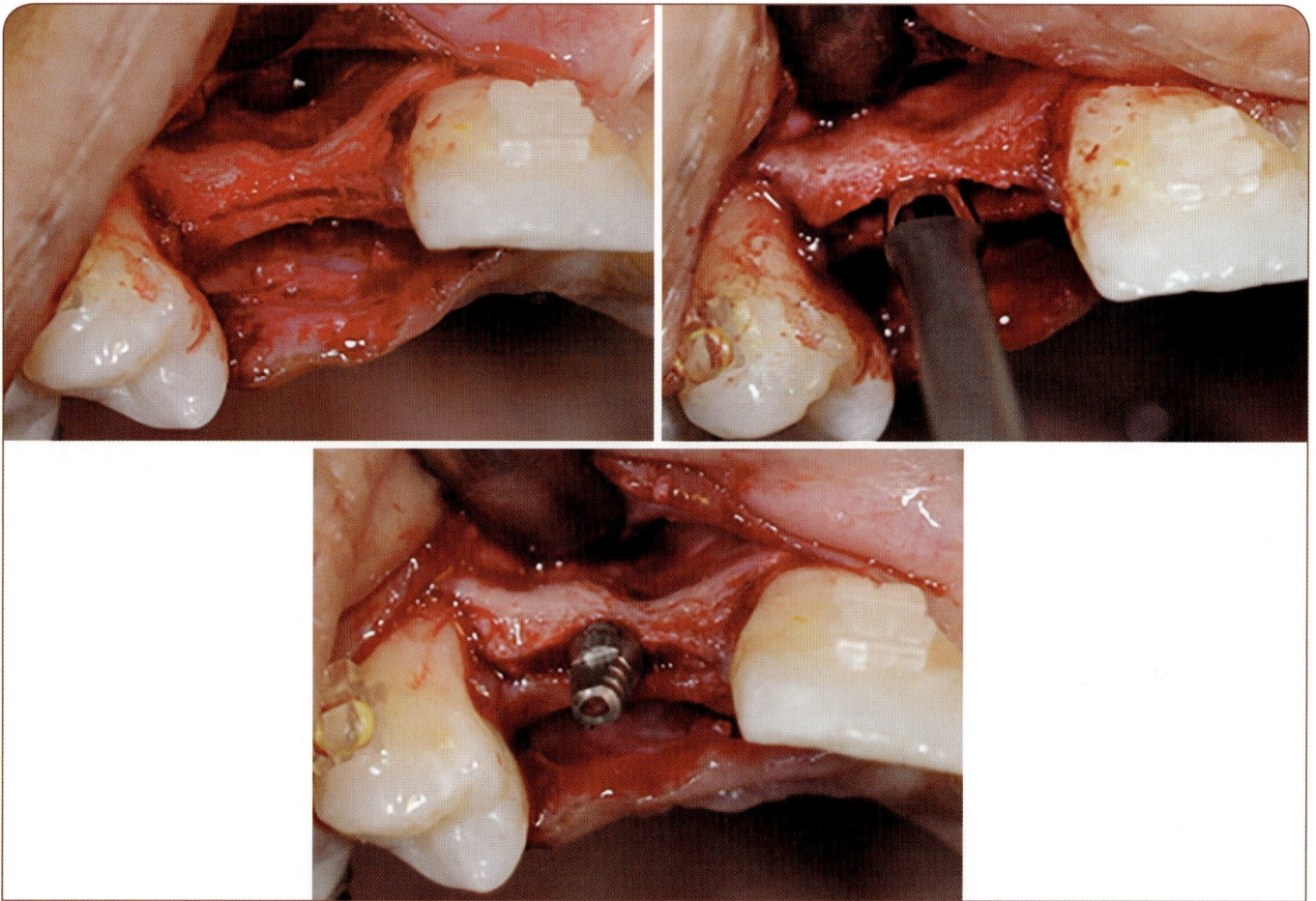

Fig. 3

Narrow ridge undergoing a bone-splitting procedure to place a one-piece implant. Separation and expansion of the labial and palatal cortical plates. Insertion of a one-piece implant to restore a missing lateral incisor **(Fig. 3)**.

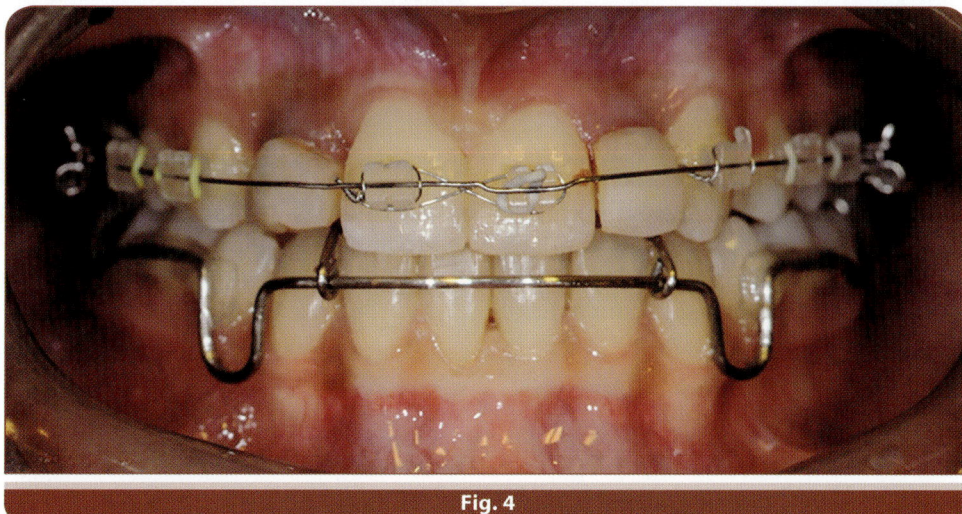

Fig. 4

Temporary acrylic crowns on implants while orthodontic treatment is completed **(Fig. 4)**.

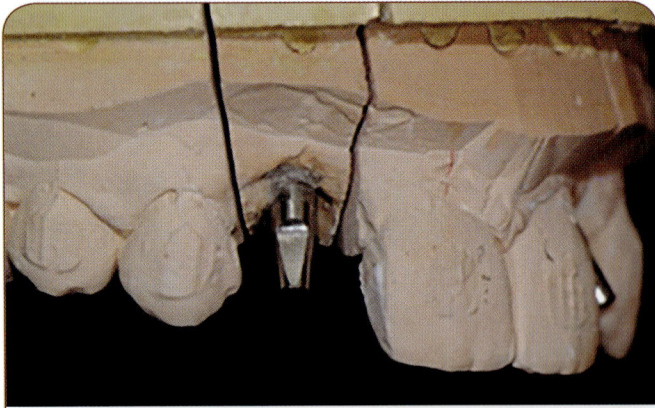

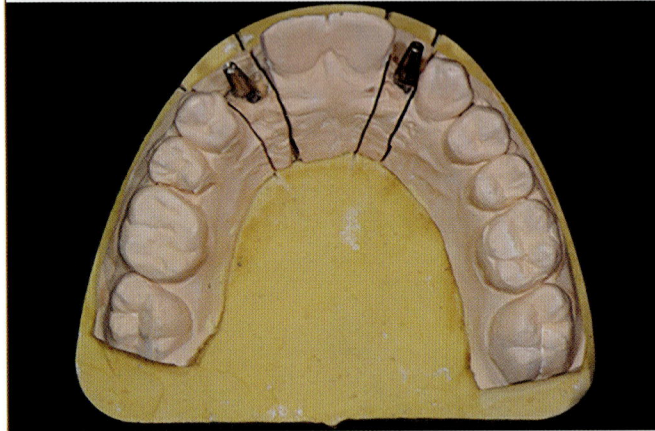

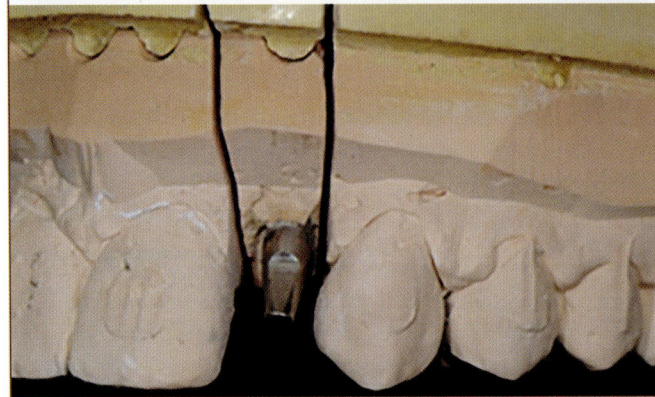

Fig. 5

Fig. 6

Layered Zirconia crowns cemented on one-piece implant **(Fig. 6)**.

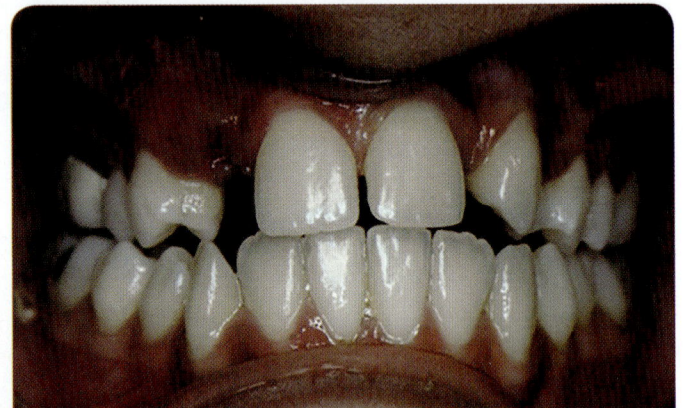

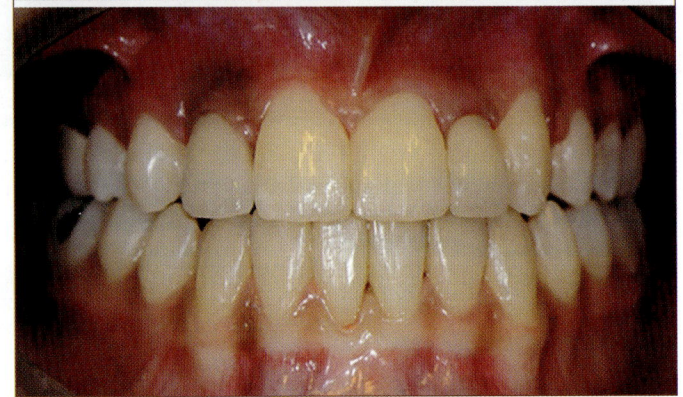

Fig. 7

Right lateral view of working model showing abutment head of one-piece implant. Occlusal view of working model showing both abutment heads in the ideal position. Left lateral view of working model showing abutment head of one-piece implant **(Fig. 5)**.

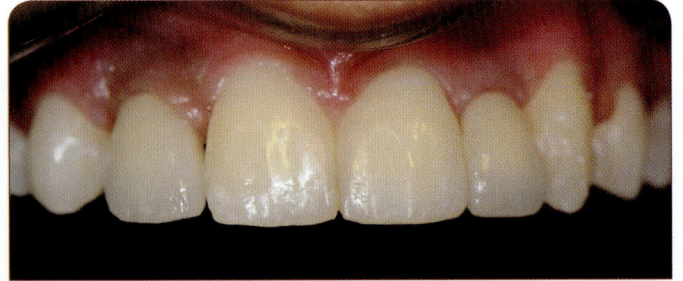

Before/After: Note that the upper right premolar has been contoured to resemble a maxillary canine **(Fig. 7)**.

SECTION 2

Immediate Implantation into Extracted Socket

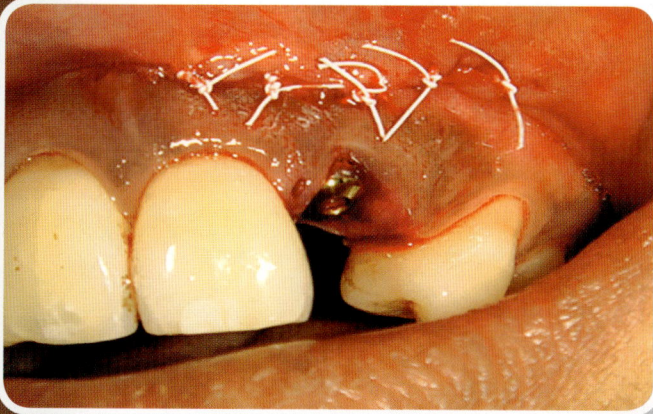

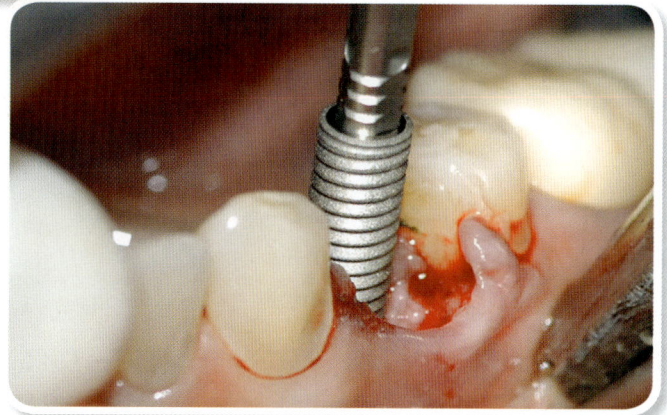

Lanka Mahesh

IMMEDIATE IMPLANTS ROOT SUBMERGENCE INTRA/EXTRA SOCKET GBR AND SOFT TISSUE MANIPULATION FOR A MAXILLARY ANTERIOR THREE UNIT PROSTHESIS

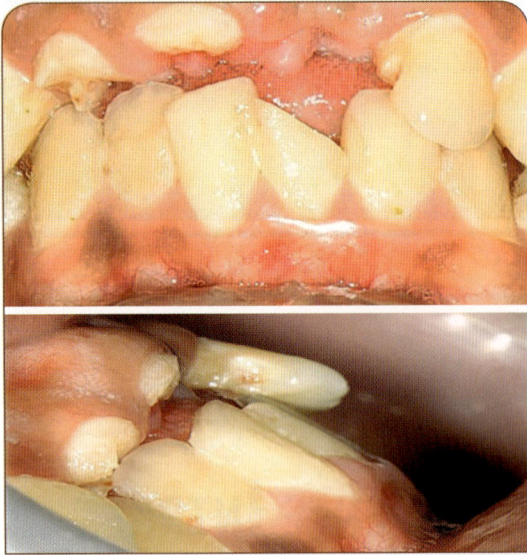

Fig. 1

A 22-year-old patient with history of trauma with fractured teeth # 11, 12 and avulsed tooth #21. Lateral view showing diminished interocclusal space. Treatment plan included implant placement in tooh #21 and tooth #12 and root submergence of tooth #11 along with GBR **(Fig. 1)**.

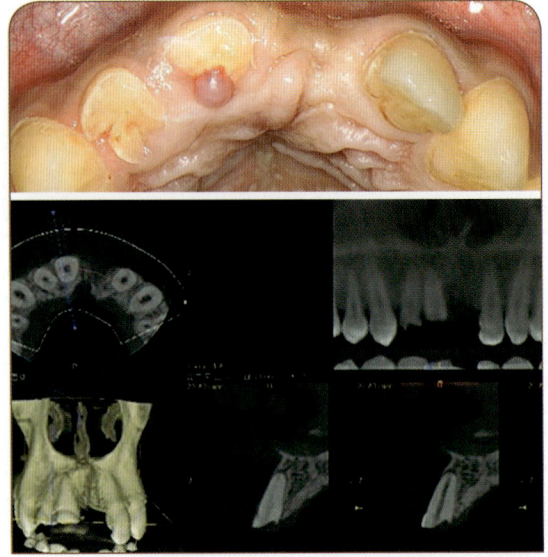

Fig. 2

Occlusal view showing reduced tissue volume at region of tooth #21. CBCT sections showing deficient facial plate in the area of concern **(Fig. 2)**.

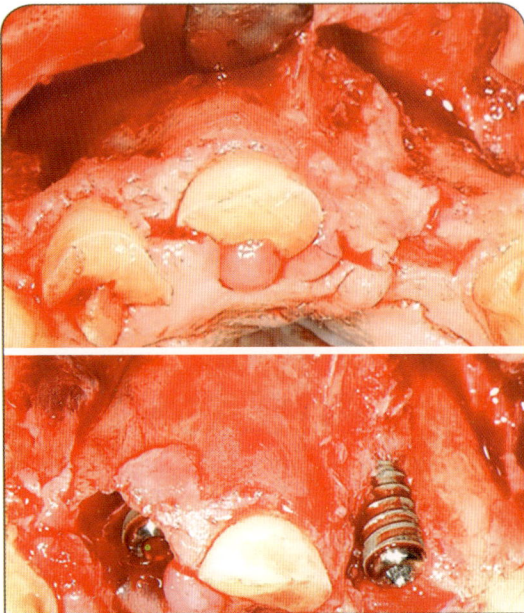

Fig. 3

Full thickness mucoperiosteal flap reflected to attain adequate visibility of the surgical site. 3.5/11.5 DM (Bioner Implant) implants placed in the region of 12 and 21. Deficiency in bone volume clearly evident and exposed implant treads visible **(Fig. 3)**.

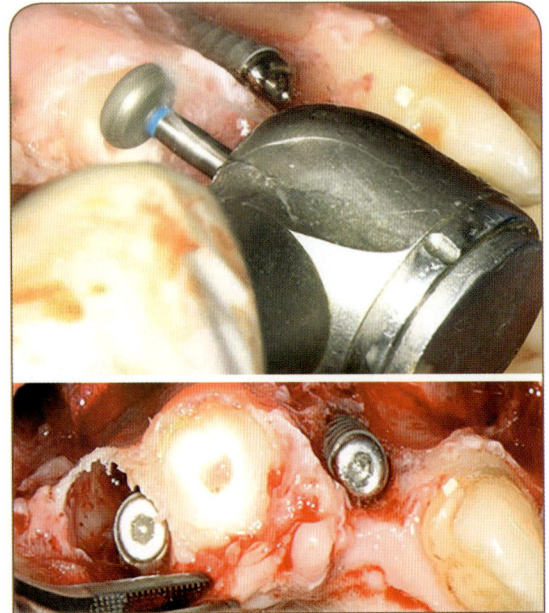

Fig. 4

Root submergence of tooth #11 with help of diamond wheel bur on high speed air rotter. Occlusal view showing the deficient site, large jumping distance in relation to tooth #12. Submerge root of tooth #11 is left vital **(Fig. 4)**.

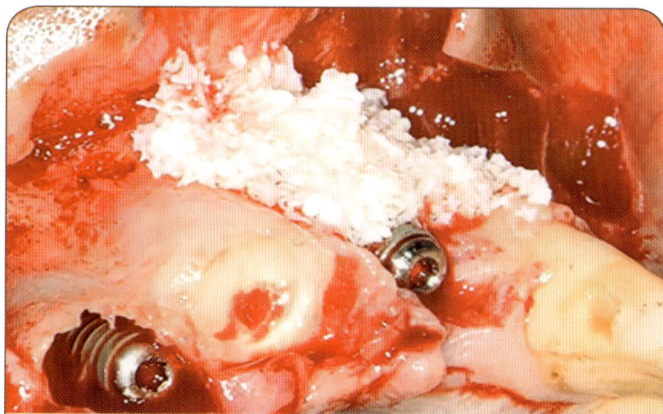

Fig. 5

Bone grafting with cerabone (Botis). Over contouring with the graft material for ridge augmentation to achieve bulk **(Fig. 5)**.

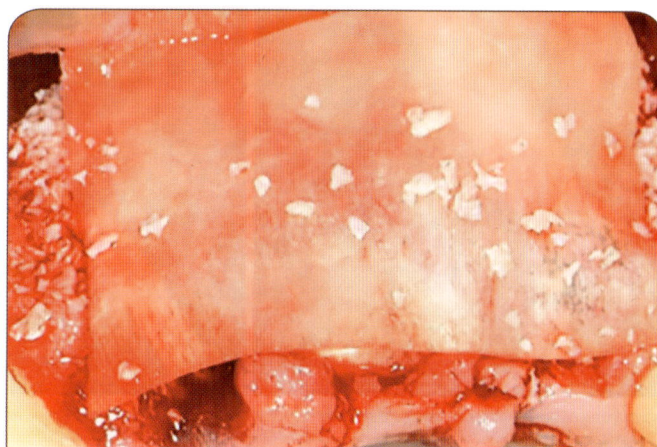

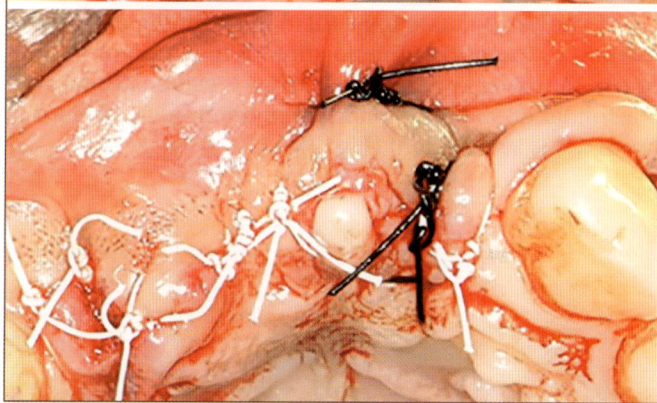

Fig. 6

Placement of Jason pericardium membrane. After adequate periosteal relief, wound closer is achieved with horizontal mattress sutures with 3–0 polyamide and interrupted sutures with 3–0 cytoplast (Ostogenics) **(Fig. 6)**.

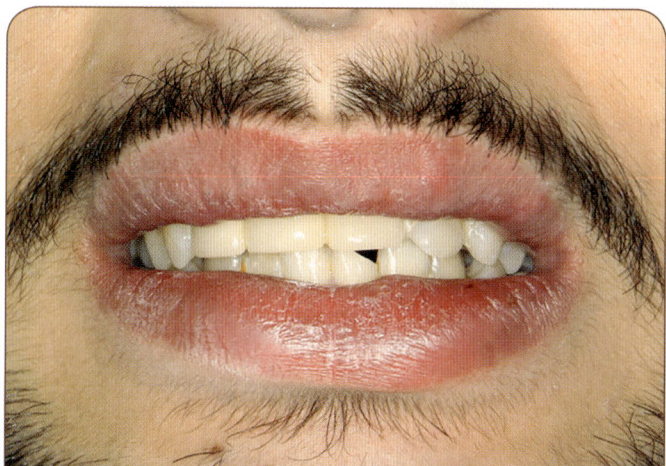

Fig. 7

Temporary Maryland Prosthesis given **(Fig. 7)**.

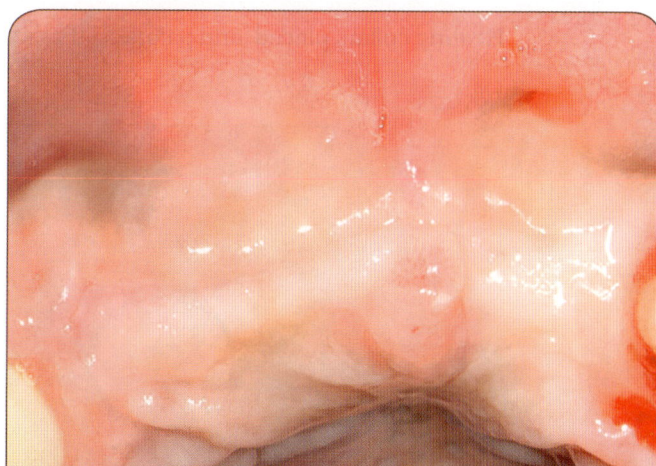

Fig. 8

Clinical view of the site, 5 months postoperative. After removal of Maryland Bridge showing adequate bulk **(Fig. 8)**.

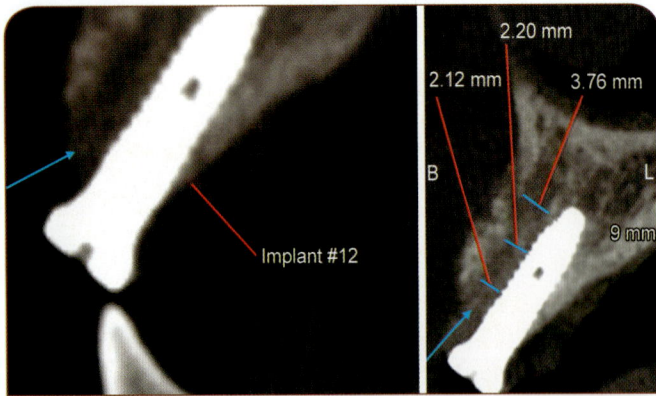

Fig. 9

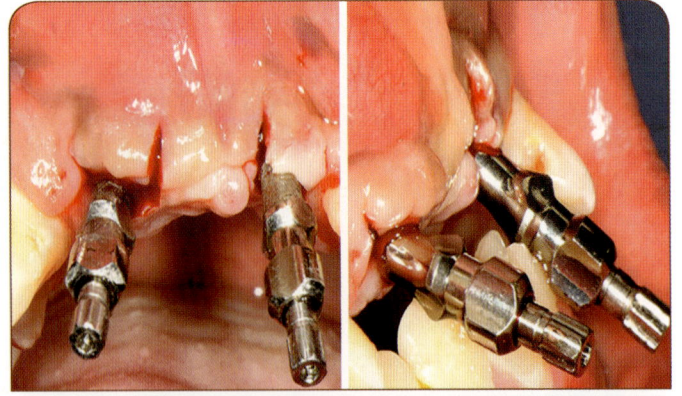

Fig. 10

CBCT shows adequate bone fill in the jumping distance in relation to tooth #12. The position of the implant in relation to the lower anterior incisal edge is evident. Bone graft consolidation and bulk build up in relation to implant in tooth #21 is also evident **(Fig. 9)**.

Minimal flap reflection for implant exposure and taking a submerged implant impression.

The position of implant can be appreciated in the lateral view **(Fig. 10)**.

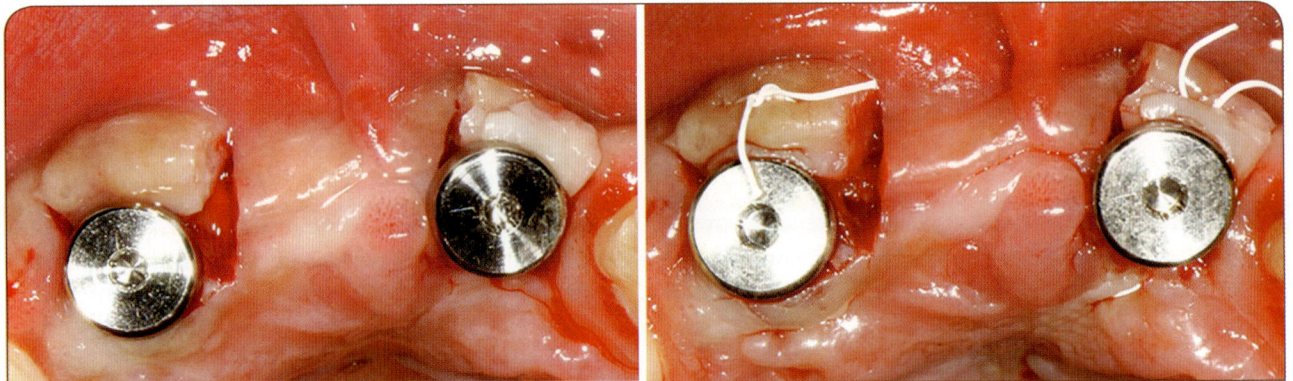

Fig. 11

Healing collars placed and palatal roll tissue stabilized with 3–0 cytoplast sutures **(Fig. 11)**.

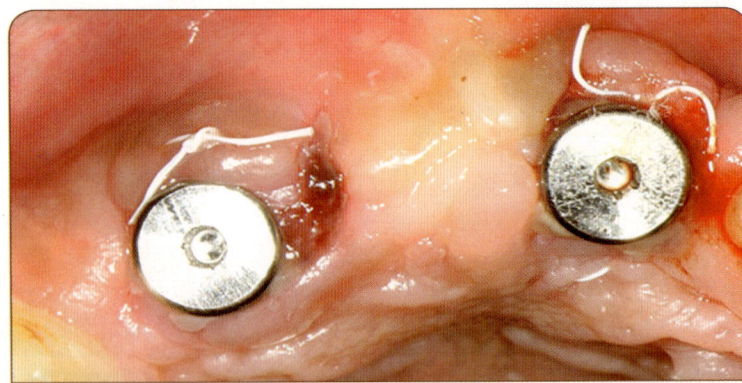

Fig. 12

Three days postoperative after healing collar placement **(Fig. 12)**.

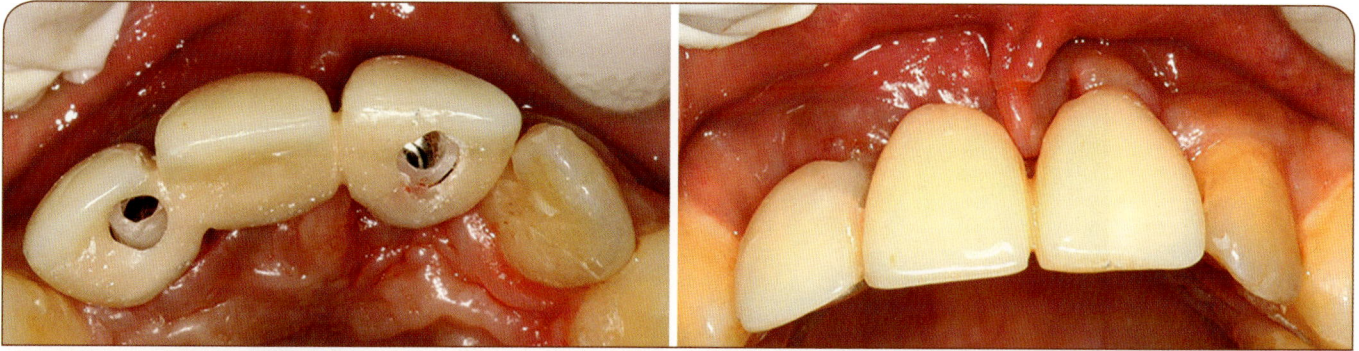

Fig. 13

Screw retained temporary composite prosthesis placed for soft tissue contouring **(Fig. 13)**.

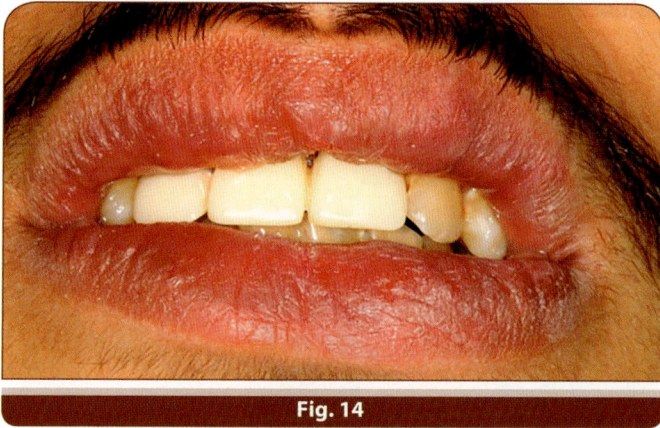

Fig. 14

Resting lip position **(Fig. 14)**.

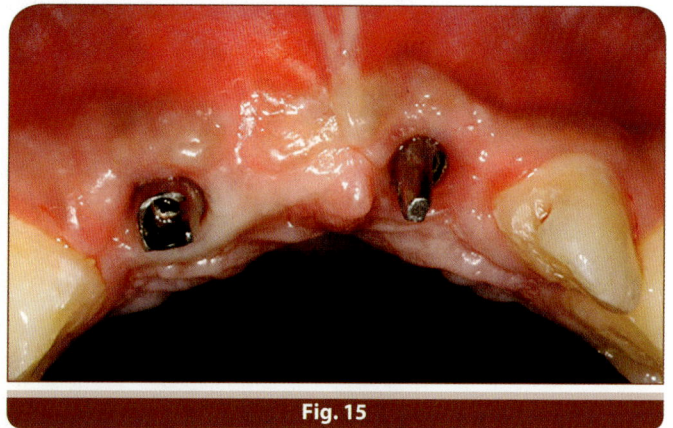

Fig. 15

After removal of temporary bridge and placement of final abutments thick tissue and adequate bone regeneration is evident **(Fig. 15)**.

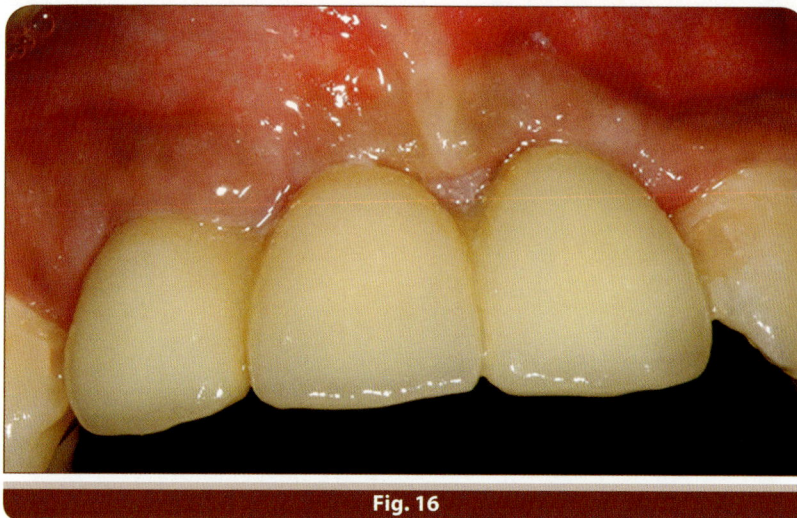

Fig. 16

Final zirconia prosthesis fixed with temporary non-eugenol cement for a period of 16 weeks to allow further soft tissue maturation. Tooth #22 has received a composite filling **(Fig. 16)**.

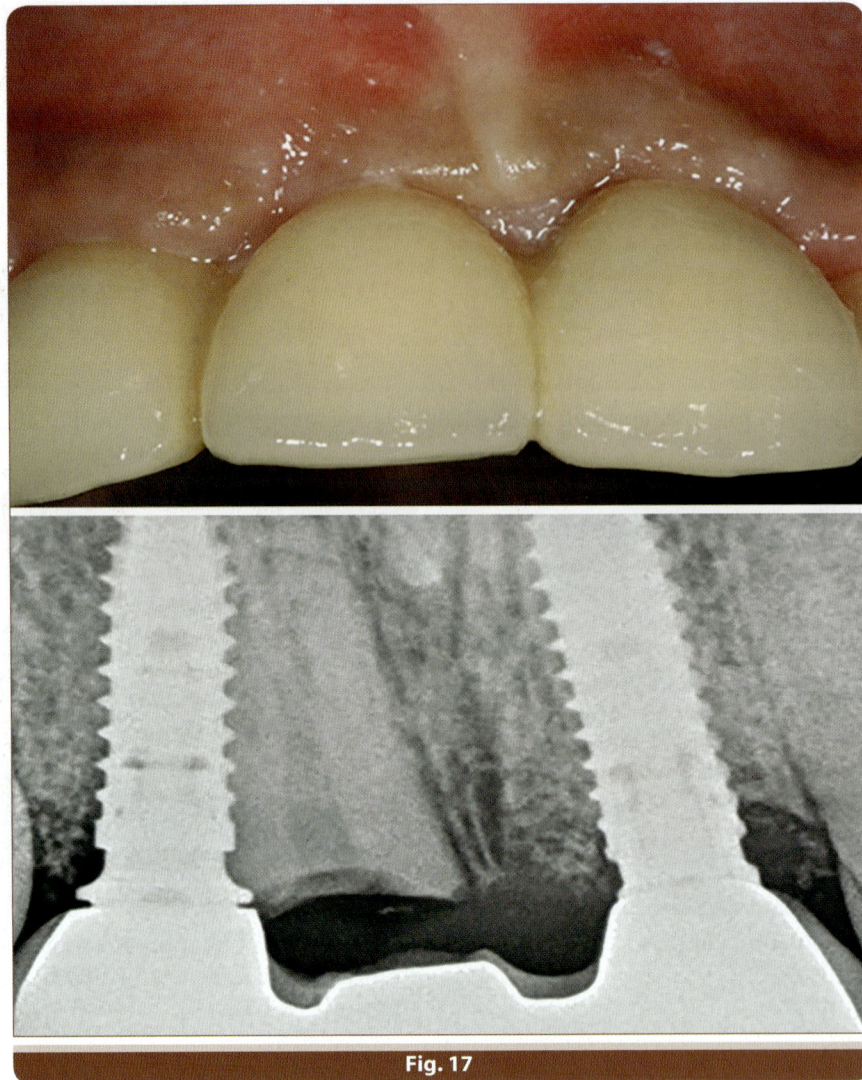

Fig. 17

Two years recall clinical and radiographic views of a successful GBR procedure and root submergence **(Fig. 17)**.

Lanka Mahesh, Vishal Gupta

ATRAUMATIC EXTRACTION USING THE 'BENEX EXTRACTOR' AND IMMEDIATE IMPLANT PLACEMENT IN THE ESTHETIC ZONE

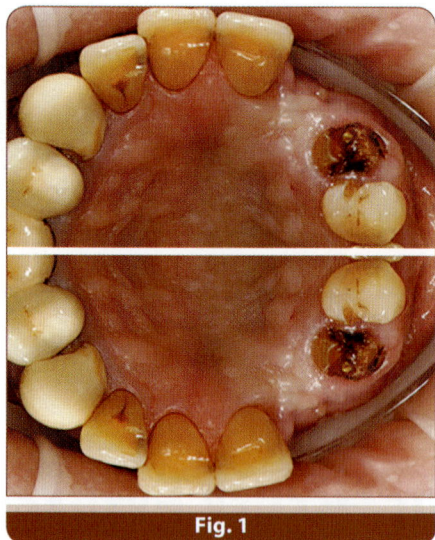

Fig. 1

Preoperative view of fracture of tooth #23 with GBR and simultaneous implant placement in relation to tooth #22 three months prior to the fracture of 32 **(Fig. 1)**.

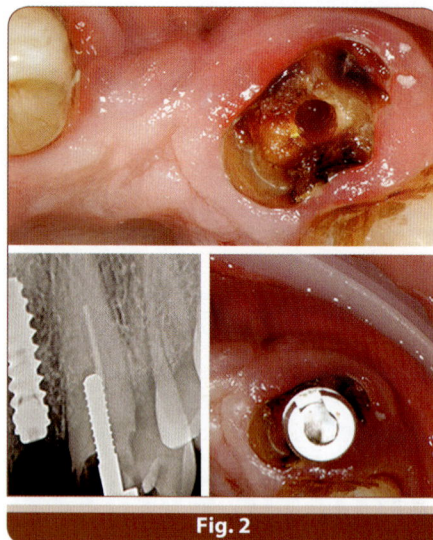

Fig. 2

After the pilot bur and the number 3 drill provided in the kit, the anchor is screwed into the tooth (care must be taken to keep the drill within the confines of the middle of the canal thereby preventing in advertent fractures of the root fragment). An X-ray verifies the final position of the anchor **(Fig. 2)**.

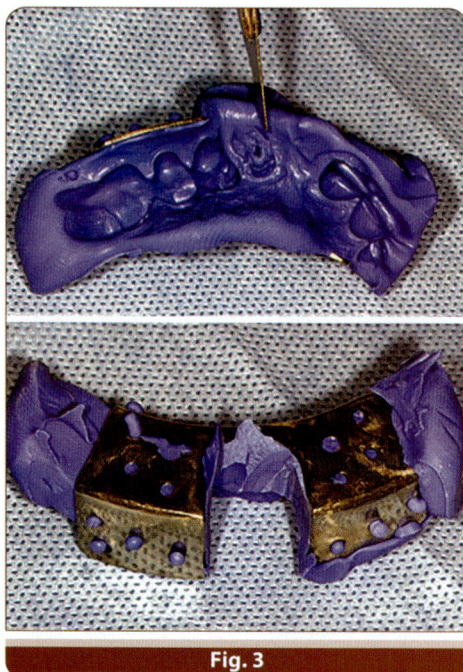

Fig. 3

The quadrant tray that is part of the instrument kit is loaded with PVS impression material. After impression recorded and the excess is cutout with a number 15 Bard Parker blade **(Fig. 3)**.

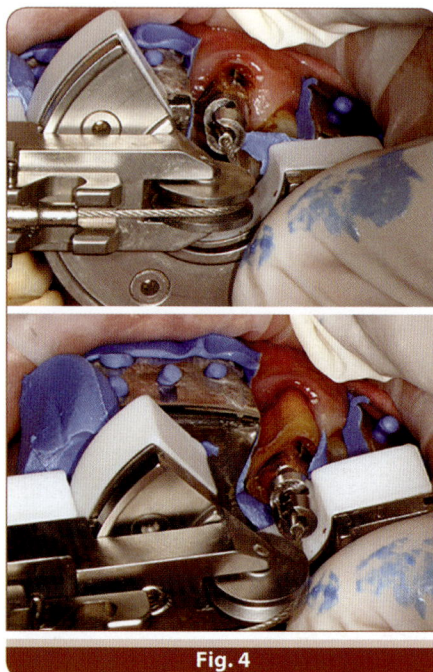

Fig. 4

The tray is placed back intraorally and the Benex extractor is placed with the wire engaging the anchor. Slow clockwise turns on the end of the extractor gently luxates the root fragment without damage to any adjacent anatomic structures **(Fig. 4)**.

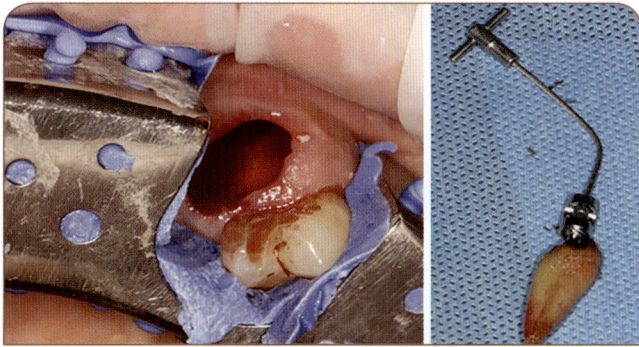

Fig. 5

The extraction socket immediately postextraction, and the extracted root fragment alongwith the wire and the anchor screw **(Fig. 5)**.

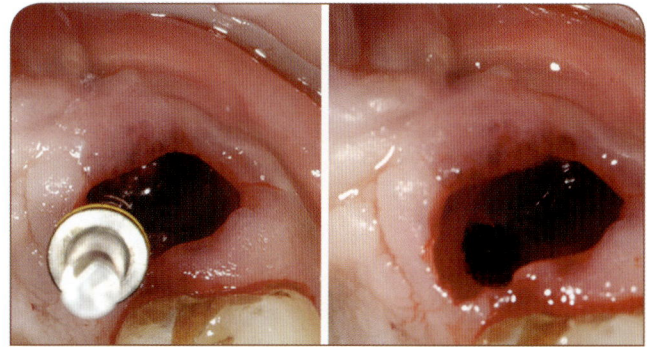

Fig. 6

Palatal osteotomy preparation initiation. The final osteotomy site (the original extraction socket is clearly visible) **(Fig. 6)**.

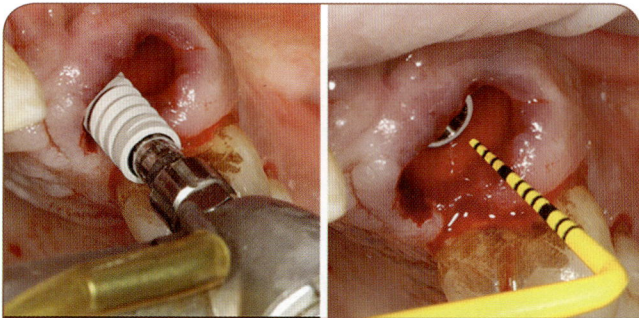

Fig. 7

The implant is placed at 40 Ncm with a handpiece at 30 rpm. A periodontal probe is used to measure the future abutment height (3 mm height in this case) **(Fig. 7)**.

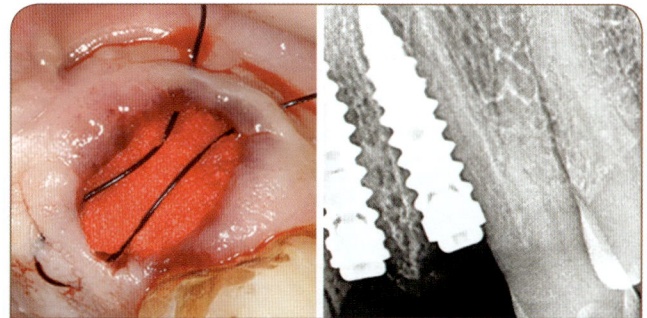

Fig. 8

The socket is closed with a collaplug (Zimmer dental) and the wound is closed with a horizontal mattress suture. Radiographic image of the implant in the final position **(Fig. 8)**.

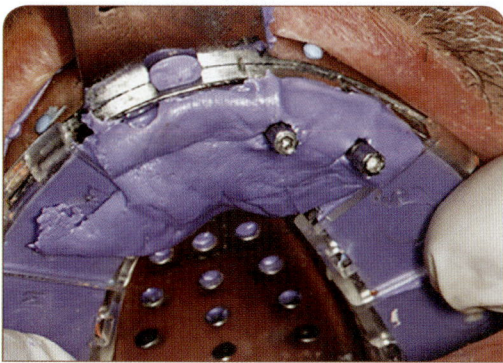

Fig. 9

Open tray impressions taken in impregum PVS (3 M). Special implant trays are used for all implant impressions (Cor Implant) **(Fig. 9)**.

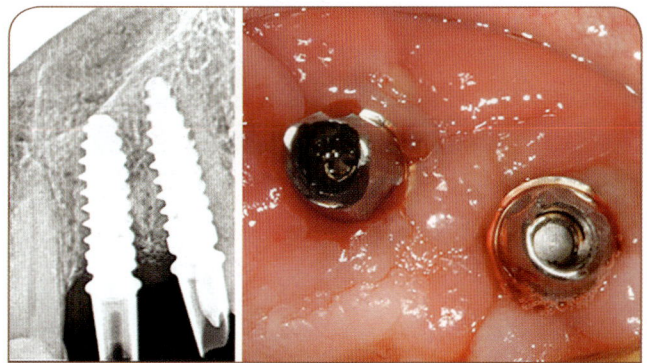

Fig. 10

Final abutments are placed and after an X-ray verification. The abutments are torqued to 30 Ncm and sealed with Teflon tape and temporary cement. Immediate post-cementation clinical view **(Fig. 10)**.

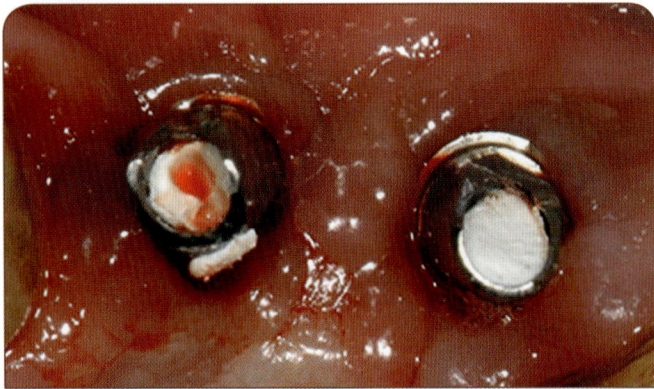

Fig. 11

The abutments ready to receive the final zirconia crowns (any excess cement as seen should be removed to prevent an ingress of the material into the gingival sulcus) **(Fig. 11)**.

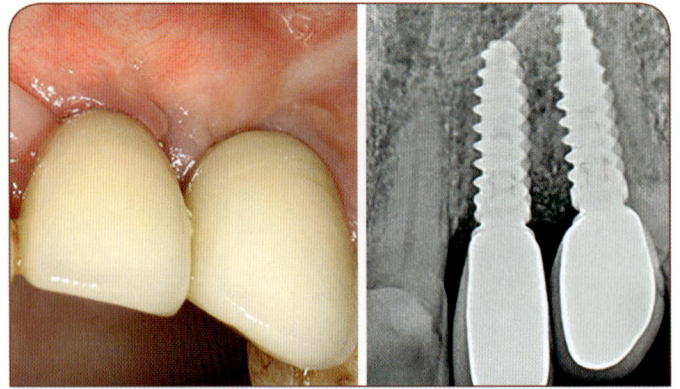

Fig. 12

Immediate postcementation clinical view of the zirconia crowns and radiographic view of the fixtures and crowns **(Fig. 12)**.

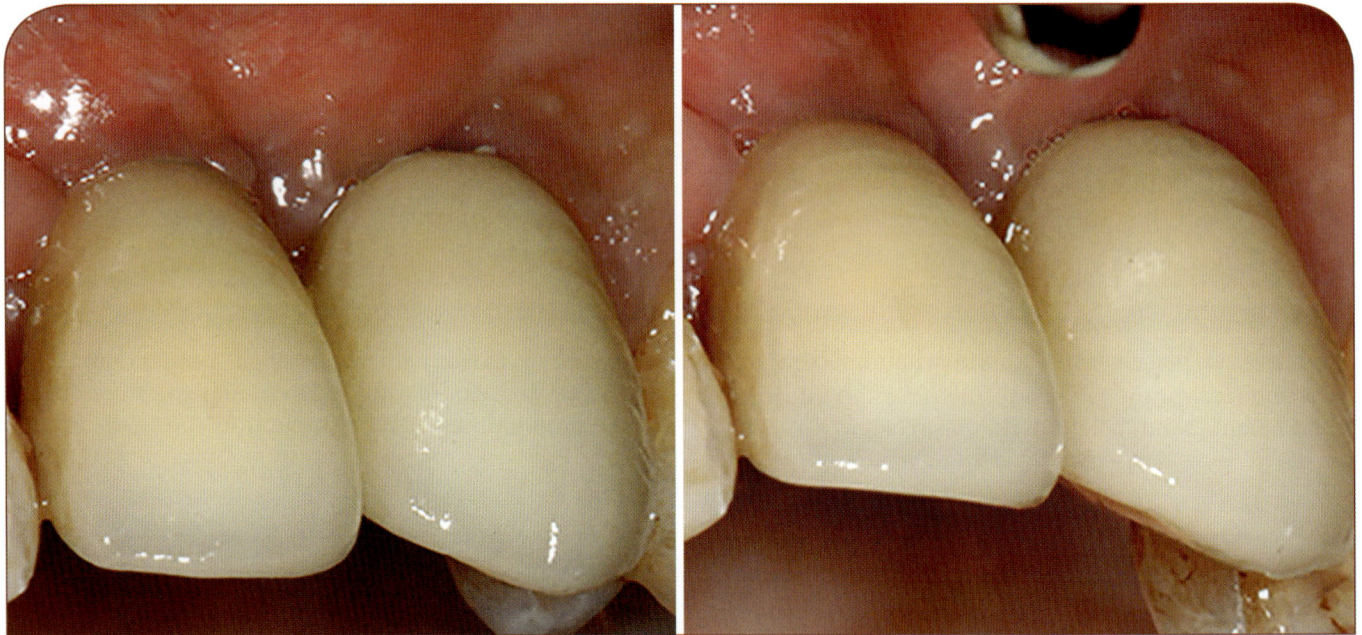

Fig. 13

Two-year recall. Clinical view showing stable tissue levels **(Fig. 13)**.

Praful Bali

Correcting Anterior Angulation after Immediate Extraction and Implant Placement with ASC Abutment

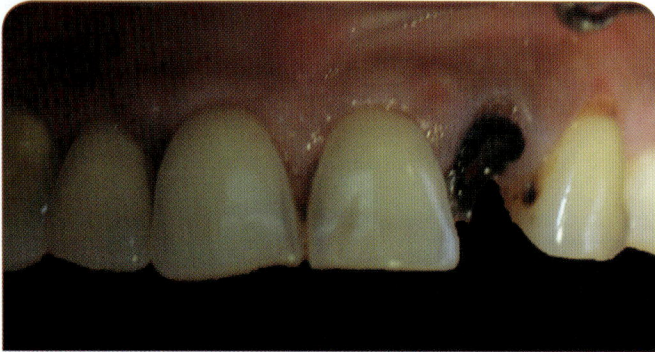

Fig. 1

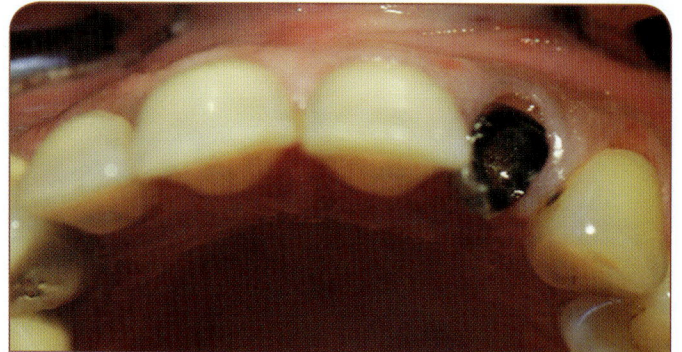

Fig. 2

A 55-year-old female patient wants replacement of unsalvageable tooth #22. Implant treatment is explained to the patient but the patient persists not to get bone or soft tissue augmentation. Wants to get work done in the very situation. Note the gingival contour of the lateral incisor root piece is slightly above the adjacent central incisor **(Fig. 1)**.

The occlusal view shows reasonable bony architecture around the root piece of tooth # 22 suggesting of a decent buccal bone **(Fig. 2)**.

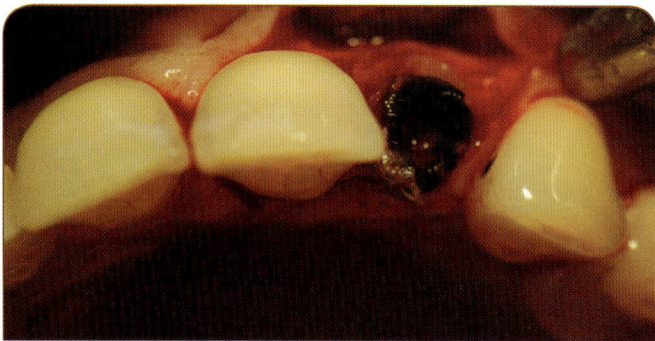

Fig. 3

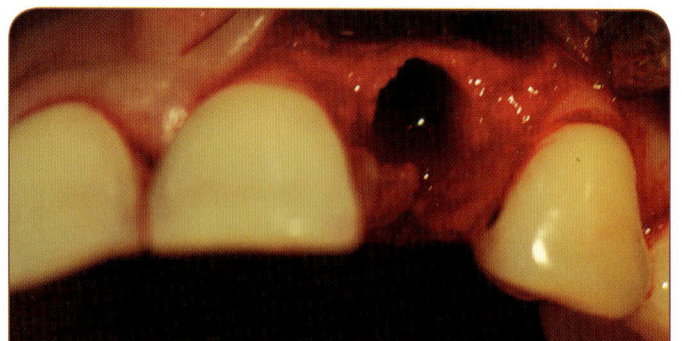

Fig. 4

Minimal flap reflection is done to expose the root piece of tooth # 22 and buccal bone **(Fig. 3)**.

Atraumatic extraction done with the help of periotomes. Care taken not to disturb the buccal bone **(Fig. 4)**.

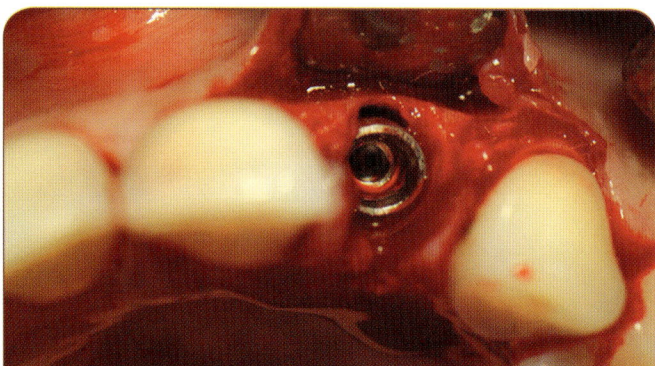

Fig. 5

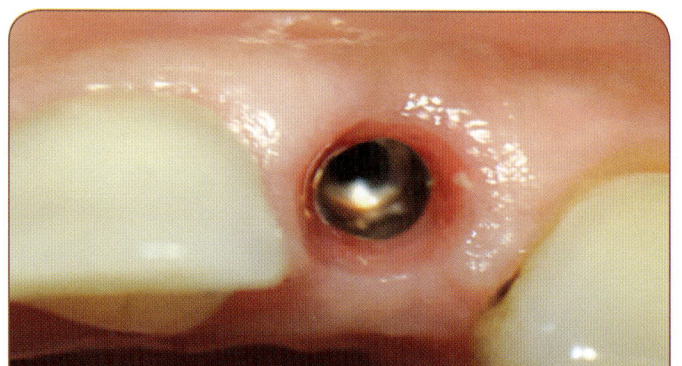

Fig. 6

A 4.3/13 Nobel parallel implant (Nobel Biocare) is placed and Novabone Putty to take care of the jumping distance **(Fig. 5)**.

The occlusal view of the healed site after 3 months. Nice buccal bone and tissue support visible **(Fig. 6)**.

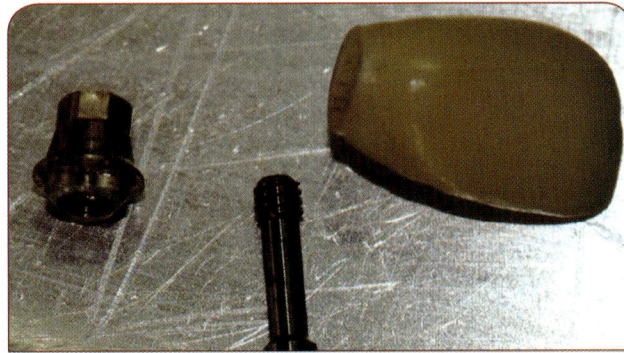

Fig. 7

Nobel ASC (Angulated Screw Channel) abutment to correct the angulation and a zirconia crown which is under contoured at the cervical area to support the soft tissue and maintain a proper emergence profile **(Fig. 7)**.

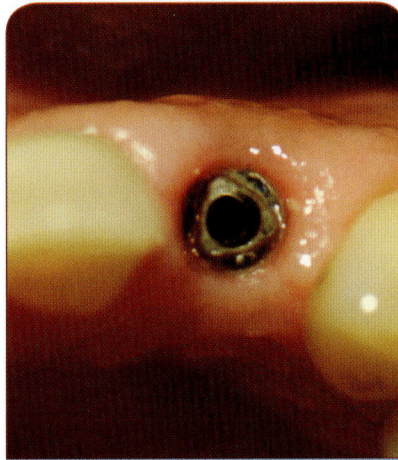

Fig. 8

The occlusal view of the ASC abutment **(Fig. 8)**.

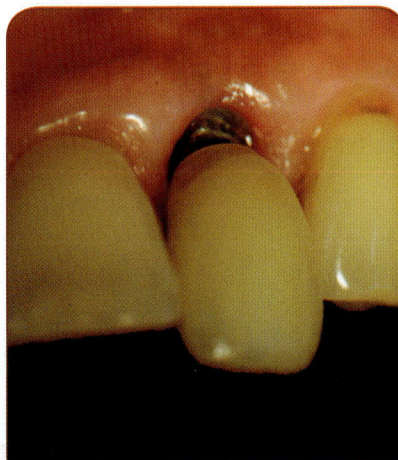

Fig. 9

The ASC abutment. Note the under contoured crown will support the soft tissue and maintain a proper emergence profile **(Fig. 9)**.

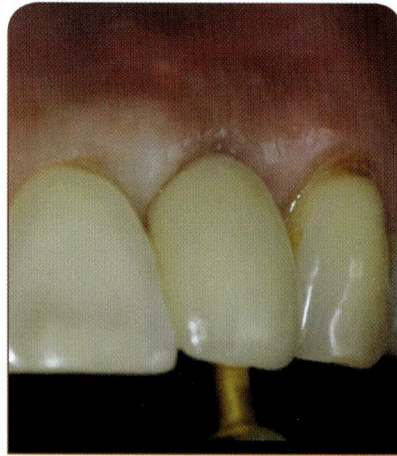

Fig. 10

The screw channel is palatal as a result of using the ASC abutment achieving an esthetic outcome. Note the emergence profile has not changed at all as care was taken to preserve every bit of hard and soft tissue that was available **(Fig. 10)**.

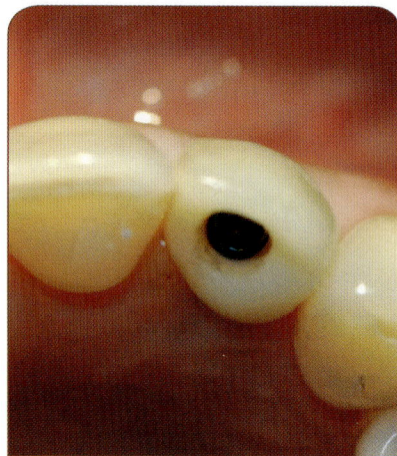

Fig. 11

The occlusal view shows the palatal screw channel **(Fig. 11)**.

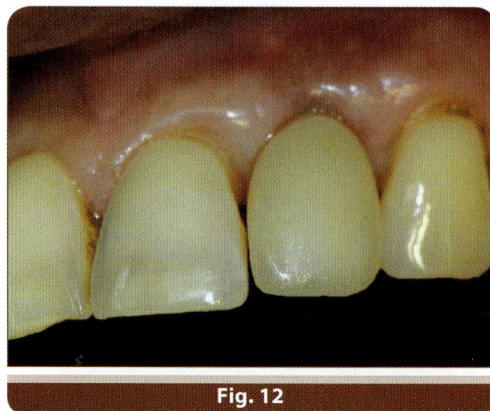

Fig. 12

Final result: Hard and soft tissue maintained **(Fig. 12)**.

Shweta Gupta, Praful Bali

Atraumatic Flapless Implant Placement for Central Incisor after Disinfection using Laser Therapy: A 4-year Follow-up

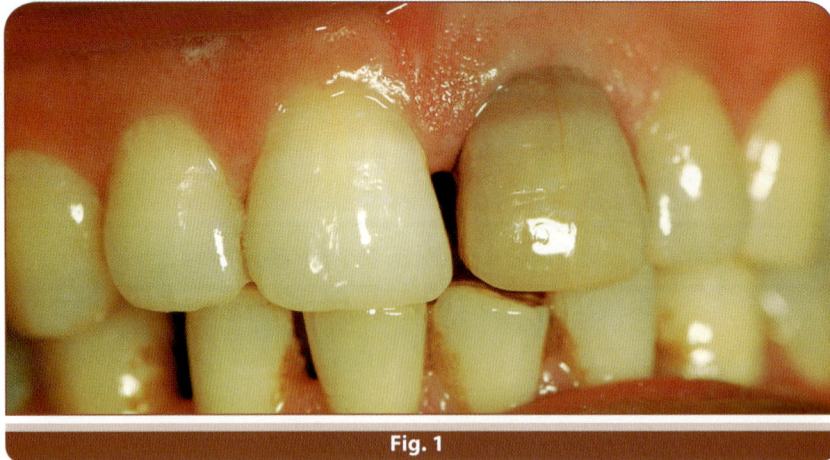

Fig. 1

Preoperative facial view—nonvital tooth # 21 with a history of trauma. Grade 2 mobility present with the tooth **(Fig. 1)**.

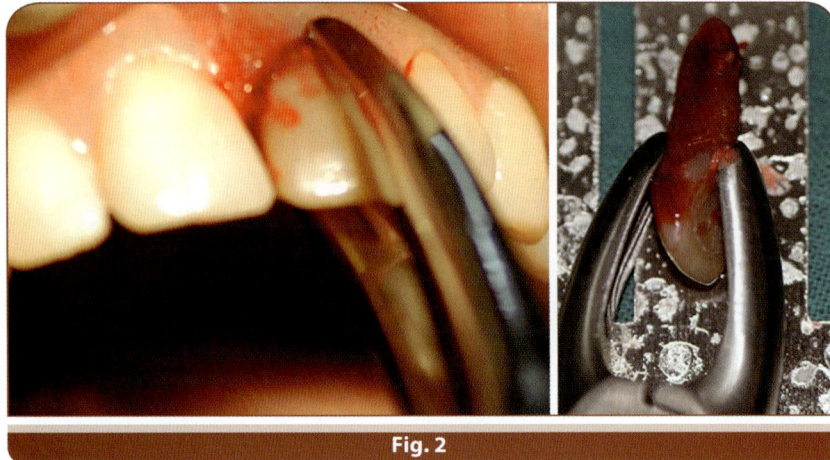

Fig. 2

Atraumatic extraction done using osteotoms and forceps with care taken to preserve the buccal bone anatomy **(Fig. 2)**.

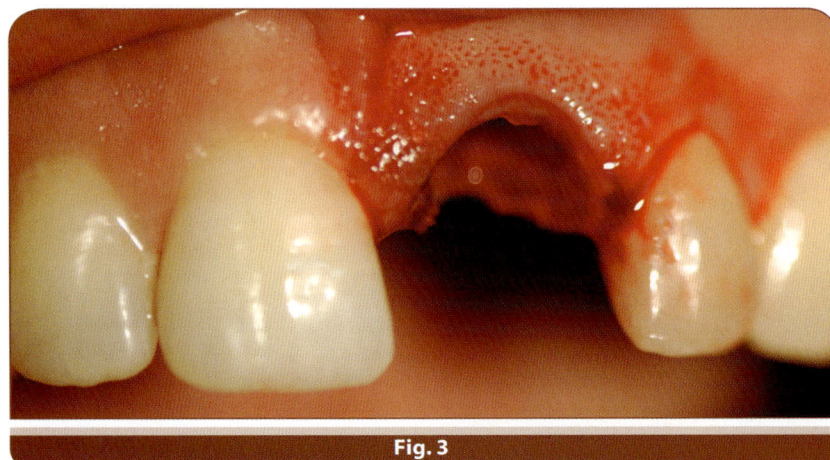

Fig. 3

Soft and hard tissue preserved after extraction **(Fig. 3)**.

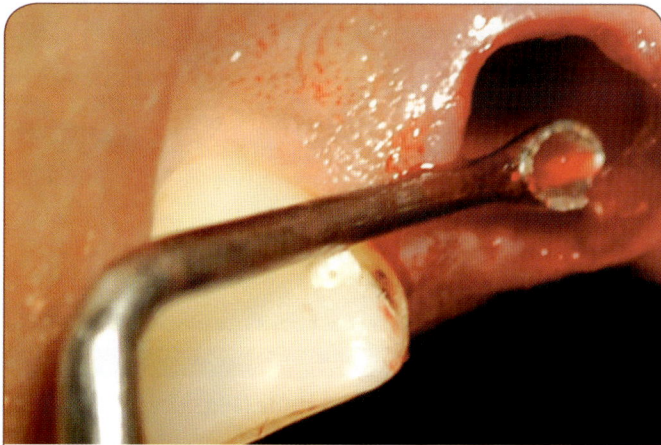

Fig. 4

Extensive curettage done and asepsis of the socket achieved by soft tissue Diode laser **(Fig. 4)**.

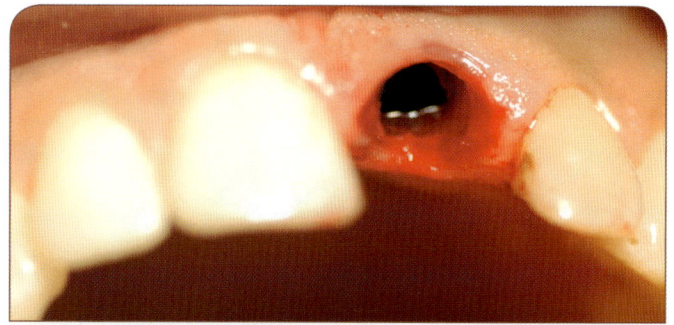

Fig. 5

3D implant placement (vertical—2–3 mm). A 5/15 Nobel biocare implant placed **(Fig. 5)**.

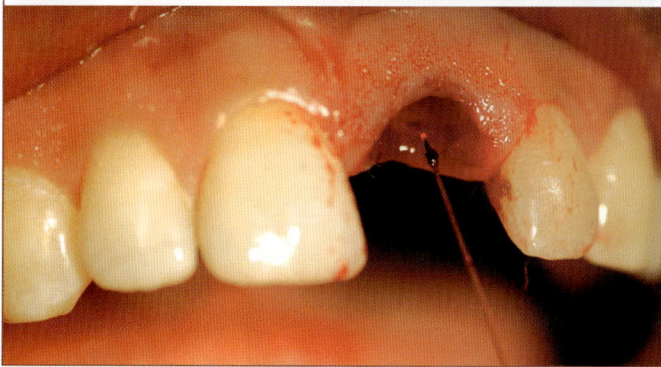

Fig. 6

3D implant placement (vertical—2–3 mm) **(Fig. 6)**.

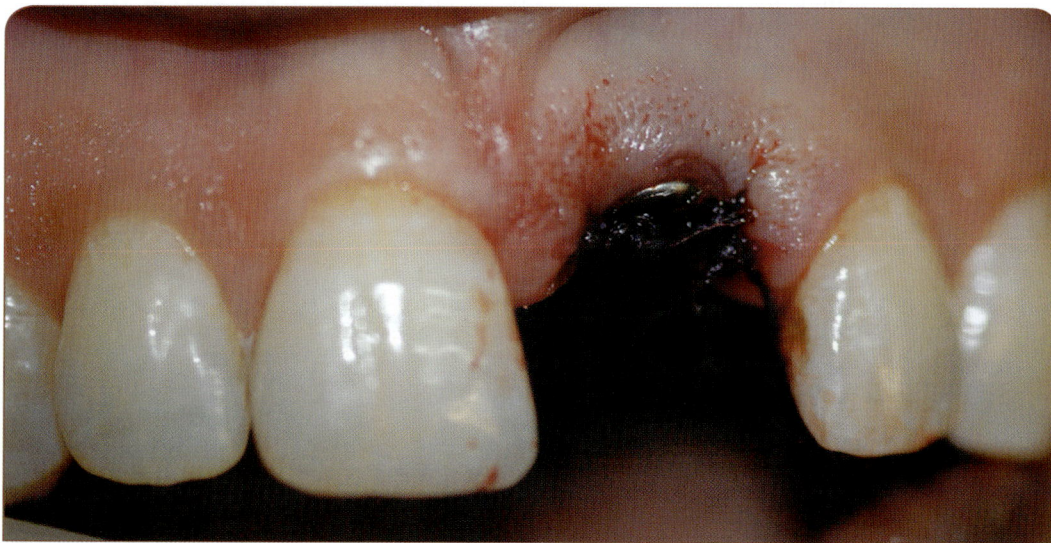

Fig. 7

A 3 mm gingival former torqued onto the implant at 15 N/cm^2 and bone graft done in the jumping distance. Suturing done with 3-0 sutures around the gingival former. The patient is temporised with a Maryland type of final prosthesis **(Fig. 7)**.

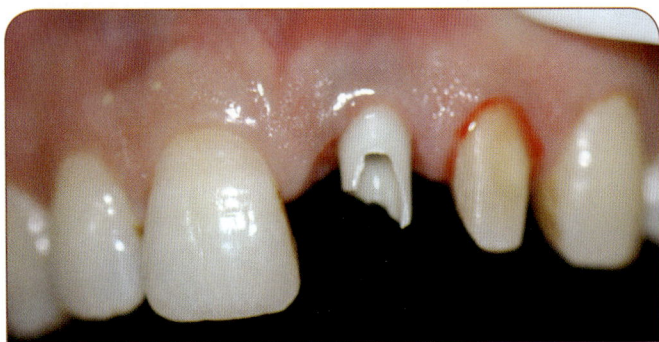

Fig. 8

Four months postoperative: Zirconia abutment is customised and torqued to 35 N/cm^2 **(Fig. 8)**.

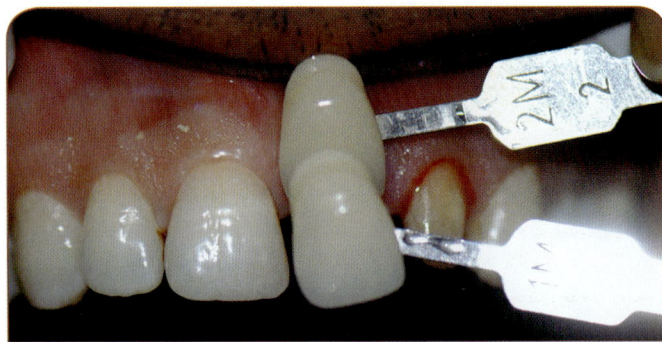

Fig. 9

Shade selection done (Fig. 9).

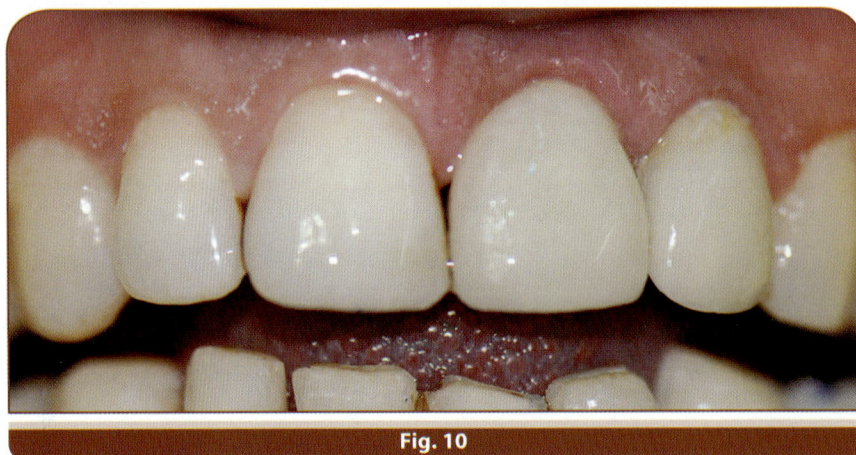

Fig. 10

Optimal result achieved by E-max all ceramic crown on teeth #21, 22 **(Fig. 10)**.

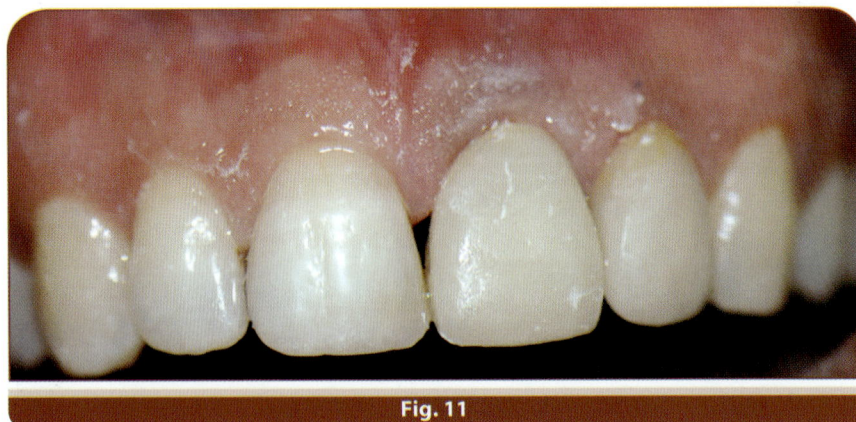

Fig. 11

Four years follow-up. Note the good architecture of bone and soft tissue. Also, tooth #22 (endodontically treated) is also tooth prepared for receiving a crown **(Fig. 11)**.

Praful Bali, Shweta Gupta

SOFT TISSUE ENGINEERING TO ACHIEVE NATURAL PONTIC SITE ESTHETICS FOR A 3 UNIT ANTERIOR BRIDGE ON 2 IMPLANTS

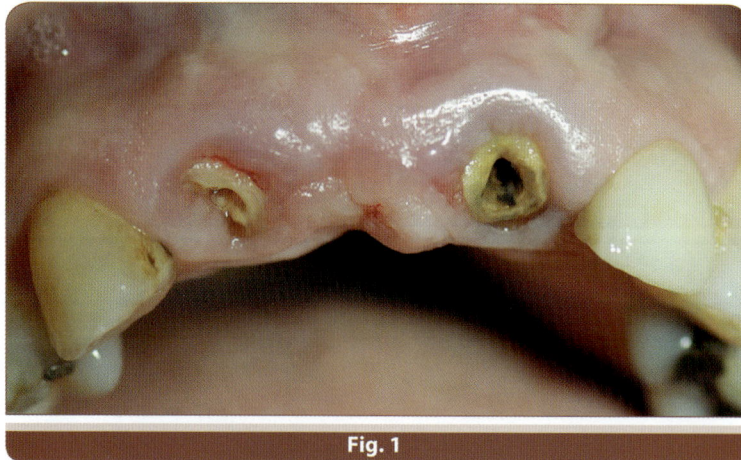

Fig. 1

Patient presents with an hopeless situation with 3 unit bridge on teeth no.#12 and 21 breaks down and immediate extraction and implant placement needed **(Fig. 1)**.

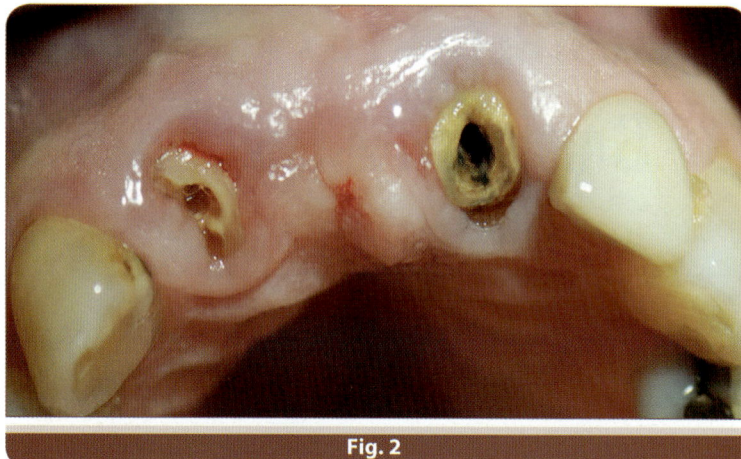

Fig. 2

Preoperative—occlusal view **(Fig. 2)**.

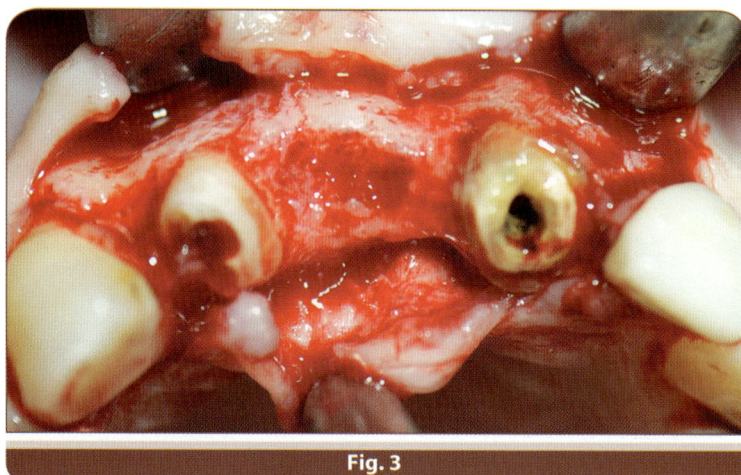

Fig. 3

Full thickness flap reflection done, note the slight deficient buccal bone on tooth #21 **(Fig. 3)**.

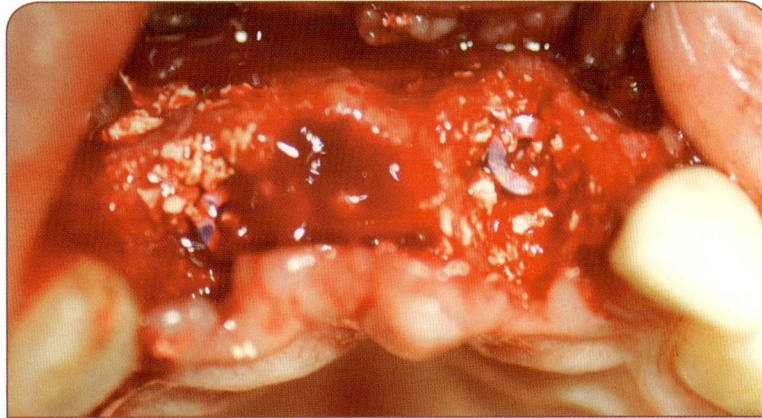

Fig. 4

Implant placement and bone graft to fill the jumping distance and to regenerate the buccal bone defect **(Fig. 4)**.

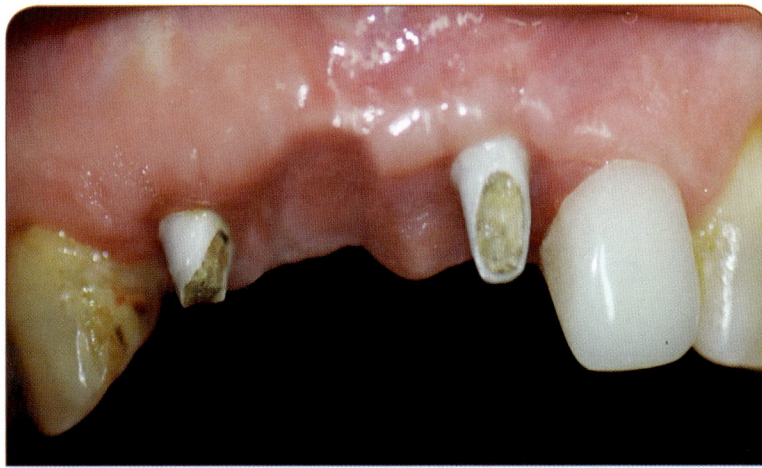

Fig. 5

Soft tissue engineering—repeated pressure is applied on the pontic region to train the soft tissue **(Fig. 5)**.

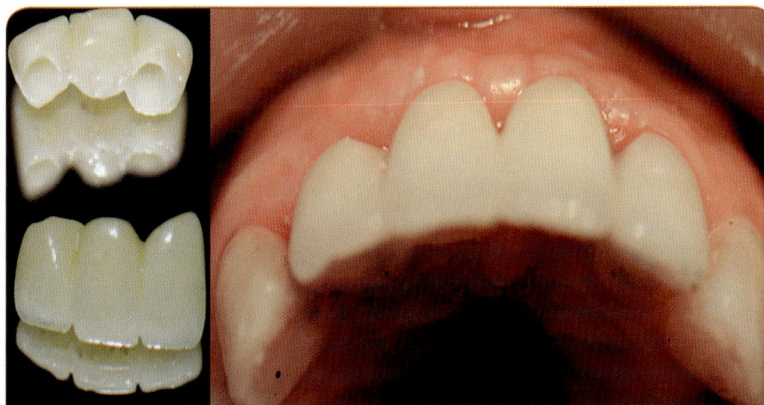

Fig. 6

Procera permanent 3 unit bridge **(Fig. 6)**.

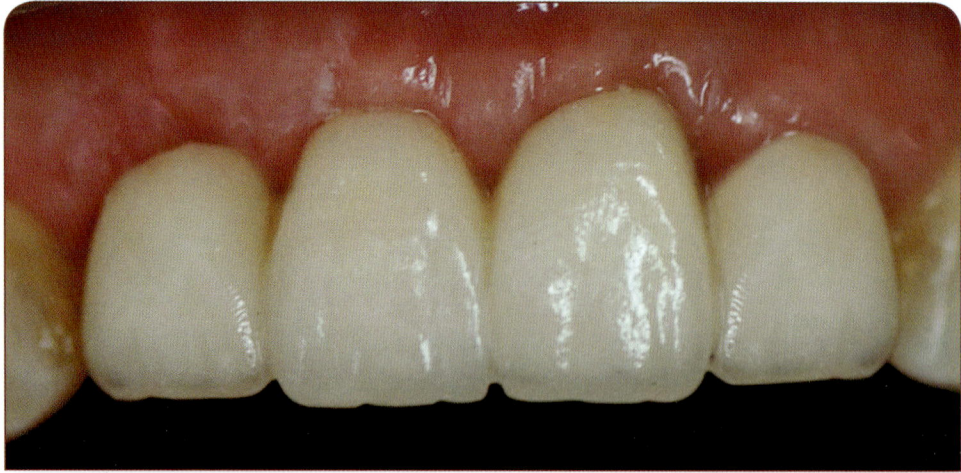

Fig. 7

Final restoration on implants. Note the excellent soft tissue esthetics **(Fig. 7)**.

Praful Bali, Sushil Nijhawan

IMMEDIATE EXTRACTION IMPLANT OF AN UPPER LATERAL INCISOR WITH ABSENCE OF BUCCAL BONE

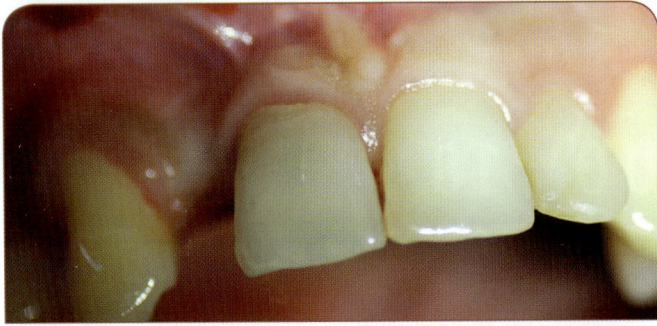
Fig. 1

A 31-year-old male patient presented a missing lateral incisor in the first quadrant. Clinical examination warranted a sequential reclamation of the adrifted labial cortex in a deficient buccolingual space for the final prosthesis **(Fig. 1)**.

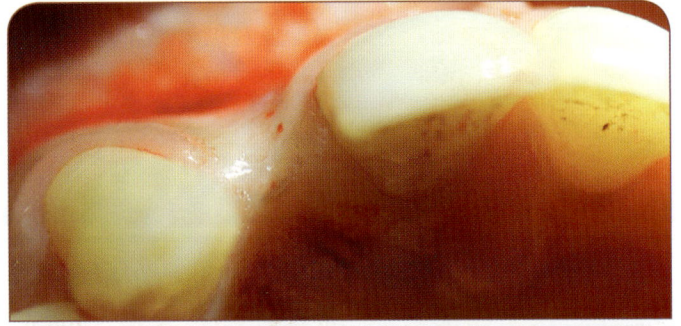
Fig. 2

A preoperative exam depicted a loss in the buccal cortex, exhibiting a possible knife like ridge. There was a remnant root piece left by the doctor extracting the tooth **(Fig. 2)**.

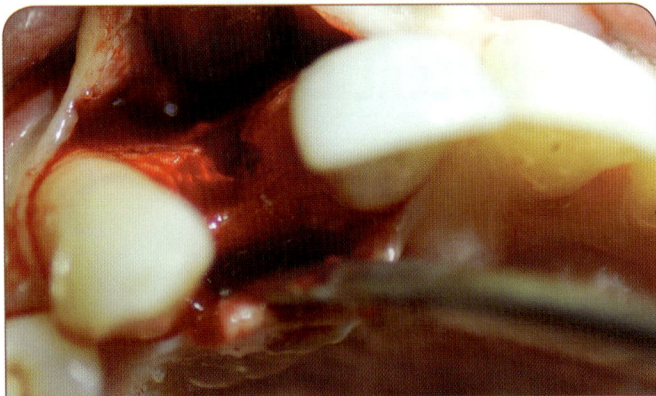
Fig. 3

An exalted full thickness mucoperiosteal flap reveals a labial cortical cleave after extraction of tooth #12 **(Fig. 3)**.

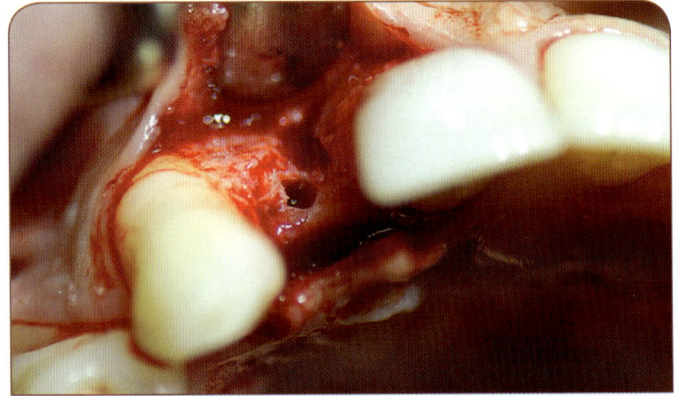
Fig. 4

The osteotomy site was prepared with sufficient circumspection and sequentially enlarged, to the required diameter at the 3D position **(Fig. 4)**.

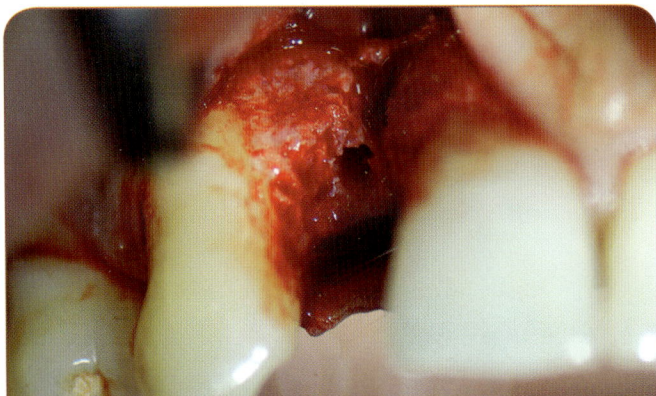
Fig. 5

A close-up contemplation of the prepared site keeping the labial defect separate than the osteotomy **(Fig. 5)**.

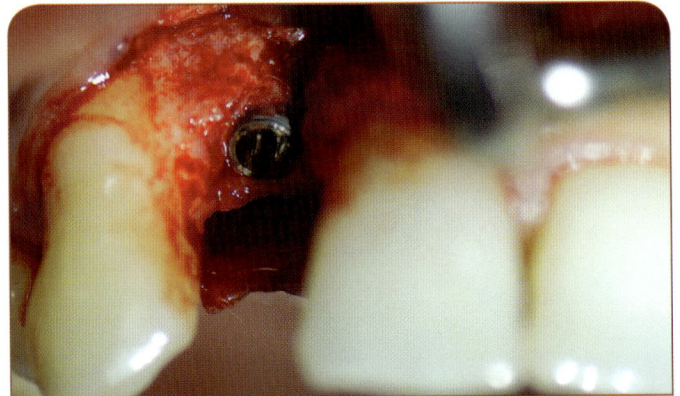
Fig. 6

The endosseous implant pinpointed in place **(Fig. 6)**.

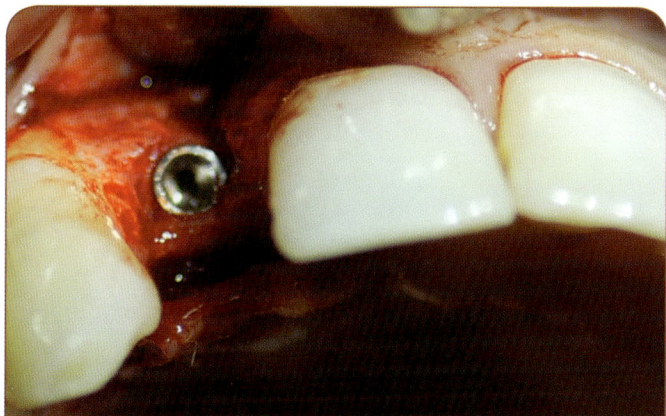
Fig. 7

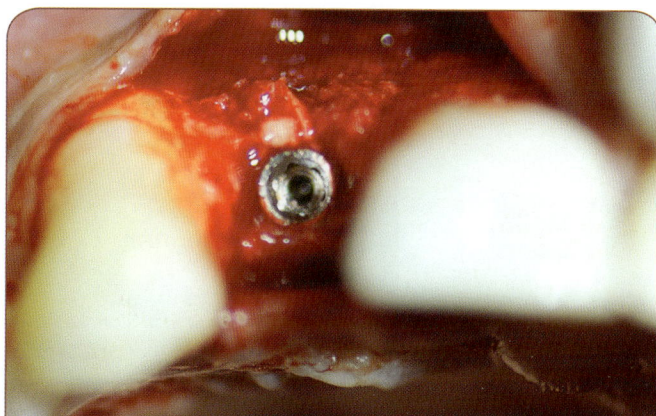
Fig. 8

Occlusal view of the implant in situ. The buccal bone is absent and a decision is made to do GBR to enhance the bone structure (Fig. 7).

A autogenous bone graft slurry dispensed liberally on the osteal cleave (Fig. 8).

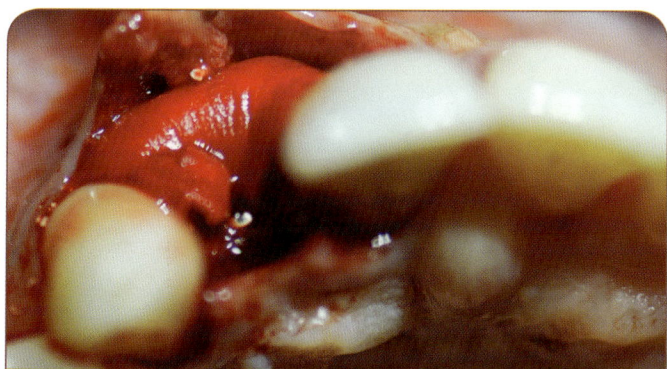
Fig. 9

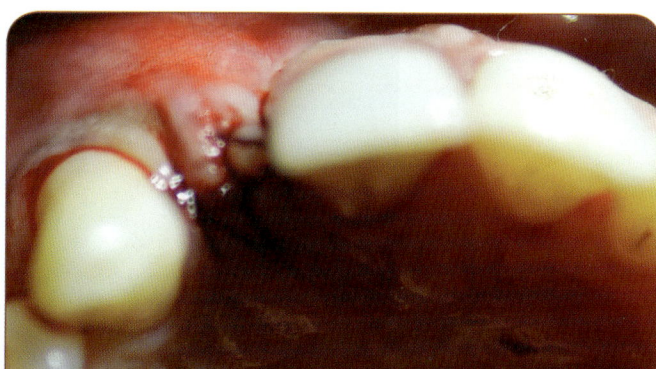
Fig. 10

Resorbable membrane after final grafting to complete the GBR (Fig. 9).

Resorbable matrices sutures given (Fig. 10).

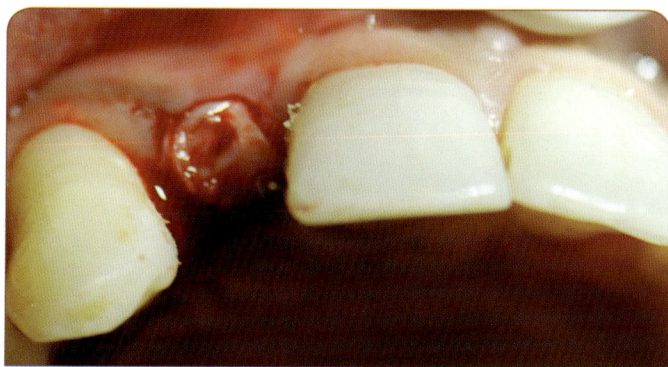
Fig. 11

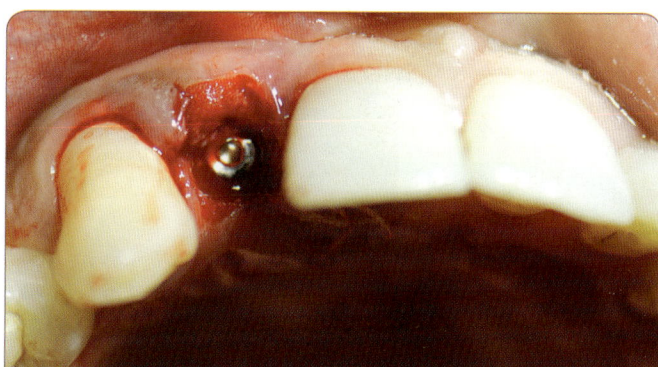
Fig. 12

Stage II initiation of the rehabilitation: roll on soft tissue graft (Fig. 11).

Surgical exposure of the integrated implant, with an archetypal circumforaneous osseous regeneration and soft tissue esthetic ensued after roll on graft (Fig. 12).

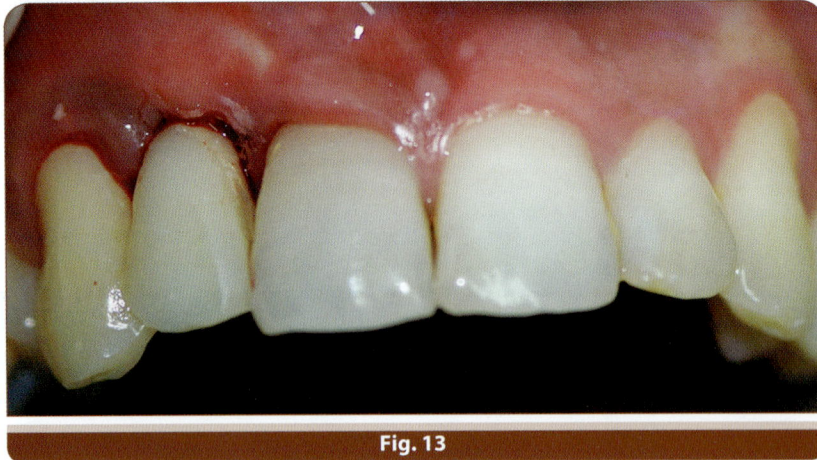
Fig. 13

An interim crown affixed for gingival recontouring. The prototypes are changed till final esthetics of gingival is achieved (Fig. 13).

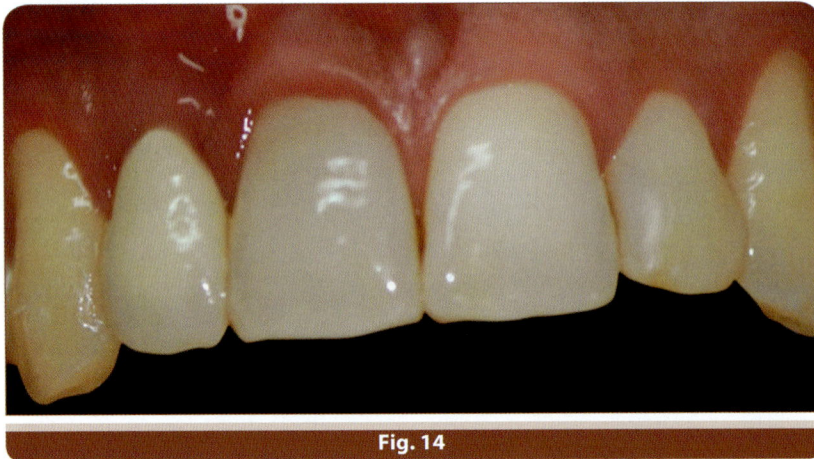
Fig. 14

Final Zirconia crown cemented with GIC: Note the excellent papilla fill (Fig. 14).

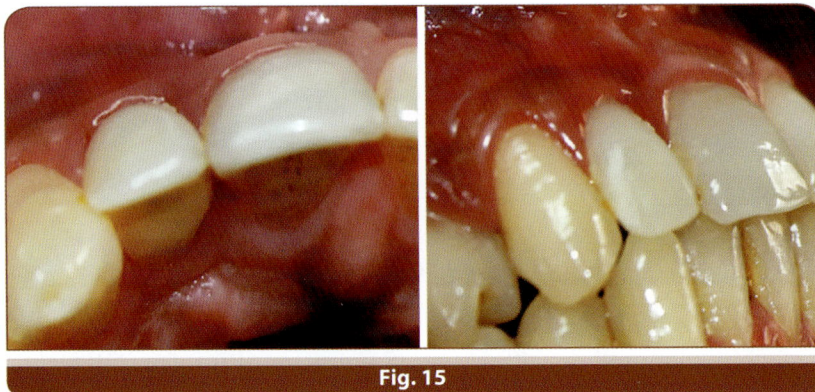
Fig. 15

The occlusal and side view shows the hard and soft tissue integration (Fig. 15).

Bassam F Rabie

MANAGING EXTRACTION SITE IN THE ESTHETIC ZONE BY PROPER PLANNING AND UTILIZATION OF DIFFERENT BIOLOGICS, TECHNIQUES AND TECHNOLOGY

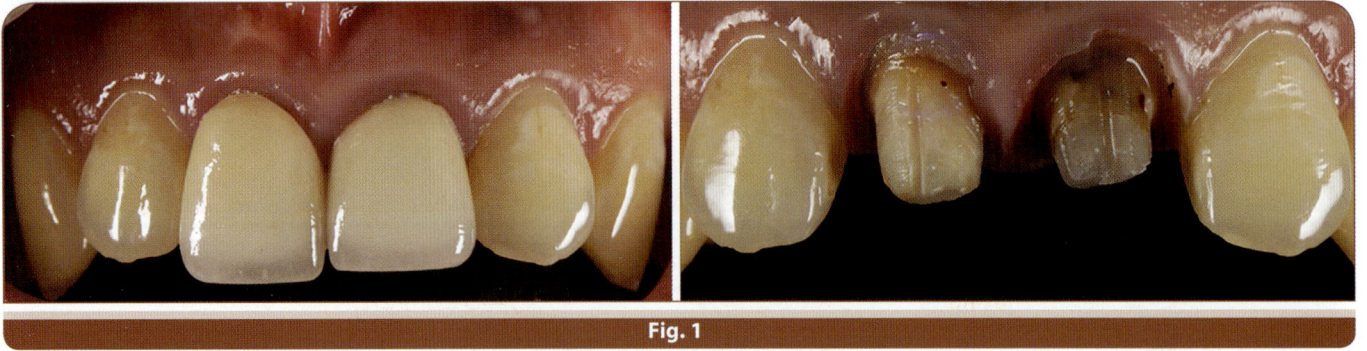

Fig. 1

Old upper 2 ceramo metal crowns on teeth #11, 21 **(Fig. 1)**.

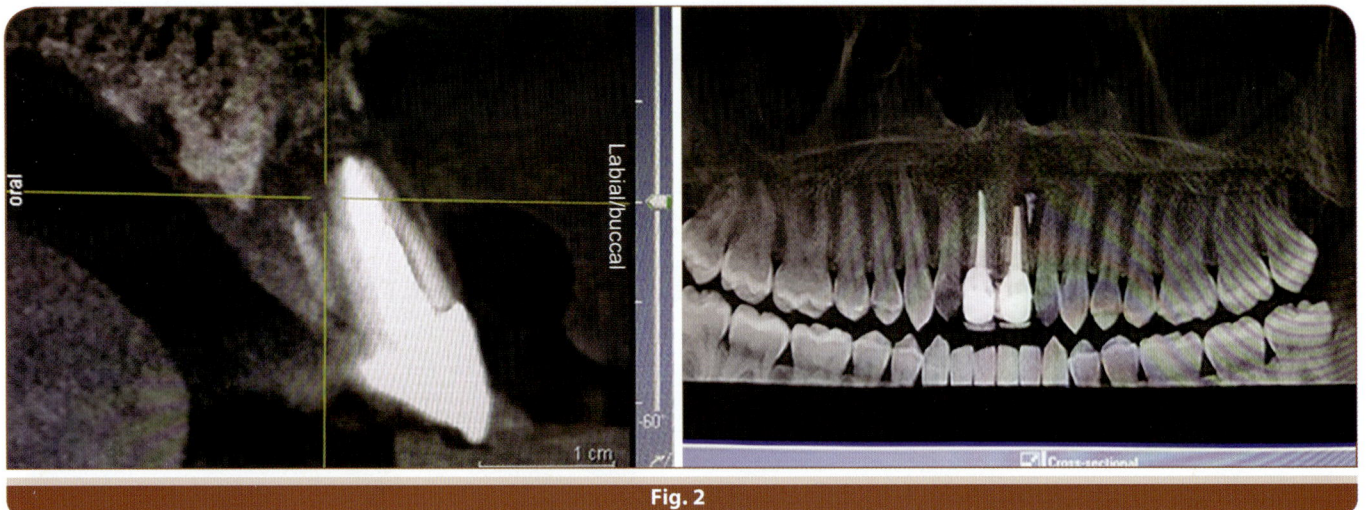

Fig. 2

CBCT **(Fig. 2)**.

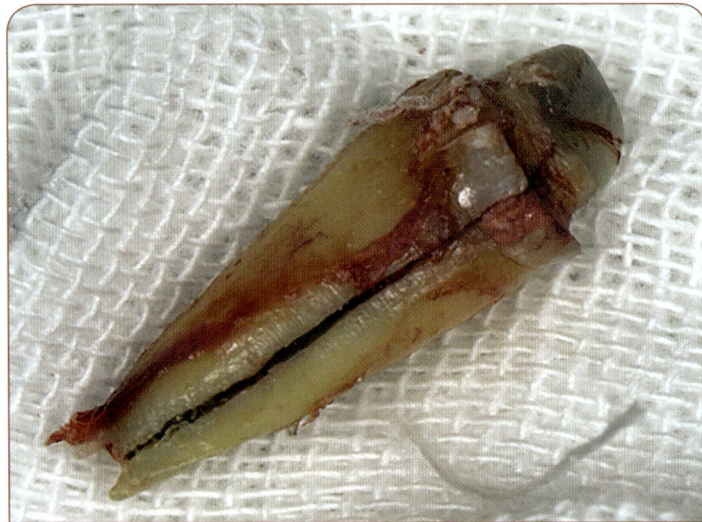

Fig. 3

Vertical fracture of tooth #21 **(Fig. 3)**.

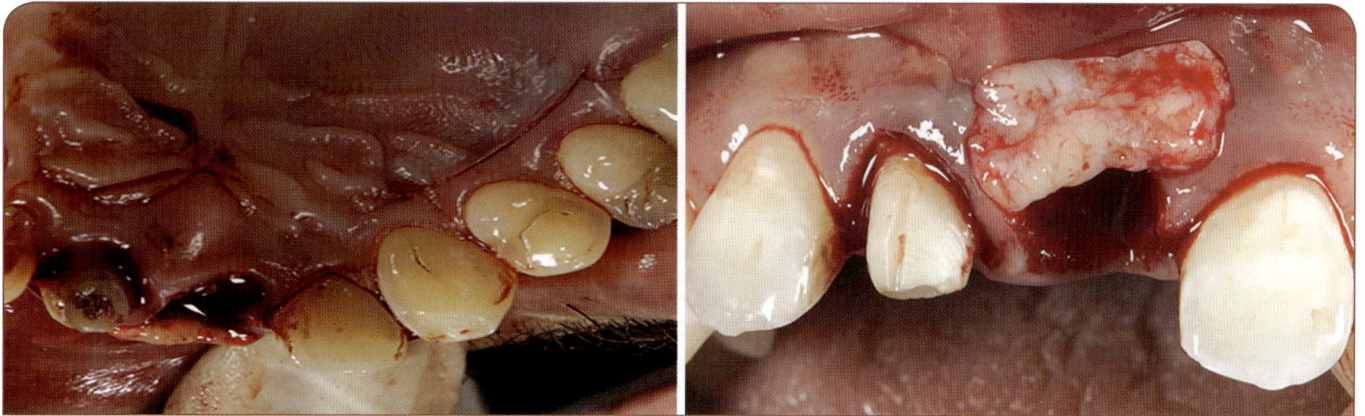

Fig. 4

Connective tissue graft **(Fig. 4)**.

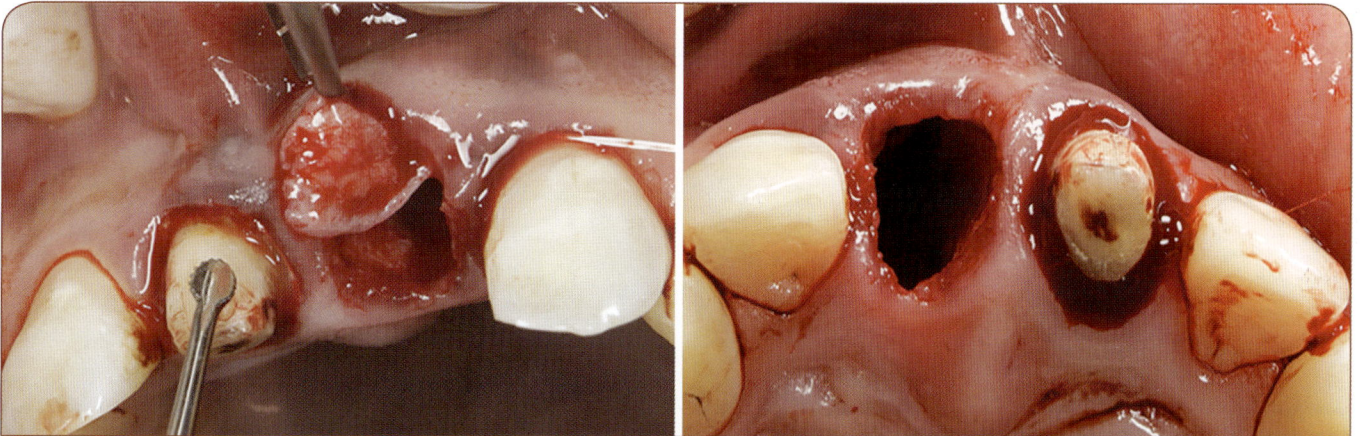

Fig. 5

Tunneling and placement of the connective tissue **(Fig. 5)**.

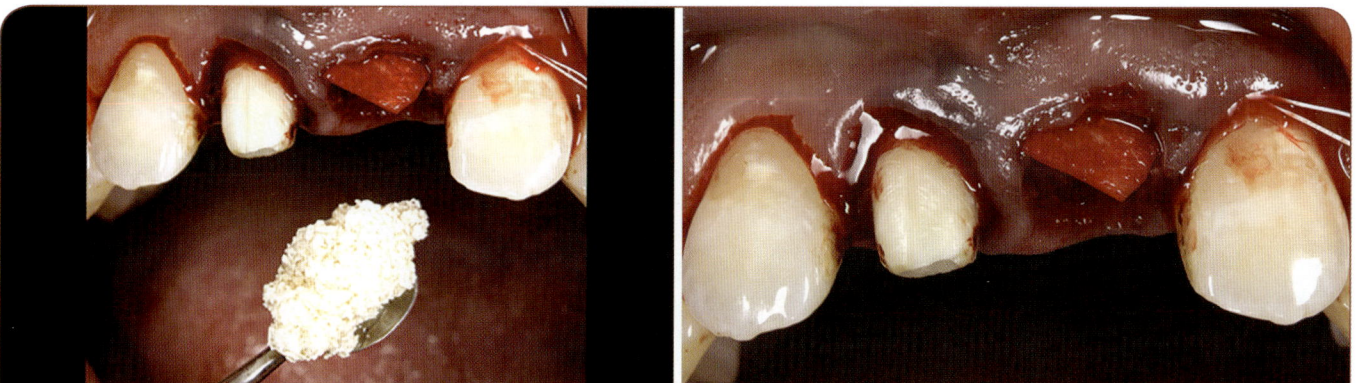

Fig. 6

Placement of a slow resorbing collagen membrane inside the socket labially to act as a barrier wall in front of the labial fenestration **(Fig. 6)**.

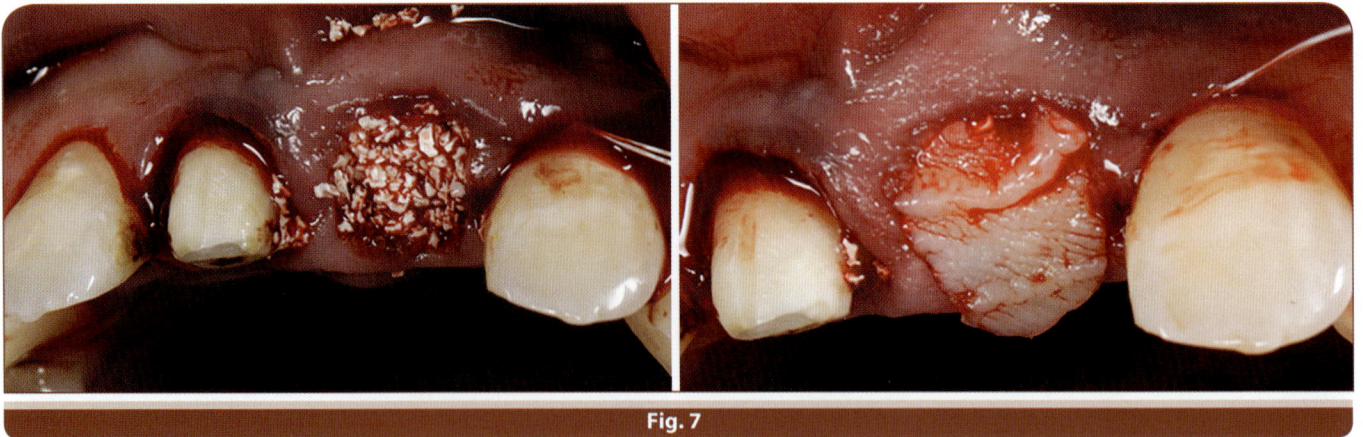

Fig. 7

Bovine bone graft placement and covered by a free gingival graft from the palate to completely close the grafted socket and to enhance quality and vertical quantity of the future implant site soft tissue **(Fig. 7)**.

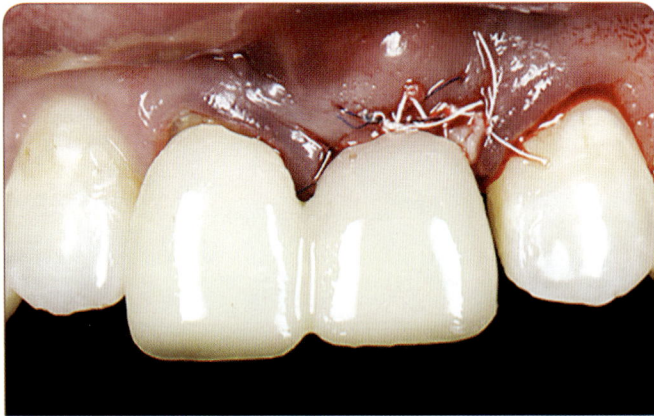

Fig. 8

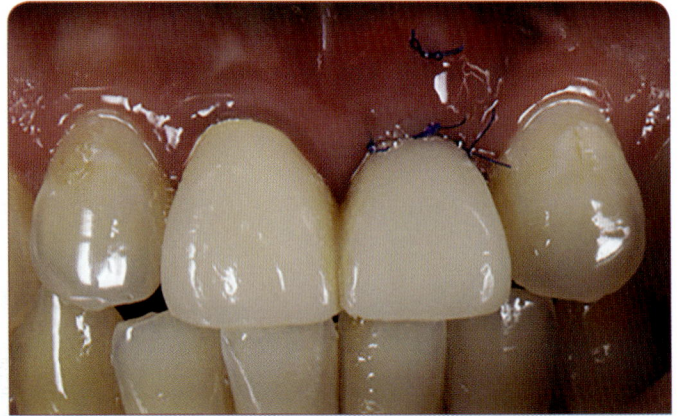

Fig. 9

Immediate conventional temporization on the adjacent central root canalled tooth with a cantilever pontic above the surgical site **(Fig. 8)**.

After 7 days of the surgery a new CAD CAM temporary was fabricated and placed with proper ovate pontic design **(Fig. 9)**.

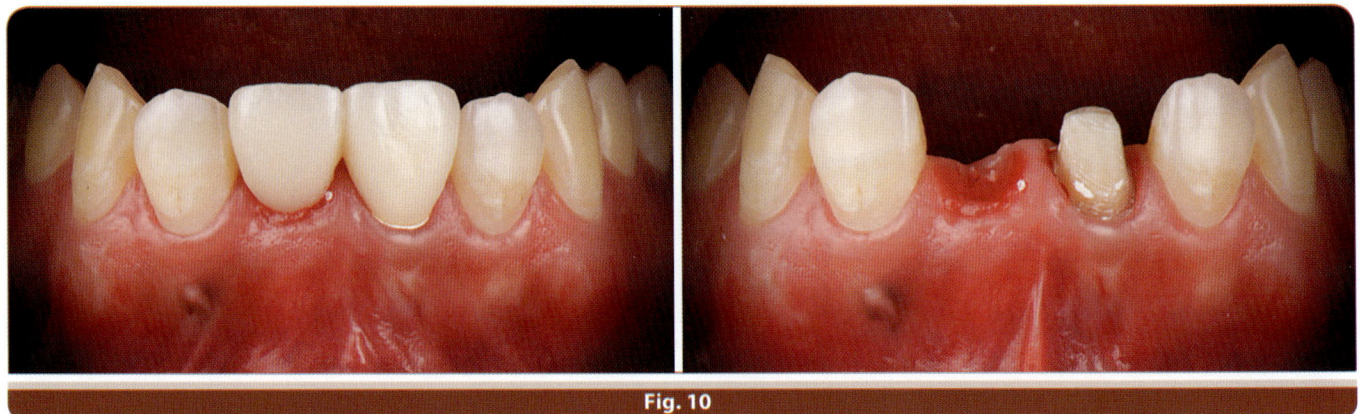

Fig. 10

After 7 month, notice the soft tissue scalloping and guided shape **(Fig. 10)**.

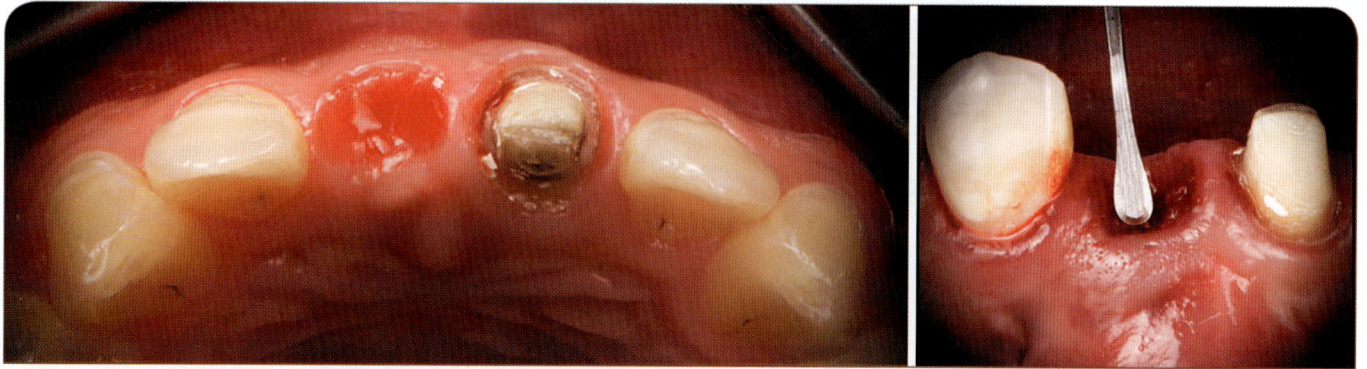

Fig. 11

Small mimicked opening to place the implant and using micro tunneling blade to create a tunnel for extra soft tissue grafting to enhance labially the soft tissue **(Fig. 11)**.

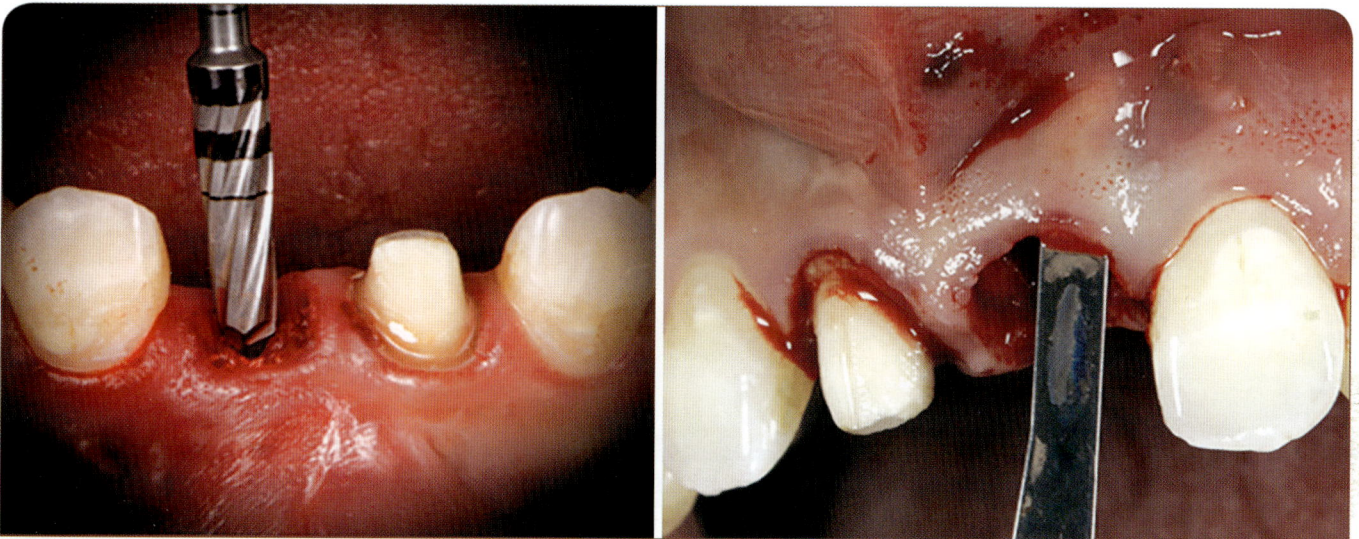

Fig. 12

Use of osseodensification drills to further enhance bone osteotomy **(Fig. 12)**.

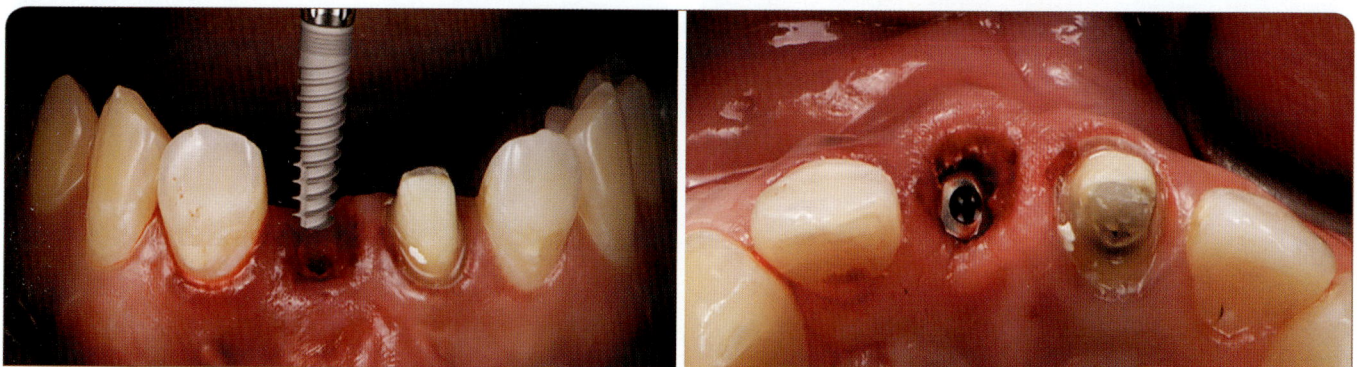

Fig. 13

Implant placement **(Fig. 13)**.

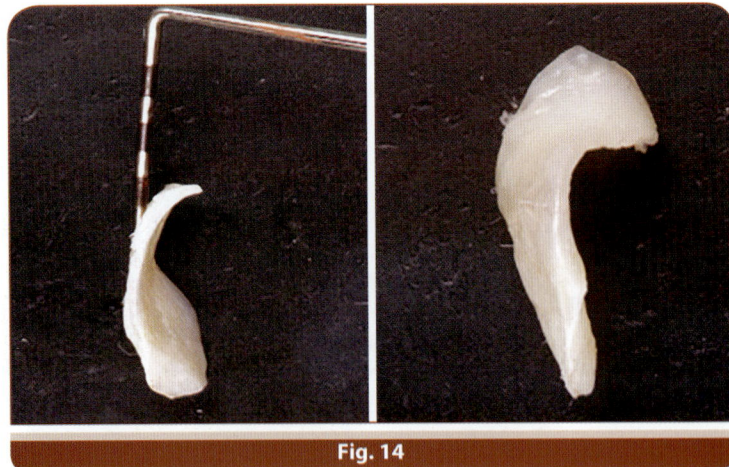

Fig. 14

Free gingival graft harvested from the palate to where the epithelium will be removed (Zucchelli) to have pure good quality connective tissue with no fatty and glandular tissue **(Fig. 14)**.

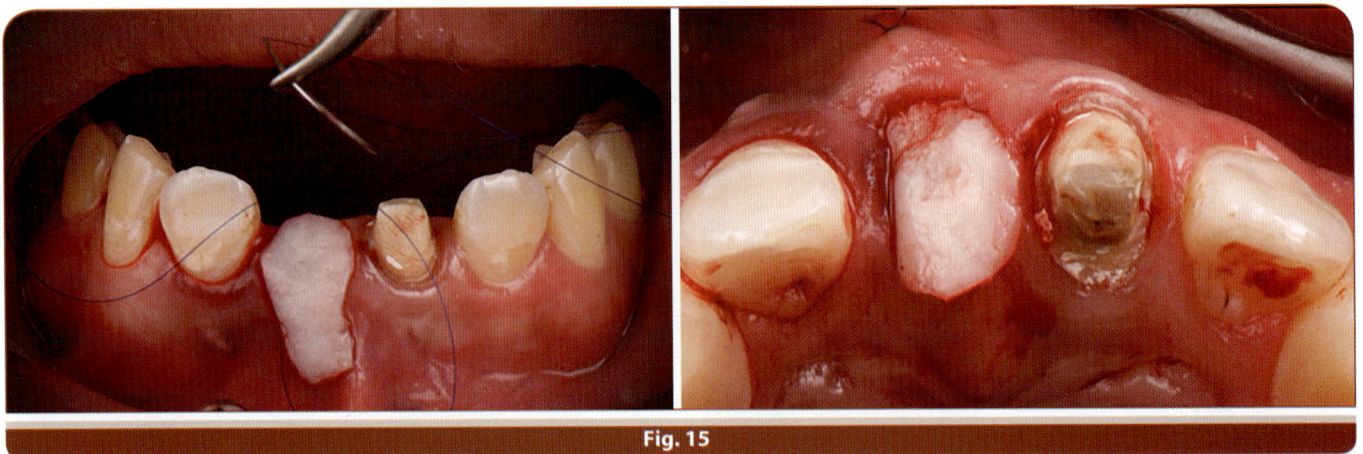

Fig. 15

Note part of the graft is de-epithelialized while the remaining part that will be closing on top of the implant has still the epithelium, to act as a free gingival seal graft **(Fig. 15)**.

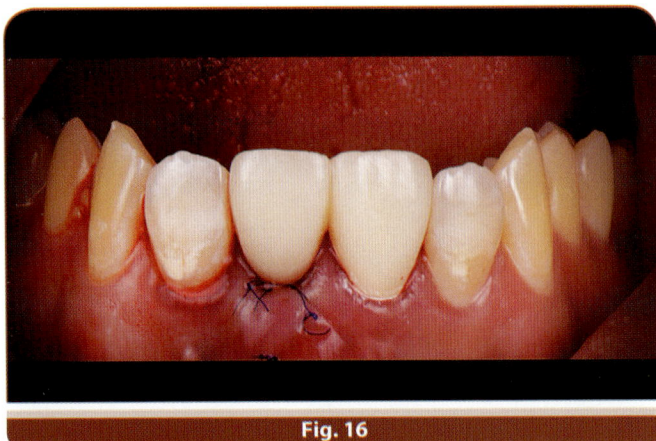

Fig. 16

CAD CAM temporary back on **(Fig. 16)**.

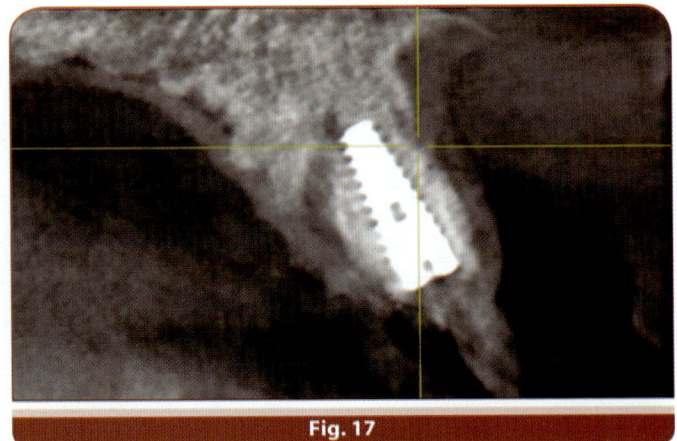

Fig. 17

CT scan showing nice placement **(Fig. 17)**.

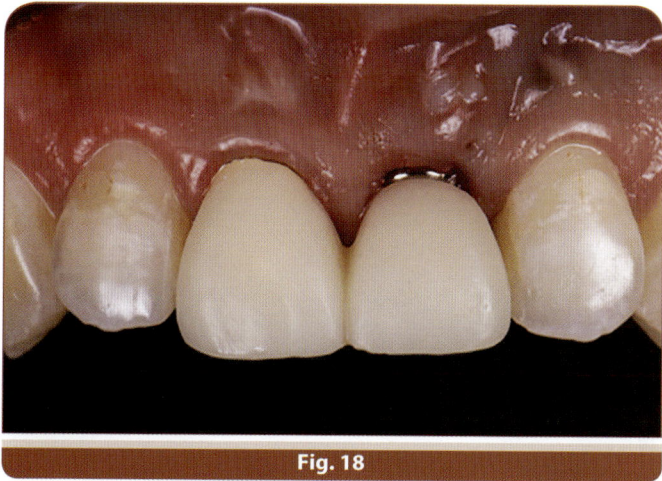

Fig. 18

After 3 months **(Fig. 18)**.

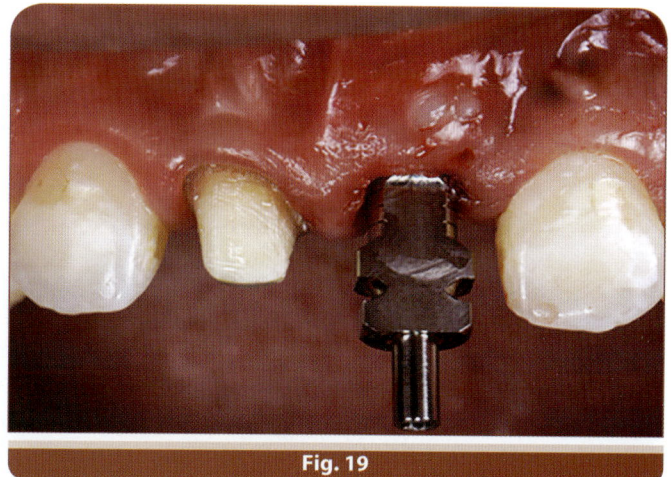

Fig. 19

Minimally invasive opening on top of the implant and direct impression to fabricate a screw retained immediate temporary **(Fig. 19)**.

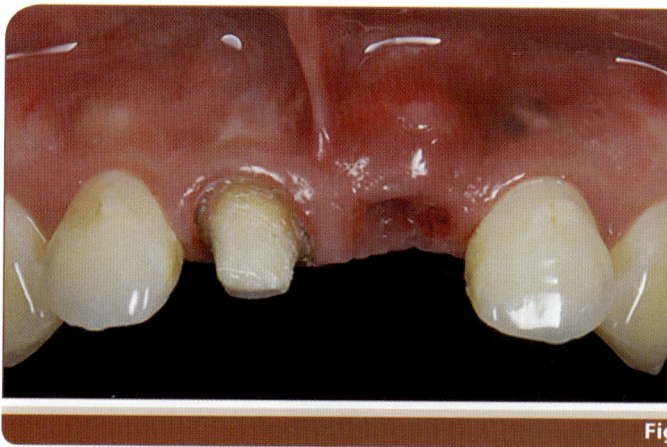

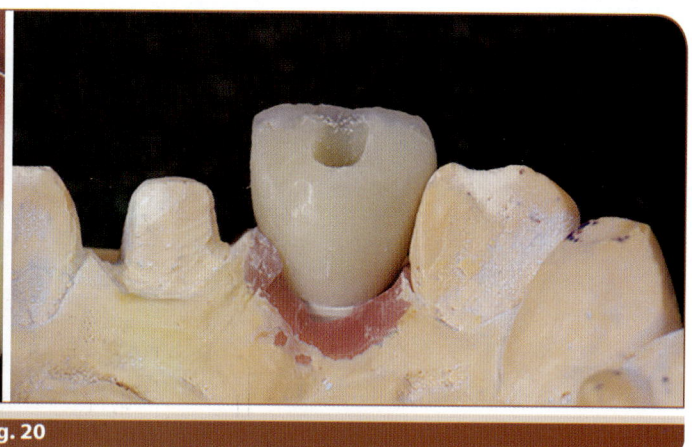

Fig. 20

Screw retained fabricated on a plastic PEEK abutment **(Fig. 20)**.

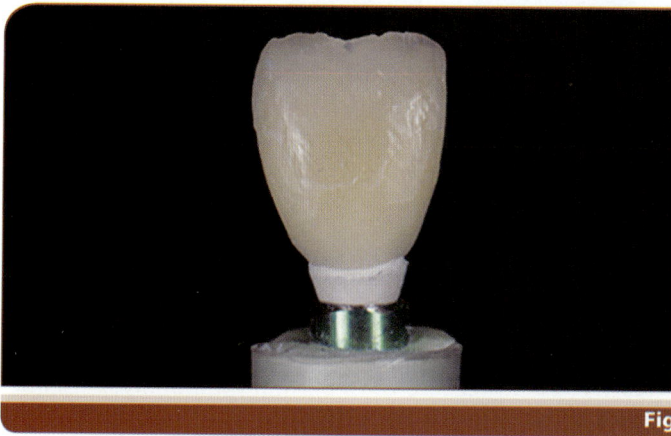

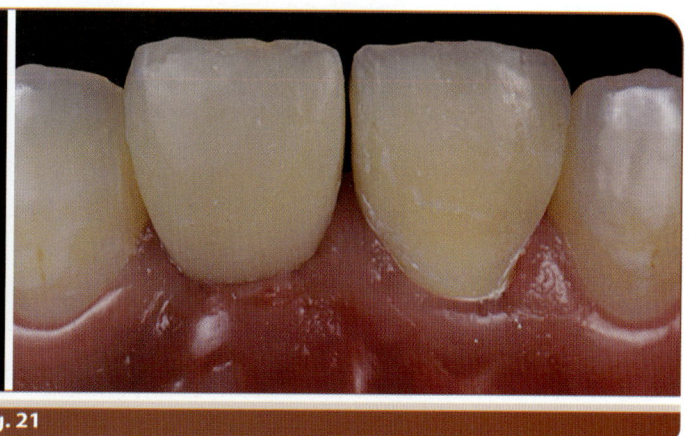

Fig. 21

Cementation of the temporary on the root canalled tooth while the temporary on the implant is screwed **(Fig. 21)**.

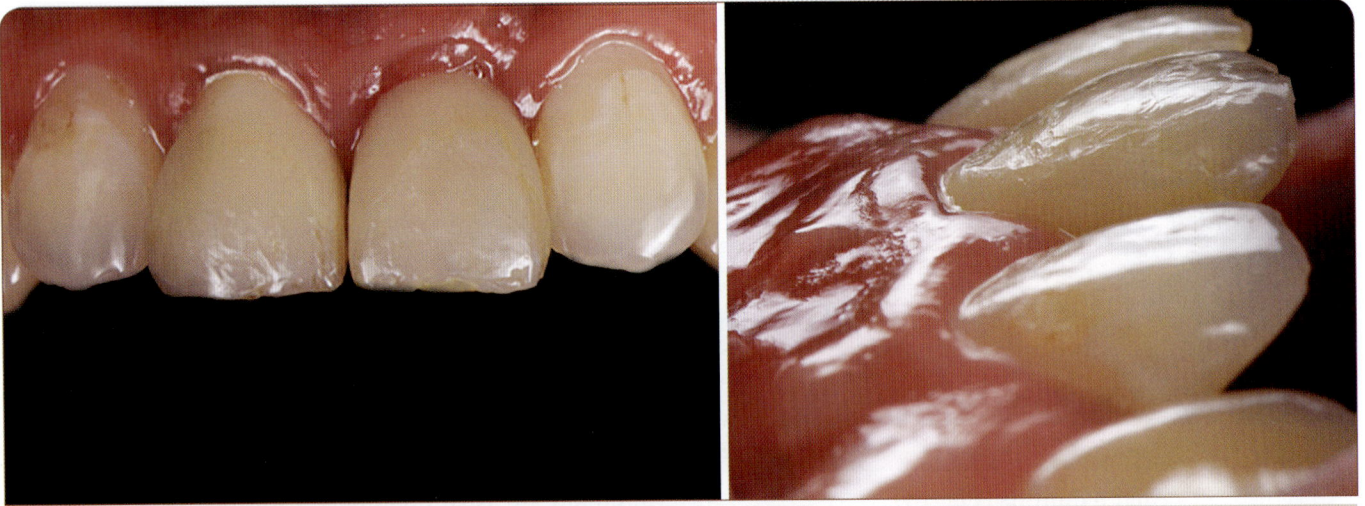

Fig. 22

Temporaries in place for 3 weeks **(Fig. 22)**.

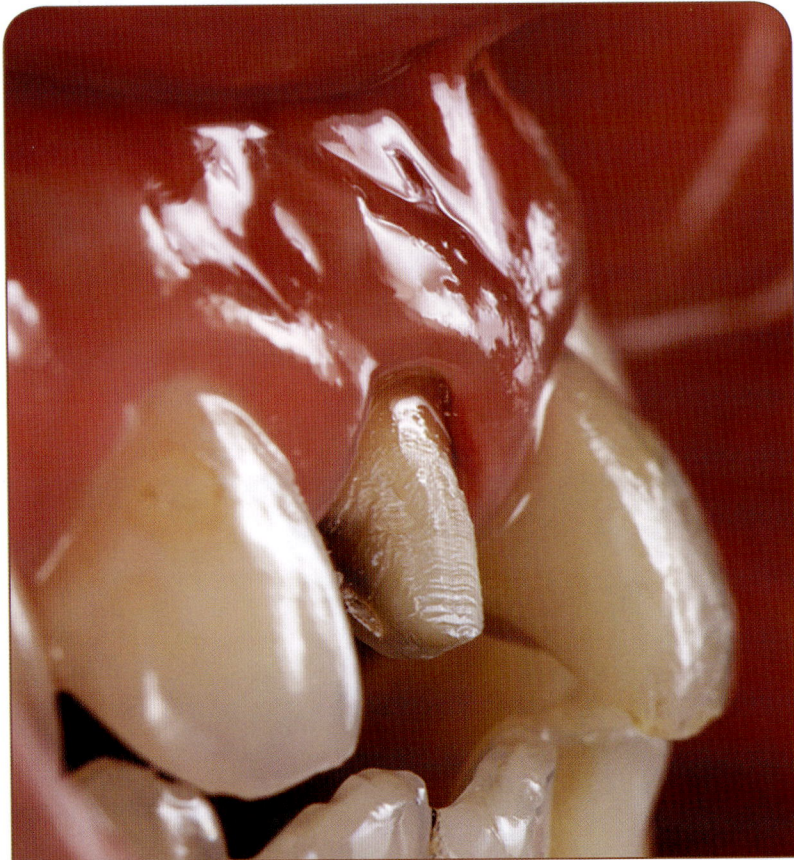

Fig. 23

Note the soft tissue around the temporary implant crown **(Fig. 23)**.

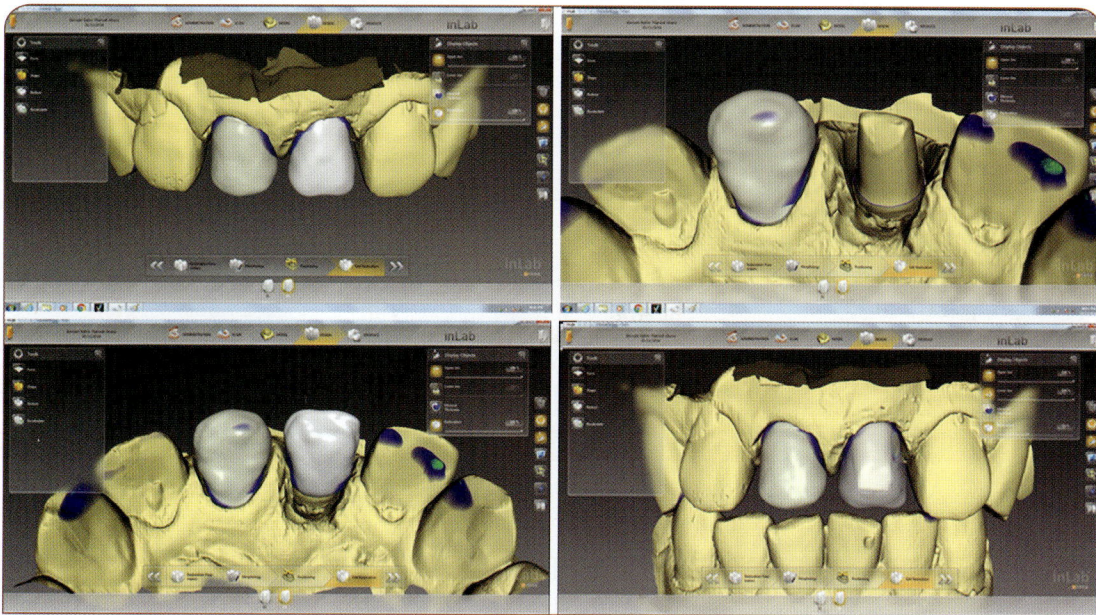

Fig. 24

CAD CAM Sirona designing **(Fig. 24)**.

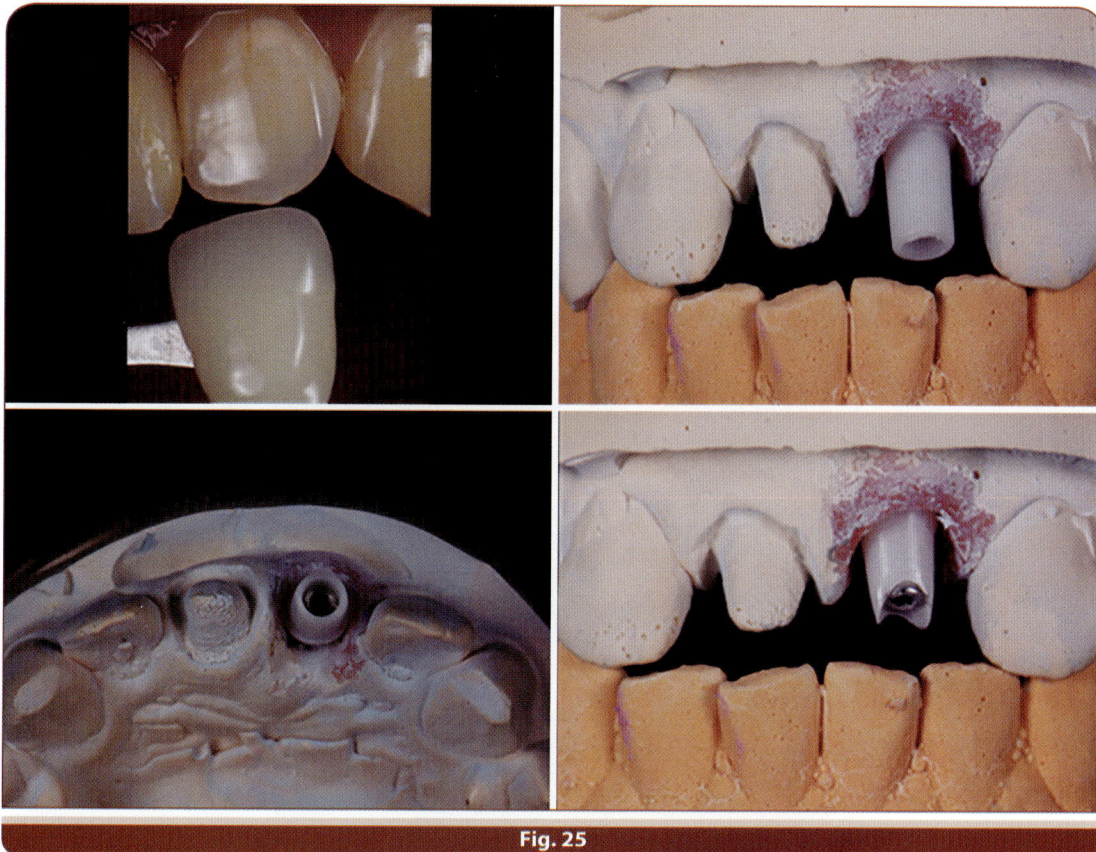

Fig. 25

AA zirconium abutment is used **(Fig. 25)**.

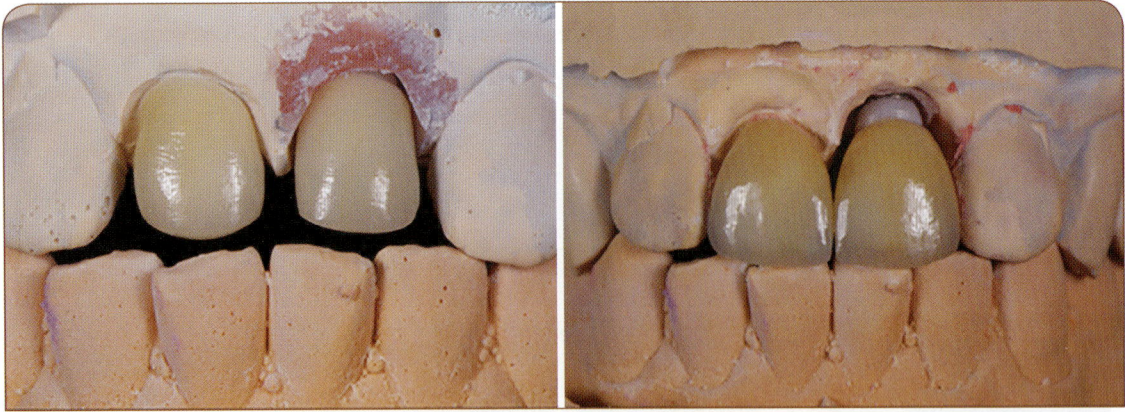

Fig. 26

E MAX CAD CAM milled and cut back crowns to be layered and characterized **(Fig. 26)**.

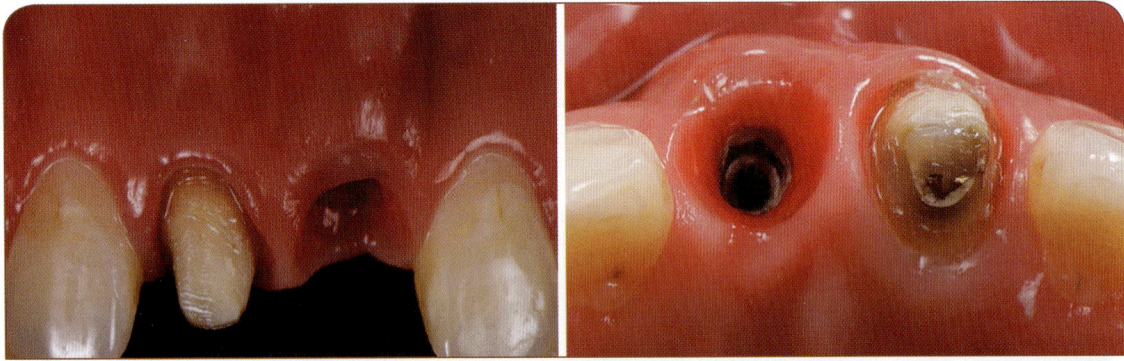

Fig. 27

Again note the soft tissue quality and quantity and the emergence profile and the intact papilla **(Fig. 27)**.

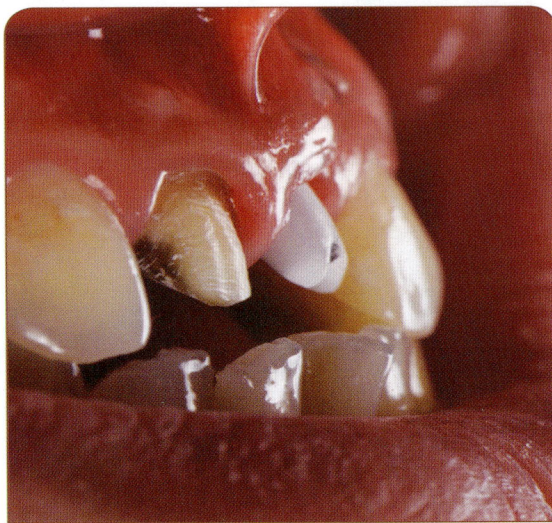

Fig. 28

Side view: Note the soft tissue **(Fig. 28)**.

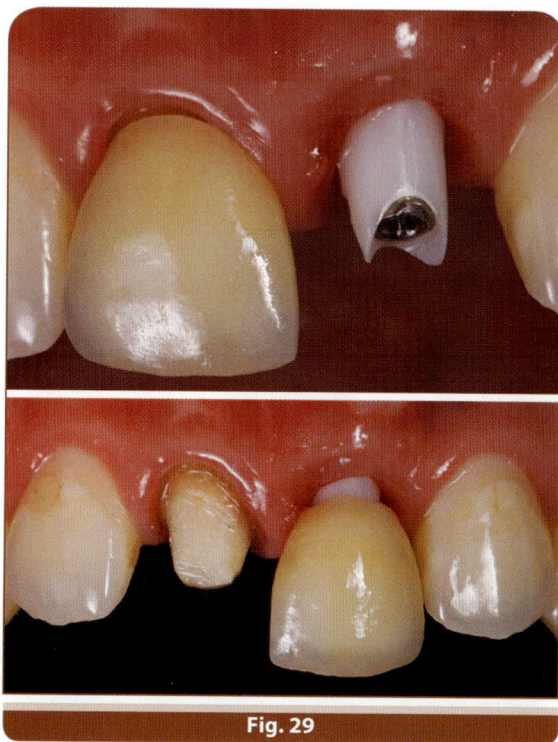

Fig. 29

Try ins **(Fig. 29)**.

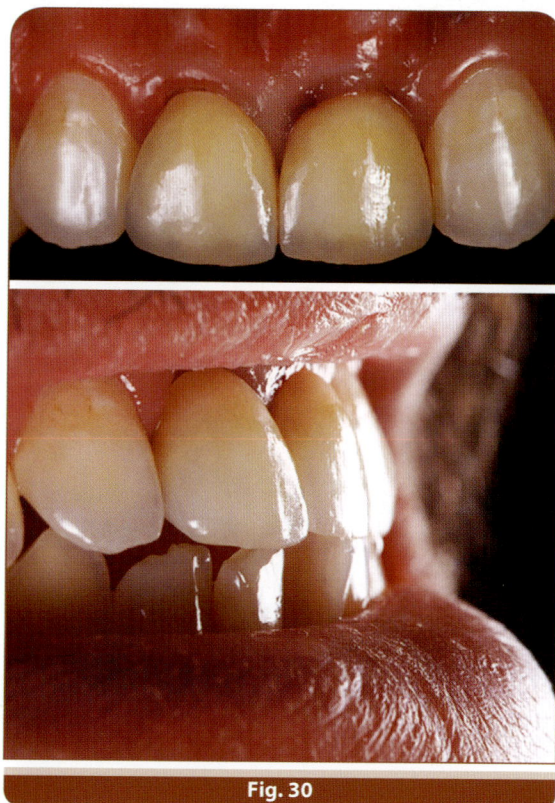

Fig. 30

Final cementation of both crowns **(Fig. 30)**.

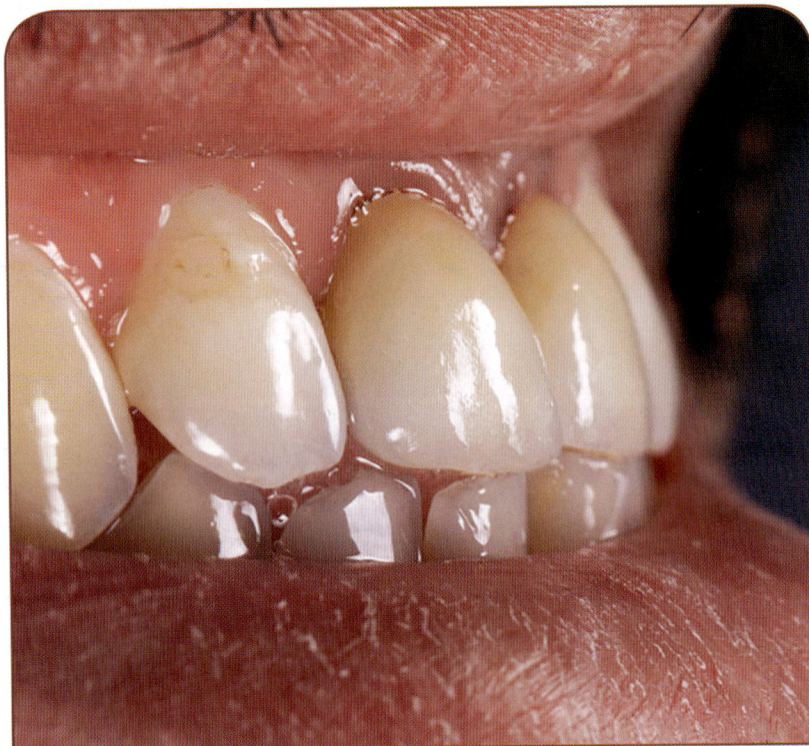

Fig. 31

Final optimal esthetic result **(Fig. 31)**.

Lanka Mahesh, Nitika Poonia

IMMEDIATE IMPLANT PLACEMENT AND RESTORATION WITH A CAD/CAM ABUTMENT AND PFM CROWN FOR AN UPPER MOLAR

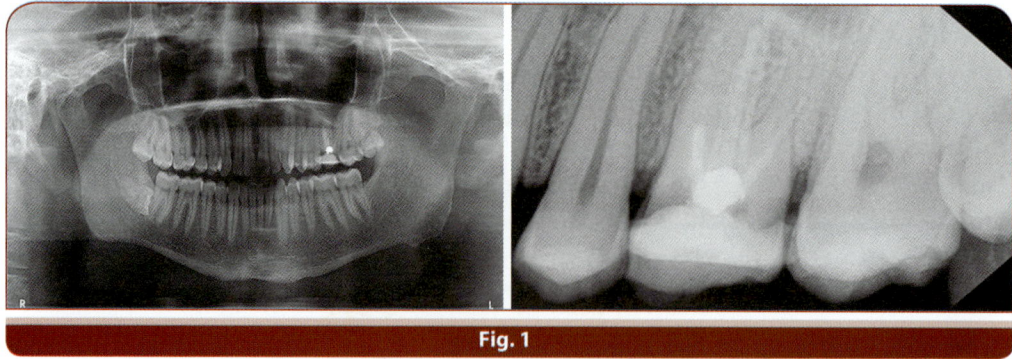

Fig. 1

A 26-year-old male patient with a chief complaint of constant pain in the upper left molar. No relevant medical history. Panorex and IOPA X-rays revealed a fractured 26 in an endodontically treated tooth. Treatment plan included an immediate implant placement with a "smart" abutment and a PFM crown **(Fig. 1)**.

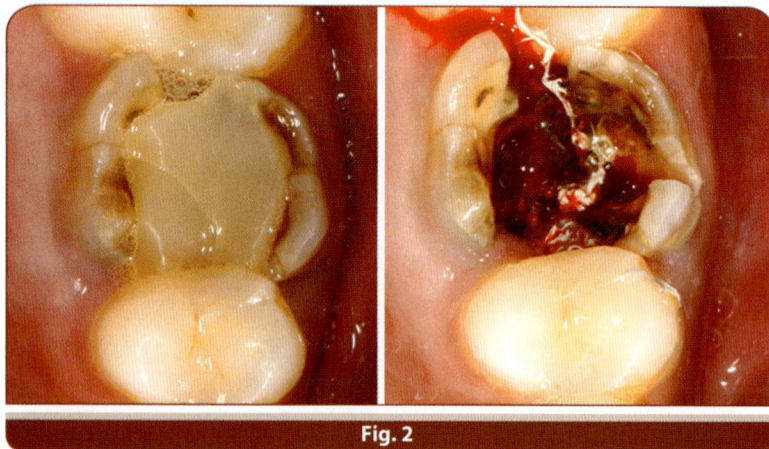

Fig. 2

Occlusal view of the tooth to be extracted. Gentle sectioning of the crown with a long shank bur on an airotor **(Fig. 2)**.

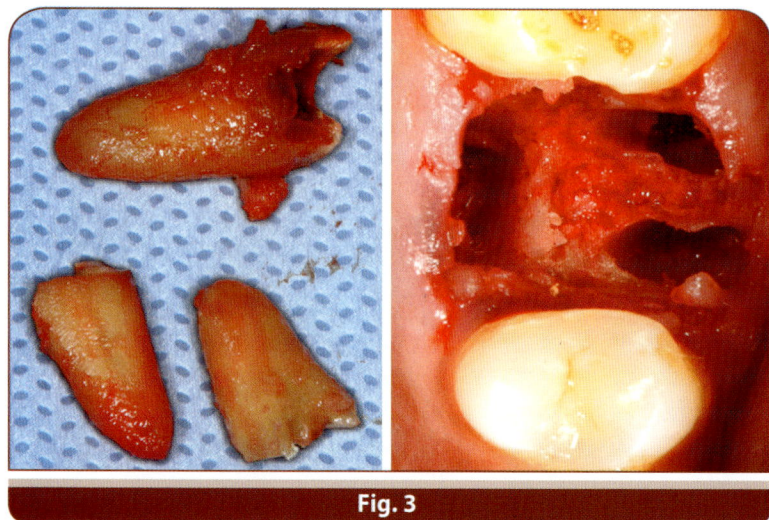

Fig. 3

Careful extraction thereby preserving the alveolus. After the roots are sectioned they are gently luxated with the use of luxators **(Fig. 3)**.

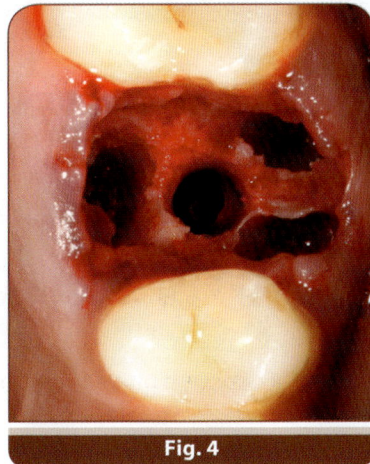

Fig. 4

Incremental drilling is done at slow speed to get adequate tactile sensation. The sinus lining is clearly visible without any tears or rupture **(Fig. 4)**.

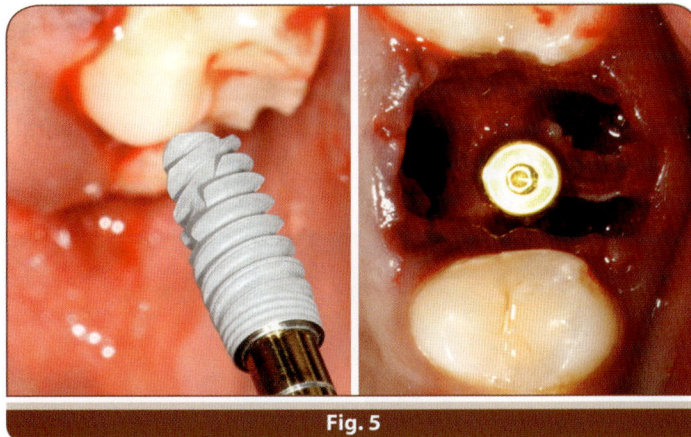

Fig. 5

A nobel biocare active implant of 4.3/11.5 is placed in the correct position within the confines of the interradicular bone. The implant is placed at 45 Ncm insertion torque. No bone graft material has been placed **(Fig. 5)**.

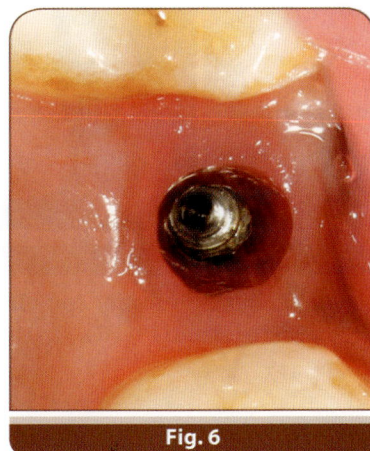

Fig. 6

Healing of soft tissue at 4 months following removal of the healing collar demonstrating adequate soft tissue maturation **(Fig. 6)**.

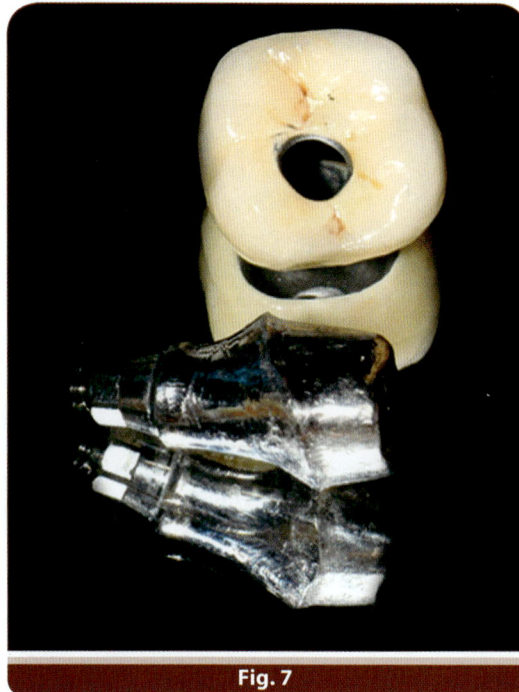

Fig. 7

The smart abutment and the final PFM prosthesis with an occlusal vent to allow extraoral cementation thereby preventing any extra cement in the gingival sulcus **(Fig. 7)**.

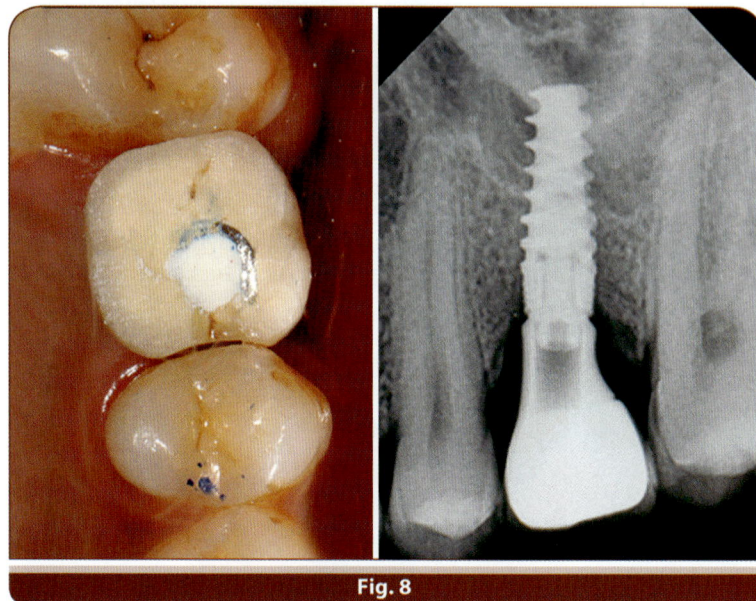

Fig. 8

Prosthesis at insertion. The access hole is sealed with glass ionomer cement (GIC). One year recall IOPA X-ray. Clearly indicating bone fill in the sinus and stable crestal bone levels **(Fig. 8)**.

CASE STUDY 21

Praful Bali, Mandeep Grewal

Socket Shield, a Viable Solution for Preservation of Hard and Soft Tissue in Anterior Zone

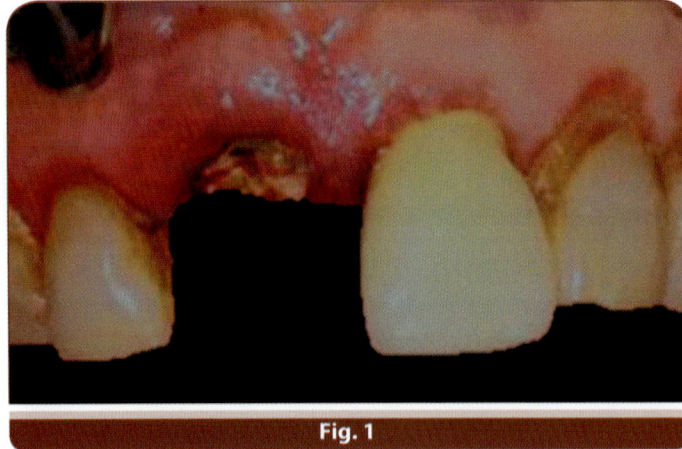

Fig. 1

Preoperative view of failed endodontics and fracture of tooth #11. Patient is an elderly lady and has periodontal health but she insists of having an implant done. The risks involved are explained to the patient **(Fig. 1)**.

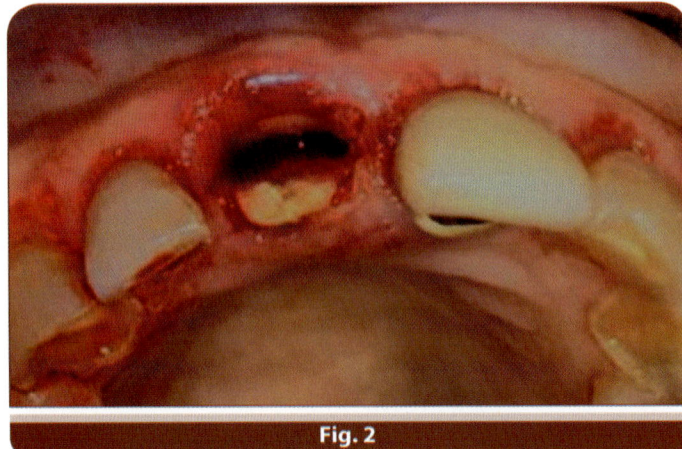

Fig. 2

The root is sliced vertically–mesiodistally to split the root into 2 pieces **(Fig. 2)**.

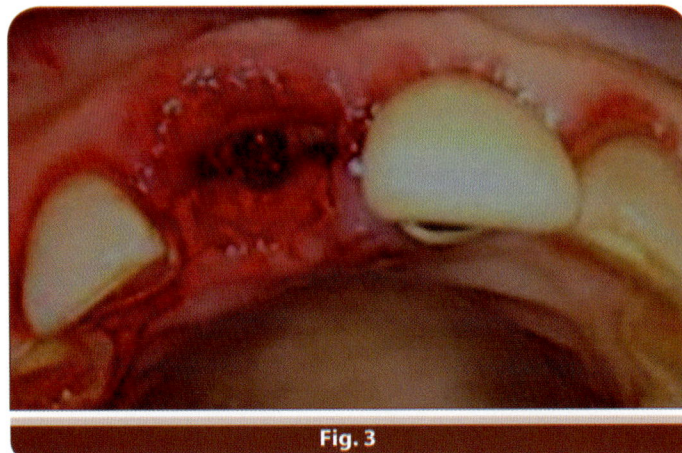

Fig. 3

The palatal portion of the root is removed. Buccal shield is left to maintain buccal contour. The buccal shield is made very thin the purpose being to supprt the buccal cortical plate **(Fig. 3)**.

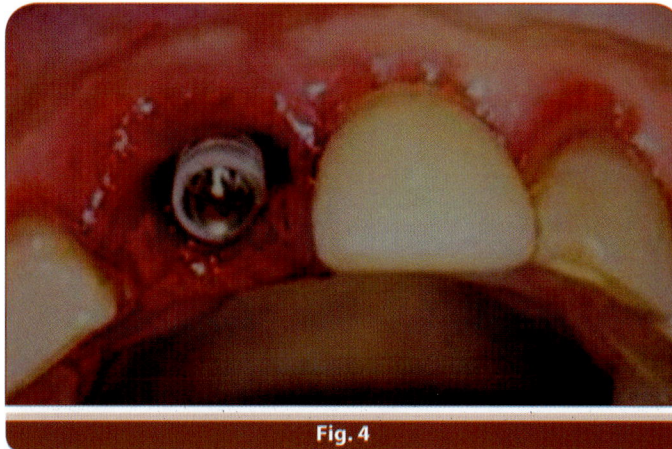

Fig. 4

4/13 Top DM implant (Bioner) placed 2–3 mm below the CE junction. The space between the implant and buccal root piece is augmented with Novabone putty **(Fig. 4)**.

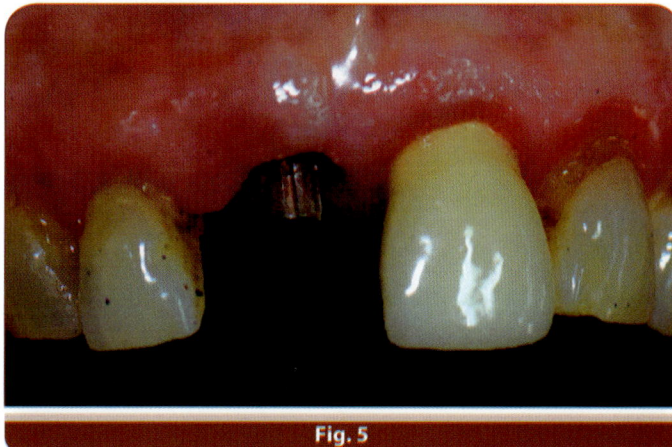

Fig. 5

Permanent abutment torqued at 35 Ncm on the same surgical visit **(Fig. 5)**.

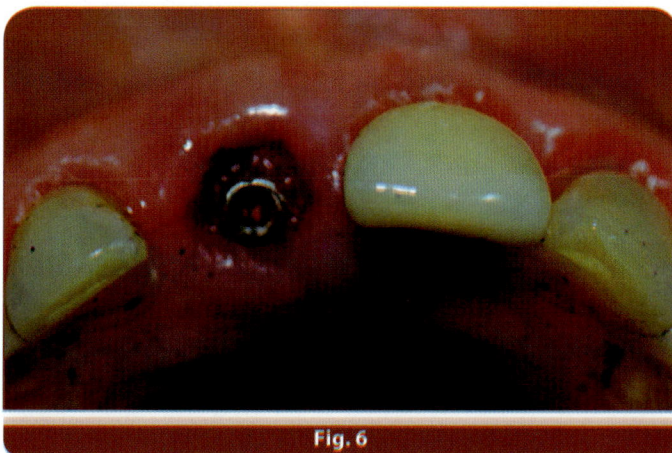

Fig. 6

Occlusal view of the implant. Note the buccal hard and soft tissue contour is maintained **(Fig. 6)**.

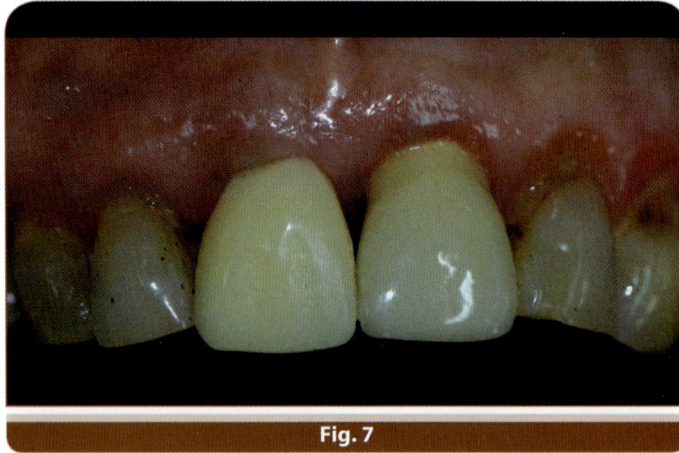

Fig. 7

A temporary crown is cemented and made out of occlusion. The crown is shaped so that the papilla fill is achieved during healing **(Fig. 7)**.

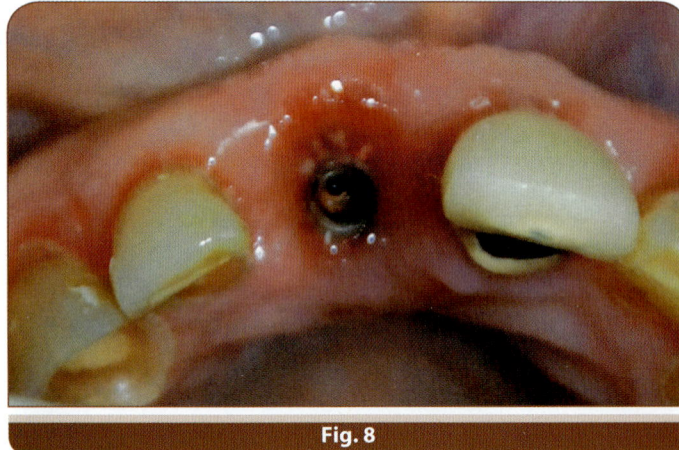

Fig. 8

Occlusal view of the healed situation 3 months after the implant placement. There is absolutely no change in the buccal contour and this is the main advantage of doing the socket shield **(Fig. 8)**.

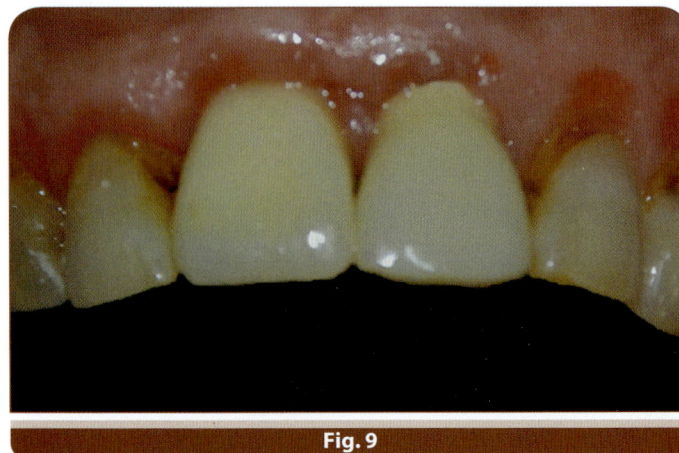

Fig. 9

Final metal ceramic crown on 11. Nice soft tissue coverage and papilla fill **(Fig. 9)**.

Lanka Mahesh, Nitika Poonia

IMPACTED CANINE REMOVAL AND SIMULTANEOUS PLACEMENT OF ADJACENT IMPLANTS WITH GBR IN THE ESTHETIC ZONE

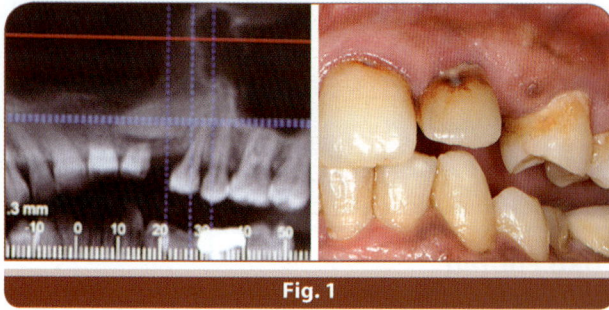

Fig. 1

Preoperative CBCT view depicting a horizontally impacted canine with extensive resorption of teeth #21 and #22 in a 40-year-old male. Clinical view of the same site **(Fig. 1)**.

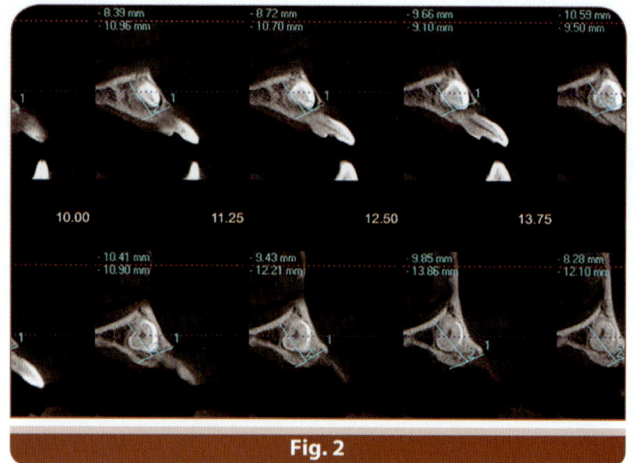

Fig. 2

Cross-sections reveal the contact with the facial plate which entails bone removal. Thereby causing loss of the bony housing which would entail a large GBR procedure. Such cases may be treated in a staged manner with GBR followed by uneventful healing or simultaneous implant placement, if adequate primary stability is achieved.

The latter approach was performed in this case **(Fig. 2)**.

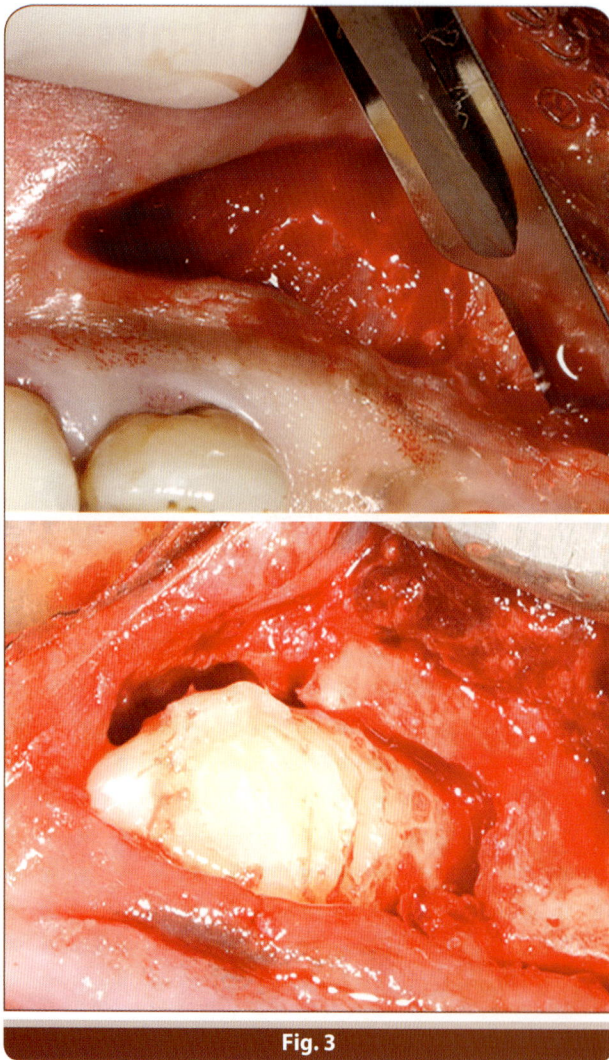

Fig. 3

A horizontal incision is made in the attached gingiva without disturbing the papillary mucosa (which limits stress on the suture line). The canine is exposed with a fissure bur on a high speed straight handpiece **(Fig. 3)**.

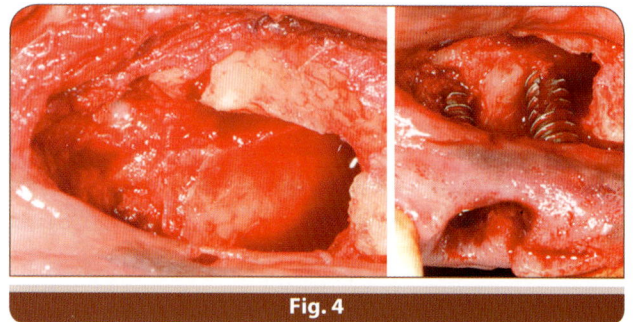

Fig. 4

A large defect is evident after the canine is removed. Two implant fixtures are threaded into place with adequate bicortical anchorage **(Fig. 4)**.

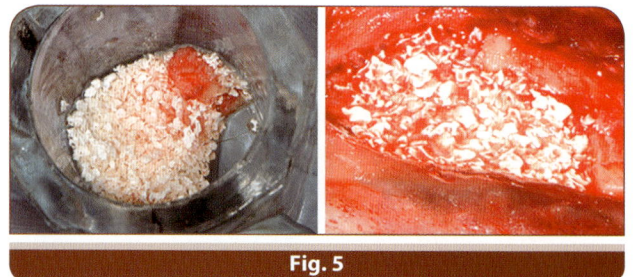

Fig. 5

Medium particle size DBBM (0.5–1 micron) (Ti-Oss) is used to fill up the defect completely. Excellent handling properties of the bone graft material are one of the most important aspects in selecting a bone graft **(Fig. 5)**.

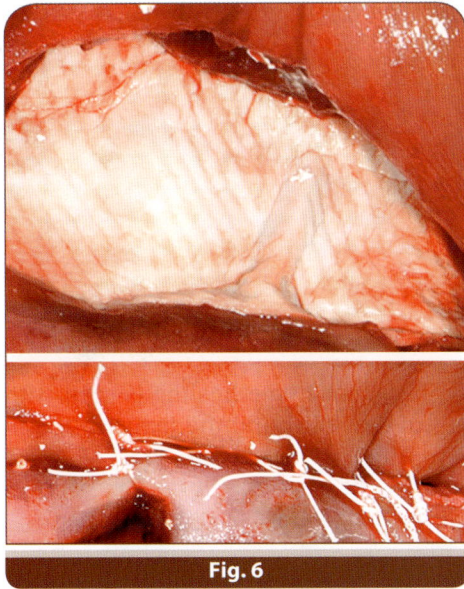
Fig. 6

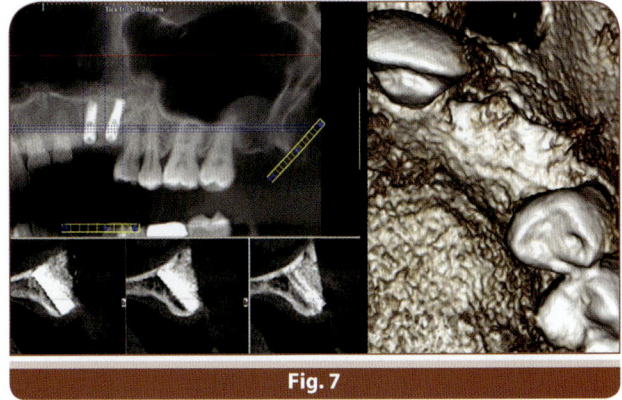
Fig. 7

CBCT views at 5 months showing excellent bone regeneration (**Fig. 7**).

The surgical site is covered with a resorbable membrane (Ossix Plus, Datum Dental). The site is closed with 3-0 cytoplast interrupted sutures (**Fig. 6**).

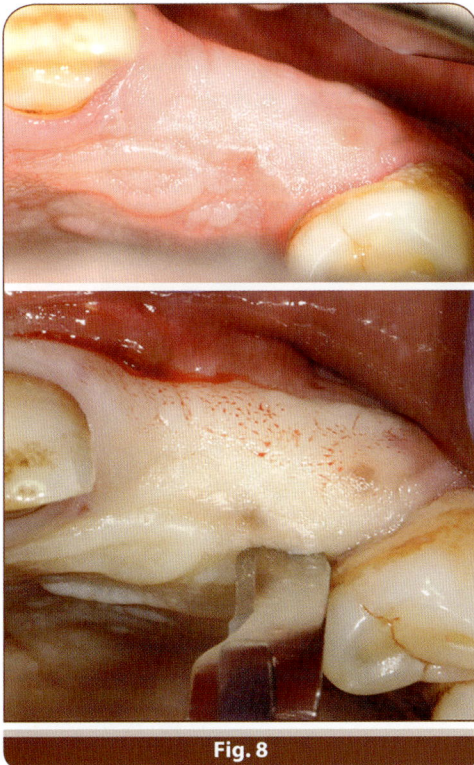
Fig. 8

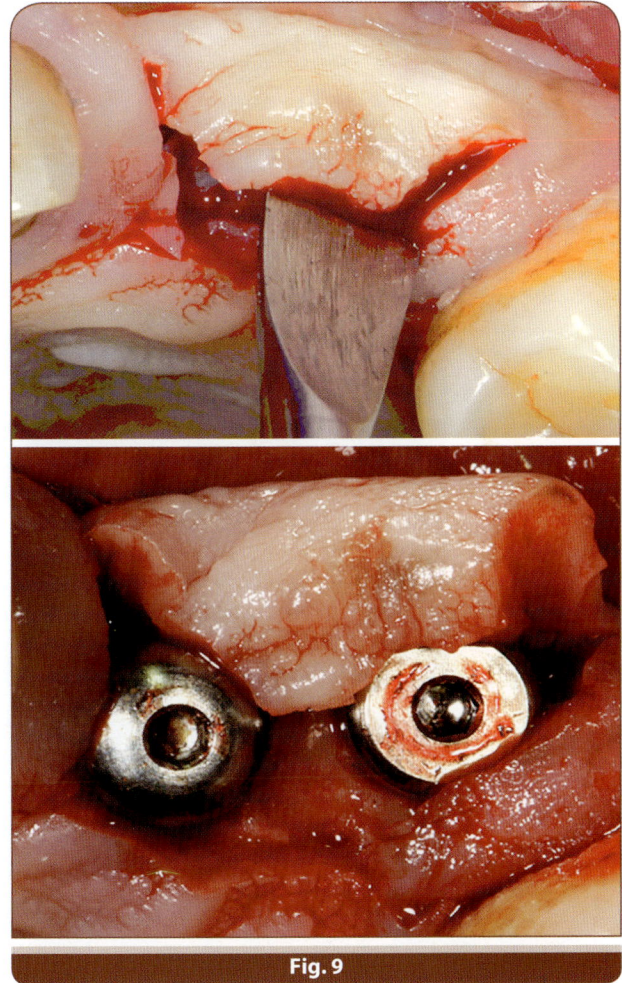
Fig. 9

Clinical appearance after 5 months of undisturbed healing. A flap with a palatal biased design is created to full depth (partial thickness flaps in such cases may cause sloughing, though have been used successfully in literature) (**Fig. 8**).

The flap is elevated gently in one stroke without causing too much trauma to the tissue. The elevated flap is rotated buccally and supported by the healing collars (**Fig. 9**).

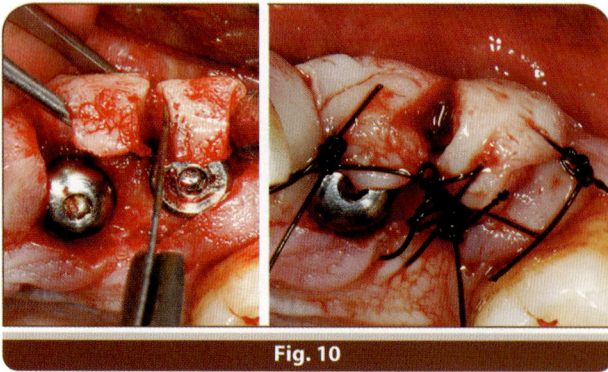

Fig. 10

The flap is split in the middle and the pedicles are created. The pedicles are sutured with 4-0 polyamide sutures around the healing collars **(Fig. 10)**.

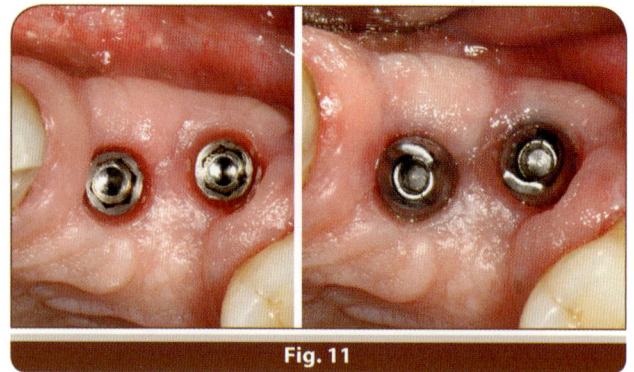

Fig. 11

At 3 weeks excellent tissue healing is seen with an adequate band of tissue around the fixtures. The final abutments are torqued into place **(Fig. 11)**.

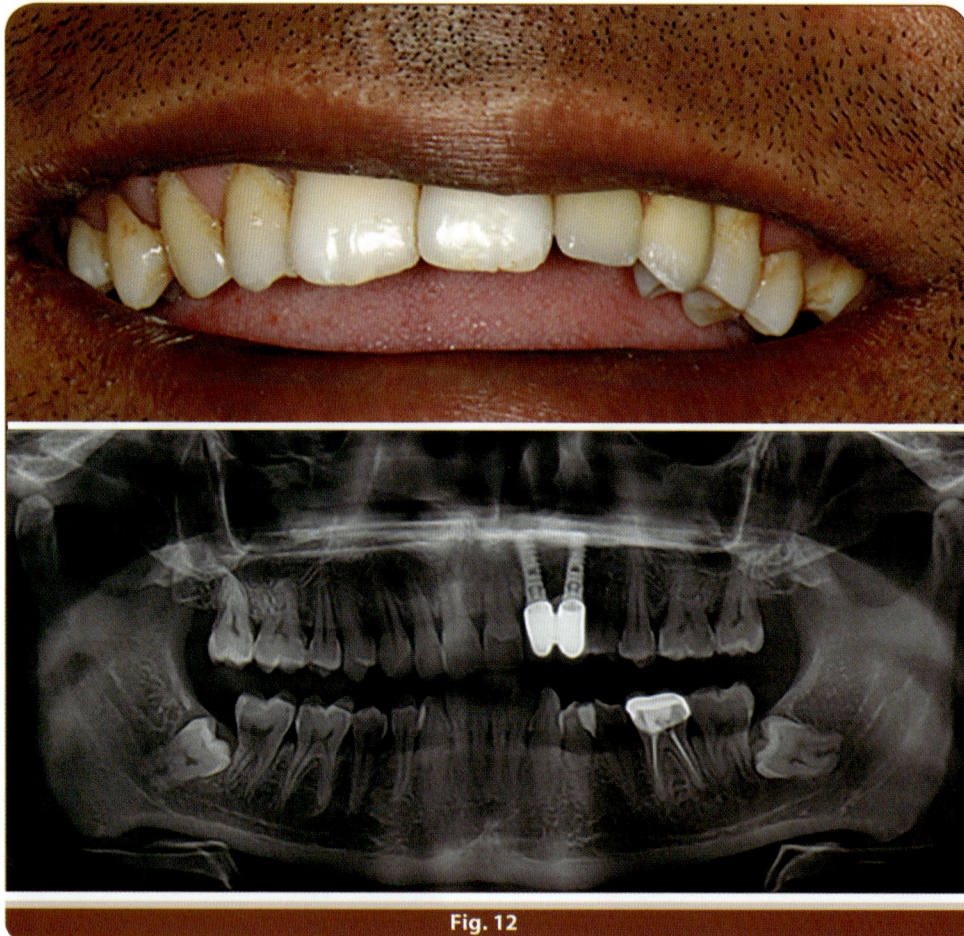

Fig. 12

The final smile line of the splinted zirconia crowns in an esthetically pleasing outcome. Postoperative panorex depicts stable bone and a very favorable crown implant ratio **(Fig. 12)**.

Praful Bali

SIMULTANEOUS IMMEDIATE EXTRACTION AND INDIRECT SINUS LIFT OF A FIRST PREMOLAR

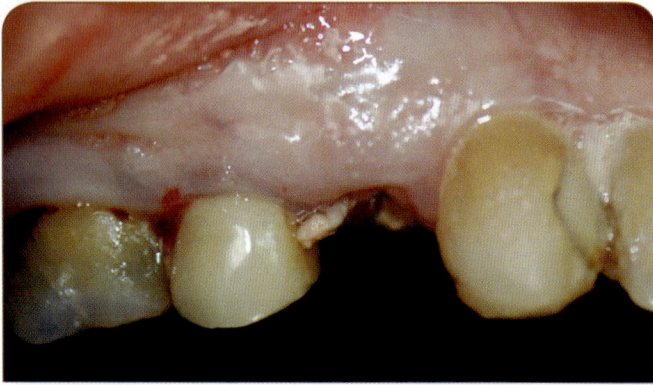

Fig. 1

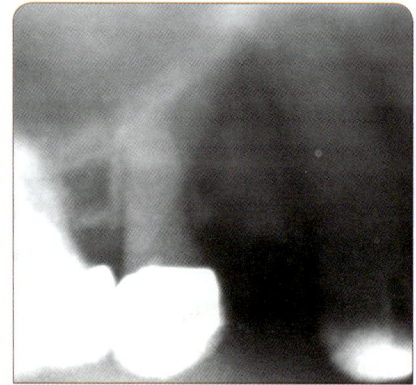

Fig. 2

Preoperative clinical view shows a grossly decayed, fractured tooth #14. There are more dental issues but the patient insists to have immediate attention to this broken tooth as it hampers her smile **(Fig. 1)**.

Preoperative X-ray reaffirms our diagnosis regarding tooth #14. Immediate extraction of the root, scoring and evaluating the socket and possible immediate implantation is suggested to the patient **(Fig. 2)**.

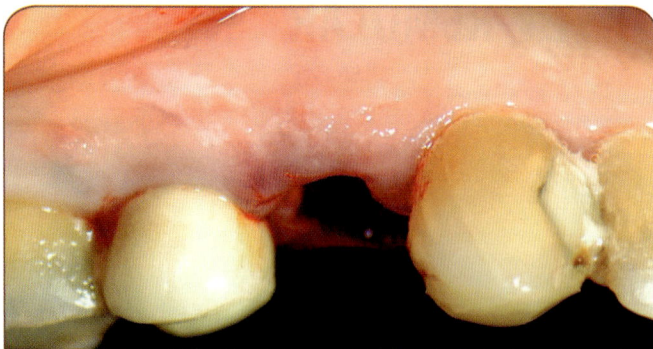

Fig. 3

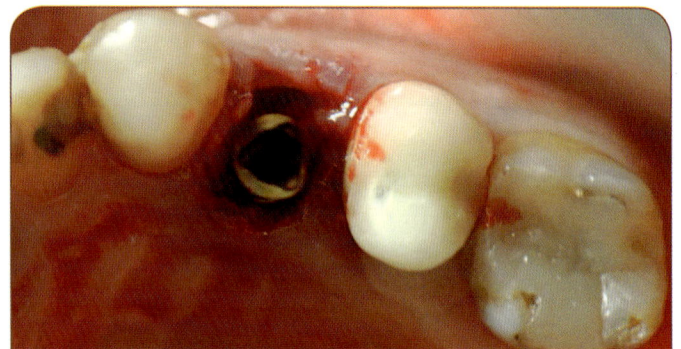

Fig. 4

Atraumatic extraction is achieved with the help of periotomes taking care not to disturb and destroy the papillas. Flapless surgery done to maintain the biology of the hard and soft tissue **(Fig. 3)**.

4.3/13 nobel groovy implant is placed taking prime stability from the palatal bone and by performing indirect sinus lift procedure. A torque of 70+ Ncm achieved **(Fig. 4)**.

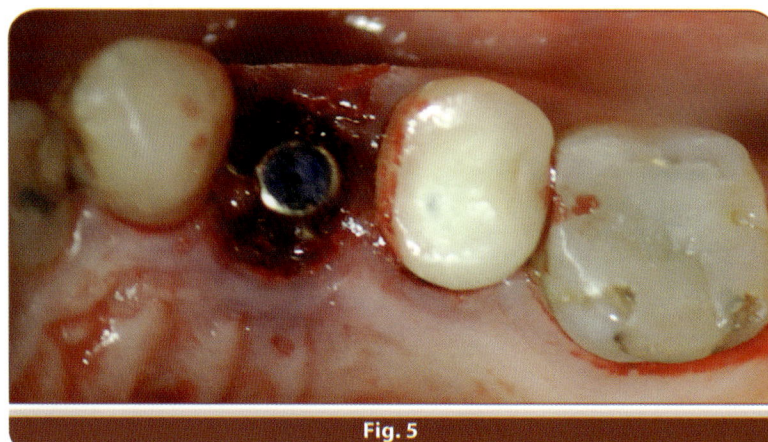

Fig. 5

1–1.5 mm jumping distance protects the buccal bone plate from compression. Nova bone is added in the socket defect **(Fig. 5)**.

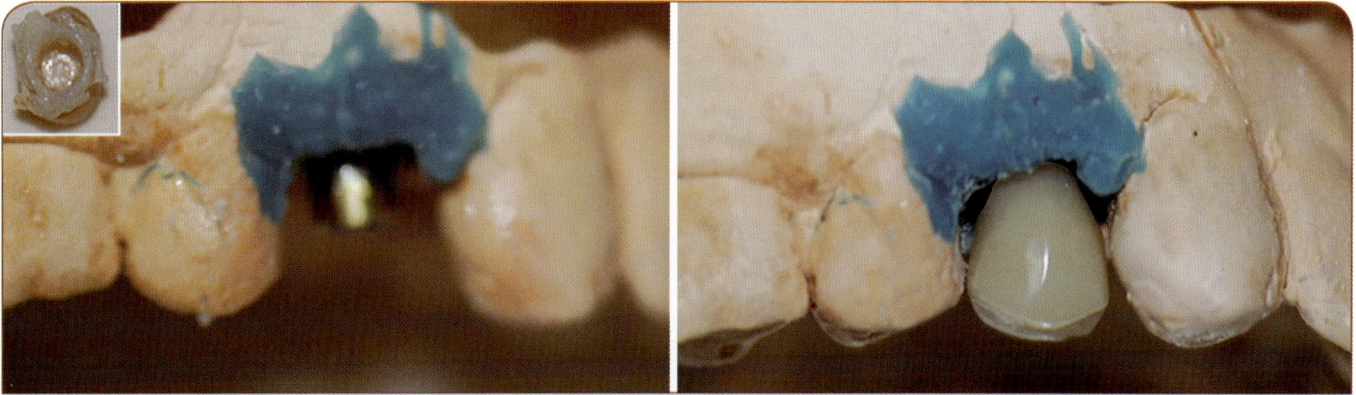

Fig. 6

An acrylic temporary is made in the lab immediately on a separate stock abutment and it is adjusted and then relined with Protemp intraorally **(Fig. 6)**.

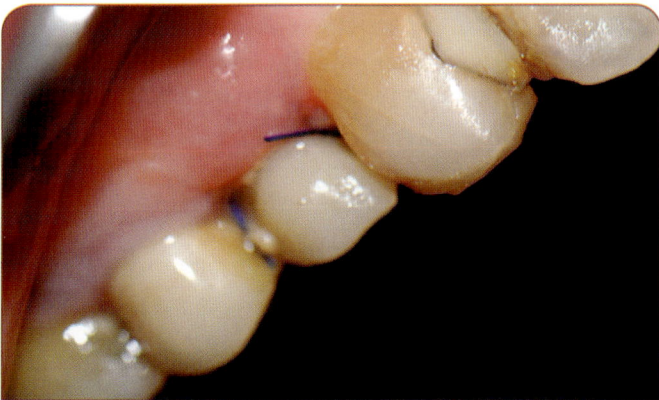

Fig. 7

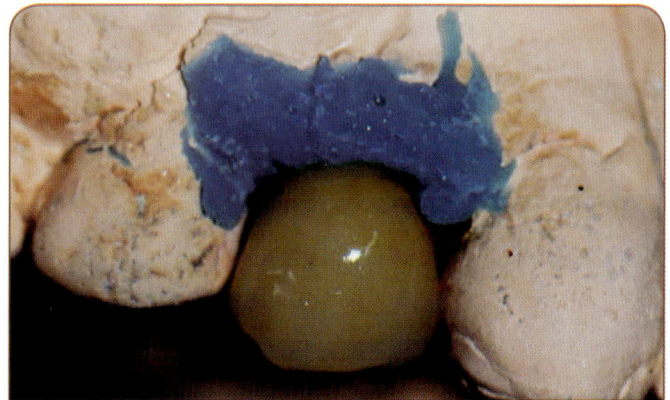

Fig. 8

Temporary crown cemented with temporary cement. Careful occlusal adjustments made. The implant crown is made slightly out of occlusion **(Fig. 7)**.

Final porcelain fused to metal crown fabricated after 3 months of healing **(Fig. 8)**.

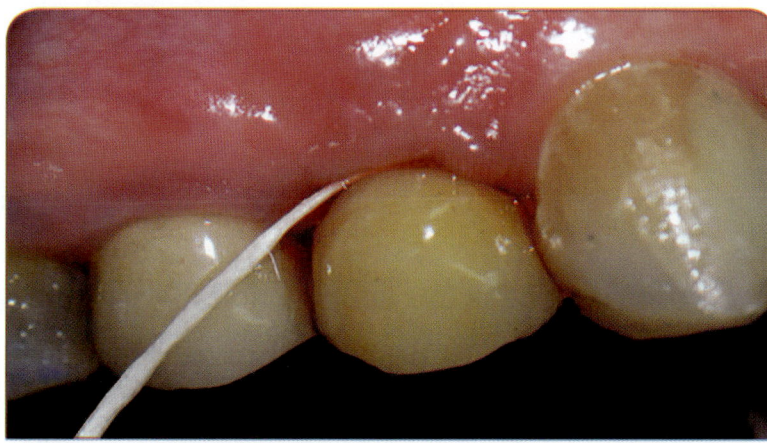

Fig. 9

Patient is instructed and taught use of inter dental aid to keep the area clean and maintain the architecture of the tissues **(Fig. 9)**.

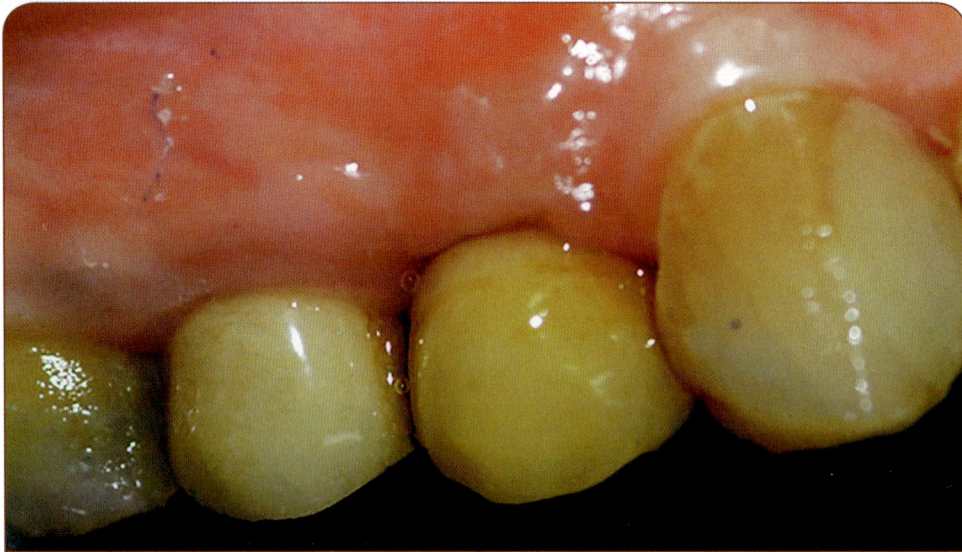

Fig. 10

Final porcelain fused to metal crown cemented with GIC. The hard and soft tissue maintained at the same level as when we started the case. Supplementary dental treatment like a composite restoration in tooth #13 also done **(Fig. 10)**.

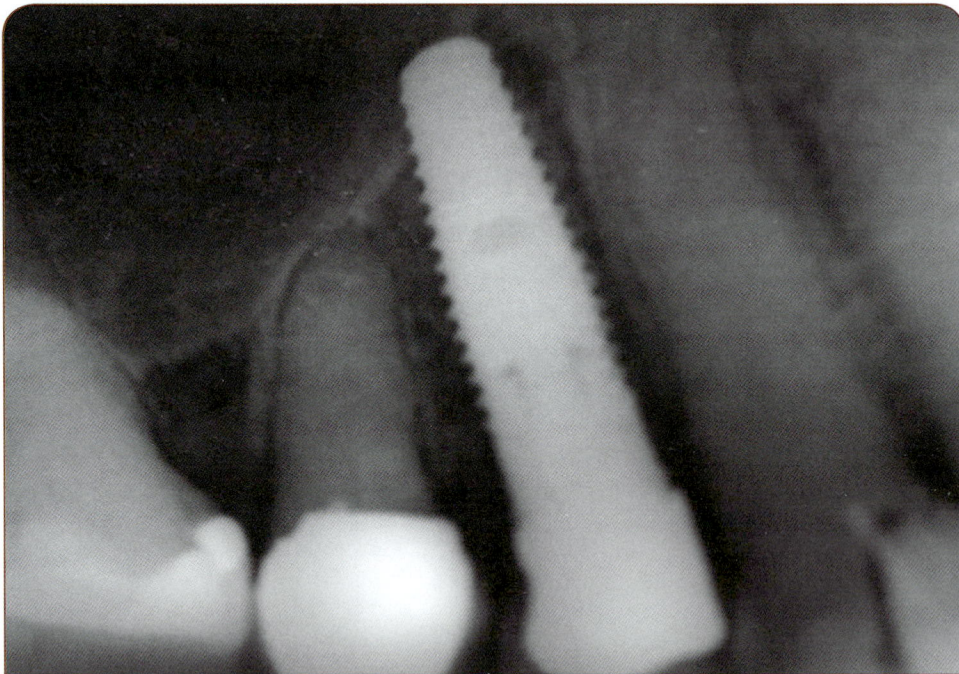

Fig. 11

Five year postoperative X-ray shows bone level maintenance with just slight remodeling but overall a satisfactory end result **(Fig. 11)**.

Socket Shield and Osseodensification:
Filling in the Gaps

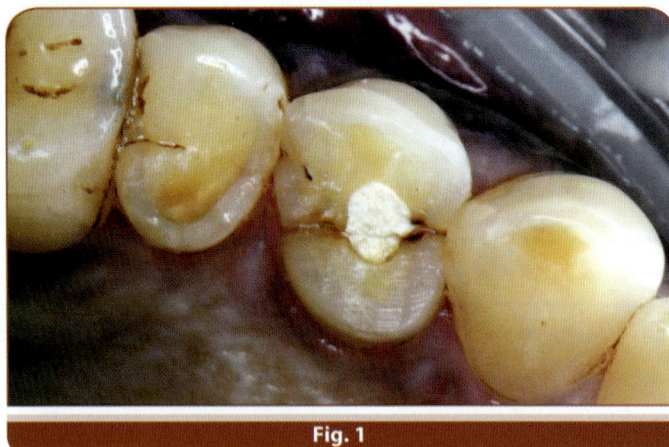

Fig. 1

Preoperative clinical view with cracked tooth #24 of a 51-year-old male with an emergency caused due to fracture of the tooth **(Fig. 1)**.

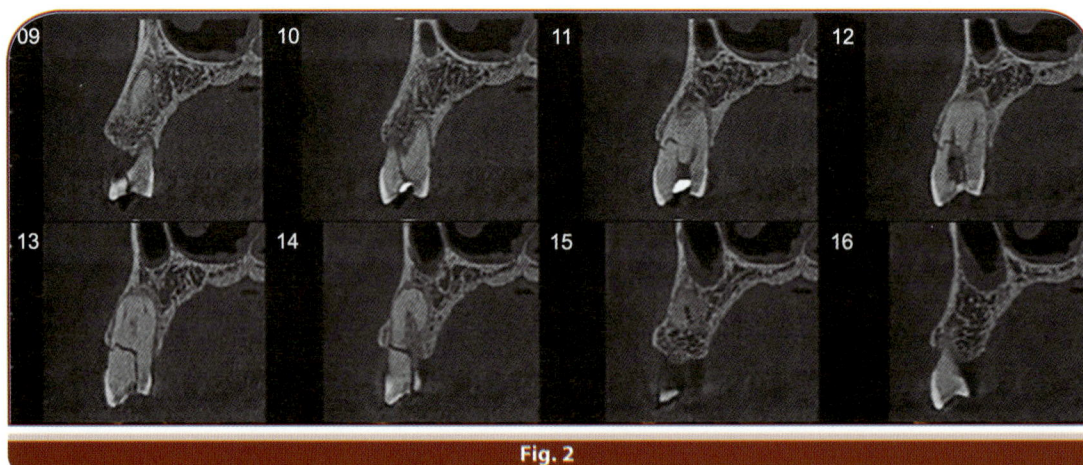

Fig. 2

Preoperative CBCT **(Fig. 2)**.

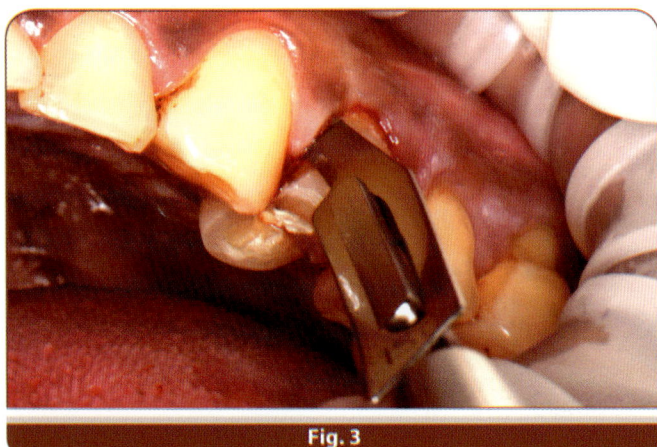

Fig. 3

Sulcular incision to separate soft tissue attachment of the fragment **(Fig. 3)**.

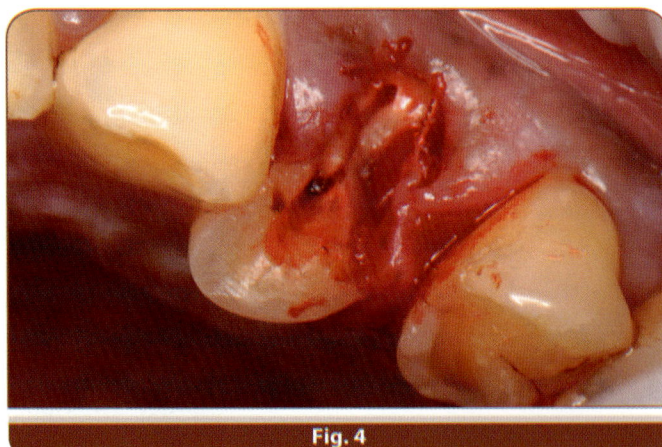

Fig. 4

Removal of facial fragment **(Fig. 4)**.

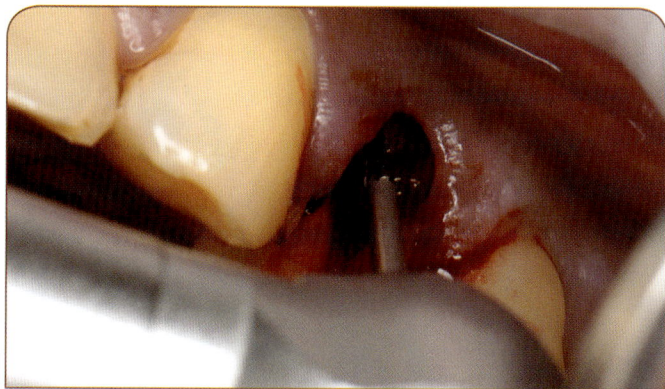
Fig. 5

Long shank airotor bur to section the tooth in a mesio-distal direction **(Fig. 5)**.

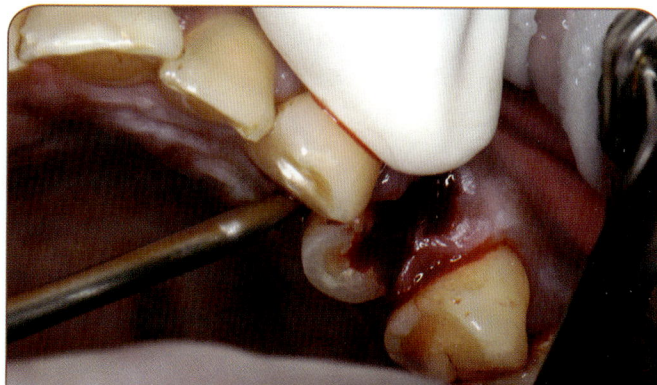
Fig. 6

Extraction of the palatal half **(Fig. 6)**.

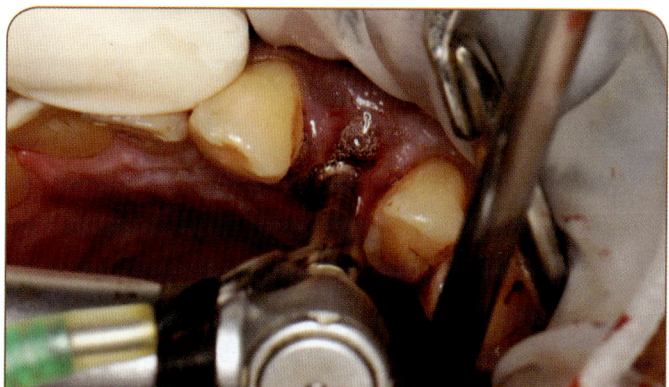
Fig. 7

Osteotomy preparation using Densah burs **(Fig. 7)**.

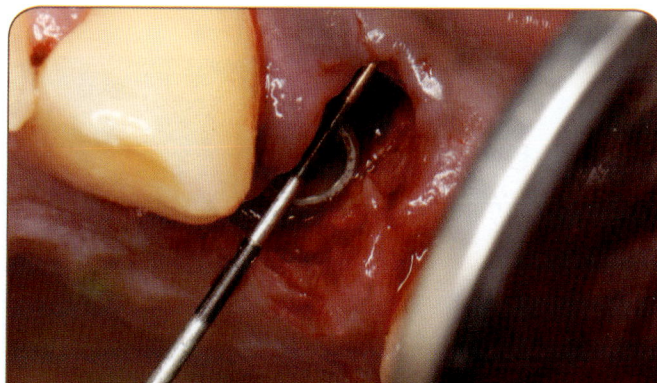
Fig. 8

Implant in position, showing the gap from the facial plate **(Fig. 8)**.

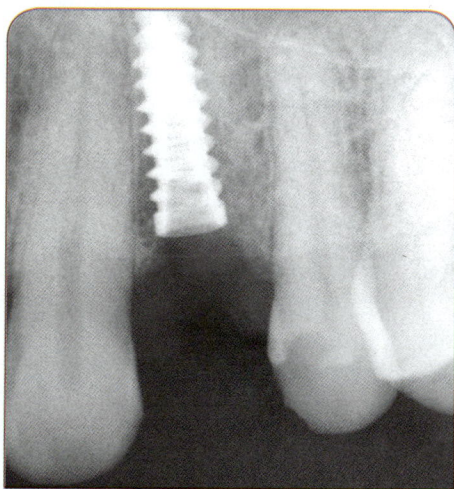
Fig. 9

Postoperative radiograph **(Fig. 9)**.

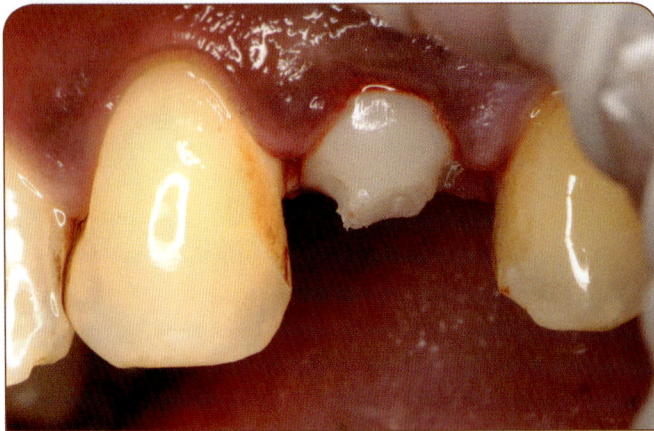

Fig. 10

Fig. 11

Postoperative photograph showing custom healing abutment utilizing a metal base castable abutment **(Fig. 10)**.

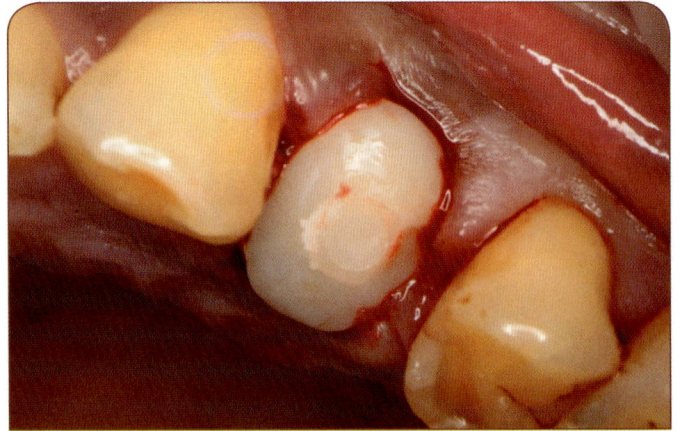

Another view of the custom healing abutment **(Fig. 11)**.

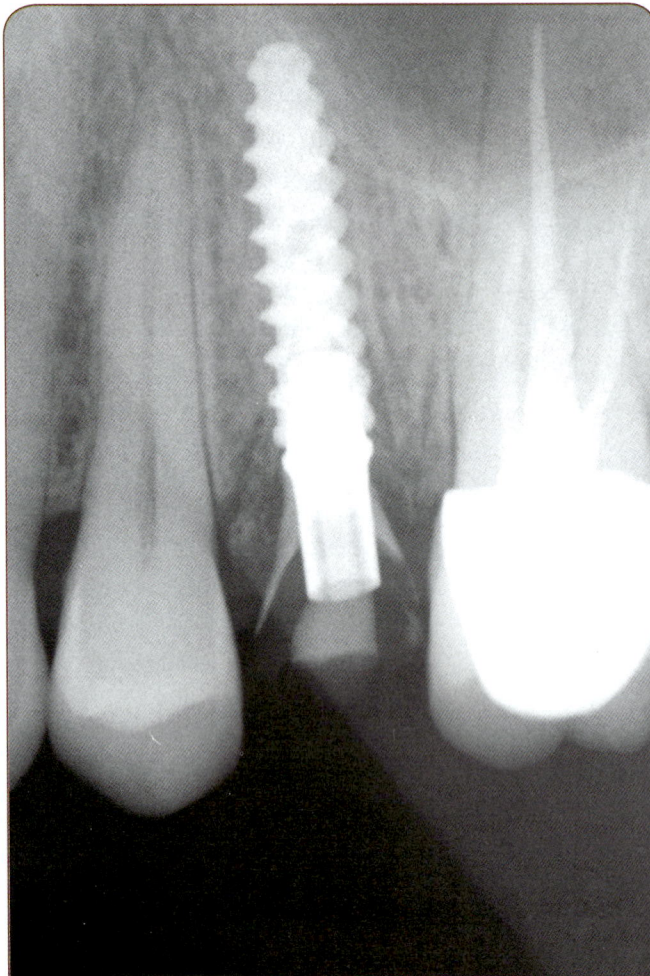

Fig. 12

Fig. 13

Radiograph with custom healing abutment **(Fig. 12)**.

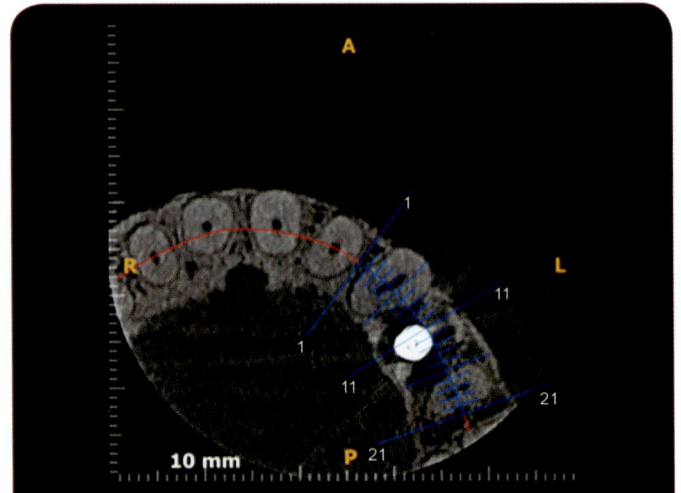

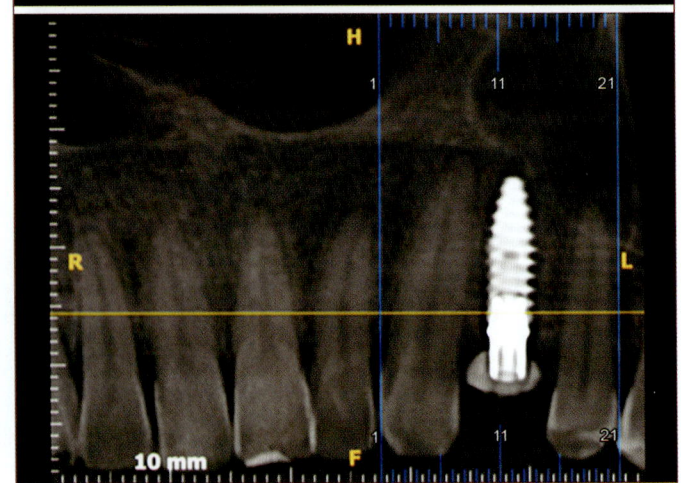

Postoperative CBC T **(Fig. 13)**.

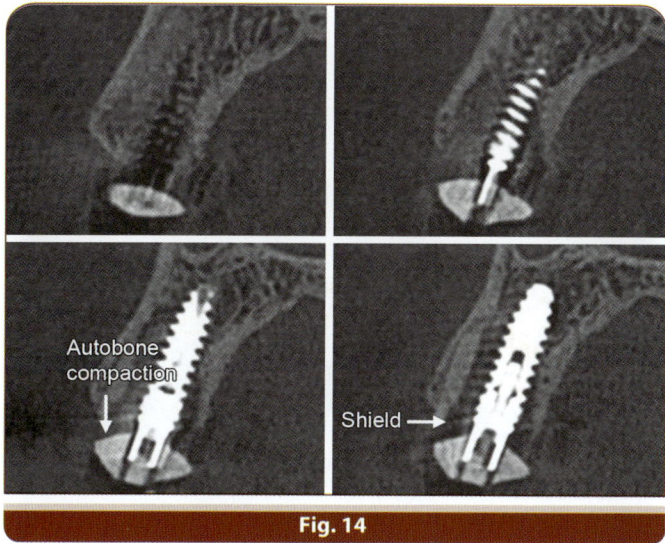

Fig. 14

Postoperative CBCT **(Fig. 14)**.

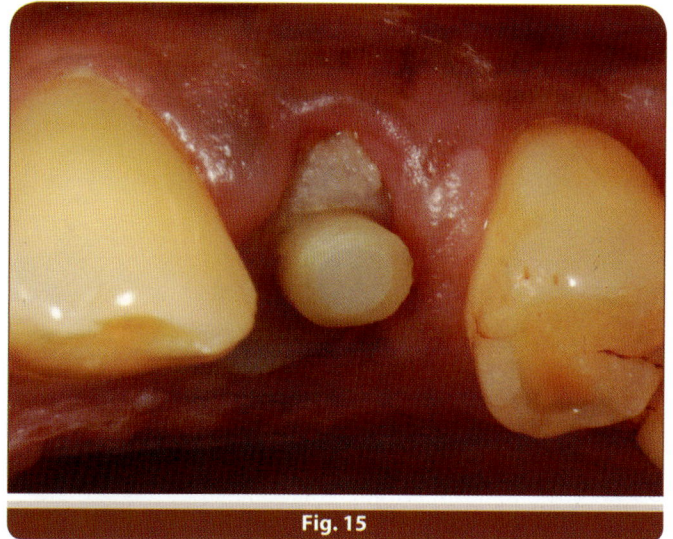

Fig. 15

The bonding between the composite and the plastic sleeve seems to have come loose in the 4 months and the composite had sunk a little **(Fig. 15)**.

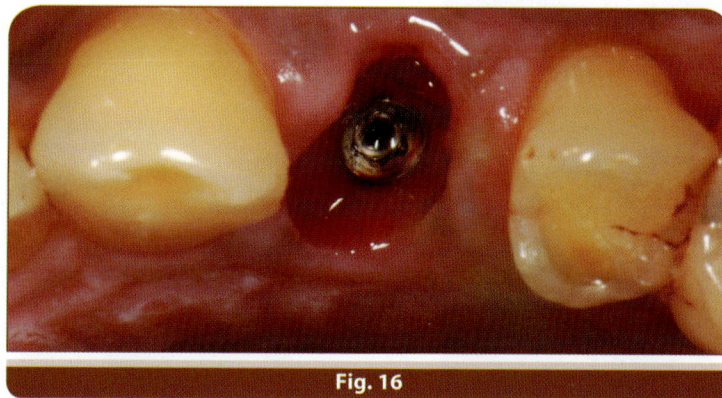

Fig. 16

Took off the custom healing, abutment, made impressions and installed a regular healing abutment **(Fig. 16)**.

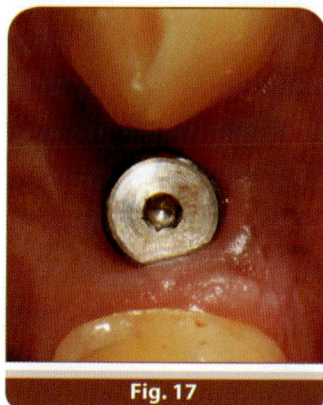

Fig. 17

Replaced custom healing abutment with standard healing abutment after impressions **(Fig. 17)**.

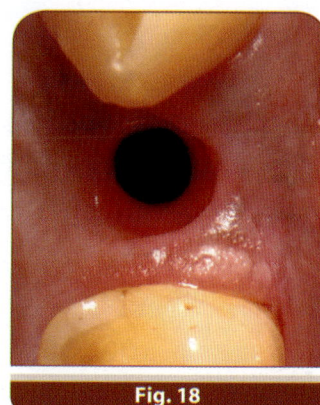

Fig. 18

Two weeks later at Crown insertion appointment **(Fig. 18)**.

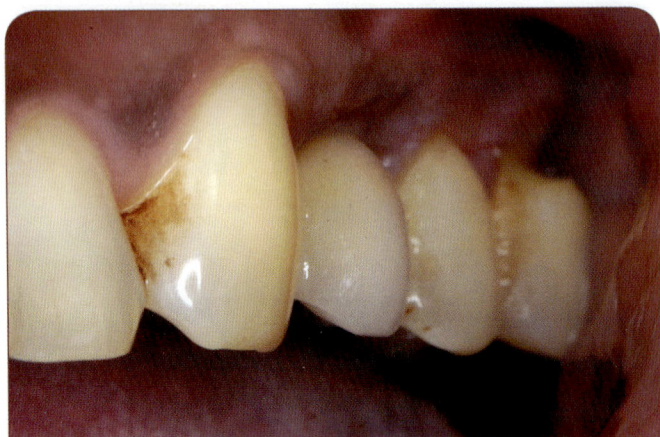

Fig. 19

Screw retained crown delivered. Buccal view of final crown **(Fig. 19)**.

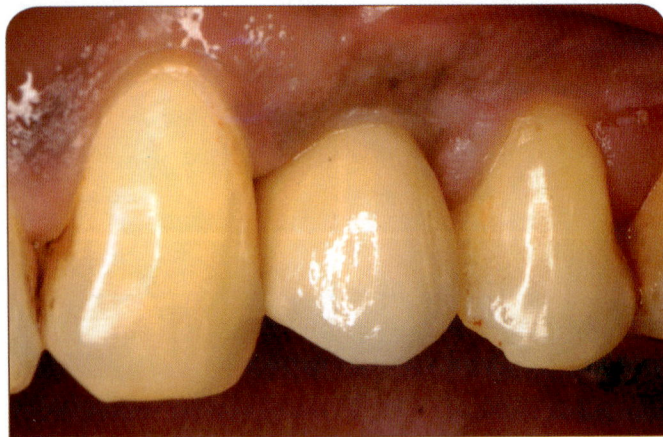

Fig. 20

Lateral view of final crown **(Fig. 20)**.

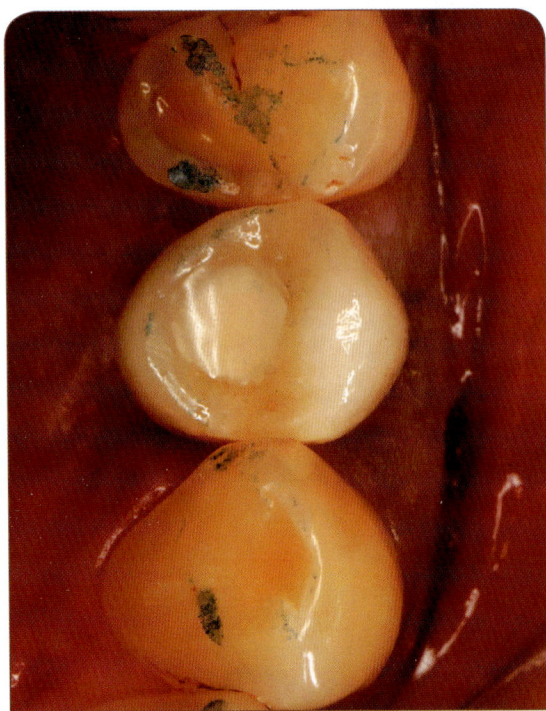

Fig. 21

Occlusal view of final crown **(Fig. 21)**.

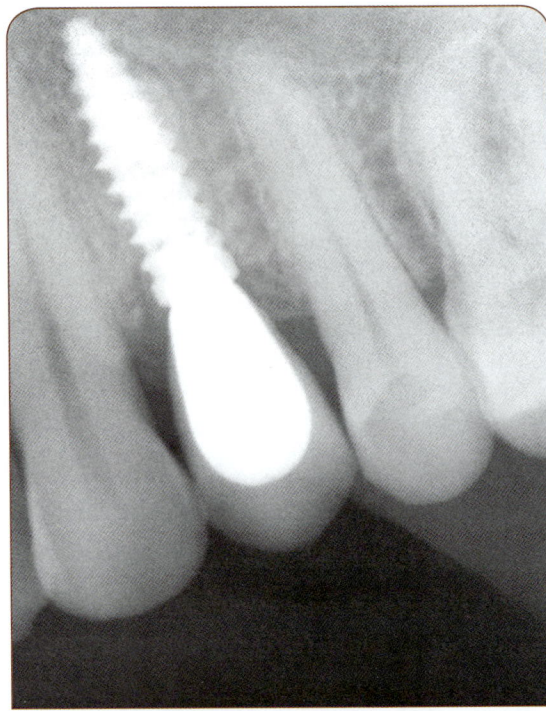

Fig. 22

Final postoperative X-ray **(Fig. 22)**.

Praful Bali, Shweta Gupta

IMMEDIATE EXTRACTION OF A LOWER PREMOLAR WITH IMMEDIATE TEMPORIZATION

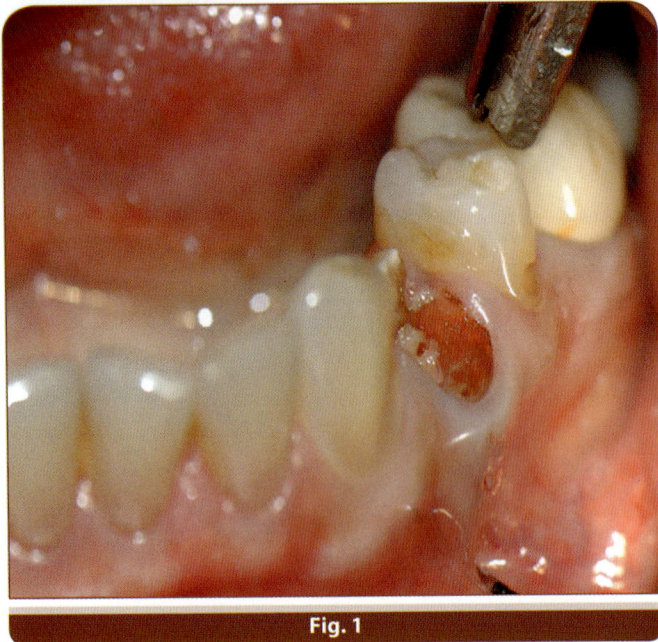

Fig. 1

Preoperative clinical view shows nonrestorable fractured tooth no #34. The supporting tissues are nice and healthy and immediate implantation into the extracted socket is planned **(Fig. 1)**.

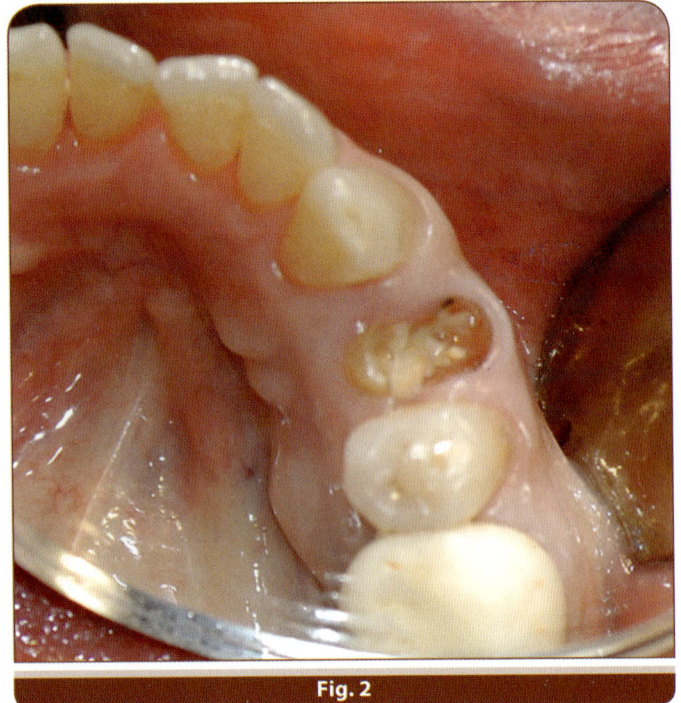

Fig. 2

Preoperative occlusal view (mirror image) shows intact buccal cortical plate and healthy soft tissue **(Fig. 2)**.

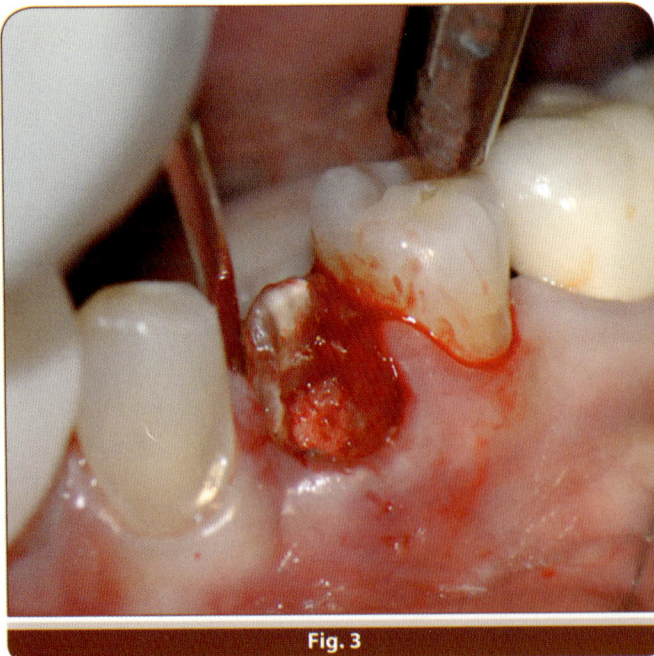

Fig. 3

Use of periotome to extract the tooth as atraumatically as possible ensuring no disturbance to underlying bone and covering soft tissue **(Fig. 3)**.

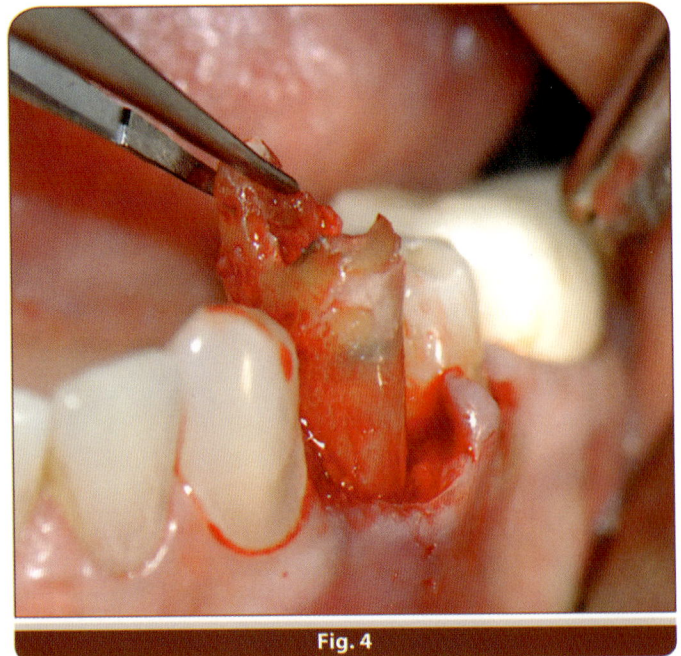

Fig. 4

Atraumatic extraction is achieved keeping all surrounding anatomy intact **(Fig. 4)**.

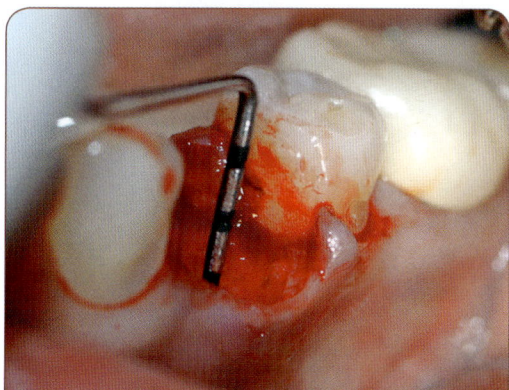

Fig. 5

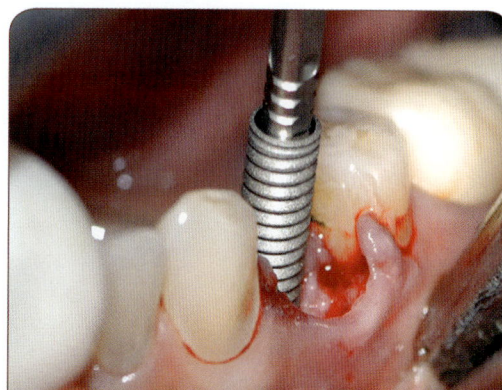

Fig. 6

Bone sounding is done to make sure all walls of the socket are intact and immediate implantation can be achieved **(Fig. 5)**.

4/12 anthogyr implant is placed taking prime stability from the lingual bone. A torque of 50+Ncm achieved **(Fig. 6)**.

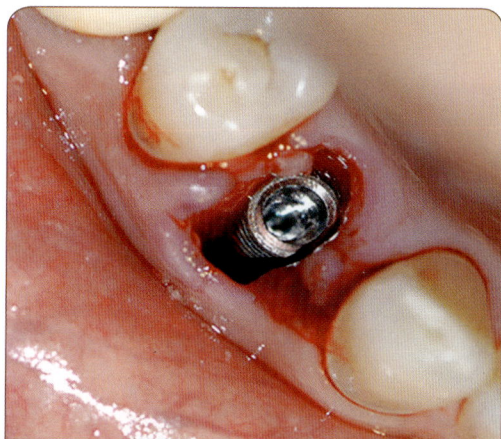

Fig. 7

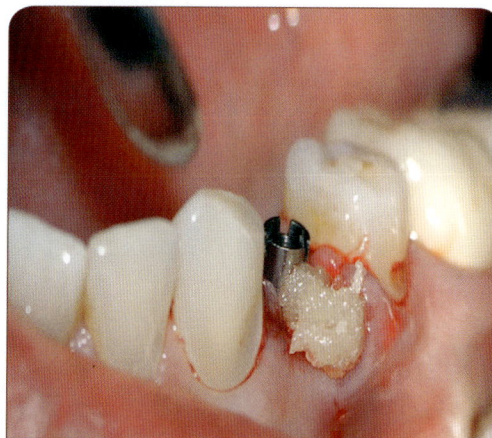

Fig. 8

2.5-3 mm jumping distance protects the buccal bone plate from compression **(Fig. 7)**.

Nova bone is added in the socket defect **(Fig. 8)**.

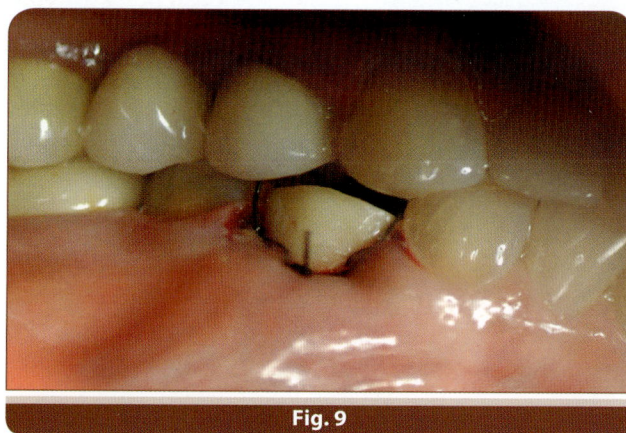

Fig. 9

Temporary crown cemented with temoprary cement. Careful occlusal adjustments made. The implant crown is made out of occlusion **(Fig. 9)**.

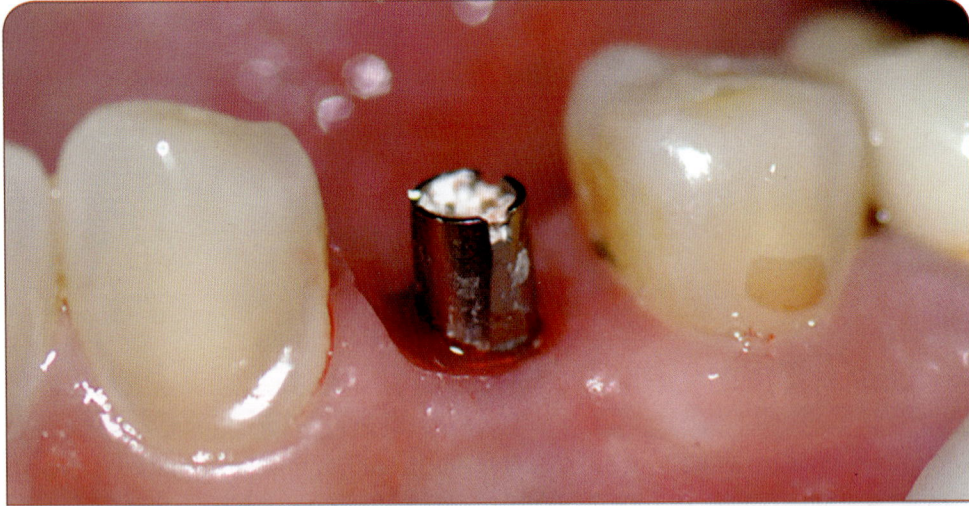

Fig. 10

A series of temporary crowns shape the soft tissue well and create a wonderful emergence **(Fig. 10)**.

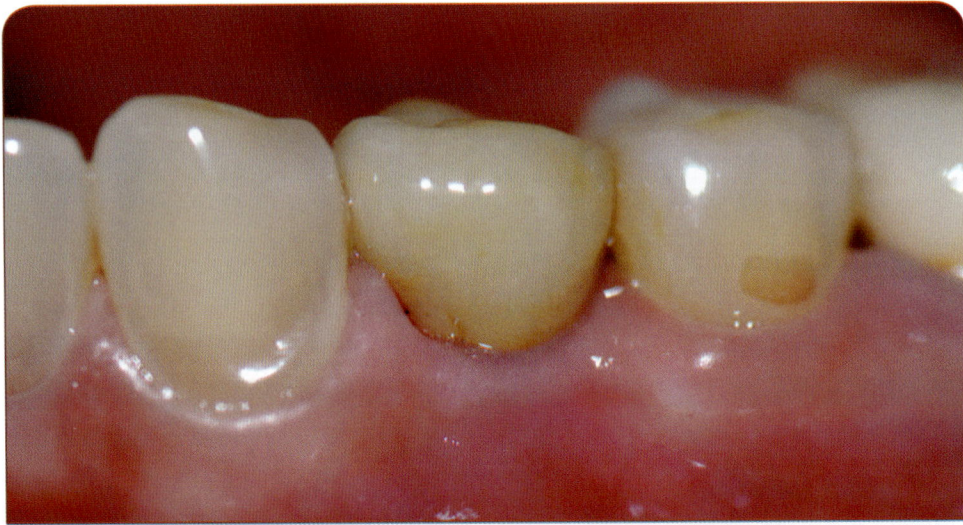

Fig. 11

Final porcelain fused to metal crown cemented with GIC. The hard and soft tissue maintained at the same level as when we started the case **(Fig. 11)**.

Jin Y Kim

IMMEDIATE IMPLANT PLACEMENT WITH IMMEDIATE LOAD/ PROVISIONALIZATION AND CORRECTION OF SOFT/HARD TISSUE DEFECTS IN THE UPPER CENTRAL INCISOR REGION

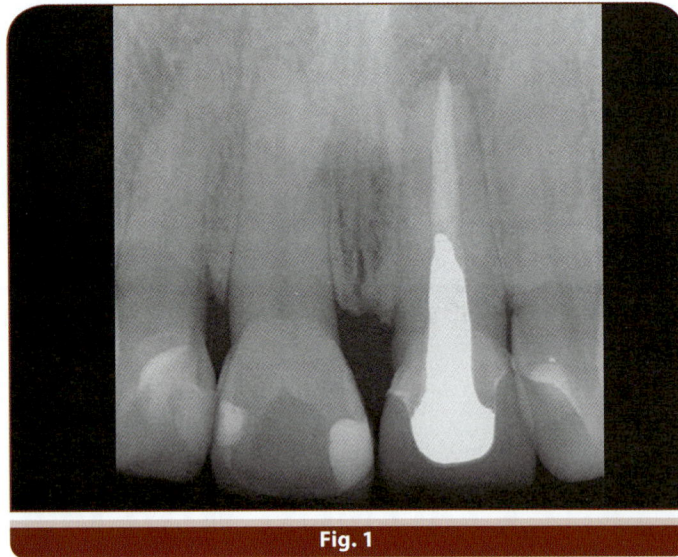

Fig. 1

Healthy 47-year-old female presented with a fractured upper left central incisor. The tooth had previous history of endodontic treatment, retrograde endodontic filling, and cast post and core restoration. Preoperative radiograph **(Fig. 1)**.

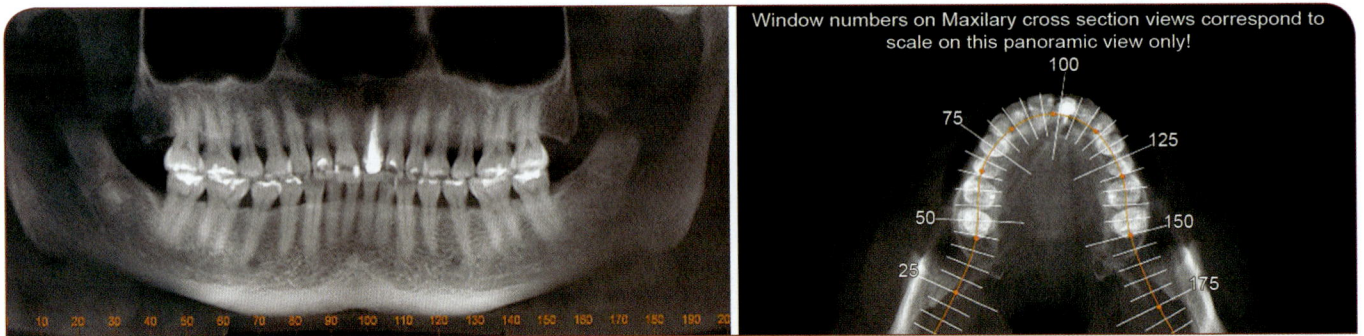

Fig. 2

CBCT revealed significant apical bone defect, and missing facial plate, except for a thin bridge of bone at the alveolar crest **(Fig. 2)**.

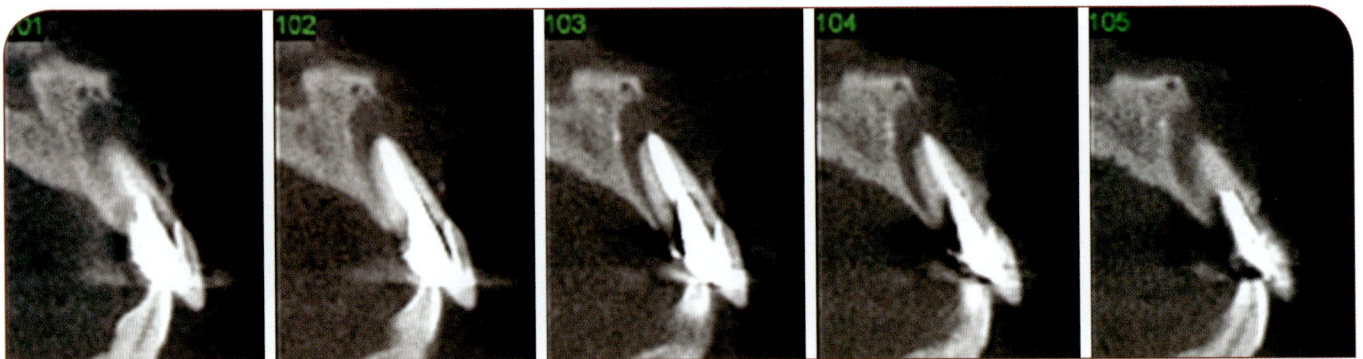

Fig. 3

Image showing thin buccal cortical plate **(Fig. 3)**.

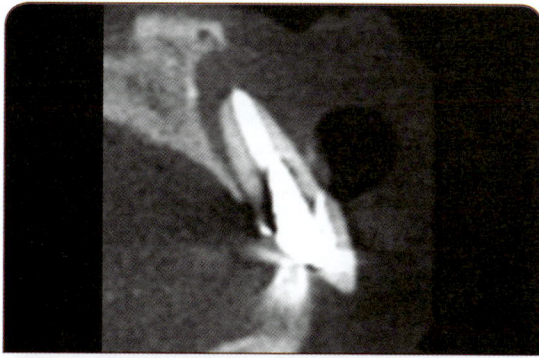

Fig. 4

Lateral bone resorption and pathology associated with labial perforation **(Fig. 4)**.

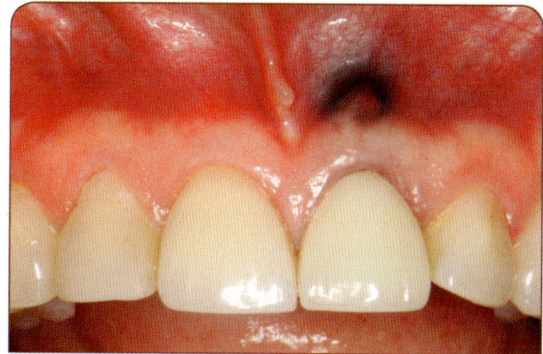

Fig. 5

Amalgam tattoo in relation to tooth #21 **(Fig. 5)**.

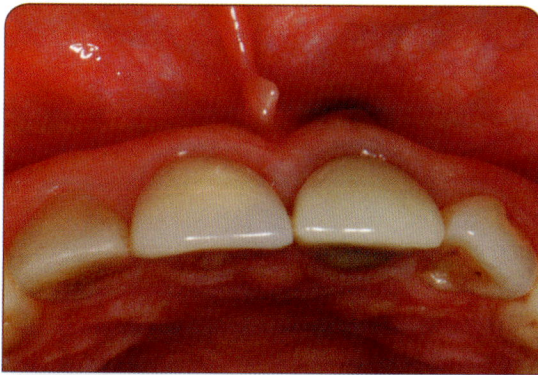

Fig. 6

Image showing thin soft tissue biotype and amalgam showing out **(Fig. 6)**.

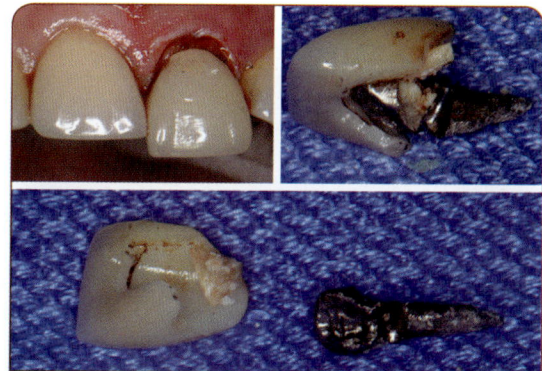

Fig. 7

Treatment plan consisted of careful removal of the tooth, immediate placement of implant, as well as immediate nonfunctional implant provisional tooth delivery.

The porcelain jacket crown was carefully preserved to be used as a shell for the immediate nonfunctional implant tooth (NFIT) **(Fig. 7)**.

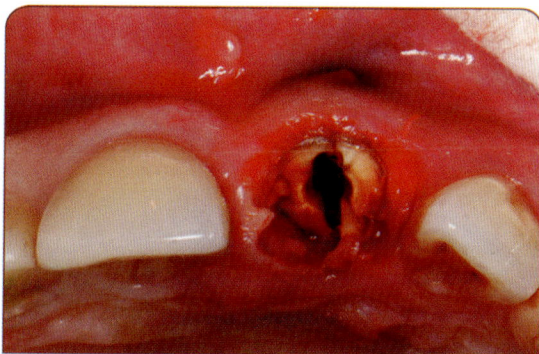

Fig. 8

In order to preserve the facial band of bone, the tooth root was sectional **(Fig. 8)**.

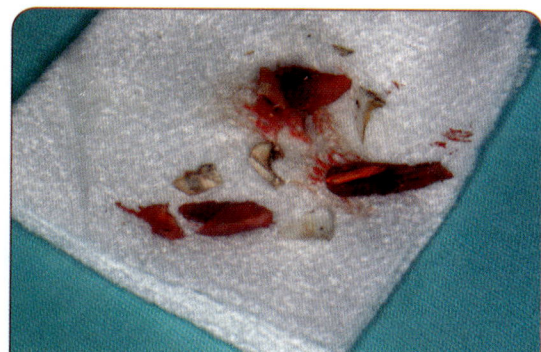

Fig. 9

Removal of fractured and small segments of root **(Fig. 9)**.

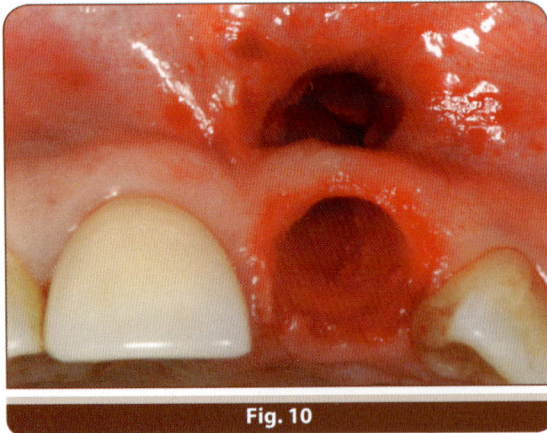

Fig. 10

Facial band of bone preserved (Fig. 10).

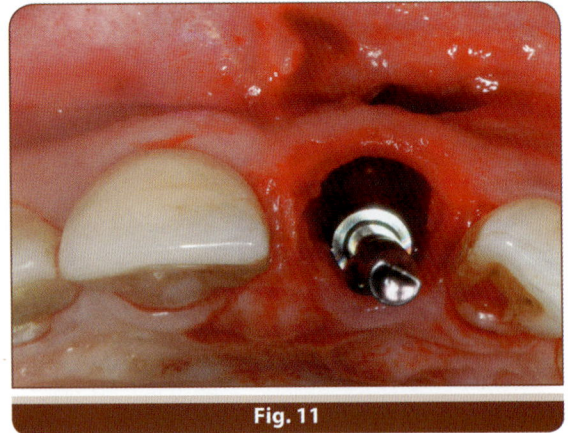

Fig. 11

The thin facial band of bone was preserved, and osteotomy was initiated on the palatal aspect of the socket defect wall **(Fig. 11)**.

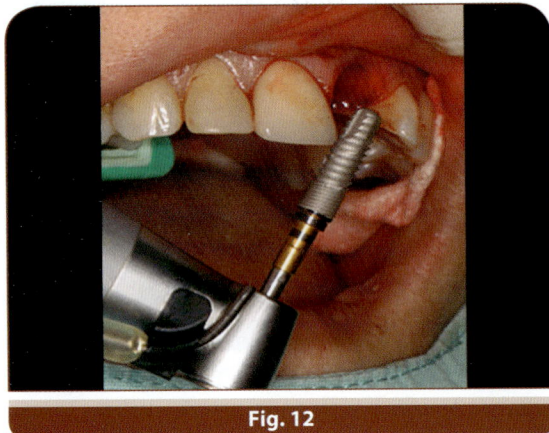

Fig. 12

A Dentis implant was placed into the slightly underprepared osteotomy to gain maximal initial stability **(Fig. 12)**.

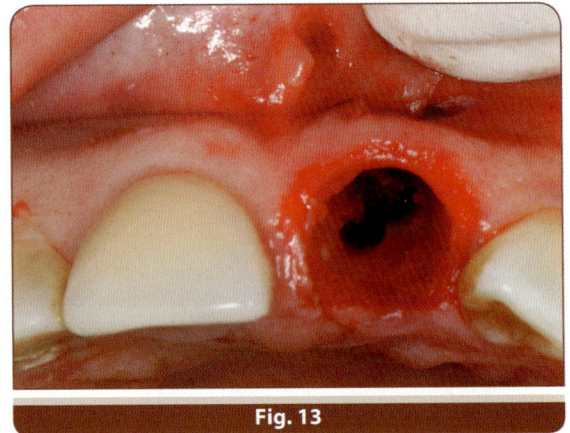

Fig. 13

Osteotomy prepared on the palatal aspect of the socket wall **(Fig. 13)**.

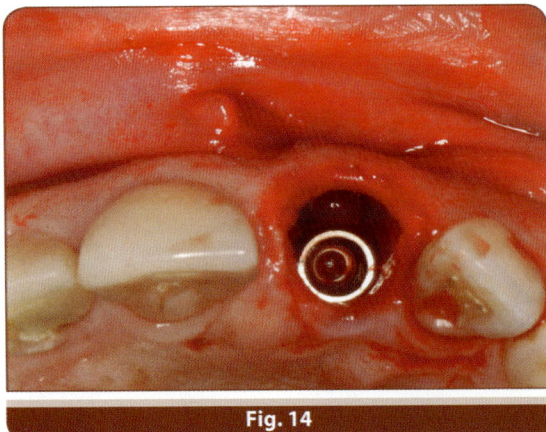

Fig. 14

Implant in position (Fig. 14)

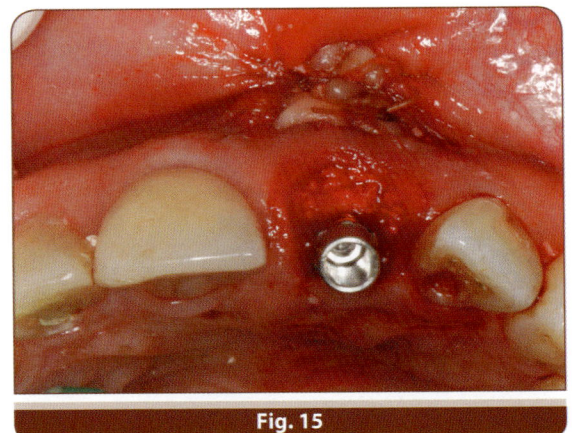

Fig. 15

The socket defect was grafted with sticky bone compromising of mineralized allograft and Sintered Bovine xenograft and autologous fibrin clot **(Fig. 15)**.

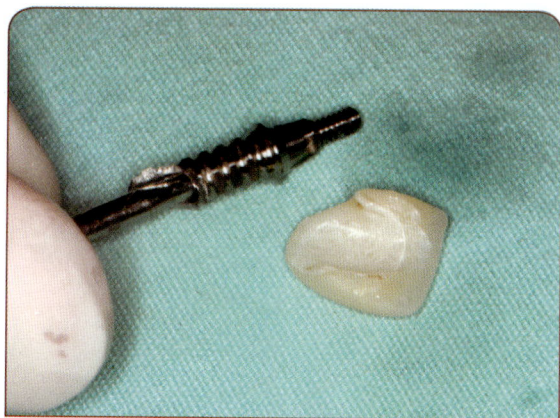
Fig. 16

The shell of the retrieved porcelain crown was shaped and directly bonded to titanium temporary abutment **(Fig. 16)**.

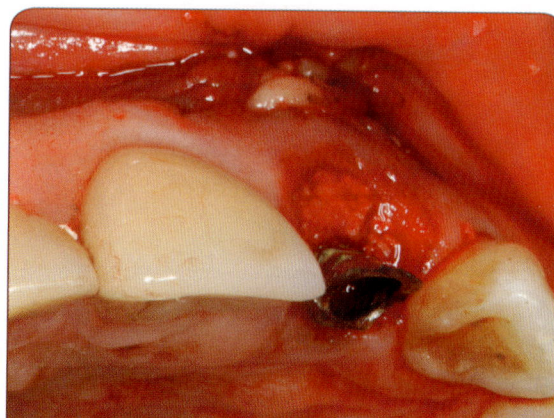
Fig. 17

Titanium temporary abutment torqued to the implant **(Fig. 17)**.

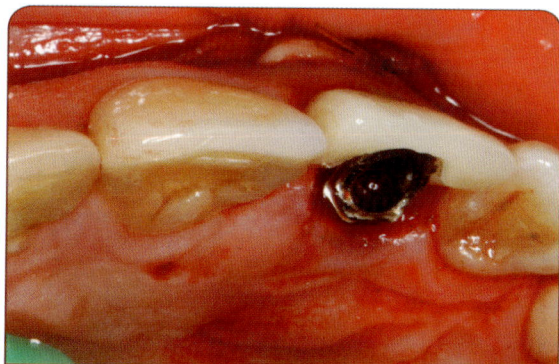
Fig. 18

Screw retained nonfunctional implant tooth fabricated intraorally **(Fig. 18)**.

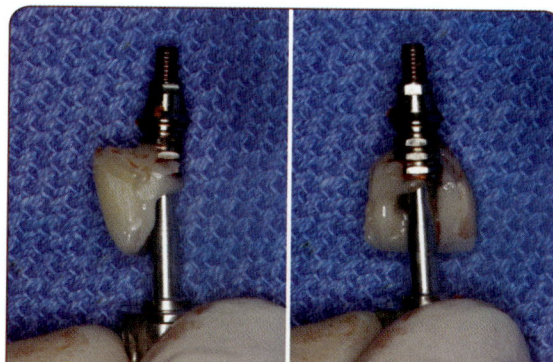
Fig. 19

An ideal emergence profile was built into the nonfunctional implant tooth. This contour is critical in the future development of the crestal soft and hard tissue interface, that determines contour and seal of the implant junction **(Fig. 19)**.

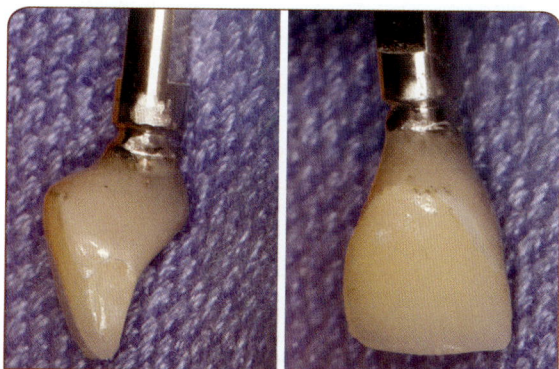
Fig. 20

The prepared nonfunctional implant tooth was installed by tightening the abutment screw **(Fig. 20)**.

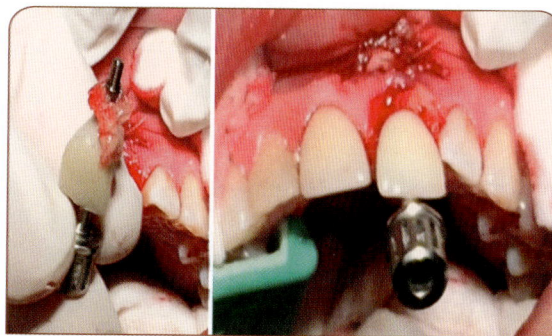
Fig. 21

A layer of pressed concentrated growth factors (CGF also known as PRF) was inserted between the restoration and socket defect also known as Poncho technique **(Fig. 21)**.

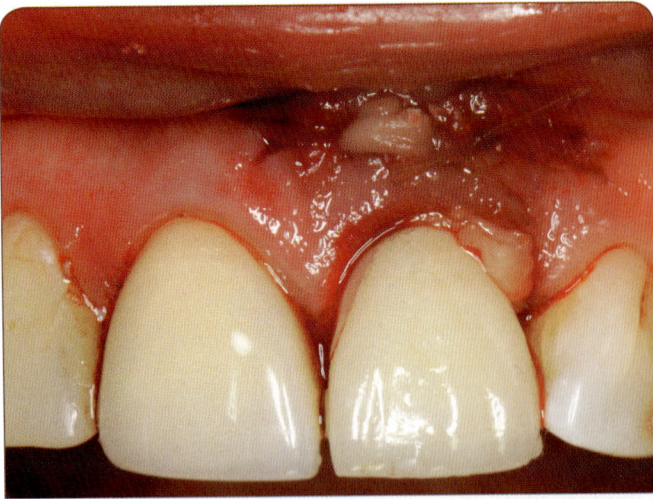

Fig. 22

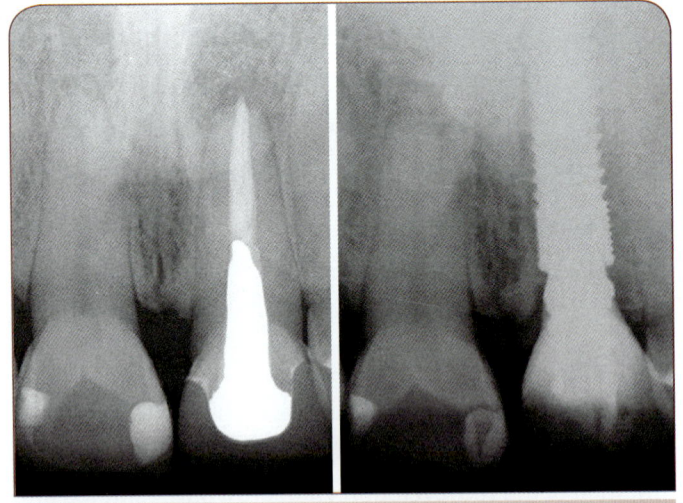

Fig. 23

The apical bone and soft tissue defect was made larger after the amalgam tattoo was removed for esthetic reasons, as per patient's request. The defect was grafted with layers of pressed concentrated growth factors (CGF) using resorbable sutures (4.0 chromic gut) Corp **(Fig. 22)**.

Preoperative and post implantation and temporization **(Fig. 23)**.

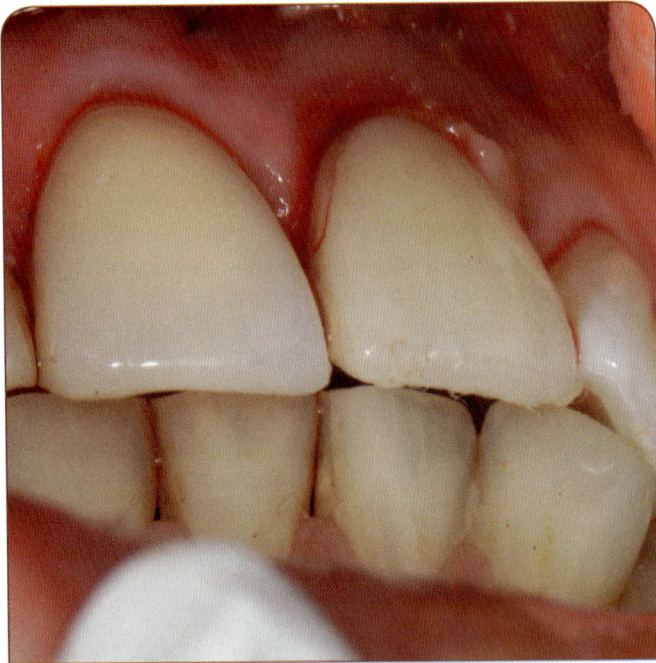

Fig. 24

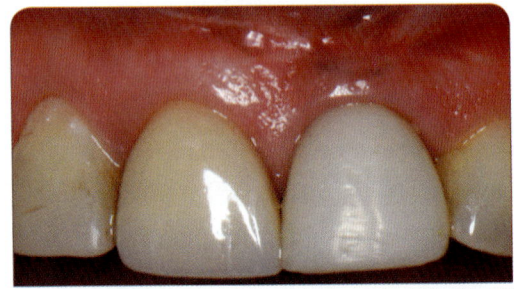

Fig. 25

Healing at 4 months **(Fig. 25)**.

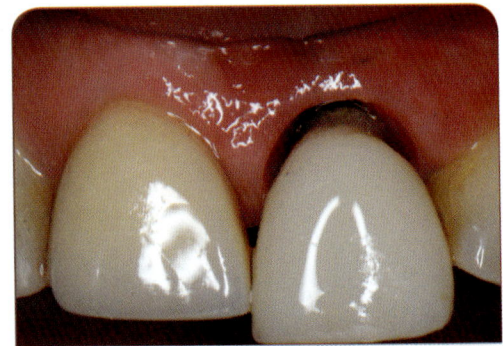

Fig. 26

The nonfunctional implant tooth was taken out of function completely by relieving the occlusal and proximal contacts. Patient was strictly instructed to avoid any physical contact with the restoration for minimum of two full months, including mastication **(Fig. 24)**.

The implant successfully osseointegrated at 4 months, producing the ideal emergence profile that was capable of supporting newly created gingival papillae **(Fig. 26)**.

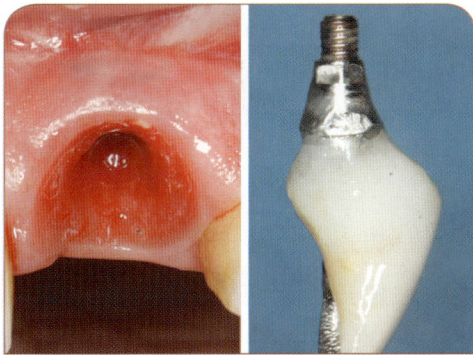
Fig. 27

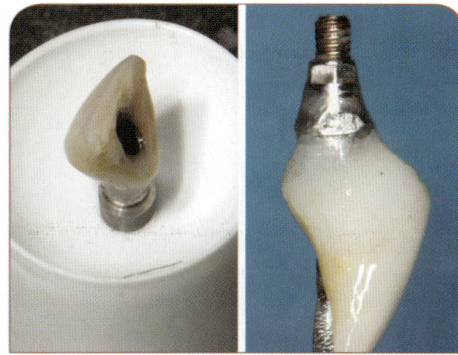
Fig. 28

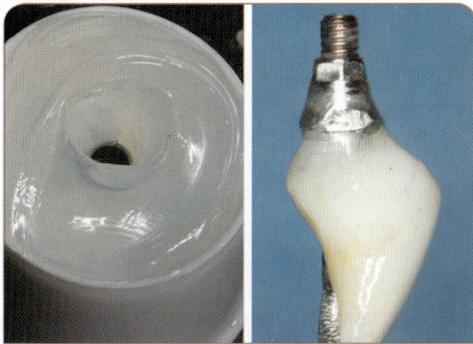
Fig. 29

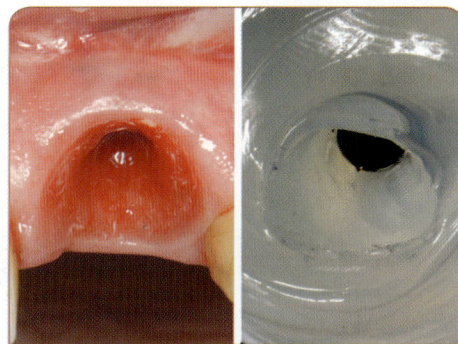
Fig. 30

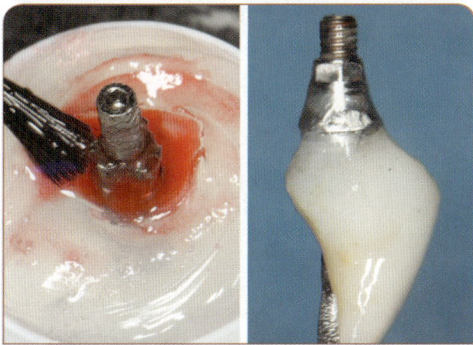
Fig. 31

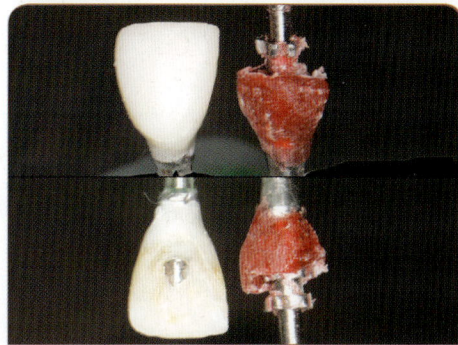
Fig. 32

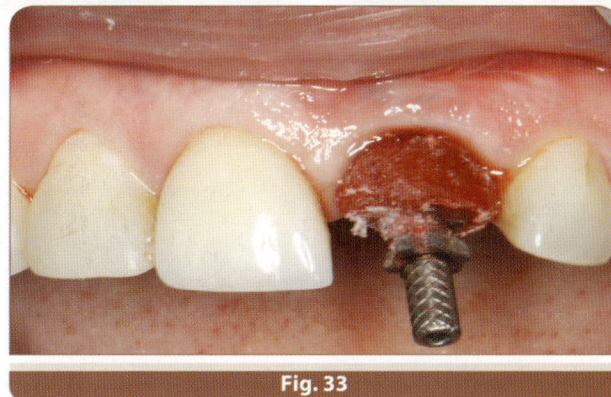
Fig. 33

A custom impression technique was employed to transfer the newly created soft tissue profile to the laboratory **(Figs. 27 to 33).**

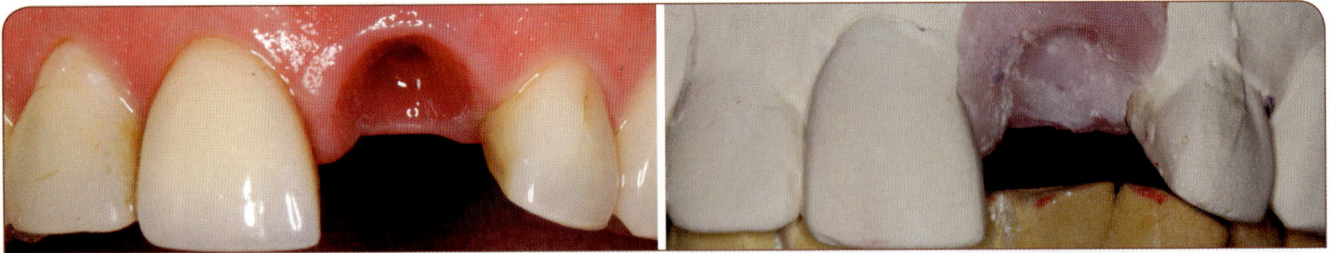

Fig. 34

Successfully transferred the newly created soft tissue profile **(Fig. 34)**.

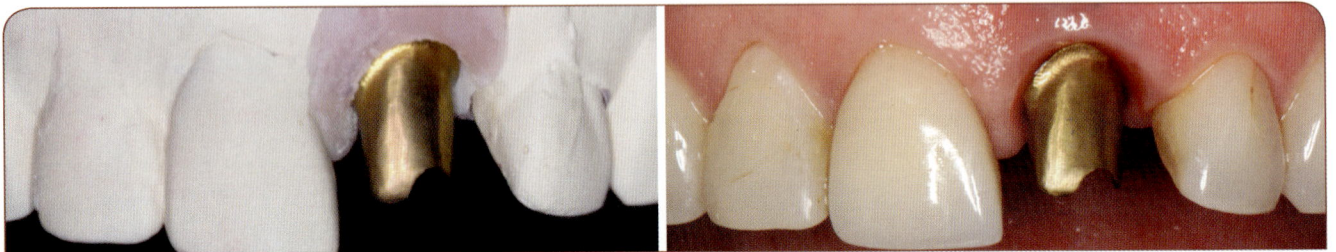

Fig. 35

A milled titanium custom abutment was fabricated and installed falial and occlusal view on cast and intraorally **(Fig. 35)**.

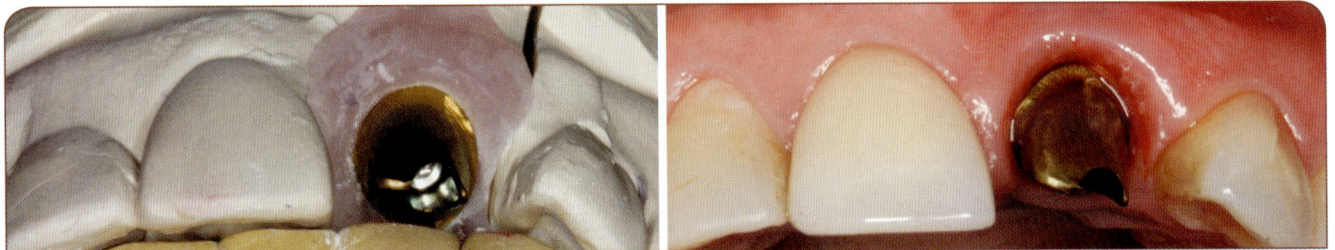

Fig. 36

Occlusal view of the milled abutment **(Fig. 36)**.

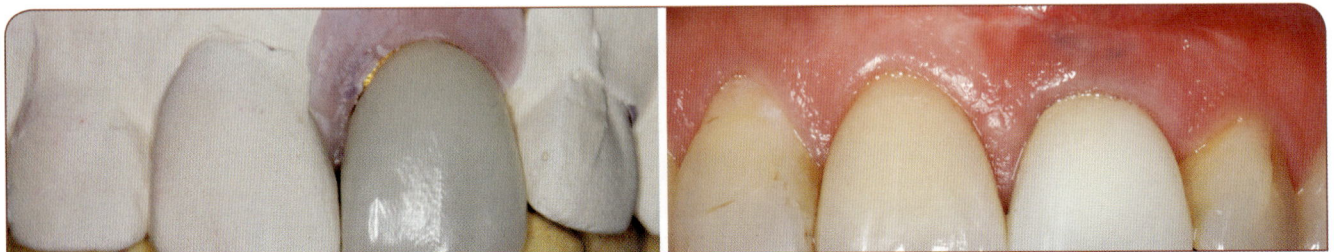

Fig. 37

Final restoration fabricated and tried **(Fig. 37)**.

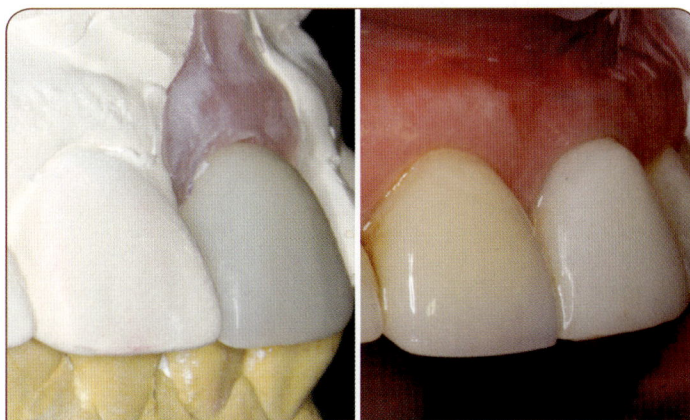
Fig. 38

Checked lateral profile of the permanent restoration **(Fig. 38)**.

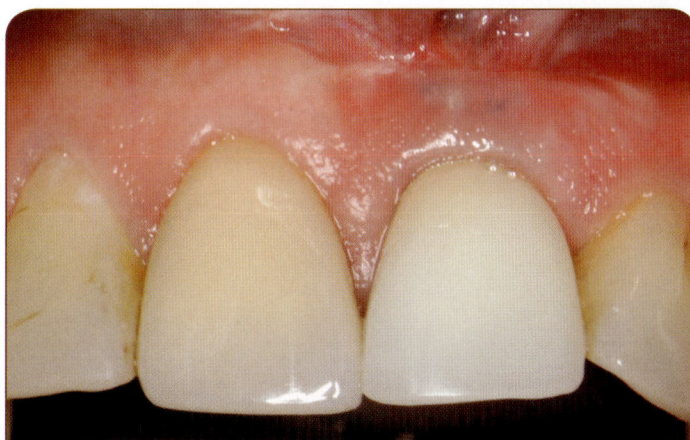
Fig. 39

Healing at 7 months **(Fig. 39)**.

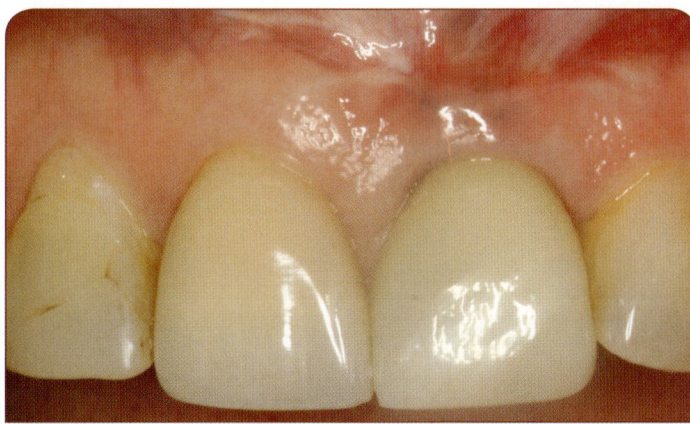
Fig. 40

Definitive restoration at 11 months postsurgery. The facial soft and hard tissue defect is completely healed, and regenerated **(Fig. 40)**.

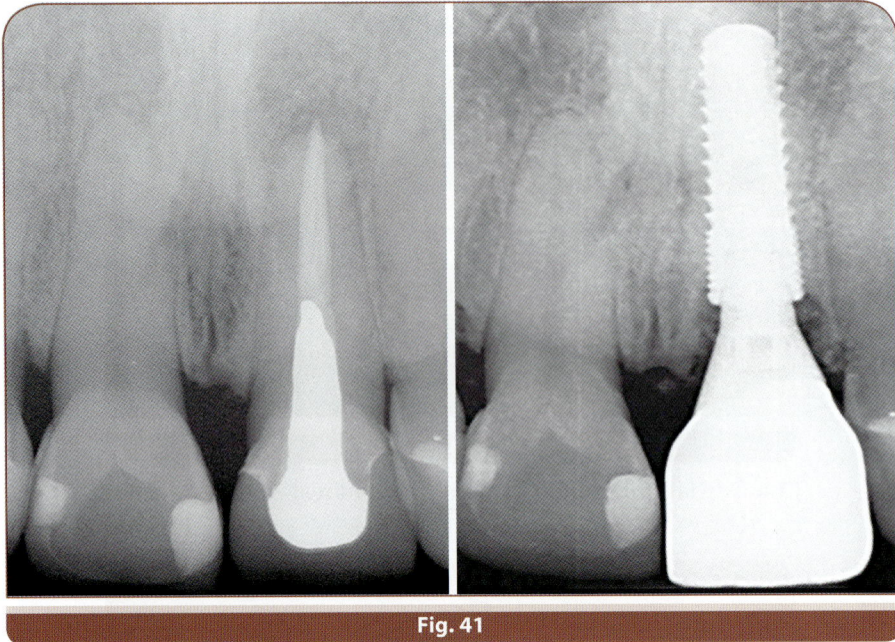

Fig. 41

Periapical radiograph at 11 months post surgery, immediate post-restoration **(Fig. 41)**.

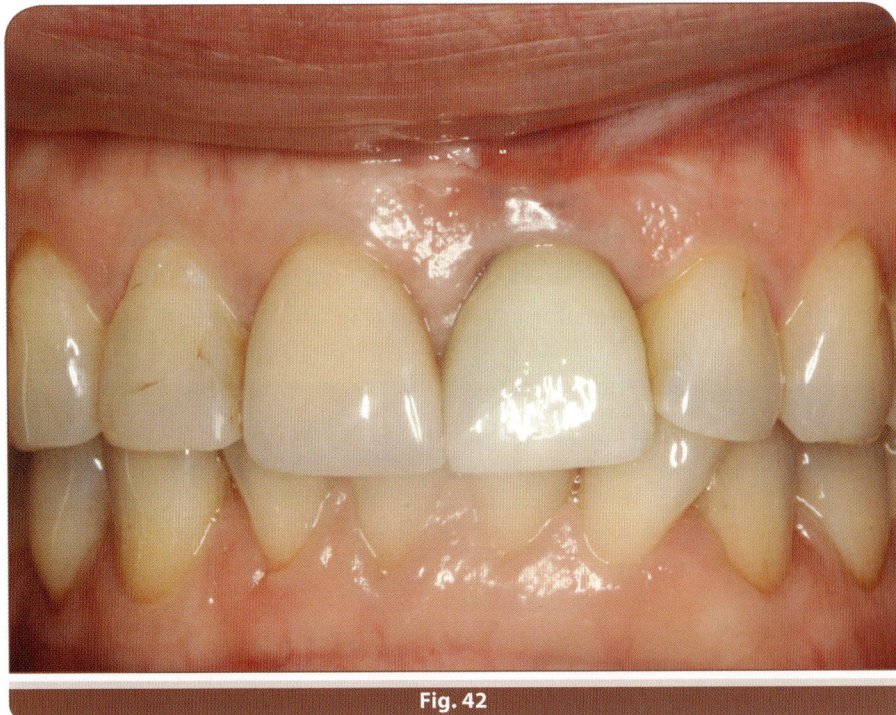

Fig. 42

Full facial view **(Fig. 42)**.

Praful Bali, Sunil Datta

SOCKET SHIELD TECHNIQUE FOR AN ESTHETIC CENTRAL INCISOR

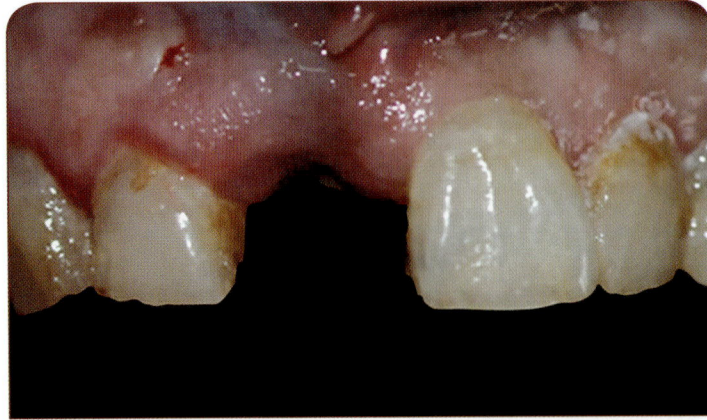

Fig. 1

Preoperative view of fractured tooth #11 **(Fig. 1)**.

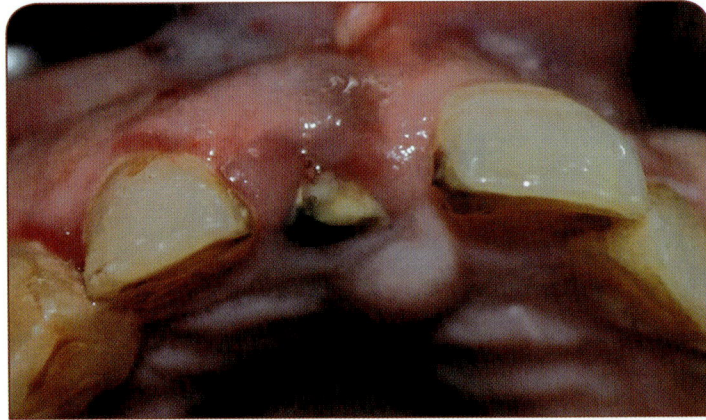

Fig. 2

Occlusal view showing remnant root piece and soft tissue coverage. Socket shield technique is planned to maintain thickness of buccal cortical plate **(Fig. 2)**.

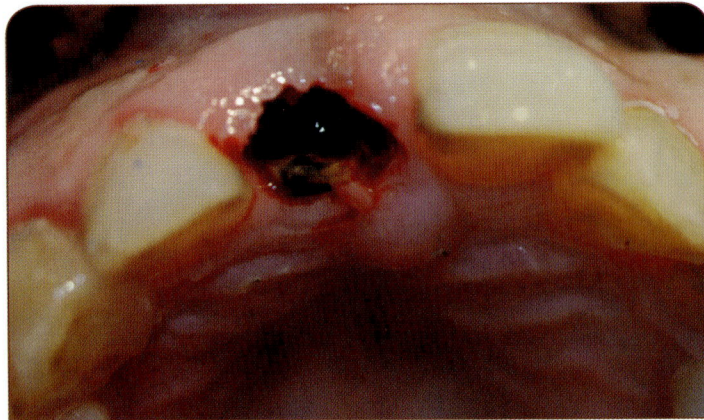

Fig. 3

Root piece is vertically split mesiodistally into buccal and palatal portions **(Fig. 3)**.

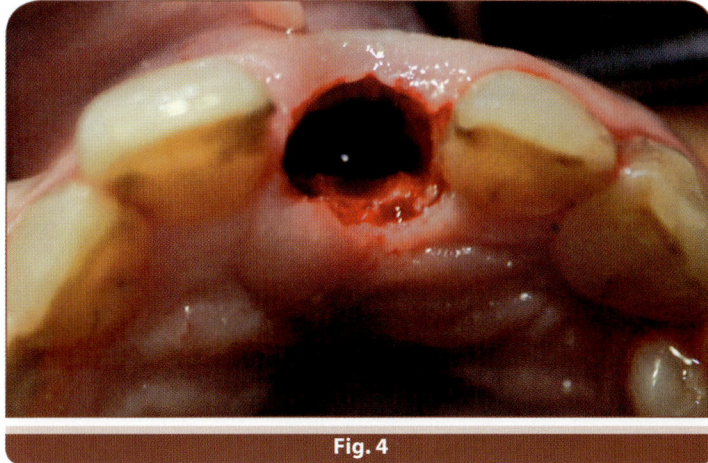

Fig. 4

Palatal portion of root removed. Buccal shield left to maintain buccal contour. The buccal root piece is trimmed 2–3 mm below the gingival margin **(Fig. 4)**.

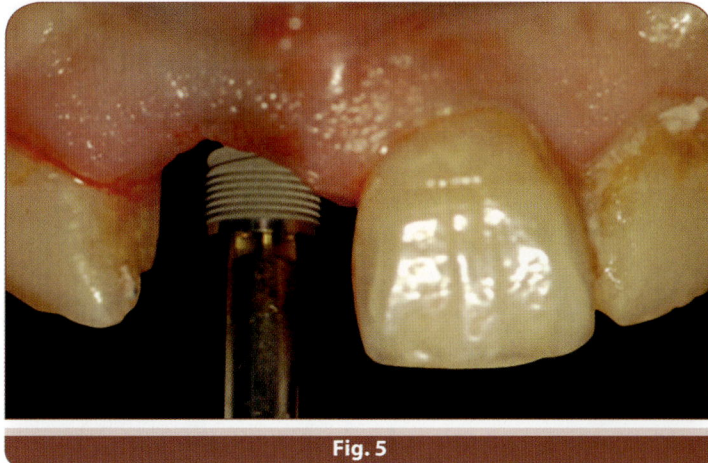

Fig. 5

Placement of Blue SKY 4/14 implant (Bredent) palatally in extracted socket **(Fig. 5)**.

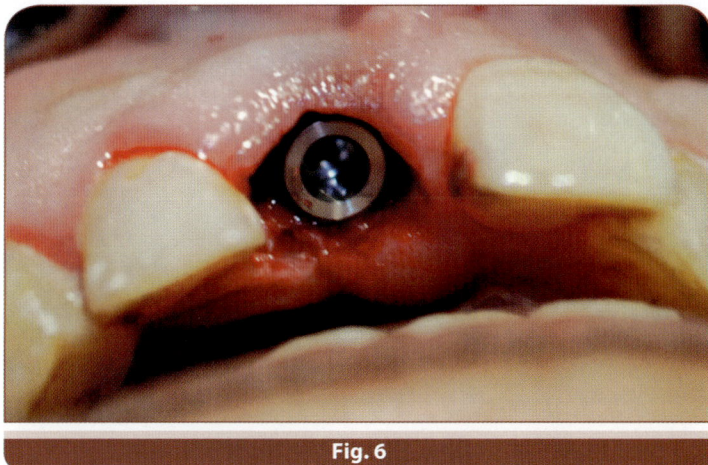

Fig. 6

Occlusal view of the implant. Note the buccal hard and soft tissue contour is maintained **(Fig. 6)**.

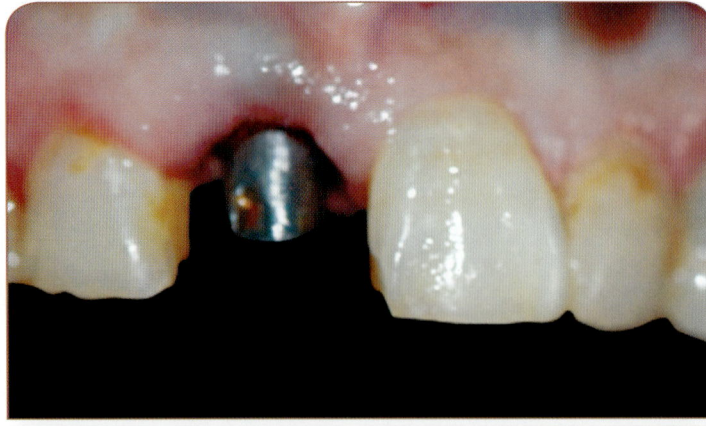

Fig. 7

Blue Sky Exo –abutment is shaped and torqued at 35 N cm **(Fig. 7)**.

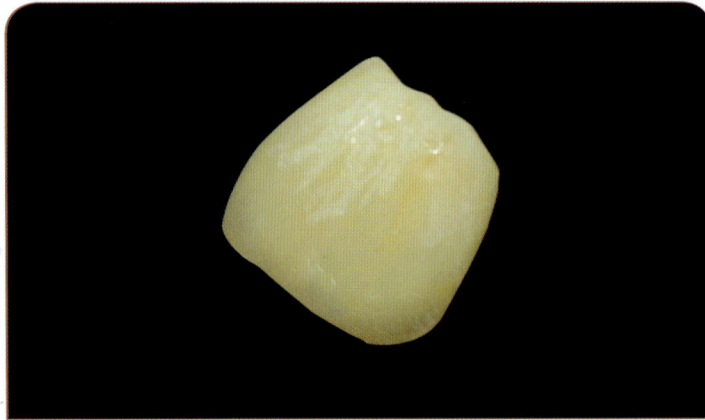

Fig. 8

Long-term temorization with Visiolign veneering material **(Fig. 8)**.

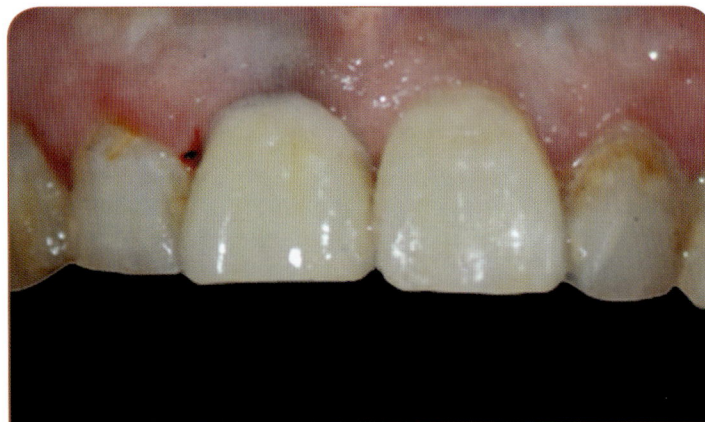

Fig. 9

One week postoperative facial view: Note that the socket shield technique has preserved the buccal cortical plate as well as maintained the soft tissue profile **(Fig. 9)**.

Jin Y Kim

IMMEDIATE IMPLANT PLACEMENT WITH IMMEDIATE LOAD/ PROVISIONALIZATION AND CORRECTION OF SOFT/HARD TISSUE DEFECTS IN THE UPPER CENTRAL INCISOR REGION

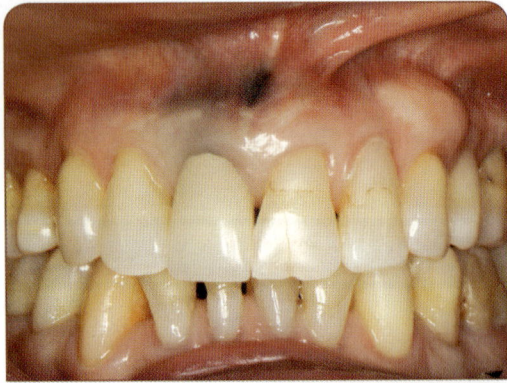

Fig. 1

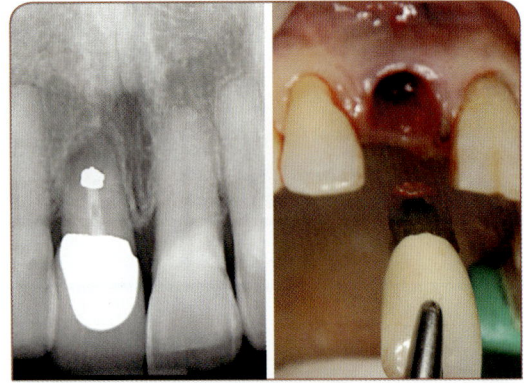

Fig. 2

Healthy 72-year-old female presented with loose and hopeless upper right (UR) central incisor. The tooth has history of conventional endodontic therapy, followed by peri-apical endodontic surgery. Tooth loosened progressively, and patient was unsatisfied with darkness showing through the root surface, as well as the "amalgam tattoo" at the root apex site **(Fig. 1)**.

External tooth resorption evident in X-ray and clinically **(Fig. 2)**.

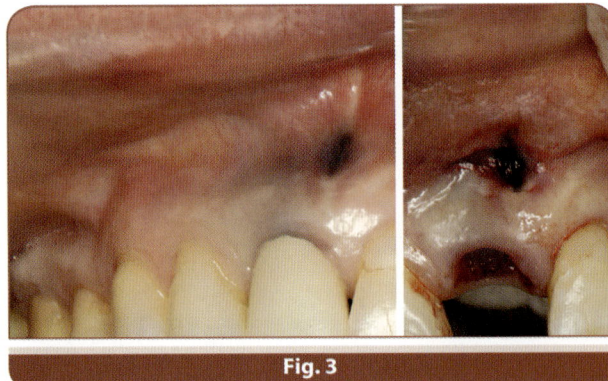

Fig. 3

The central incisor was removed with laying a soft tissue flap **(Fig. 3)**.

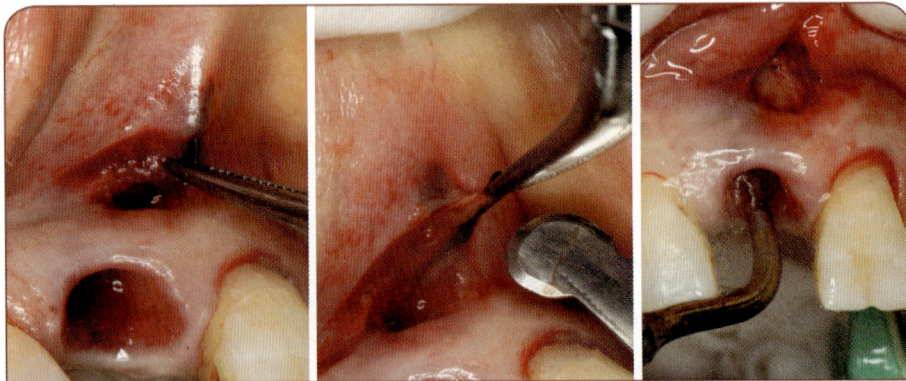

Fig. 4

Amalgam fragments and the subsequent melanin formation in the soft tissue extended all the way to periosteum. The pigments were dissected out with blades and with dermabrasion with high speed diamond rotary instruments, and with piezoelectric surgical device **(Fig. 4)**.

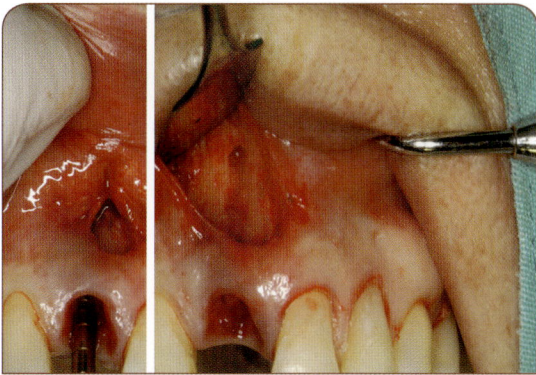

Fig. 5

Osteotomy for implant placement was carried out with ultrasonic piezoelectric surgery device (SurgyBone)™ **(Fig. 5)**.

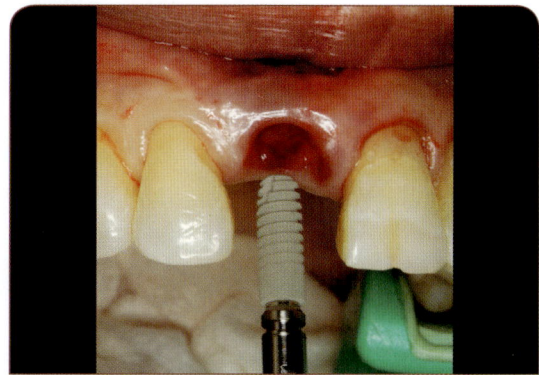

Fig. 6

Osteotomy for implant placement was completed to ensure precise implant placement, but, also in preparation for hard and soft tissue regeneration **(Fig. 6)**.

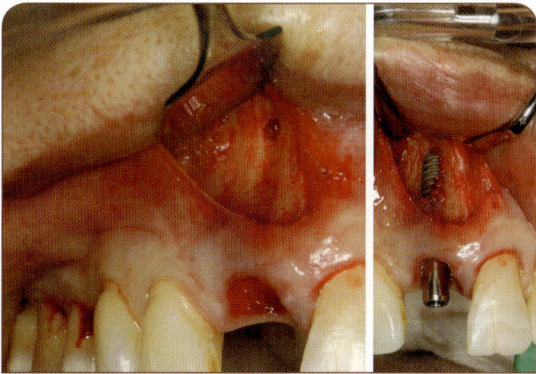

Fig. 7

Implant is in the correct position that allows for screw access in the cingulum. The resulting fenestration of the implant surface needs to be grafted with hard tissue. implant utilized is an Ankylos 3.5 mm × 11.5 mm **(Fig. 7)**.

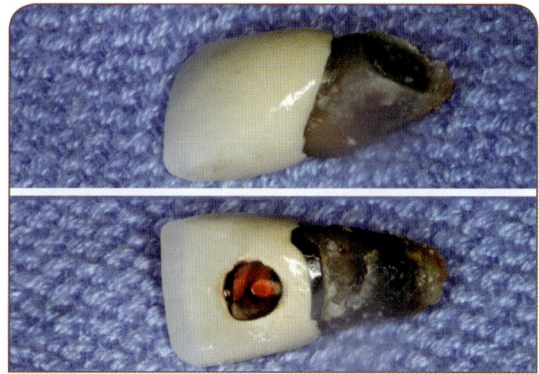

Fig. 8

Extended tooth #11 **(Fig. 8)**.

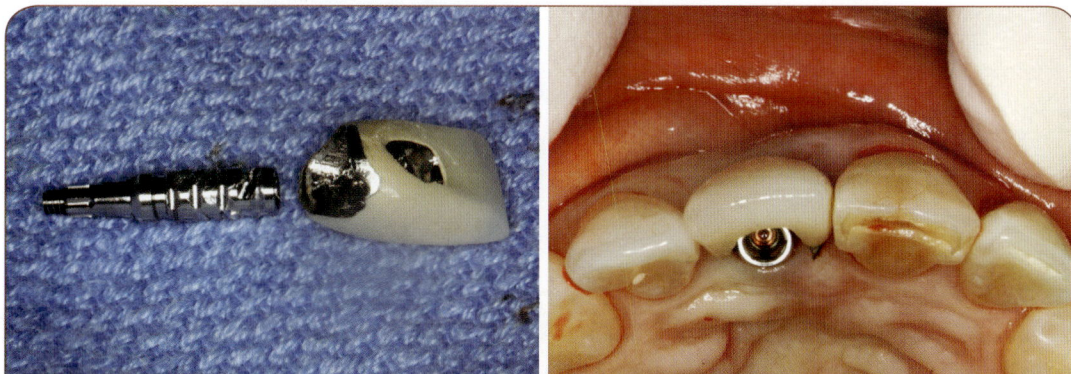

Fig. 9

The ceramo-metal restoration from the extracted tooth was carefully adjusted to act as a nonfunctional immediate implant restoration, supported by the implant just placed **(Fig. 9)**.

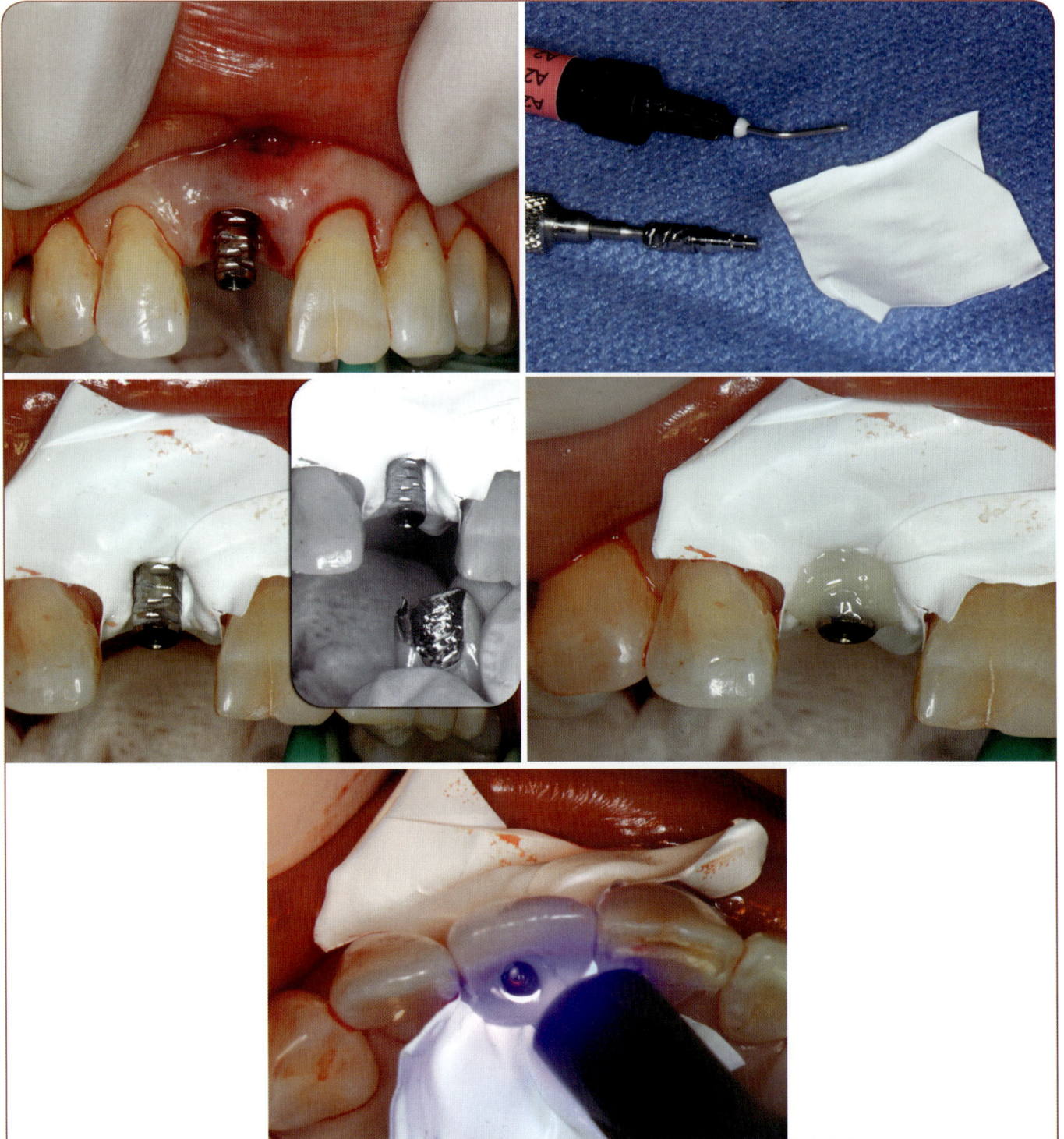

Fig. 10

In order to replicate the ideal emergence profile, light cured composite was utilized with a screw-retained temporary titanium abutment. A layer of thick teflon membrane (heavy duty 4-mm thick Polytetrafluoroethylene (PTFE) industrial sealing tape, autoclaved before use) was used to prevent resin from flowing into the socket defect **(Fig. 10)**.

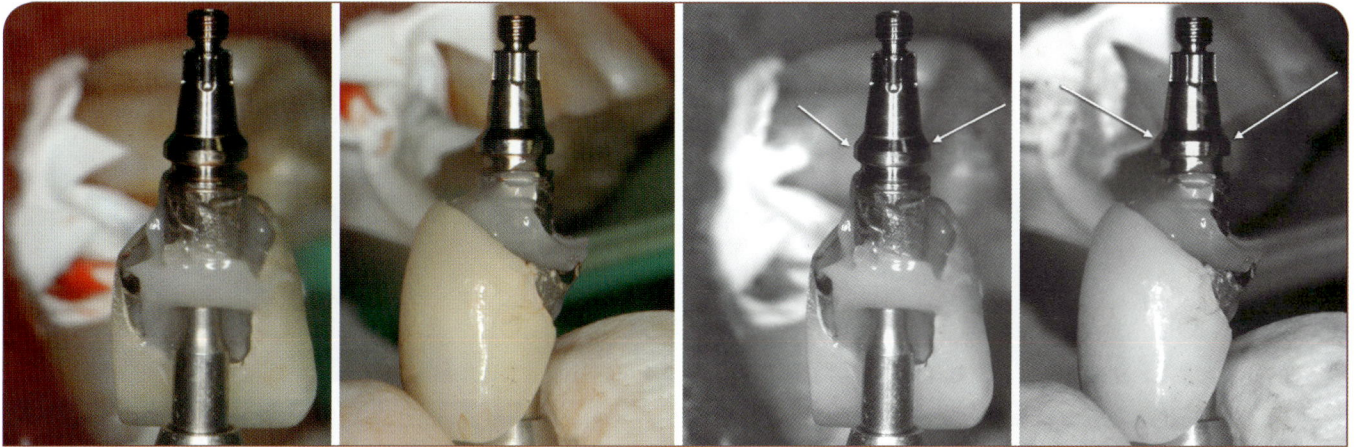

Fig. 11

Composite used to join temporary abutment with patients old crown to make screw retained prosthesis **(Fig. 11)**.

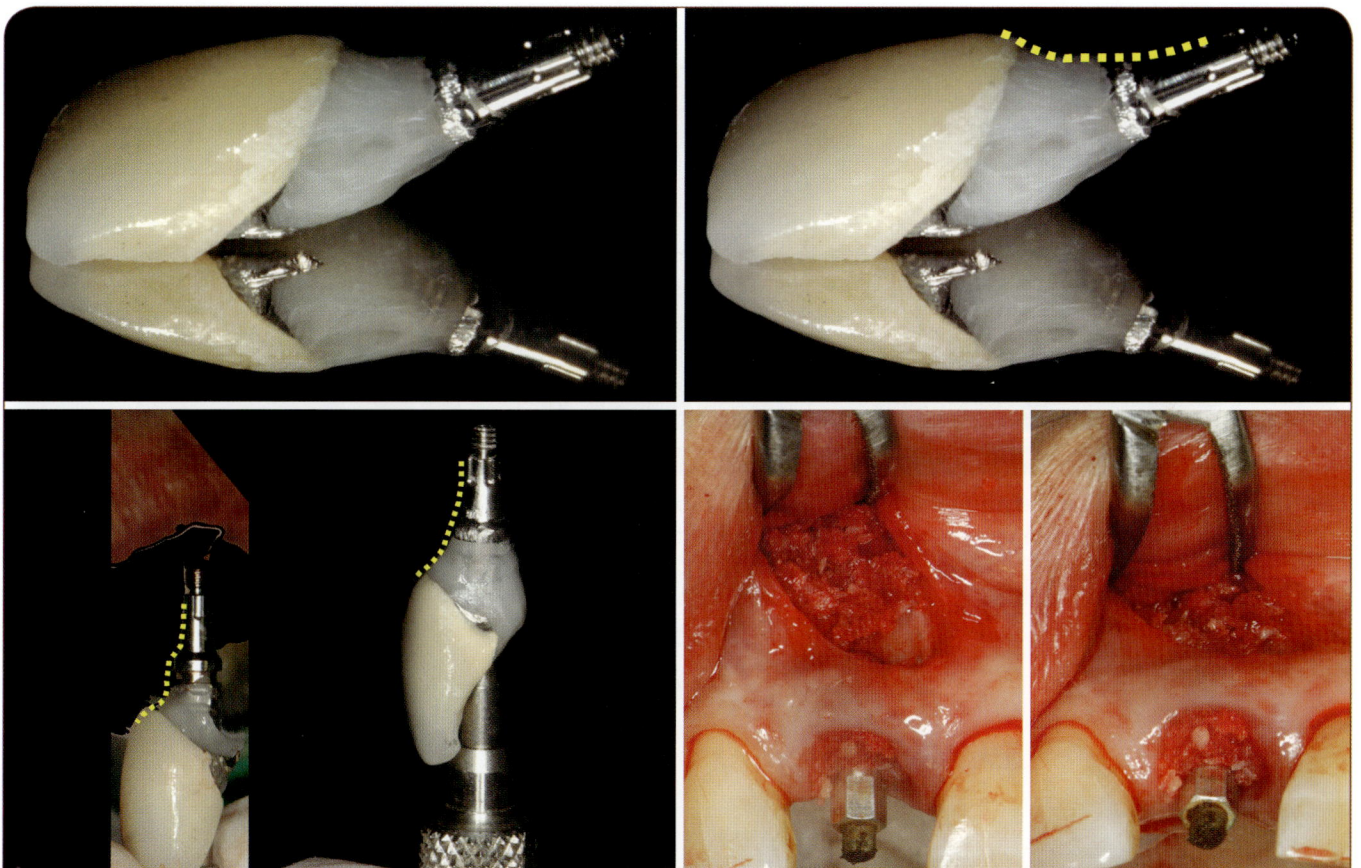

Fig. 12

The nonfunctional implant restoration (NFIR) was completed with the appropriate contours, by adding and curing resin, and removing unnecessary contours on the abutment. The subgingival contours should be under contoured as to allow more soft and hard tissue to form during the initial healing period **(Fig. 12)**.

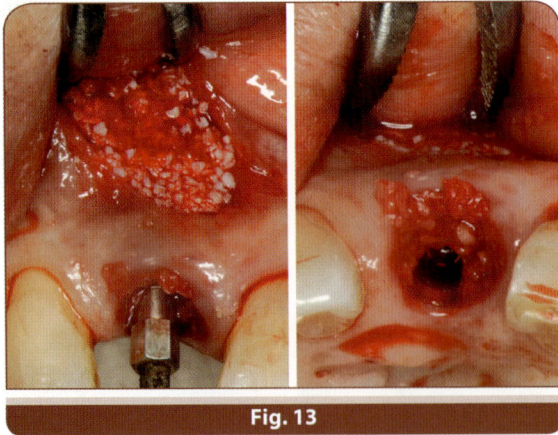

Fig. 13

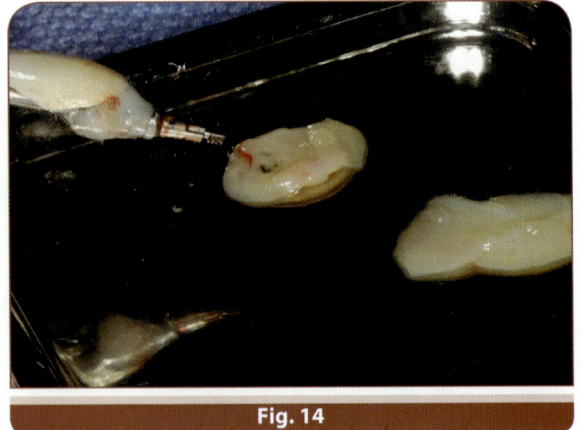

Fig. 14

The facial and apical bone defect was grafted in two layers of "sticky bone." The first layer is cancellous particulate of mineralized freeze-dried bone allograft coagulated in autologous fibrin glue (AFG) obtained by centrifuging venous blood in centrifuge, that forms the gel-like "sticky bone." **(Fig. 13)**.

The second layer is composed of inorganic bovine particulate graft material coagulated in autologous fibrin glue (AFG) **(Fig. 14)**.

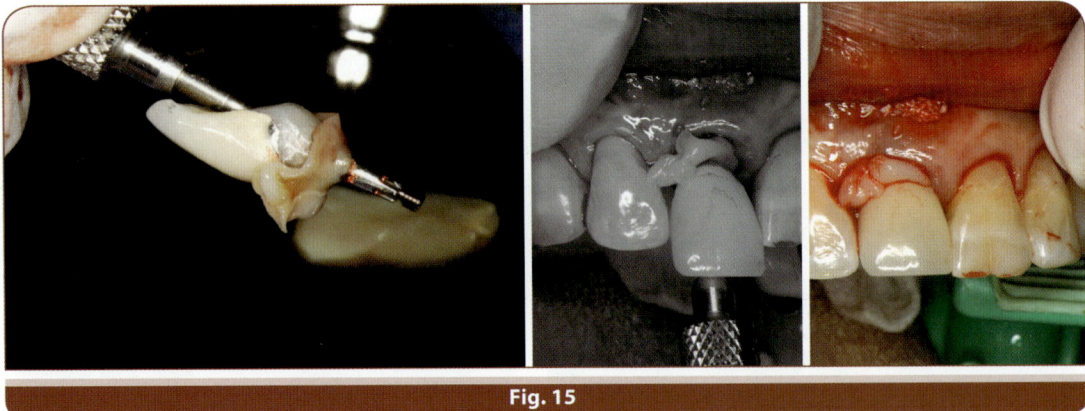

Fig. 15

The NFIR is secured onto the immediately placed dental implant by tightening the retention screw. A double layer of pressed concentrated growth factors with a hole created in the center is placed with the restoration in what is known as "Poncho" technique **(Fig. 15)**.

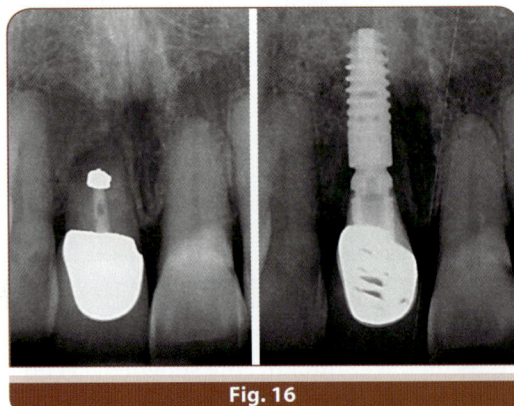

Fig. 16

Preoperative and postoperative radiograph **(Fig. 16)**.

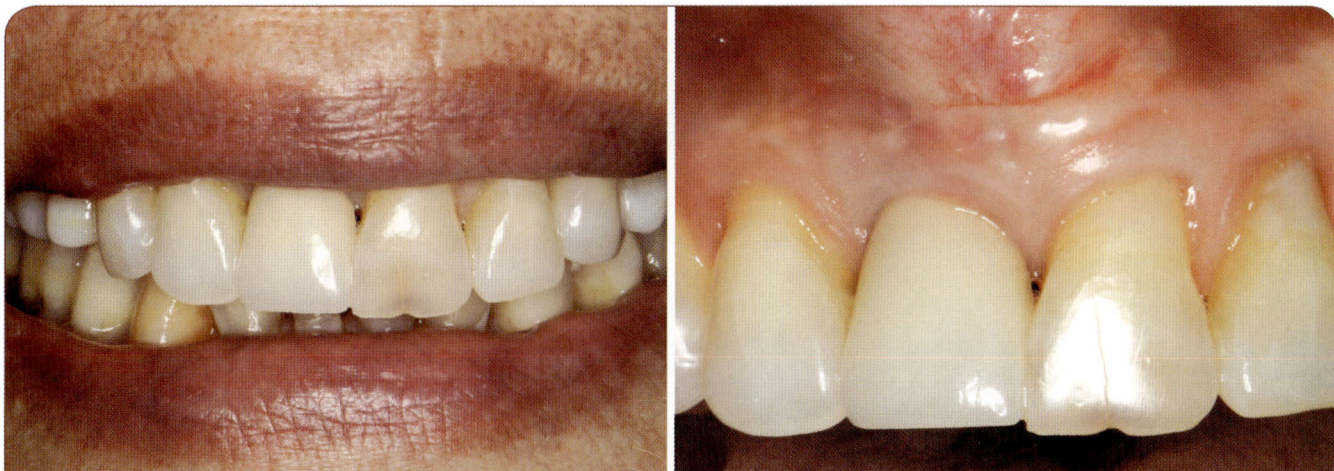

Healing at 3 months (Fig. 17).

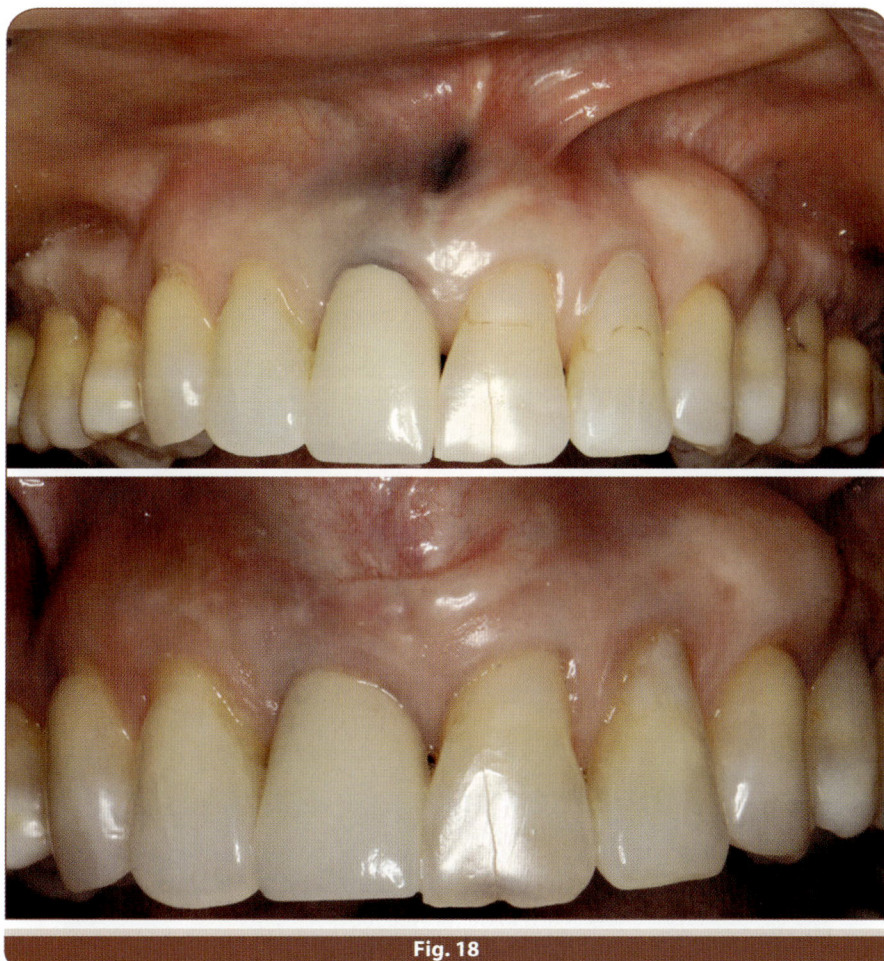

Preoperative and 3 months post temporization (Fig. 18).

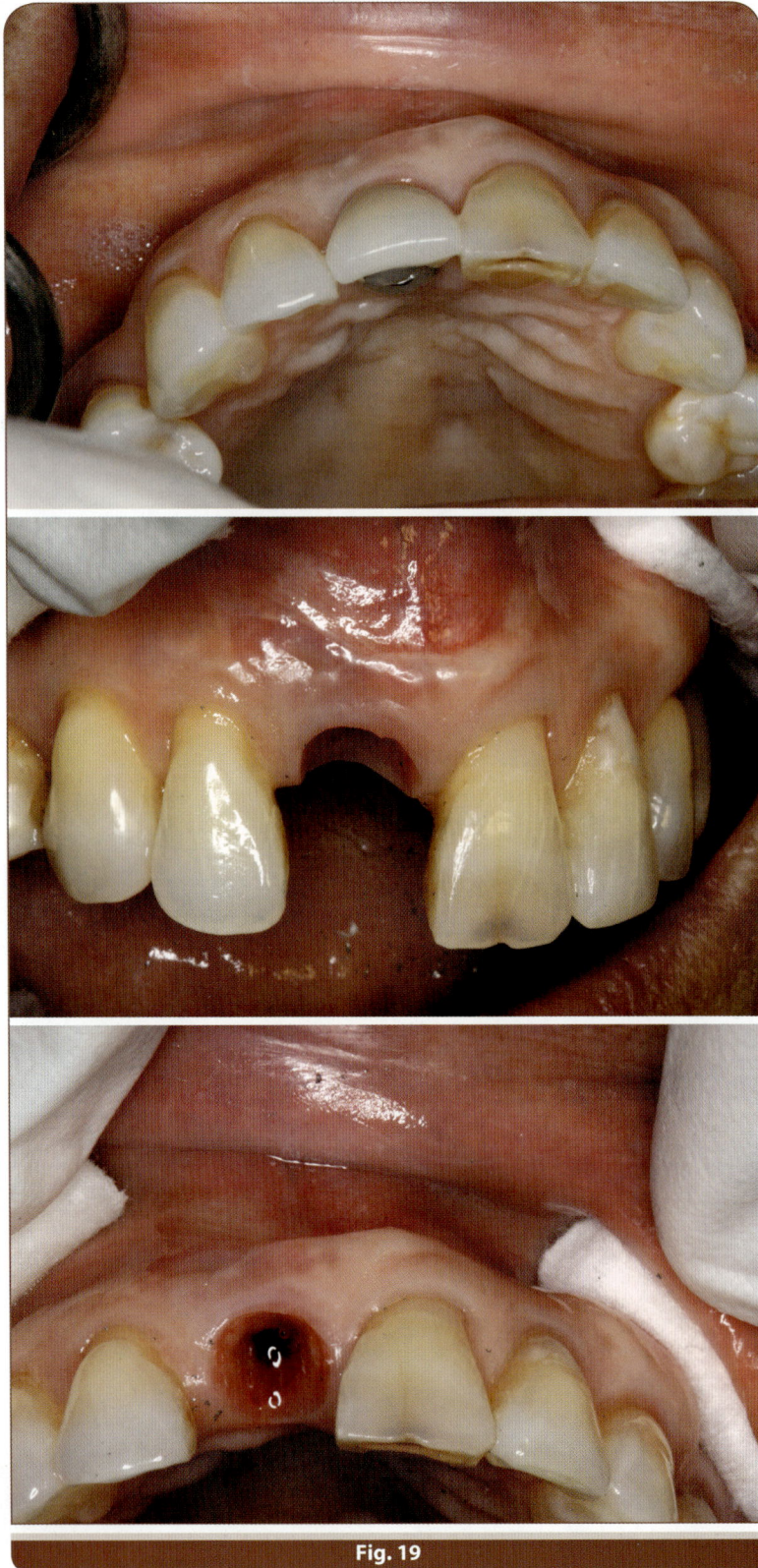

Fig. 19

At 3 months, the amalgam pigmentation was completely unrecognizable. Tissue overlying the previous defect seems to be adequate, both functionally and esthetically **(Fig. 19)**.

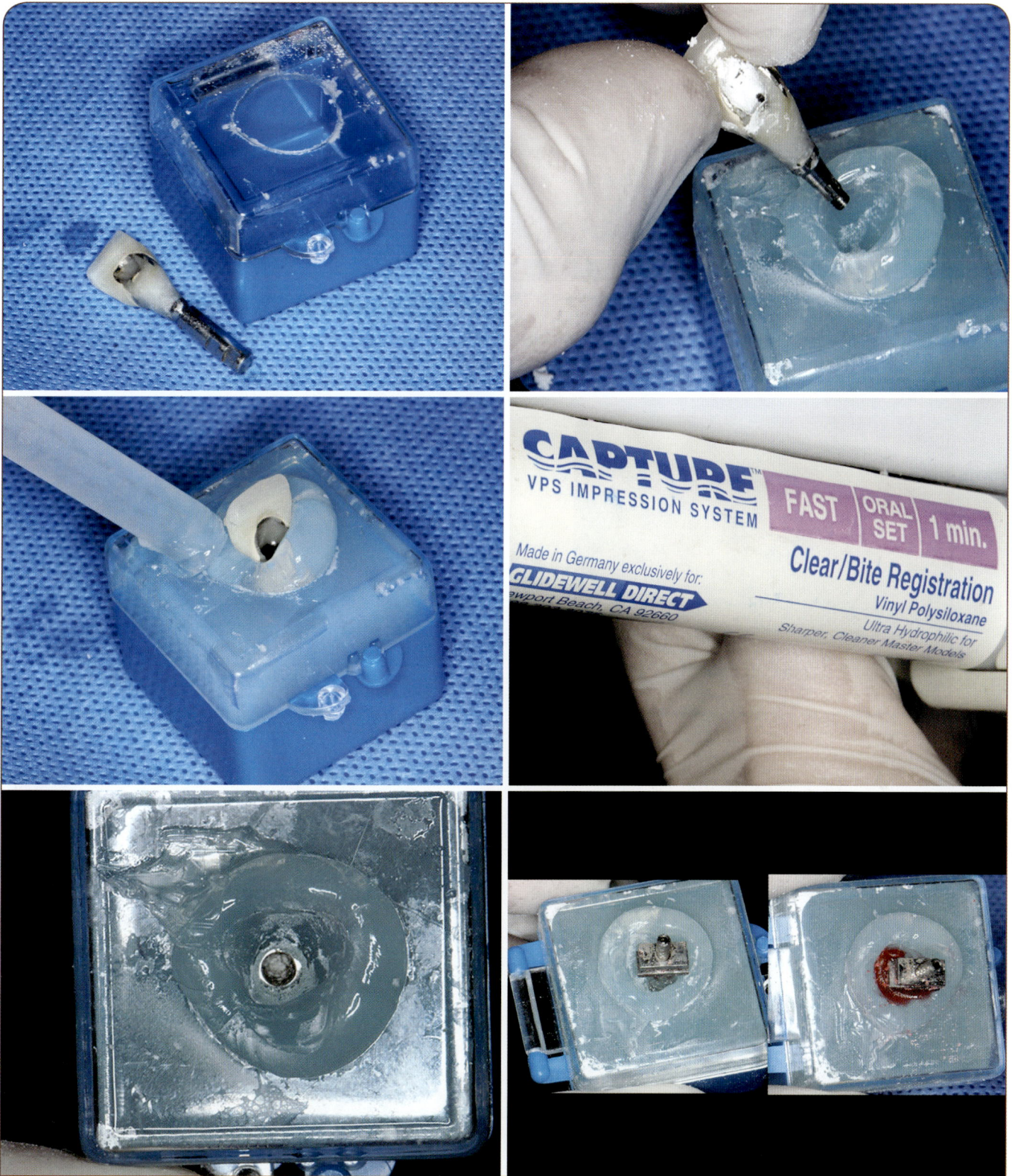

Fig. 20

The existing provisional restoration was utilized to duplicate the peri-implant tissue contours (**Fig. 20**).

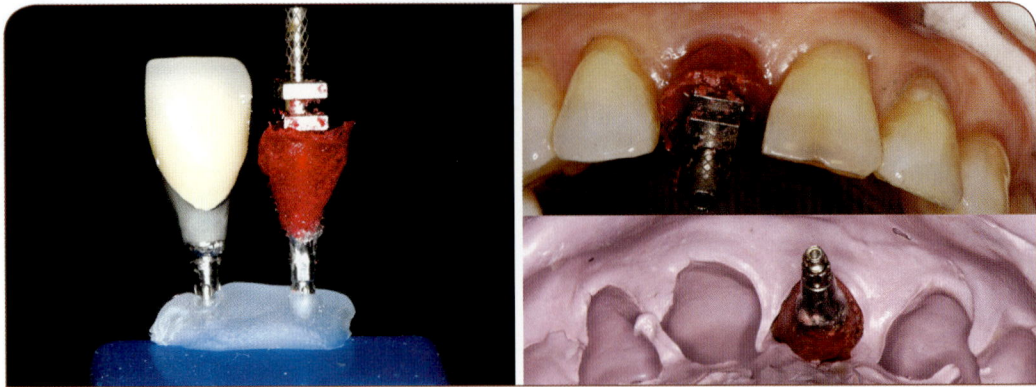

Fig. 21

A custom impression coping was fabricated as a duplicate of the existing provisional restoration. This impression coping is used to pick-up the precise soft tissue contour to be communicated to the dental laboratory (Kim 2004) **(Fig. 21)**.

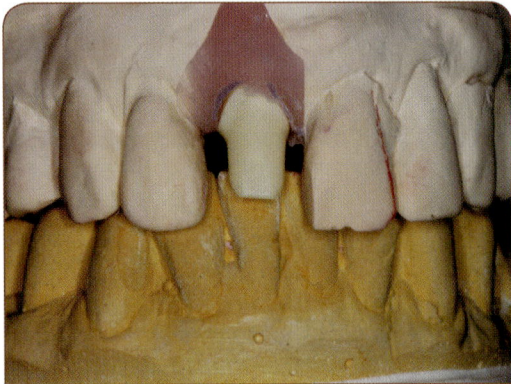

Fig. 22

Custom made zirconia abutments **(Fig. 22)**.

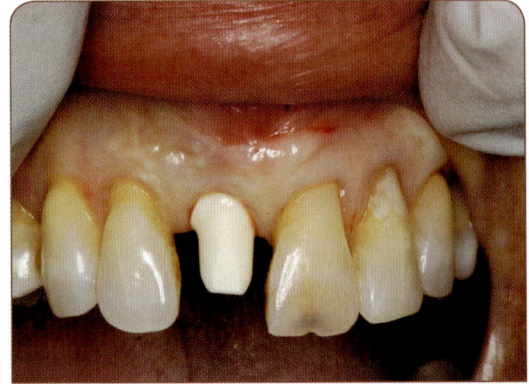

Fig. 23

A custom milled abutment was fabricated out of zirconia, to the exact soft tissue profile provided by the custom impression technique **(Fig. 23)**.

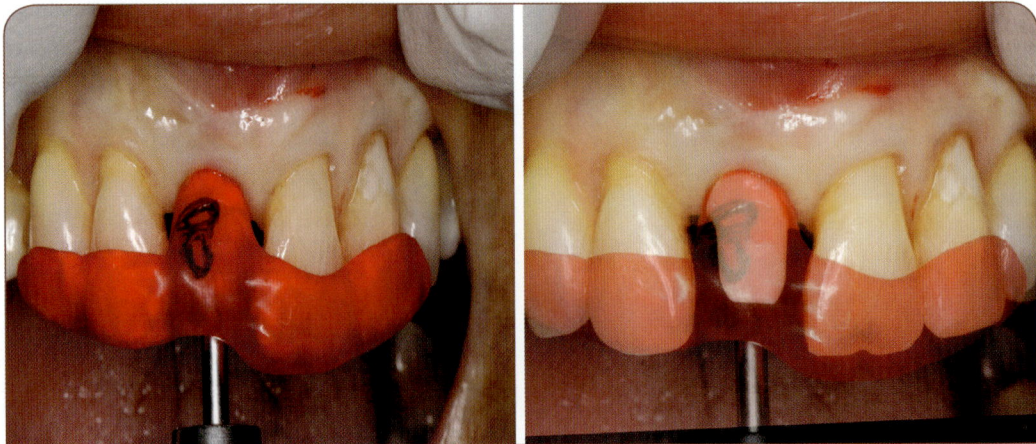

Fig. 24

Pattern resin by used to index the abutment **(Fig. 24)**.

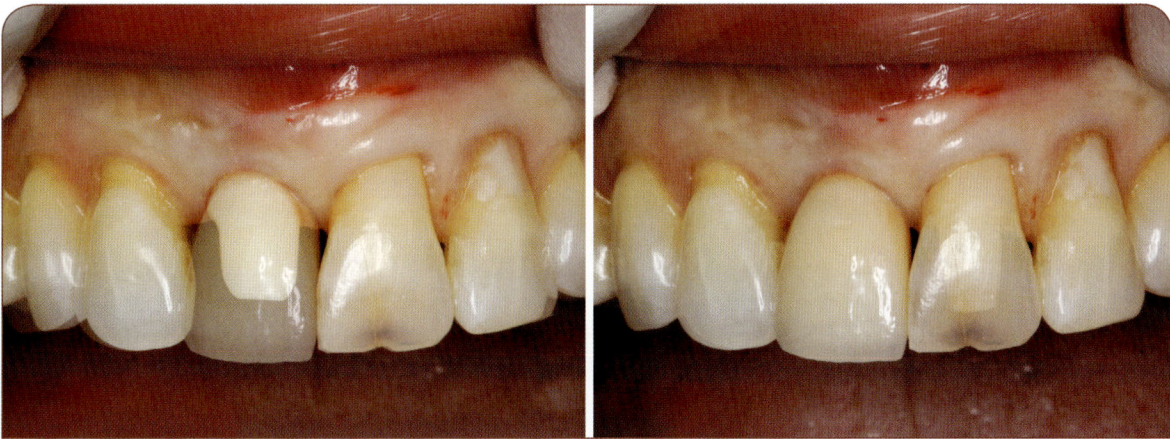

Fig. 25

E-Max crown tried on abutment in tooth #11 region **(Fig. 25)**.

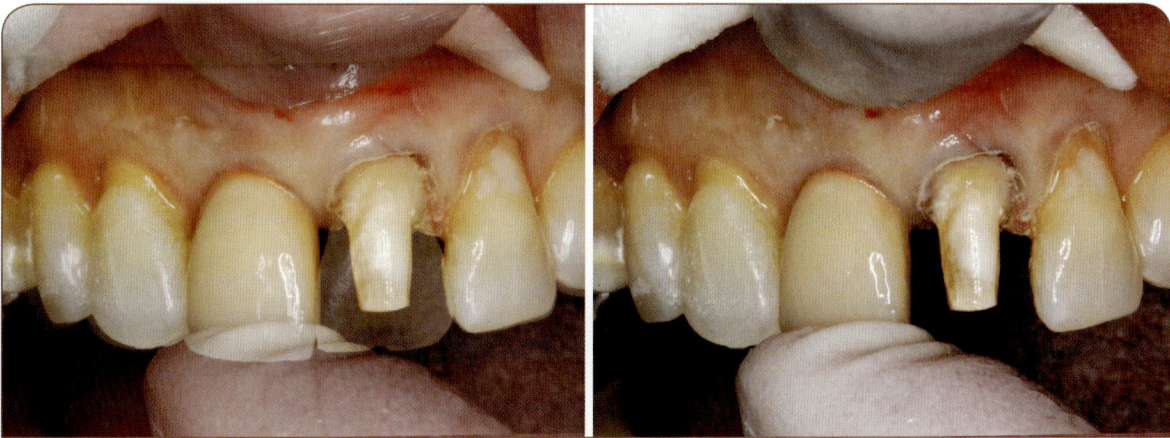

Fig. 26

Crown preparation of tooth #21 done corresponding to tooth#11 crown for E-Max crown restoration **(Fig. 26)**.

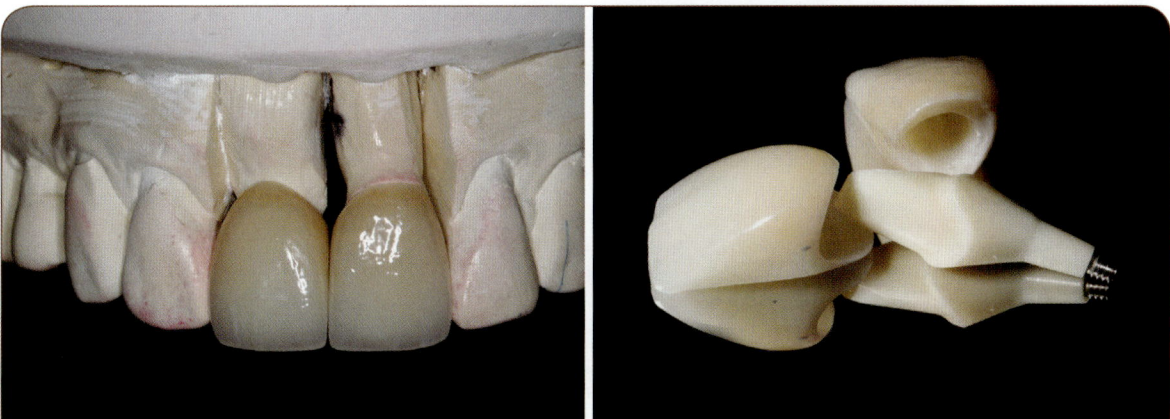

Fig. 27

Screw retained ceramic abutment on implant in tooth #11 region and E-Max crowns on implant abutment and tooth #21 **(Fig. 27)**.

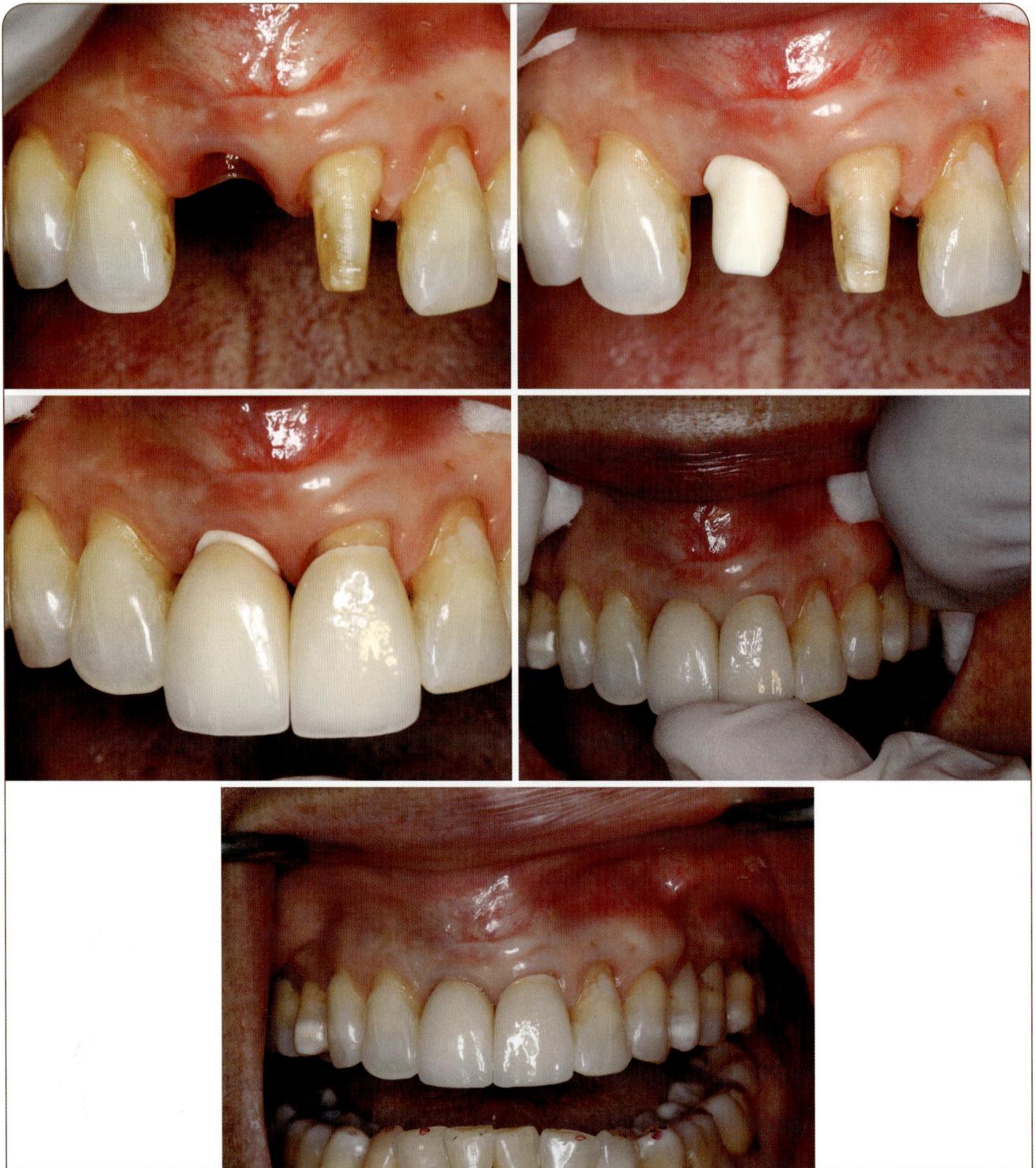

Fig. 28

Screw-retained ceramic abutment with cemented EMAX™ restoration was utilized in the implant site. The cementable restoration was cemented in the mouth, and the cement junction cleaned and smoothened outside the mouth by unscrewing the restoration. Upper left central incisor, a natural tooth, received an EMAX™ full coverage restoration for esthetics and for symmetry **(Fig. 28)**.

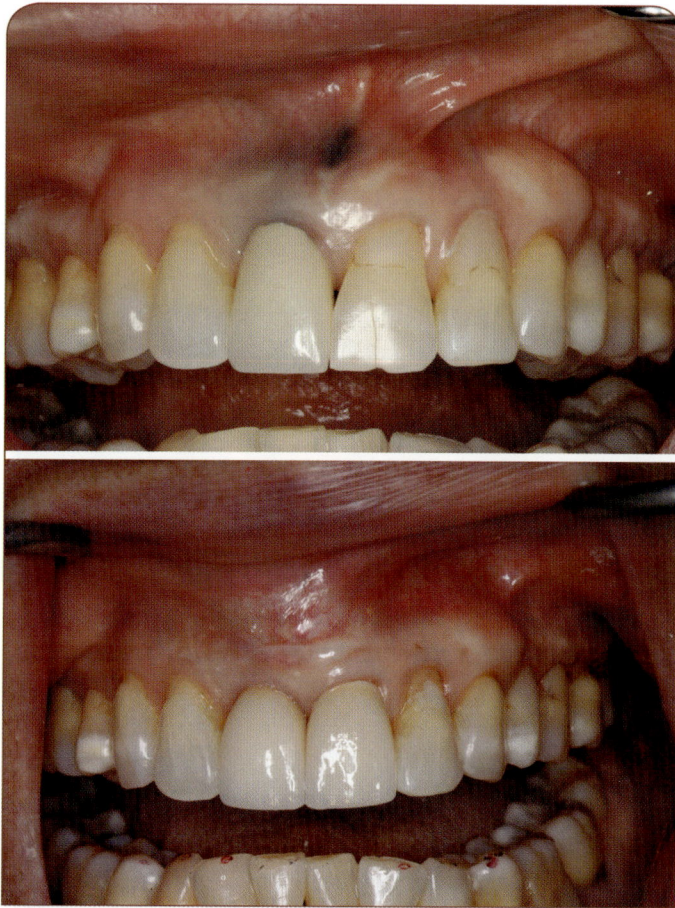

Fig. 29

Preoperative and postoperative images **(Fig. 29)**.

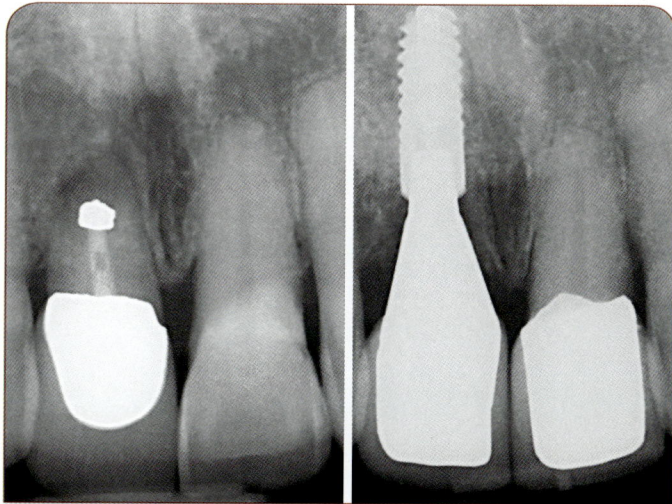

Fig. 30

Preoperative and postoperative radiographs **(Fig. 30)**.

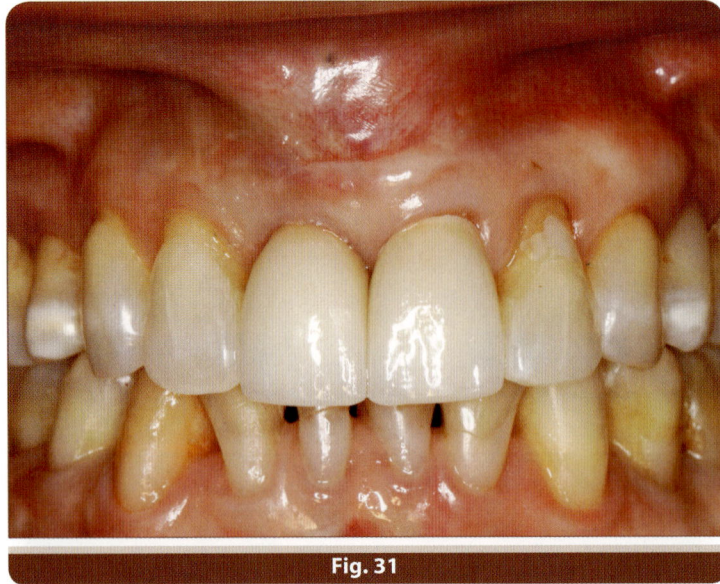

Fig. 31

Follow up at 6 months post restorations. The amalgam tattoo is not evident, as a result of surgical debridement, and concurrent grafting with soft and hard tissue, in a single operation—utilizing the autologous sticky augmentation protocol (ASAP) procedure **(Fig. 31)**.

Amit Gulati

IMMEDIATE EXTRACTION IMPLANT PLACEMENT HARD AND SOFT TISSUE MANAGEMENT PROSTHETIC DESIGN FOR TOOTH AND IMPLANT SUPPORTED PROSTHESIS

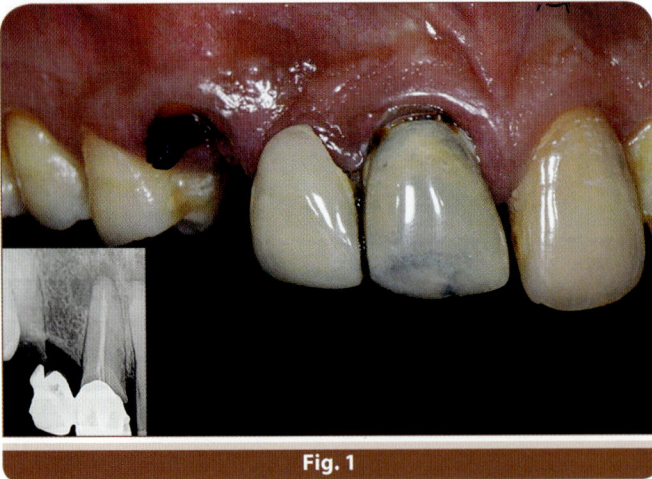

Fig. 1

Tooth #13 Root fragment, tooth #12 cantilever on tooth #11 **(Fig. 1)**.

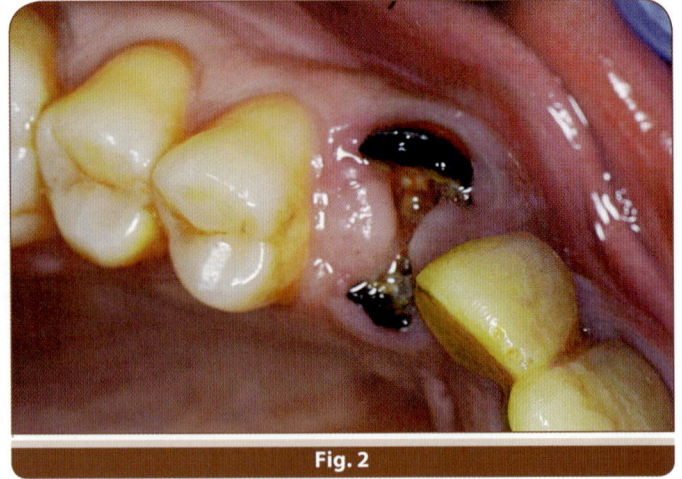

Fig. 2

Baseline—Occlusal view **(Fig. 2)**.

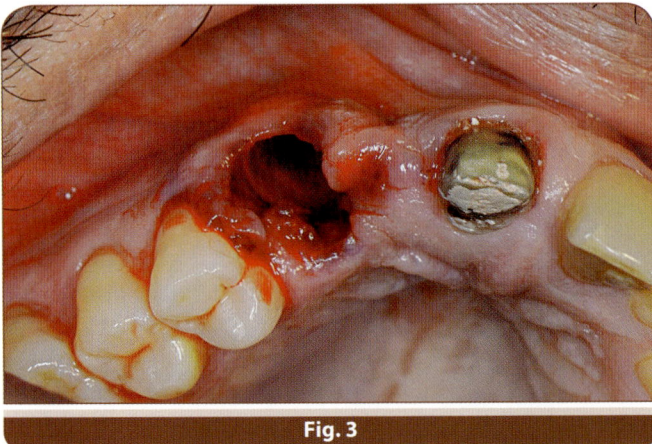

Fig. 3

Tooth #13 extraction with periotomes and luxators **(Fig. 3)**.

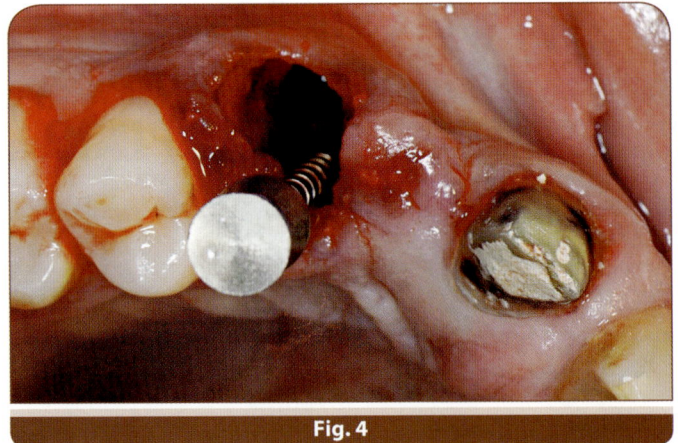

Fig. 4

Osteotomy—Palatally in the socket **(Fig. 4)**.

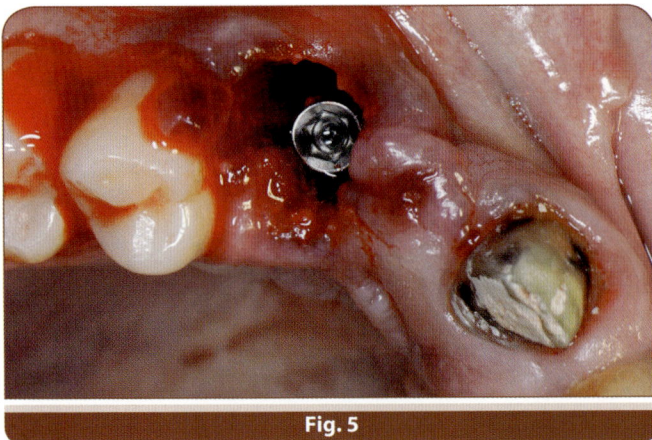

Fig. 5

Implant placement **(Fig. 5)**.

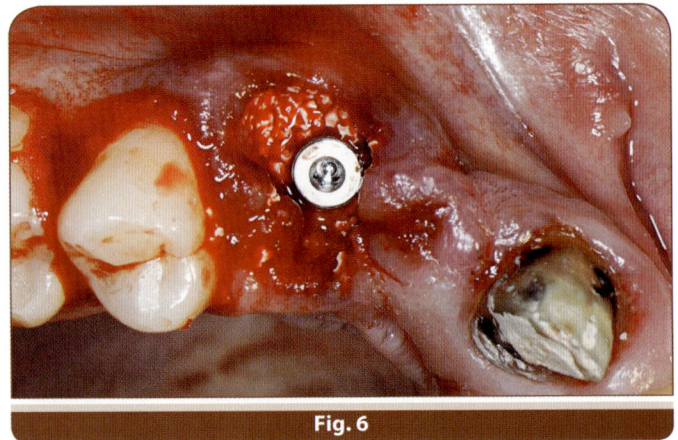

Fig. 6

Bovine bone + Autogenous mix around the implant. Dual-zone grafting **(Fig. 6)**.

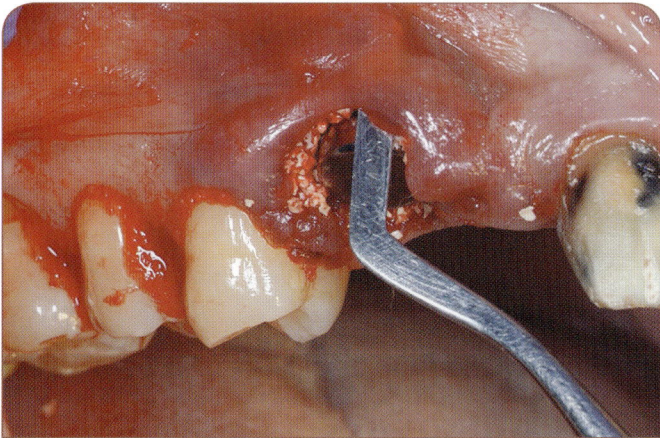

Fig. 7

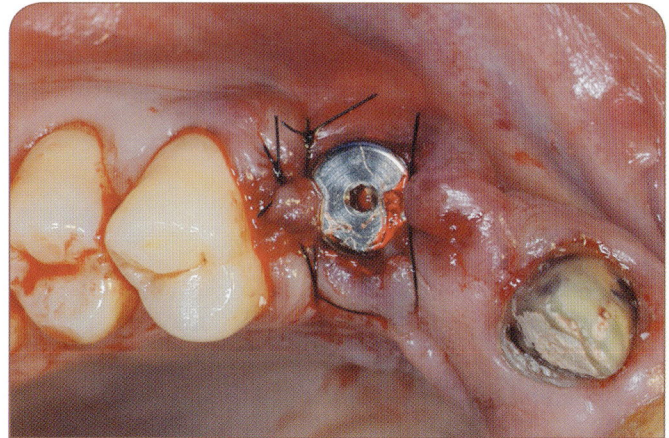

Fig. 8

Slight facial release to facilitate some closure (Fig. 7).

Wide gingival former for a soft tissue seal. Closure with 5-0 nylon (Fig. 8).

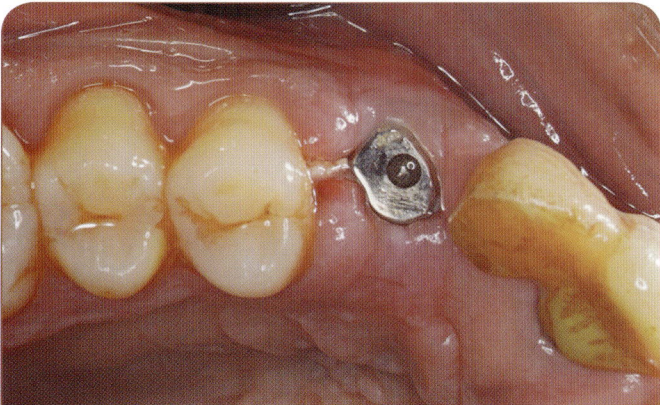

Fig. 9

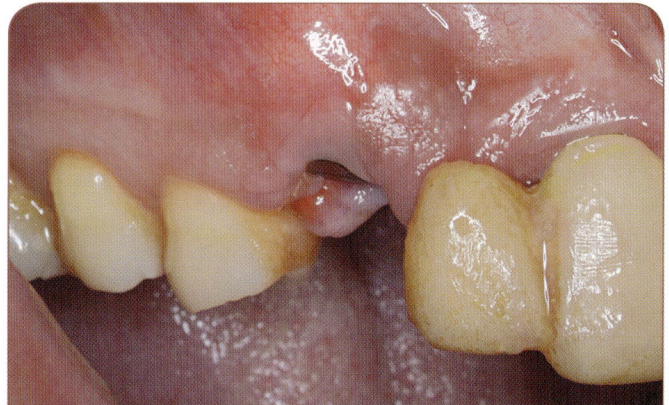

Fig. 10

Recall at 4 weeks. Tissue migrating over the gingival former (Fig. 9).

Recall at 4 weeks. Soft tissue height maintained (Fig. 10).

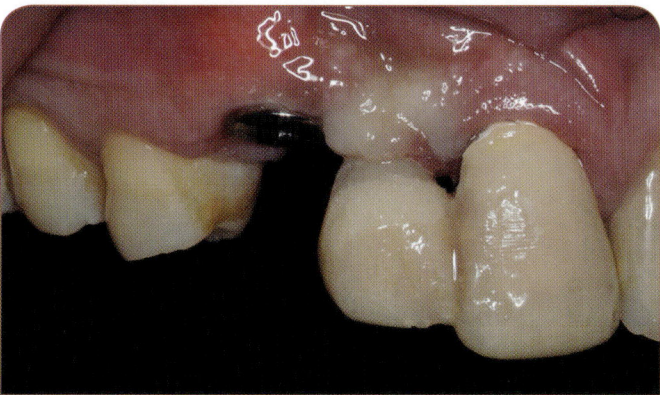

Fig. 11

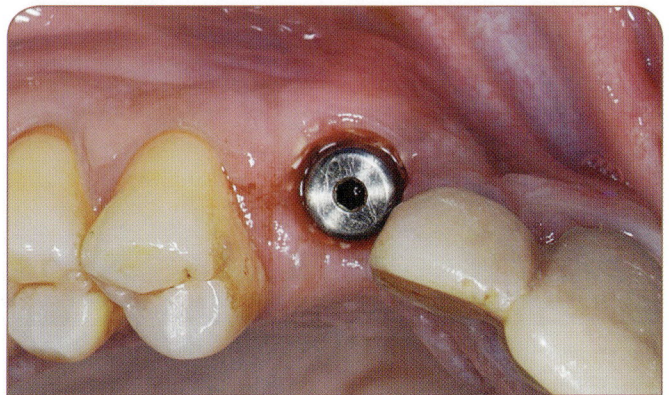

Fig. 12

Pontic site creation for tooth #12. Pontic modified to ovate form by adding Composite (Fig. 11).

Switching to narrow former to allow coronal migration of soft tissue margin (Fig. 12).

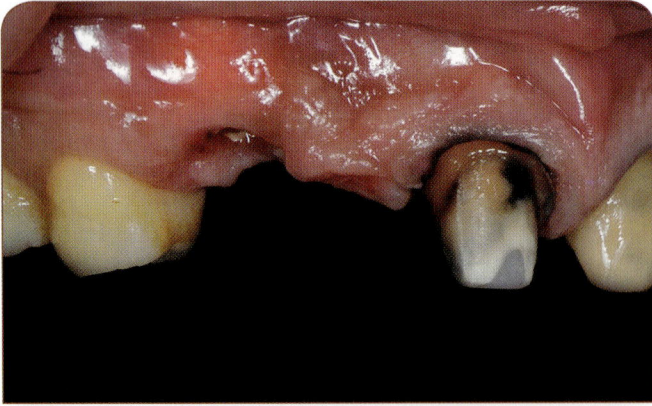

Fig. 13

Ready for making impressions **(Fig. 13)**.

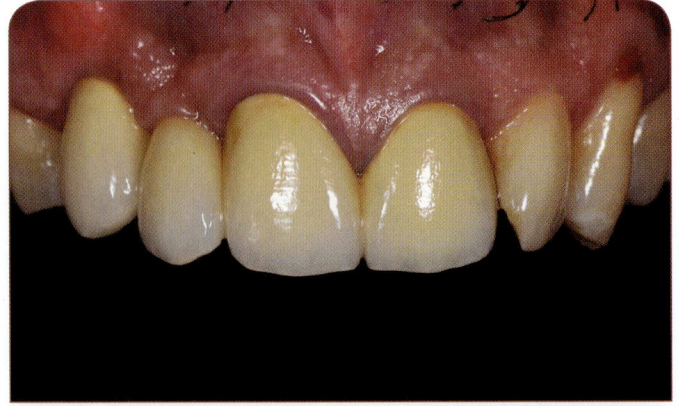

Fig. 14

Tooth #13 implant crown. Teeth #12–#21 convetional FPD with tooth#12 cantilever and a rest on tooth #13. Ovate pontic tooth #12 **(Fig. 14)**.

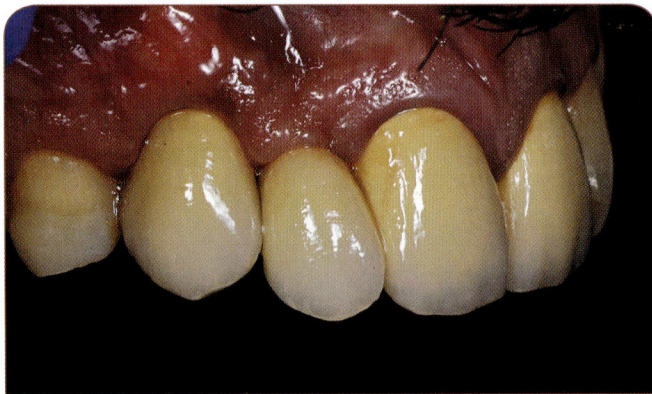

Fig. 15

Lateral view (Fig. 15).

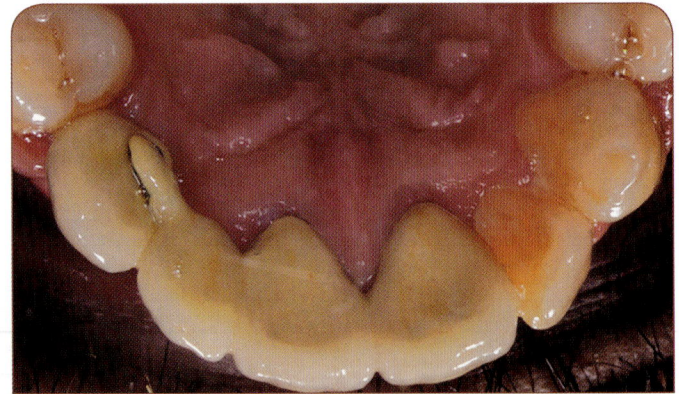

Fig. 16

Occlusal view (Fig. 16).

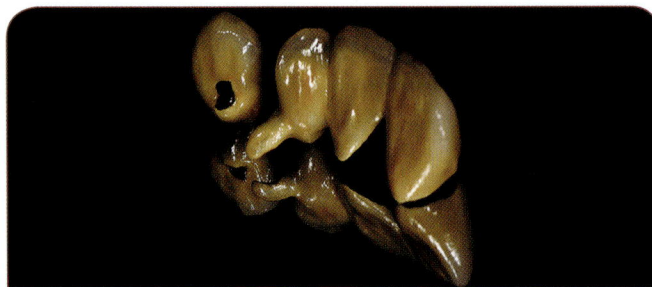

Fig. 17

Tooth #13 implant crown **(Fig. 17).** Tooth #12–#21 Convetional FPD.

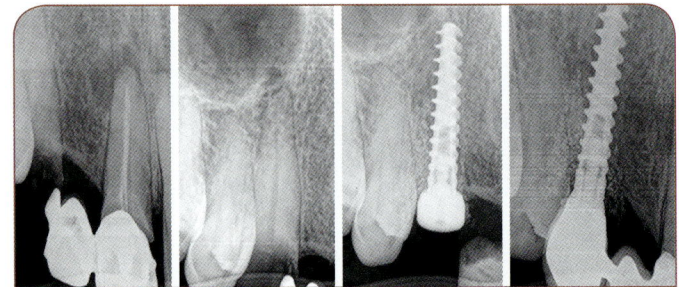

Fig. 18

Comparative radiographs **(Fig. 18)**.

Praful Bali, Sumit Datta

PROSTHETIC MANAGEMENT OF TWO CENTRAL INCISORS WITH HUGE DIASTEMA

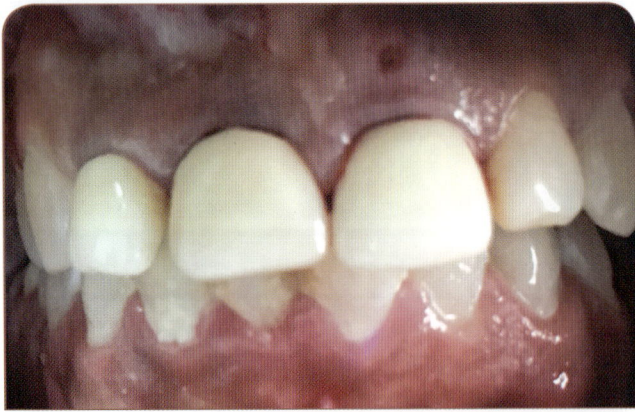
Fig. 1

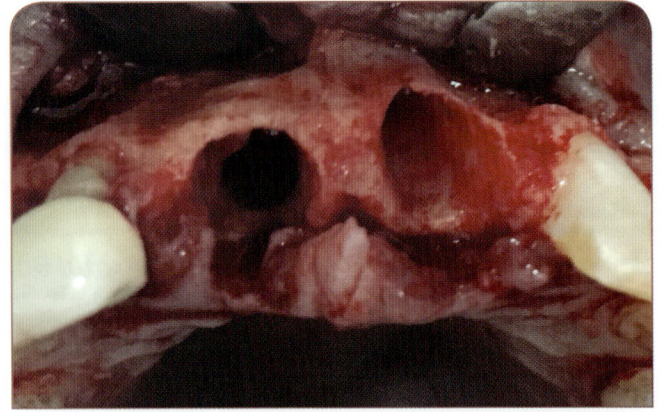
Fig. 2

Patient presents with grade 3 mobility of teeth # 11, 21. Patient desires immediate treatment **(Fig. 1)**.

Teeth #11, 21 extracted with care so that the remaining buccal cortical plate is preserved **(Fig. 2)**.

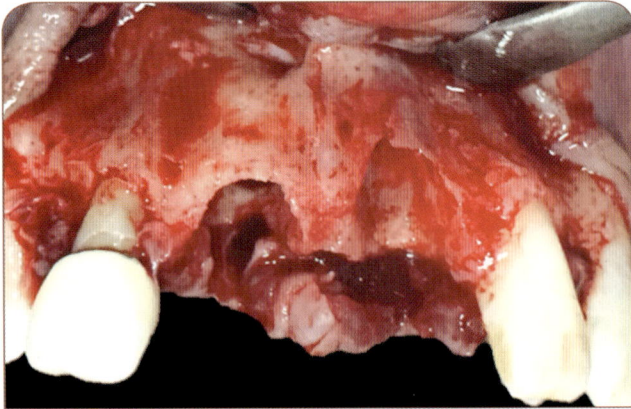
Fig. 3

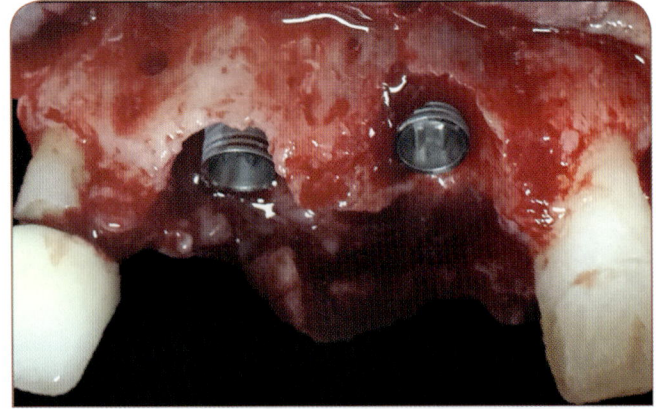
Fig. 4

But due to mobility of the teeth and associated periodontal pathology, there is deficient bone in the buccal aspect **(Fig. 3)**.

2–3.5/11.5 Nobel active (Nobel biocare) implants are done according to the surgical stent **(Fig. 4)**.

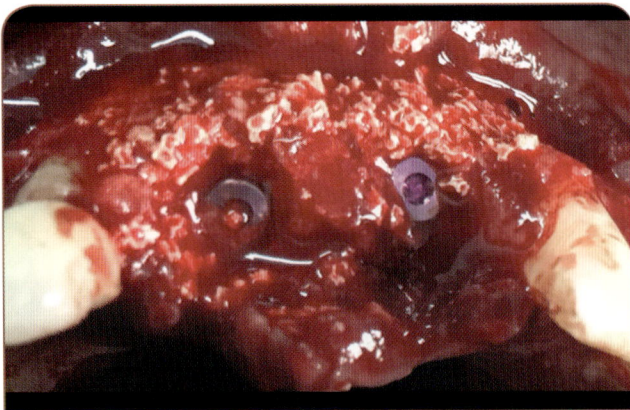
Fig. 5

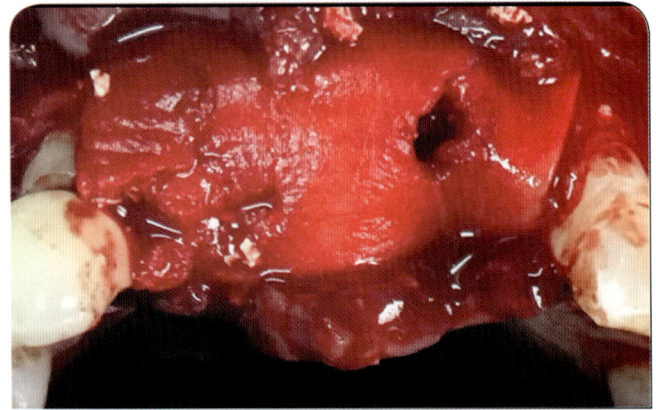
Fig. 6

GBR done around the implants with Bio-Oss **(Fig. 5)**.

Collagen membrane—Nobel biocare done **(Fig. 6)**.

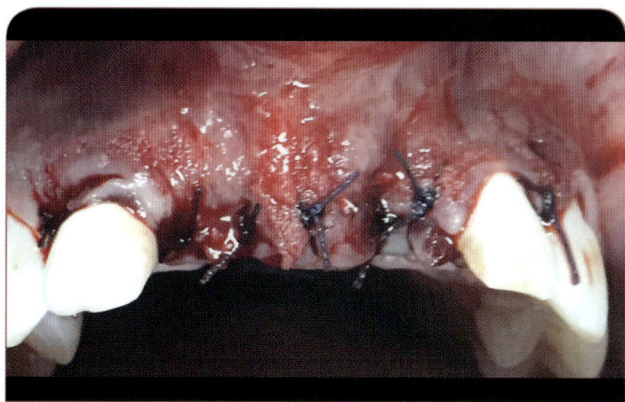

Fig. 7

Suturing done and the site is left to heal for 5 months **(Fig. 7)**.

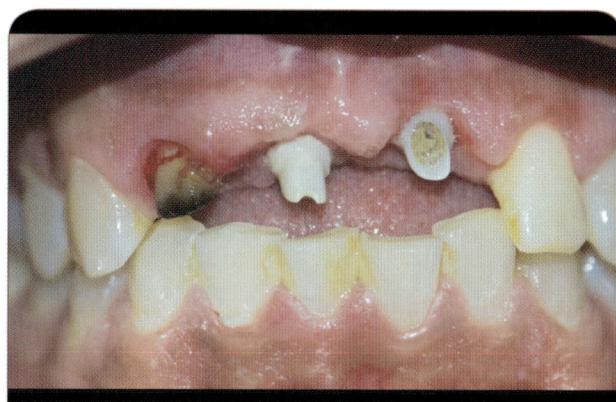

Fig. 8

Zirconia procera abutments torqued at 35 Ncm **(Fig. 8)**.

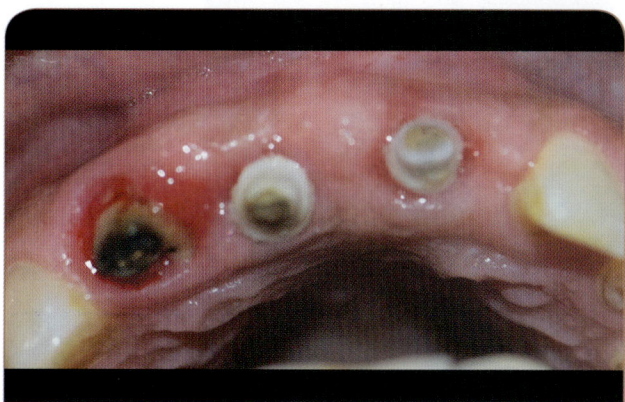

Fig. 9

Occlusal view clearly shows the success of GBR. Good integration around implants **(Fig. 9)**.

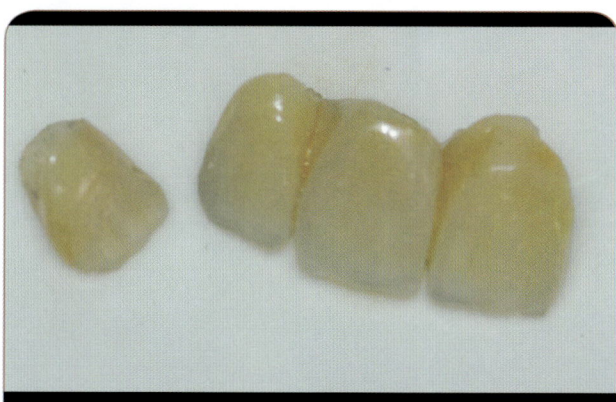

Fig. 10

Two individual crowns were tried but they were looking quite unesthetic. So a decision was made in consultation of the patient to make a 3 unit bridge on 2 implants and give 2 lateral incisors—one on the implant bridge and one on tooth #12 which is endo treated **(Fig. 10)**.

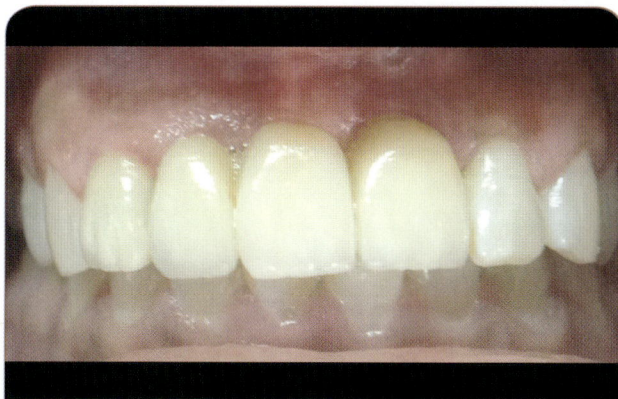

Fig. 11

Final all ceramic work on the implants and tooth #2 **(Fig. 11)**.

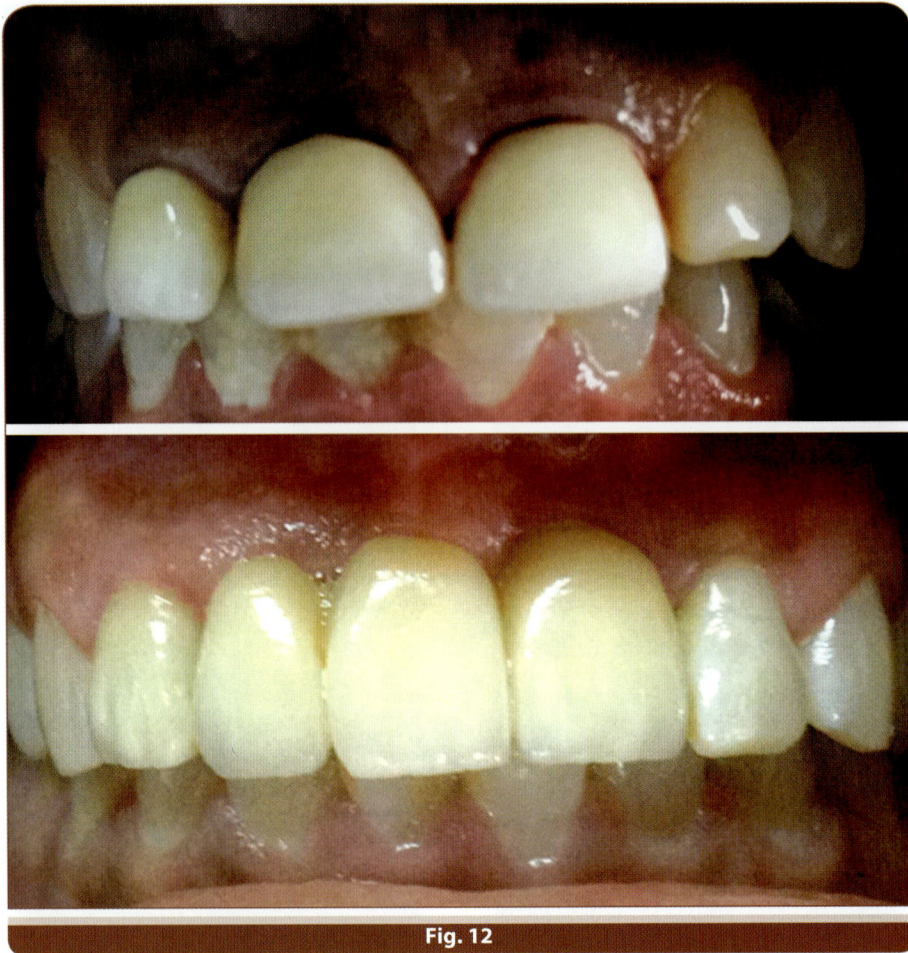

Fig. 12

Pre- and Post-comparison: Our decision to make a 3 unit bridge made the overall result better for sure **(Fig. 12)**.

Narayan TV

IMMEDIATE IMPLANT AND DUAL ZONE GRAFTING WITH IMMEDIATE PROVISIONAL

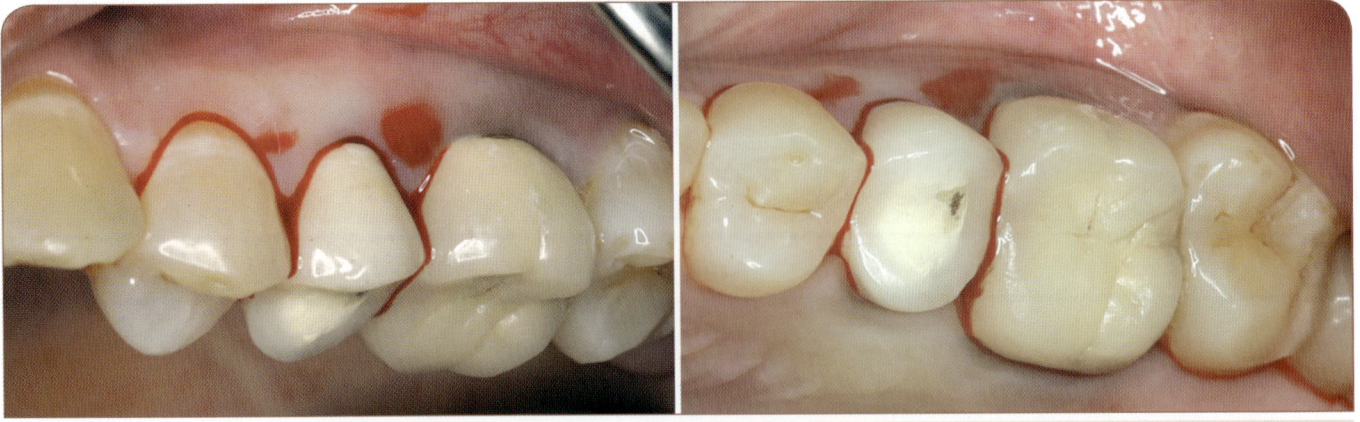

Fig. 1

This case deserves a descriptive history: A 53-year-old female came to me for an opinion on the replacement of tooth # 16, after being told by 2 dentists that to have a bridge done because she was averse to sinus grafting. In the course of her consult, she also expressed that she had trouble with the root canal treated and crowned tooth # 25, which she had repeatedly pointed out to her old dentists, and was dismissed as being nothing by both. Upon percussion, there was a vague tenderness and mobility not commensurate with the bone levels on the radiograph. She already had her entire maxilla scanned but this tooth had not been looked at, having got lost in the discussions on replacement of 16 **(Fig. 1)**.

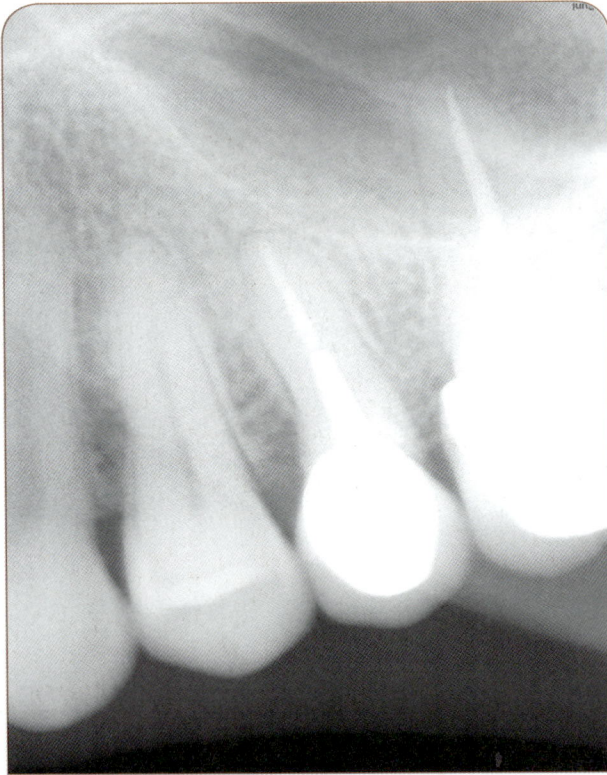

Fig. 2

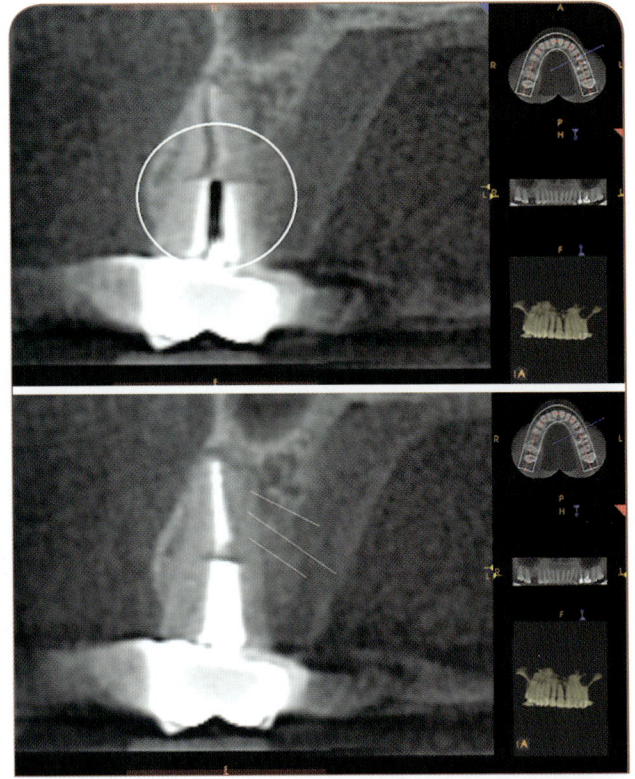

Fig. 3

Largely unremarkable in light of the symptoms, other than the distal crown margin. Interdental peaks and periapex seem alright **(Fig. 2)**.

A close look at the CBCT at middle third, missed palatal canal noted **(Fig. 3)**.

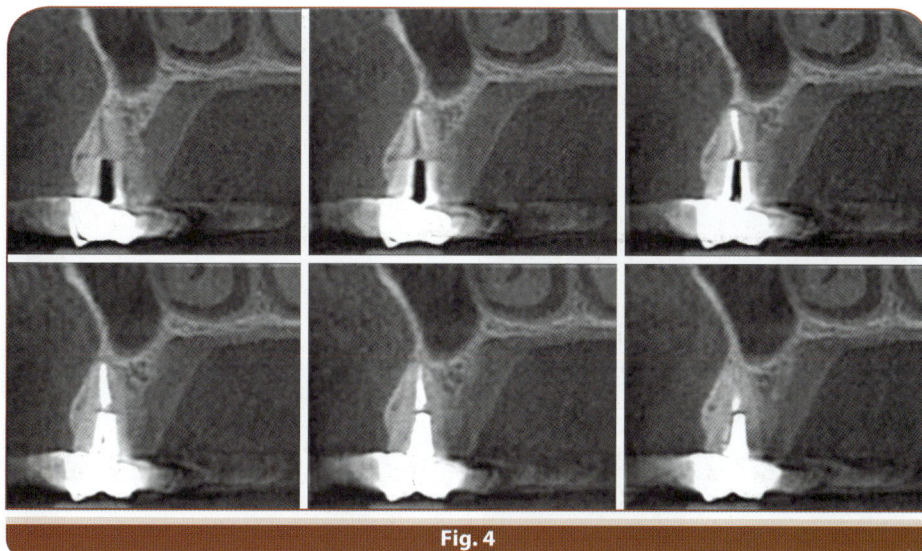

Fig. 4

I spoke to her about exploring after crown removal, and the possibility of immediate placement. Explained to her about the proximity to the sinus and she was insistent that she did not want a sinus lift/graft in the sinus. On looking closer at the CBCT, you can see that there is a very narrow window of bone palatal to the root apex to engage the implant for stability and this was a little more in the mesiopalatal corner of the socket than any other. Proceeded with the proviso that, if I was not comfortable going forward, I would abort the procedure **(Fig. 4)**.

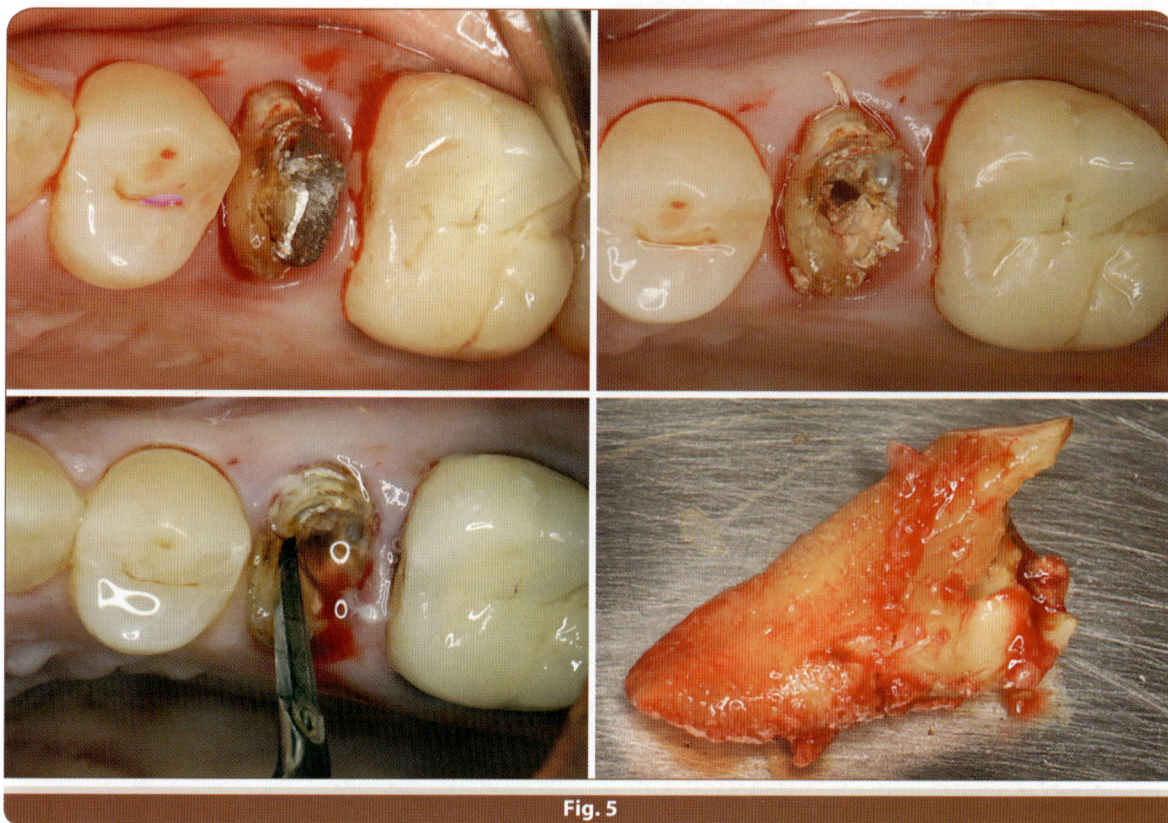

Fig. 5

Failed post and core, fracture crown and root with secondary caries noted. Extraction of tooth # 15 done using Piezo **(Fig. 5)**.

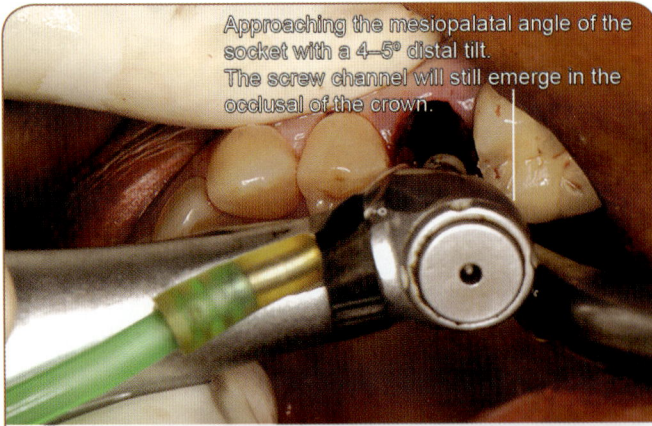

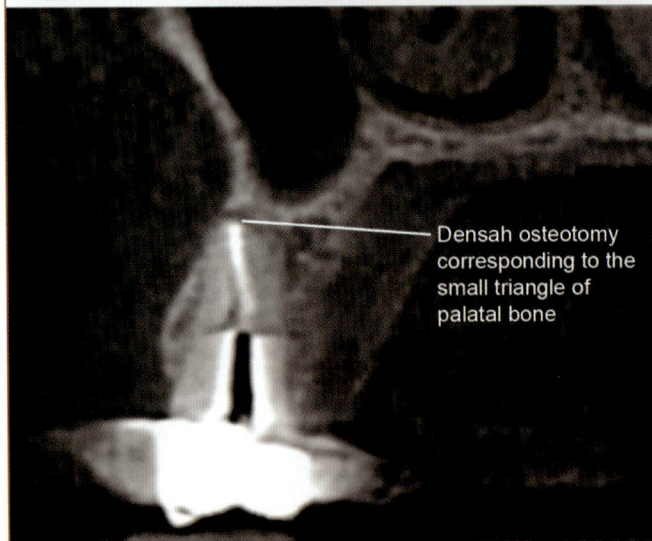

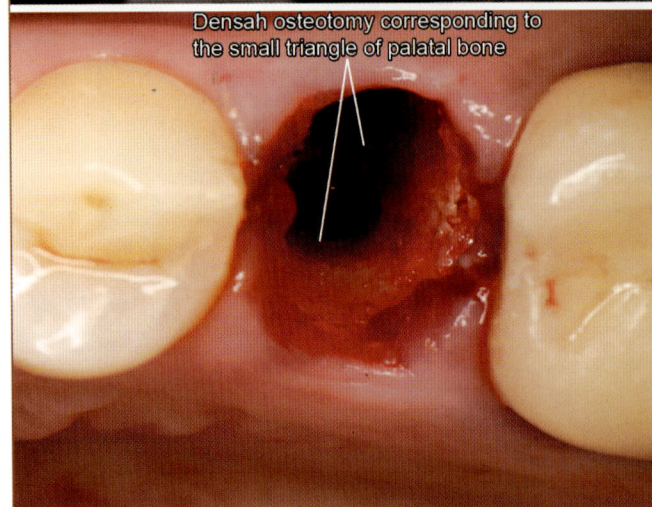

Approaching the mesiopalatal angle of the socket with a 4–5° distal tilt. The screw channel will still emerge in the occlusal of the crown.

Densah osteotomy corresponding to the small triangle of palatal bone

Densah osteotomy corresponding to the small triangle of palatal bone

Fig. 6

Fig. 7

Implant osteotomy preparation in the distopalatal corner of the socket using osseodensification burs from Densah **(Fig. 6)**.

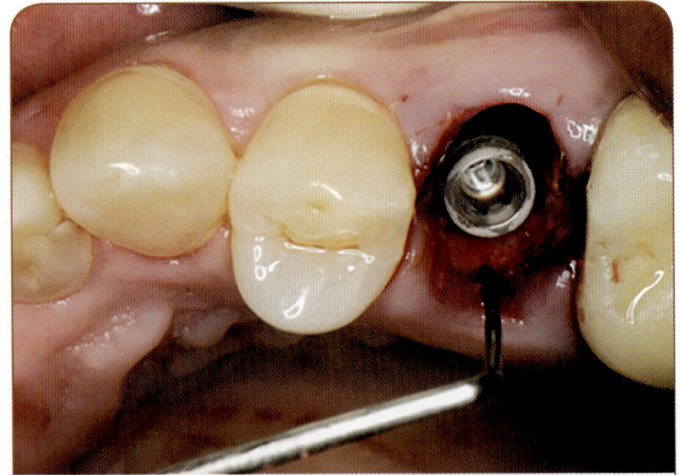

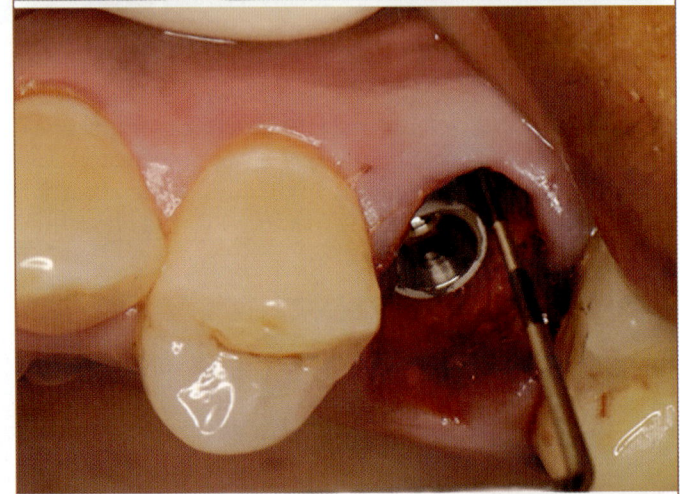

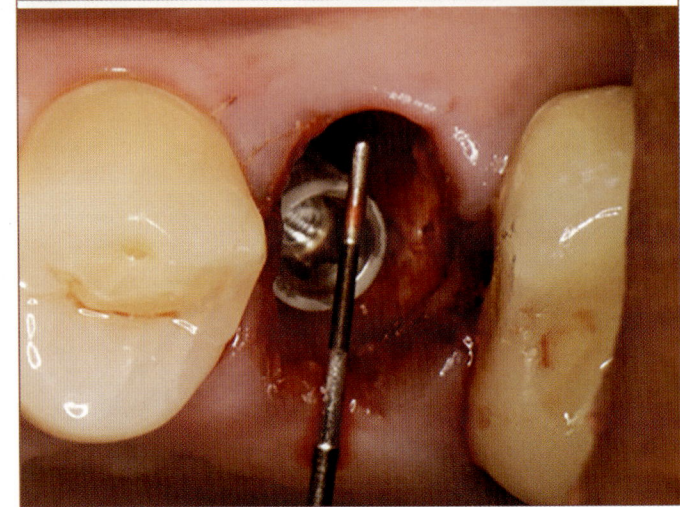

3D implant position:
4 × 11.5 Bioner DM >45 Ncm insertion torque.
>2 mm apical to palatal crest.
~2 mm apical to buccal crest. ~3 mm jump gap **(Fig. 7)**.

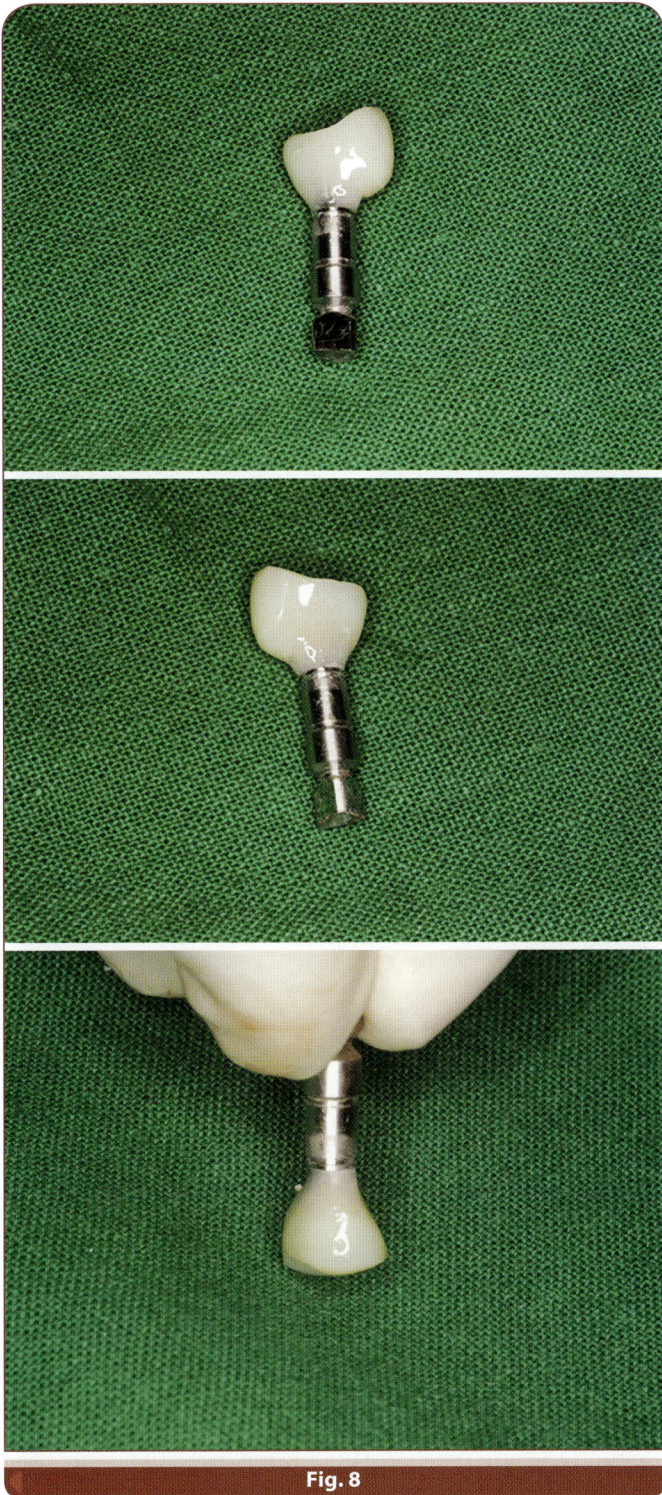

Fig. 8

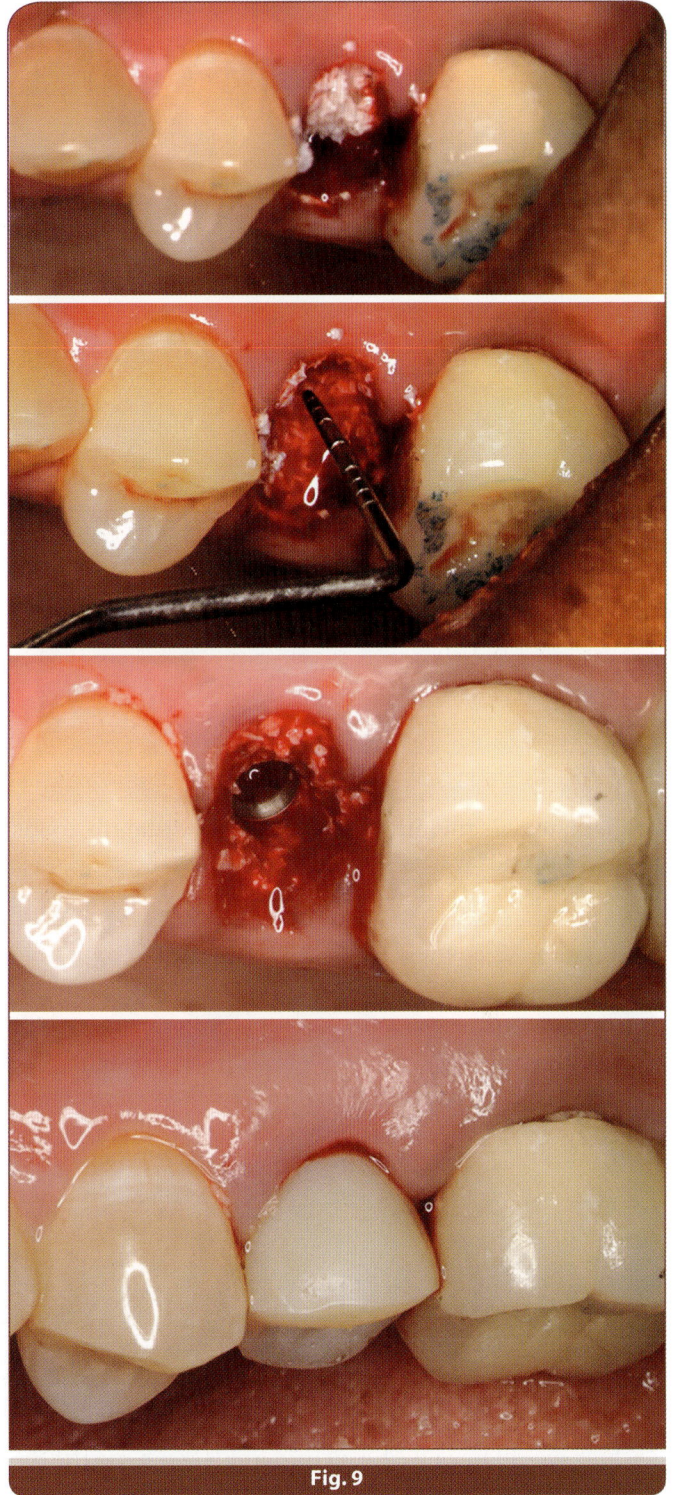

Fig. 9

Screw retained Protemp provisional **(Fig. 8)**.

Bio-Oss in the gap. Use a thin instrument like a perio probe to gently push the material in, not pack it in.

Have the Bio-Oss extend into the soft tissue zone (dual zone) and seal it in with provisional restoration screwed to 25 Ncm **(Fig. 9)**.

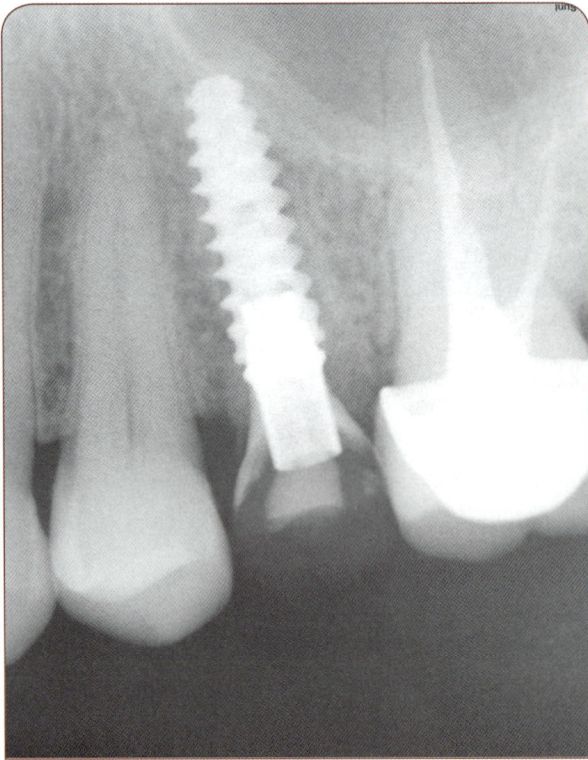

Fig. 10

Immediate postoperative: Note the slight distal tilt, to just kiss the anterior wall of the sinus **(Fig. 10)**.

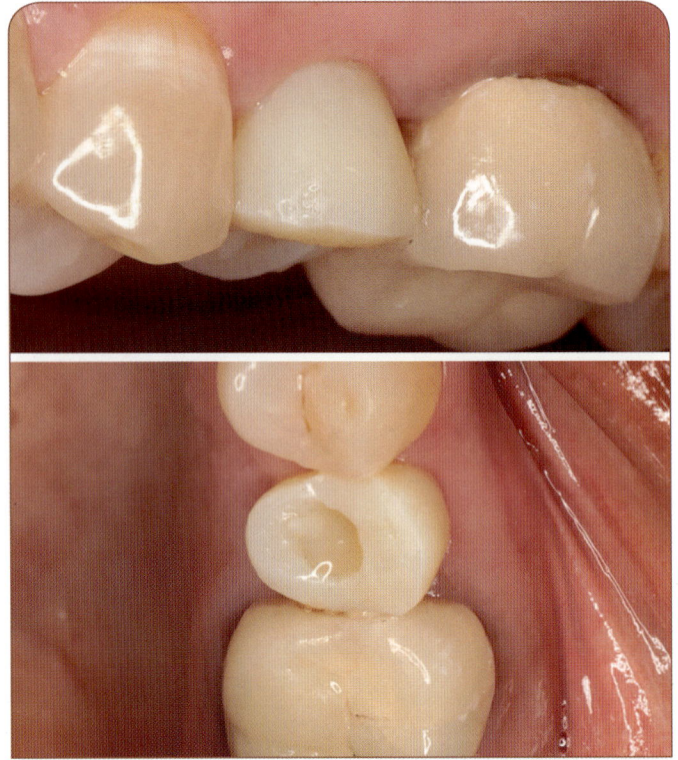

Fig. 11

3-week recall **(Fig. 11)**.

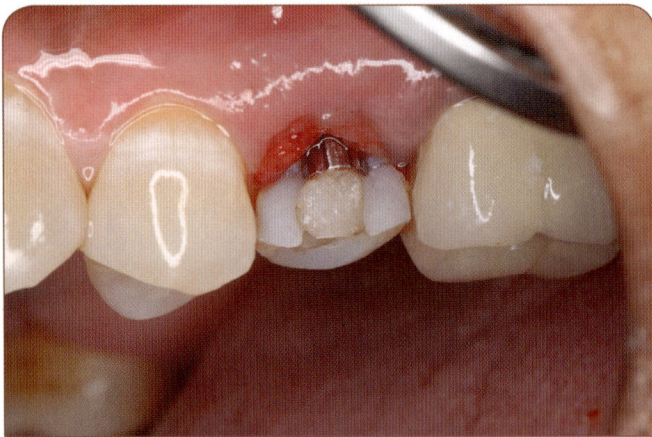

Fig. 12

As luck would have it, she bit into a chicken bone the day she was traveling abroad, and came to me in an emergency a few hours before her flight so did a quick repair and sent her off, since I was seeing her between patients on a packed day. This was 3 months after implantation. Fractured provisional restoration at 3 months post implantation **(Fig. 12)**.

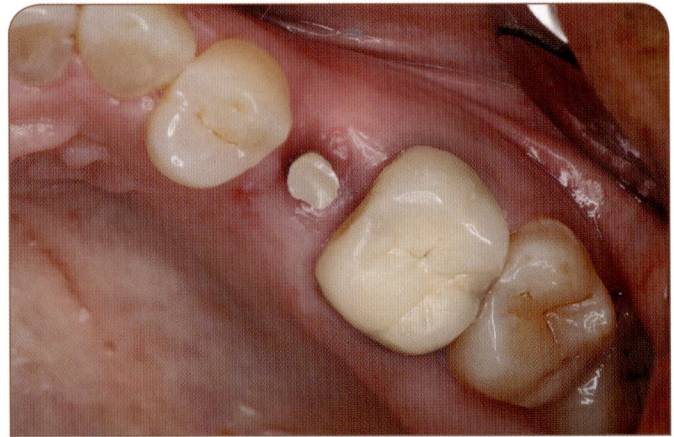

Fig. 13

By the time she reached Hong Kong, it was all gone, and this is how she came back from Japan 3 weeks later. 3 weeks after restoration fracture **(Fig. 13)**.

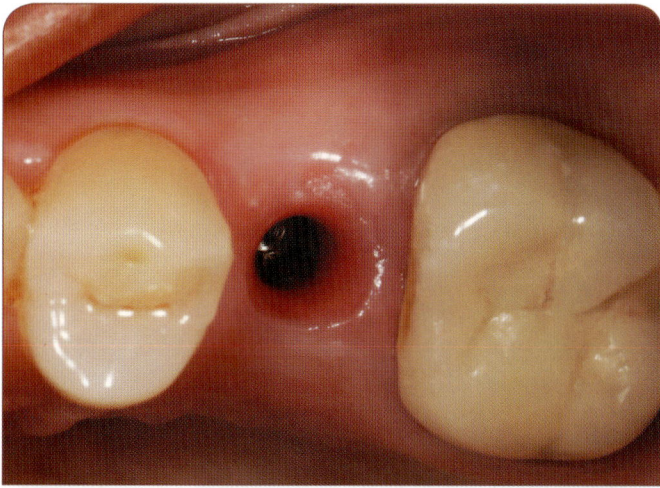

Fig. 14

Changed to a healing abutment after making her impressions. This is on the day of crown insertion (Fig. 14).

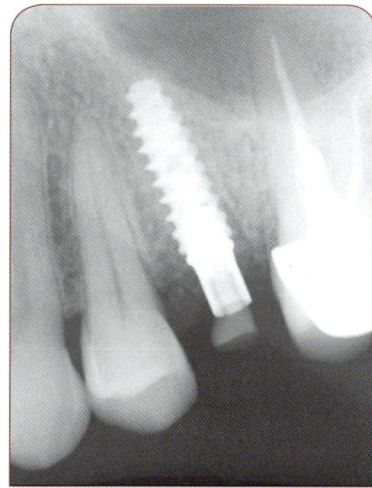

Fig. 15

Radiograph at 4 months (Fig. 15).

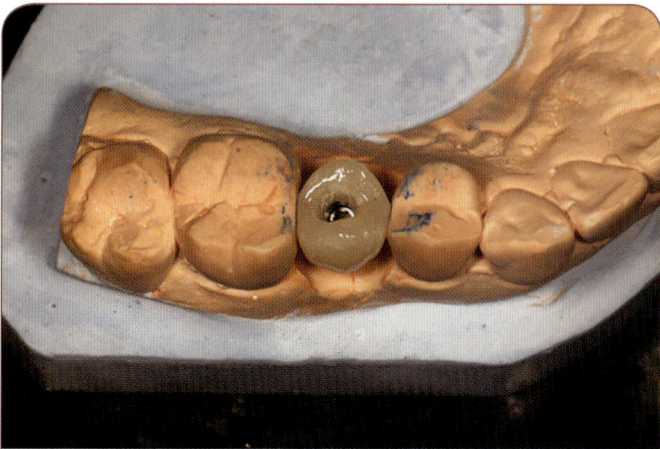

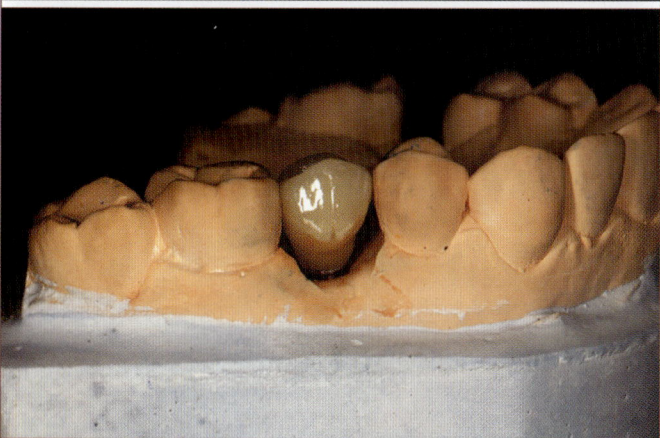

Fig. 16

E-max bonded to Ti base. Final screw retained crown in PFM (Fig. 16).

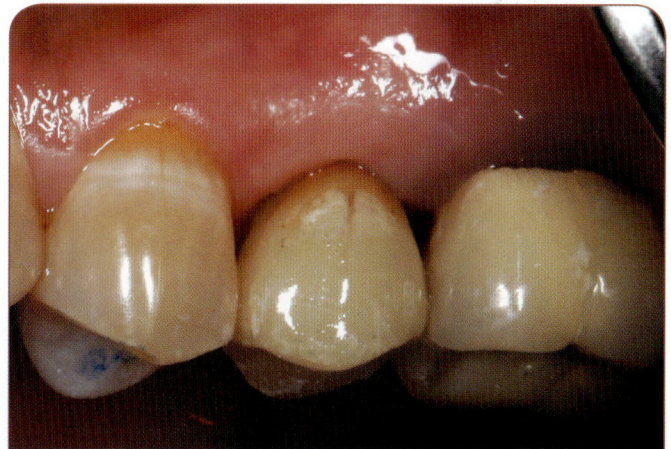

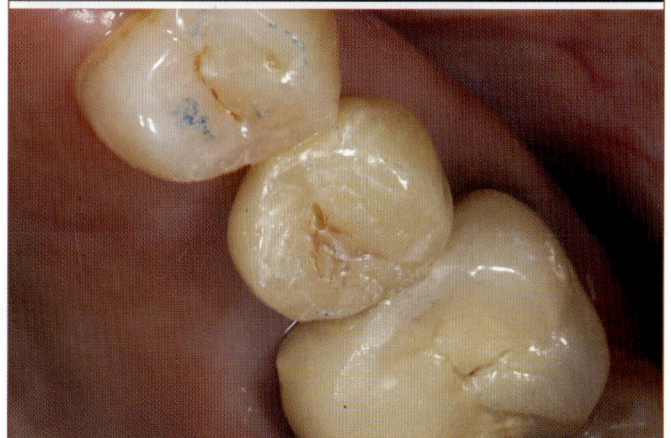

Fig. 17

Immediate post insertion (Lateral and occlusal view) (Fig. 17).

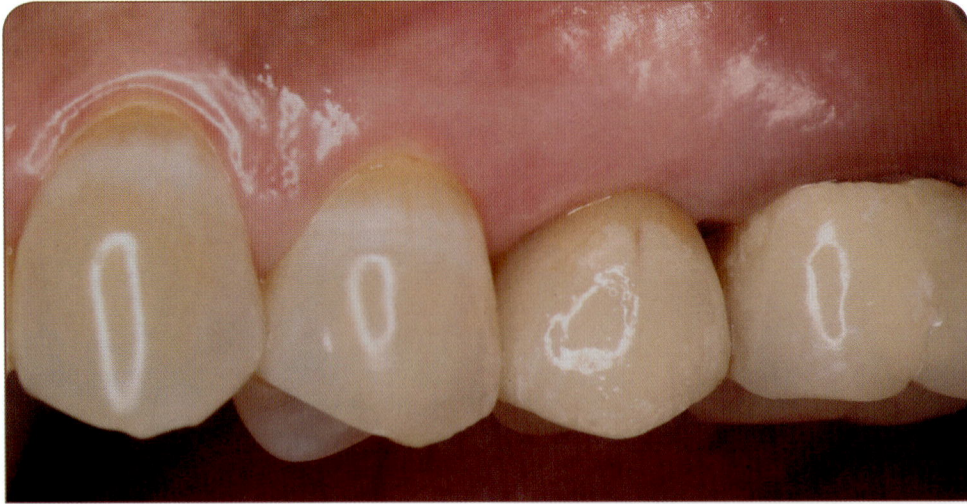

Fig. 18

Ten days postinsertion. I expect some creep of the distal papilla. Now she does not like the way the molar crown looks and wants to change it **(Fig. 18)**.

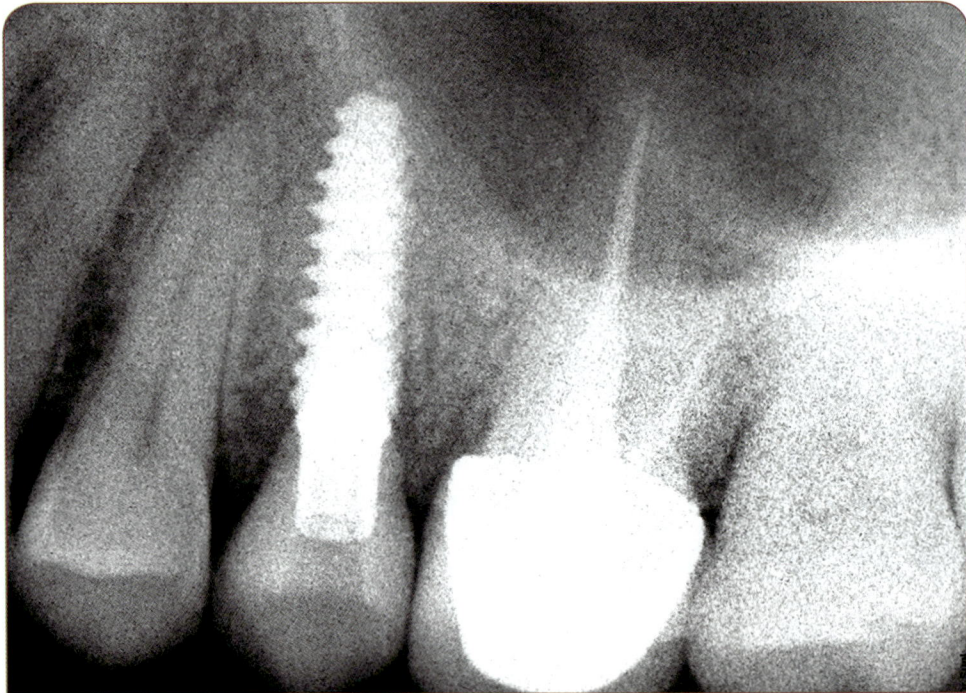

Fig. 19

Final radiograph **(Fig. 19)**.

Saj Jivraj

GUIDED SURGERY PLANNING FOR
FAILING CENTRAL INCISORS

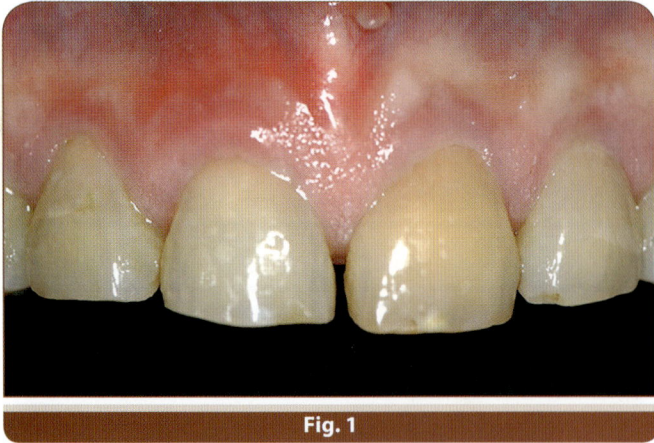

Fig. 1

Preoperative 2 centrals failing **(Fig. 1)**.

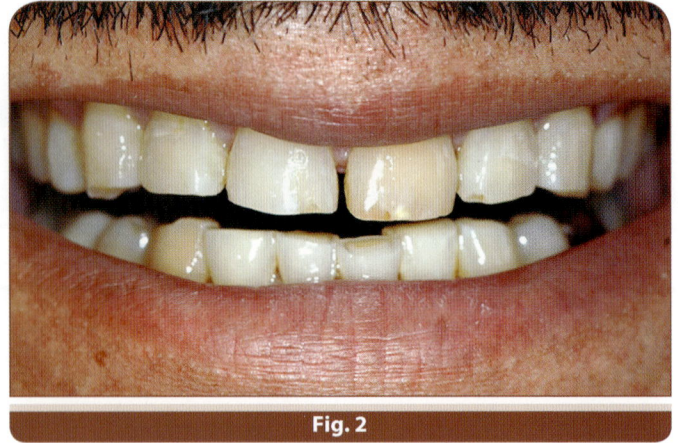

Fig. 2

Preoperative smile **(Fig. 2)**.

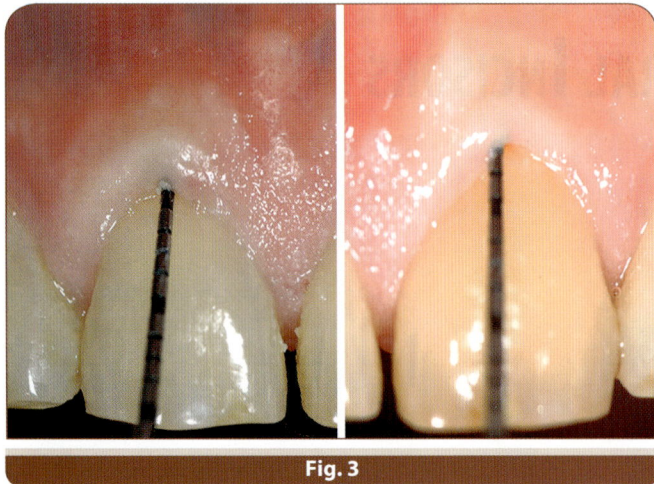

Fig. 3

Probing to determine crest position **(Fig. 3)**.

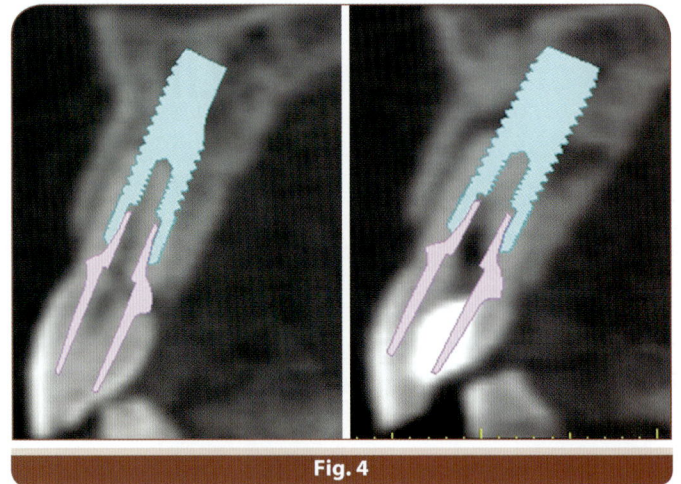

Fig. 4

Guided surgery planning **(Fig. 4)**.

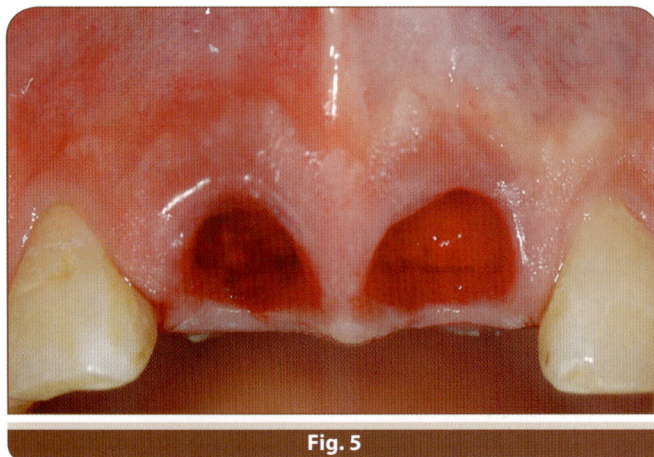

Fig. 5

Teeth atraumatically extracted. Integrity of buccal plate evaluated **(Fig. 5)**.

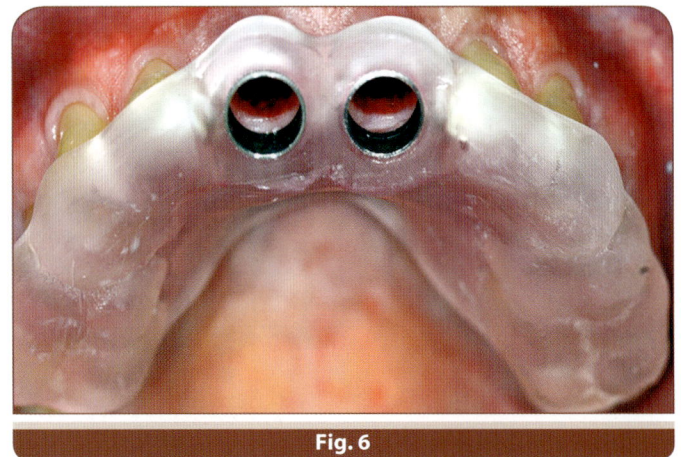

Fig. 6

Implants placed using guide **(Fig. 6)**.

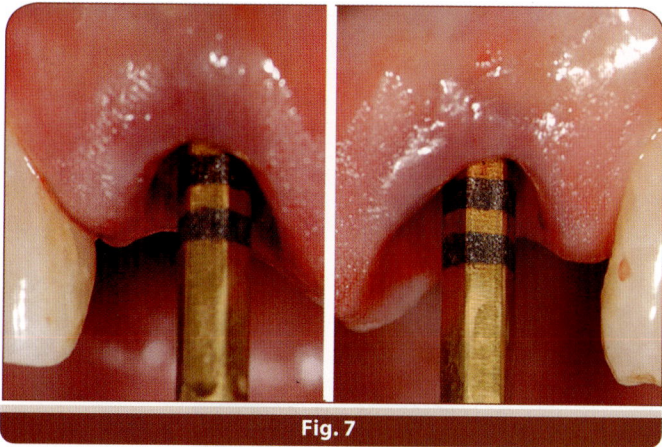

Fig. 7

Implant depth evaluation (Fig. 7).

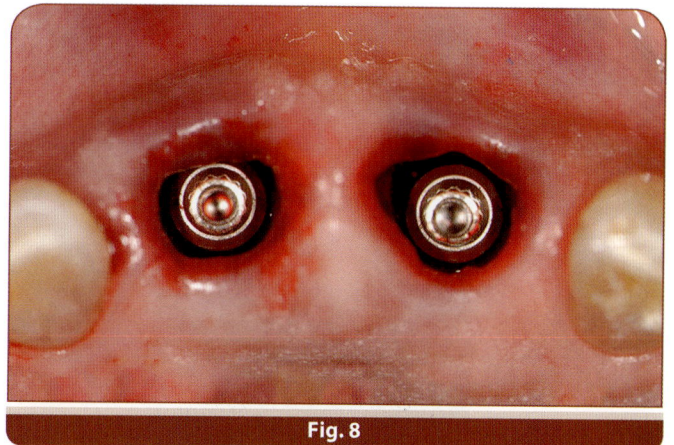

Fig. 8

Primary stability achieved to 50 Ncm (Fig. 8).

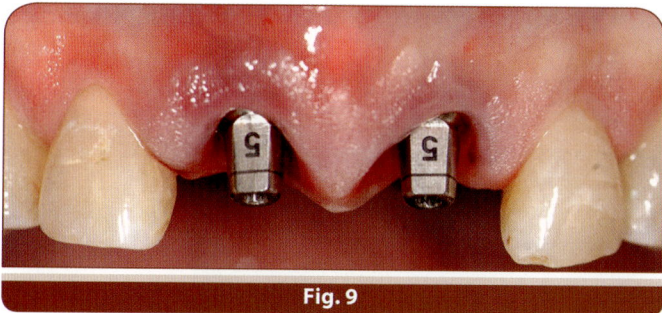

Fig. 9

Stock abutments placed (Fig. 9).

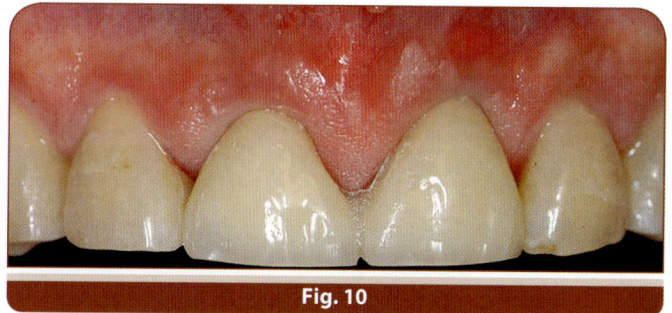

Fig. 10

Implants immediately loaded with undercontoured provisionals. No cement used, friction fit (Fig. 10).

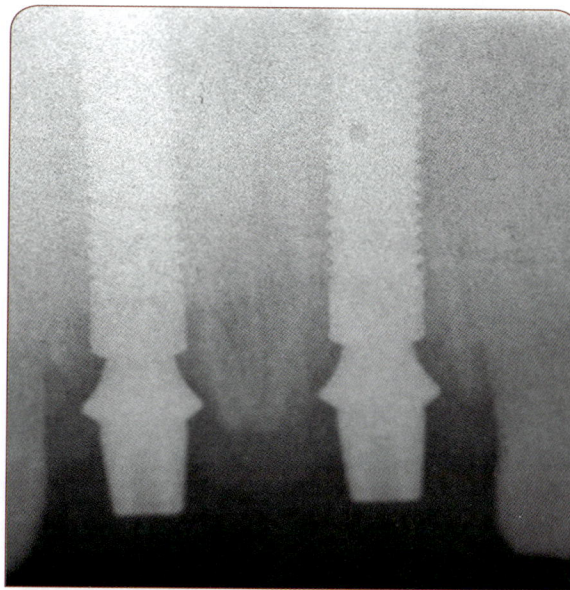

Fig. 11

Radiograph to verify seating of abutments (Fig. 11).

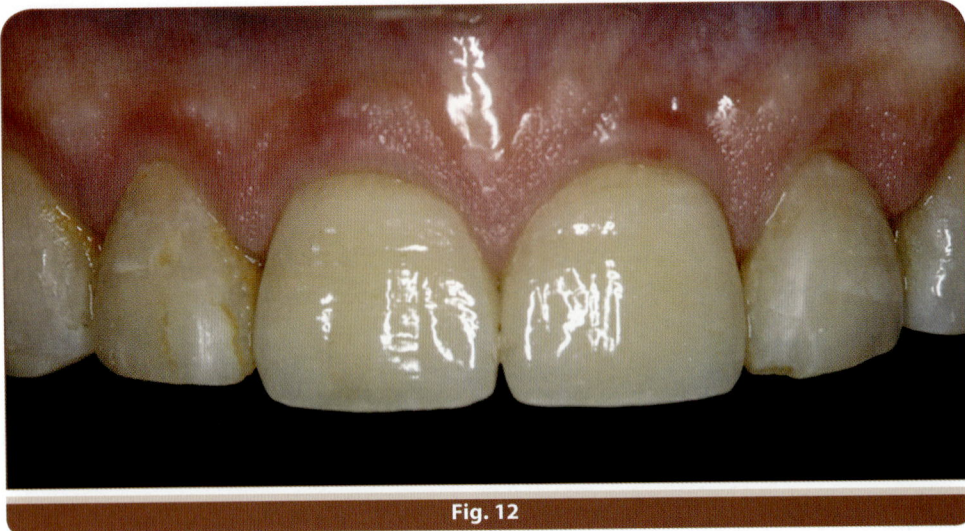

Fig. 12

Definitive restorations, Zirconia-based cemented restorations. Cement line must follow contour of gingiva and be 0.5 mm subgingival. Minimal cement is used for cementation **(Fig. 12)**.

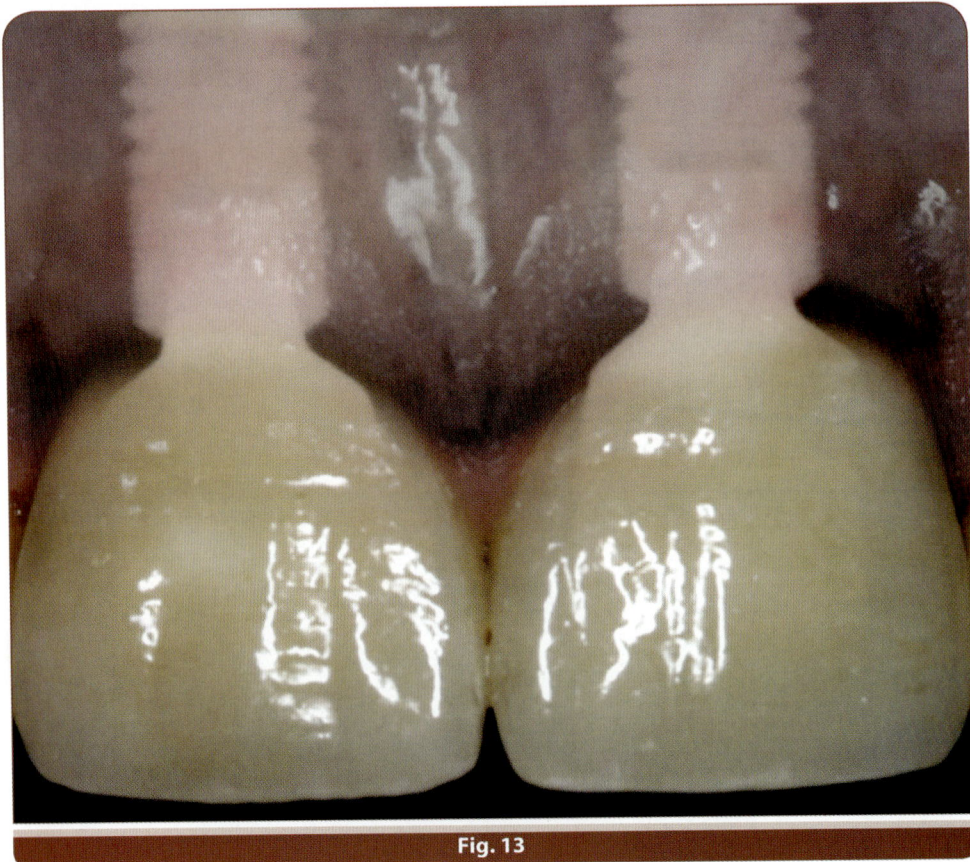

Fig. 13

Superimposition to show bone and papilla **(Fig. 13)**.

Saj Jivraj

Two Failing Central Incisors: Immediate Implantation and Provisionalization

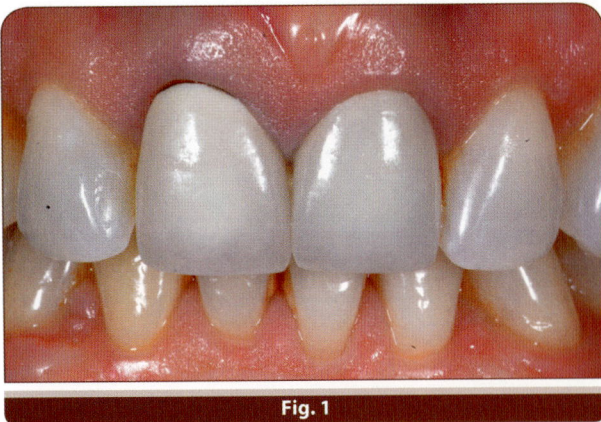

Fig. 1

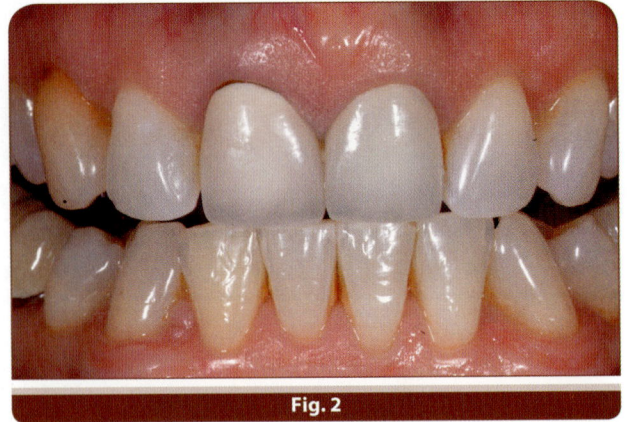

Fig. 2

Two centrals endodontically failing. Deep vertical overlap, two-step occlusion, thick tissue, high smile line, gingival margin same as laterals **(Fig. 1)**.

Timing of placement, type of implants, how do we provisionalize? Patient does not want to be without teeth. Deep vertical overlap. Patient refuses orthodontics **(Fig. 2)**.

Timing of placement: Extraction and immediate placement. Type of Implants: 2 implants (Internal connection with aggressive threads). How do we provisionalize? Fixed screw retained provisionals same day. Effect on papilla? We will lose 1–1.5 mm of papilla. Nightguard.

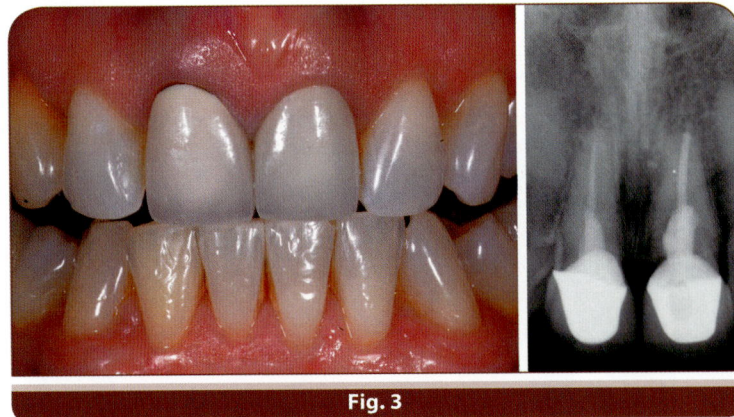

Fig. 3

Endodontically failing central incisors. Patient's treatment planned for dental implants with immediate provisional restorations **(Fig. 3)**.

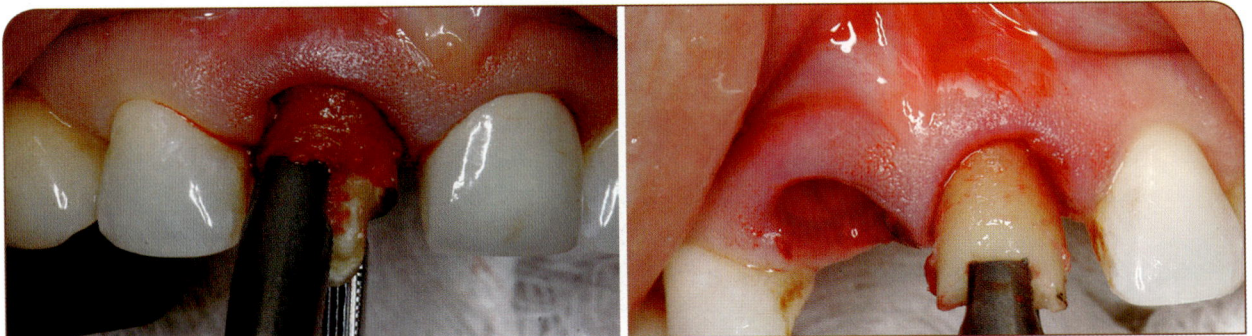

Fig. 4

Teeth atraumatically extracted **(Fig. 4)**.

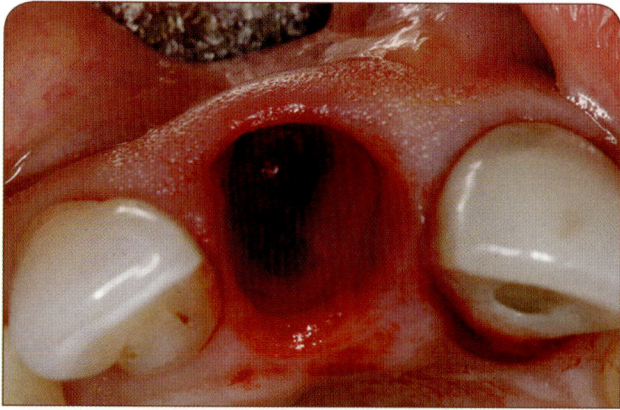

Fig. 5

Buccal plate intact **(Fig. 5)**.

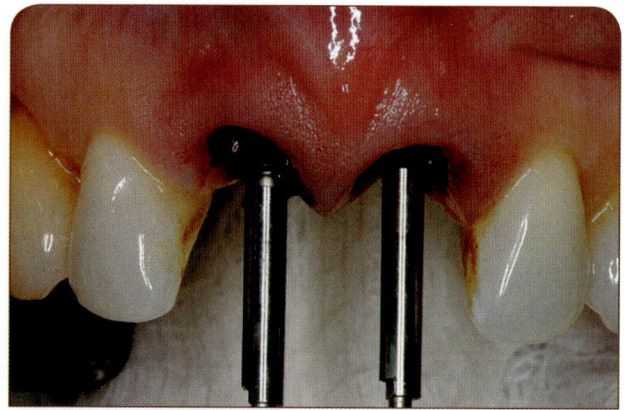

Fig. 6

Placed as far palatally as possible **(Fig. 6)**.

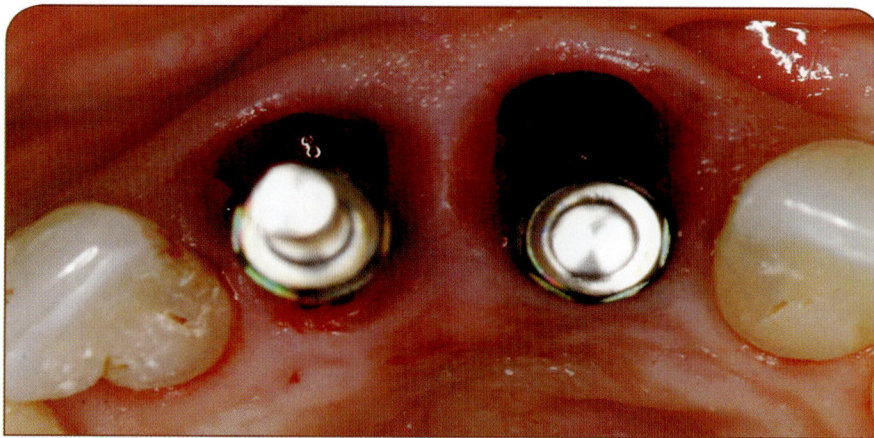

Fig. 7

Bone grafted buccal to implants **(Fig. 7)**.

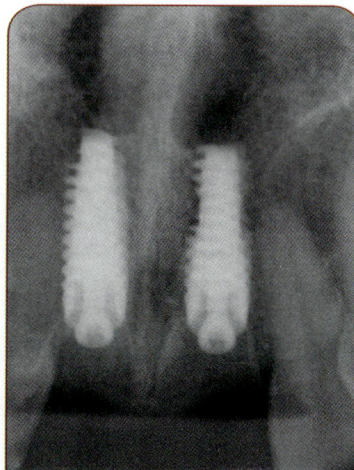

Fig. 8

IOPA X-ray **(Fig. 8)**.

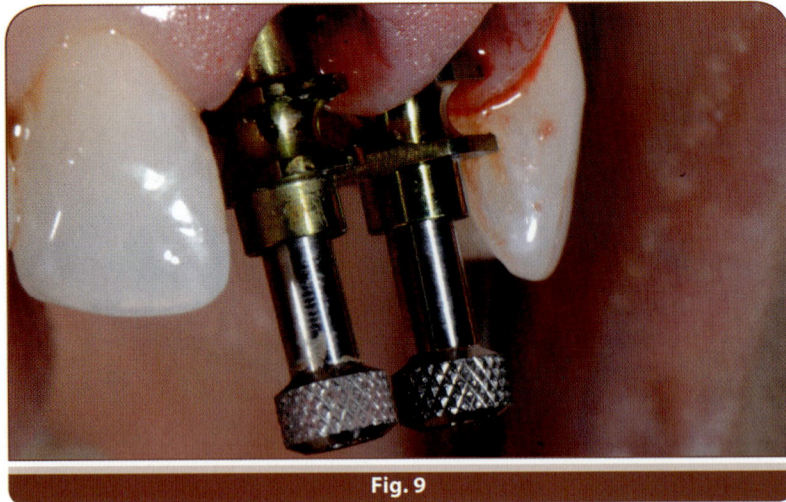

Fig. 9

Flapless placement with insertion torque of more than 50 N/cm^2 **(Fig. 9)**.

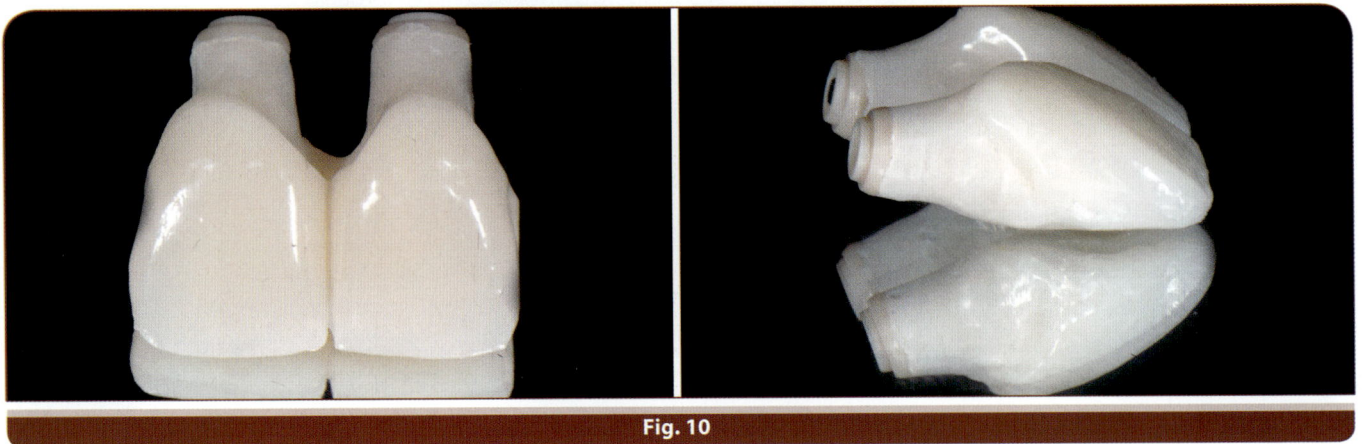

Fig. 10

Maximize soft tissue splinted screw retained. Crowns with undercontoured subgingival architecture **(Fig. 10)**.

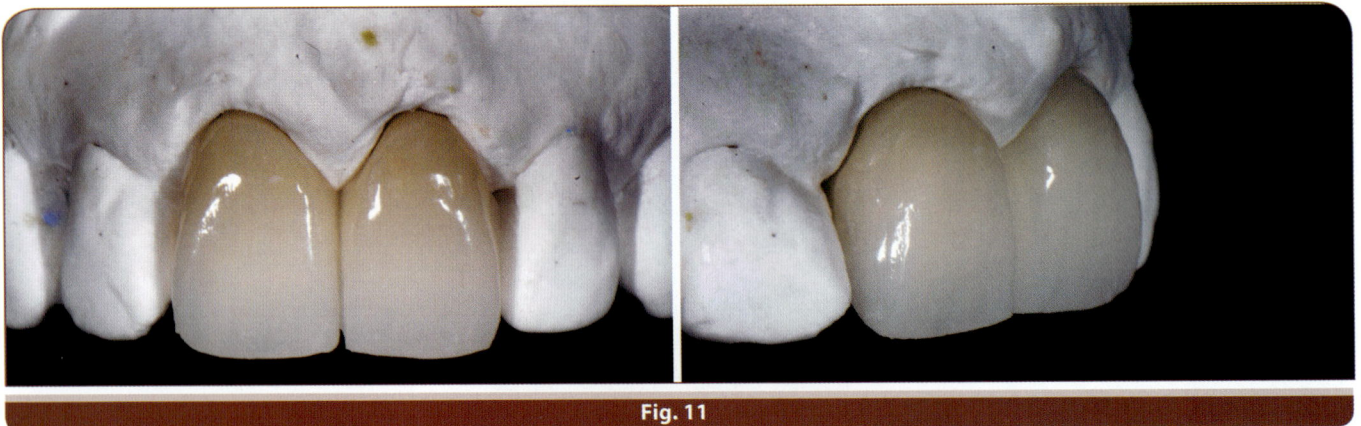

Fig. 11

Provisional restorations in laboratory **(Fig. 11)**.

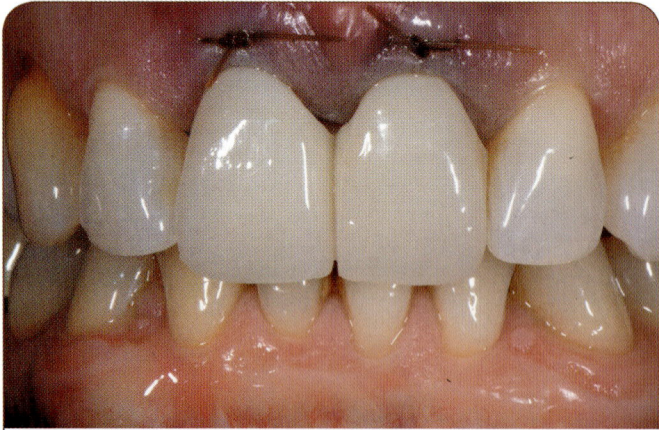

Provisional restorations in situ (**Fig. 12**).

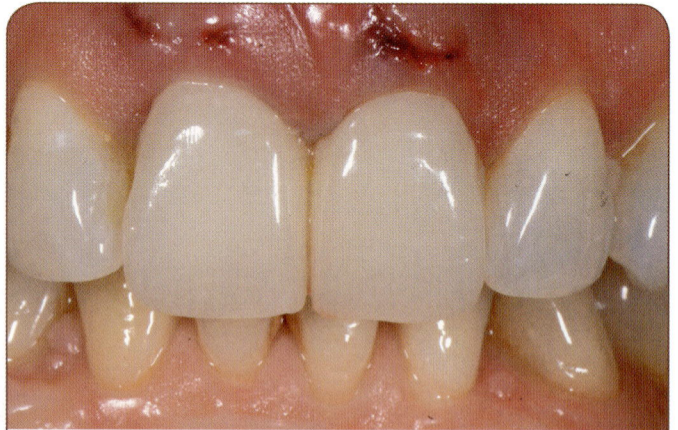

One week postoperative (**Fig. 13**).

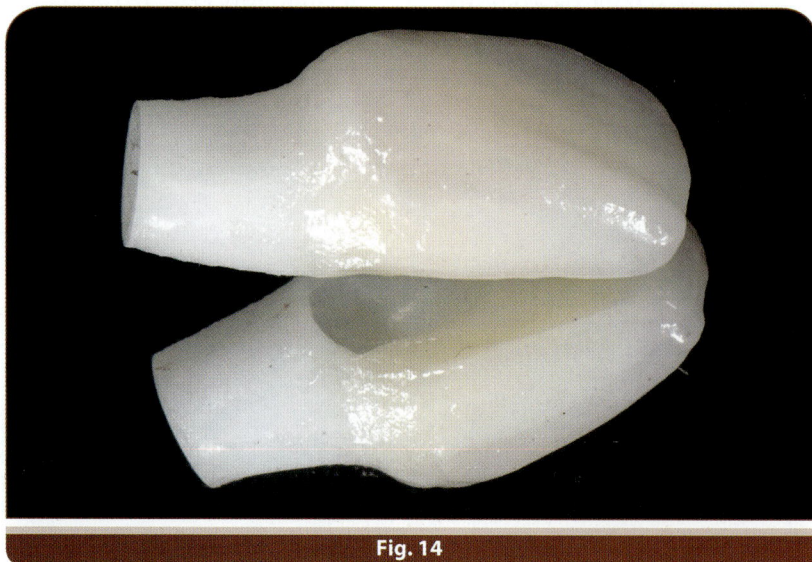

Concave subgingival contours: Use of altered screw channel to correct angle (**Fig. 14**).

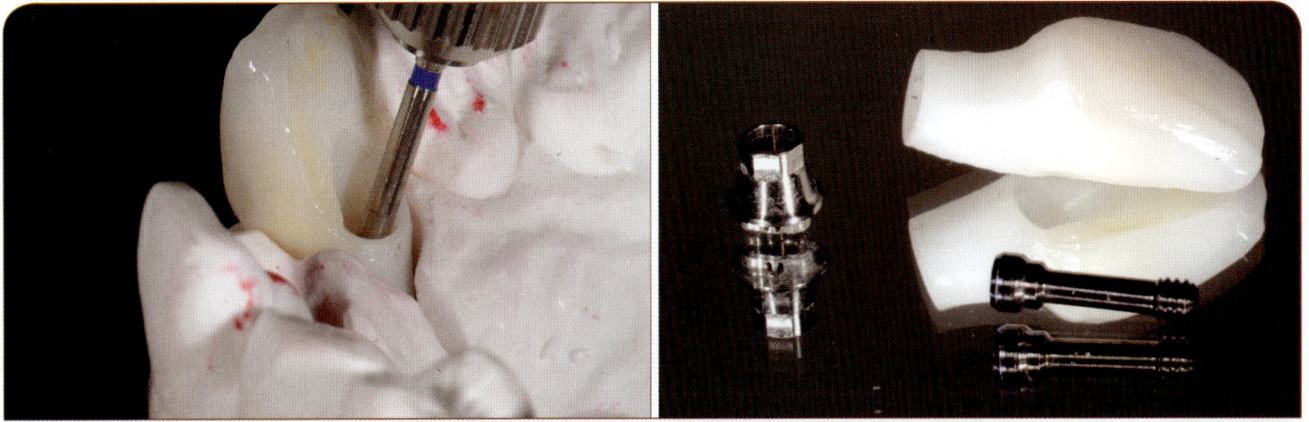

Fig. 15

Three piece, requires specific screw driver, can correct up to 25° **(Fig. 15)**.

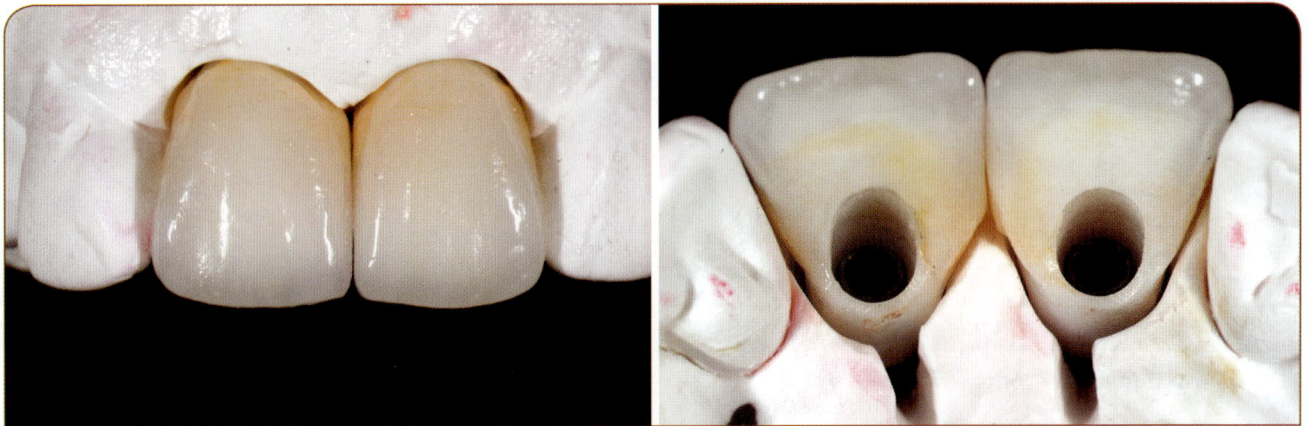

Fig. 16

Zirconia-based restorations in laboratory **(Fig. 16)**.

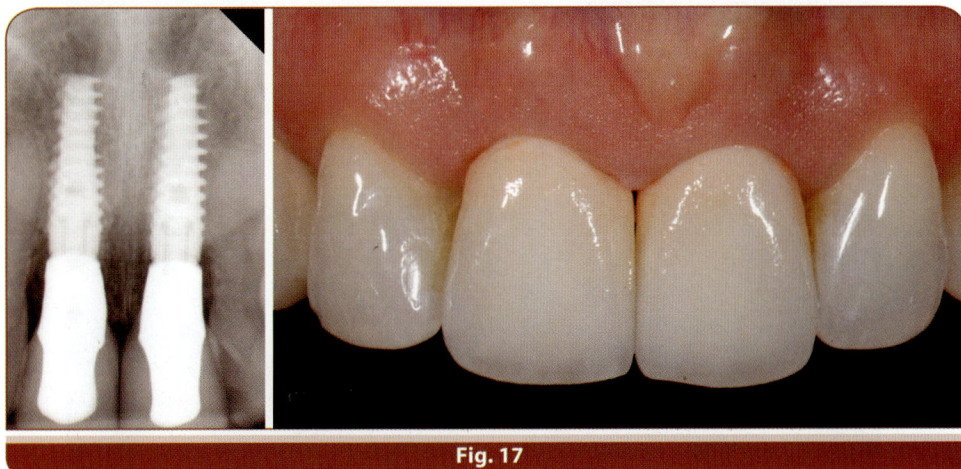

Fig. 17

Intraoral view of definitive restorations. Intraoral periapical radiograph showing good seat of abutments with final restoration and healthy crestal bone **(Fig. 17)**.

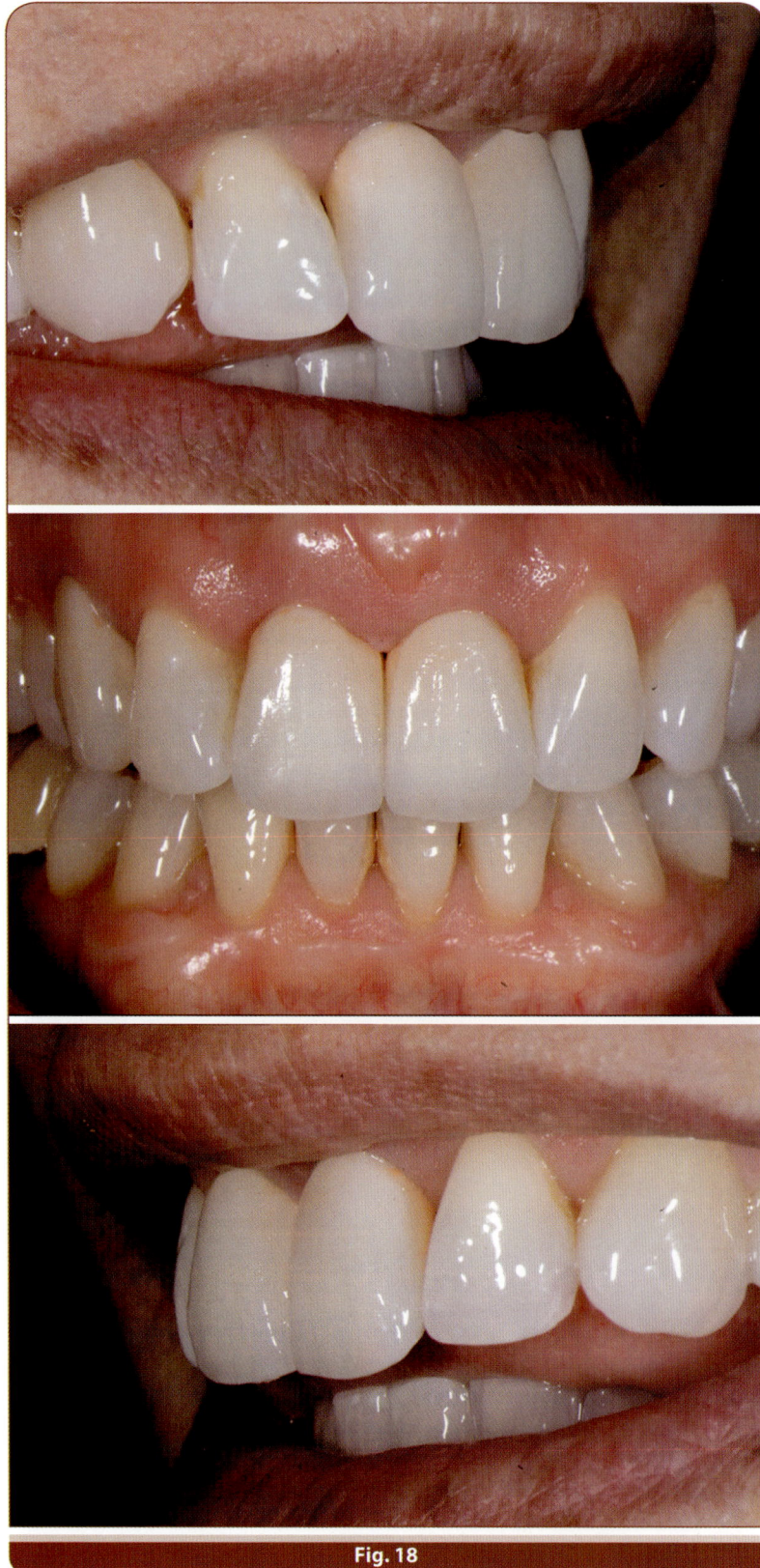

Fig. 18

One week postoperative **(Fig. 18)**.

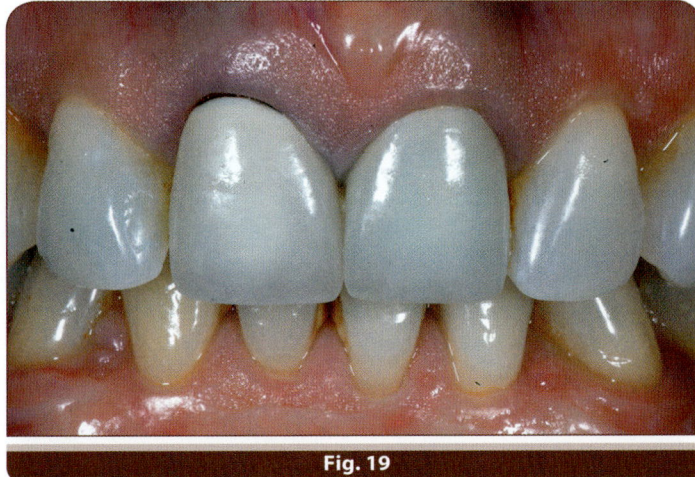

Fig. 19

Preoperative intraoral view **(Fig. 19)**.

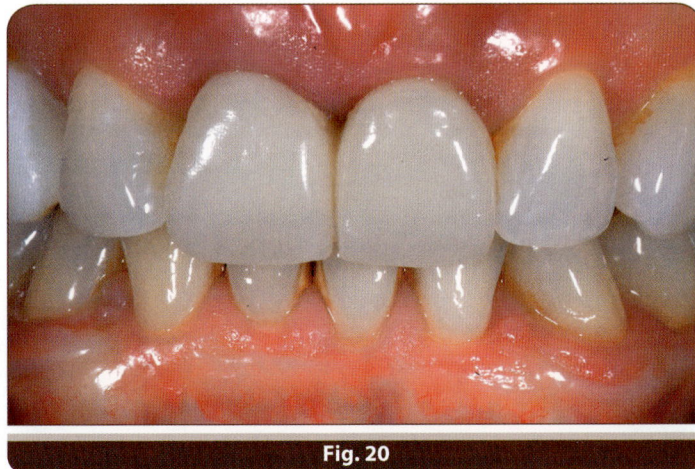

Fig. 20

Provisional crowns on tooth #11 and tooth #21 **(Fig. 20)**.

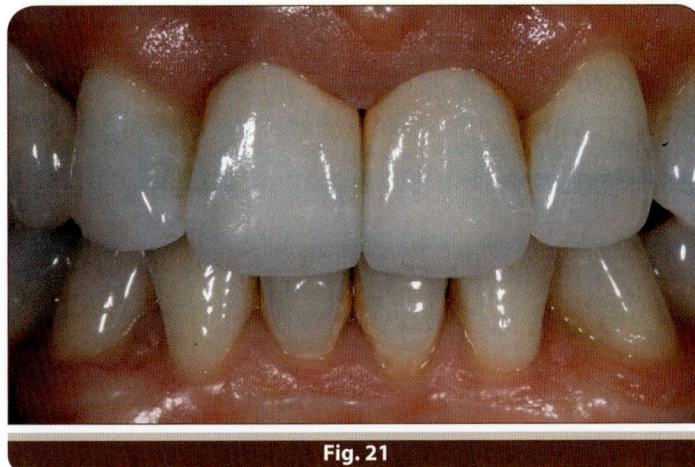

Fig. 21

Final restoration in place **(Fig. 21)**.

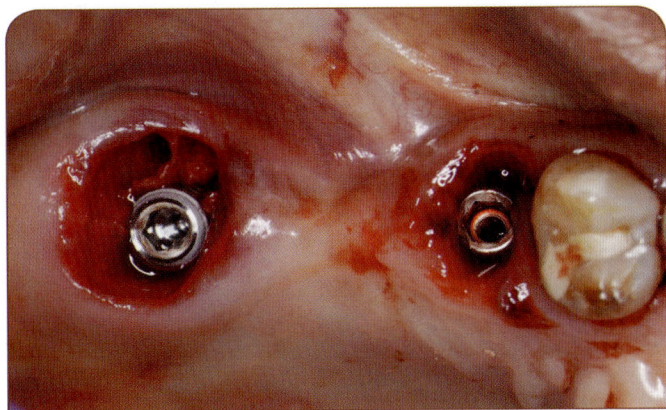

Fig. 7

Both implants achieved insertion torque of about 40 Ncm **(Fig. 7)**.

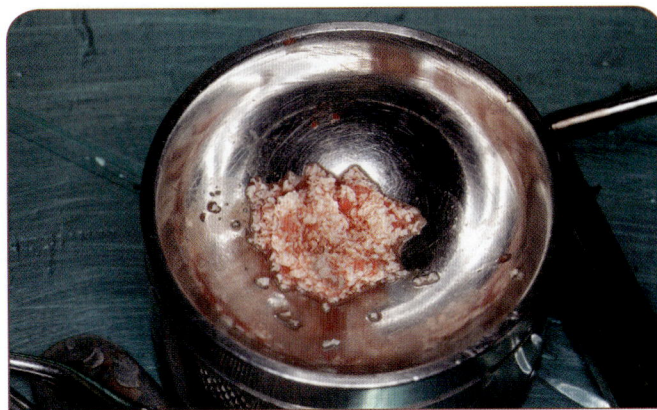

Fig. 8

Graft mix of autogenous and bovine bone **(Fig. 8)**.

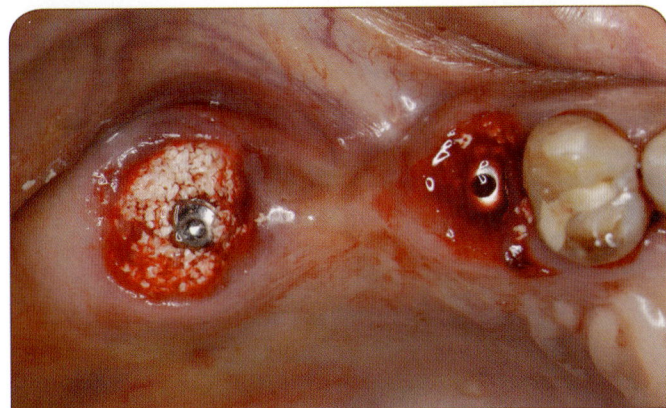

Fig. 9

Grafting around implants with cover screws in place **(Fig. 9)**.

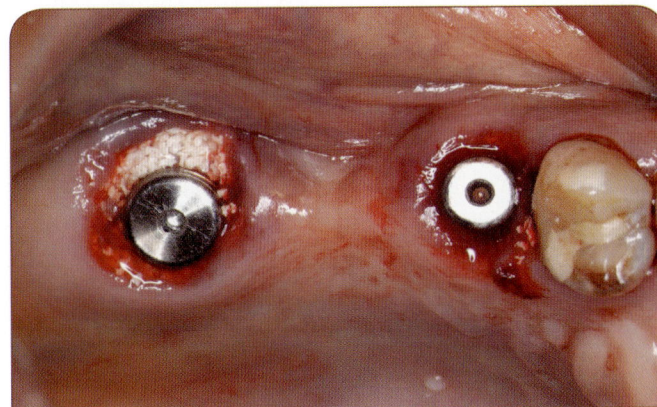

Fig. 10

Cover screws replaced with healing collars **(Fig. 10)**.

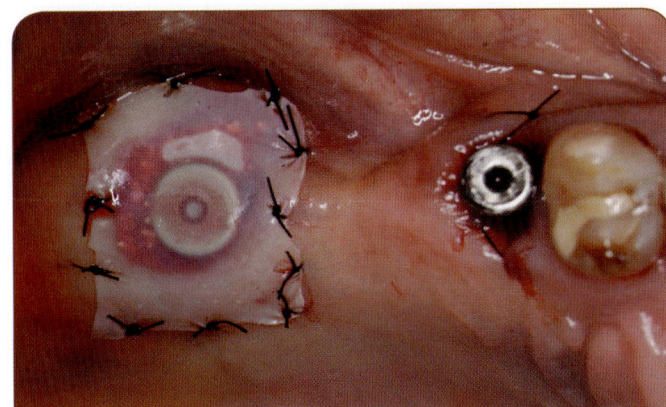

Fig. 11

Latex bandage to protect tooth #27. Optimum closure achieved around tooth #25 **(Fig. 11)**.

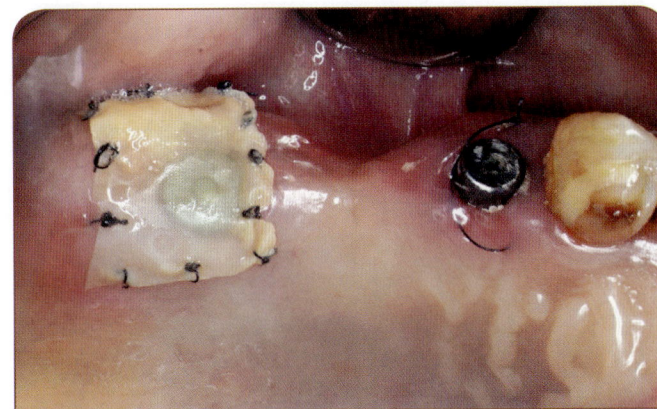

Fig. 12

One week recall **(Fig. 12)**.

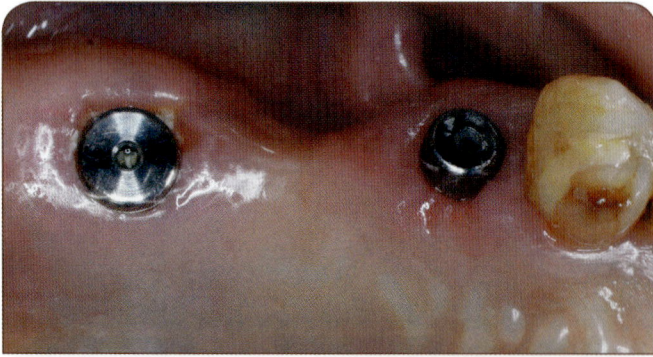
Fig. 13

One week recall—after suture and bandage removal and a chlorhoxidine (CHX) swab **(Fig. 13)**.

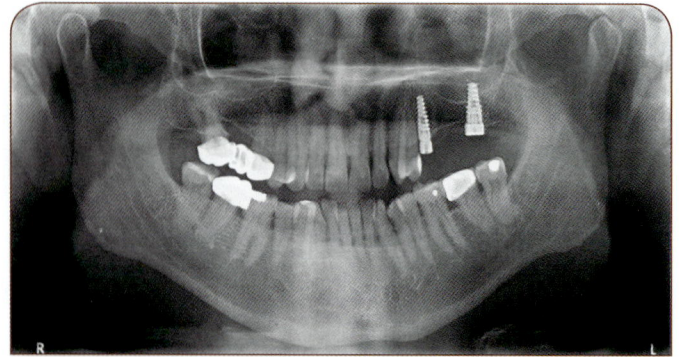
Fig. 14

Postsurgical **(Fig. 14)**.

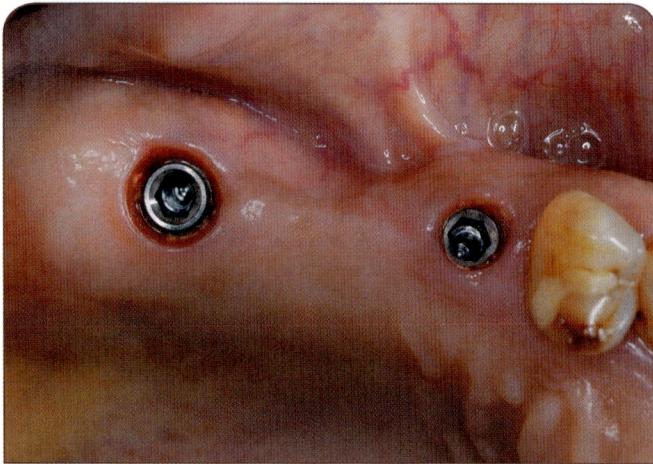
Fig. 15

Five months **(Fig. 15)**.

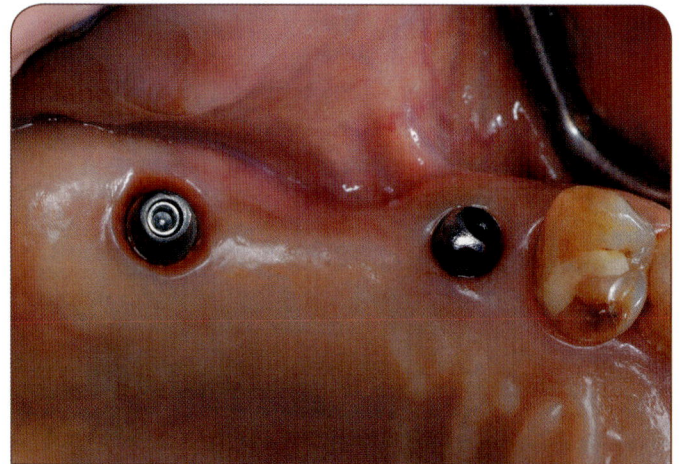
Fig. 16

Milled abutments in place **(Fig. 16)**.

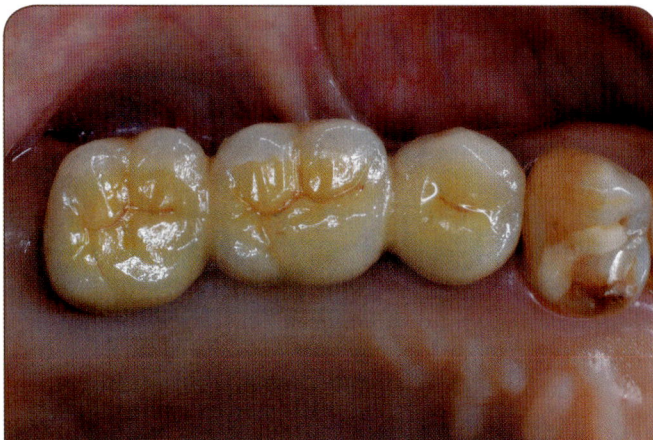
Fig. 17

Final prosthesis in place occlusal view **(Fig. 17)**.

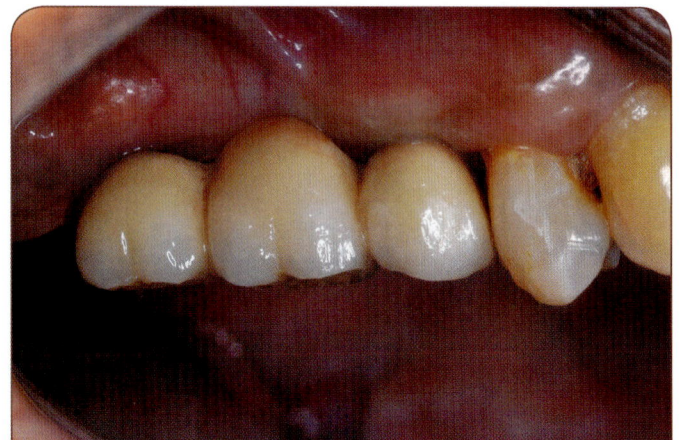
Fig. 18

Final prosthesis in place. Lateral view **(Fig. 18)**.

CASE STUDY 35

Amit Gulati

Immediate Extraction Implant Placement with Simultaneous GBR Double Poncho Technique

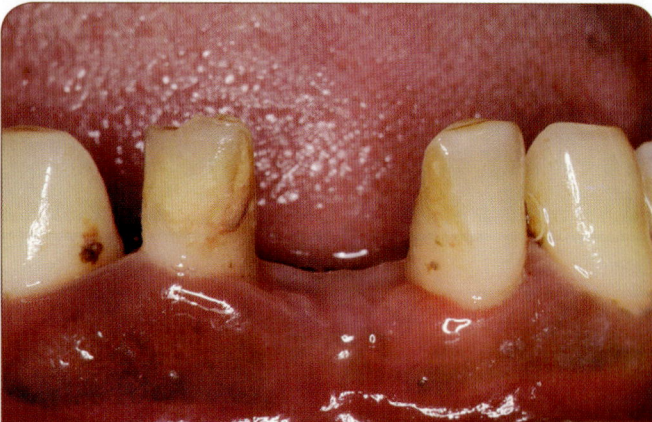

Fig. 1

Teeth #41, #31 lost few months back. Teeth #42, #32 Grade II mobile **(Fig. 1)**.

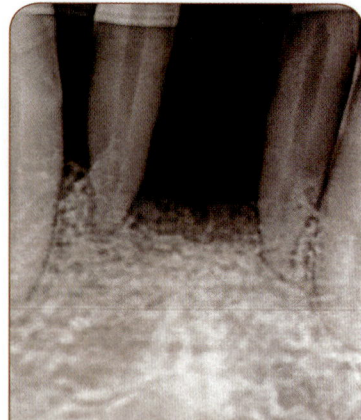

Fig. 2

Baseline intraoral periapical radiograph **(Fig. 2)**.

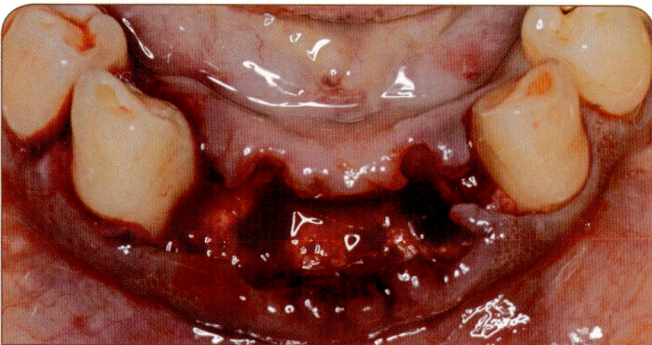

Fig. 3

Extraction of tooth #42, #32. Sockets curetted and irrigated with metronidazole IV solution **(Fig. 3)**.

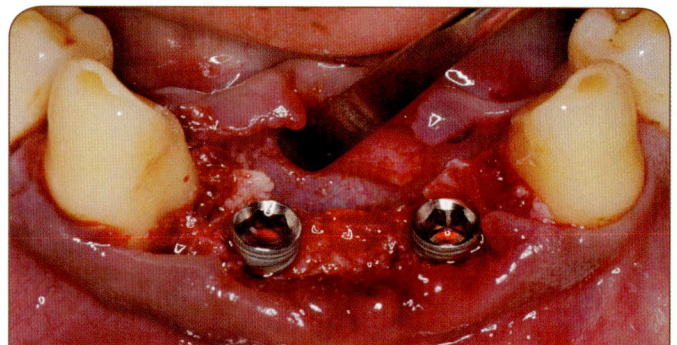

Fig. 4

Implants in position after preparing osteotomies. Implant head positions above the level of the native bone **(Fig. 4)**.

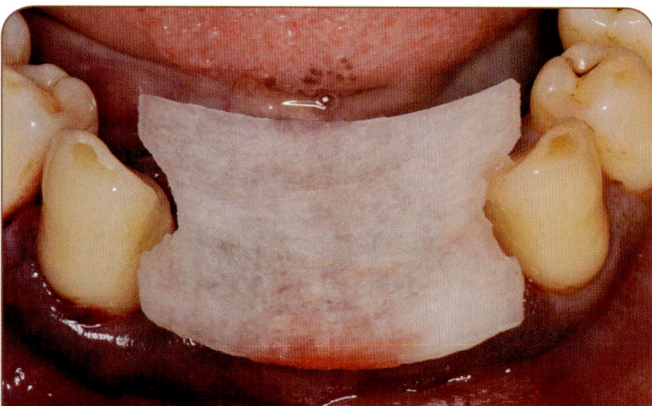

Fig. 5

Cytoplast—resorbable collagen membrane. Shaped to size **(Fig. 5)**.

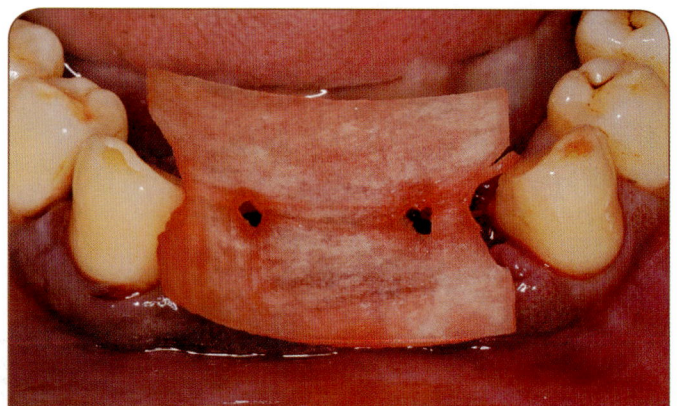

Fig. 6

Double Poncho technique **(Fig. 6)**.

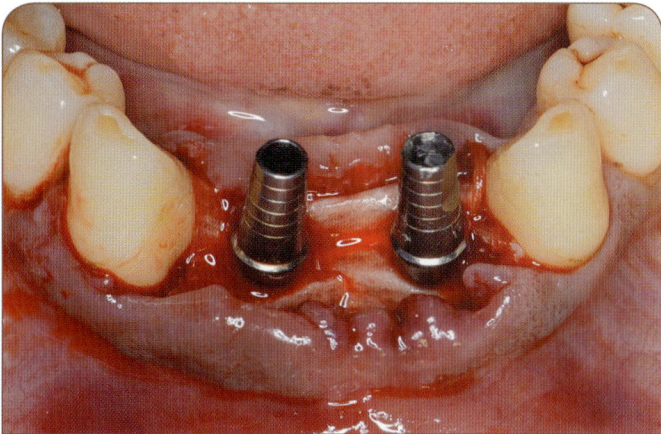

Fig. 7

Abutments stabilizing the membrane **(Fig. 7)**.

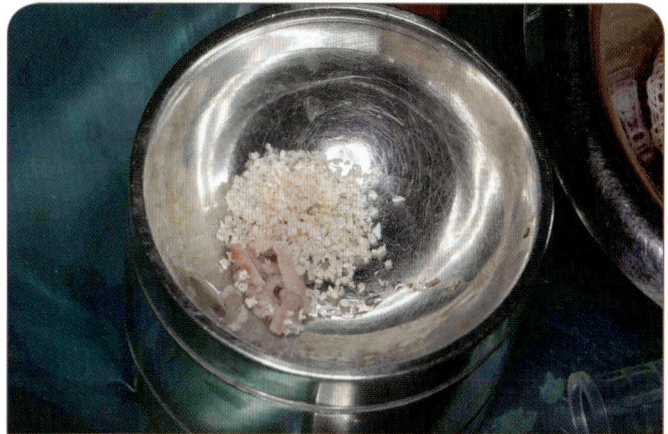

Fig. 8

Autogenous + cerabone **(Fig. 8)**.

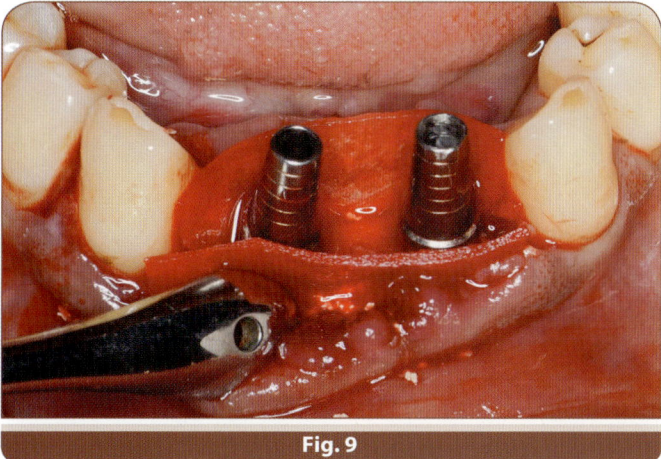

Fig. 9

Composite graft to augment the defect **(Fig. 9)**.

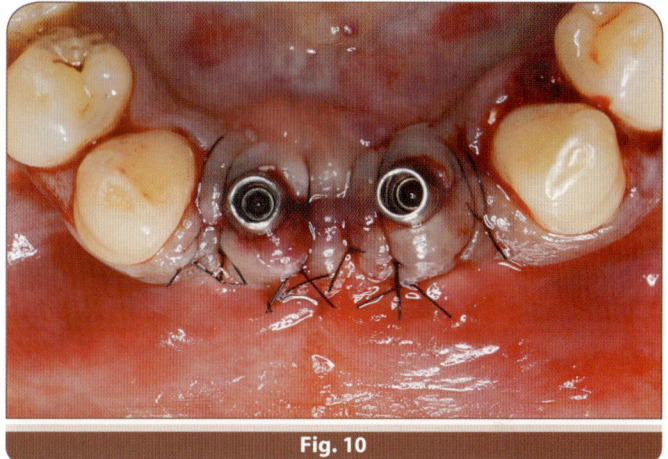

Fig. 10

Watertight closure achieved with 5-0 nylon **(Fig. 10)**.

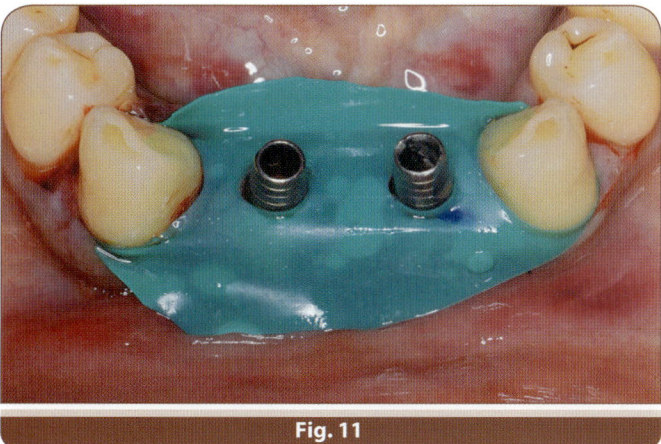

Fig. 11

Rubber dam isolation **(Fig. 11)**.

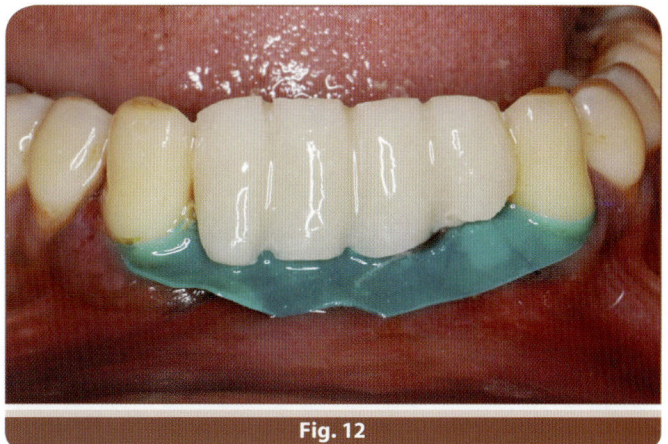

Fig. 12

Temporary fabricated with indirect technique using BIS-GMA resin **(Fig. 12)**.

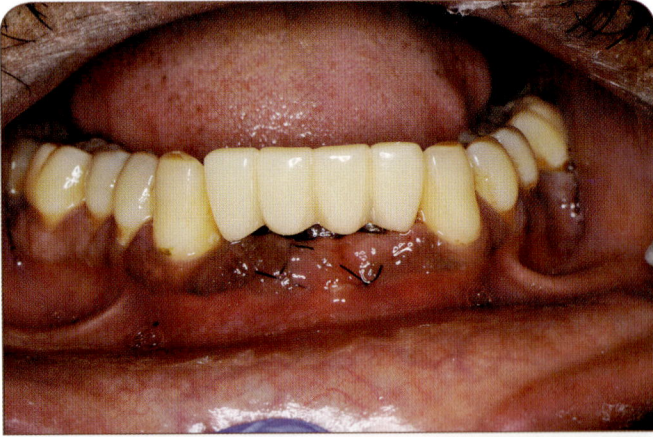
Fig. 13

Recall at 10 days postsurgery (**Fig. 13**).

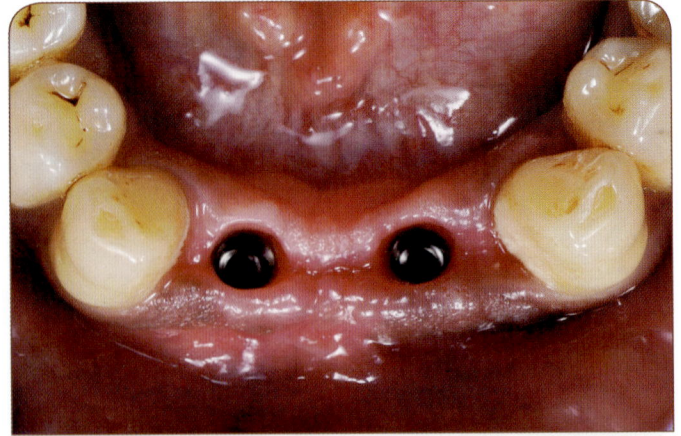
Fig. 14

Recall at 4 months postsurgery occlusal view (**Fig. 14**).

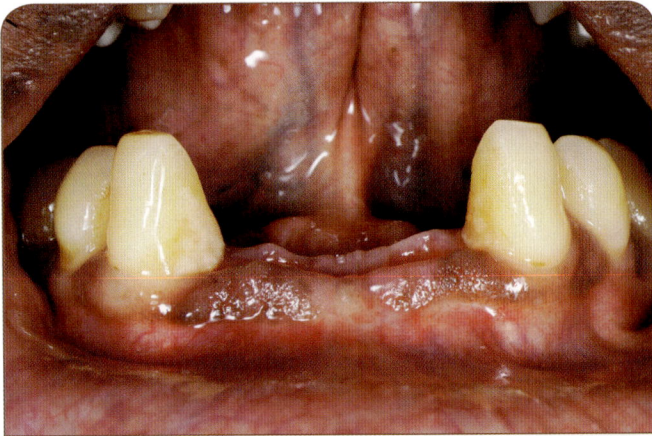
Fig. 15

Recall at 4 months postsurgery frontal view (**Fig. 15**).

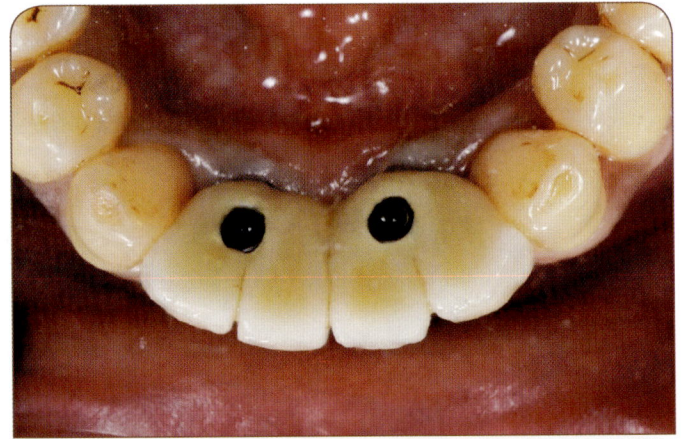
Fig. 16

Final screw retained PFM prosthesis—occlusal view (**Fig. 16**).

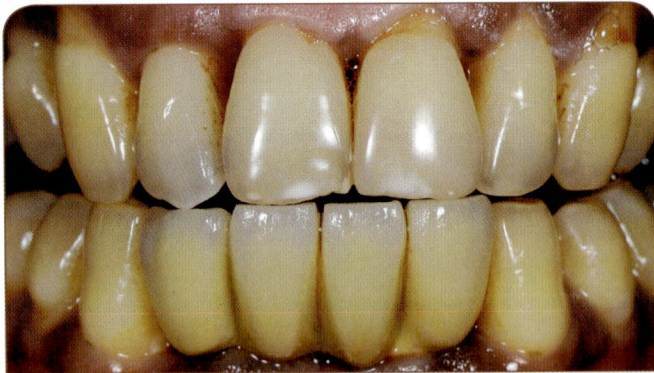
Fig. 17

Final screw retained PFM prosthesis—facial view (**Fig. 17**).

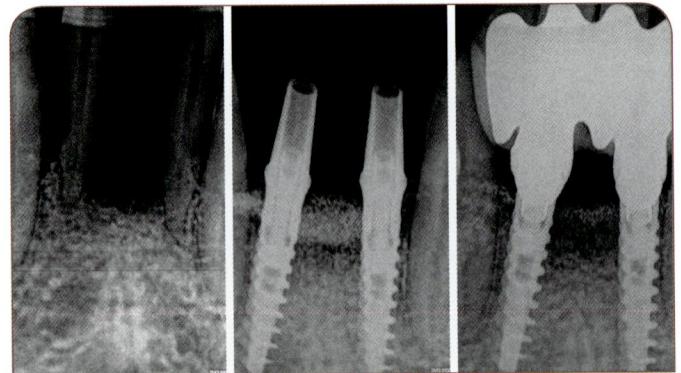
Fig. 18

Comparison of preoperative and postoperative radiographs (**Fig. 18**).

Praful Bali

SMILE DESIGNING ALONG WITH IMMEDIATE EXTRACTION OF A LATERAL INCISOR

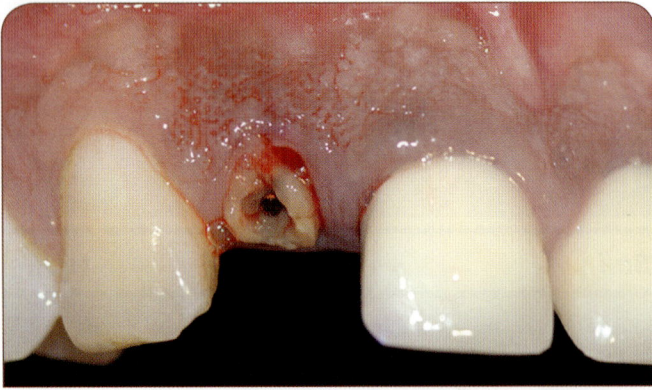

Fig. 1

Patient presents with fractured post and core on tooth #12. The tooth is planned for an implant therapy **(Fig. 1)**.

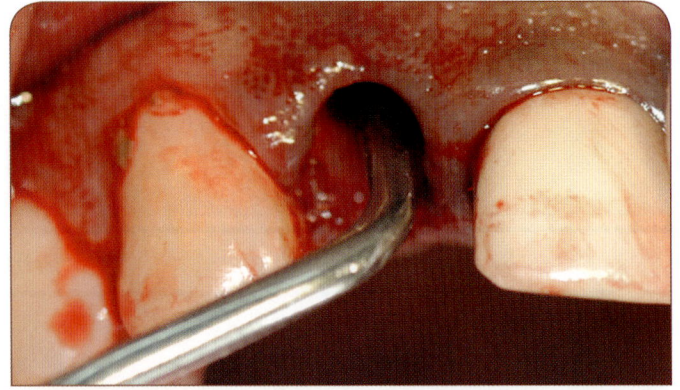

Fig. 2

Tooth is extracted atraumatically with the help of periotomes and the possibility of flapless surgery is evaluated by scoring all socket walls **(Fig. 2)**.

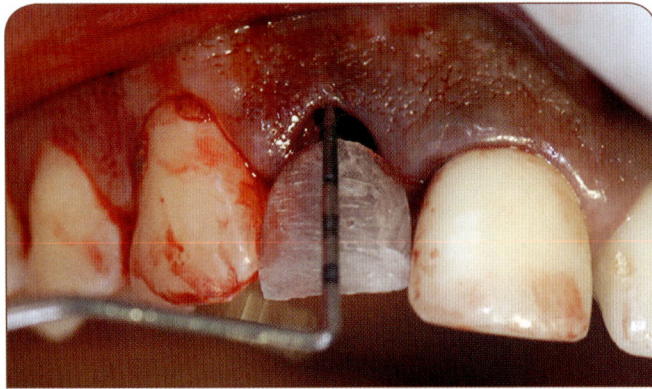

Fig. 3

3.5/13 Nobel replace implant is placed with the help of a surgical guide to achieve a 3D implant position **(Fig. 3)**.

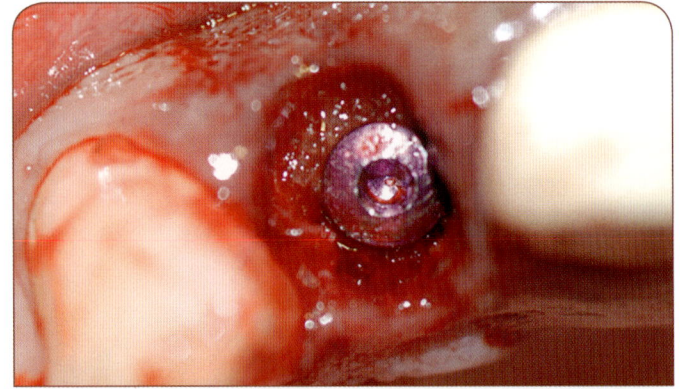

Fig. 4

The Jumping distance is grafted with Calcium Phosphosilicate (Novabone) **(Fig. 4)**.

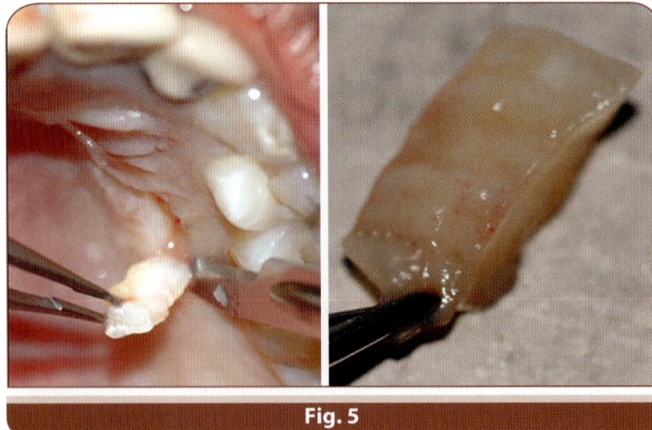

Fig. 5

A free gingival graft is taken from the palate **(Fig. 5)**.

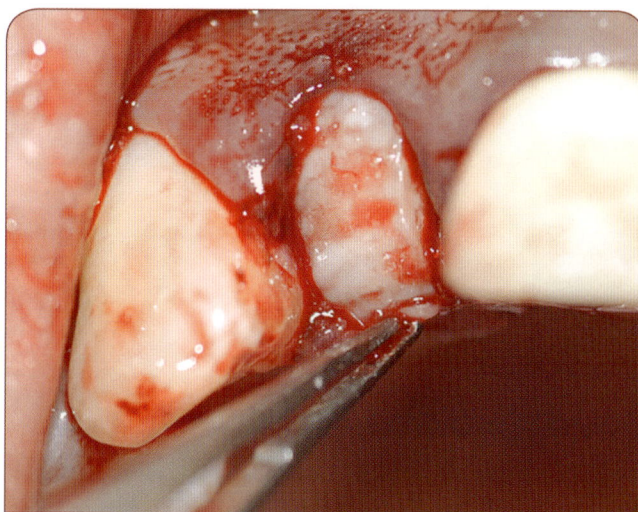

Fig. 6

A free gingival graft is placed over the socket defect and sutured around it **(Fig. 6)**.

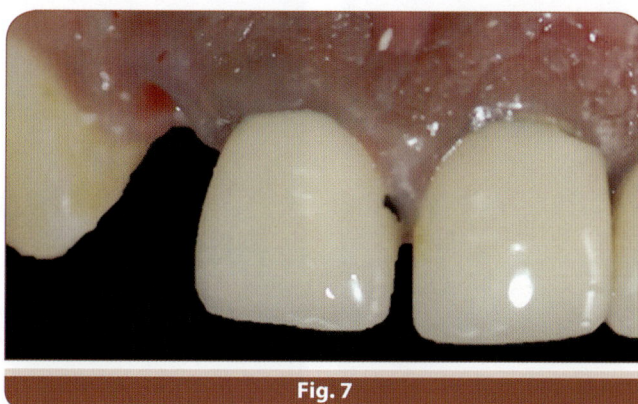

Fig. 7

Four months postoperatively, stage II surgery is done. Note the formation of the papilla and soft tissue integration **(Fig. 7)**.

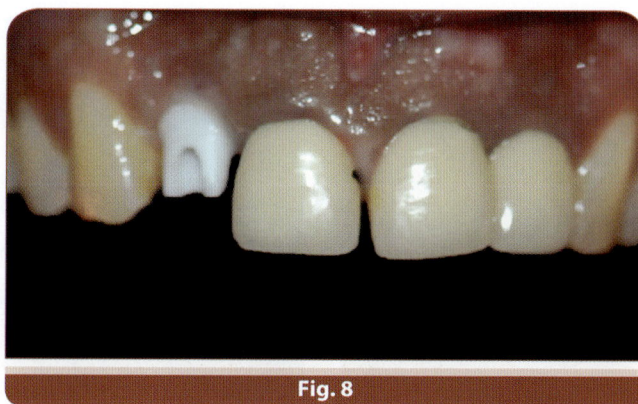

Fig. 8

A milled Procera abutment is torqued at 35 Ncm
At this moment it is suggested to the patient to get the old metal ceramic crowns on teeth # 11,21,22 also changed. Endo treatment of these teeth has already been done. The patient agrees for a smile makeover **(Fig. 8)**.

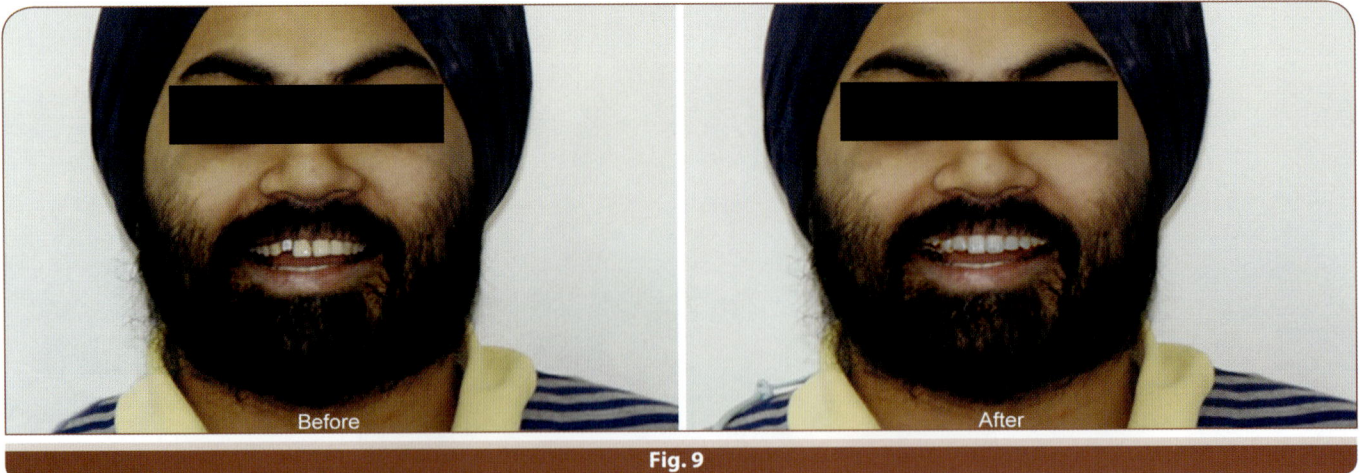

Fig. 9

The GPS software is used to build up a waxup and immediately shown to the patient. The patient gets convinced for eliminating the diastema and the smile makeover immediately **(Fig. 9)**.

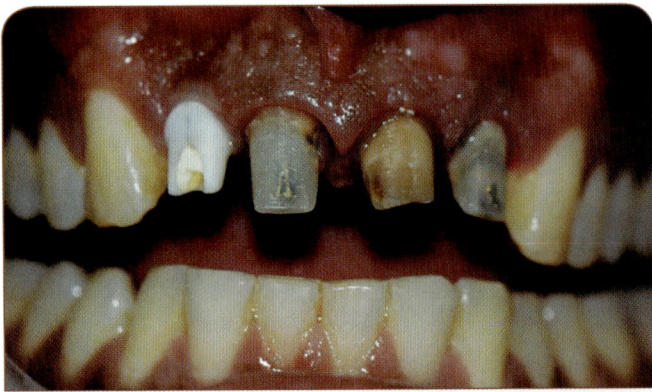

Fig. 10

Teeth preparation done for individual all ceramic crowns on teeth #11,21,22 and an all ceramic on implant too **(Fig. 10)**.

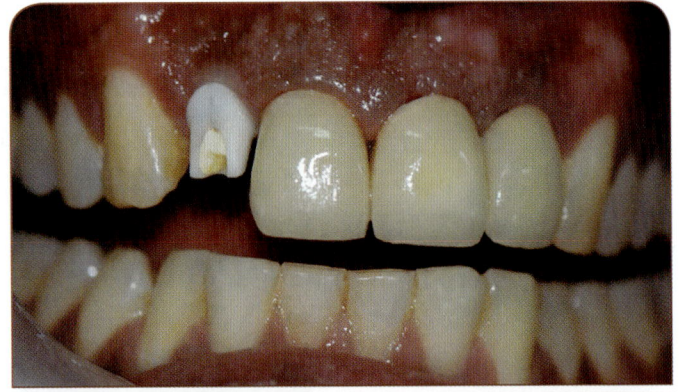

Fig. 11

The E max crowns are cemented on the teeth **(Fig. 11)**.

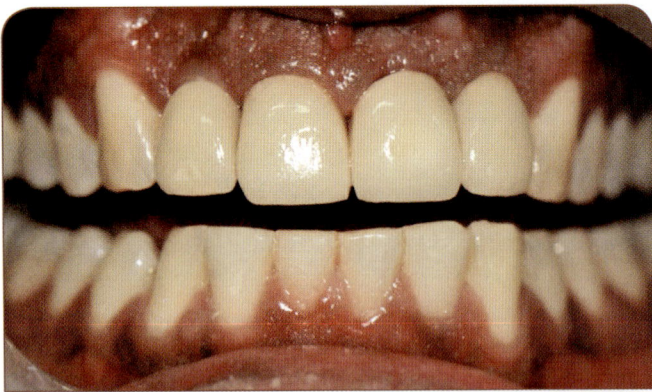

Fig. 12

E-Max crown on the implant also completing the anterior esthetic work **(Fig. 12)**.

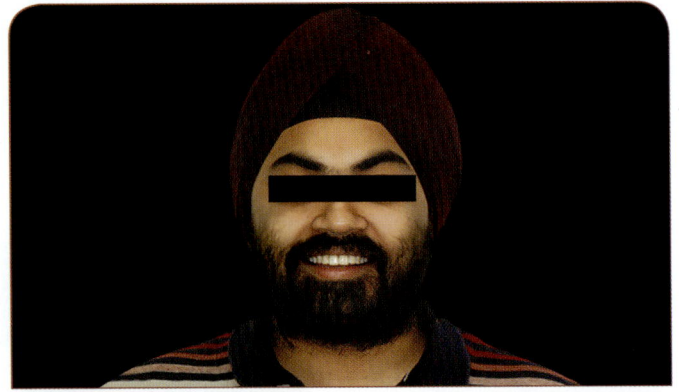

Fig. 13

Smile makeover of the patient **(Fig. 13)**.

Sujit Bopardikar

EXTRACTION AND IMMEDIATE IMPLANT PLACEMENT WITH IMMEDIATE PROVISIONAL AND ALL PORCELAIN RESTORATION

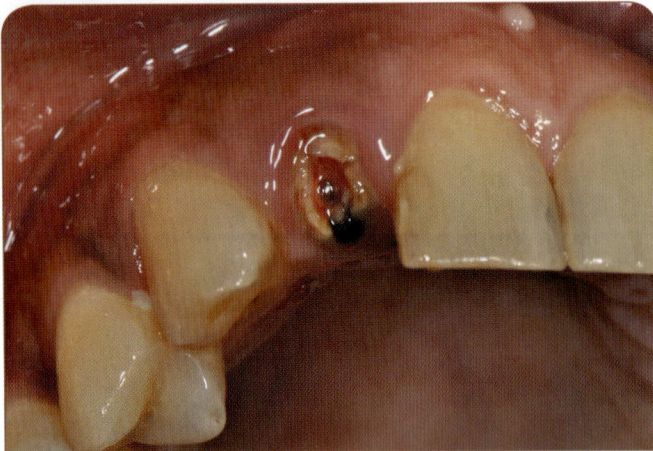

Fig. 1

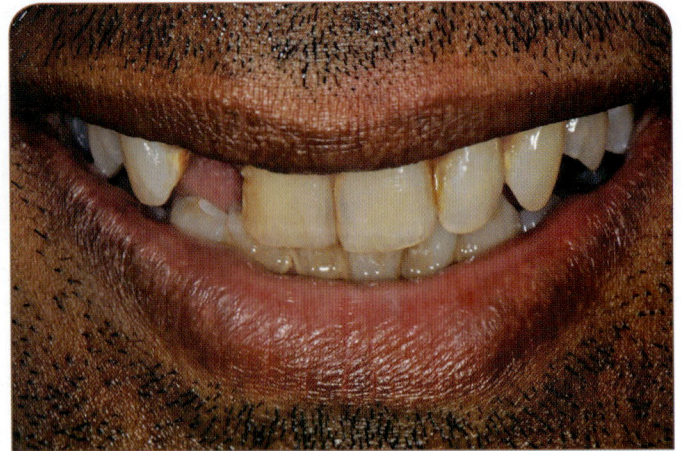

Fig. 2

A 30-year-old patient with a complain of a fractured and decemented post on tooth #12.

Chief complain was esthetic. Patient could not go about his daily chores without the tooth. Patient desired a tooth immediately.

Fractured tooth #12 a post and core previously done. The root piece was too small and a ferrule was not possible and given the root configuration, it was decided to extract the tooth **(Fig. 1)**.

The smile was moderate where the Gingiva were not visible. Patient had discolored composite restorations on other teeth which he did not want to touch.

Patient had a very deep bite with very little space for the missing tooth.

It was decided to do an extraction and an immediate implant and provisional followed by a zirconia screw retained abutment with a Lithium disilicate (Emax) veneer for esthetic.

Preoperative smile **(Fig. 2)**.

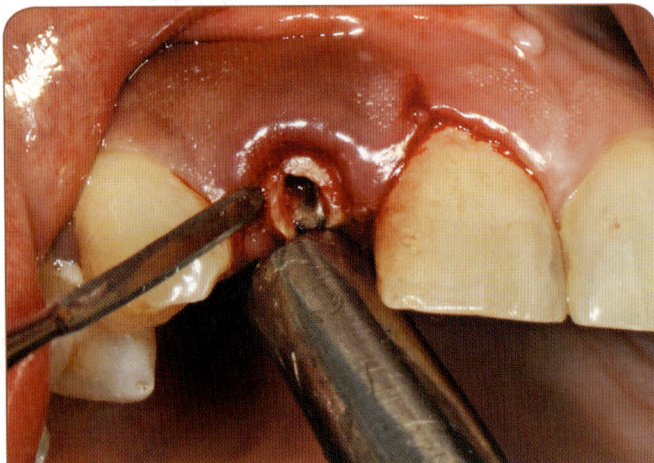

Fig. 3

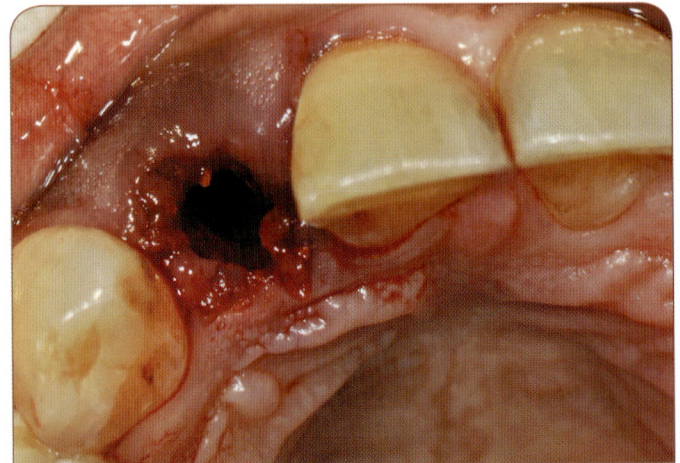

Fig. 4

Extraction carried out atraumatically using periotomes and luxators without damaging the buccal cortex.

Suspicion of buccal plate involvement prompted the course of reflecting the gingiva and placemen of implant **(Fig. 3)**.

Preserved socket post extraction possible buccal cortex breach **(Fig. 4)**.

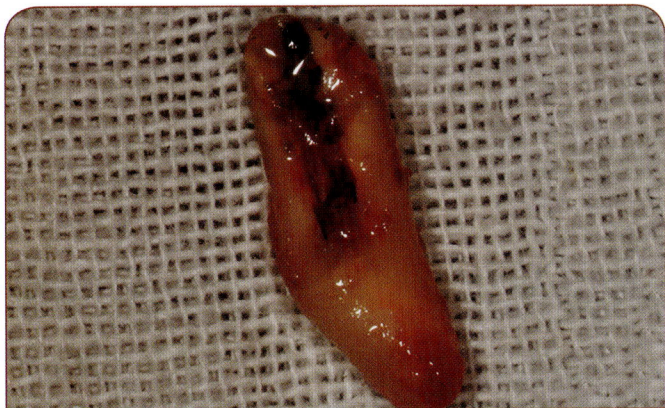
Fig. 5

Extracted root piece **(Fig. 5)**.

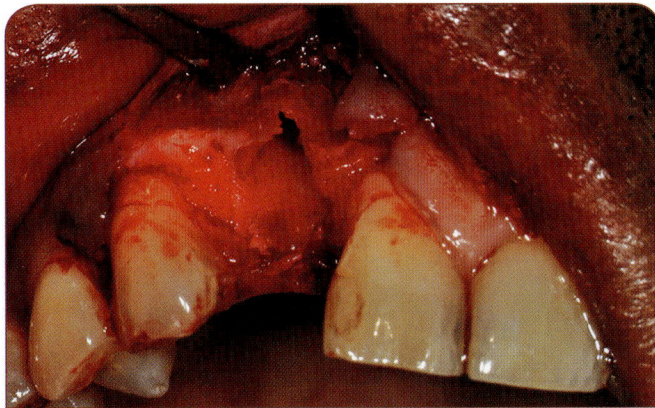
Fig. 6

Minimal reflection of the buccal mucosa to visually inspect the buccal cortex **(Fig. 6)**.

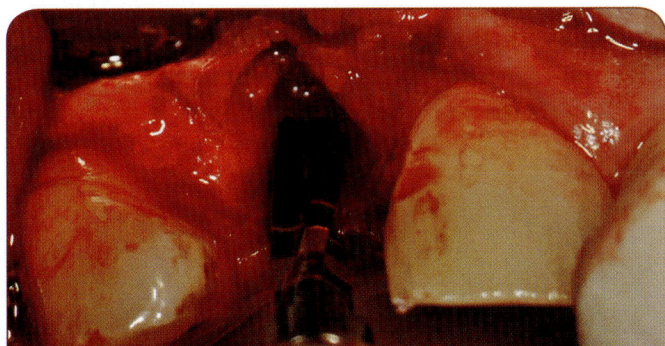
Fig. 7

Fresh osteotomy made along the palatal wall of the socket keeping the biologic placement angulation in mind. The implant was placed along the cinglium of the adjacent tooth **(Fig. 7)**.

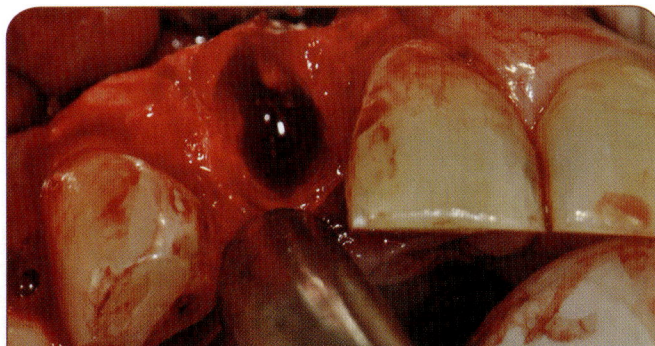
Fig. 8

Fresh osteotomy site prepared along the palatal wall of the socket and ensuring there is no pressure on the buccal cortex **(Fig. 8)**.

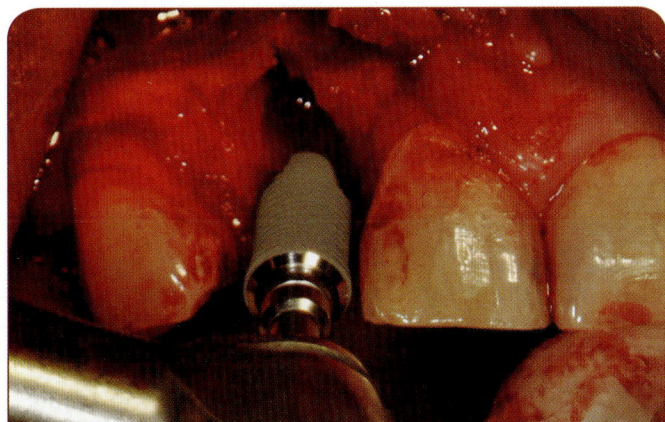
Fig. 9

4.00 mm diameter and a 12 mm length Dentium implant sandblasted large grit and acid-etched (SLA) coated placed **(Fig. 9)**.

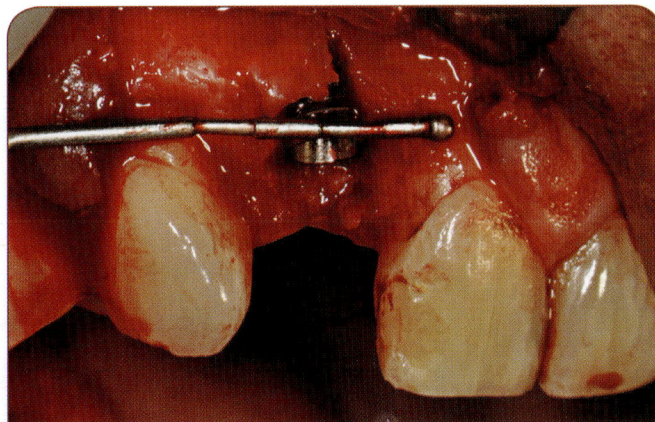
Fig. 10

Apico coronal position of the implant 2 mm higher than the adjacent CEJ **(Fig. 10)**.

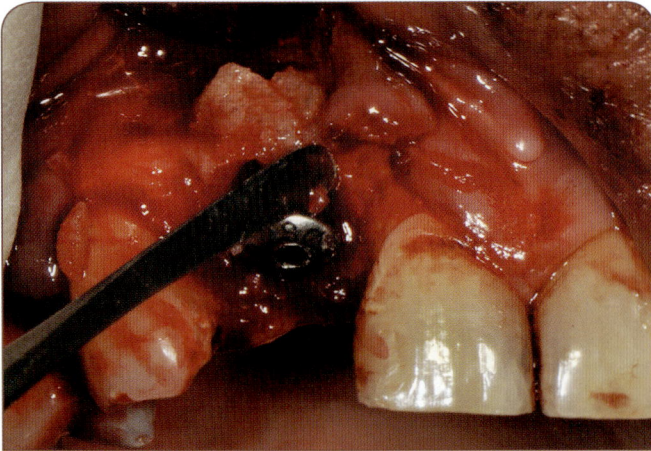

Fig. 11

Bone grafting with a mixture of autogenous and zenograft **(Fig. 11)**.

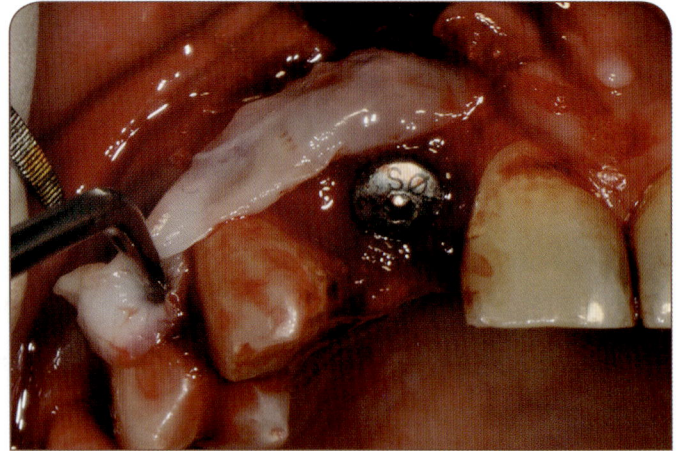

Fig. 12

Placement of a resorbable collagen membrane covered by plasma rich in growth factors (PRGF) membrane **(Fig. 12)**.

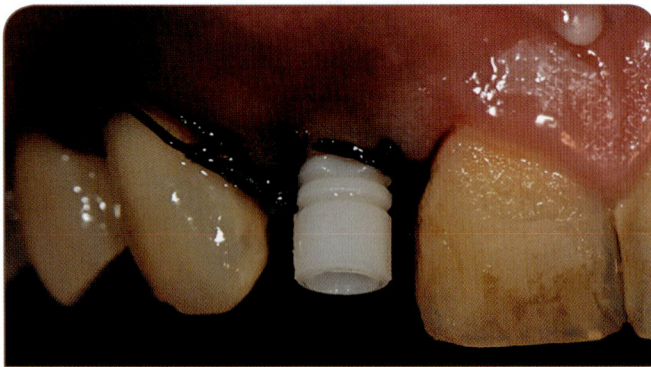

Fig. 13

Suturing and placement of a temporary abutment for the fabrication of an immediate provisional **(Fig. 13)**.

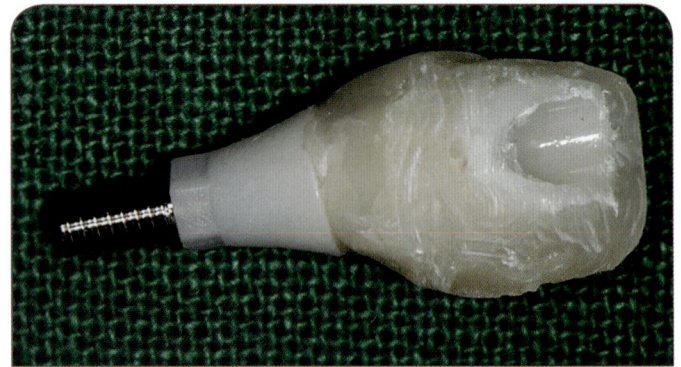

Fig. 14

Composite provisional fabricated **(Fig. 14)**.

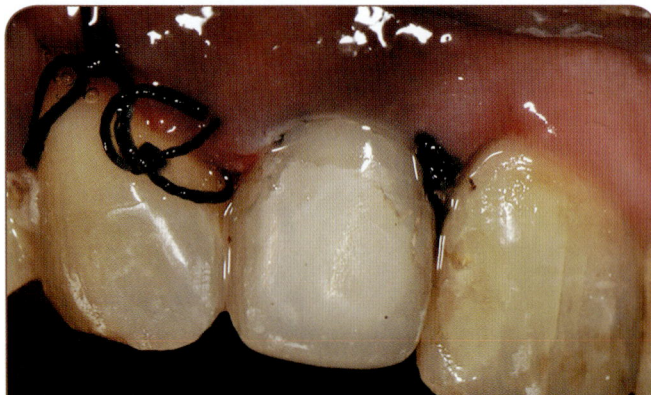

Fig. 15

Composite provisional screwed in position and access hole blocked **(Fig. 15)**.

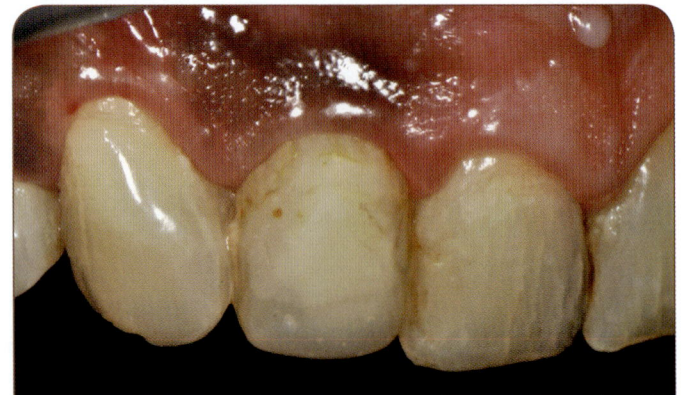

Fig. 16

Healing post one week **(Fig. 16)**.

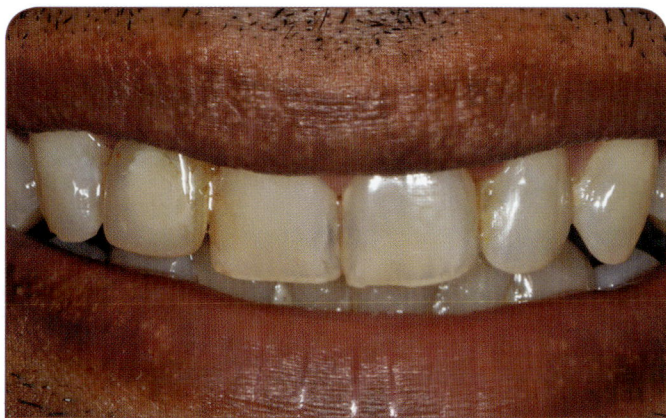
Fig. 17

Provisional smile **(Fig. 17)**.

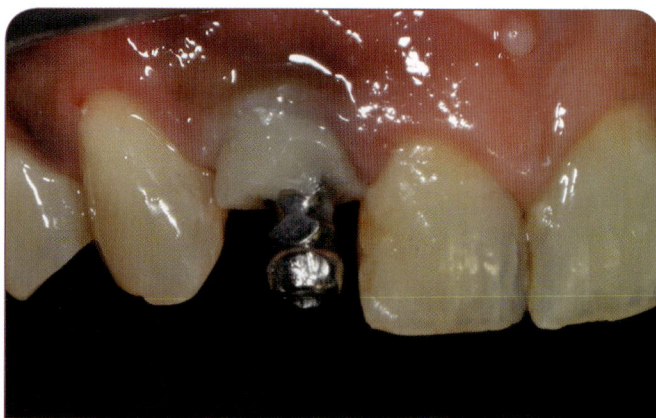
Fig. 18

Impression post customized for gingival support **(Fig. 18)**.

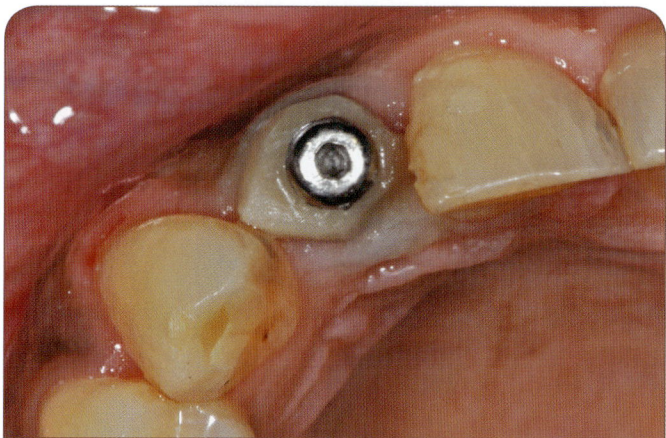
Fig. 19

Occlusal view of the impression post **(Fig. 19)**.

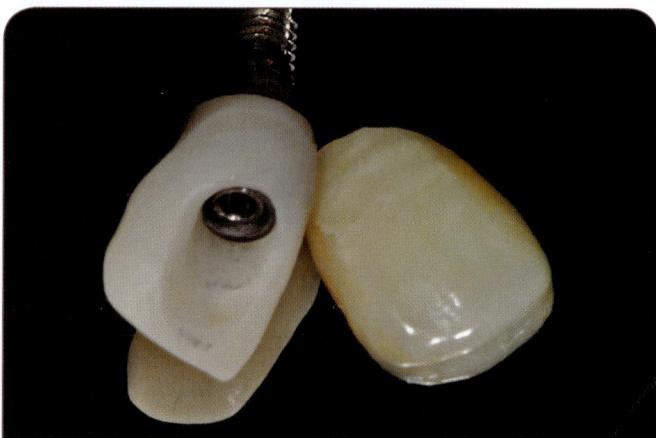
Fig. 20

Customized Zirconia abutment and lithium disilicate veneer **(Fig. 20)**.

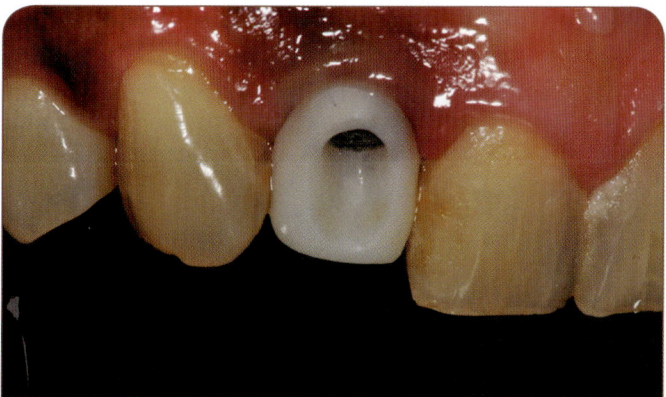
Fig. 21

Zirconia abutment placed in the mouth **(Fig. 21)**.

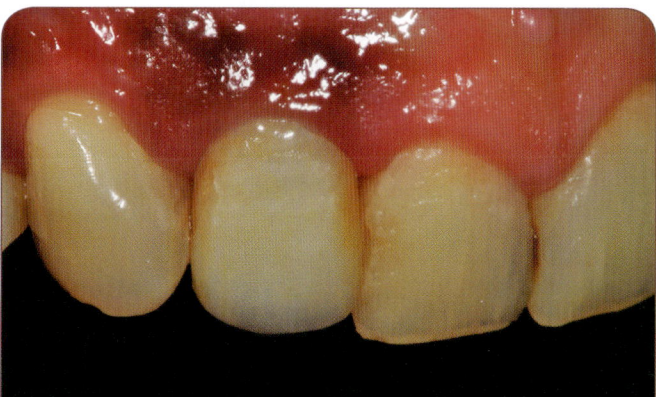
Fig. 22

Lithium disilicate veneer placed **(Fig. 22)**.

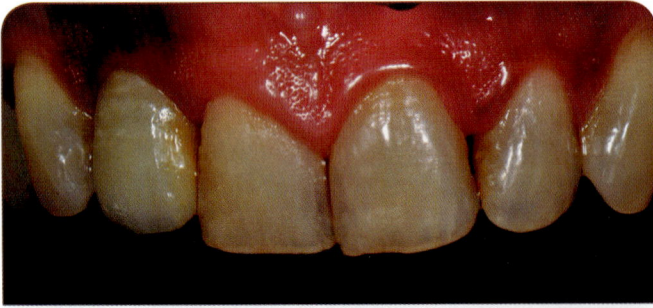

Fig. 23

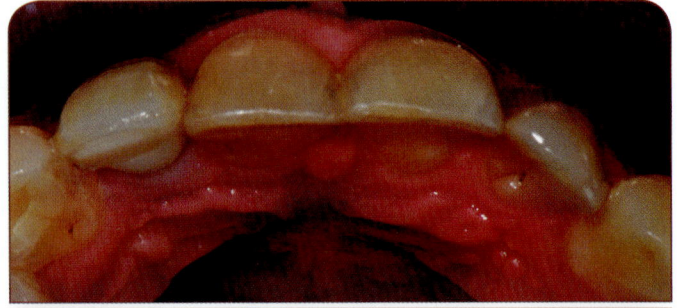

Fig. 24

Intraoral picture post cementation of the Veneer **(Fig. 23)**.   Occlusal view **(Fig. 24)**.

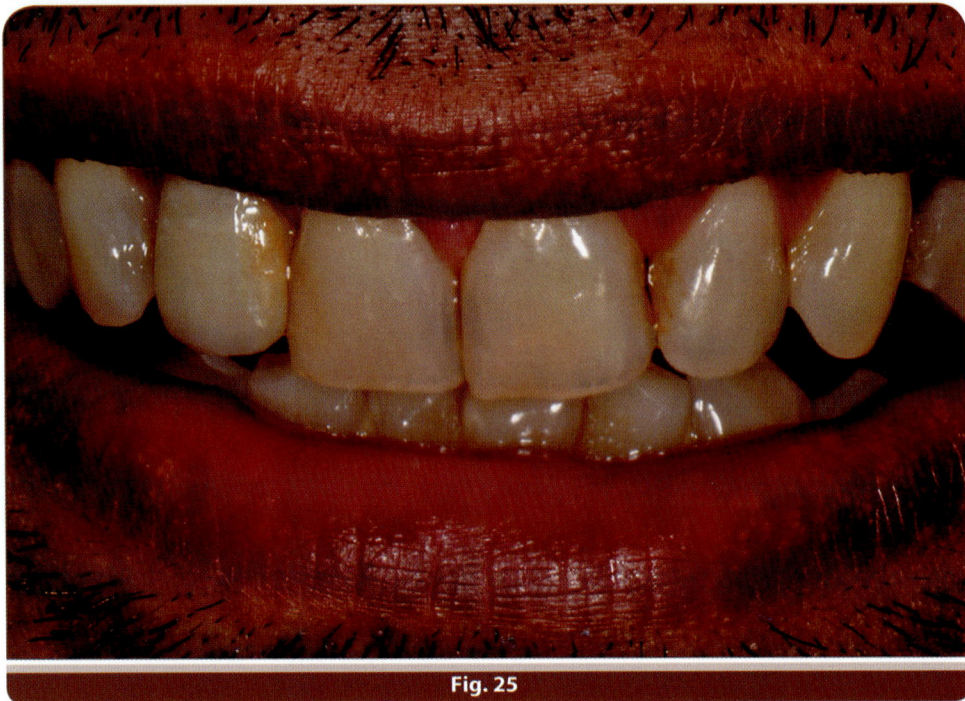

Fig. 25

Smile. Postoperative with prosthesis in place **(Fig. 25)**.

Narayan TV

Maxillary Canine Socket Shield, Custom Healing Abutment and Final Restoration

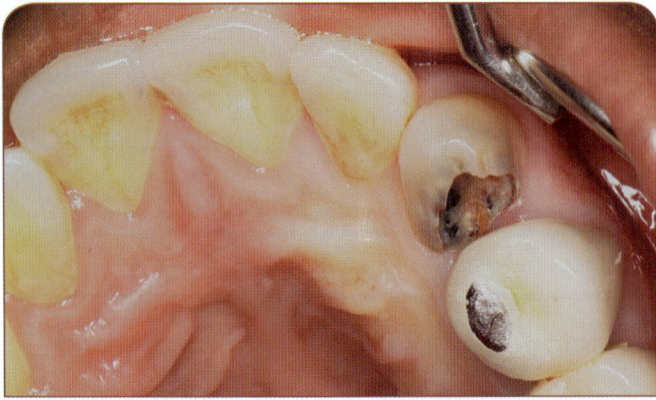

Fig. 1

A 40-year-old male with deeply decayed left maxillary canine **(Fig. 1)**.

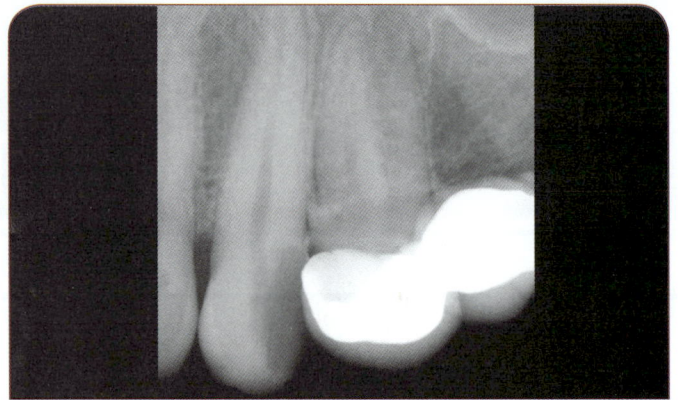

Fig. 2

Preoperative X-ray **(Fig. 2)**.

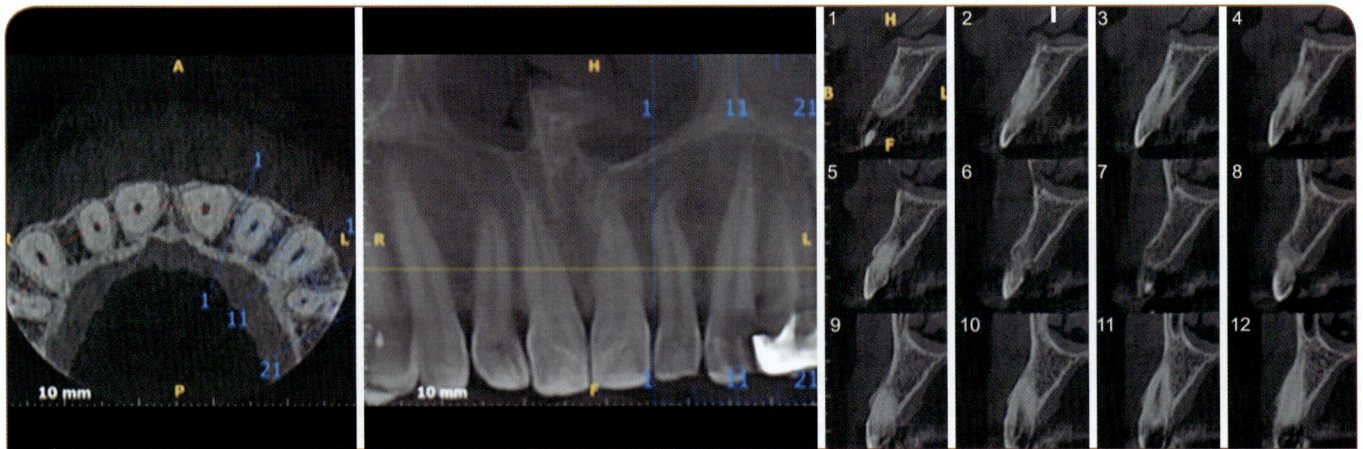

Fig. 3

Preoperative CBCT. The barely visible labial plate (10,11,12), prominent and long root **(Fig. 3)**.

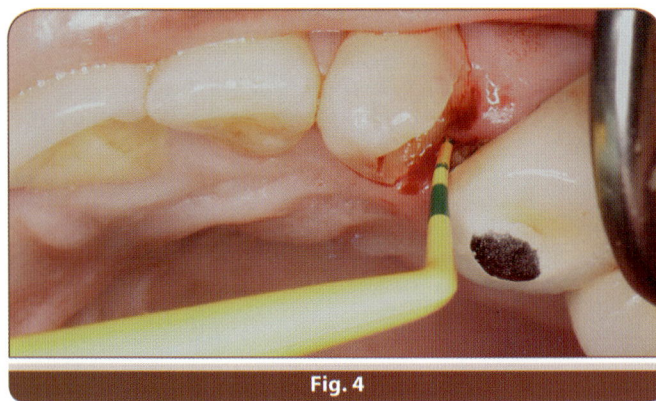

Fig. 4

Bone sounding to check relation to apical extent of caries. Crown lengthening procedure (CLP) option offered to the patient. Patient preferred the implant option, having had several earlier failures of root canals and crowns **(Fig. 4)**.

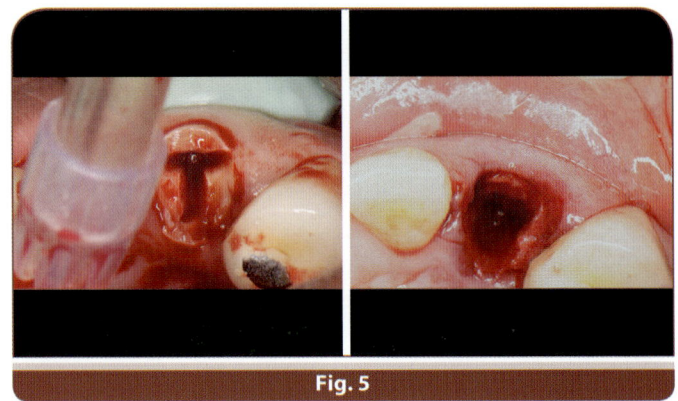

Fig. 5

Root sectioned in a "T" shape to facilitate easy extraction. Socket shield attached to facial plate **(Fig. 5)**.

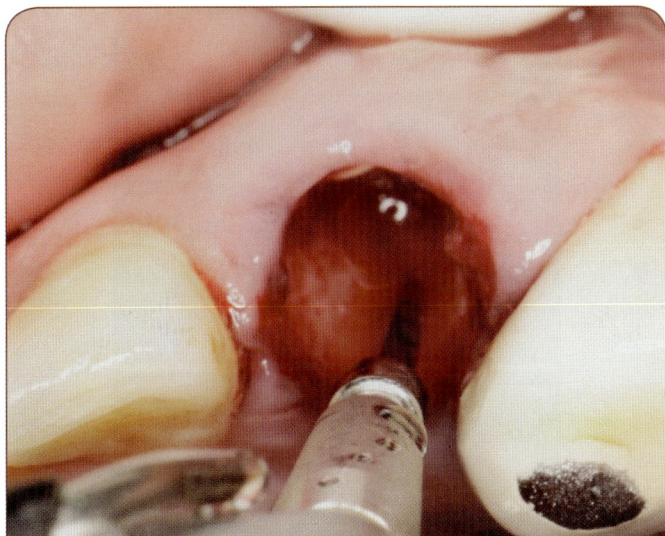
Fig. 6

Osteotomy on the palatal plate **(Fig. 6)**.

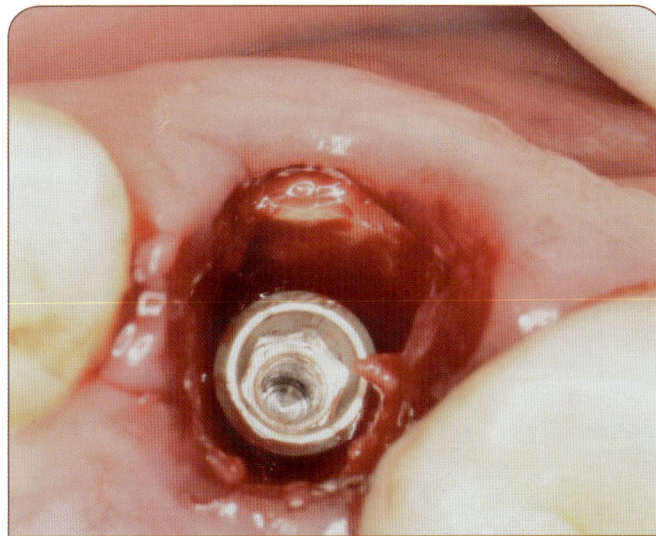
Fig. 7

4 × 13 Bioner DM Implant placed with buccal gap **(Fig. 7)**.

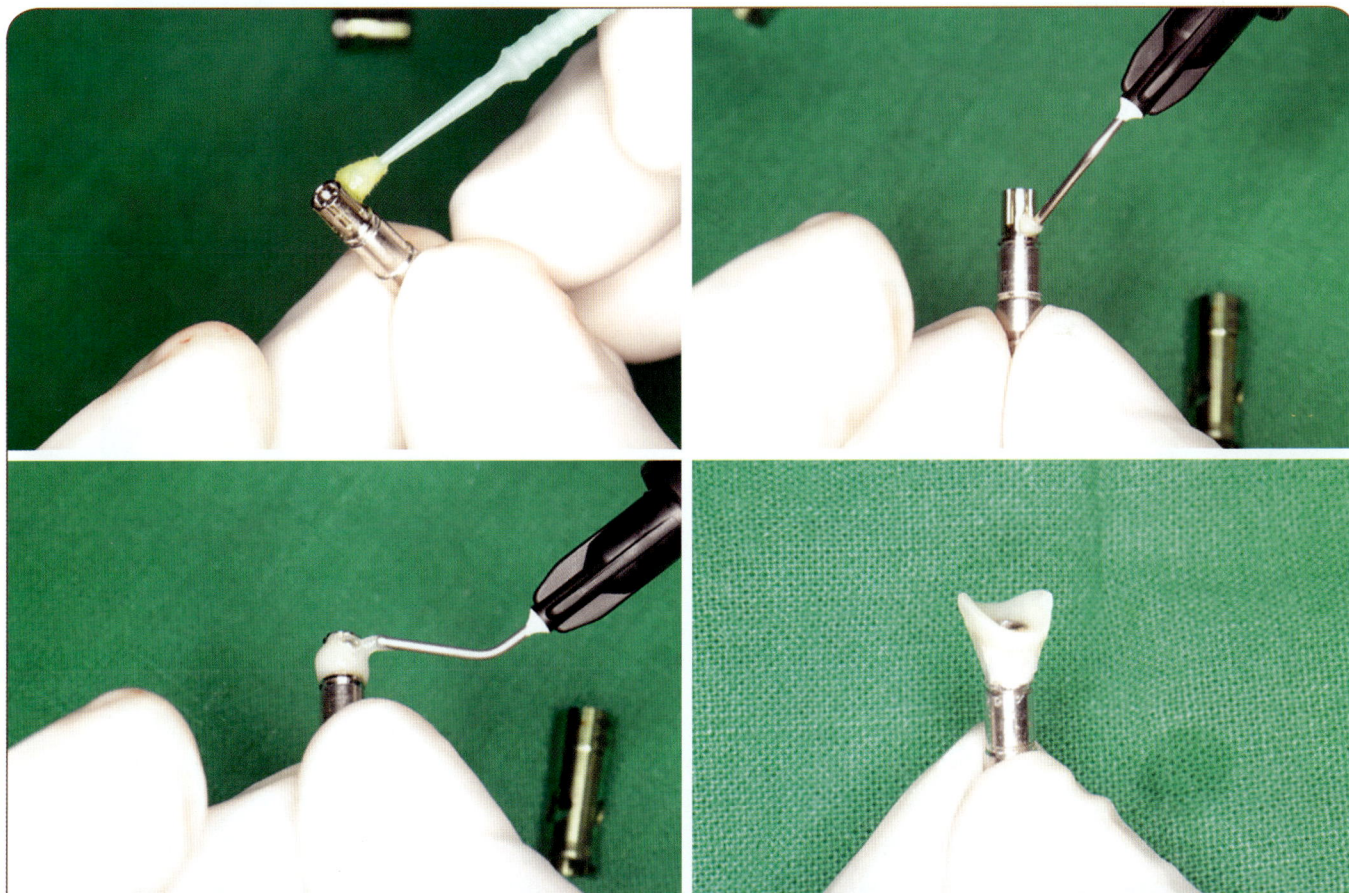
Fig. 8

Custom healing abutment **(Fig. 8)**.

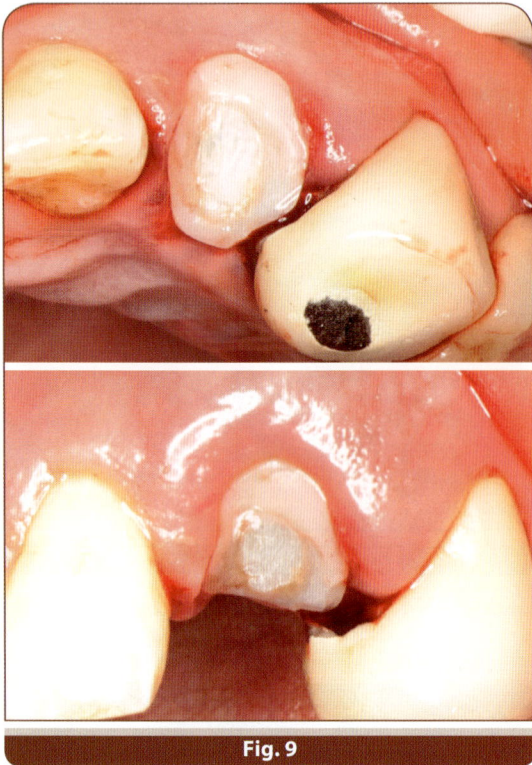

Fig. 9

Custom healing abutment **(Fig. 9)**.

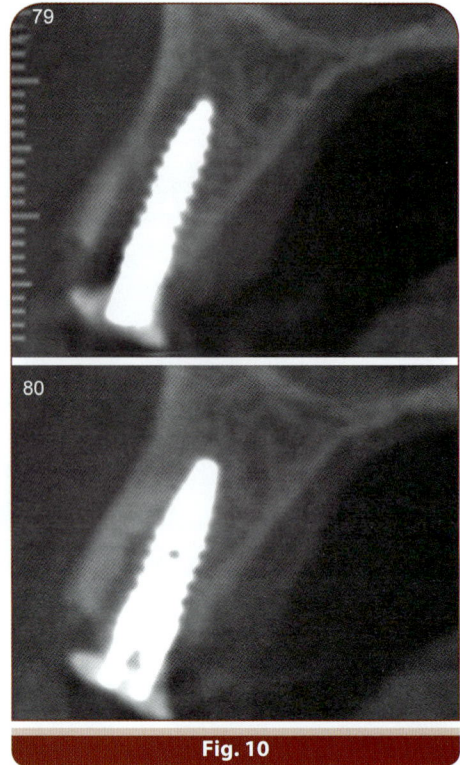

Fig. 10

About 2 months later. Needed to image the 2nd premolar region for implant evaluation, so had the canine region imaged as well, there is clearly no contact between the shield and the implant and there's woven bone intervening **(Fig. 10)**.

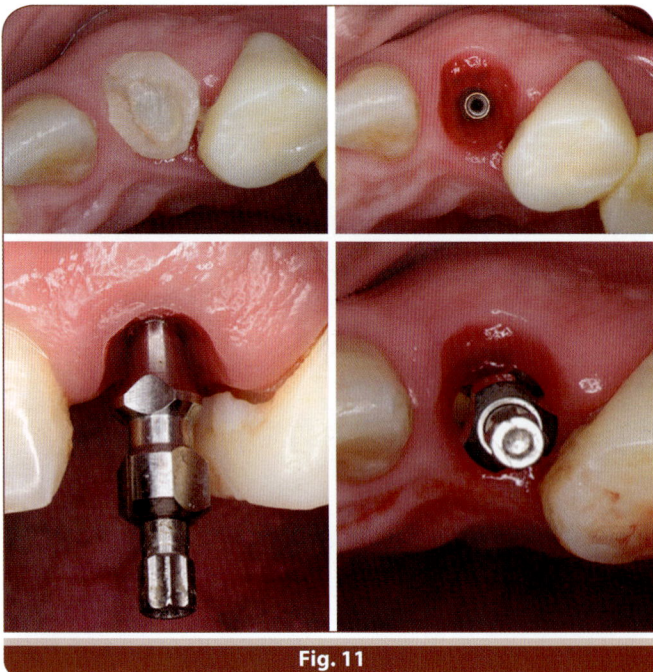

Fig. 11

4 months later **(Fig. 11)**.

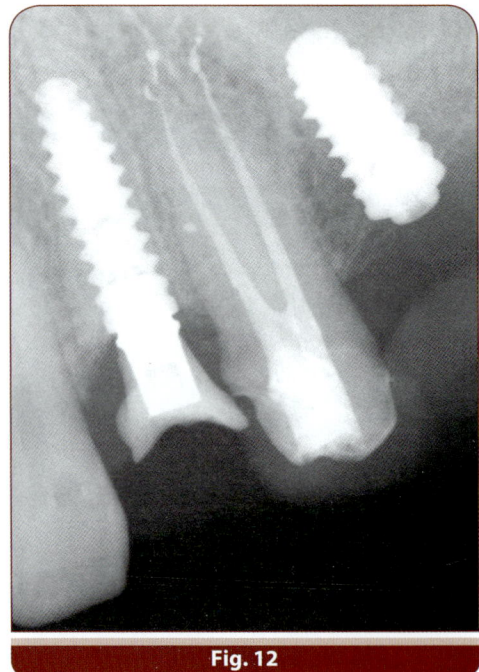

Fig. 12

Immediate postoperative X-ray **(Fig. 12)**.

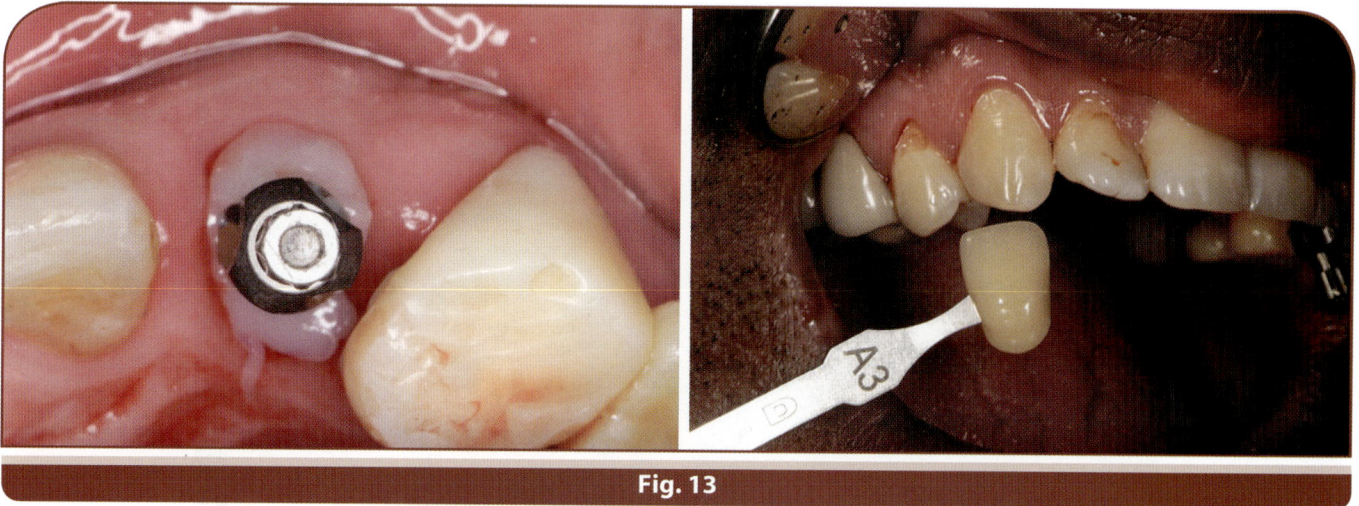

Fig. 13

Custom impression coping and shade selection (**Fig. 13**).

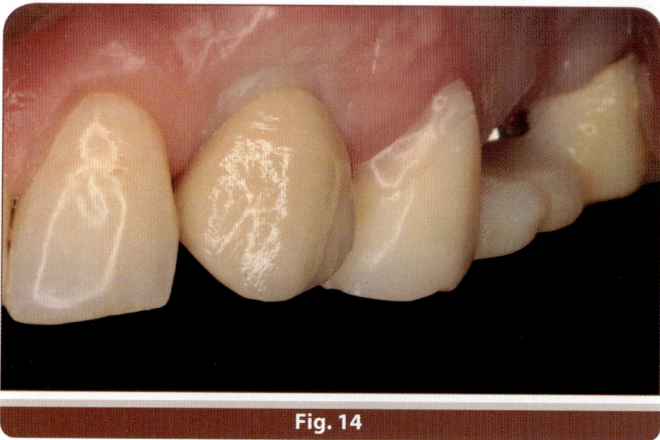

Fig. 14

Final restoration (**Fig. 14**).

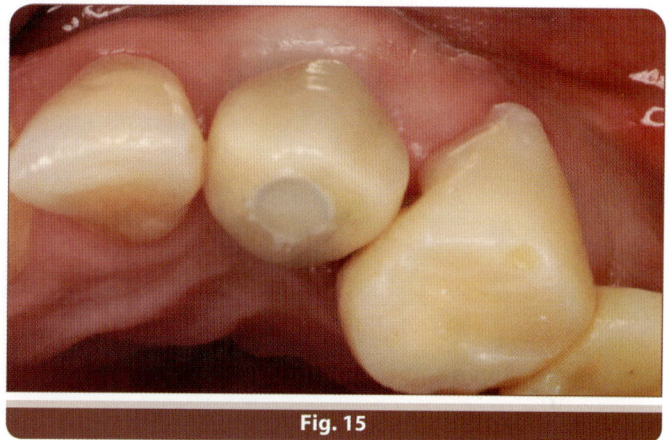

Fig. 15

Final restoration (**Fig. 15**).

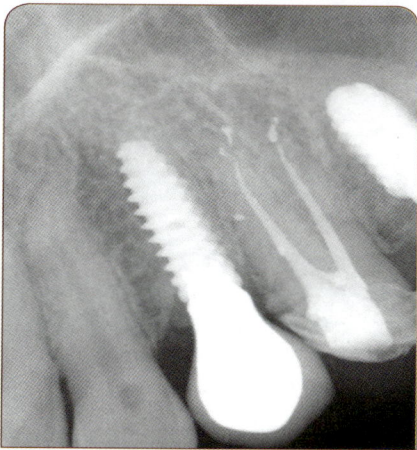

Fig. 16

X-ray with final restoration (**Fig. 16**).

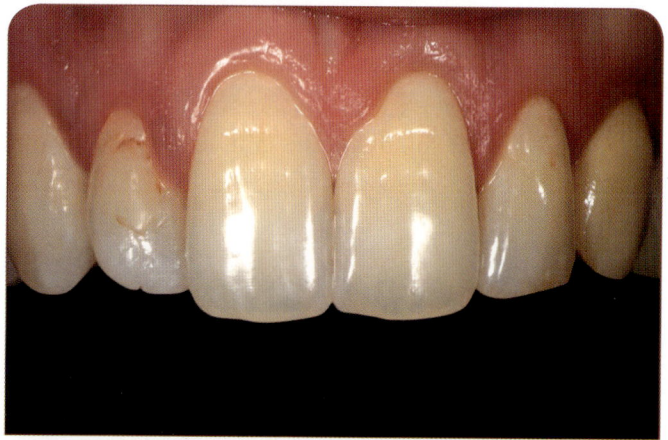

Fig. 17

Final restoration after 24 hours (**Fig. 17**).

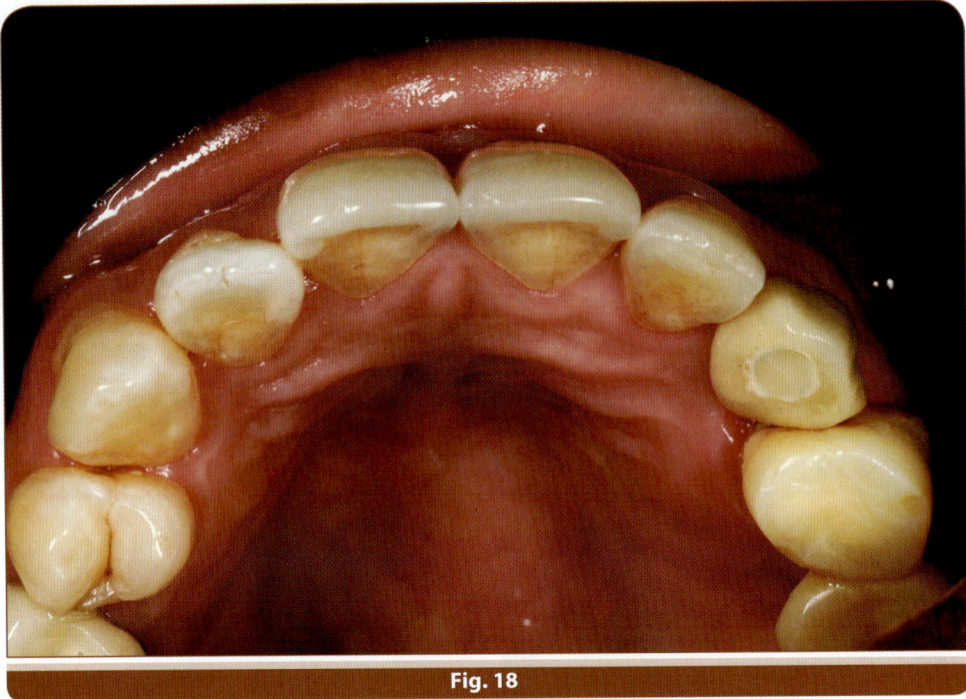

Final restoration after 24 hours **(Fig. 18)**.

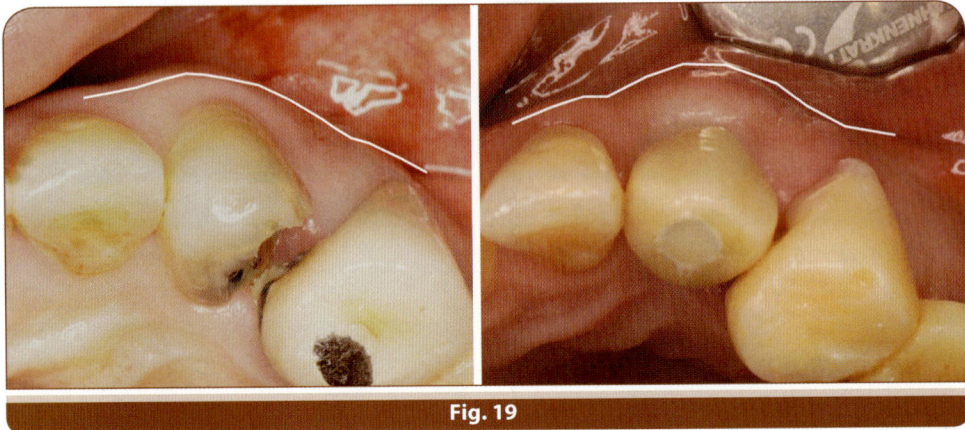

Note the soft tissue integration around the implant crown using socket shield technique **(Fig. 19)**.

Praful Bali, Sourabh Nagpal

SOCKET SHIELD TO PRESERVE THE BUCCAL CORTICAL PLATE FOR AN ESTHETIC OUTCOME

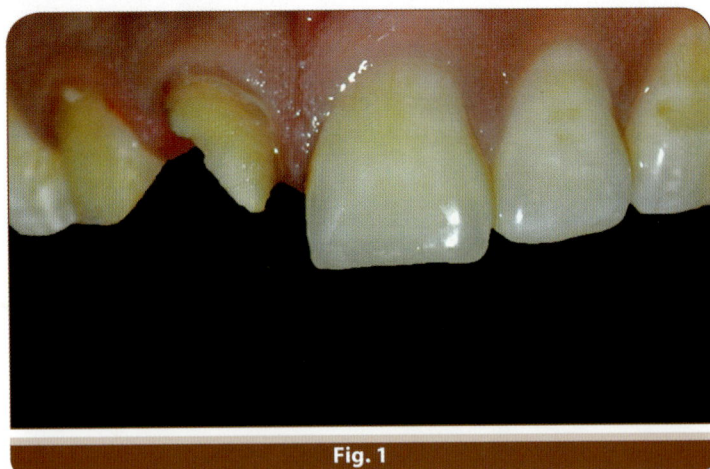

Fig. 1

Preoperative view of failed endodontics and fracture of tooth #11 **(Fig. 1)**.

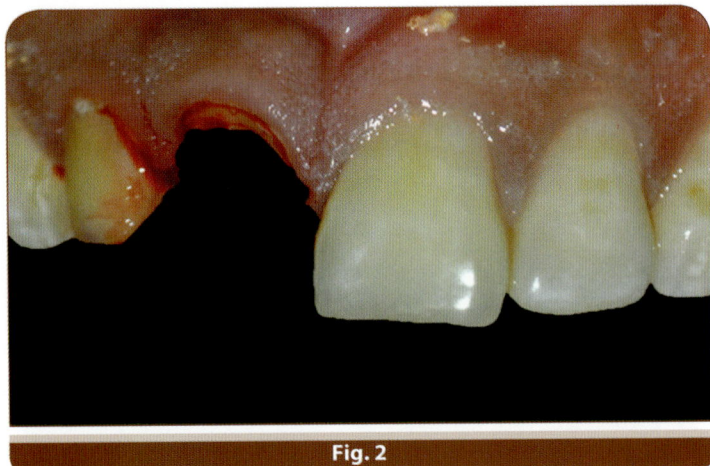

Fig. 2

The tooth is trimmed till the gingival level before vertically slicing the tooth **(Fig. 2)**.

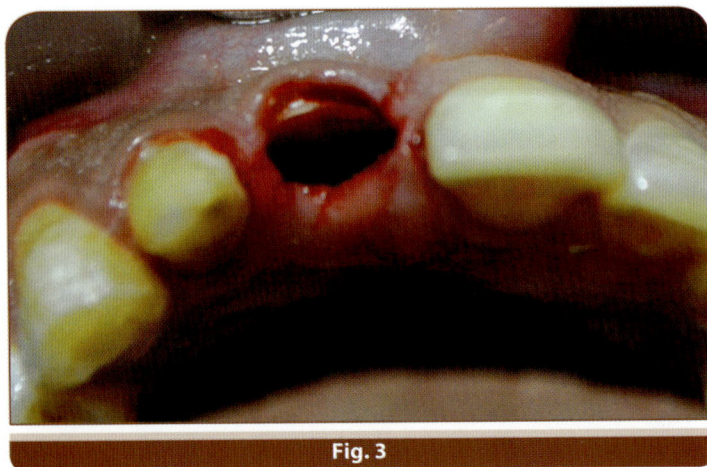

Fig. 3

The root is sliced vertically – mesiodistally to split the root into 2 pieces. Palatal portion of root is removed. Buccal shield is left to maintain buccal contour **(Fig. 3)**.

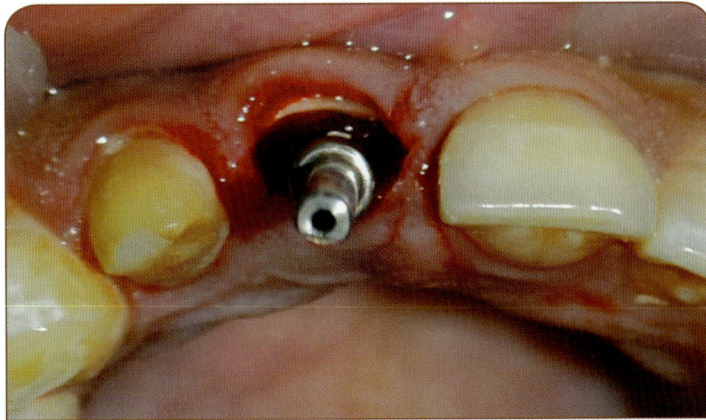

Fig. 4

Osteotomy preparation on the palatal aspect of the socket **(Fig. 4)**.

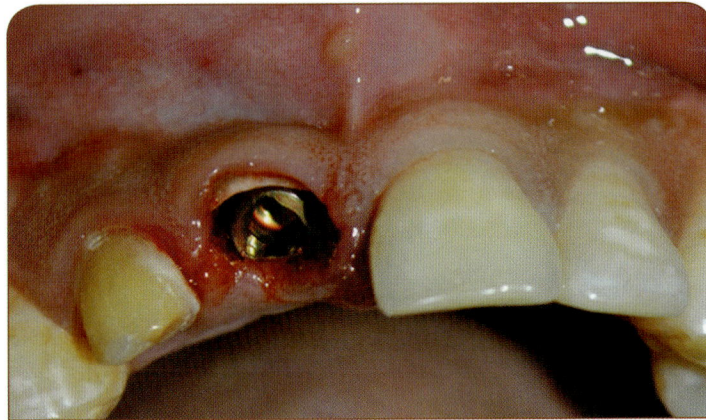

Fig. 5

4.3/13 Nobel Groovy implant (Nobel Biocare) placed 2-3 mm below the CE junction. The space between the implant and buccal root piece is augmented with Novabone putty **(Fig. 5)**.

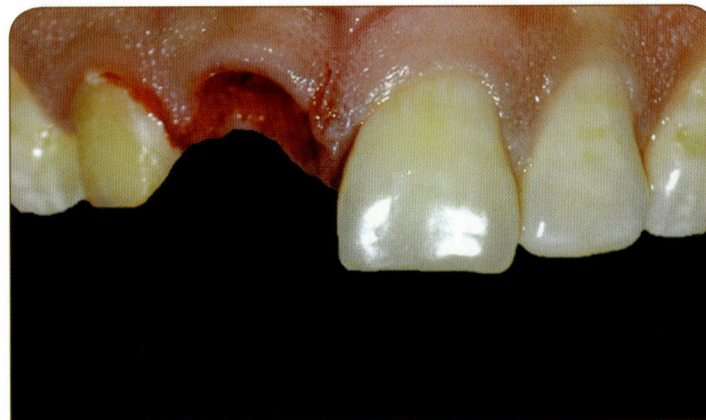

Fig. 6

The tooth is now trimmed below the gingival level **(Fig. 6)**.

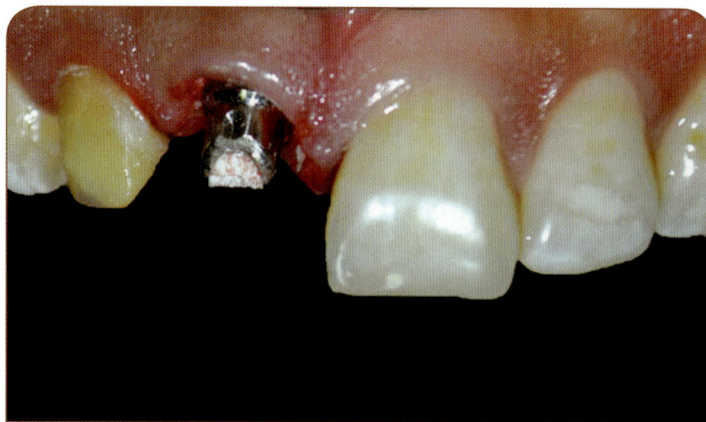

Fig. 7

Nobel snappy abutment torqued at 35N cm **(Fig. 7)**.

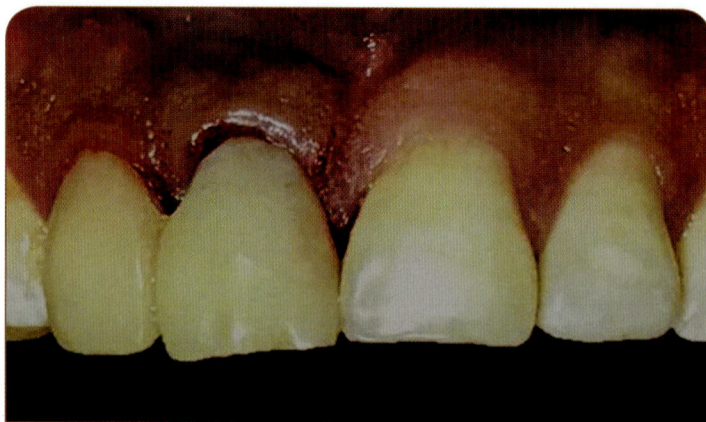

Fig. 8

Immediate temporary crowns cemented on the implant tooth and tooth #12. The crown made out of occlusion **(Fig. 8)**.

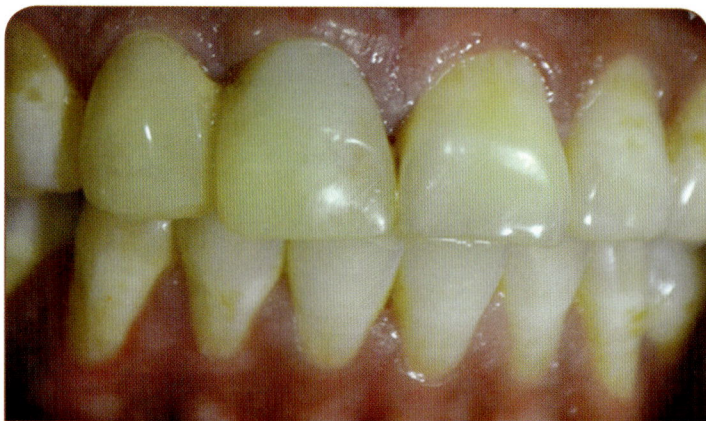

Fig. 9

One week postoperative facial view: Note that the socket shield technique has preserved the buccal cortical plate as well as maintained the soft tissue profile **(Fig. 9)**.

Amit Gulati

Immediate Extraction Placements GBR with Ti Mesh Segmental Procera Implant Bridge Prosthesis

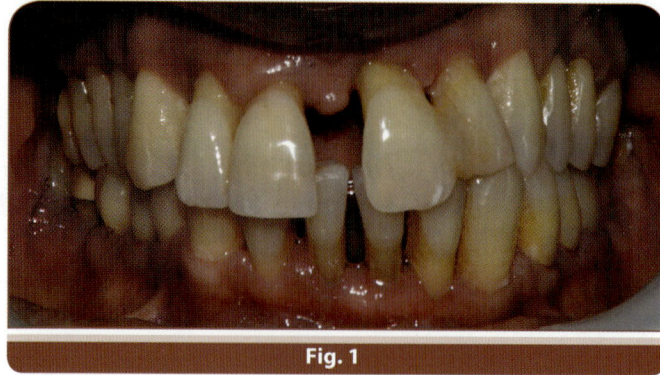

Fig. 1

Periodontally involved, grade III mobile Maxillary Anterior Dentition **(Fig. 1)**.

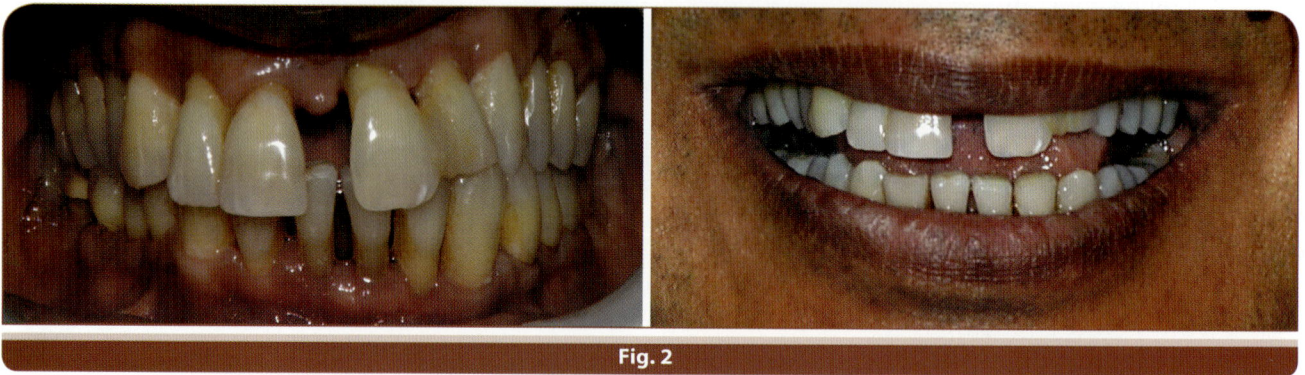

Fig. 2

Patients' main concern. Diastemas to be created in temporary and final prosthesis **(Fig. 2)**.

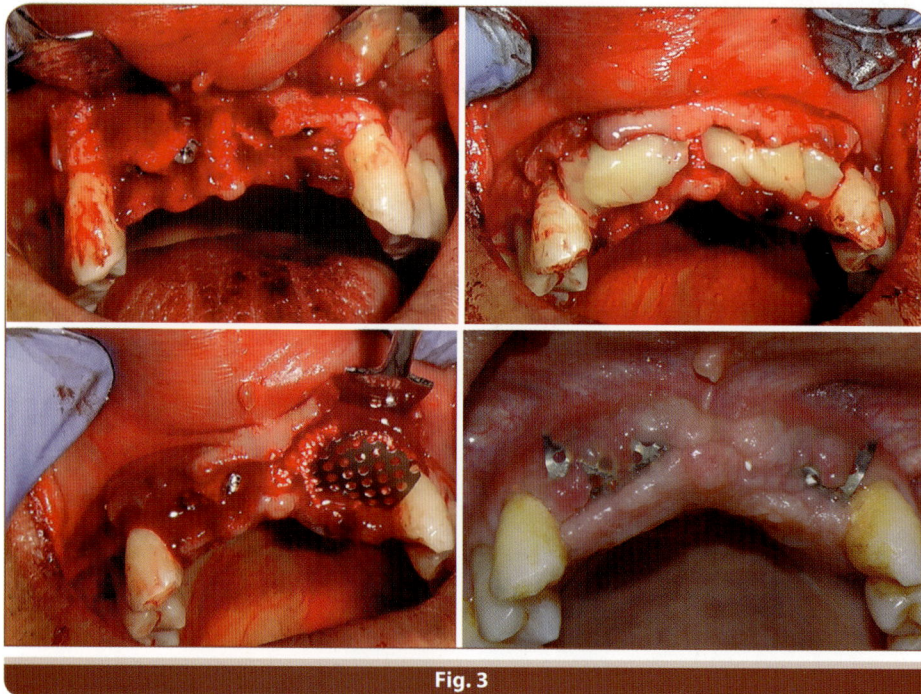

Fig. 3

Extraction of maxillary incisors done and immediate implant placement GBR with Titanum mesh. The Titanium mesh was visible after 8 weeks **(Fig. 3)**.

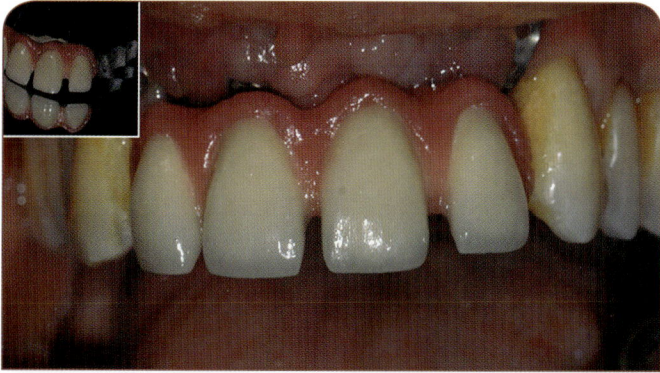

Fig. 4

Maryland temporary prosthesis **(Fig. 4)**.

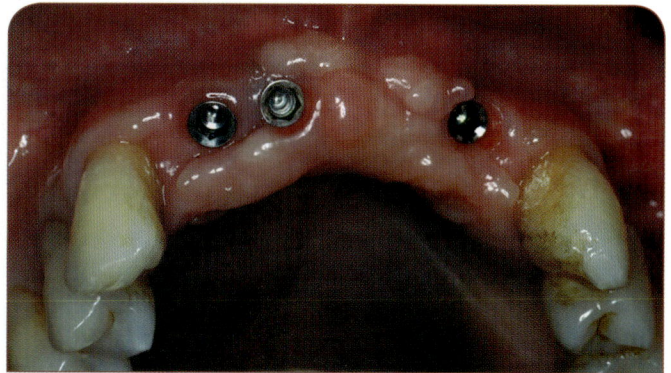

Fig. 5

After five months, 2nd stage done **(Fig. 5)**.

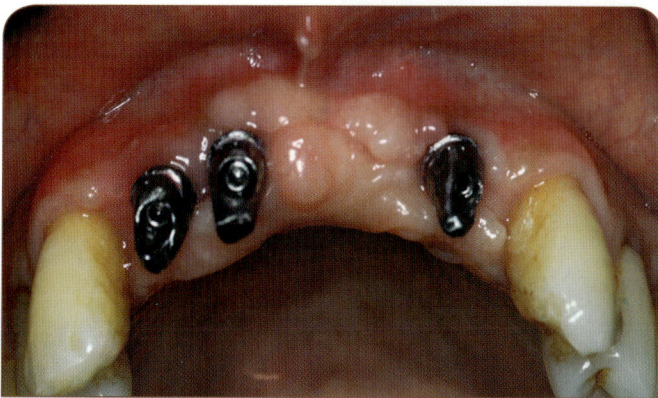

Fig. 6

Milled abutments for temporary prosthesis **(Fig. 6)**.

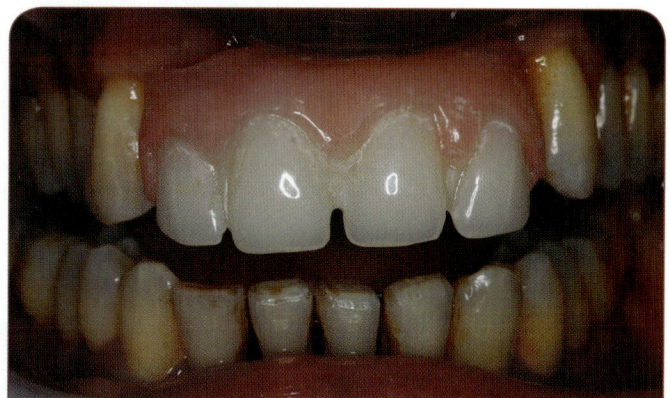

Fig. 7

Temporary prosthesis as received from lab **(Fig. 7)**.

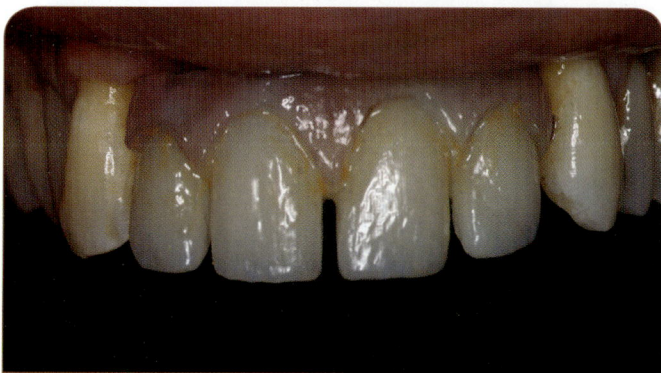

Fig. 8

Temporary prosthesis modifications **(Fig. 8)**.

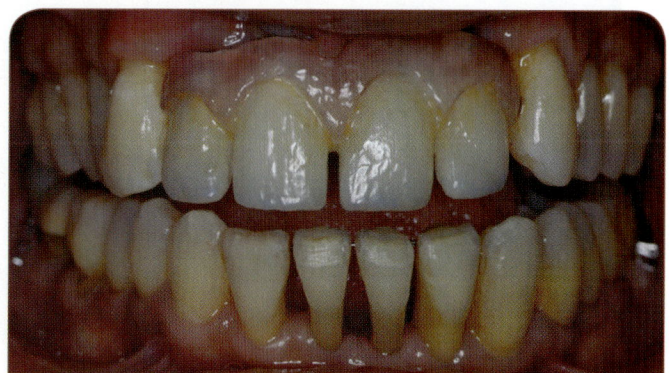

Fig. 9

Temporary prosthesis modifications **(Fig. 9)**.

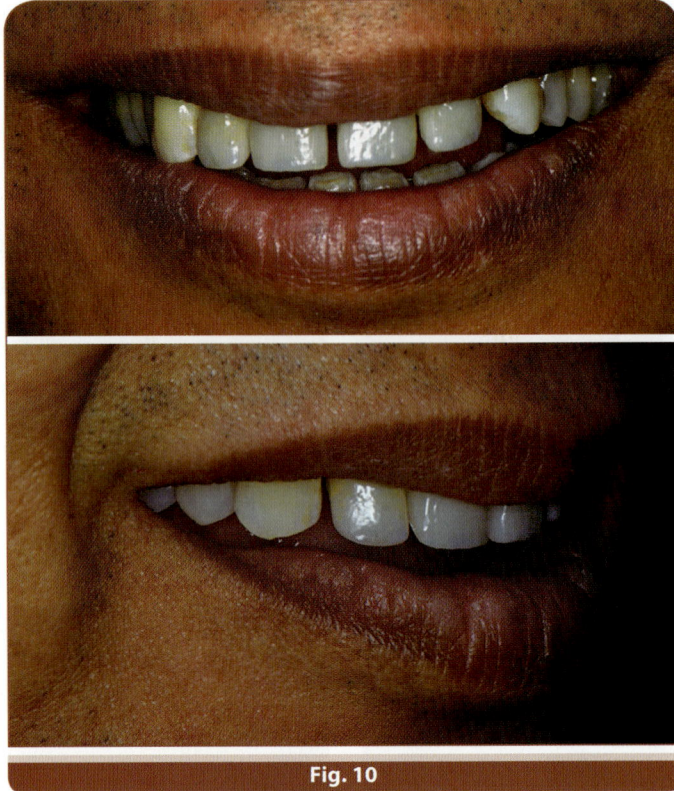

Fig. 10

Temporary prosthesis on implants **(Fig. 10)**.

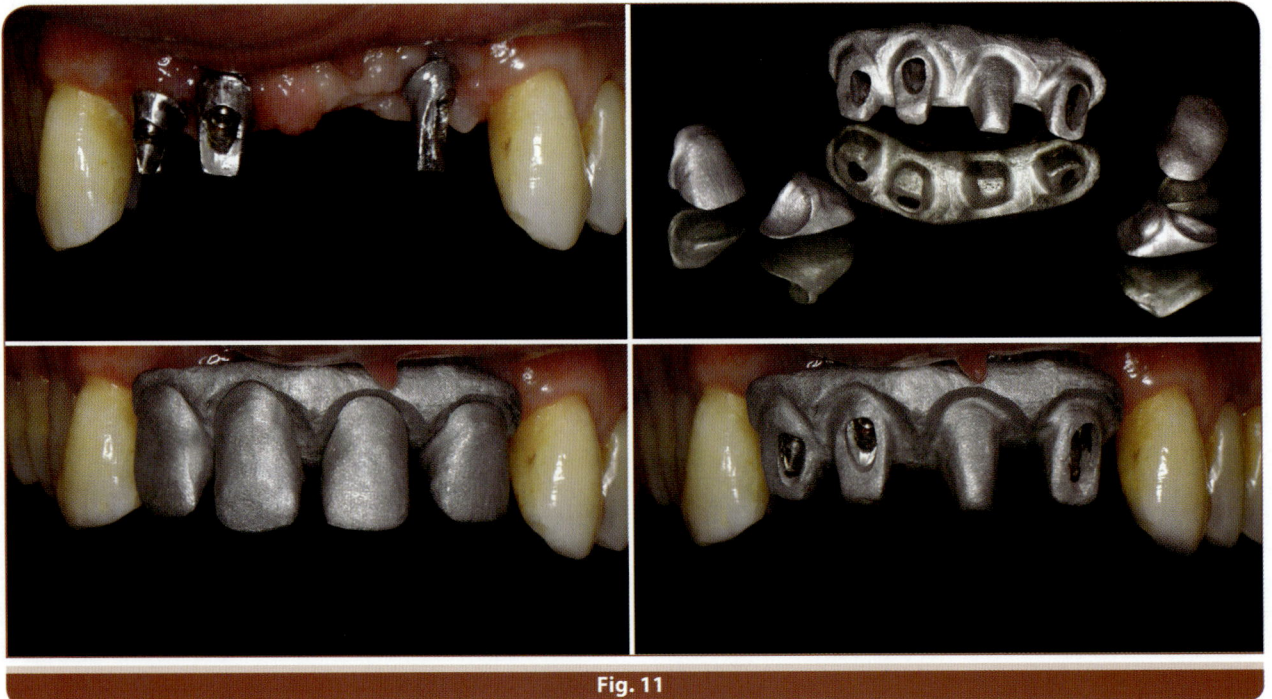

Fig. 11

Final prosthesis–coping trial, segmental procera Implant Bridge type **(Fig. 11)**.

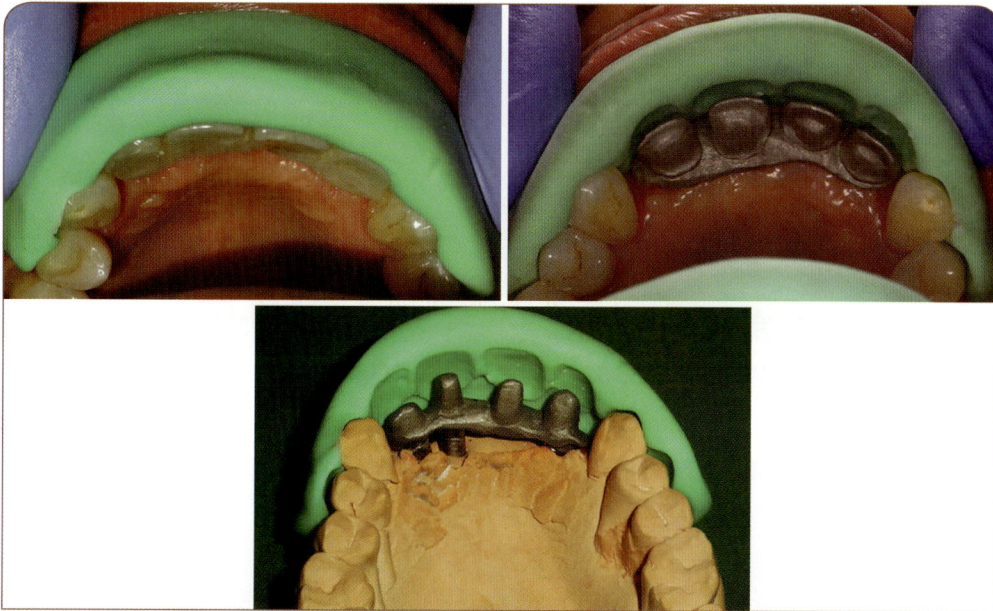

Fig. 12

Putty index of temporary prosthesis to guide ceramic layering **(Fig. 12)**.

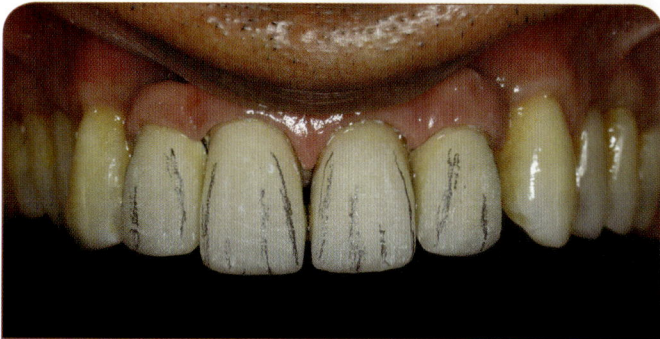

Fig. 13

Bisque trial, defining anatomy, line angles and textures **(Fig. 13)**.

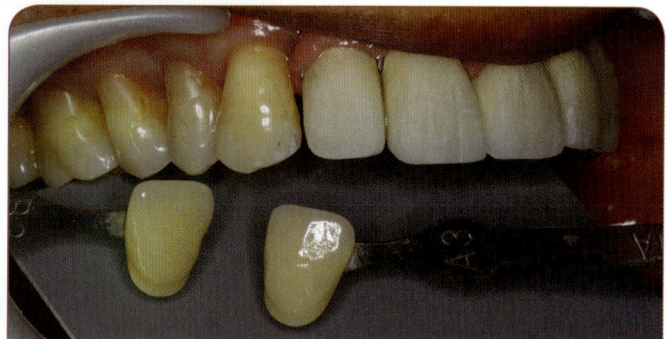

Fig. 14

Shade communication using 18% gray card **(Fig. 14)**.

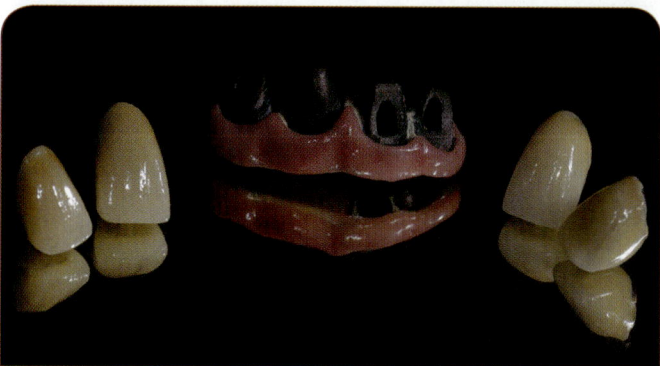

Fig. 15

Final prosthesis **(Fig. 15)**.

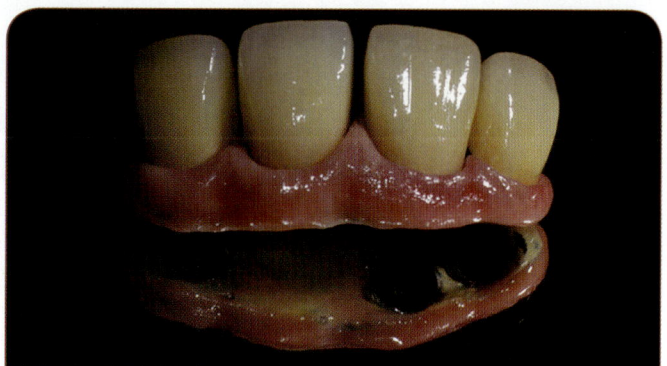

Fig. 16

Final prosthesis **(Fig. 16)**.

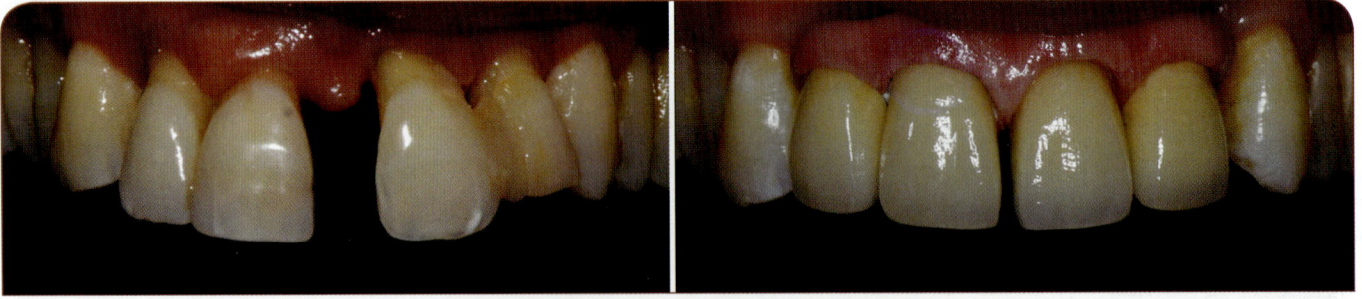

Fig. 17

Preoperative and postoperative **(Fig. 17)**.

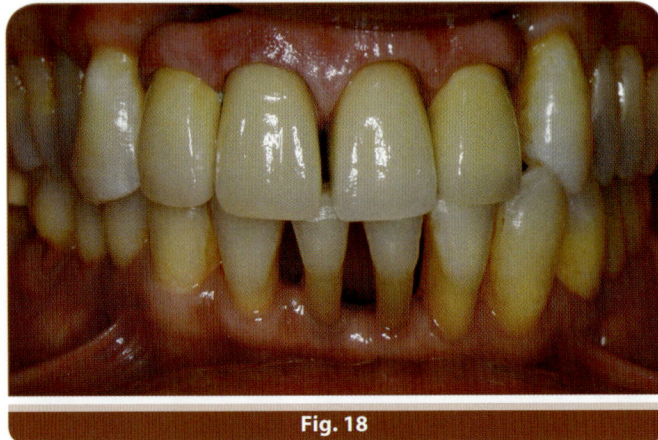

Fig. 18

Frontal view. Final prosthesis **(Fig. 18)**.

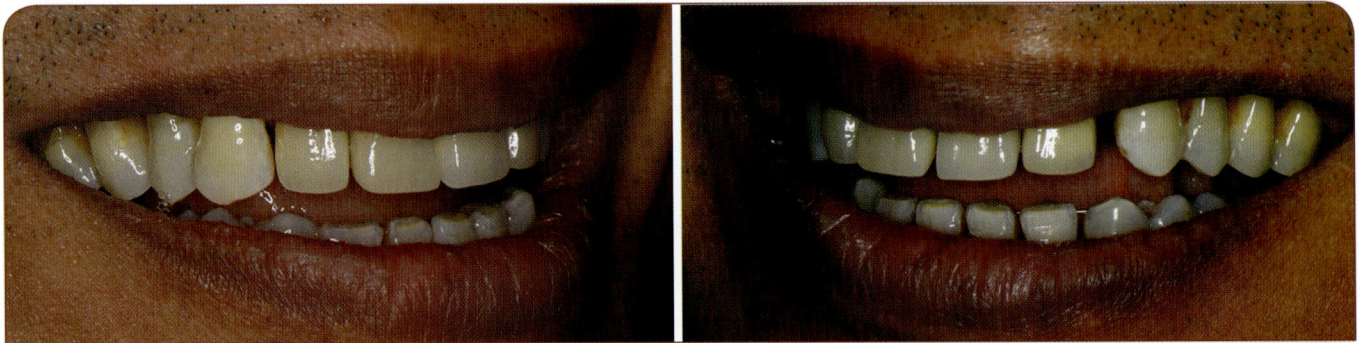

Fig. 19

Left lateral and right lateral view of final prosthesis **(Fig. 19)**.

Praful Bali

Full Mouth Rehabilitation with Immediate Implantation and Immediate Loading: Complete Rebuilt of Esthetics, Function and Occlusion

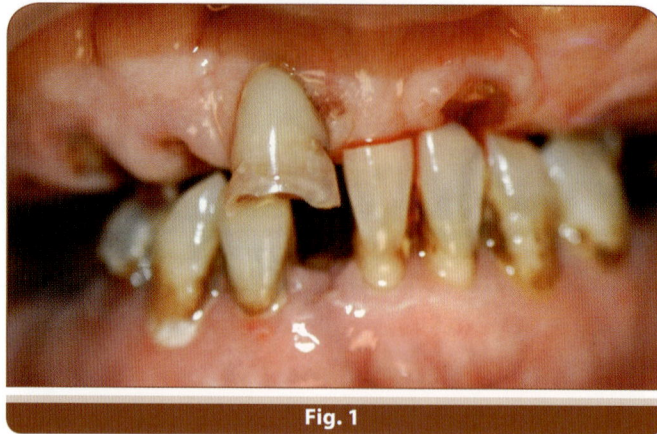

Fig. 1

Preoperative facial view of an elderly an male patient with failed dentition, multiple root stumps present, gingival inflammation and pus discharge in local areas. Patient complains of difficulty and pain while chewing and intermediate bleeding from upper front area due to trauma from lower front teeth as there is no occlusal stop **(Fig. 1)**.

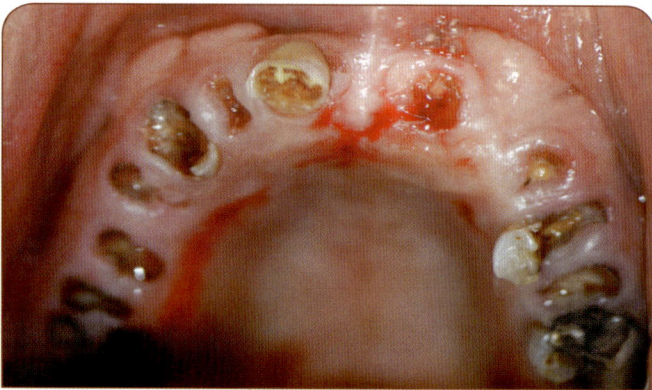

Fig. 2

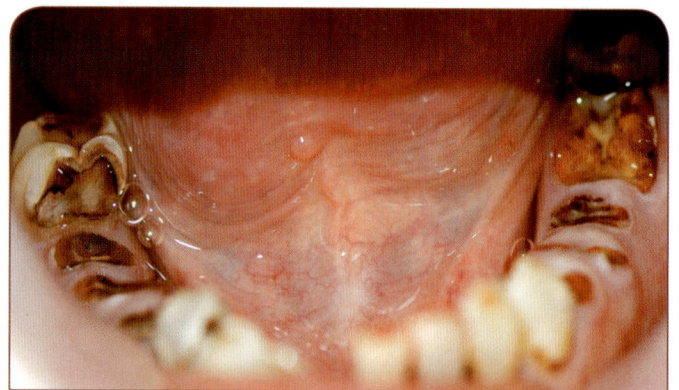

Fig. 3

Occlusal view—Multiple root stumps and grossly decayed teeth with caries and periodontal disease present in the maxillary arch **(Fig. 2)**.

Occlusal view—Similar situation in the posterior mandible too. Grossly decayed teeth and root pieces **(Fig. 3)**.

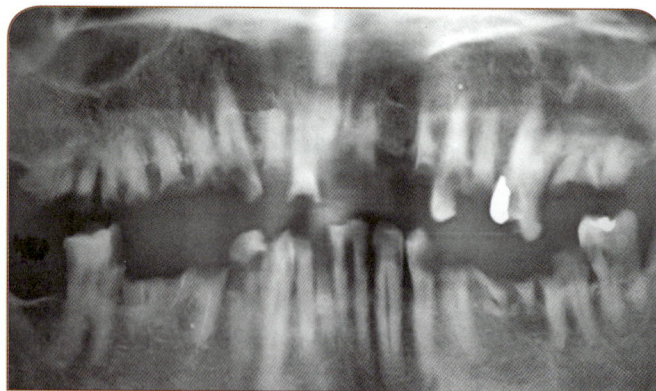

Fig. 4

OPG—X-ray showing broken teeth in both arches **(Fig. 4)**.

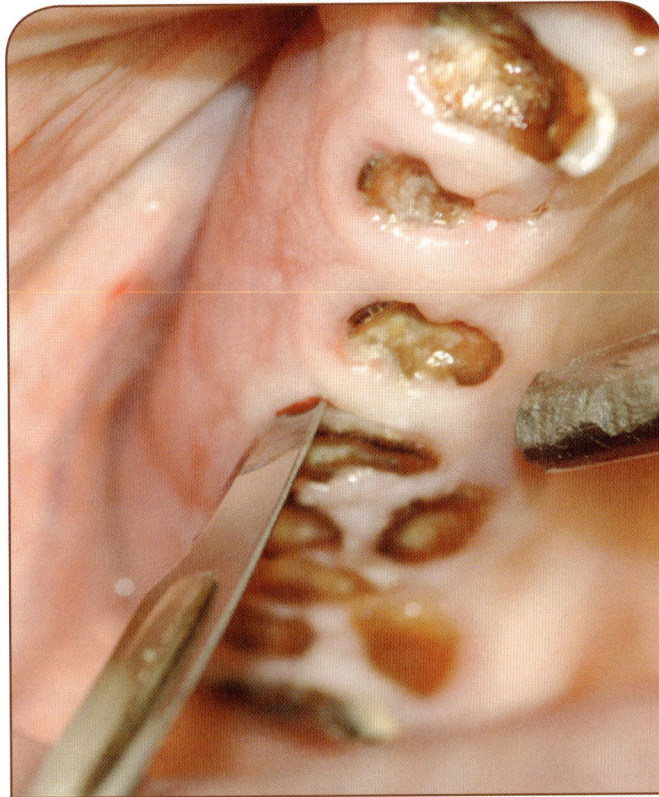

Fig. 5

Incision given all around the root pieces. A complete flap reflection is avoided **(Fig. 5)**.

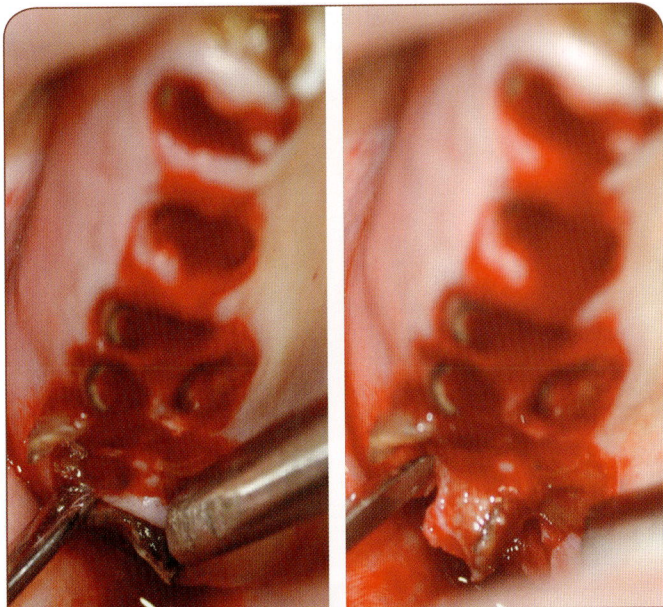

Fig. 6

Flapless surgery done, all root pieces extracted **(Fig. 6)**.

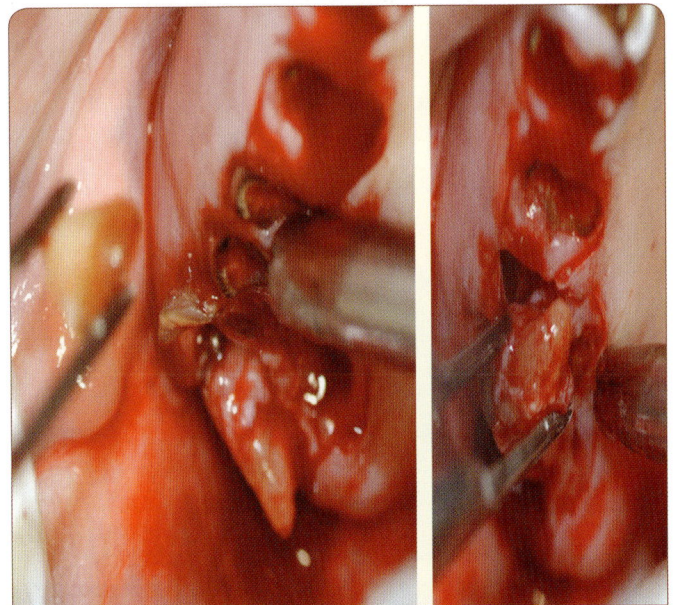

Fig. 7

Care taken to conserve remaining bone on all sides **(Fig. 7)**.

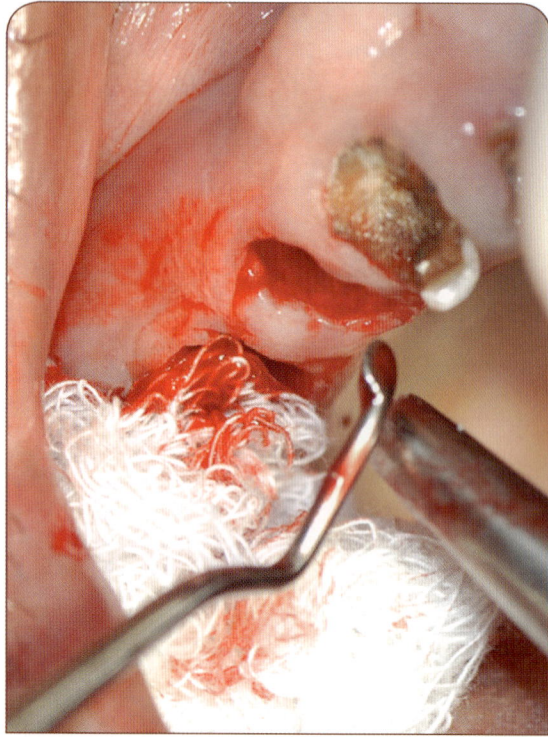

Fig. 8

The extracted sockets are cleaned properly, curetted nicely **(Fig. 8)**.

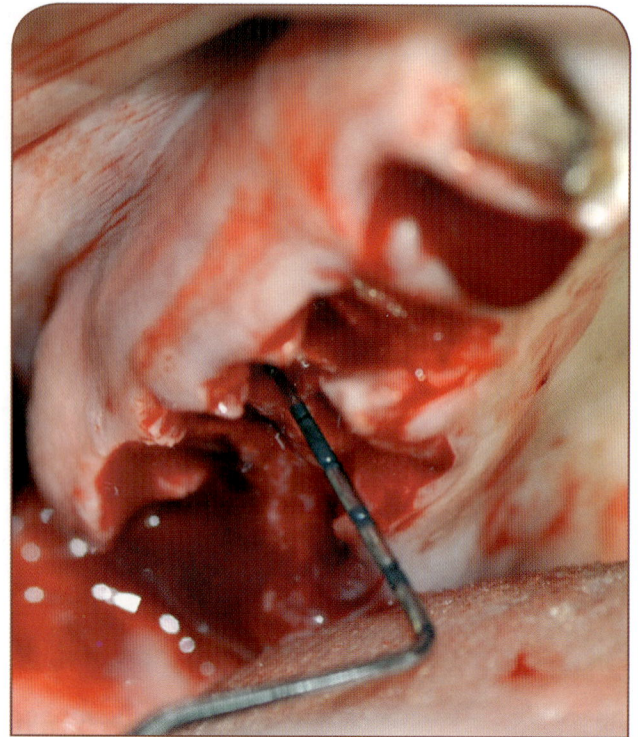

Fig. 9

Bone sounding done to check presence or absence of all walls of the socket **(Fig. 9)**.

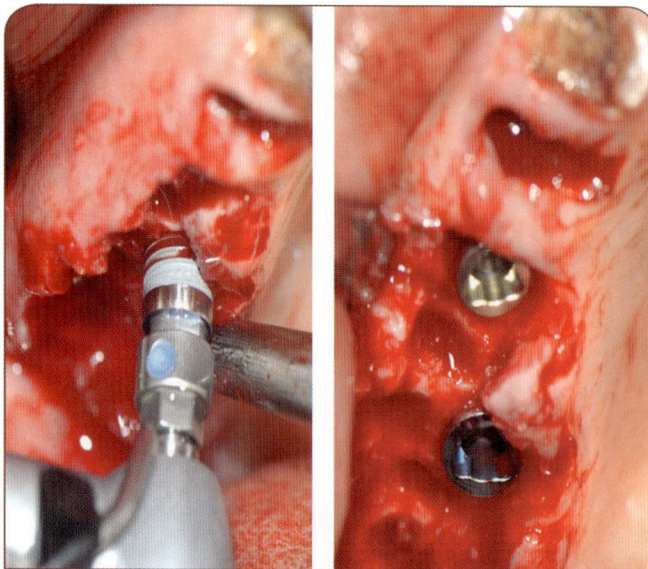

Fig. 10

Nobel groovy implants being placed in the premolar and molar region in posterior maxilla **(Fig. 10)**.

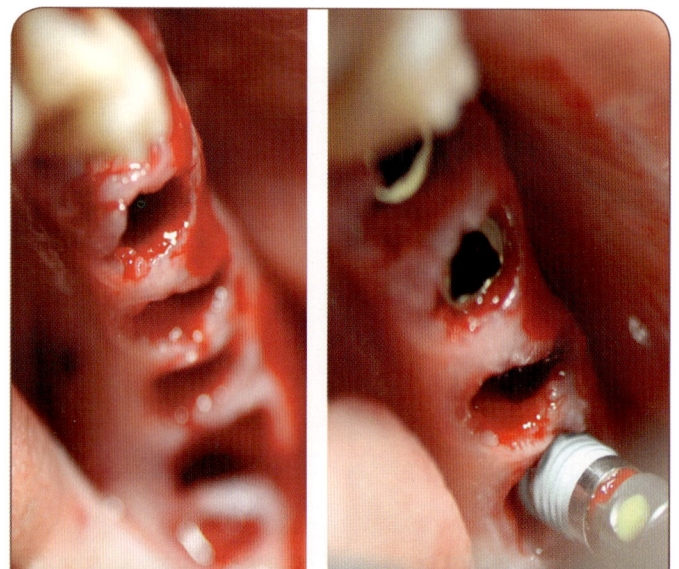

Fig. 11

Nobel groovy implants being placed in the premolar and molar region in the mandibular arch too **(Fig. 11)**.

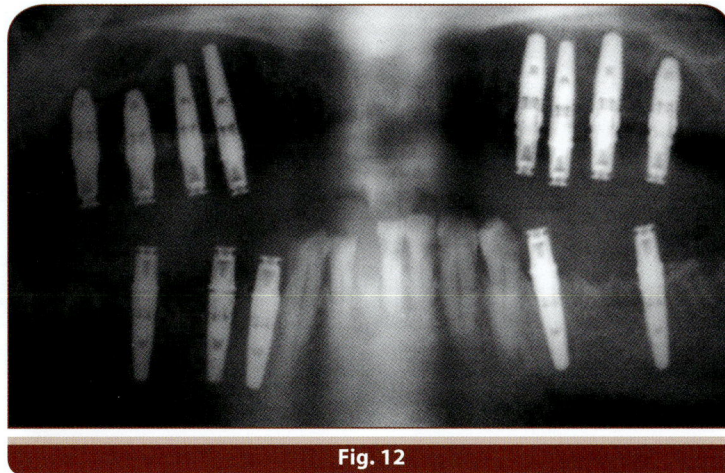

Fig. 12

Nobel groovy implants placed in the premolar and molar region on both sides of the arch. Permanent abutments also torqued in place to receive an immediate temporary prosthesis **(Fig. 12)**.

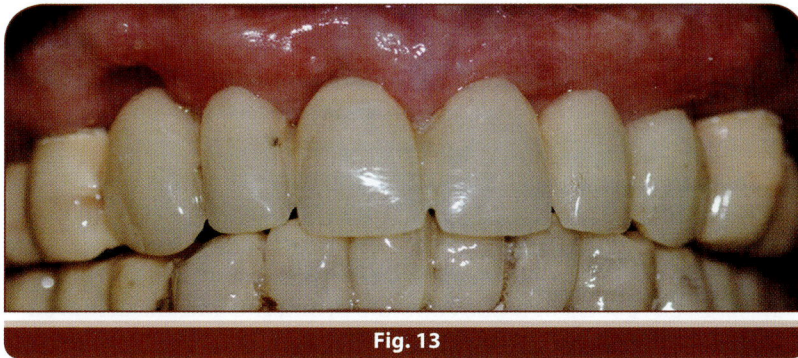

Fig. 13

Immediate temporary prosthesis is kept for 3 months after soft tissue modifications are done in the anterior pontic region **(Fig. 13)**.

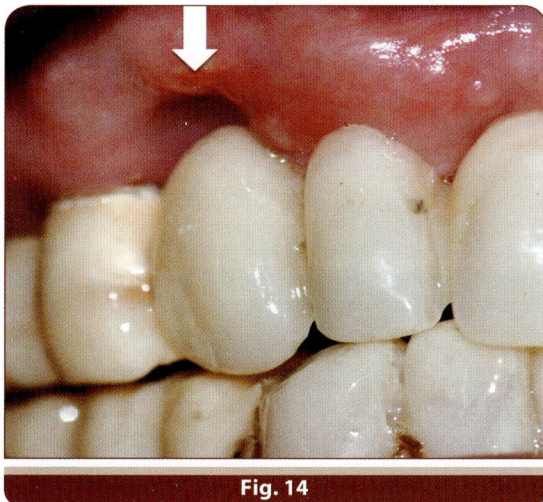

Fig. 14

There is a big bony defect in the right canine area that needs attention **(Fig. 14)**.

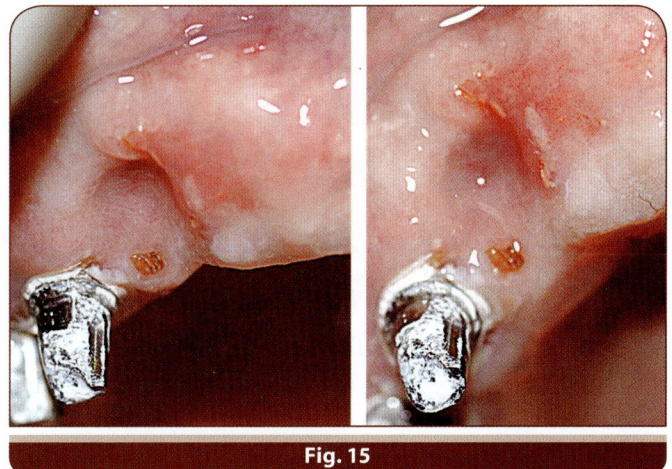

Fig. 15

Soft tissue enhancement is done in the anterior pontic region specially to correct the big defect in the right upper canine area **(Fig. 15)**.

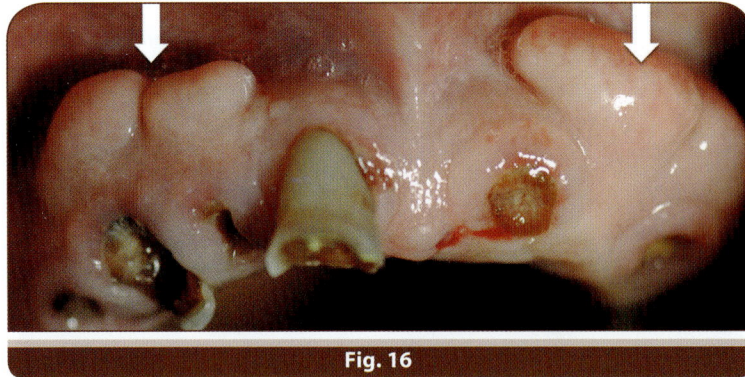

Fig. 16

The prominent bony projections on the facial anterior region as seen in the preoperative clinical photo are also flattened **(Fig. 16)**.

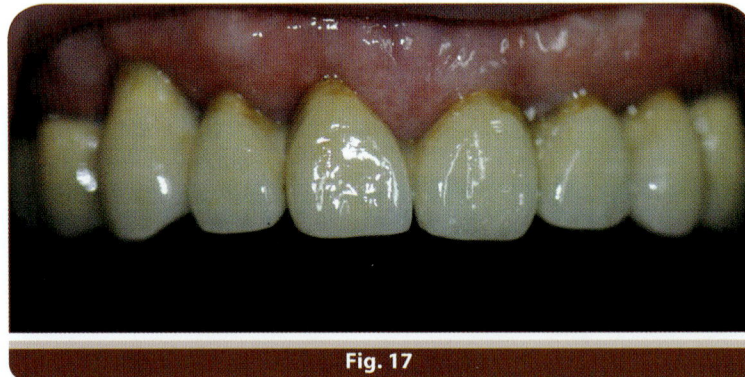

Fig. 17

Final fixed cemented prosthesis given , good soft tissue contours in anterior maxilla achieved—papilla contouring done **(Fig. 17)**.

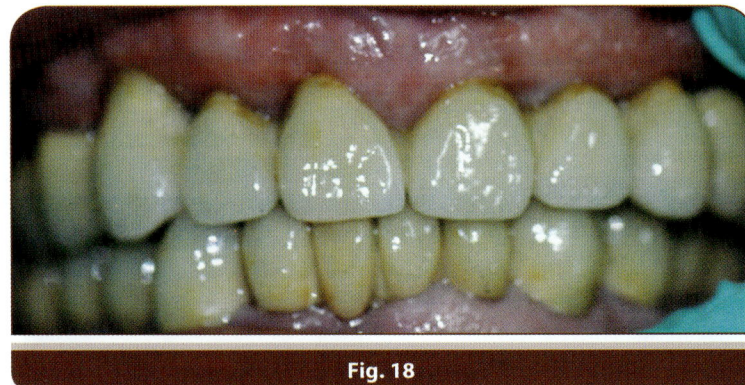

Fig. 18

Permanent fixed prosthesis in both arches with thick soft tissue type and anterior esthetics **(Fig. 18)**.

SECTION 3

Management of Posterior Maxilla including Sinus Grafting

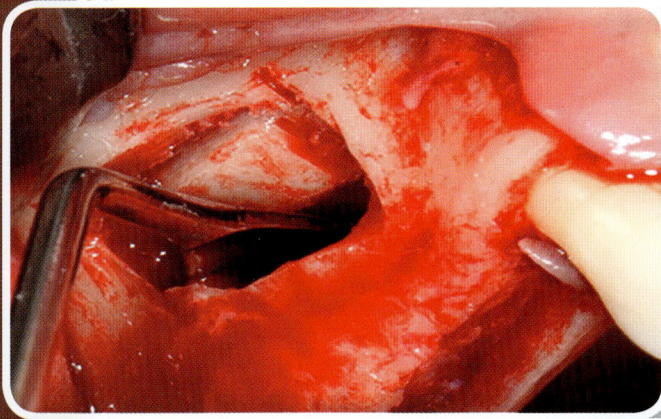

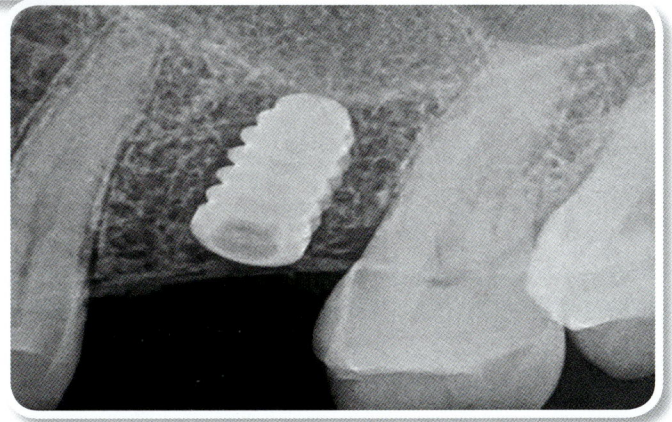

Lanka Mahesh

Direct Sinus Grafting in Minimum Height Cases (Less than 5 mm RBH)

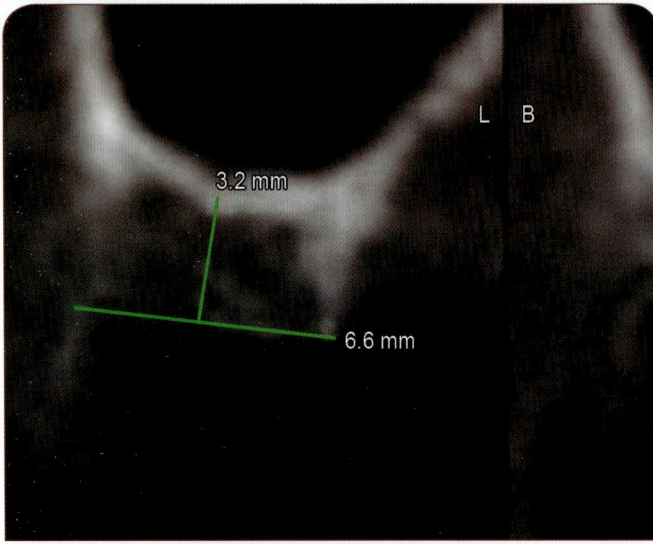

Fig. 1

A 32-year-old female patient with no relevant medical history reported to the clinic. 4 weeks old extraction site. Radiographic examination revealed height of available bone 3.2 mm (to obtain primary stability, as the rest of the extraction site has not healed. Available width 6.6 mm. Treatment plan for the case with direct sinus lift with simultaneous implant **(Fig. 1)**.

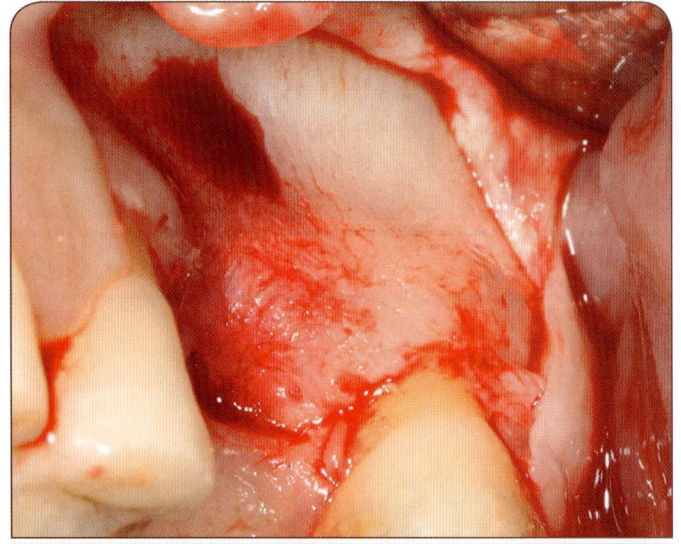

Fig. 2

Full thickness flap elevated exposing the facial wall. Ideally the incision should extend one tooth mesial and distal to the operative site to allow tension free closure and greater visibility of the operative site **(Fig. 2)**.

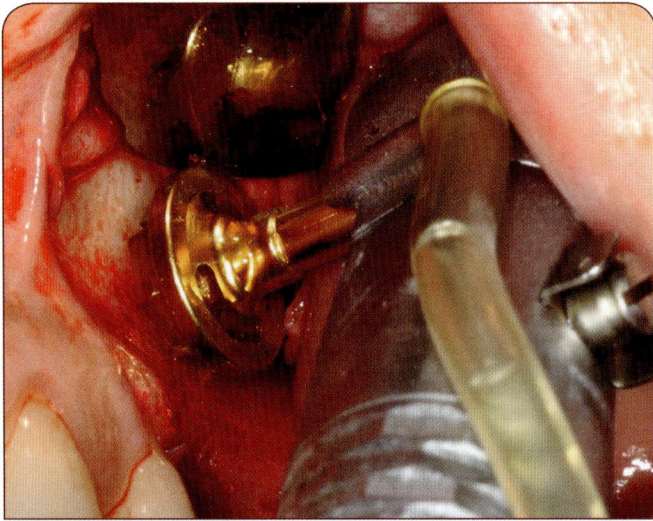

Fig. 3

The antrostomy is performed using a SLA kit (Neobiotech) AL reamer of 3 mm depth and 4 mm diameter is being used **(Fig. 3)**.

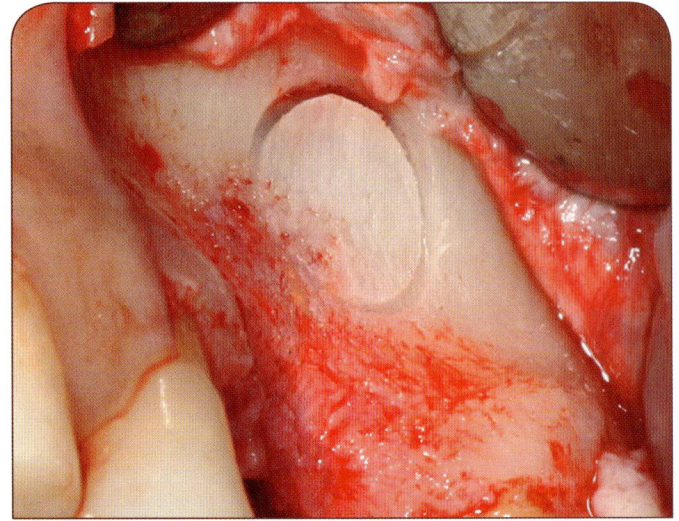

Fig. 4

Initial preparation of the antrostomy. It is ideal to get a purchase point to prevent the bur (reamer) from slipping. Ideal speed 1000–1200 rpm **(Fig. 4)**.

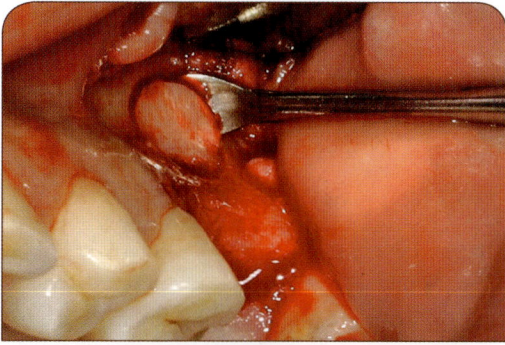

Fig. 5

The completed window preparation. The bony window should be carefully detached using a sinus curette. A cm 2/4 from Hu-Friedy is being used here **(Fig. 5)**.

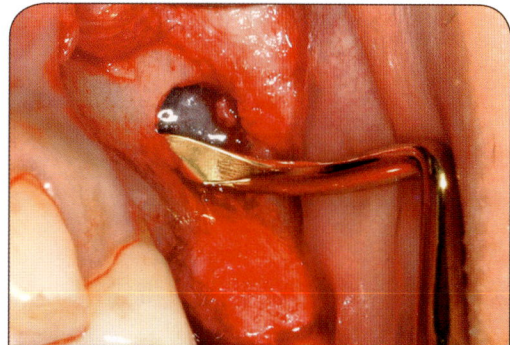

Fig. 6

Schneiderian membrane elevation is gently performed using sinus curettes starting from the most mesial aspect of the antrostomy. Care should be taken to keep the instrument in contact with bone at all times to prevent membrane perforation **(Fig. 6)**.

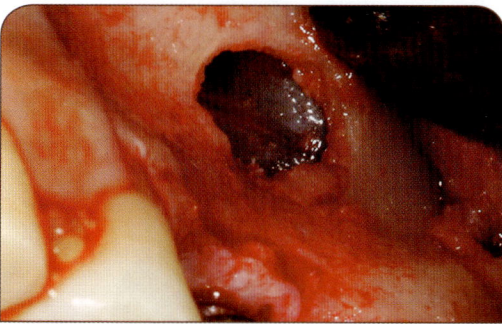

Fig. 7

An intraosseous artery is clearly evident running across the sinus membrane. Careful elevation in a circumferential manner prevents rupture of the vessel and is lifted along with the sinus membrane **(Fig. 7)**.

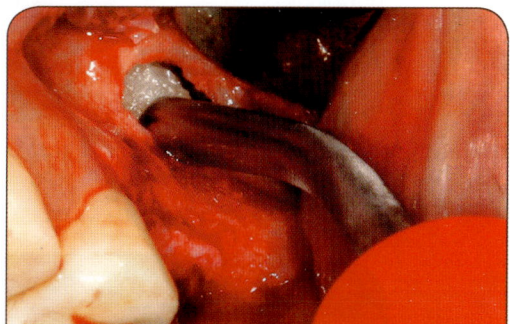

Fig. 8

After osteotomy preparation. A calcium phosphosilicate putty is being injected into the area (NovaBone) **(Fig. 8)**.

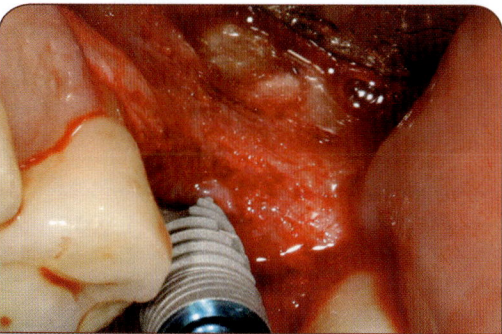

Fig. 9

An implant is seated at 30 rpm. Cortex conical implant of 4.2/11.5 mm **(Fig. 9)**.

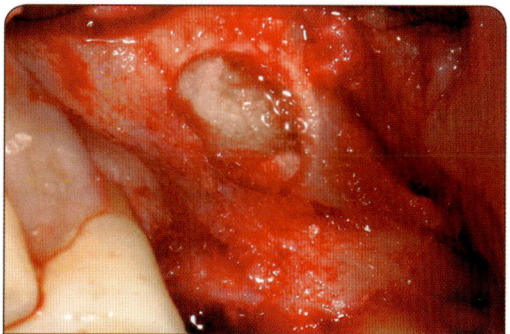

Fig. 10

More grafting material is injected over the implant to achieve a sandwich effect. A total of 1 cc graft material is used in this case **(Fig. 10)**.

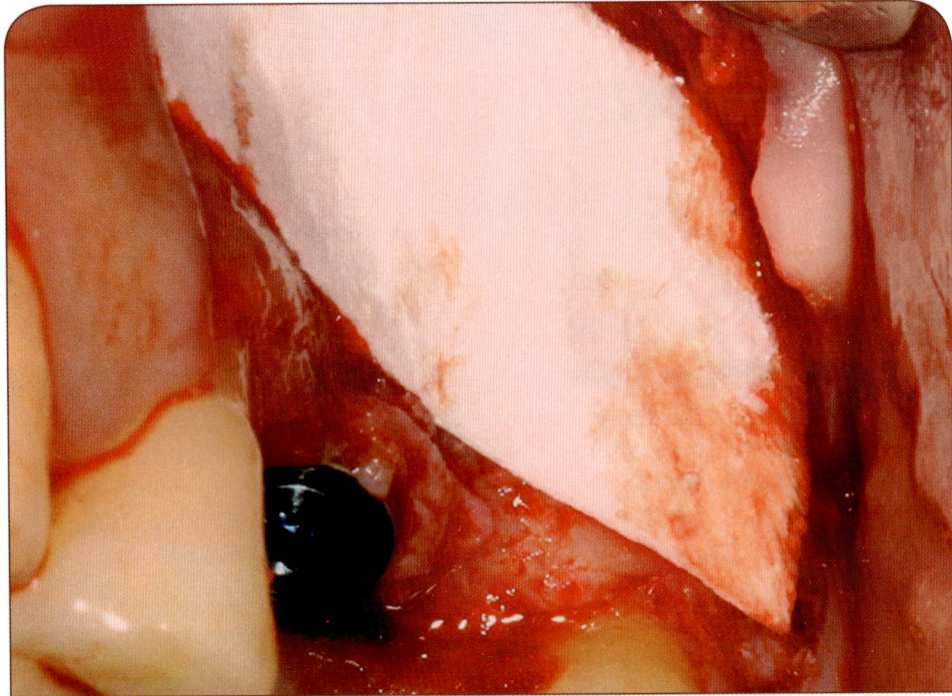

Fig. 11

A resorbable membrane is placed over the grafted area and closed with 3–0. e PTFE sutures (cytoplast-osteogenics) **(Fig. 11)**.

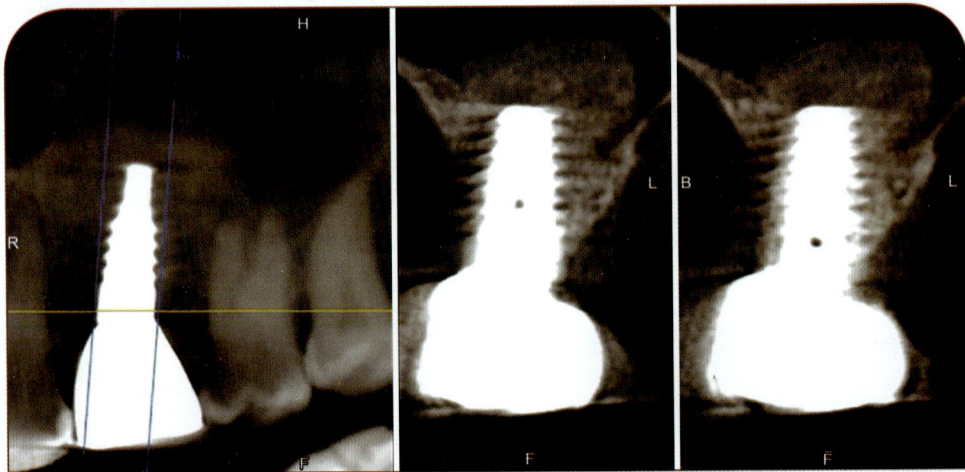

Fig. 12

One year postoperative CBCT views showing complete bone fill and graft consolidation **(Fig. 12)**.

Praful Bali

DIRECT SINUS LIFT AND SOFT TISSUE ENHANCEMENT FOR A COMPLETE ESTHETIC AND FUNCTIONAL RESULT

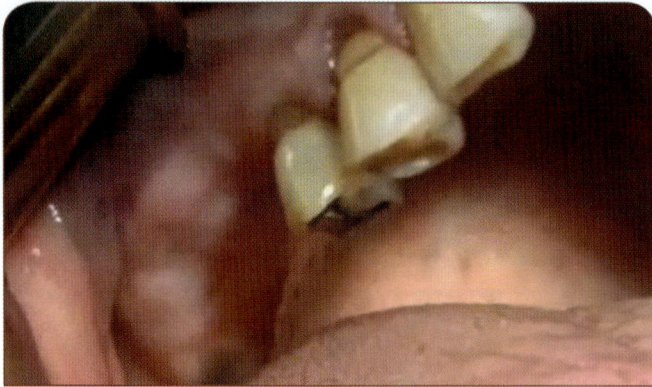

Fig. 1

Preoperative clinical view of a case of a direct sinus lift procedure. Teeth #16,17 missing **(Fig. 1)**.

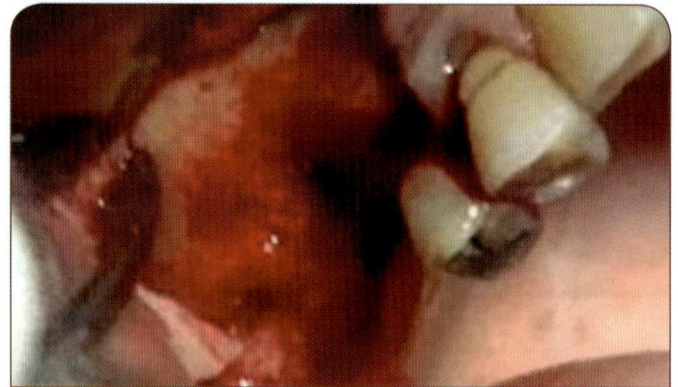

Fig. 2

Full thickness flap raised with vertical relieving incisions to expose the lateral wall of the sinus **(Fig. 2)**.

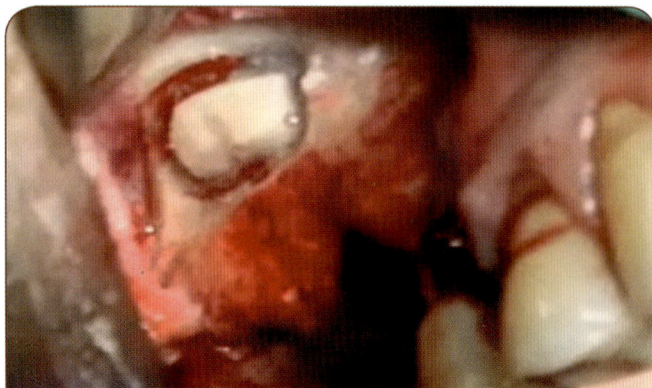

Fig. 3

Boundaries of the lateral window for the lift are defined with a round diamond bur on a straight handpiece **(Fig. 3)**.

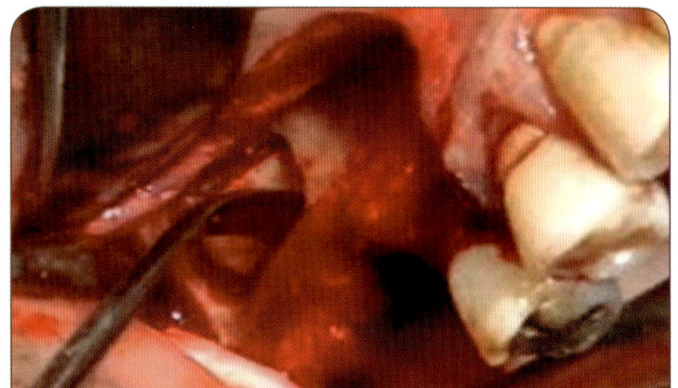

Fig. 4

Sinus membrane is manipulated with sinus curettes till the whole part is lifted uniformly **(Fig. 4)**.

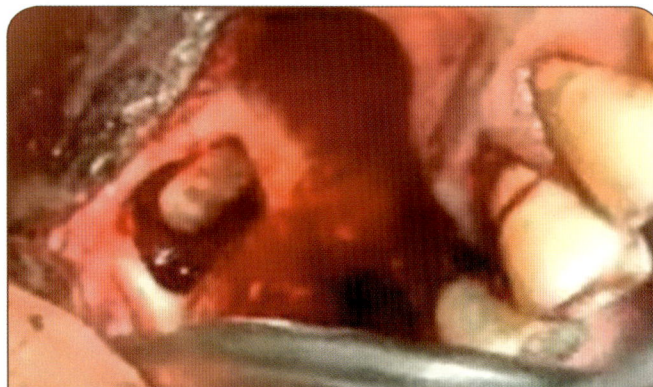

Fig. 5

Sinus lift done. Note the new floor of the sinus **(Fig. 5)**.

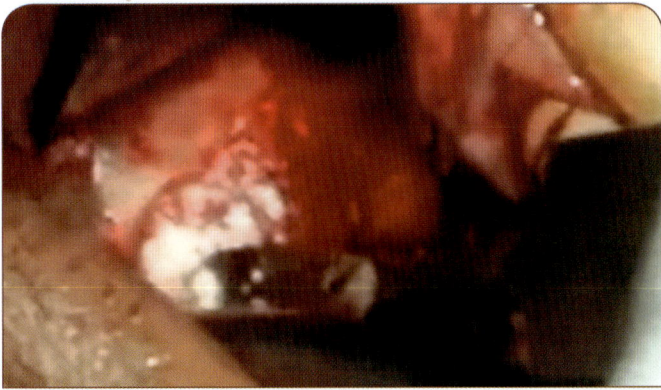

Fig. 6

The sinus is filled with Bio Oss bone graft **(Fig. 6)**.

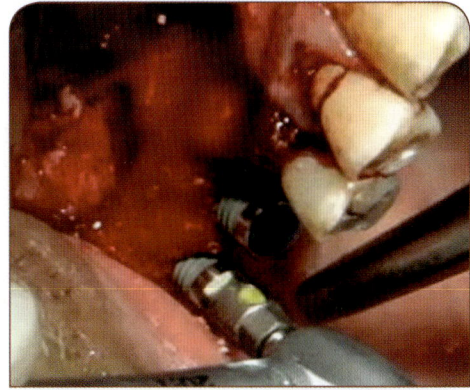

Fig. 7

2 Nobel Biocare implants, 5/11.5, 4.3/11.5 are placed **(Fig. 7)**.

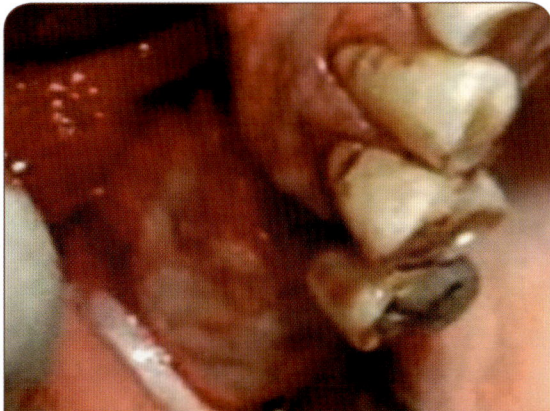

Fig. 8

A collagen membrane is used to cover the sinus window and secure the graft **(Fig. 8)**.

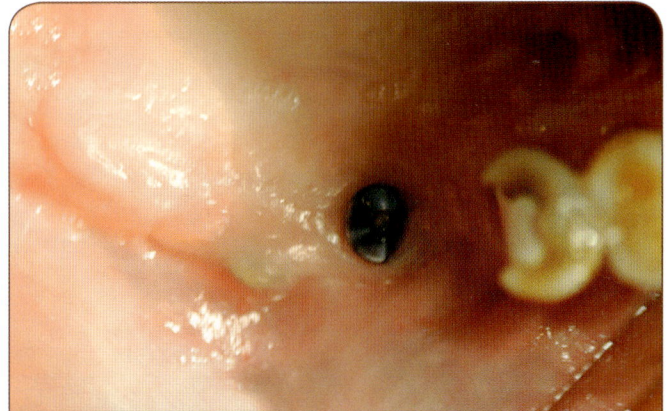

Fig. 9

3 months postoperatively there is lack of keratinized soft tissue around the implants, the cover screw of the anterior implant hence exposed due to thin gingiva **(Fig. 9)**.

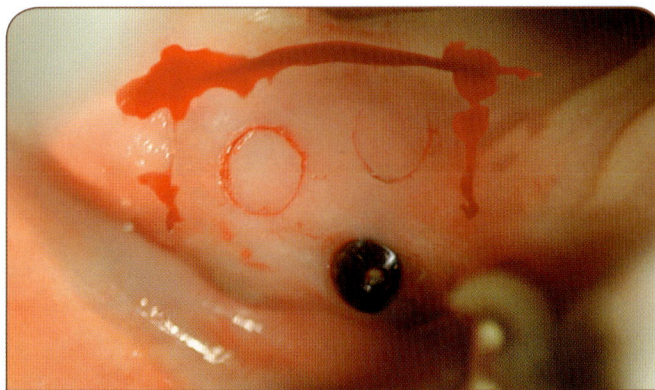

Fig. 10

To add bulk to the tissue and have healthy tissue around the implants , 2 punches are made on the palate and an incision given in the manner shown **(Fig. 10)**.

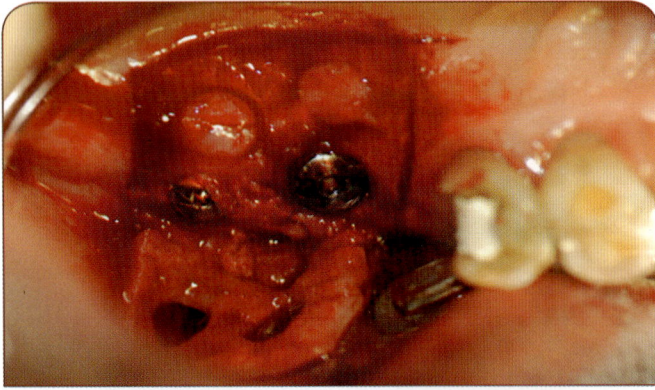

Fig. 11

A partial thickness flap raised **(Fig. 11)**.

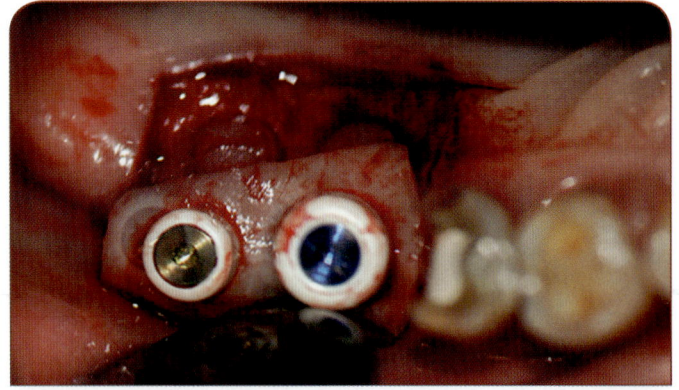

Fig. 12

The flap is moved over the implants and secured around the implants **(Fig. 12)**.

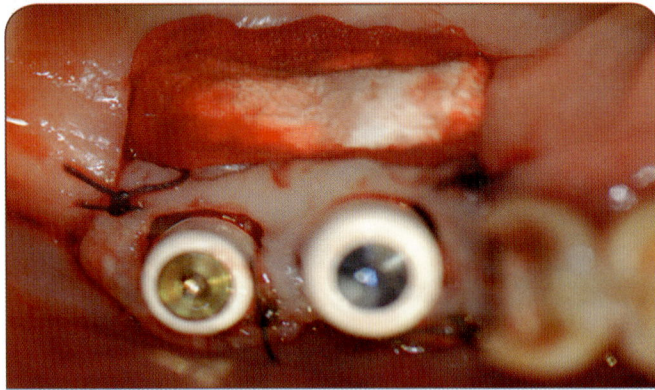

Fig. 13

The flap is sutured around the implants and the defect is packed with collatape and sealed **(Fig. 13)**.

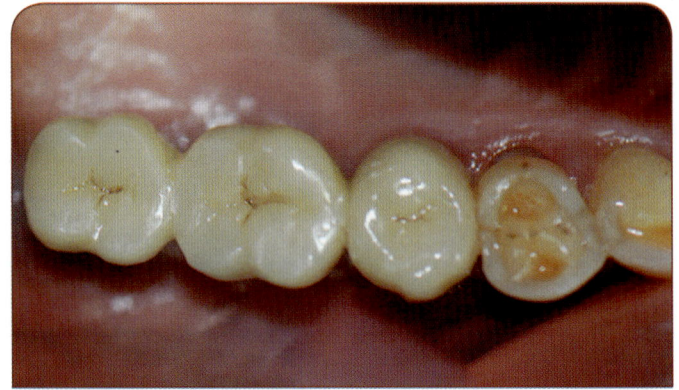

Fig. 14

Final metal ceramic restorations given. Note the thick band of tissue around the implants. Tooth #15 also receives a crown after endo treatment **(Fig. 14)**.

CASE STUDY 44

Lanka Mahesh, Vishal Gupta

DIRECT SINUS GRAFTING IN MINIMAL RBH (LESS THAN 2 MM) AND SIMULTANEOUS IMPLANT PLACEMENT

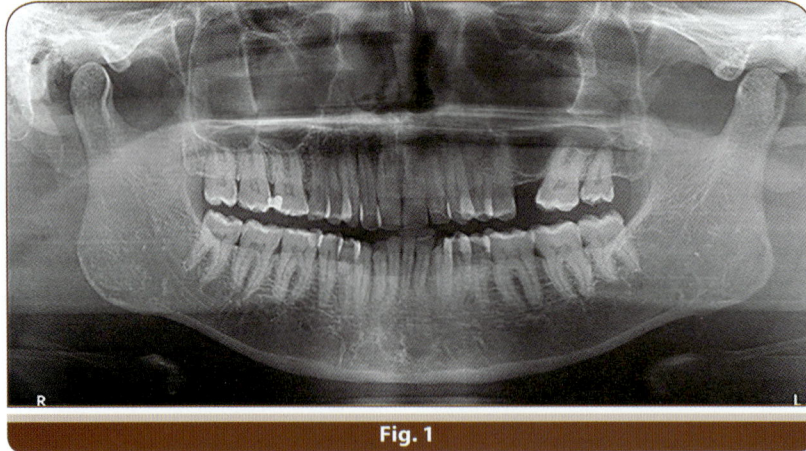

Fig. 1

Preoperative panorex of a 45-year-old male patient, desiring replacement of the left upper posterior tooth. Residual bone height is less than 2 mm and tooth # 27 has drifted mesially encroaching on the mesiodistal space of the missing 26. A direct sinus lift with simultaneous implant placement was planned **(Fig. 1)**.

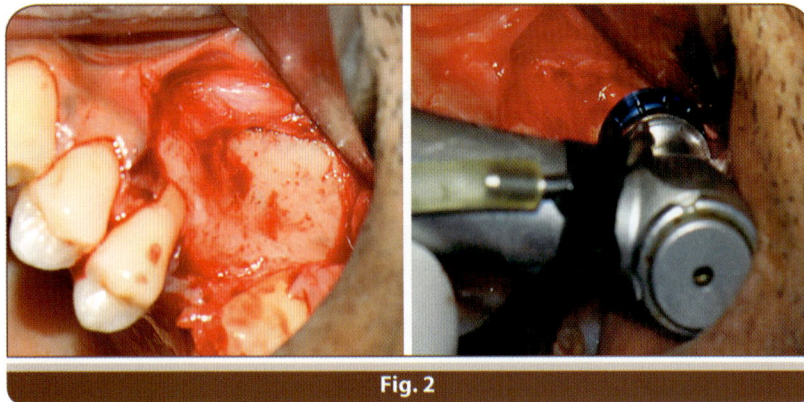

Fig. 2

A full thickness mucoperiosteal flap is elevated to expose the lateral wall of the sinus. The sinus window is prepared with a LAS-KIT (Osstem) the stopper on the bur is clearly seen **(Fig. 2)**.

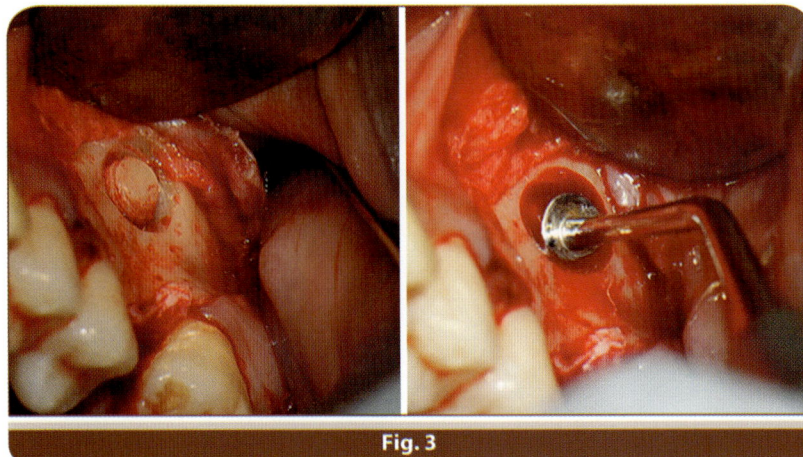

Fig. 3

Creation of the lateral wall osteotomy. An elephant foot instrument (Osung) is used circumferentially to gently tease the sinus membrane from all around the osteotomy site **(Fig. 3)**.

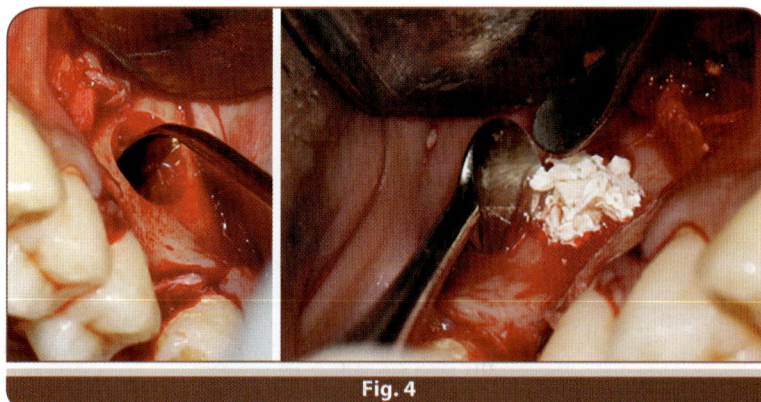

Fig. 4

A sinus curette (Osung), is introduced into the floor of the sinus and the sinus membrane is gently elevated. Bone substitute material is introduced into the sinus, cerabone (Botiss) **(Fig. 4)**.

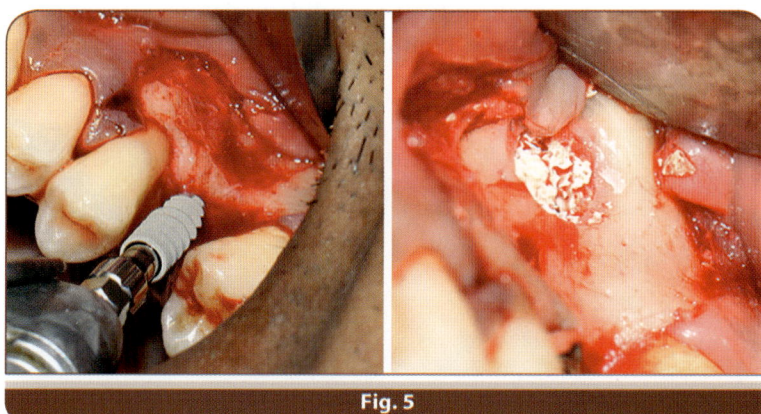

Fig. 5

A 4/11, 5 mm DM implant (Bioner) is placed at 40 ncm and more graft is placed over the lateral osteotomy to achieve a sandwich effect **(Fig. 5)**.

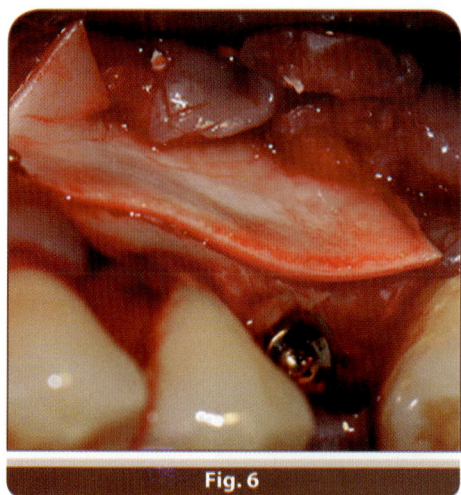

Fig. 6

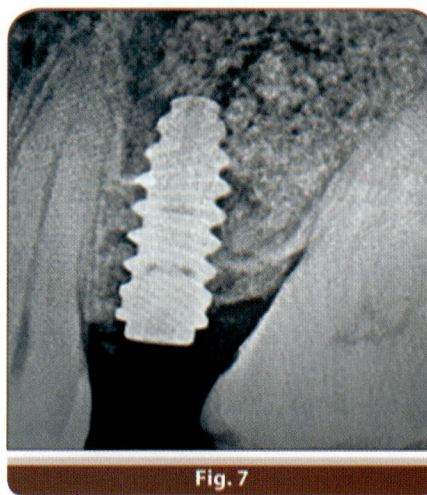

Fig. 7

The lateral window is covered with a resorbable collagen membrane (conform, ACE Surgicals) **(Fig. 6)**.

Immediate postoperative X-ray demonstrates good bone fill of the sinus. The implant is placed parallel to 25 therefore allowing for sufficient restorative space **(Fig. 7)**.

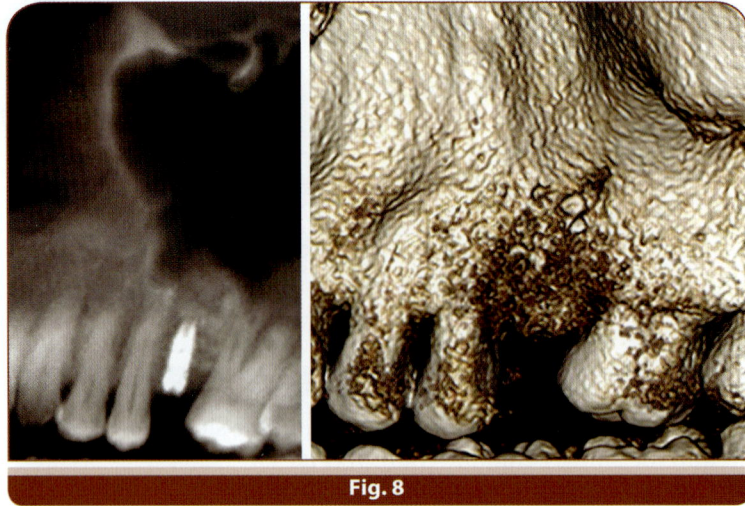

Fig. 8

A 6-month postoperative CBCT views show excellent graft consolidation and a lift that is higher than the length of the fixture placed is evident. 3D volume rendering shows complete closure of the lateral window osteotomy **(Fig. 8)**.

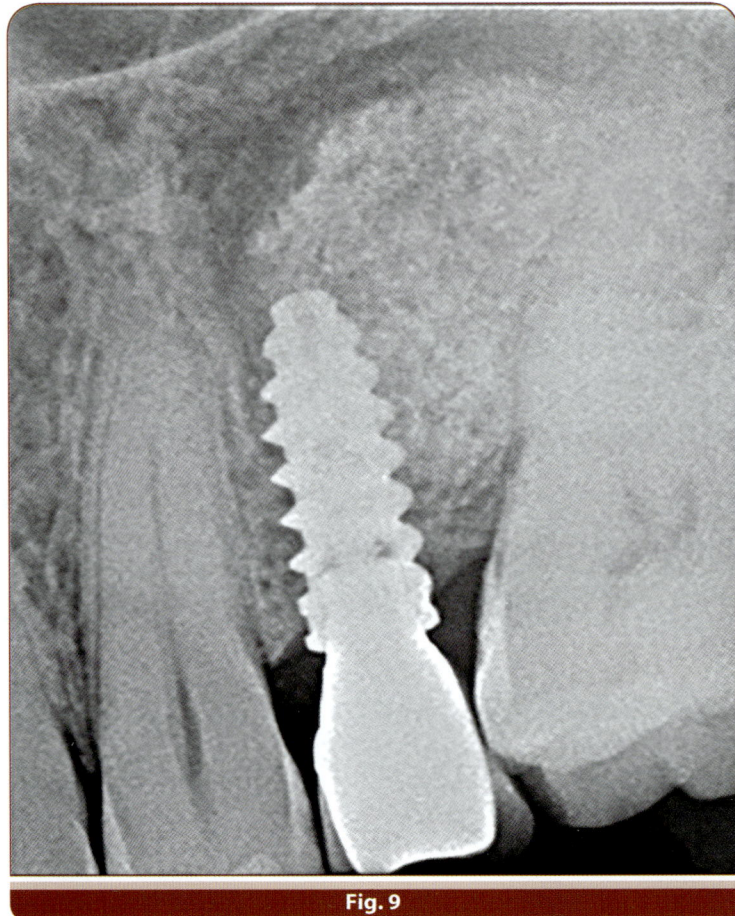

Fig. 9

A 2-year recall IOPA X-ray and clinical picture show an excellent and stable graft material and a PFM crown in a stable environment **(Fig. 9)**.

Lanka Mahesh

IMMEDIATE IMPLANT PLACEMENT WITH INDIRECT SINUS LIFT IN AN UPPER MOLAR

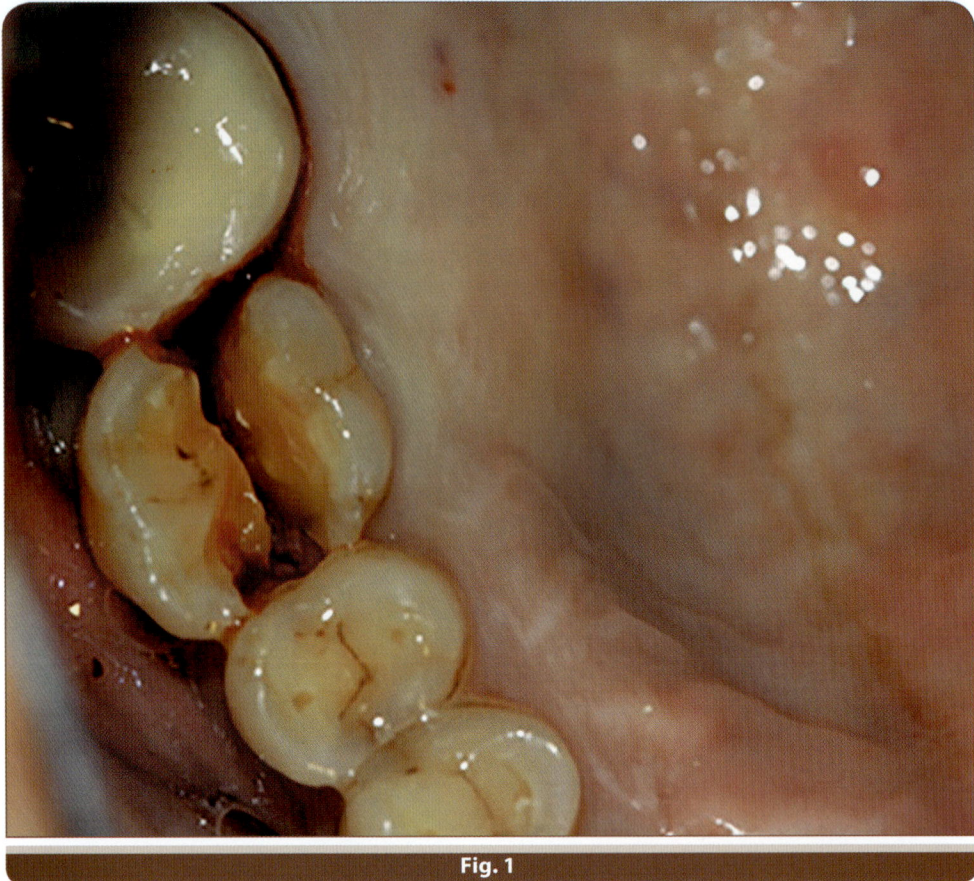

Fig. 1

A 55-year-old patient presented with a vertically fractured tooth #16 with hopeless prognosis. The treatment plan included an immediate implant in the interseptal bone along with an indirect sinus lift considering the less residual bone height (RBH) **(Fig. 1)**.

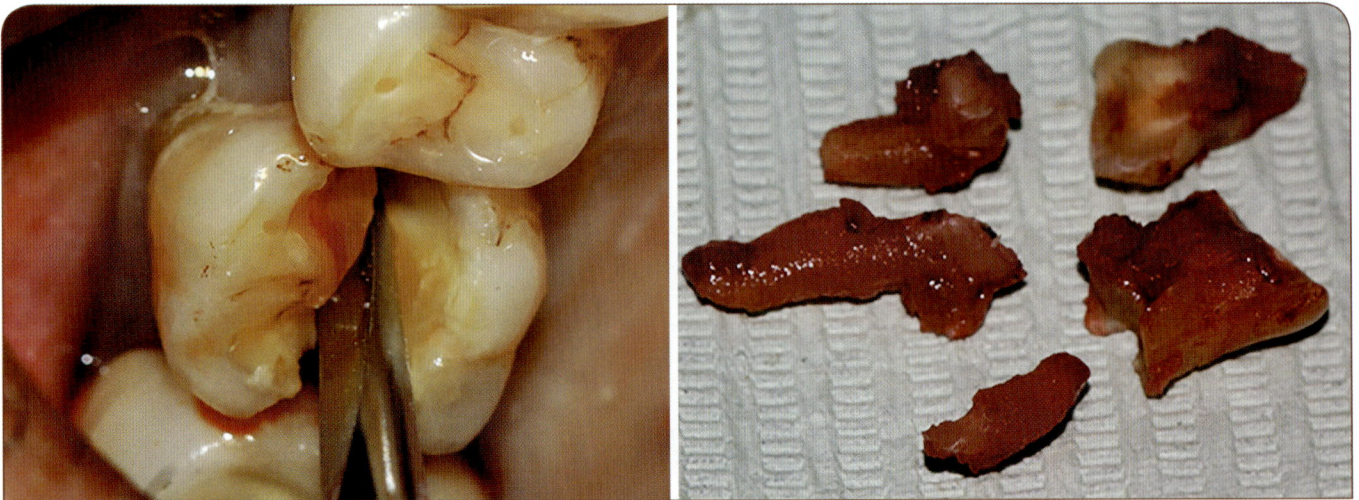

Fig. 2

The tooth is gently luxated out of the socket. Keeping all bony walls intact to facilitate an immediate implant placement **(Fig. 2)**.

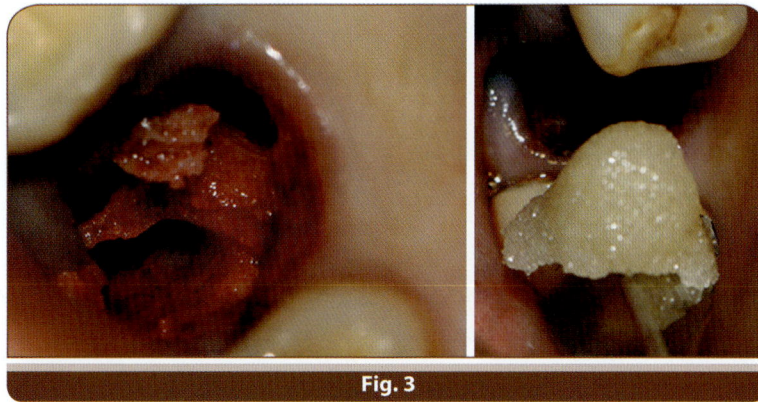

Fig. 3

The interseptal bone is clearly visible to be sound without any breach. After drilling short of the sinus floor. Till the 3.4 mm drill an osteotone of 3.8 mm is used to gently fracture the sinus floor. CPS putty (Novabone) is then inserted into the created osteotomy and gently packed with a blunt instrument **(Fig. 3)**.

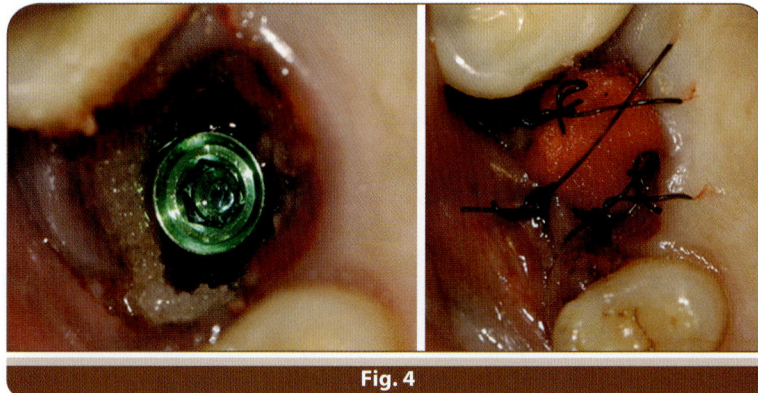

Fig. 4

A 4.6/12 mm Tapered implant (Biohorizons) is placed at 30 Rpm and 30 Ncm torque, the position of the implant hex is exactly in the position of the central fossa of the tooth it will replace. The site is sealed with CollaPlug (Zimmer Dental) and closed with cross sutures using 3-0 polyamide **(Fig. 4)**.

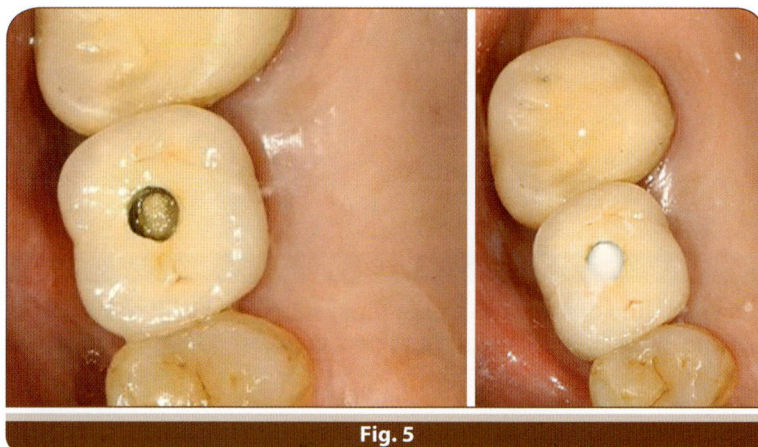

Fig. 5

The final prosthesis is cemented extraorally on the abutment and transferred intraorally. The abutment is torqued to 35 Ncm and the access hole is filled with teflon tape and sealed with glass ionomer cement **(Fig. 5)**.

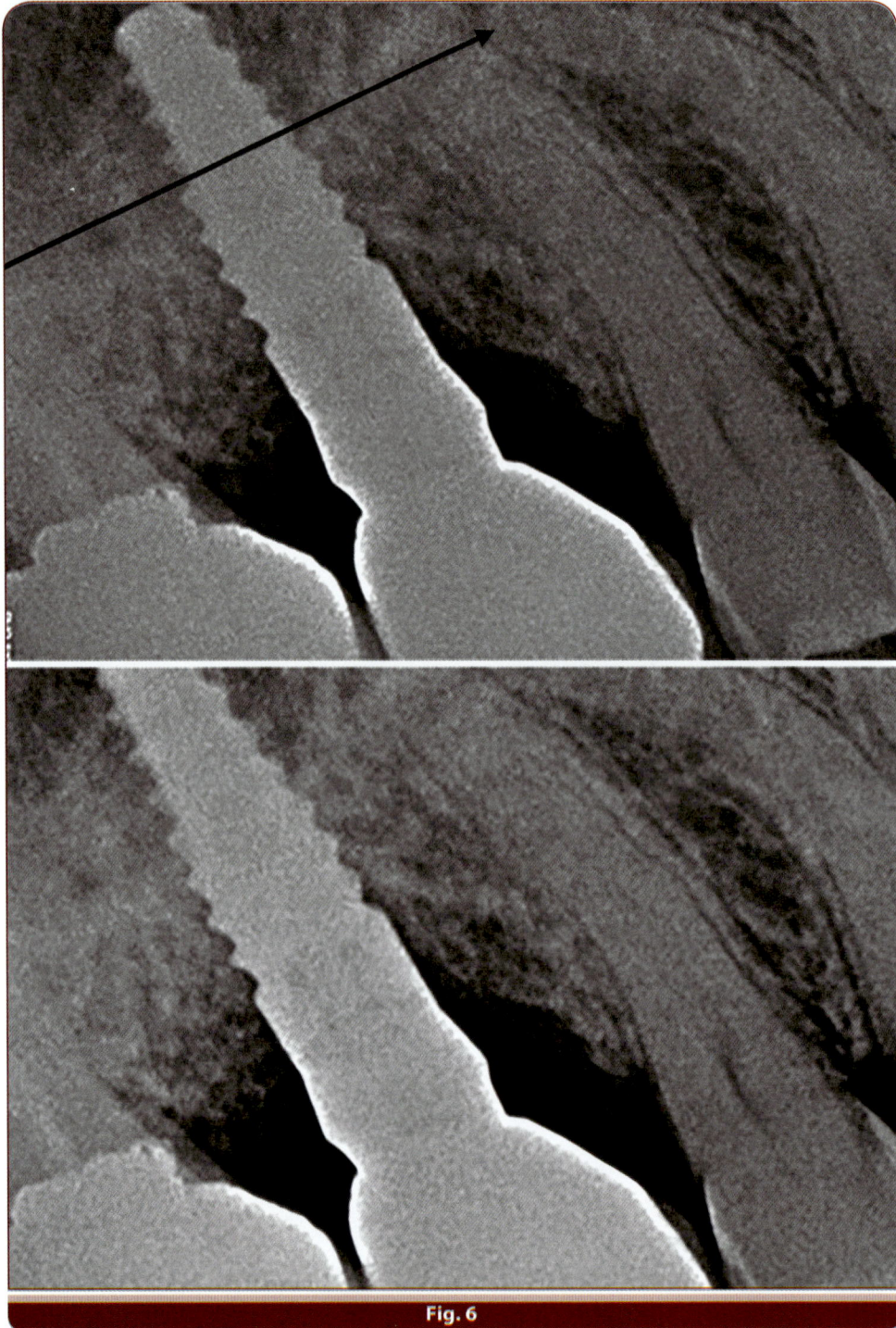

Fig. 6

IOPA X-rays at insertion (the green line demarcates the original sinus floor). Five year recall X-ray demonstrates good bone fill in the sinus, some crestal bone loss at the mesial aspect compared to the X-ray at insertion **(Fig. 6)**.

Lanka Mahesh

Lateral Wall Sinus Graft with Delayed Implant Placement using an Alloplast

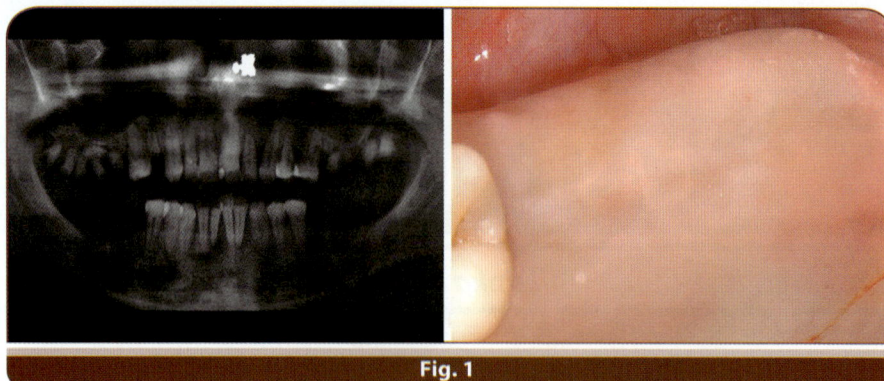

Fig. 1

Preoperative panorex of a 42-year-old lady. Treatment plan included extractions of the maxillary posterior root fragments, a 6 week healing period. Followed by lateral wall sinus lifts (direct sinus lifts) and delayed implant placement. Implant supported prosthesis in the mandibular posteriors. Clinical view of the right maxillary posterior quadrant 6 weeks following extractions **(Fig. 1)**.

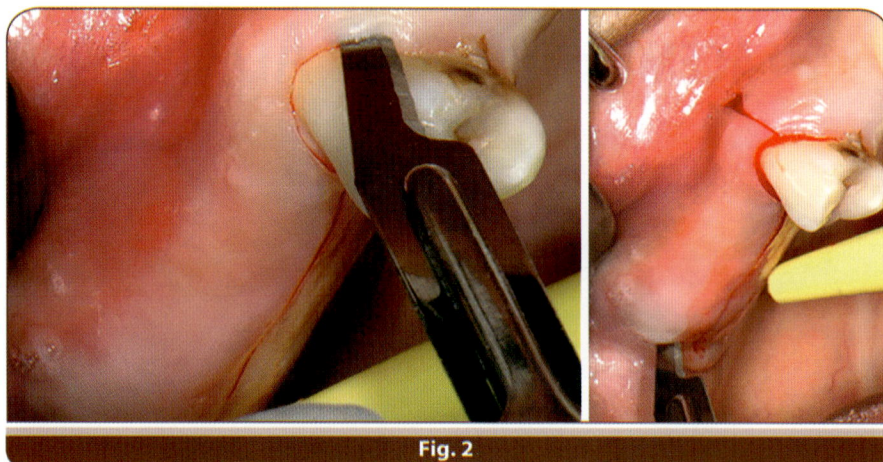

Fig. 2

The incision with 15C blade runs crestally with a distal release incision and mesially to anterior to the tooth present mesial to the operative site where it ends in a vertical release. (In case both premolars were present the incision would be extended further to the middle of 14 and 15) **(Fig. 2)**.

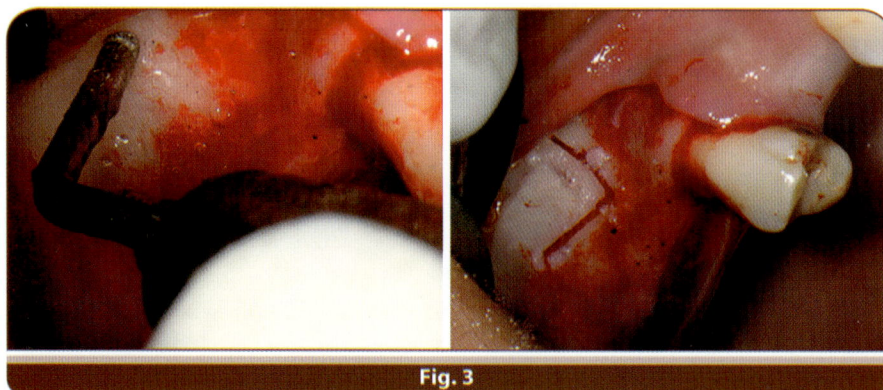

Fig. 3

After adequate flap reflection the osteotomy is initiated with a round tip. To outline the lateral window the tip is changed to a saw tip on the piezosurgery unit (Piezo Art, Dowell Dental) for completion of the window **(Fig. 3)**.

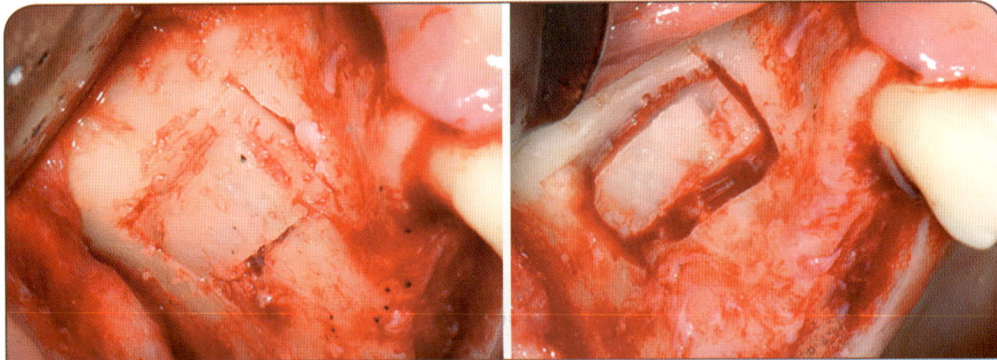

Fig. 4

Careful examination of the osteotomy is critical before attempting a membrane lift, the first picture clearly shows an incomplete cut in the superior mesial part of the window. The window should be free from all sides and verified with a blunt instrument such as a ball burnisher (**Fig. 4**).

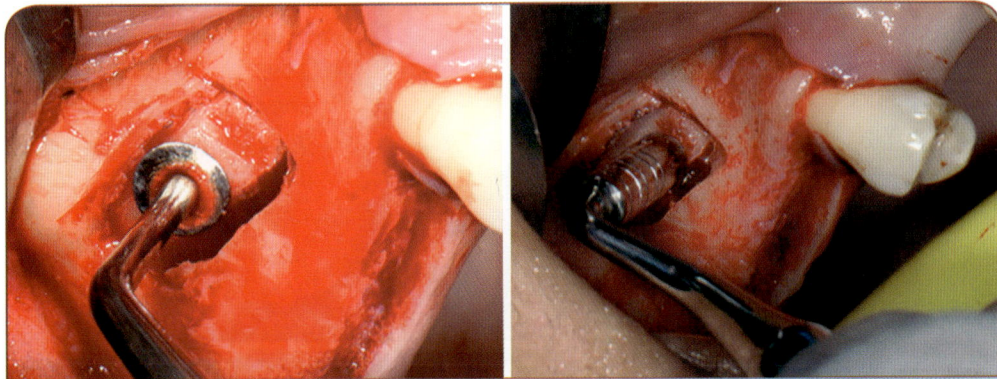

Fig. 5

An elephant foot instrument (Osung) is used very gently to push the window to check the integrity of the elasticity of the sinus lining and ensuring complete freedom from any bony ledges preventing a proper sinus elevation procedure. A large head bone plugger can be used to the same effect (**Fig. 5**).

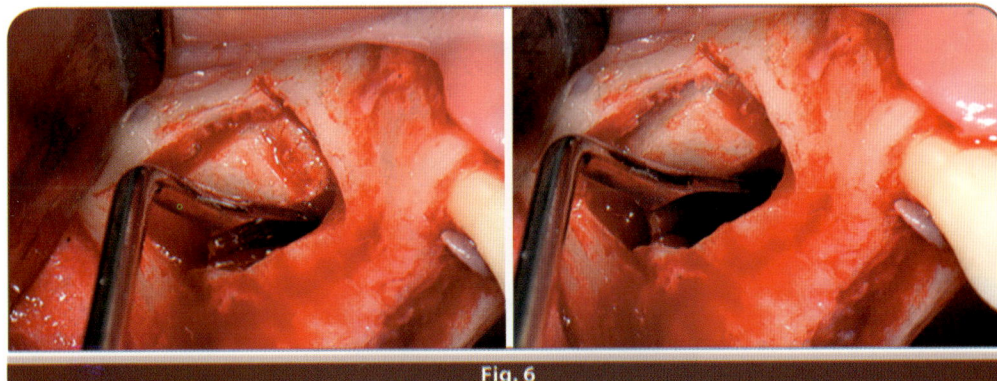

Fig. 6

An obtuse angle elevator is gently introduced into the floor of the sinus. Always keeping the instrument in contact with the bony surface to prevent membrane tears. Gradual elevation is achieved with the instrument. An acute angle elevator is used in the mesial and distal parts of the sinus to achieve a complete lift (**Fig. 6**).

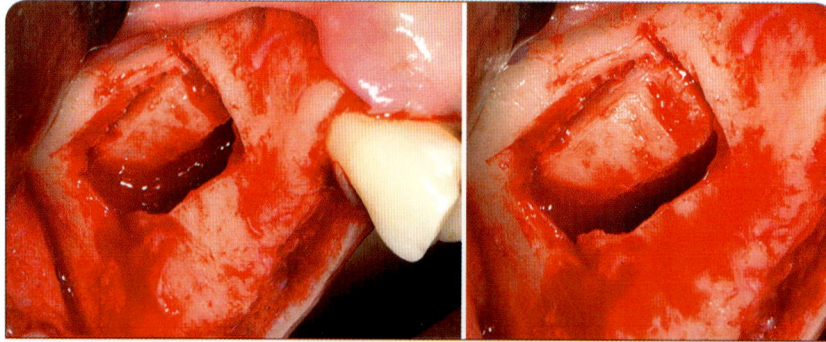

Fig. 7

Integrity of the sinus membrane is clearly evident during inhalation and exhalation. Care should be taken not to do this step too vigorously which can cause a membrane rupture by a blow out **(Fig. 7)**.

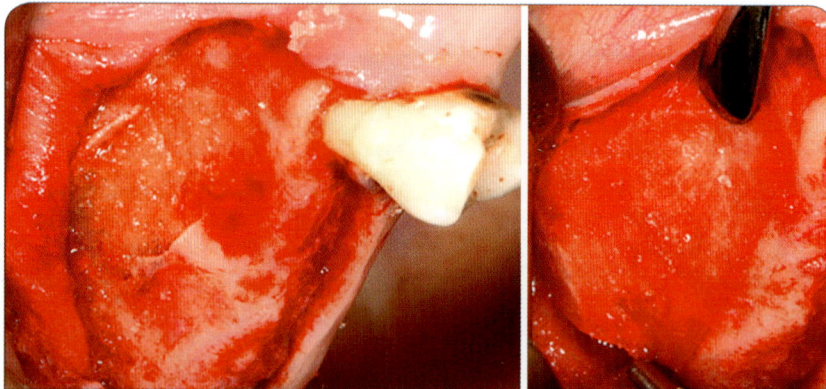

Fig. 8

The graft is packed with 1.5 cc CPS putty (NovaBone). A long resorbing equine membrane is draped over the osteotomy and saline is gently sprayed over it to make it more adaptive to the bony surface (this can be done prior to membrane placement as well) **(Fig. 8)**.

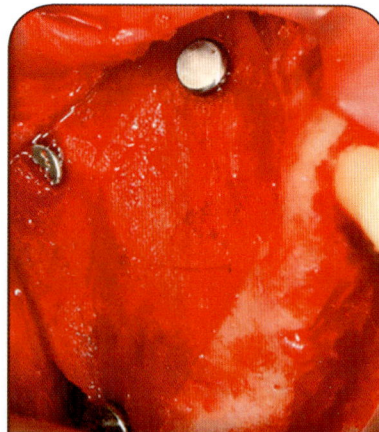

Fig. 9

The membrane is stabilized using tacs in a tripod manner to prevent any movement during the healing period. The bone tacs (Bioner, Barcelona) are fixated with gentle tapping force of a surgical mallet on the tac holding instrument **(Fig. 9)**.

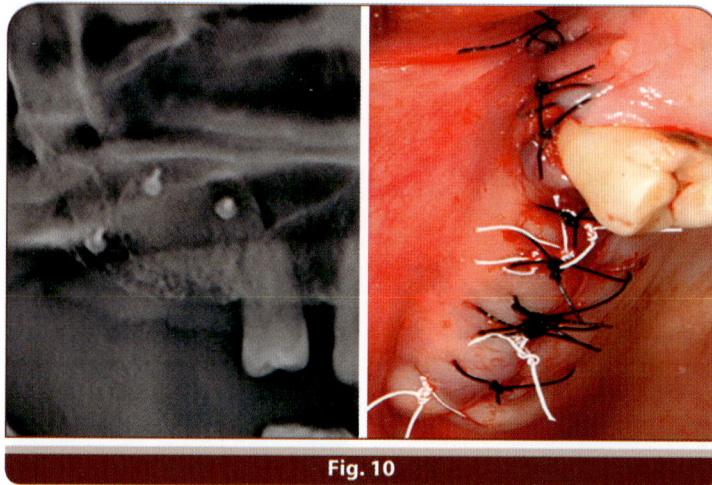

Fig. 10

Wound closure with 3–0 cytoplast sutures (osteogenics) and 3–0 polyamide, the polyamide sutures are removed in a week and the cytoplast sutures after 3 weeks. Immediate postoperative panorex clearly demonstrates adequate bone fill of the antrum **(Fig. 10)**.

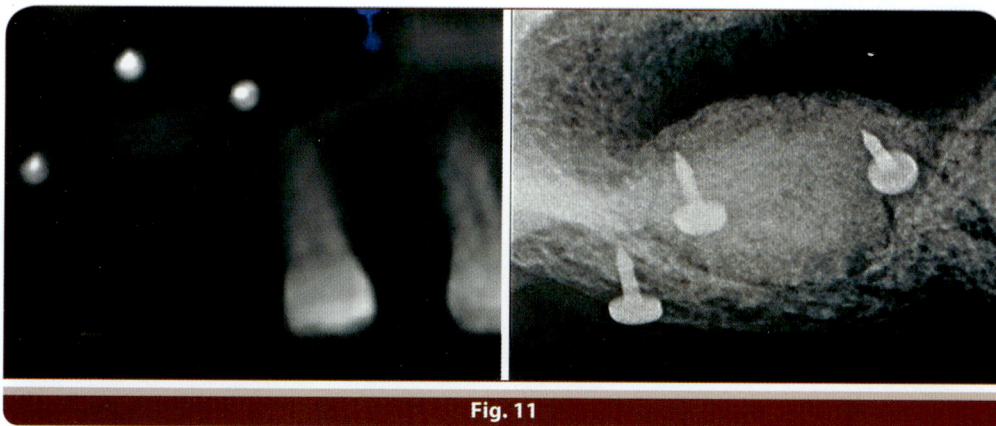

Fig. 11

CBCT view at 6 months postoperative. Intraoral X-ray view of the same site **(Fig. 11)**.

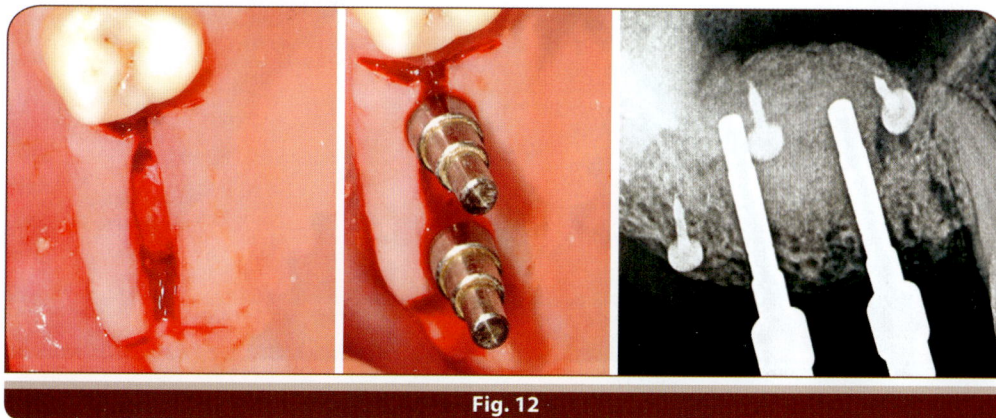

Fig. 12

After flap reflection, trephine cores are obtained, paralleling pins are placed for verification of correct mesiodistal implant placement **(Fig. 12)**.

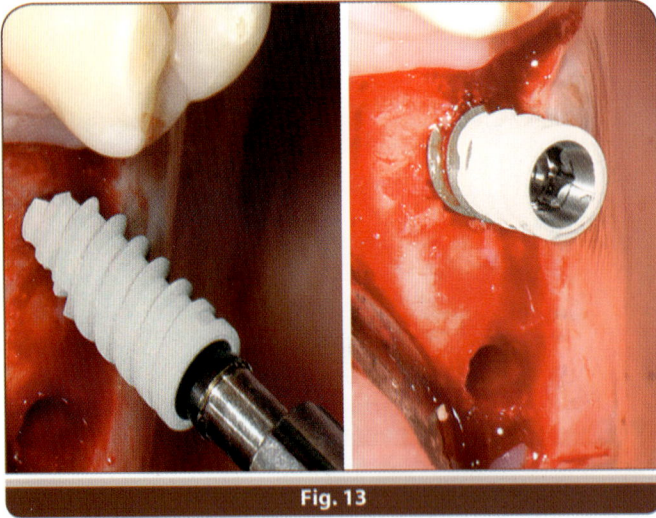

Fig. 13

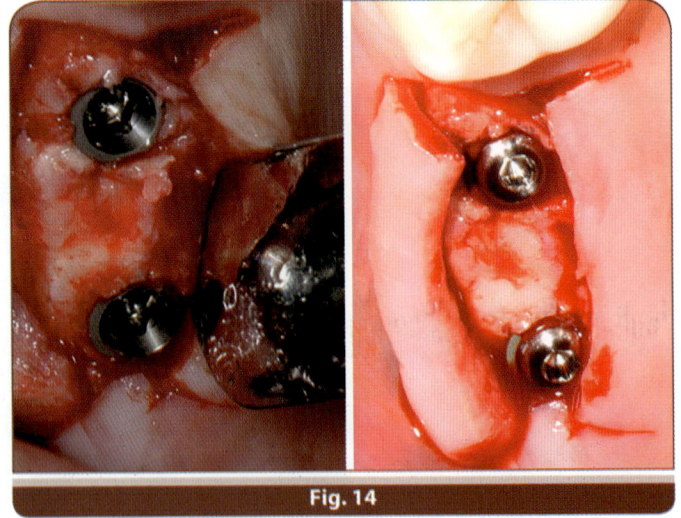

Fig. 14

After a 2.8 mm trephine core biopsy is obtained from the site two implants of 4/11.5 mm (top DM, Bioner) are inserted at 50 Ncm torque. No additional implant drills are used owing to the aggressive nature of this implant design (**Fig. 13**).

Excellent primary stability is achieved. Small conservative flaps are adequate in cases where a resorbable barrier membrane is used in the first stage surgery (**Fig. 14**).

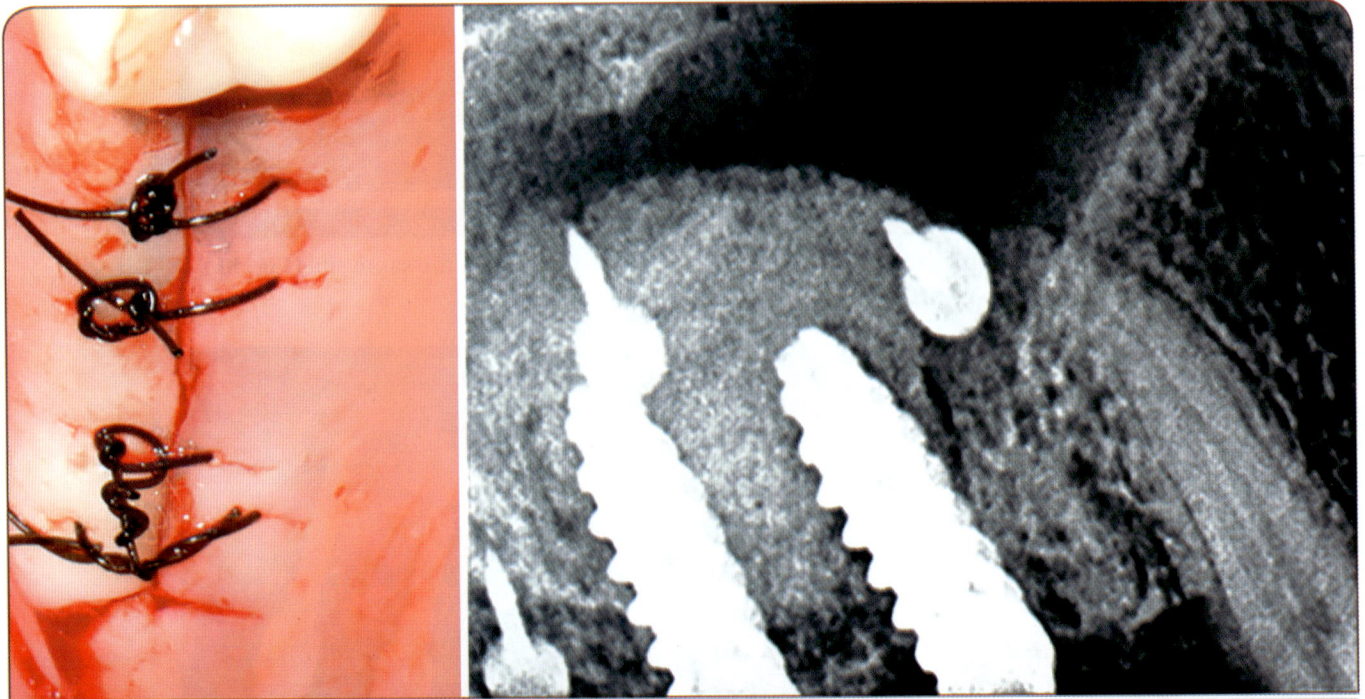

Fig. 15

Wound closure with 4-0 polyamide sutures. Intraoral radiograph showing the implants well ensconced in the grafted sinus (**Fig. 15**).

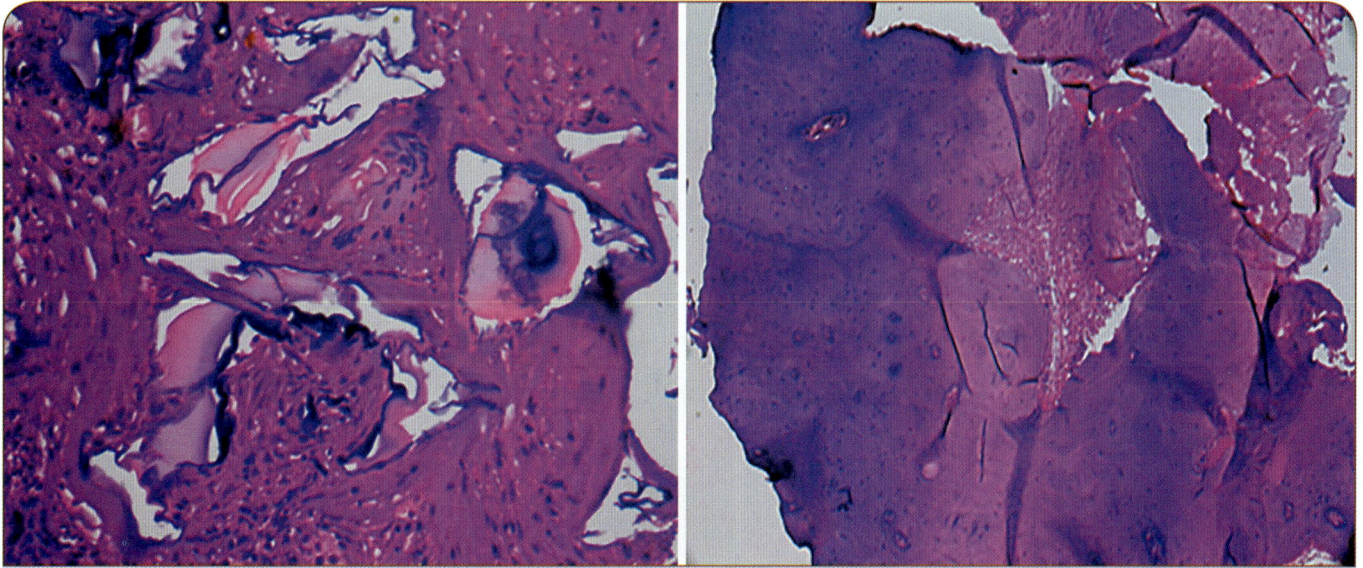

Fig. 16

The trephine biopsies were submitted for histopathological examination after being fixed in neutral buffered formalin for 24 hours. The bone was decalcified in 5% nitric acid and examined histopathologically after staining with routine Hematoxylin and eosin stain. The decalcified section of the trephine biopsy core revealed dense abundant mature vital bone with osteoblastic rimming and osteocytes within the lacunae. Multiple foci of new bone formation are seen in the section in the scaffold provided by the graft material **(Fig. 16)**.

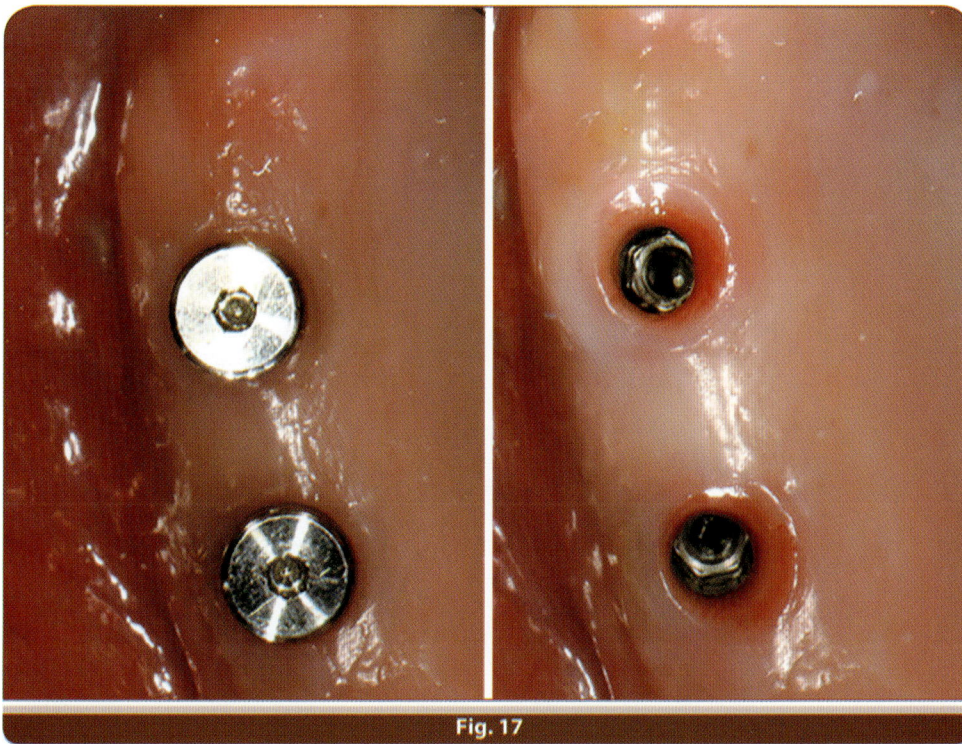

Fig. 17

Clinical view of healing collars at second stage surgery. Thick band of keratinized tissue supporting the implants is evident **(Fig. 17)**.

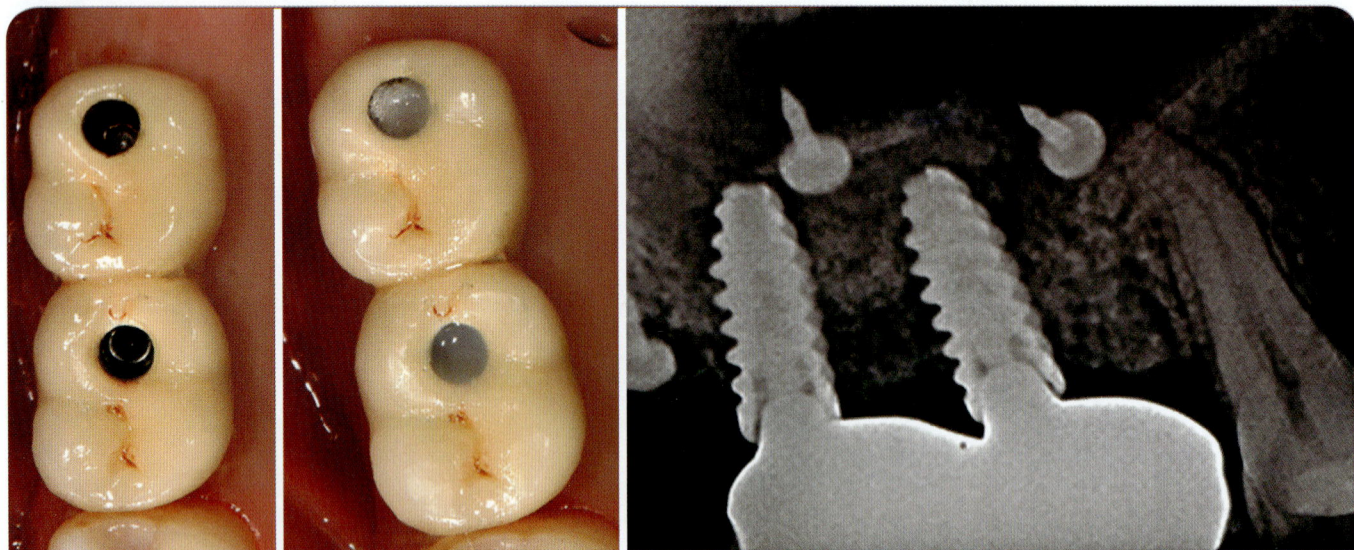

Fig. 18

Final screw retained prosthesis. The abutment screws are torqued to 30 Ncm and the access filled with temporary cement, after 6 weeks loading the cement is changed to flowable composite. Radiograph taken at 16 months **(Fig. 18)**.

Lanka Mahesh, Vishal Gupta

FLAPLESS PLACEMENT OF SHORT IMPLANTS IN THE POSTERIOR MAXILLA TO AVOID SINUS GRAFTING

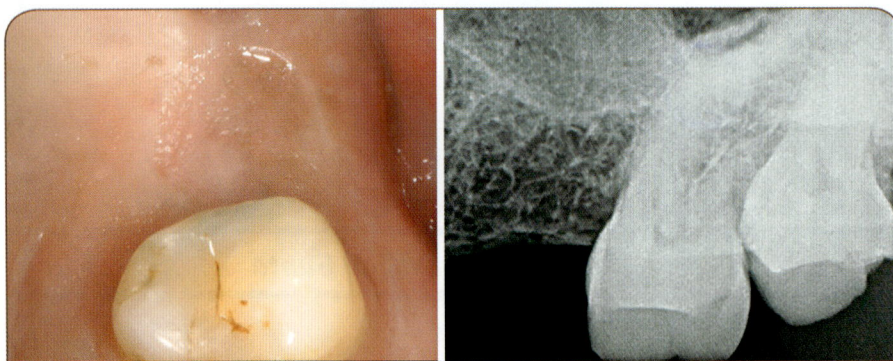

Fig. 1

A 44-year-old male patient with missing upper 26, was against any form of grafting procedures. The clinical width of the alveolus was adequate to accommodate a wide fixture placement. The IOPA X-ray revealed adequate height and mesiodistal space **(Fig. 1)**.

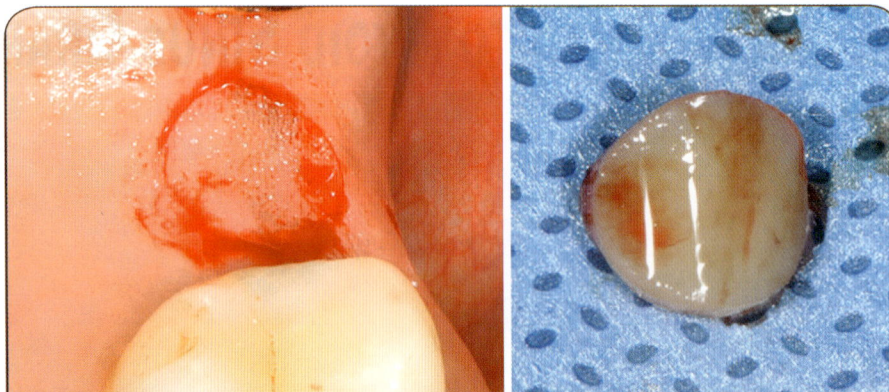

Fig. 2

A tissue punch (Stoma, GmbH) of 6 mm diameter is used in the exact fixture placement site, the size of the punch should be at least 1 mm wider than the diameter of the planned fixture diameter. The tissue is gently excised with a Buser elevator (Hu-Friedy) **(Fig. 2)**.

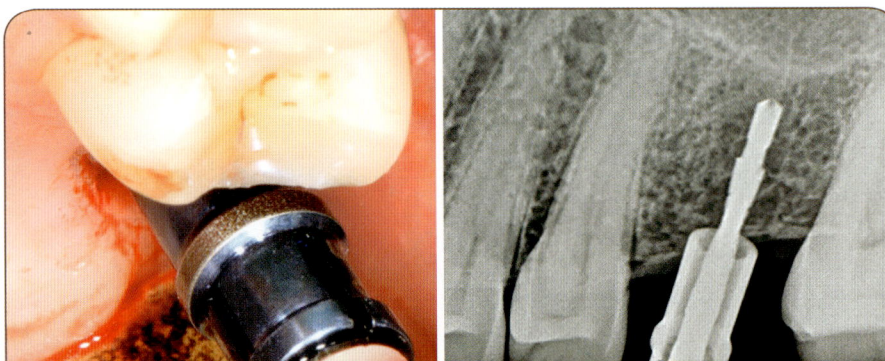

Fig. 3

The implant drill with a predetermined height stopper is used. A check X-ray at this stage is mandatory. To ensure the osteotomy is neither over or under sized **(Fig. 3)**.

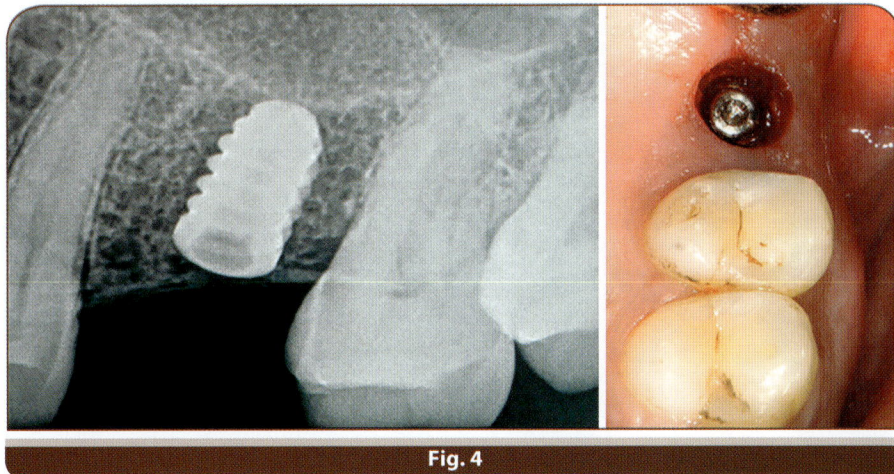

Fig. 4

Placement of a 5/8.5 mm diameter DM implant (Bioner), the implant is exactly at the floor of the antrum with no perforations, and the final clinical photograph with the cover screw (a healing collar may be placed as an option for a one stage surgery) **(Fig. 4)**.

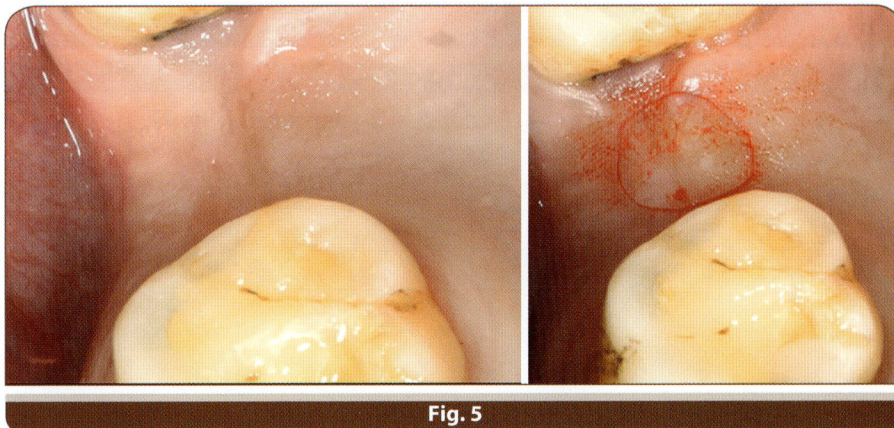

Fig. 5

The same procedure is carried out in site of 16 with a similar implant size **(Fig. 5)**.

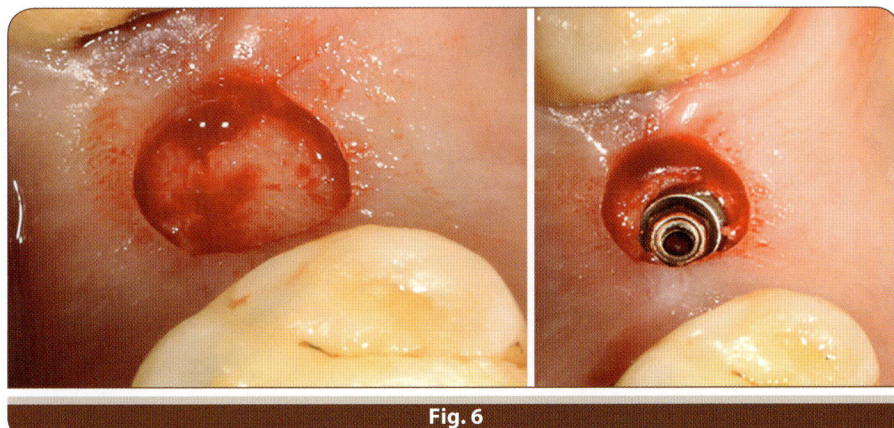

Fig. 6

Care must be taken ensuring the implant is seated completely to the level of the alveolus. It is prudent to measure the thickness of the 'punched tissue' with a probe to prevent the implant to be placed at the soft tissue level which is a common error in flapless placement especially in the posterior region **(Fig. 6)**.

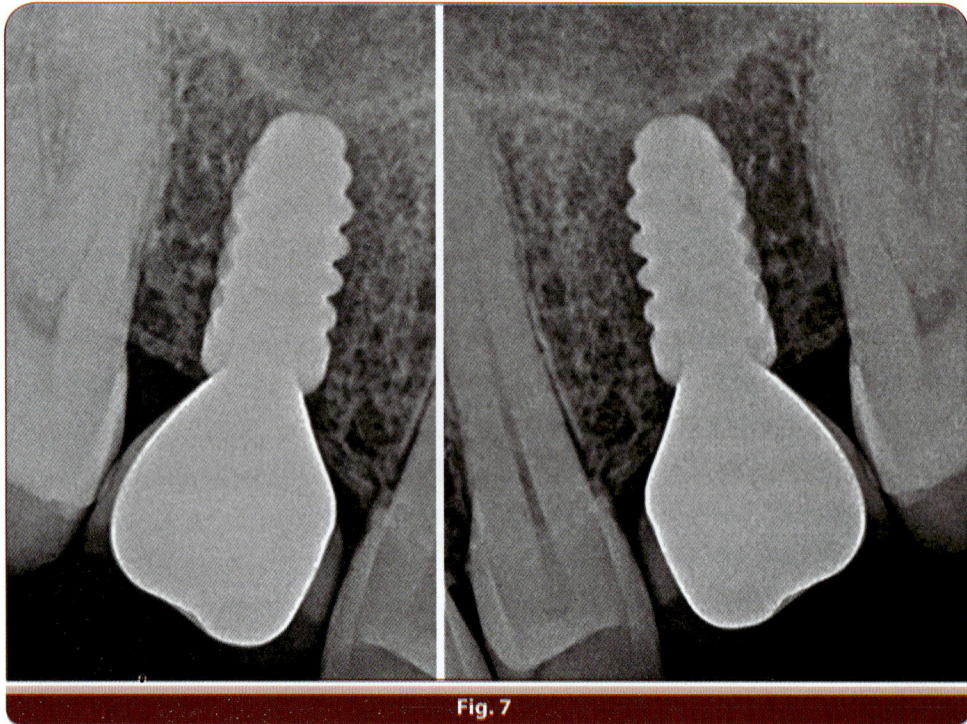

Fig. 7

X-rays of implants in 16 and 26 at 2-year recall (Fig. 7).

Lanka Mahesh

TREPHINE CORE SINUS LIFT IN A DEFICIENT MAXILLARY ARCH FOR A POSTERIOR SINGLE TOOTH RESTORATION

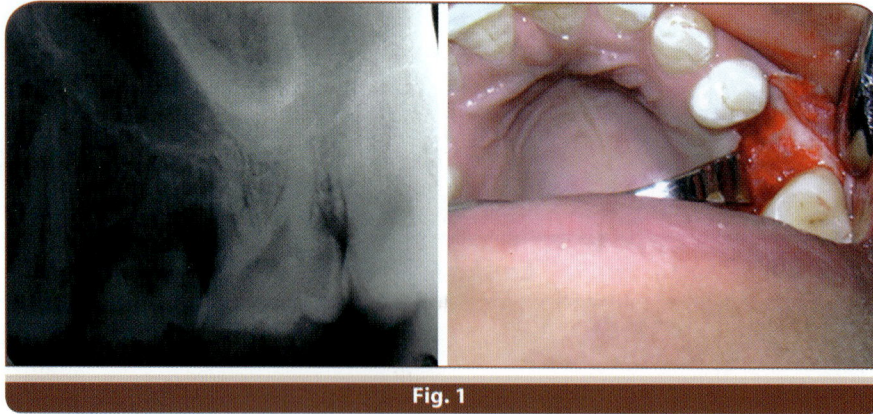

Fig. 1

A 22-year-old female patient with a retained deciduos molar. The X-ray reveals less than 5 mm of residual bone height. After extraction of the mobile tooth and flap reflection adequate width is noticed to accommodate a wide diameter fixture. A trephine core sinus lift is planned with simultaneous implant placement **(Fig. 1)**.

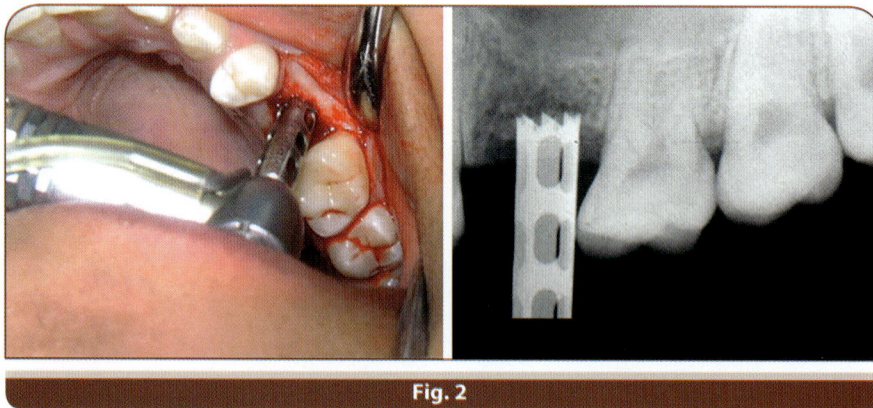

Fig. 2

A 5.2 mm diameter (stoma Gmbh) is used at 900 rpm in a counter clockwise motion to create the core of bone. An X-ray is taken at this stage to verify the correct position and depth of the trephine (the core is made 1–2 mm short of the alveolus) **(Fig. 2)**.

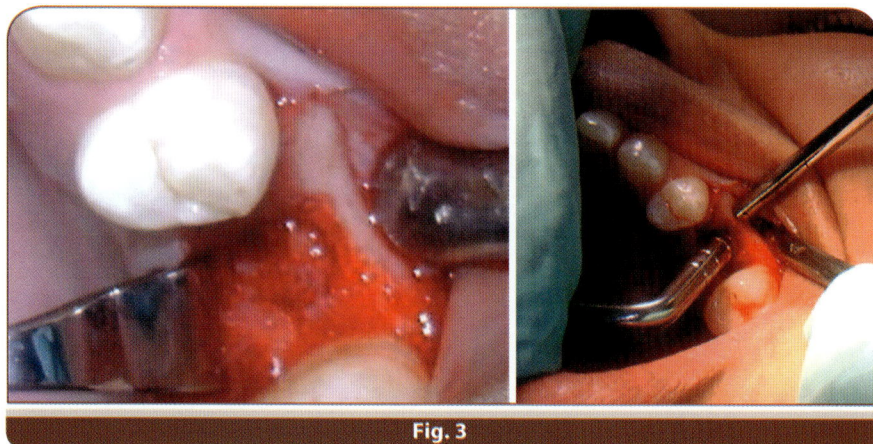

Fig. 3

The outline of the core is clearly visible. After ensuring the core is mobile circumferentially an angled osteotome is used to infracture the segment with light tapping strokes from a mallet **(Fig. 3)**.

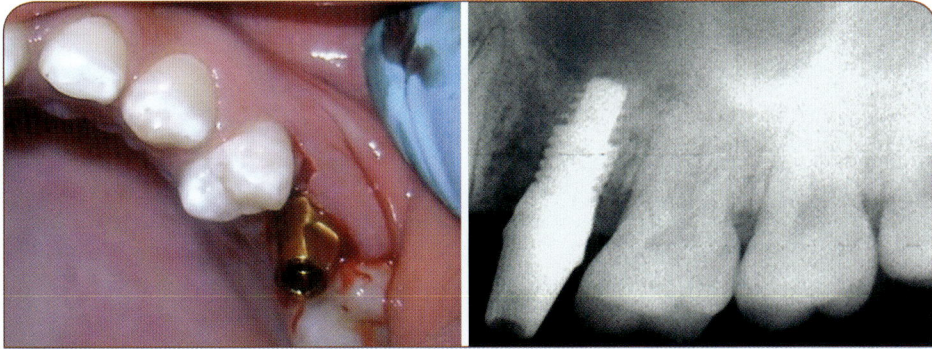

Fig. 4

A 5/10.5 mm biohorizons internal implant is placed at an insertion torque of 30 Ncm. Immediate postoperative X-ray shows the correct implant position **(Fig. 4)**.

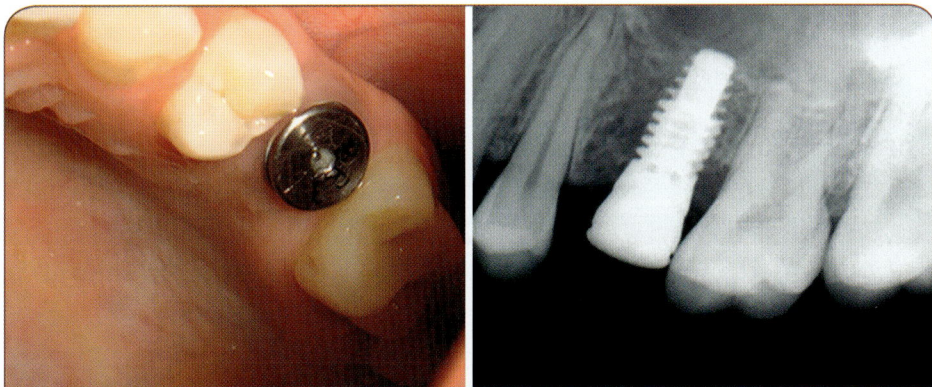

Fig. 5

After 4 months of submerged healing, a healing collar is placed. An X-ray at this stage clearly demonstrates adequate bone fill of the sinus **(Fig. 5)**.

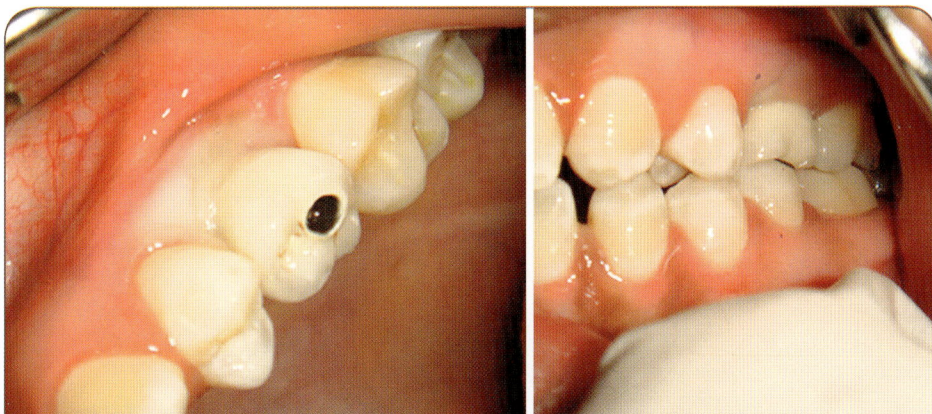

Fig. 6

The final screw retained restoration in place, the screw channel is sealed with cotton and flowable composite filling material. View of the prosthesis in occlusion **(Fig. 6)**.

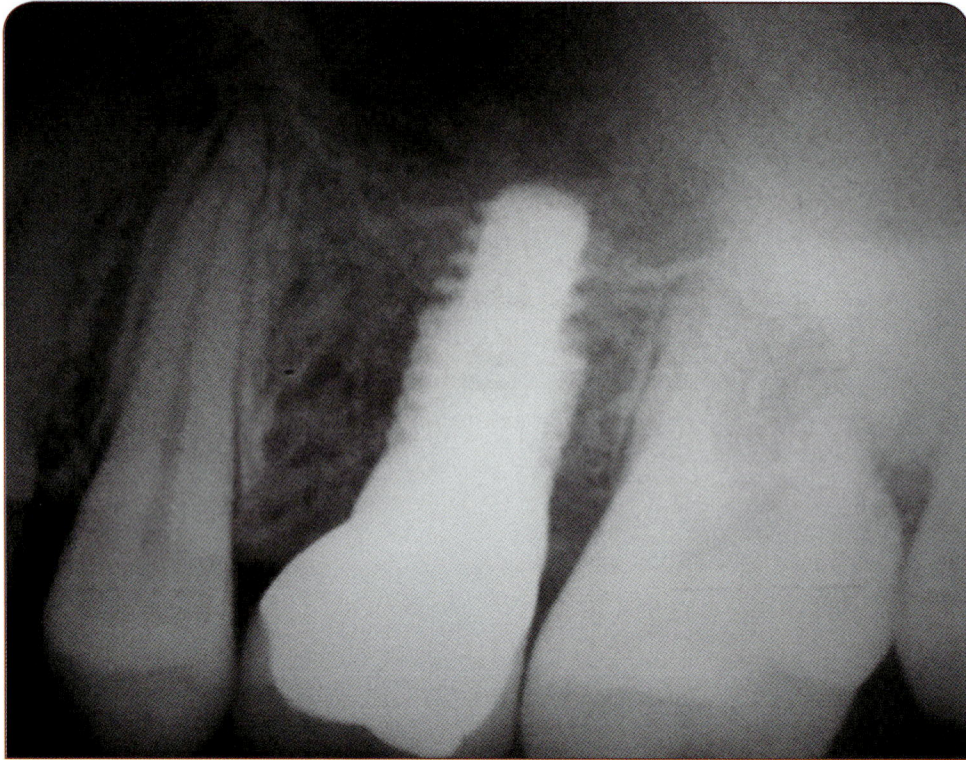

Fig. 7

A ten-year postoperative CBCT section shows stable crestal bone levels and a successful sinus lift and bone consolidation in the antrum **(Fig. 7)**.

Jin Y Kim

SINUS GRAFT IN THE SINGLE UPPER LEFT SECOND MOLAR SITE: SUCCESSFUL OUTCOME DESPITE SCHNEIDERIAN MEMBRANE TEAR

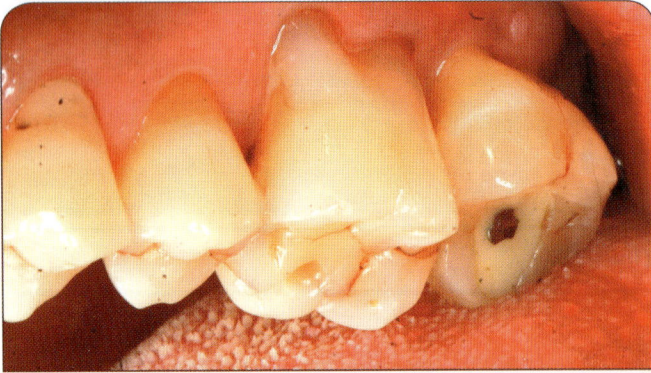
Fig. 1

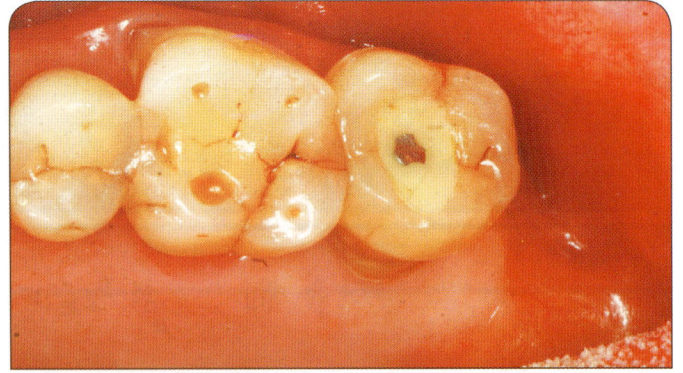
Fig. 2

A healthy 65-year-old male patient presented with periodontally damaged upper second molar (Fig. 1).

Occlusal view (Fig. 2).

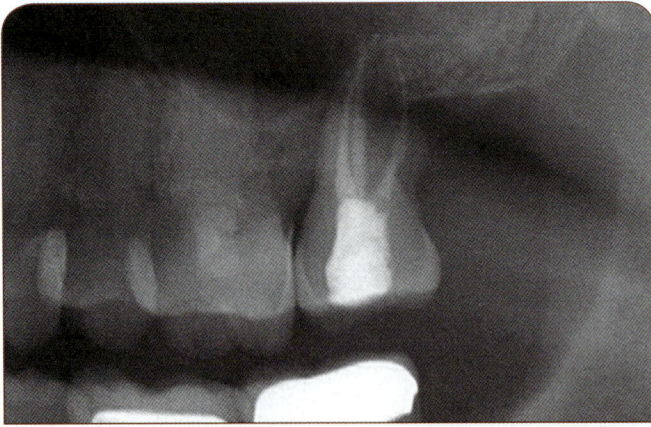
Fig. 3

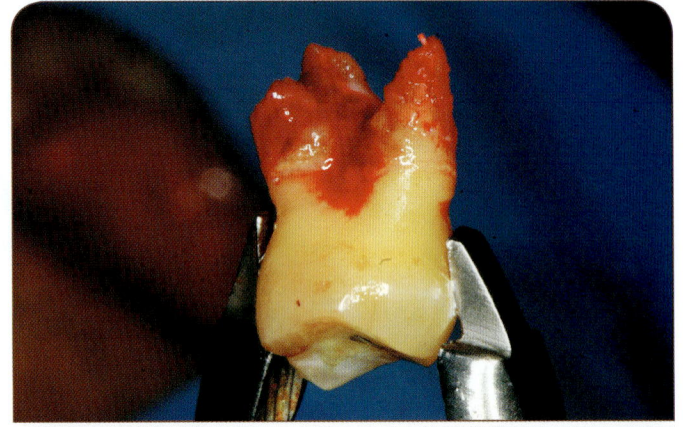
Fig. 4

IOPA X-ray (Fig. 3).

Tooth was deemed non-restorable, and was surgically extracted without raising a flap (Fig. 4).

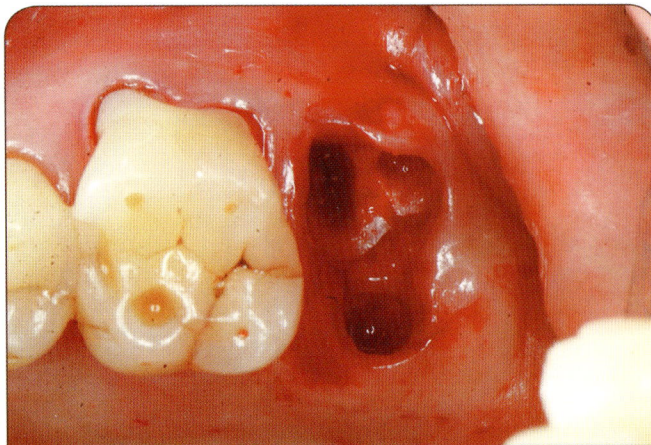
Fig. 5

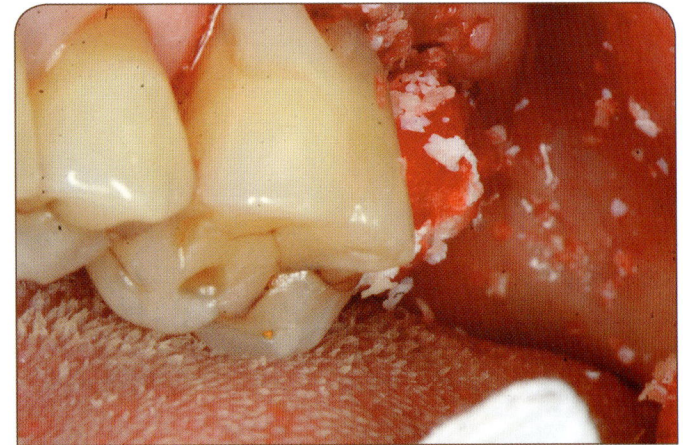
Fig. 6

The socket defect was debrided (Fig. 5), and grafted with mineralized allograft (Mine-ross, Biohorizons), (Fig. 6).

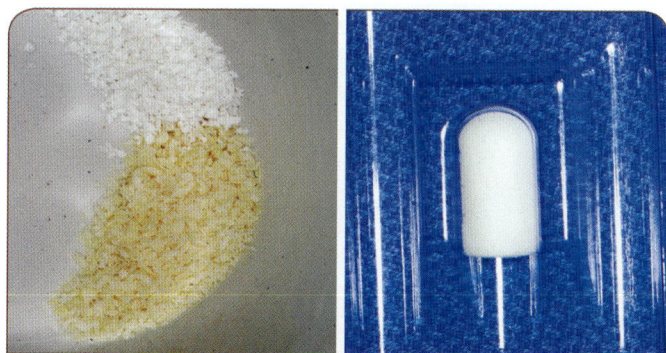

Fig. 7

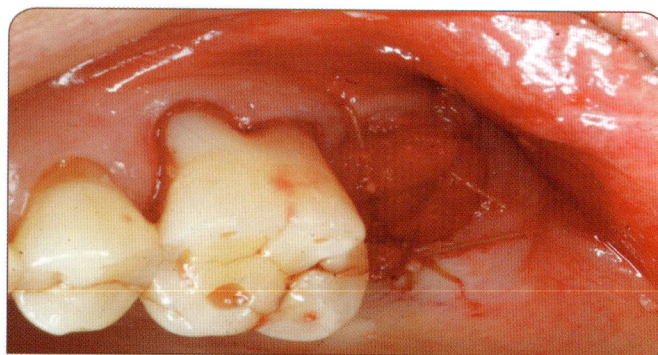

Fig. 8

The socket opening was closed with a collagen dressing **(Fig. 7)** (OraPlug, Salvin Dental Specialties), with 4.0 chromic gut suture (Surgical Specialties Corporation). No attempt was made to displace the mucoperiosteum, nor to alter the facial vestibule **(Fig. 8)**.

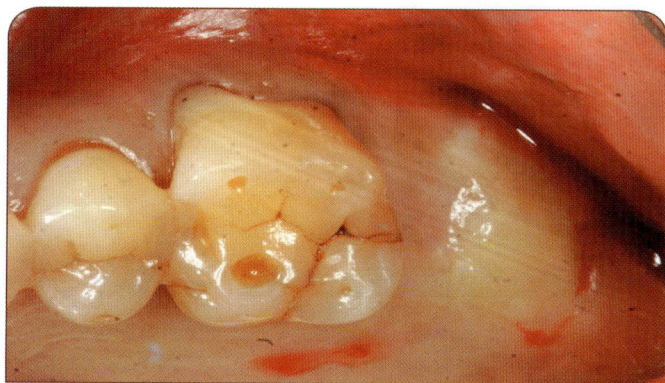

Fig. 9

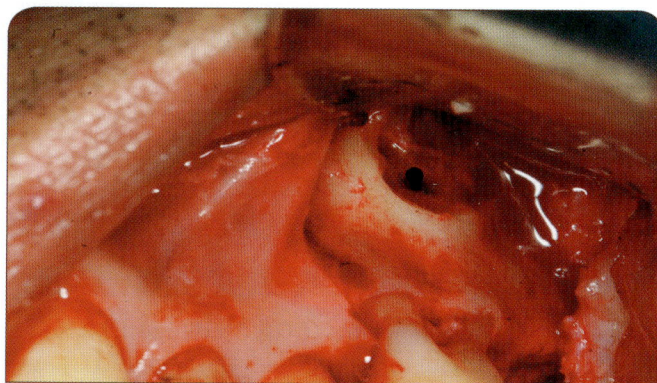

Fig. 10

Uneventful healing was noted at 4 months. The width and height of alveolar ridge was preserved. Moreover, the soft tissue over the socket is fully keratinized, and the vestibule depth was presented, and not altered **(Fig. 9)**.

During the routine lateral window approach sinus augmentation, a small tear was noted in the Schneiderian membrane **(Fig. 10)**.

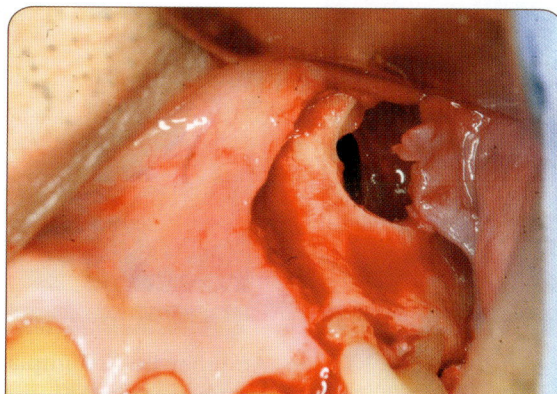

Fig. 11

Liberal release of the Schneiderian membrane was attempted, in order to lessen the tension in the perforated site. Although the tear got larger, adequate release was achieved **(Fig. 11)**.

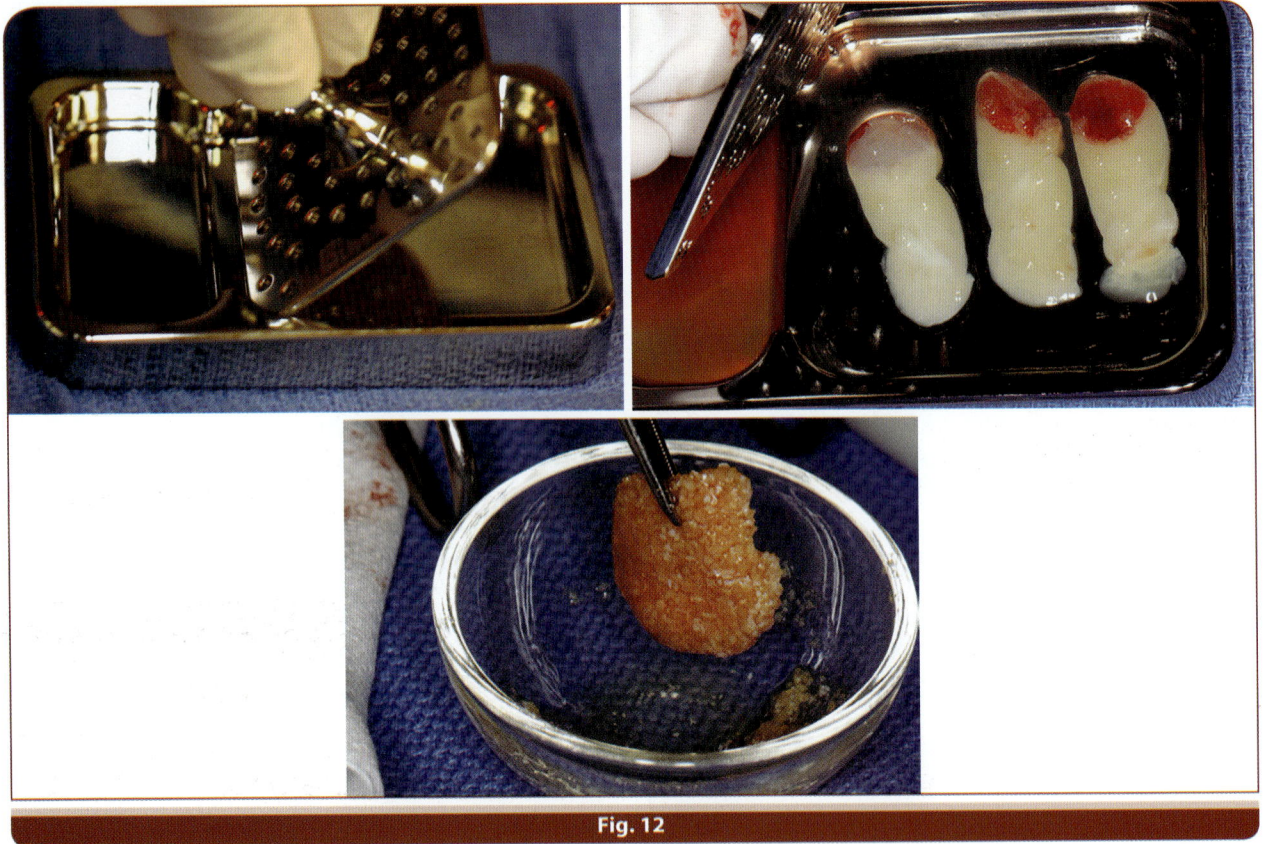

Fig. 12

Concentrated Growth Factors (CGF, Medifuge)™, also known as PRF, was prepared using patient's venous blood. CGF was flattened with a Fibrin Gel Press (LisaTech LLC), removing the platelet-poor plasma component. The biometrical was used to close the perforation in the sinus.

"Sticky Bone" was prepared using patient's venous blood, and was used to fill the sinus cavity (**Fig. 12**).

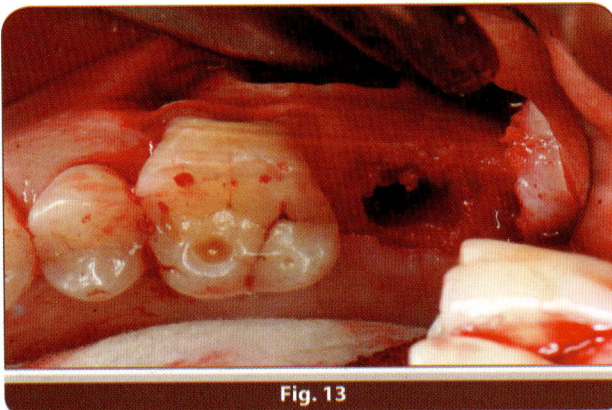

Fig. 13

Occlusal view of the osteotomy preparation (**Fig. 13**).

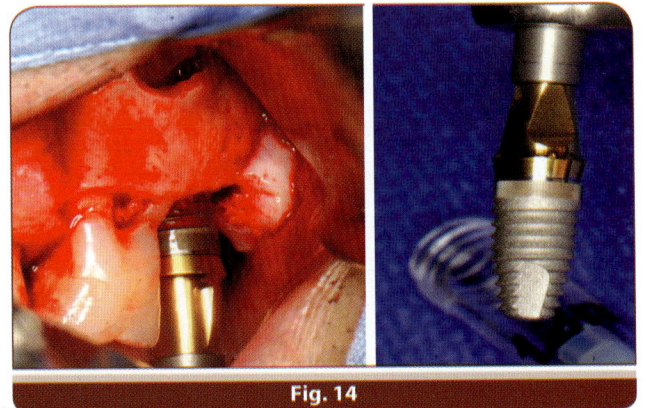

Fig. 14

An taper-bodied implant of 5.6 mm diameter, and 12 mm length, was placed into the prepared site (LaserLok, Biohorizons). Implant stability, measured by Osstell device was 70 ISQ. The implant was placed with a healing abutment (**Fig. 14**).

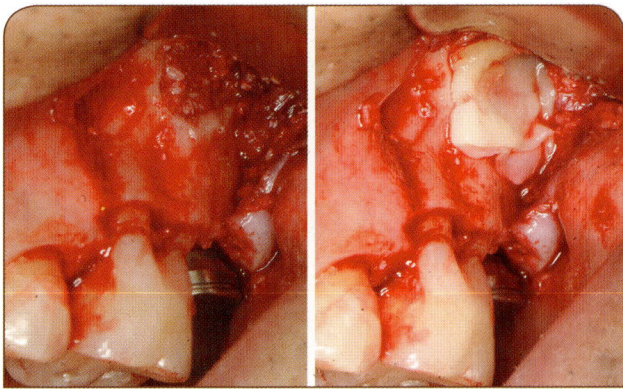

Fig. 15

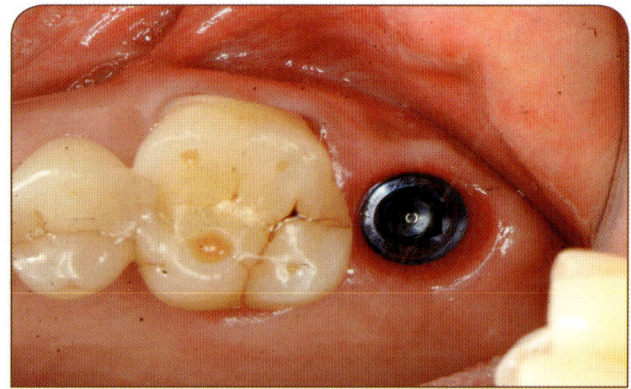

Fig. 16

Sinus was grafted with 'sticky bone' and sutured above it **(Fig. 15)**.

At 6 months, implant stability was re-measured with the Osstell device. It registered 74 ISQ, and deemed fully osseointegrated **(Fig. 16)**.

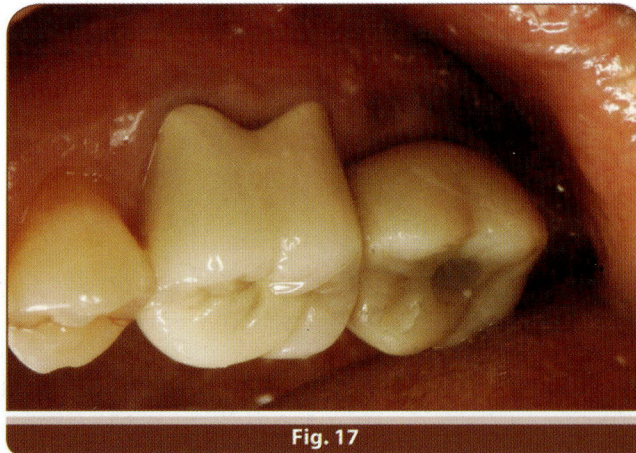

Fig. 17

A screw-retained UCLA type ceramo-metal restoration was fabricated and installed by the restorative dentist **(Fig. 17)**.

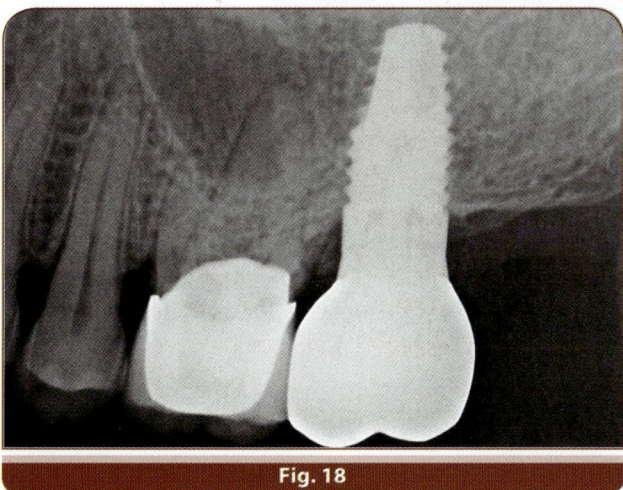

Fig. 18

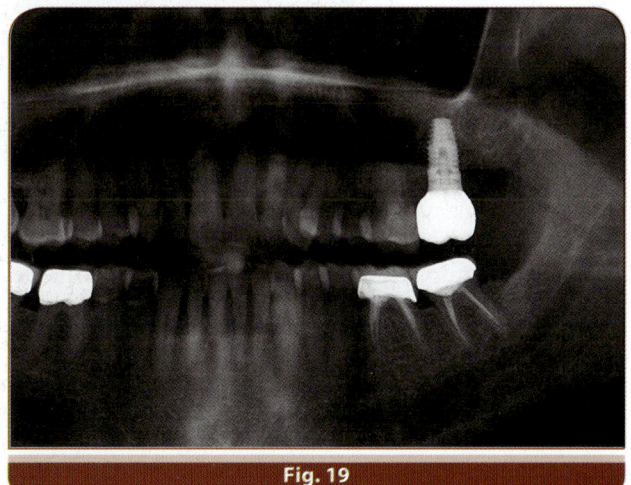

Fig. 19

Periapical film at immediate post-restoration phase **(Fig. 18)**.

Panoramic X-ray also taken **(Fig. 19)**.

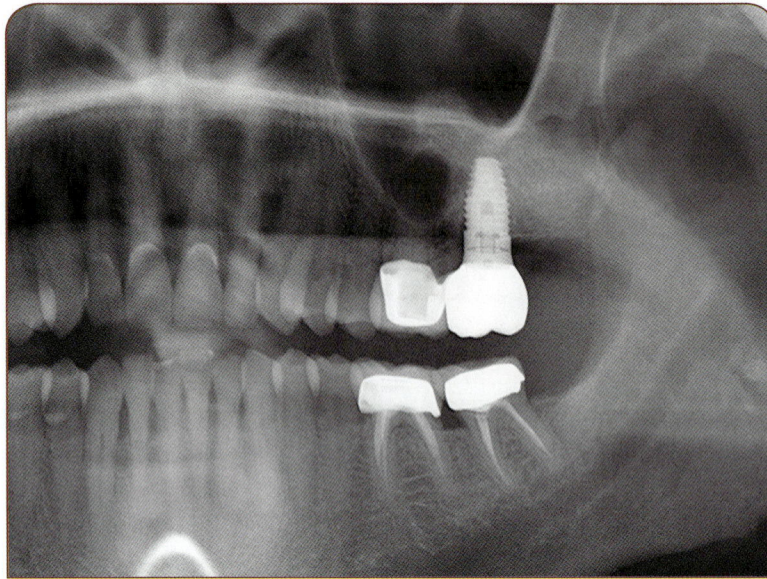

Fig. 20

Panoramic film after 4 years follow-up **(Fig. 20)**.

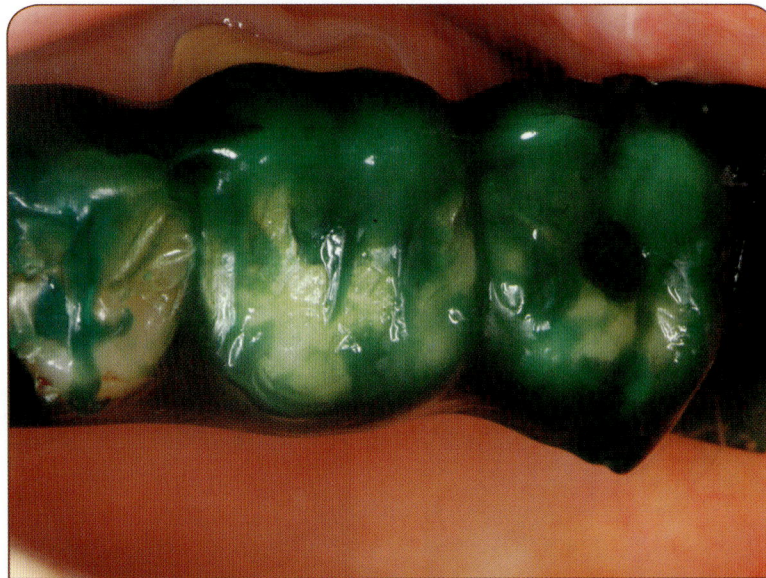

Fig. 21

At 4 years follow-up, occlusion was in good form-centric stop in the functional (palatal) cusp, with clearance for lateral excursion in the buccal cusps. This form of axial load allows for long-term stability, especially for a single molar implant in a previously grafted site **(Fig. 21)**.

Dong Seok Sohn

SINUS AUGMENTATION USING DECALCIFIED OSTEOINDUCTIVE AUTOLOGOUS TOOTH BONE

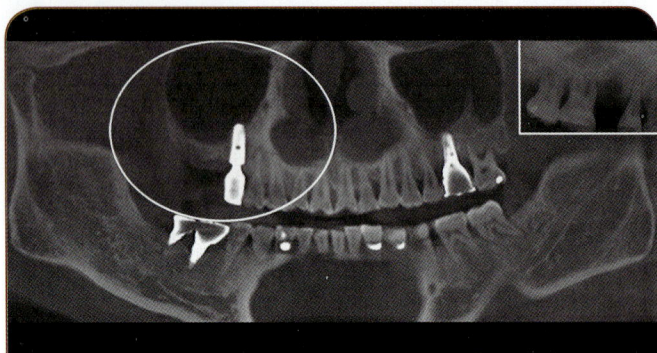

Fig. 1

A 52-year-old aged man patient visited my department to replace the periodontally hopeless teeth #16 and #17 with implant supported restoration **(Fig. 1)**.

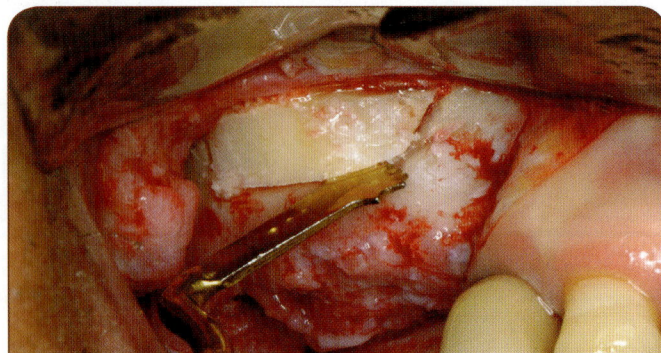

Fig. 2

Replaceable osteoinductive bony (ROB) window was prepared with saw tip connecting with piezoelectric device **(Fig. 2)**.

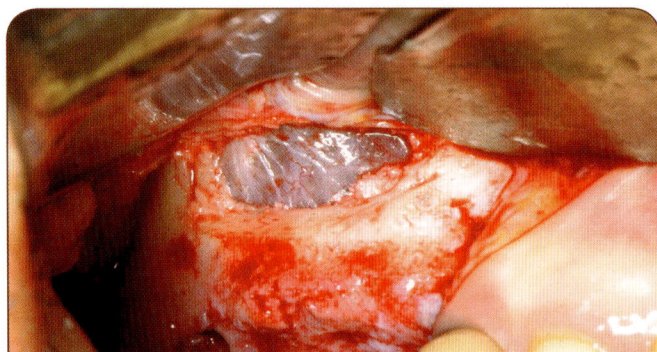

Fig. 3

Note intact sinus mucosa after detachment of ROB window after **(Fig. 3)**.

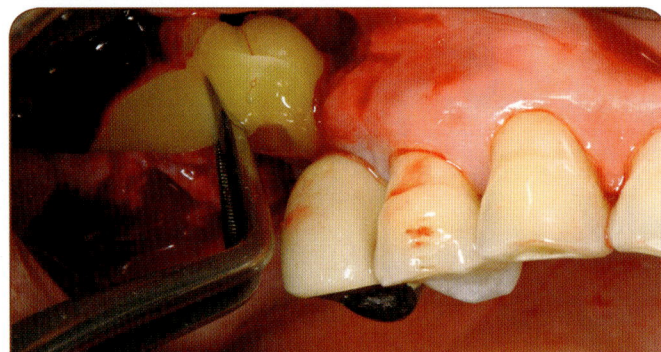

Fig. 4

After careful elevation of sinus mucosa, fibrin block with concentrated growth factors (CGF) was inserted to accelerated new bone formation in the sinus **(Fig. 4)**.

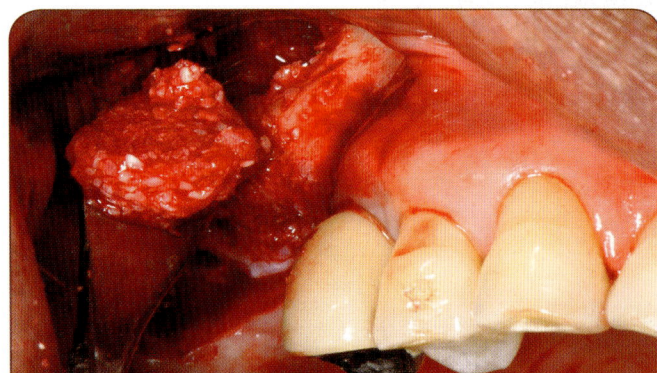

Fig. 5

The extracted teeth #16 and #17 was crushed, decalcified and sterilized to transform osteoinductive autologous tooth bone. This tooth graft was mixed with autologous fibrine glue in order to make Sticky Bone™ and this stick tooth bone was inserted in the sinus **(Fig. 5)**.

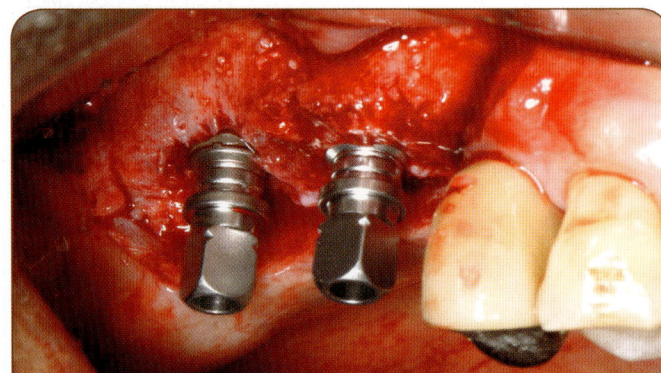

Fig. 6

Two Ankylos implants were placed simultaneously **(Fig. 6)**.

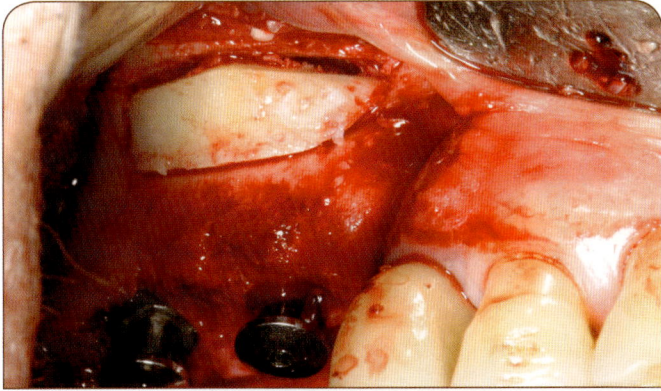

Fig. 7

ROB widnow was repositioned on the lateral window to accelerated new bone formation in the sinus and prevent soft tissue ingrowth into sinus **(Fig. 7)**.

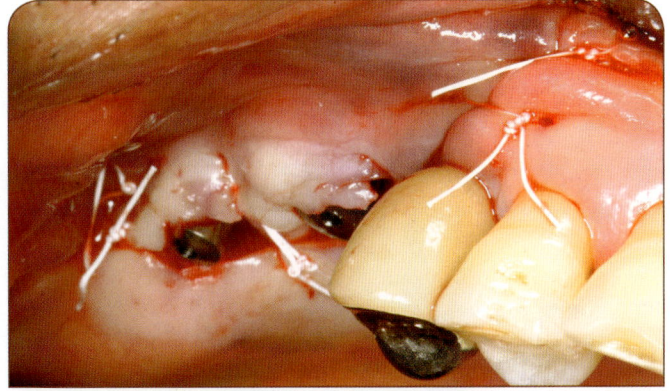

Fig. 8

One-stage procedure was done **(Fig. 8)**.

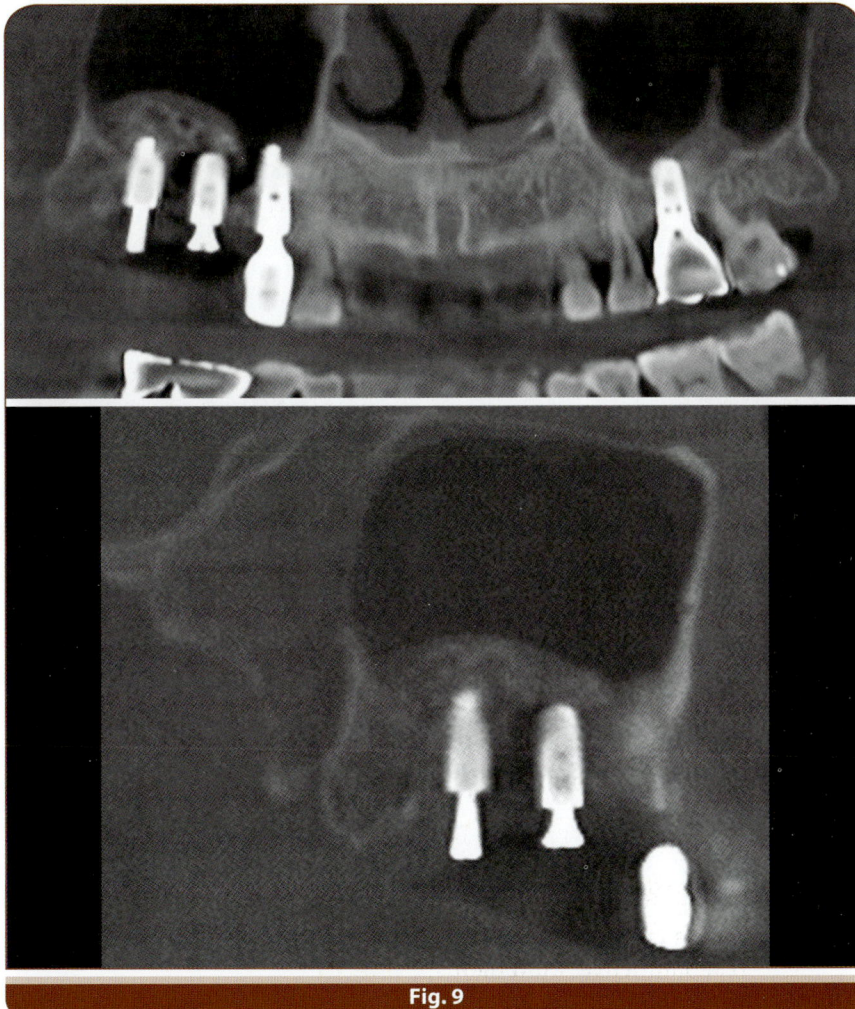

Fig. 9

Postoperative CBCT shows well augmented sinus **(Fig. 9)**.

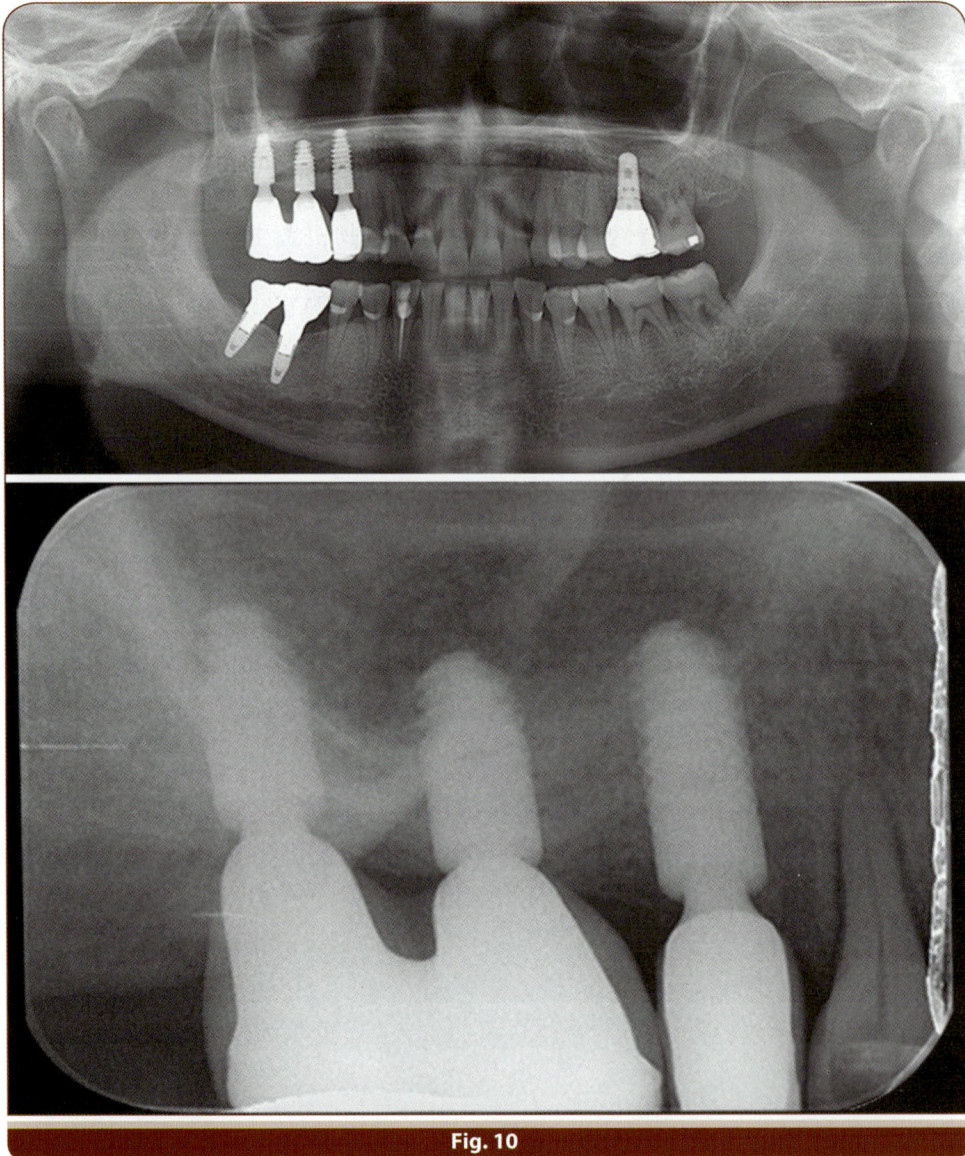

Fig. 10

Final ceramic restoration was cemented after 5 months healing. Periapical radiogram shows 5 years in function **(Fig. 10)**.

Ziv Mazor

RECONSTRUCTION OF POSTERIOR MAXILLARY DEFICIENCY WITH IMPLANTS USING OSSEODENSIFICATION FOR SUBCRESTAL SINUS AUGMENTATION

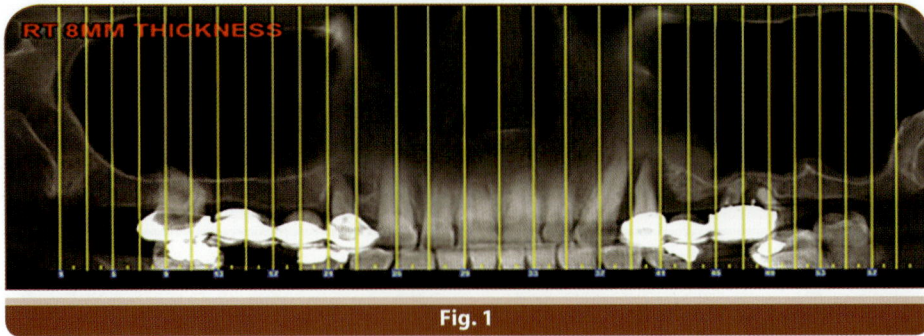

Fig. 1

Preoperative CBCT of a 40-year-old female patient with a facing bilateral upper posterior dentition **(Fig. 1)**.

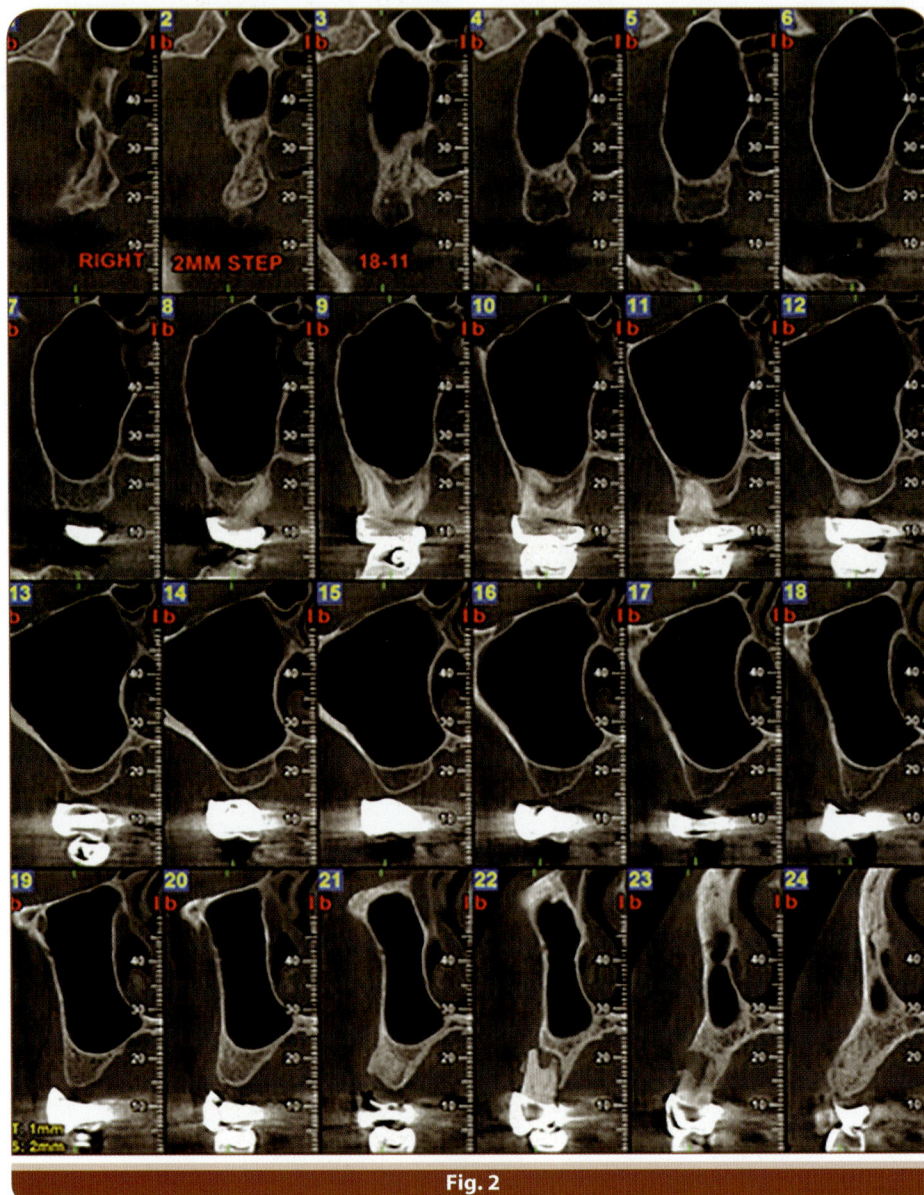

Fig. 2

CT scan revealed 3-4 mm of residual bone height between the ridge and the maxillary sinus **(Fig. 2)**.

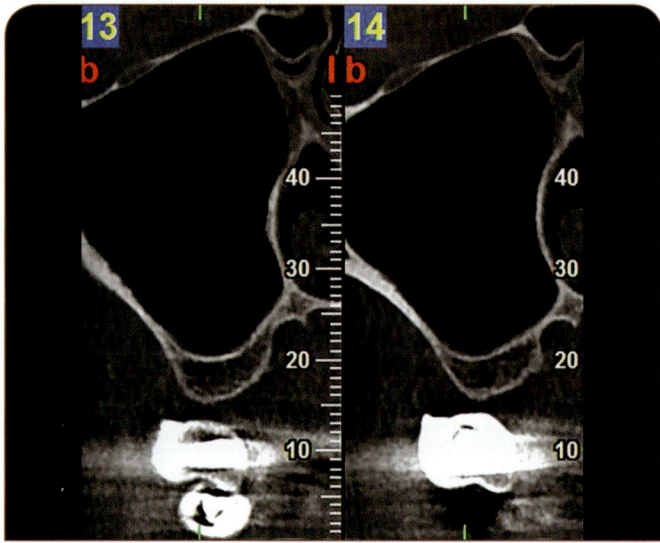

Fig. 3

CBCT shows minimal bone height **(Fig. 3)**.

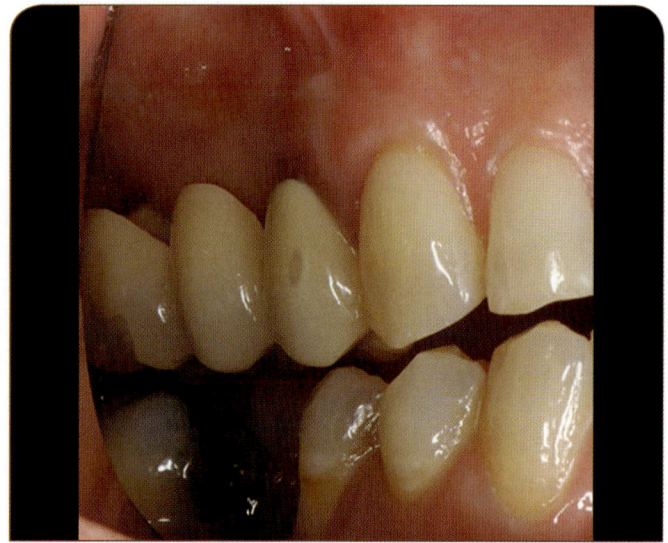

Fig. 4

Clinical view of posterior right side **(Fig. 4)**.

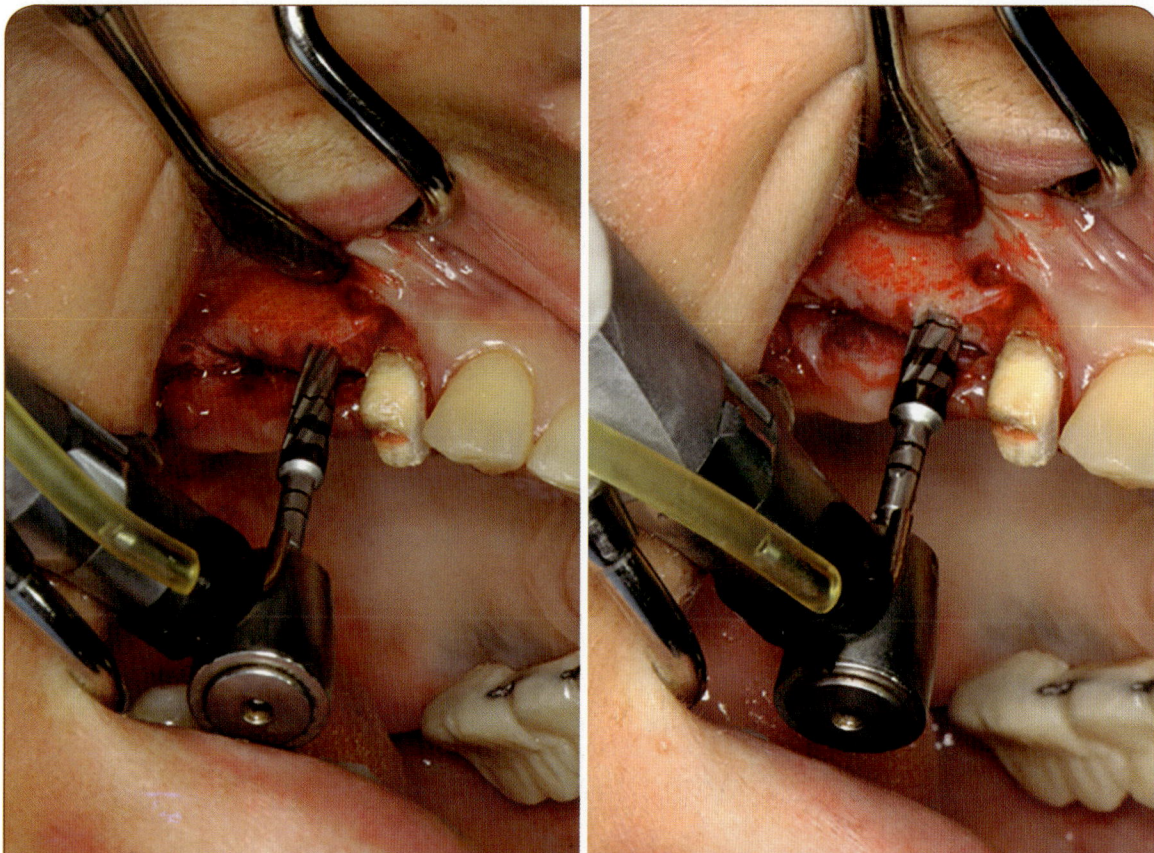

Fig. 5

Subcrestal sinus augmentation using osseodensification (Densahbur kit) **(Fig. 5)**.

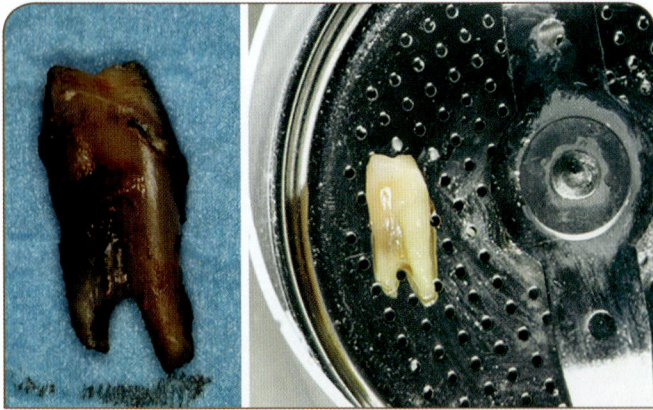

Fig. 6

Tooth grinding: Using the patient's tooth as a source for graft material (Fig. 6).

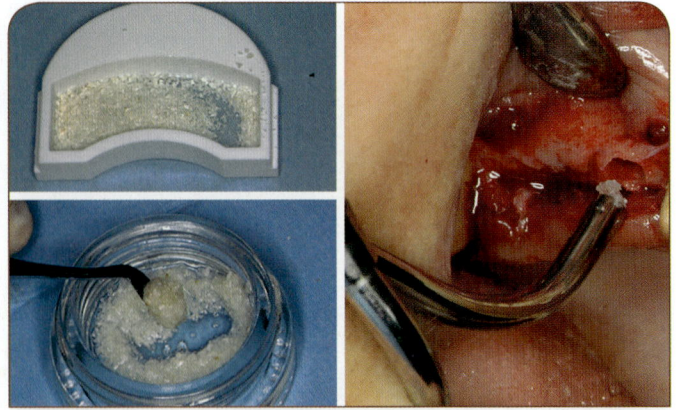

Fig. 7

Tooth#14 had been grinded and processed to be utilized as graft material (Fig. 7).

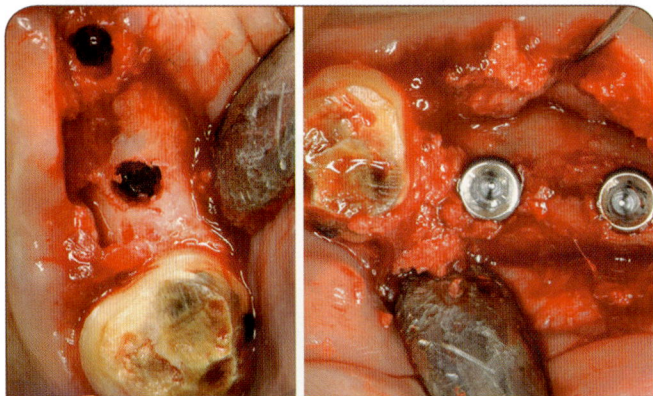

Fig. 8

Osteotomies completed and implants inserted (Fig. 8).

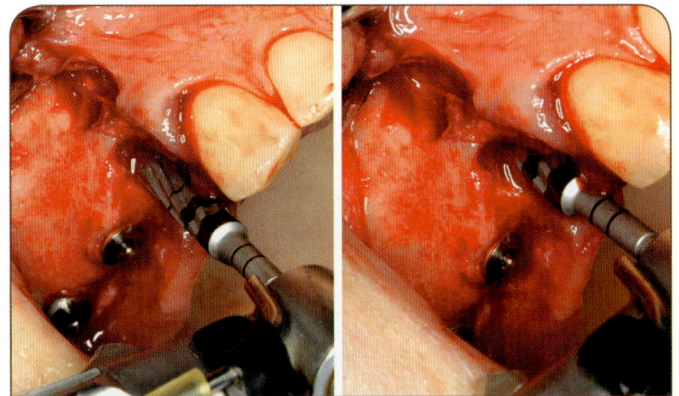

Fig. 9

Following extraction of 14 osteotomy site is prepared by osseodensification (Fig. 9).

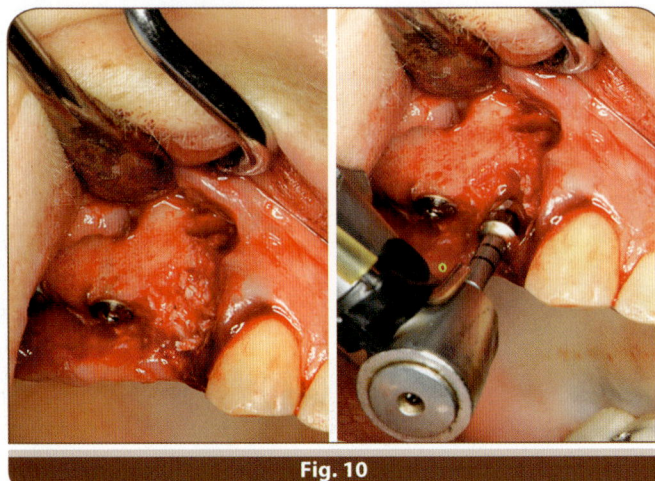

Fig. 10

Following extraction of 14 osteotomy site is prepared by osseodensification (Fig. 10).

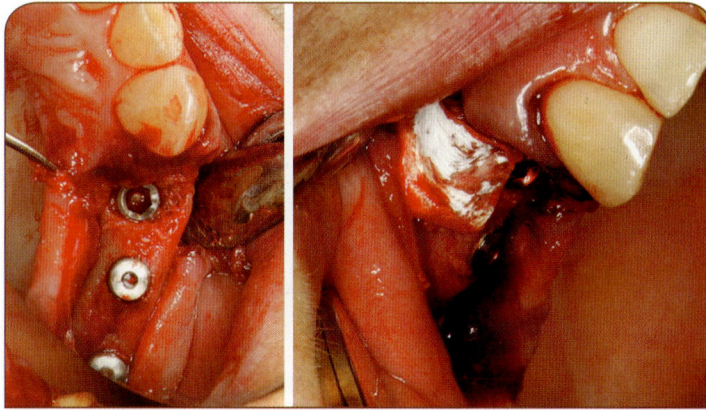

Fig. 11

Anterior implant inserted and grafted on the buccal aspect **(Fig. 11)**.

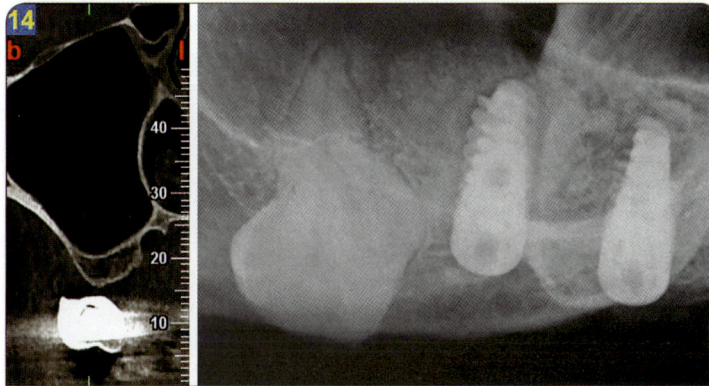

Fig. 12

CBCT and periapical X-ray immediately after treatment completion **(Fig. 12)**.

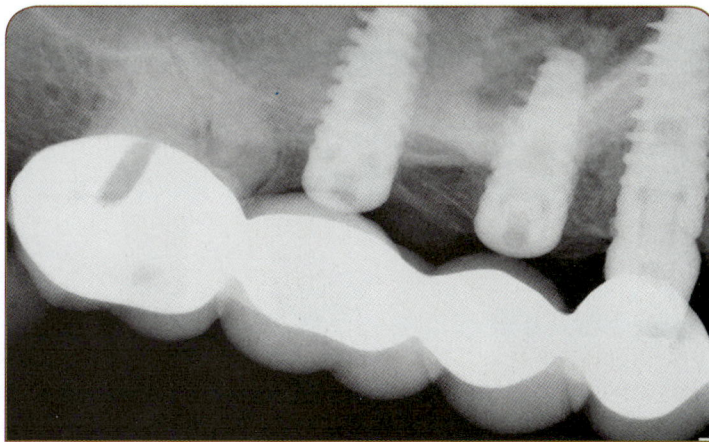

Fig. 13

Periapical X-ray 3 months postoperative **(Fig. 13)**.

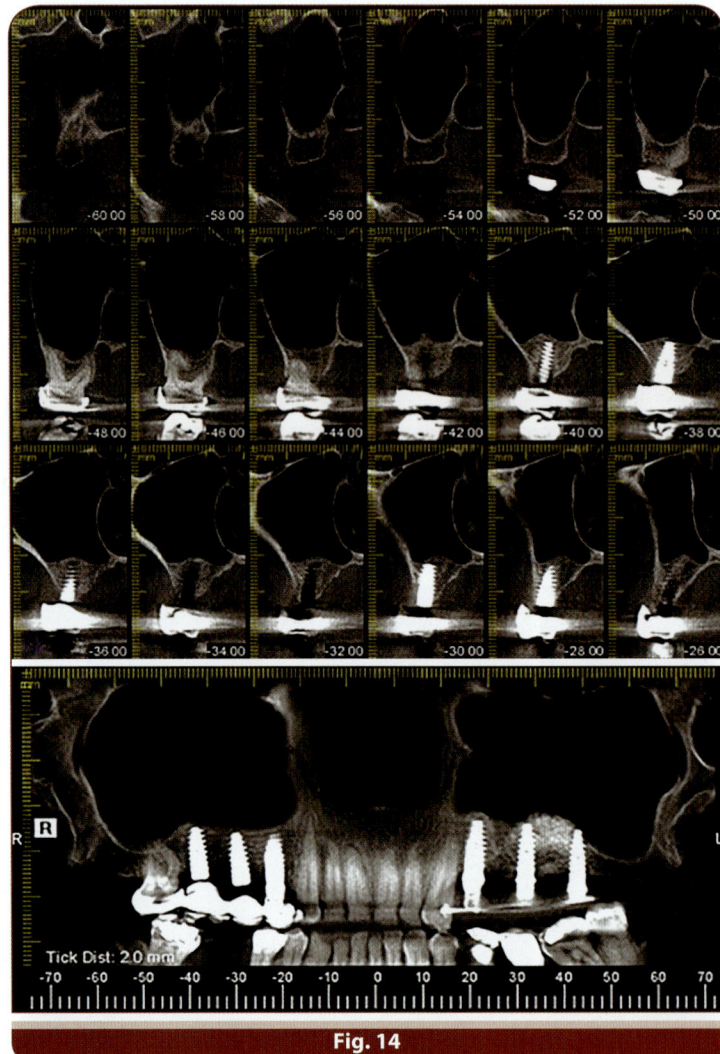

Fig. 14

Five months postoperative CBCT showing bone regeneration **(Fig. 14)**.

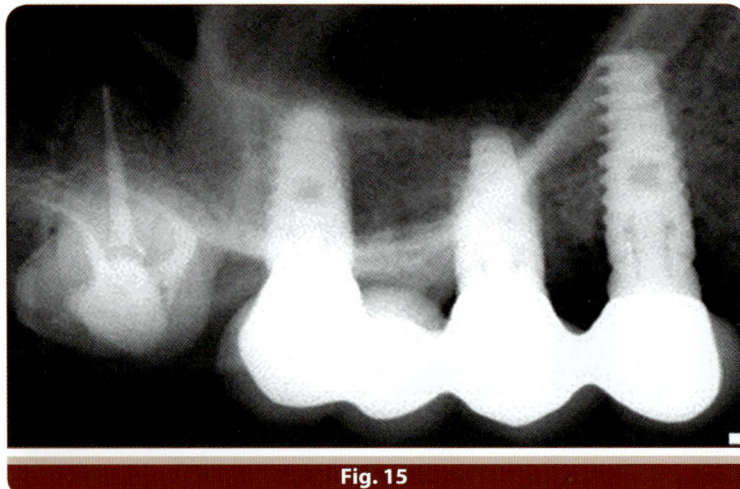

Fig. 15

Two years postoperative radiograph **(Fig. 15)**.

CASE STUDY 52

José Luis Calvo Guirado

SINGLE UNIT SINUS GRAFTING IN PNEUMATIZED SINUS

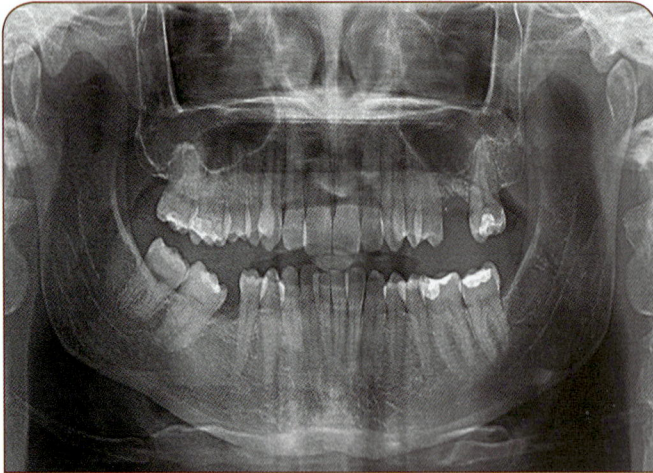

Fig. 1

A 35-year-old female, no relevant medical history, 3 years healed bone **(Fig. 1)**.

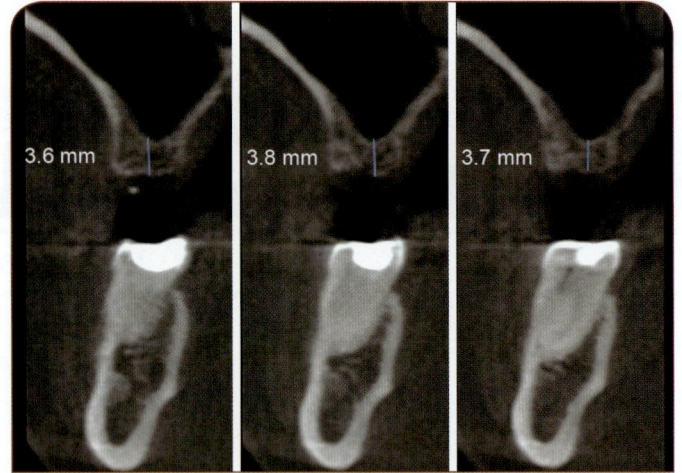

Fig. 2

Height of available bone 3.7 mm (to obtain primary stability, available width 8.0 mm, direct sinus lift with simultaneous implant placement planned **(Fig. 2)**.

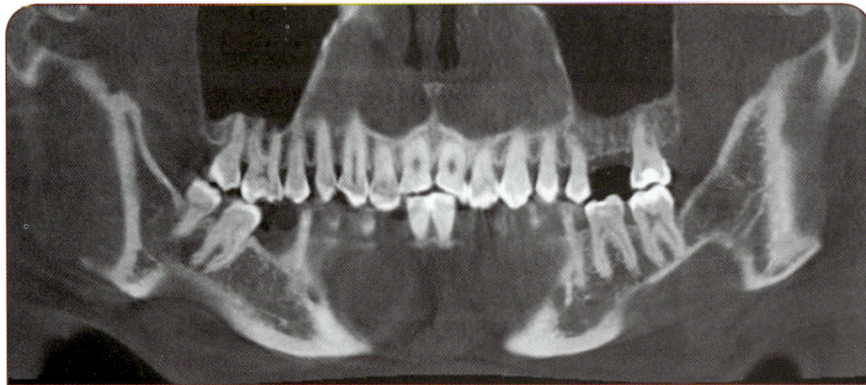

Fig. 3

Panoramic X-ray of upper left 1st molar region **(Fig. 3)**.

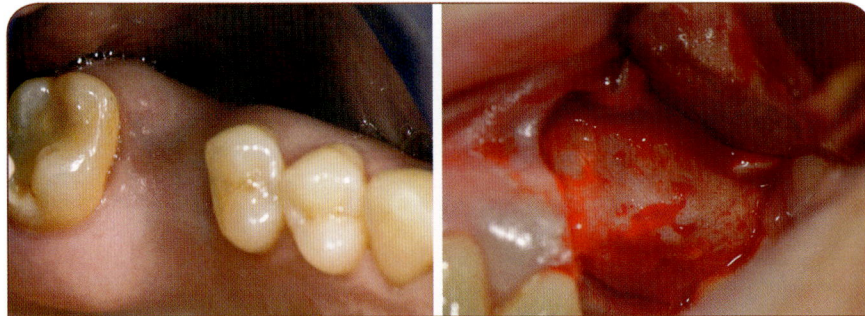

Fig. 4

10 mm width from buccal to lingual, 8 mm width from mesial to distal. Full thickness flap elevated exposing the facial wall. The incision should extend one tooth distal to the operative site to allow tension free closure and greater visibility of the operative site **(Fig. 4)**.

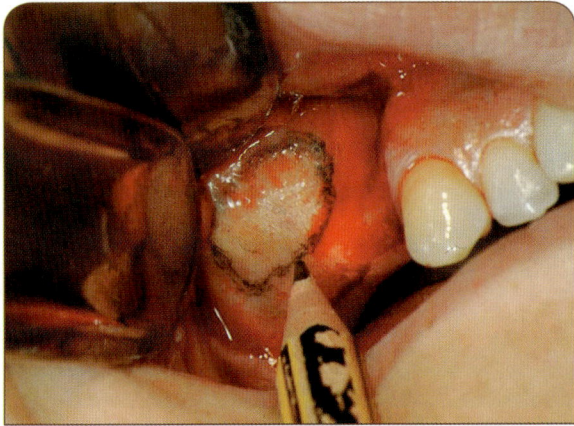

Fig. 5

The external wall was marked with graphite **(Fig. 5)**.

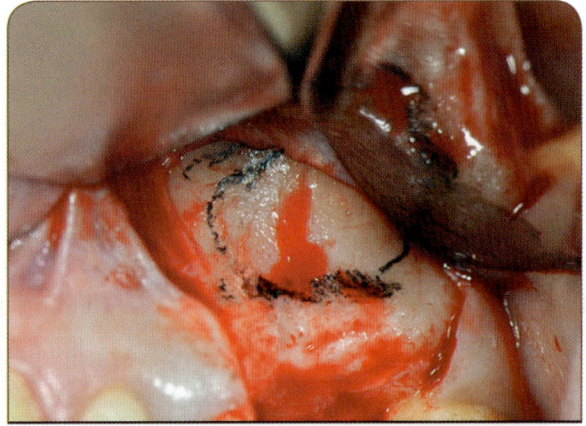

Fig. 6

Full thickness flap elevated exposing the facial wall. Ideally wall mark with some graphite **(Fig. 6)**.

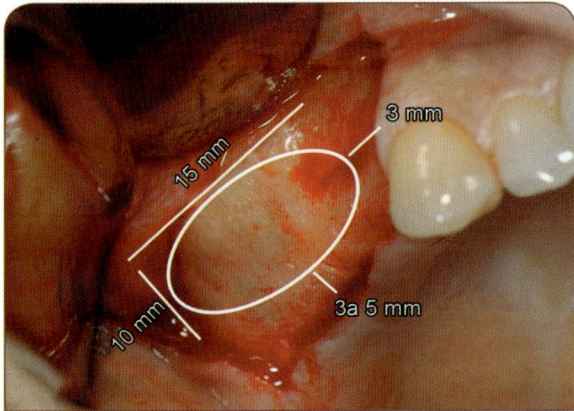

Fig. 7

Dimension of external wall **(Fig. 7)**.

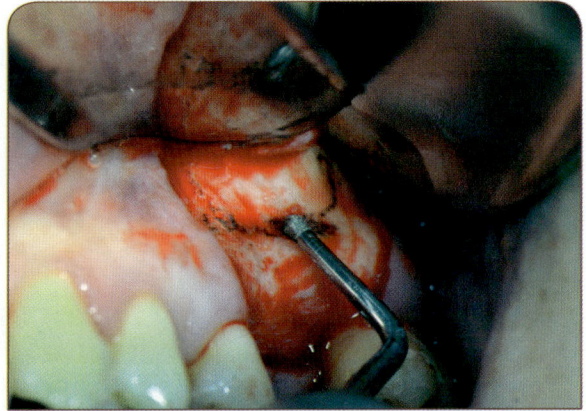

Fig. 8

Diamond bur for Piezomed grinding the wall **(Fig. 8)**.

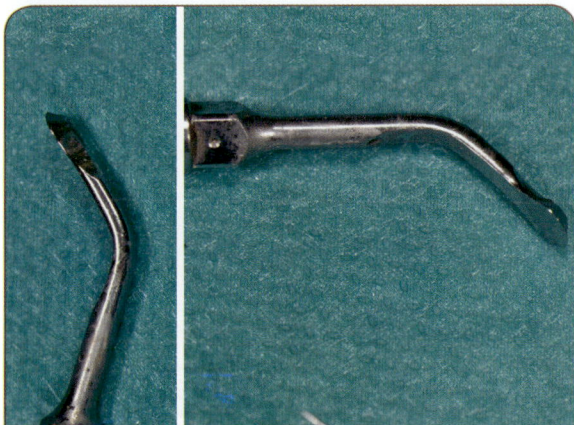

Fig. 9

Carbide tungsten bur for Piezomed grinding the wall **(Fig. 9)**.

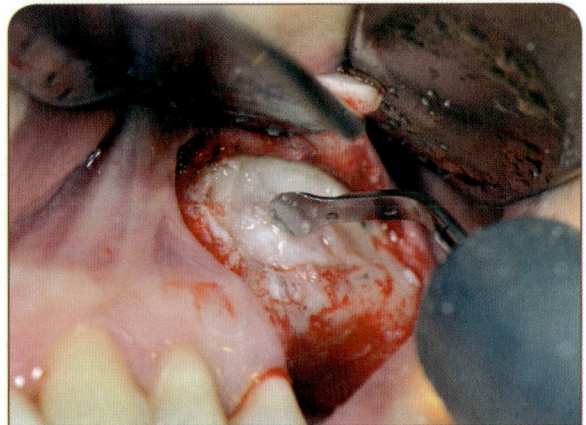

Fig. 10

External wall being grinded **(Fig. 10)**.

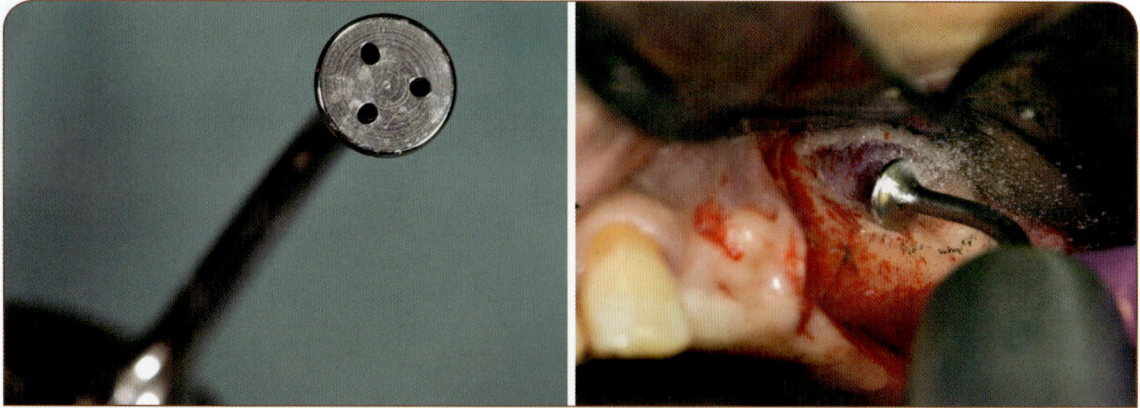

Fig. 11

Elephant feet for membrane separation **(Fig. 11)**.

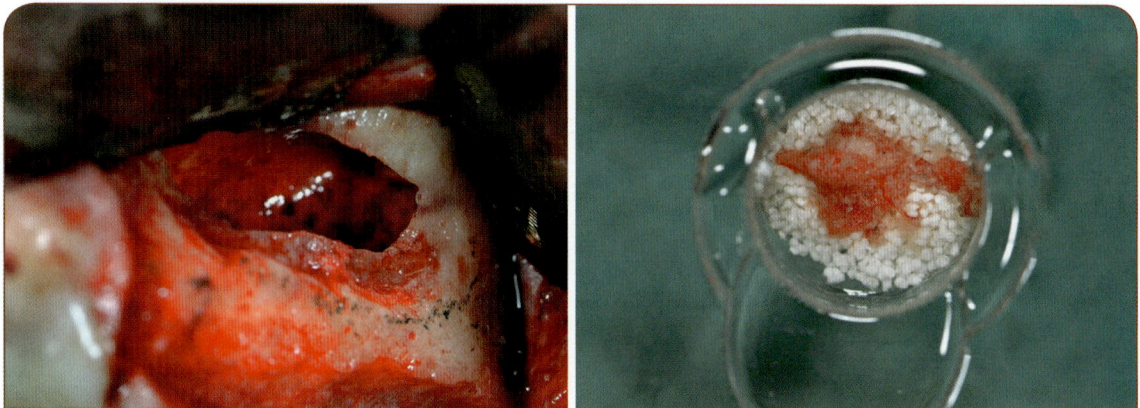

Fig. 12

Membrane elevated and Kera OS biomaterial prepared for use **(Fig. 12)**.

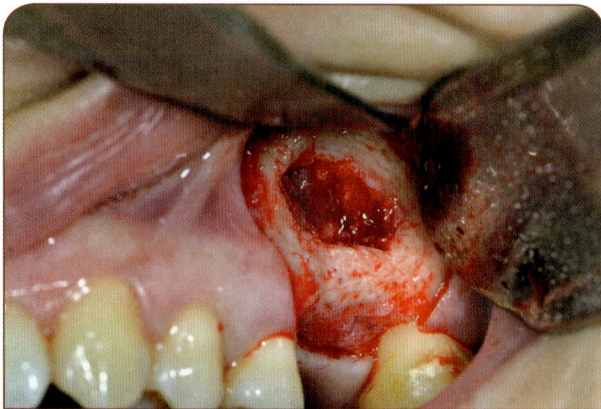

Fig. 13

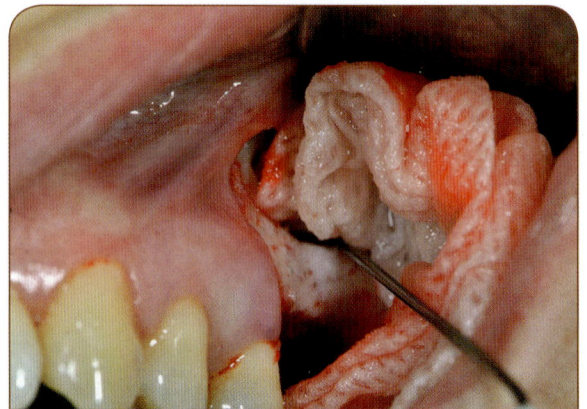

Fig. 14

Scheneiderian membrane elevation is gently performed using sinus curettes starting from the most mesial aspect of the antrostomy **(Fig. 13)**.

Hydrated gauge was used to elevate the membrane after curettes **(Fig. 14)**.

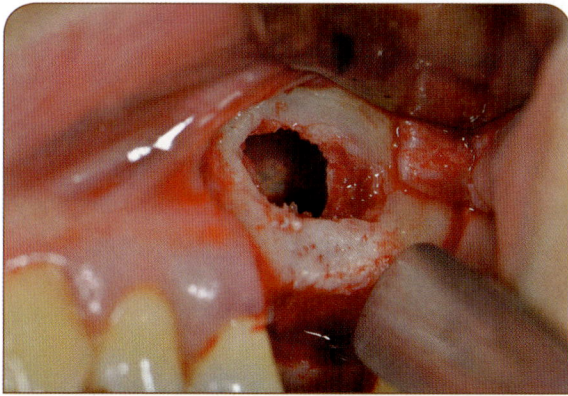

Fig. 15

Membrane elevated **(Fig. 15)**.

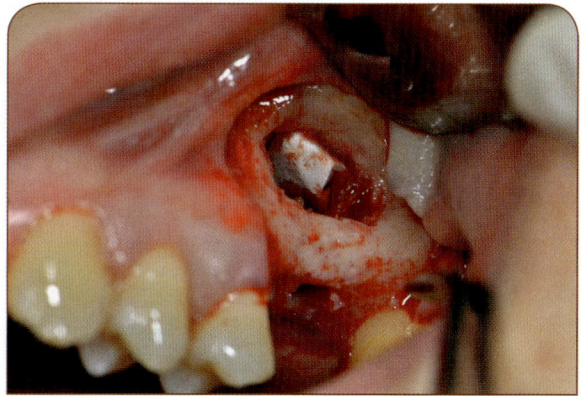

Fig. 16

Collagen membrane was placed internally protecting Schneiderian membrane **(Fig. 16)**.

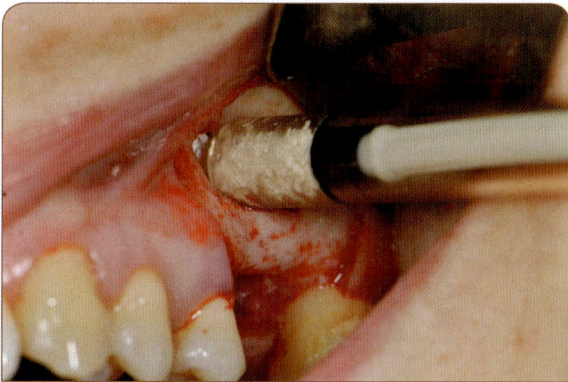

Fig. 17

Kera Os biomaterial was placed **(Fig. 17)**.

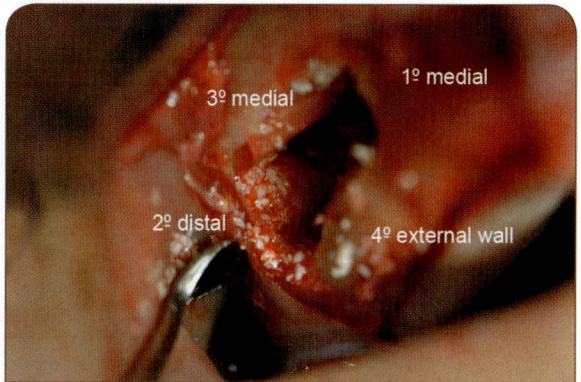

Fig. 18

How the biomaterial has to be placed **(Fig. 18)**.

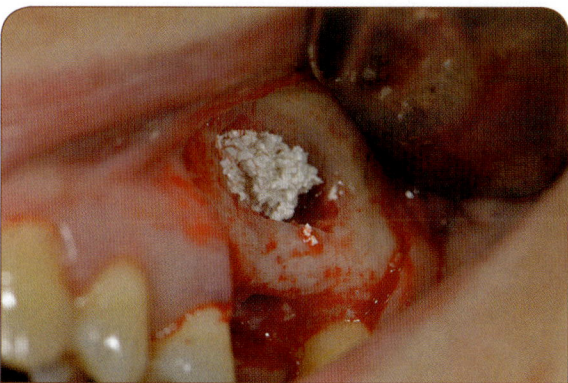

Fig. 19

More grafting material is injected over the implant to achieve a sandwich effect. A total of 2CC graft material is used in this case **(Fig. 19)**.

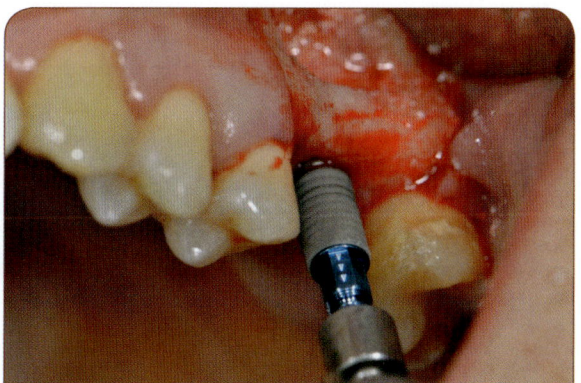

Fig. 20

More grafting material is injected over the implant to achieve a sandwich effect. Bone level Straumann 4.1 mm diameter by 12 mm length was placed **(Fig. 20)**.

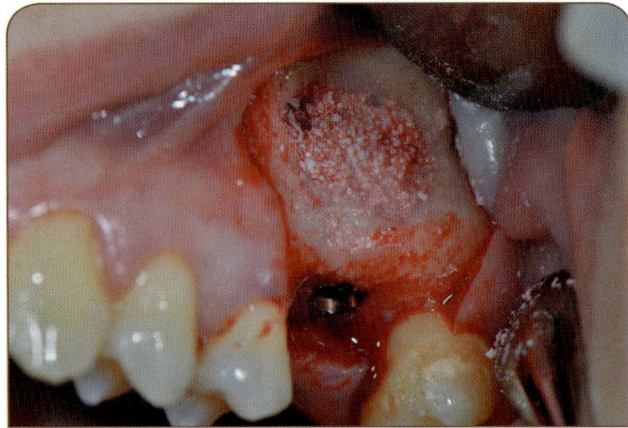

Fig. 21

Biomaterial and implant in place **(Fig. 21)**.

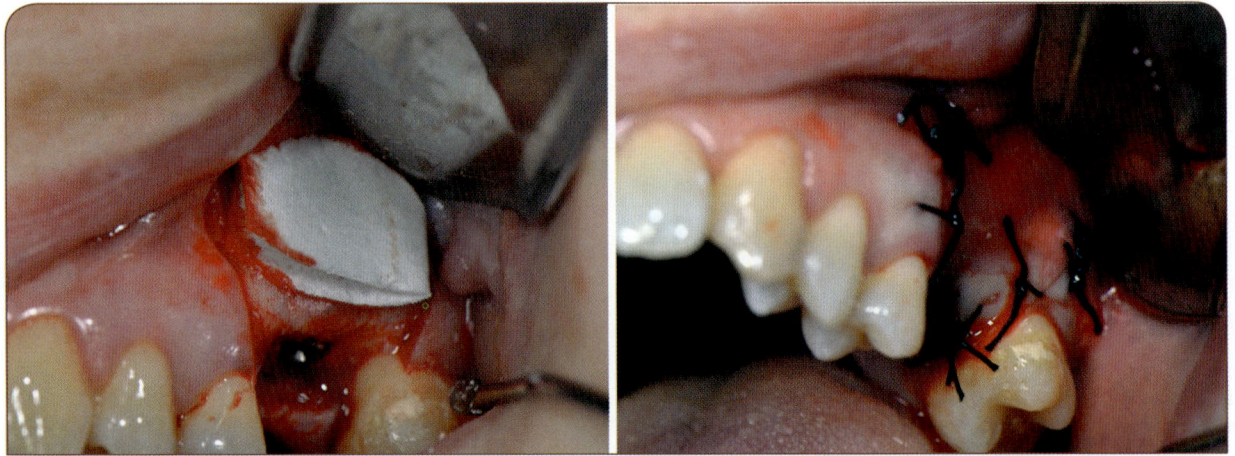

Fig. 22

Collagen membrane covering the external wall **(Fig. 22)**.

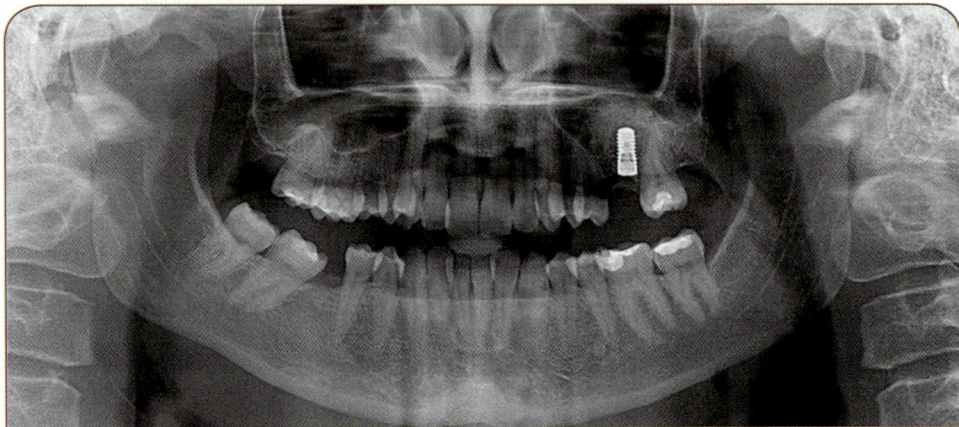

Fig. 23

Panoramic X-ray after implant placement **(Fig. 23)**.

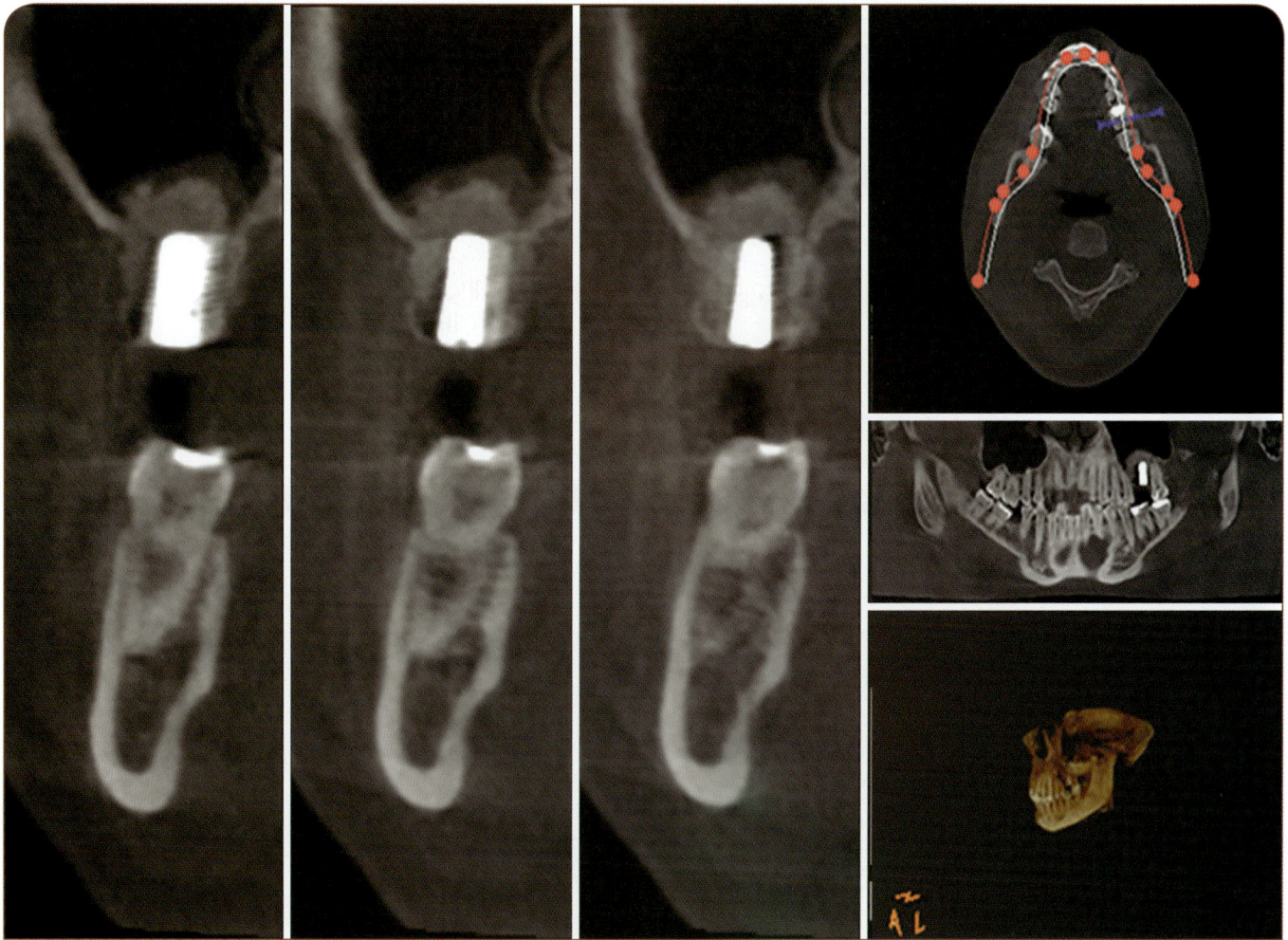

Fig. 24

CBCT scan after implant placement **(Fig. 24)**.

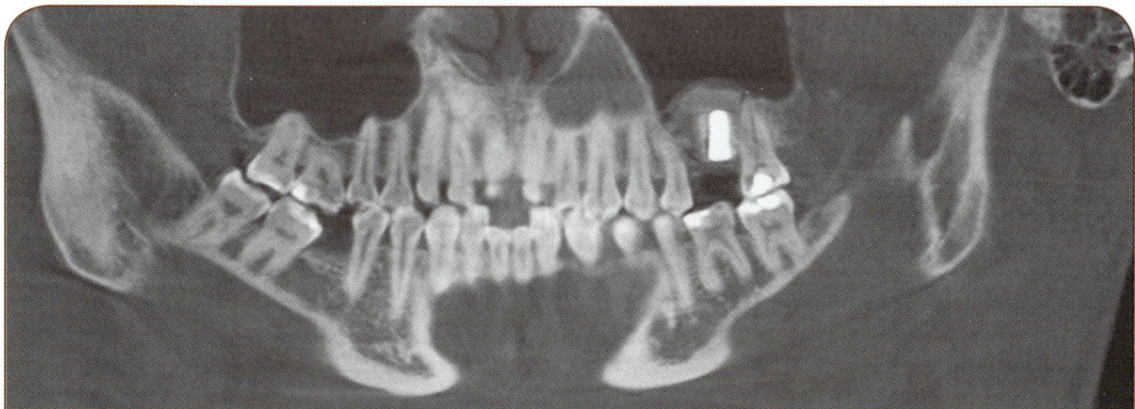

Fig. 25

A 6 month postoperative CBCT views showing complete bone fill and graft consolidation **(Fig. 25)**.

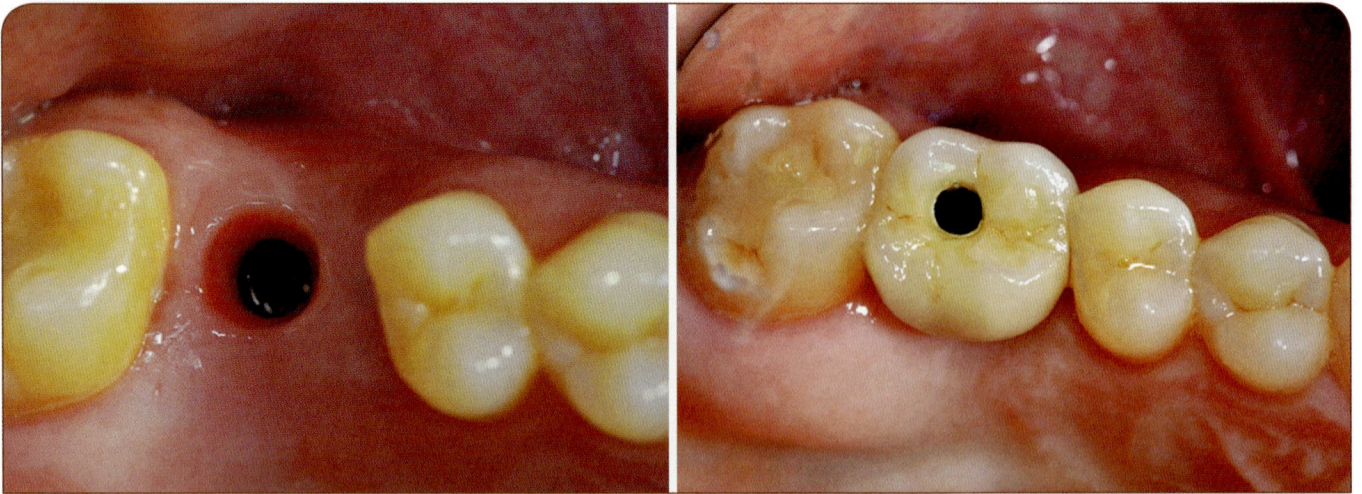

Fig. 26

Final restoration in place **(Fig. 26)**.

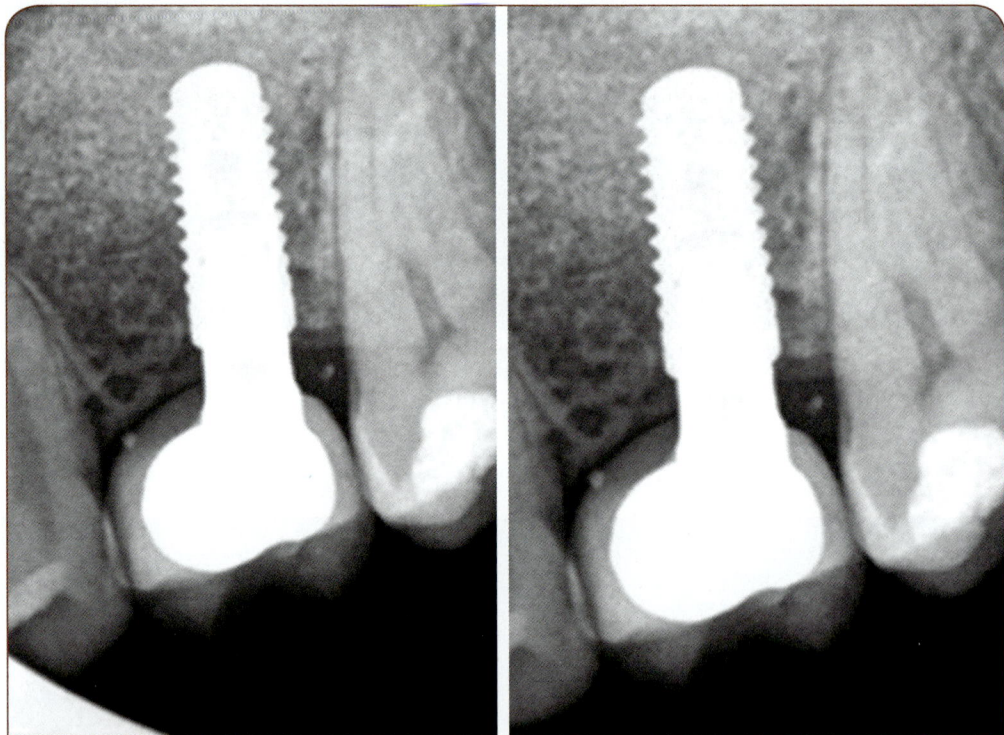

Fig. 27

Digital X-ray after crown placement, Digital RX after 1 year crown placement **(Fig. 27)**.

Ziv Mazor

Posterior Maxillary Rehabilitation of an Aggressive Periodontitis Patient using Osseodensification and Subcrestal Implants Placement

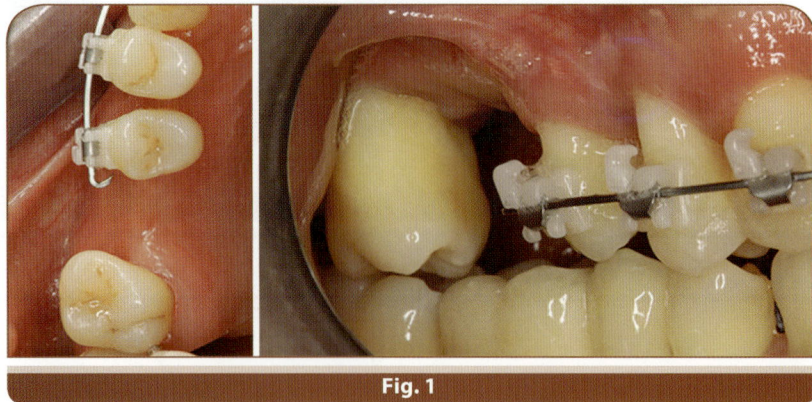

Fig. 1

Clinical view of tooth # 17. A 27-year female with aggressive periodontitis, tooth # 16 had been extracted in the past and 17 is hopeless 2 mm of available ridge height. Proposed Treatment: Subcrestal sinus augmentation using osseodensification utilizing patient's own tooth as a graft material **(Fig. 1)**.

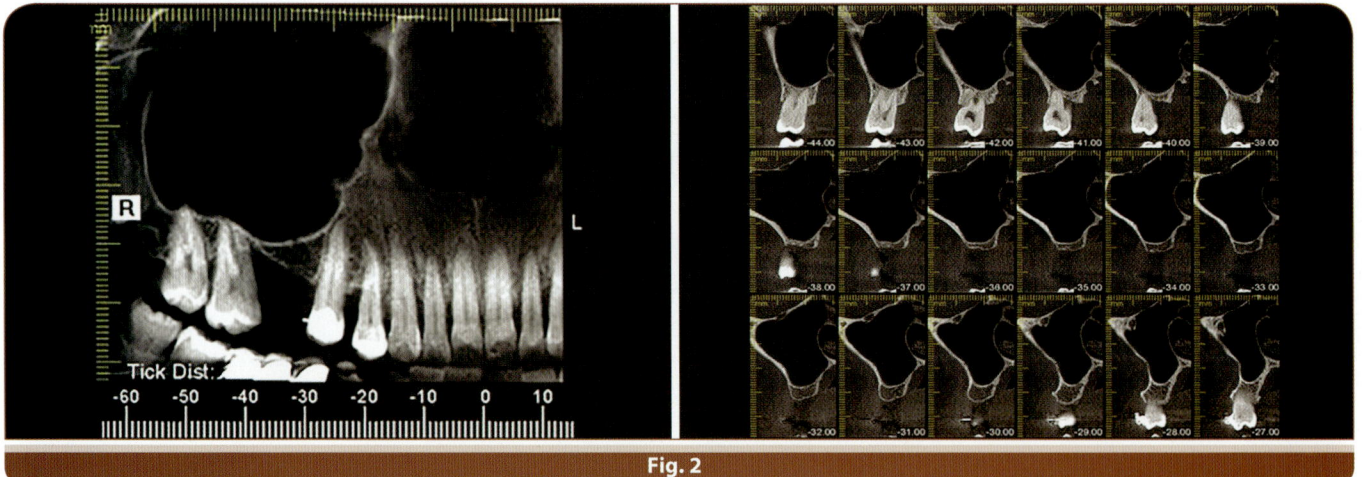

Fig. 2

CBCT demonstrating lack of alveolar ridge height **(Fig. 2)**.

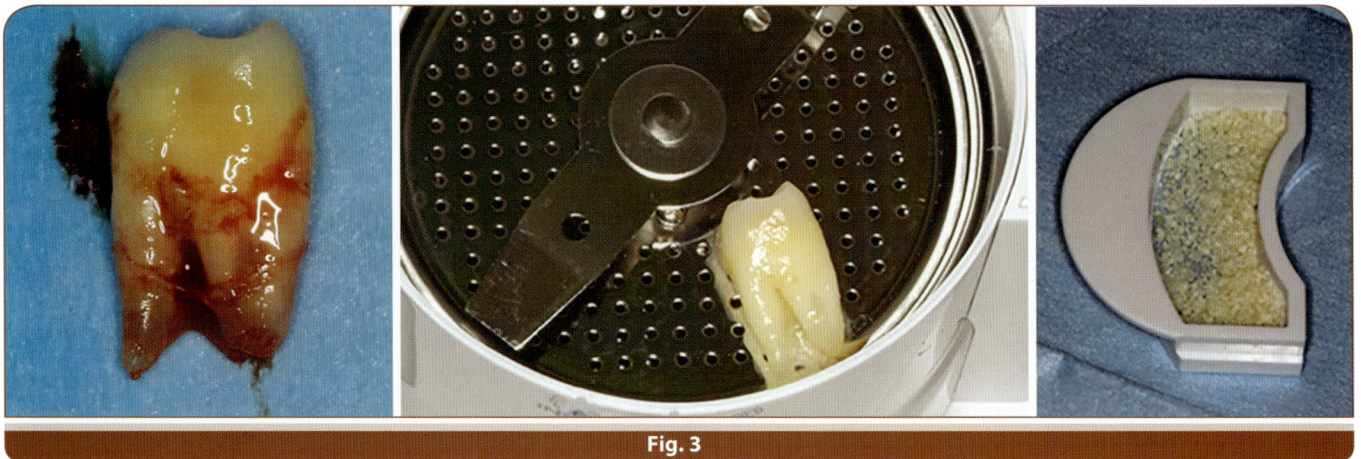

Fig. 3

Extracted tooth #17 that had been grinded to be utilized as graft material **(Fig. 3)**.

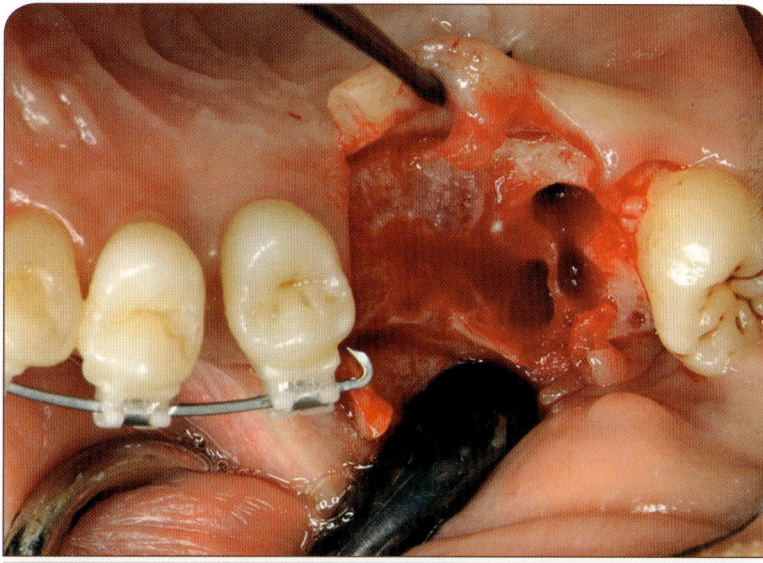

Fig. 4

Site after extraction of tooth#17 **(Fig. 4)**.

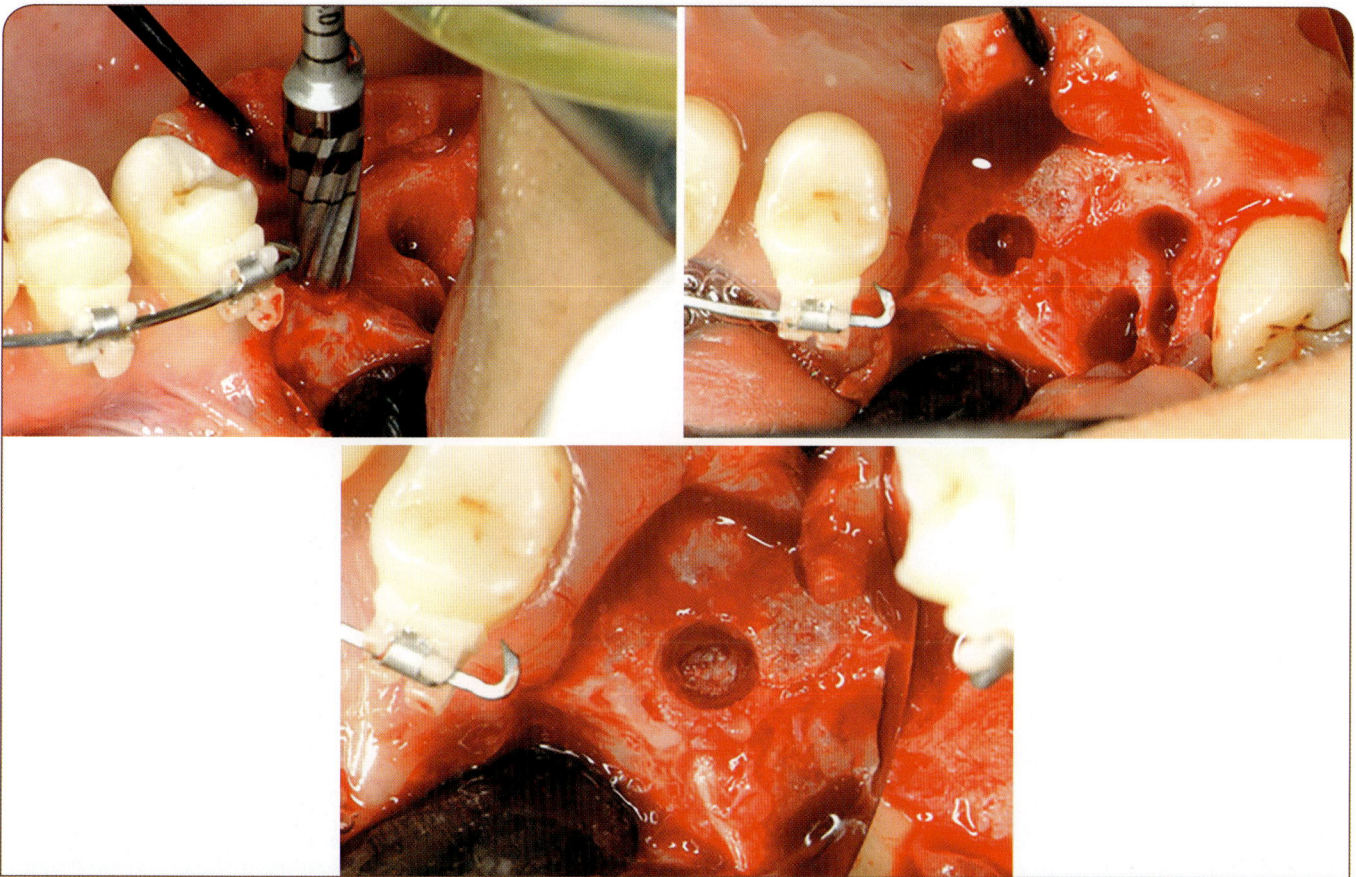

Fig. 5

Osseodensification steps with subcrestal sinus elevation **(Fig. 5)**.

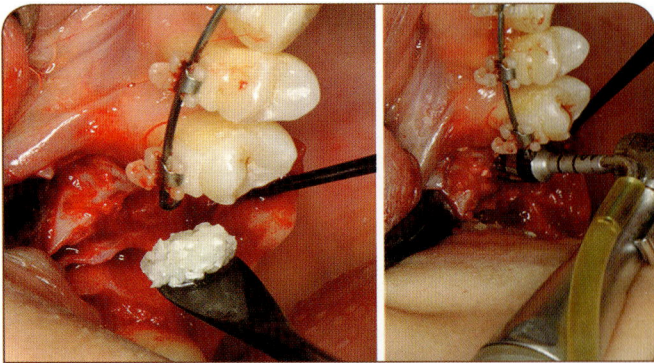

Fig. 6

Graft placement using the osseodensification drills **(Fig. 6)**.

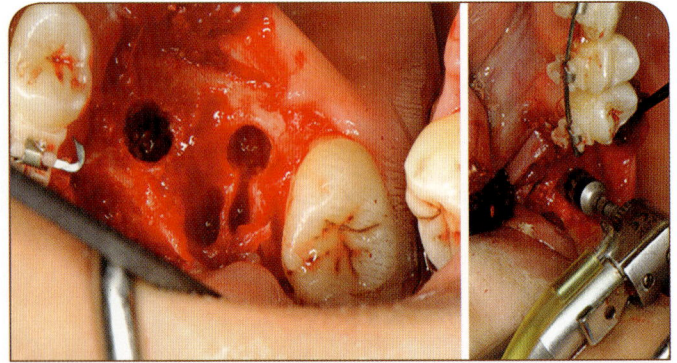

Fig. 7

Graft placement using the osseodensification drills **(Fig. 7)**.

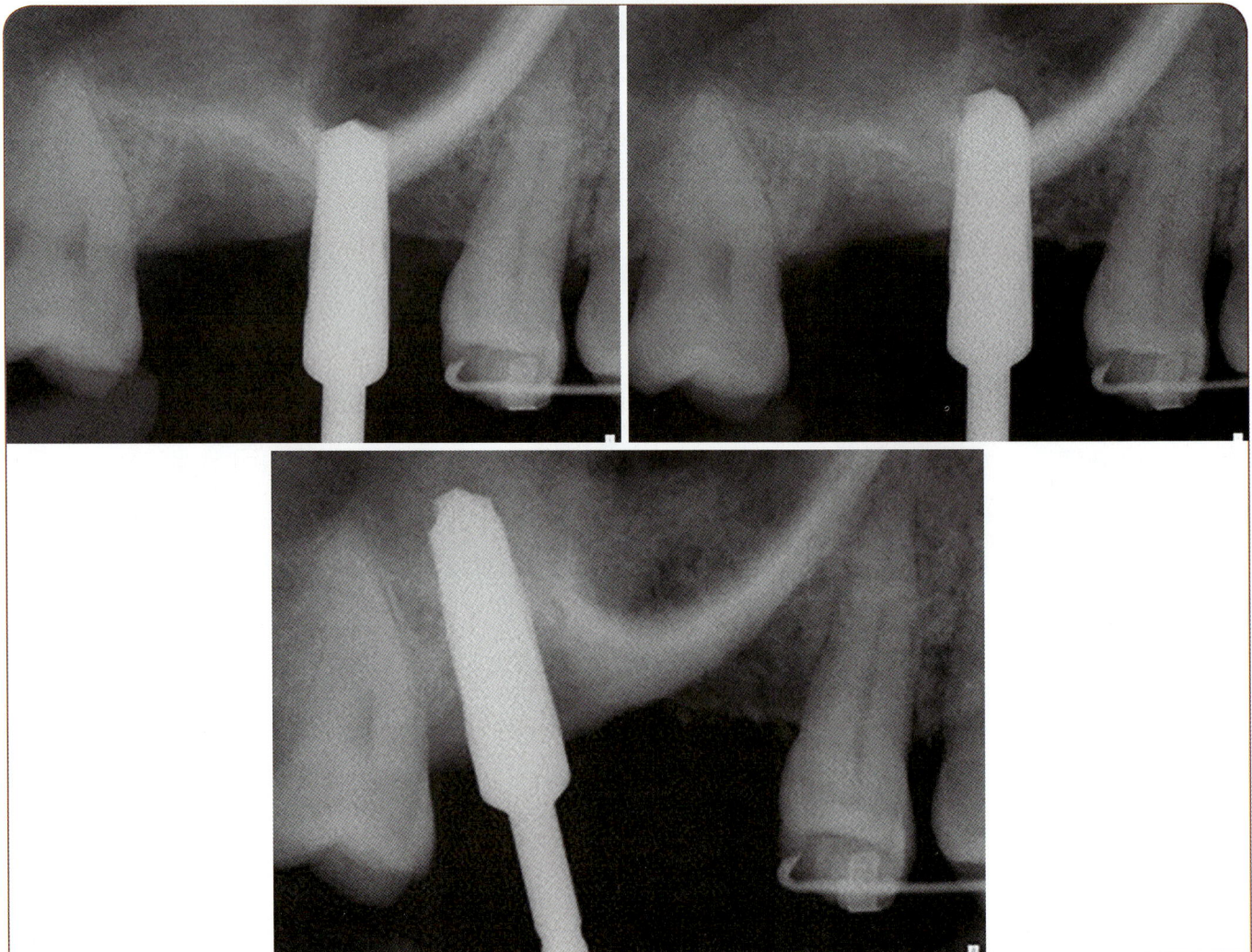

Fig. 8

Radiograph showing graft material in position and drills used for osteotomies in region of tooth # 16 and tooth # 17 **(Fig. 8)**.

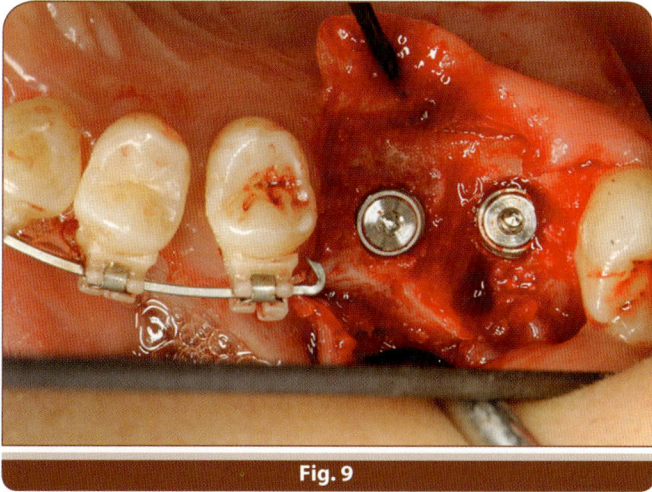

Fig. 9

Postoperative image after implant placement **(Fig. 9)**.

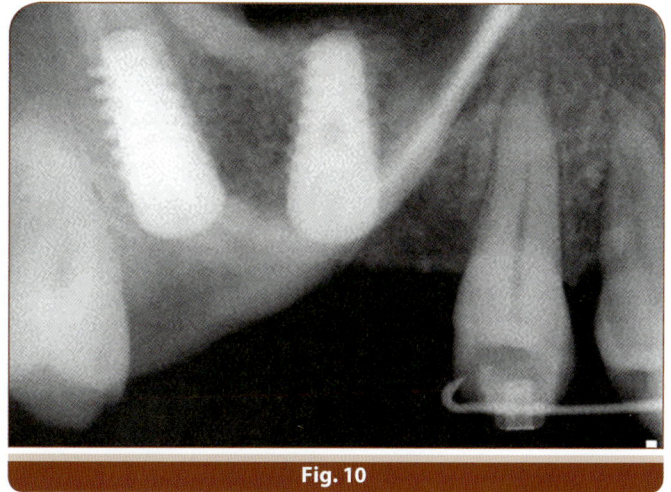

Fig. 10

Postoperative radiograph showing the 2 implants in position **(Fig. 10)**.

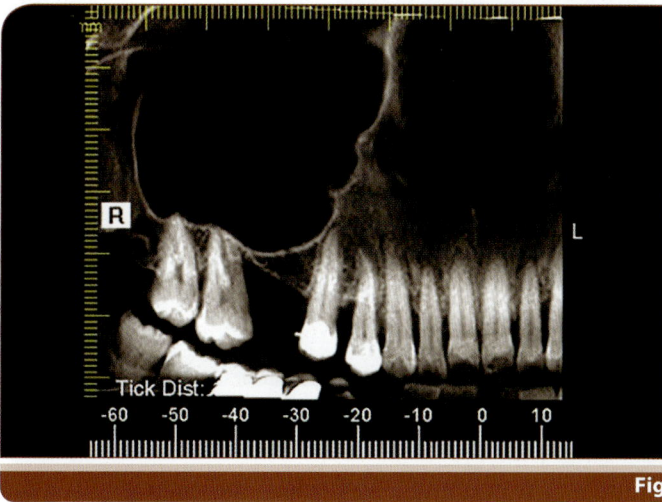

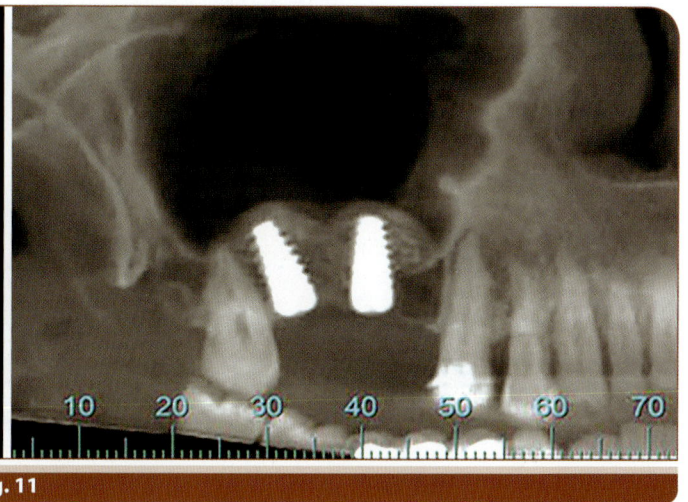

Fig. 11

Pre-vs Post-CBCTs **(Fig. 11)**.

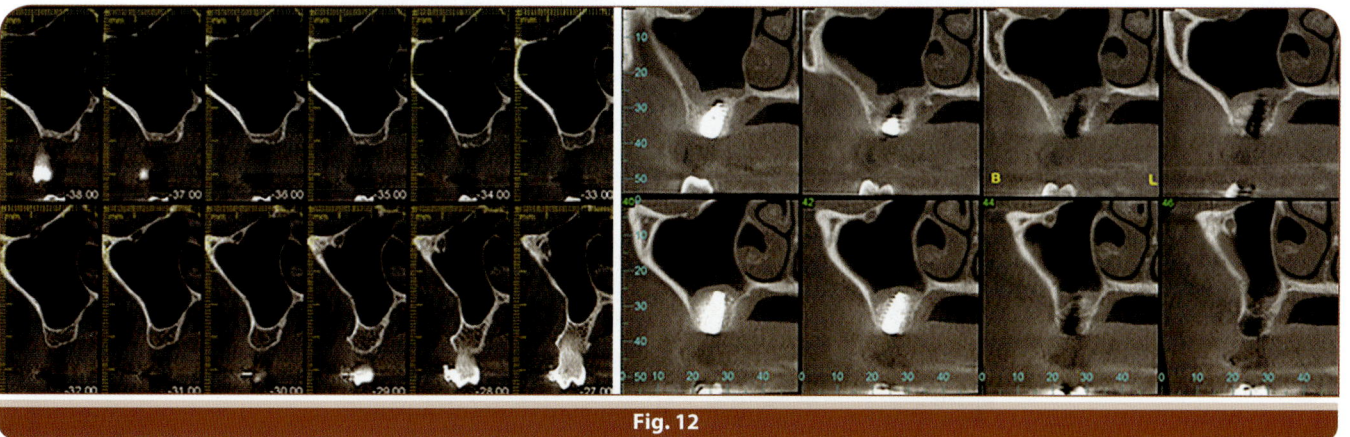

Fig. 12

Pre- vs Post-CBCTs **(Fig. 12)**.

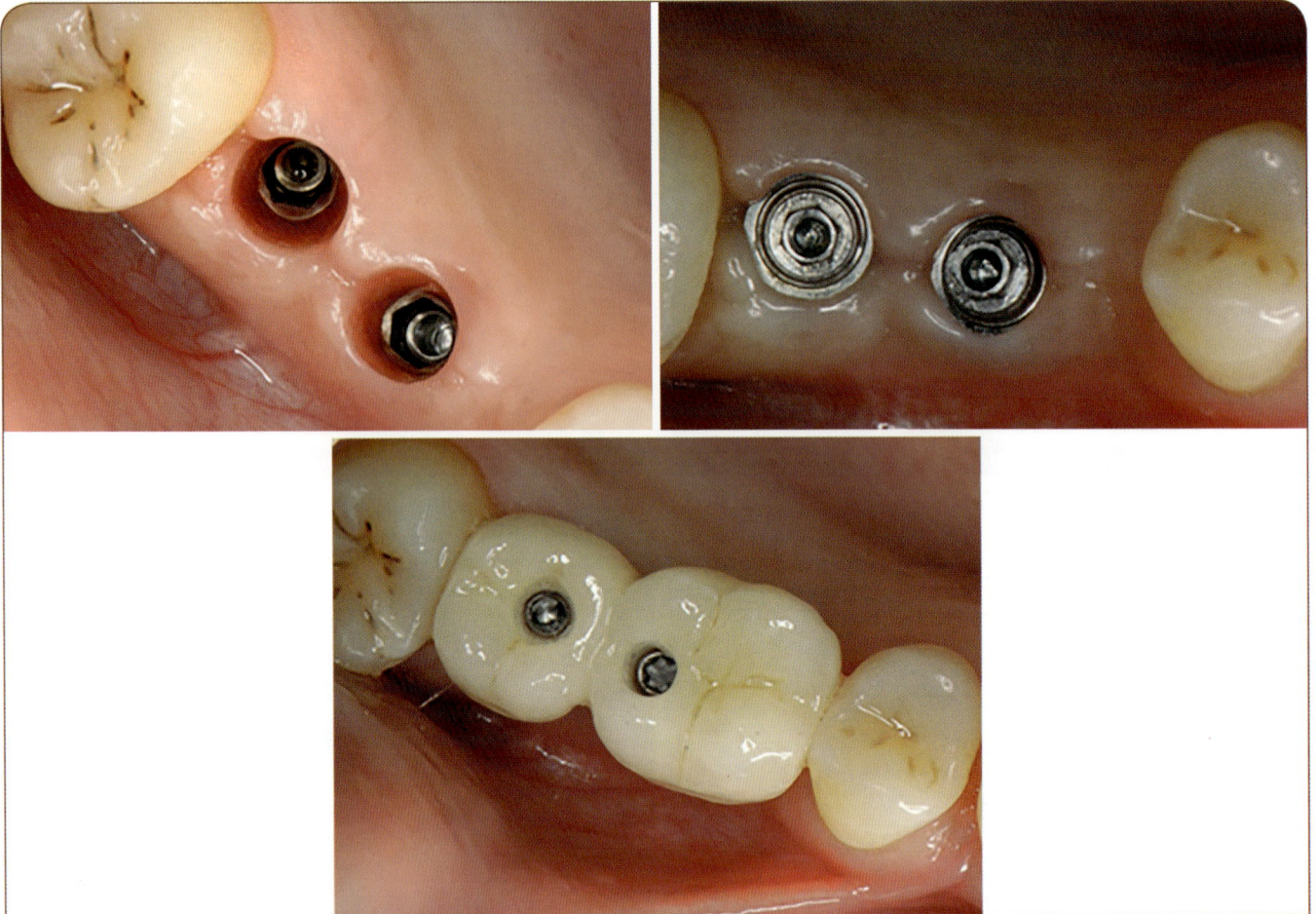

Fig. 13

Final prosthetic reconstruction using screw retained prosthesis **(Fig. 13)**.

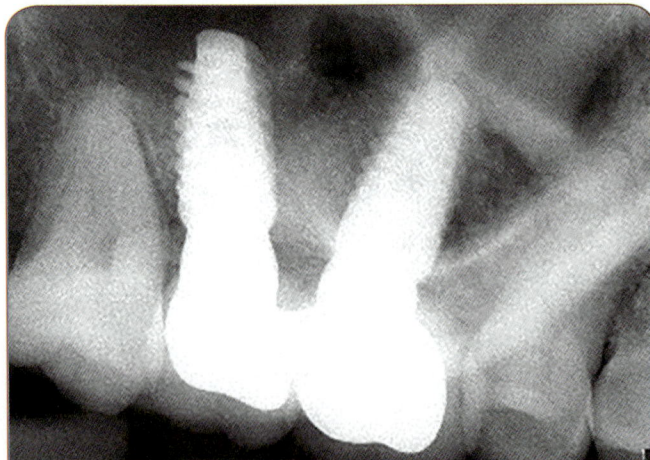

Fig. 14

Three years postoperative radiograph **(Fig. 14)**.

CASE STUDY 54

Lanka Mahesh, Nitika Poonia

OSSEODENSIFICATION WITH DENSAH BURS

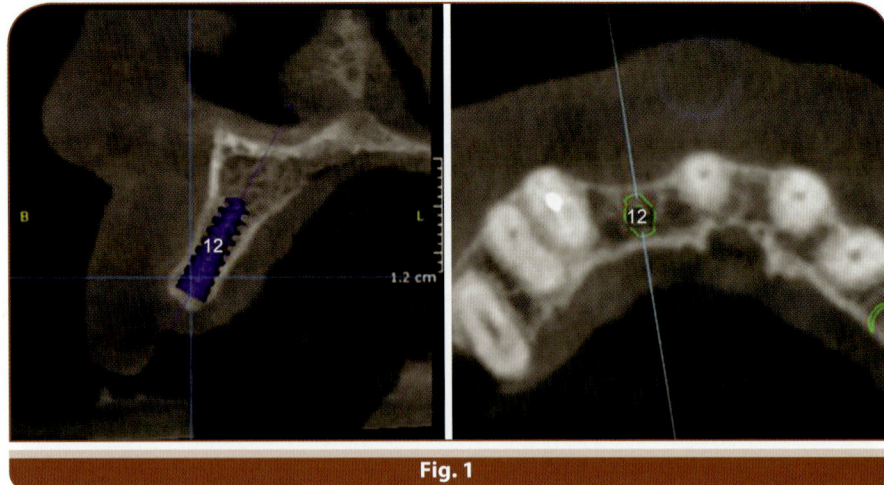

Fig. 1

A 58-year-old female patient with no systemic contraindications for surgery. Referred for implant placement in relation to teeth # 12, 23 and 25. 13 was planned for a post and core by the referring dentist hence left undisturbed **(Fig. 1)**.

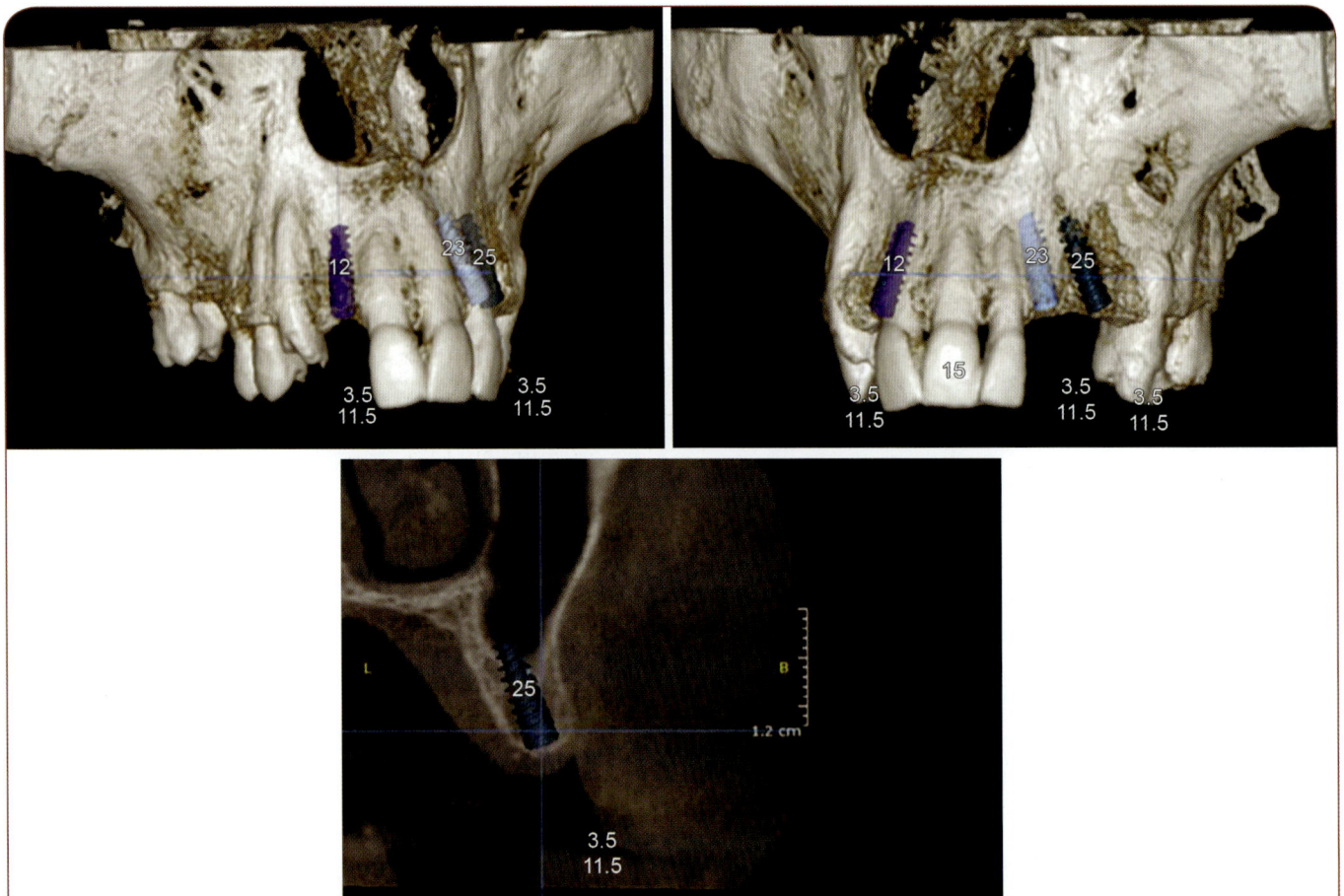

Fig. 2

The CBCT implant planning showed us all implants of 3.5 mm diameter. All implants planned 3.5/11.5 mm (on CBCT) **(Fig. 2)**.

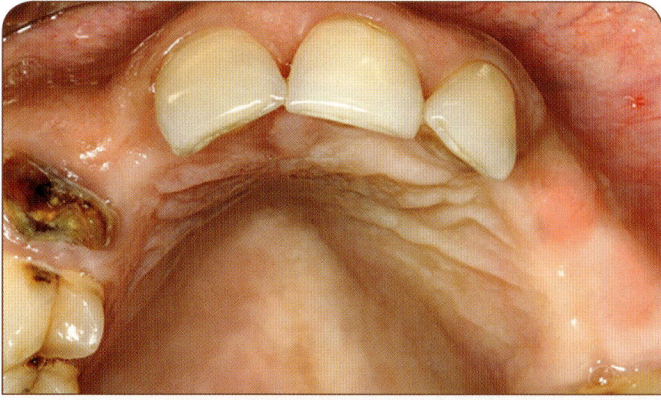

Fig. 3

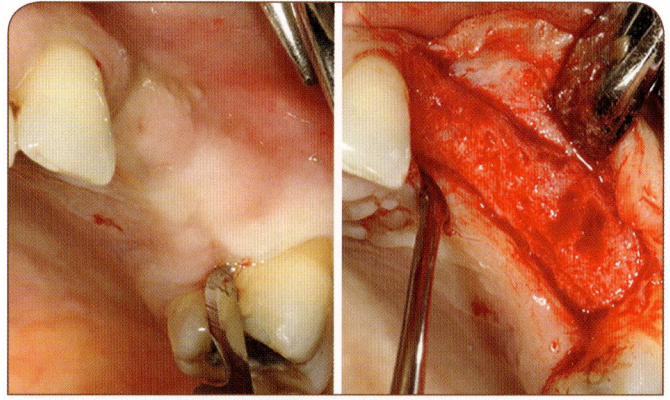

Fig. 4

Site in 12 clearly demonstrates soft tissue defect imply-ing underlying alveolar defect. Sites 23–25 appear having adequate soft tissue although the CBCT illustrates a lesser volume of bone **(Fig. 3)**.

Complete elevation and exposure of the surgical site. Nar-row bucco-palatal defect evident (23 region). Densah burs were used for osteotomies **(Fig. 4)**.

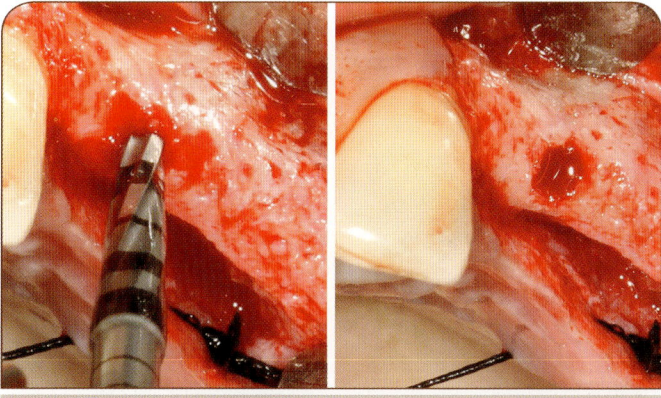

Fig. 5

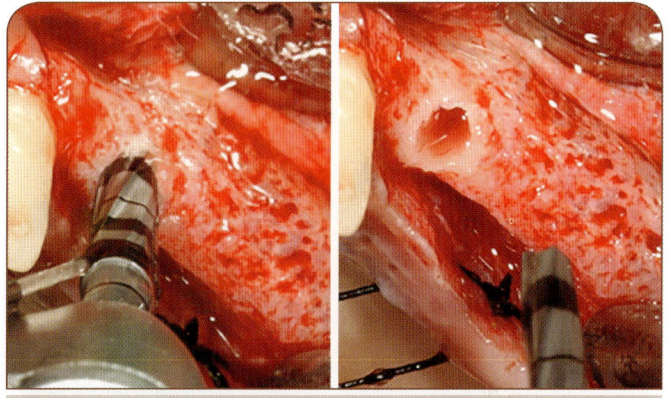

Fig. 6

1.5 mm bur 1200 rpm forward mode **(Fig. 5)**.

2.2 mm bur in reverse mode. 900 rpm **(Fig. 6)**.

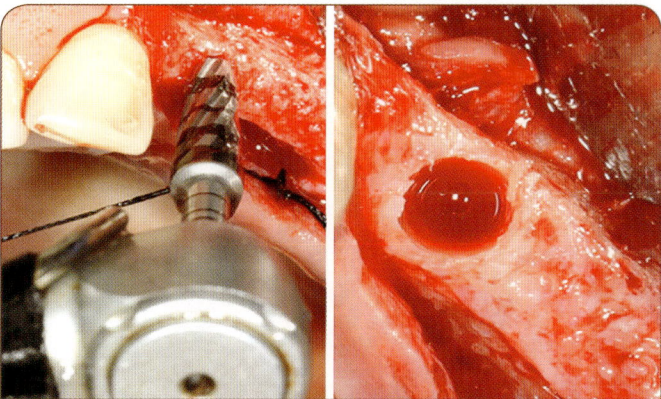

Fig. 7

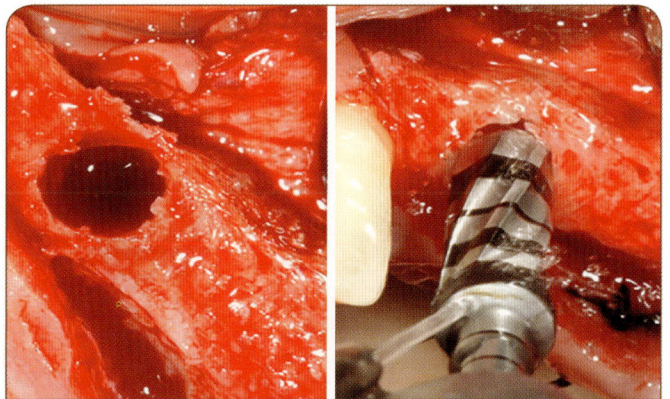

Fig. 8

2.5 mm, bur, 900 rpm in reverse mode (gradual osseoden-sification evident) **(Fig. 7)**.

3.2 mm bur, 900 rpm in reverse mode and the final osteo-tomy (note: no fenestration/dehiscence) **(Fig. 8)**.

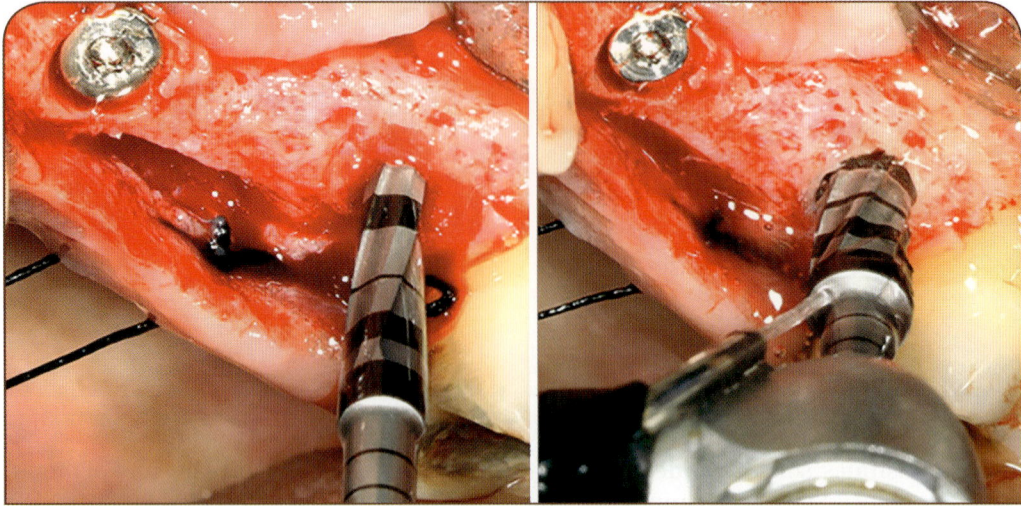

Fig. 9

Same protocol for 25 implant (RBH on CBCT, 8.5 mm) **(Fig. 9)**.

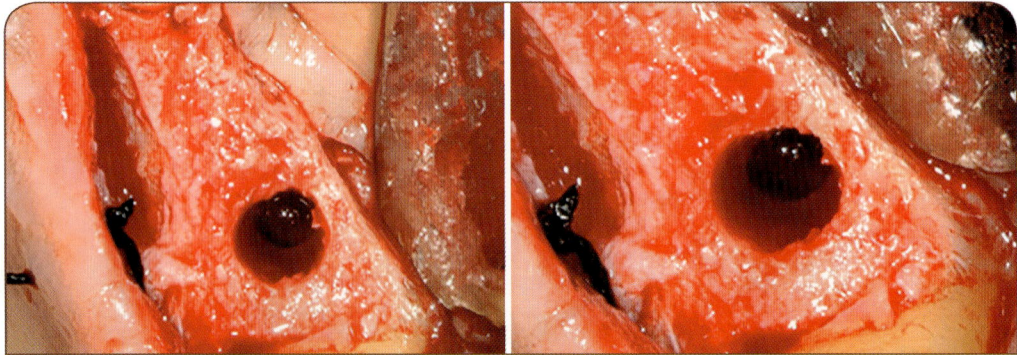

Fig. 10

Intact sinus membrane is lucid. Same frame zoomed in **(Fig. 10)**.

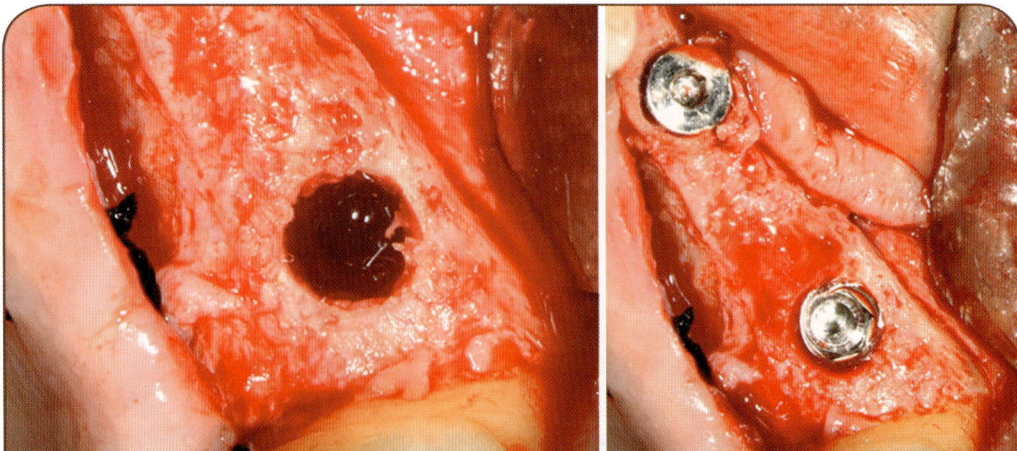

Fig. 11

Blood seeping into the osteotomy. Implants 3.75 mm/11.5 in 23 and 4.2/11.5 in 25 **(Fig. 11)**.

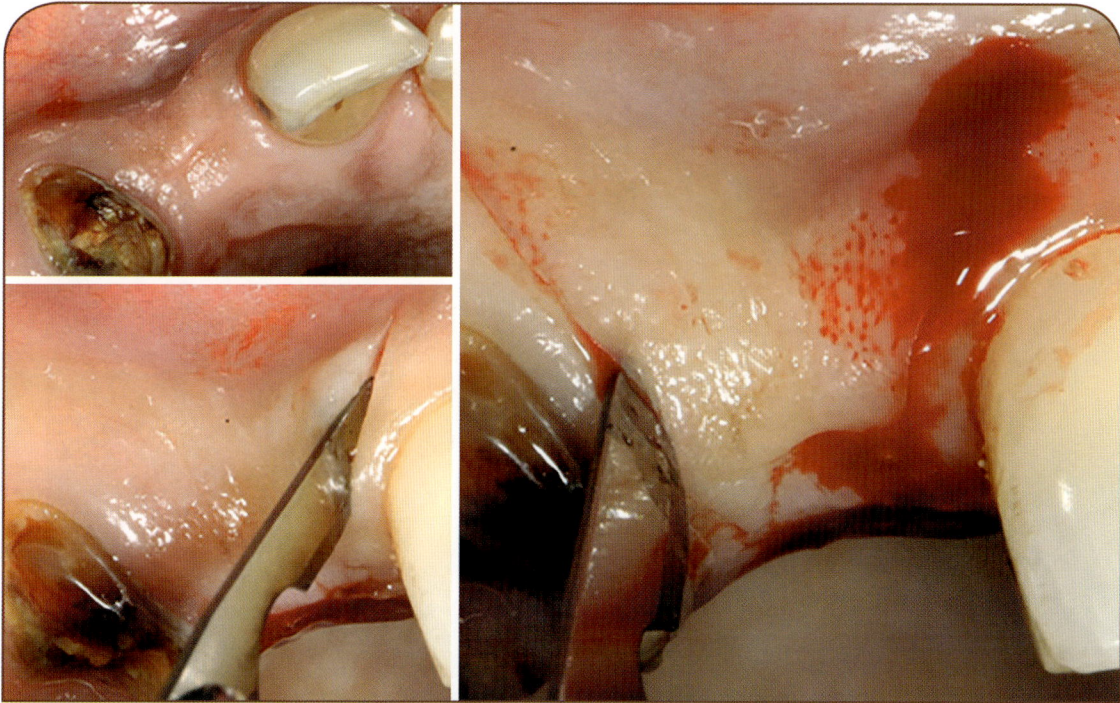

Fig. 12

Papilla preserving incision with a palatal bias at site 12 **(Fig. 12)**.

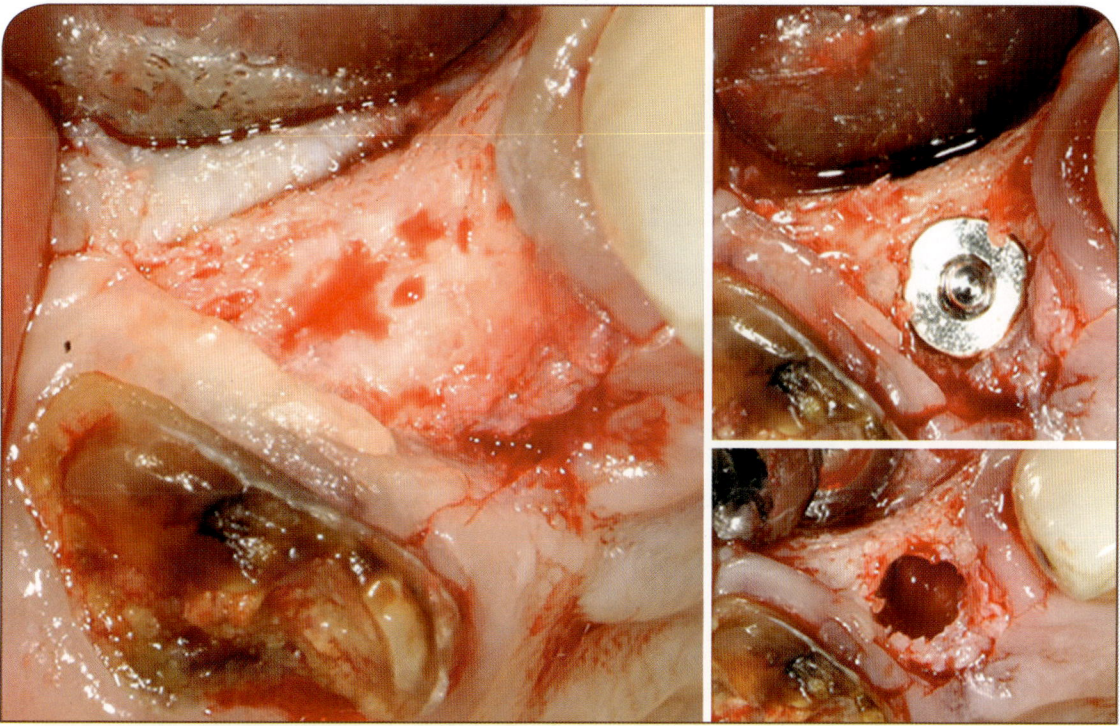

Fig. 13

Same protocol followed up to 3.2 mm bur. Implant placed 3.75/11.5 mm **(Fig. 13)**.

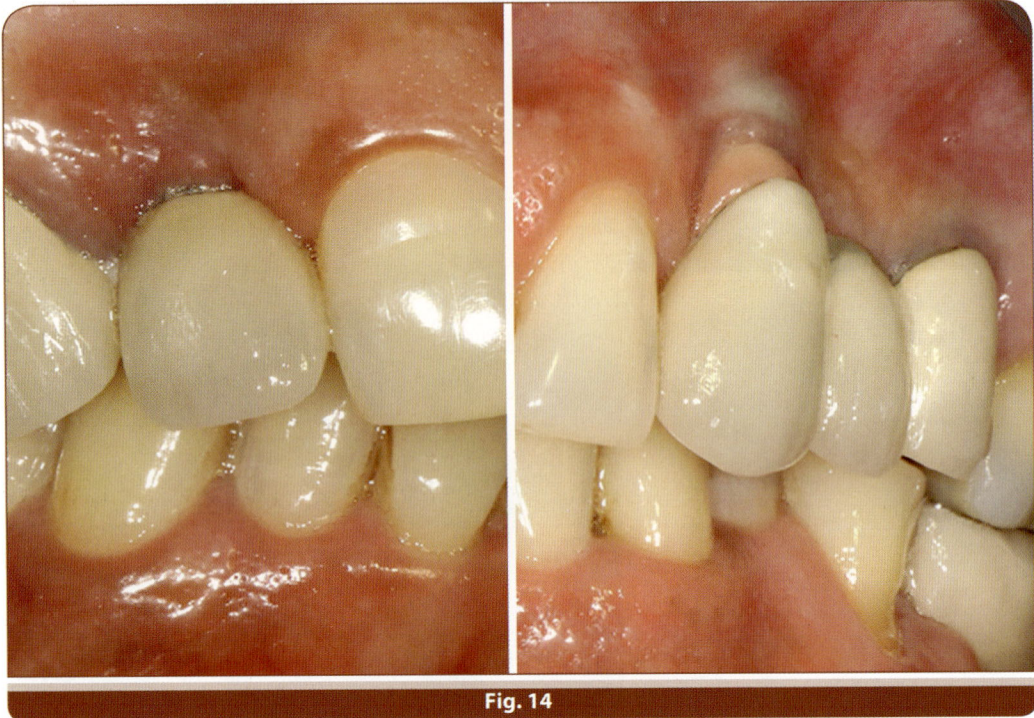

Fig. 14

Final clinical view at 14 months recall **(Fig. 14)**.

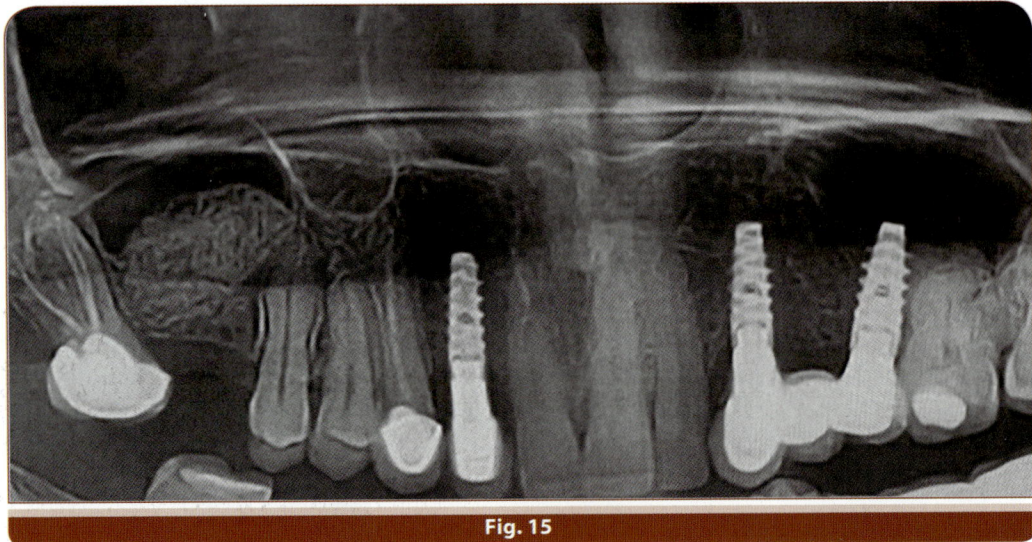

Fig. 15

Postoperative panorex at 14 months. Demonstrates adequate bone fill in the 25 region. Bone graft consolidation is also evident in the region of 16, where a direct sinus graft was performed **(Fig. 15)**.

Internal Sinus Lift (ISL) and Immediate Implant Placement

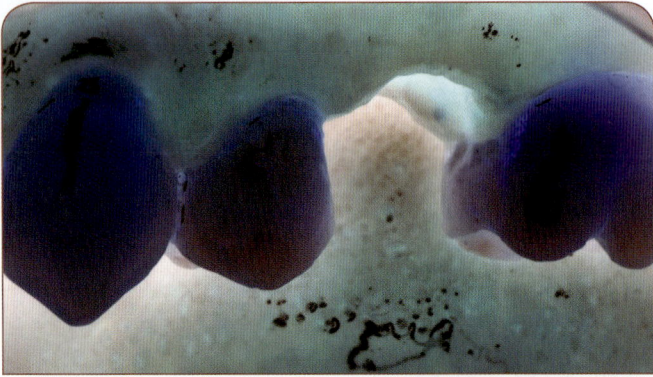

Fig. 1

Immediate extraction implant. Internal sinus lift through the socket. Custom healing abutment. Custom impression post. Screw cement retained (SCR) prosthesis **(Fig. 1)**.

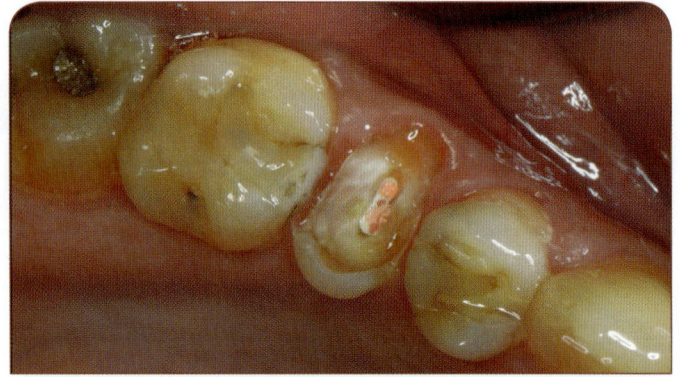

Fig. 2

Baseline **(Fig. 2)**.

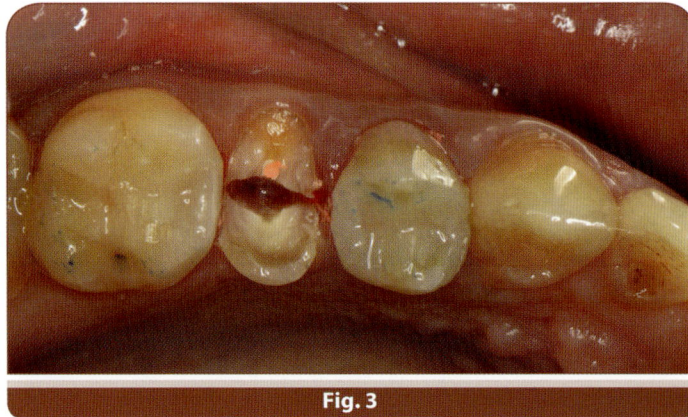

Fig. 3

The tooth is carefully split and extracted as atraumatically as possible **(Fig. 3)**.

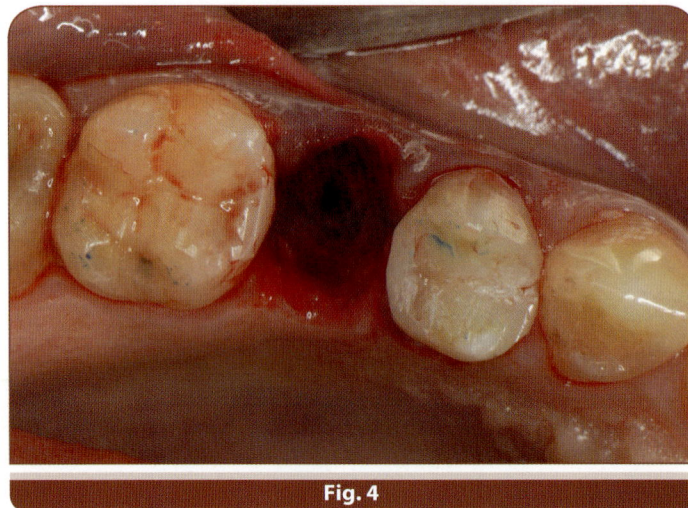

Fig. 4

Atraumatic extraction. ISL through the socket using MCT expanders **(Fig. 4)**.

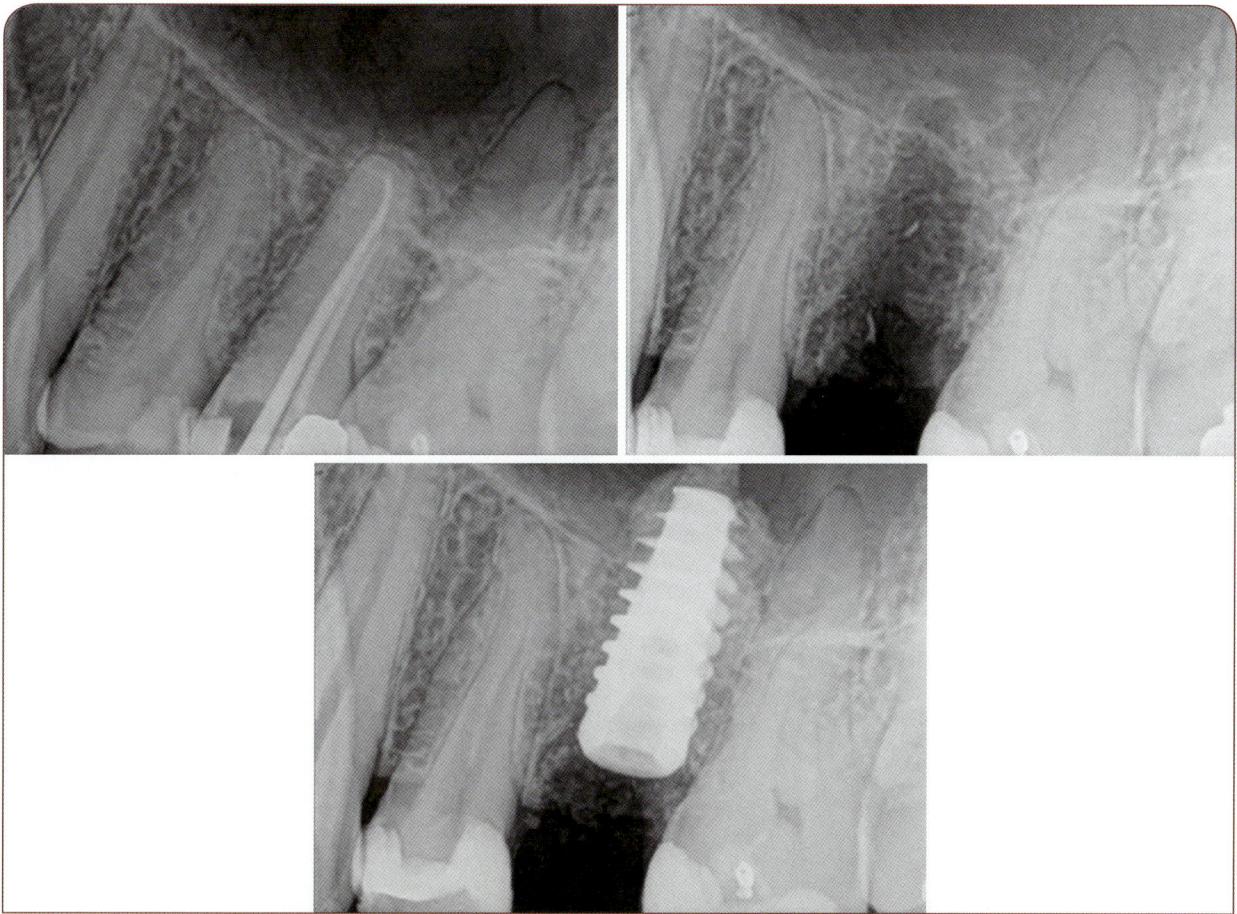

Fig. 5

ISL through the socket, immediate extraction implant placement **(Fig. 5)**.

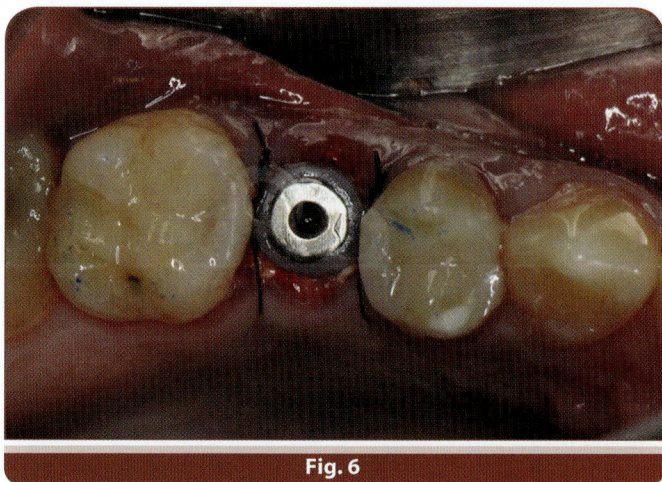

Fig. 6

Jump distance grafted with bovine-bone. Custom gingival former created by lining with composite **(Fig. 6)**.

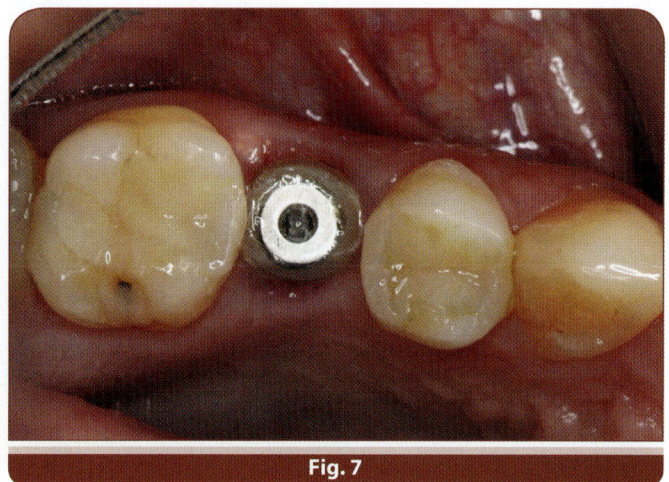

Fig. 7

Six months postoperative **(Fig. 7)**.

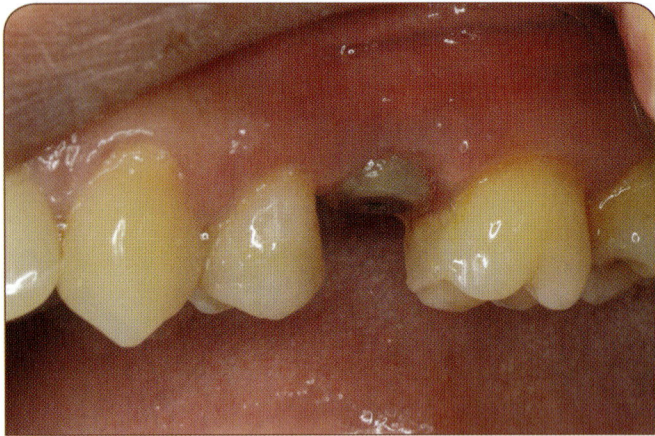

Fig. 8

Six months postoperative **(Fig. 8)**.

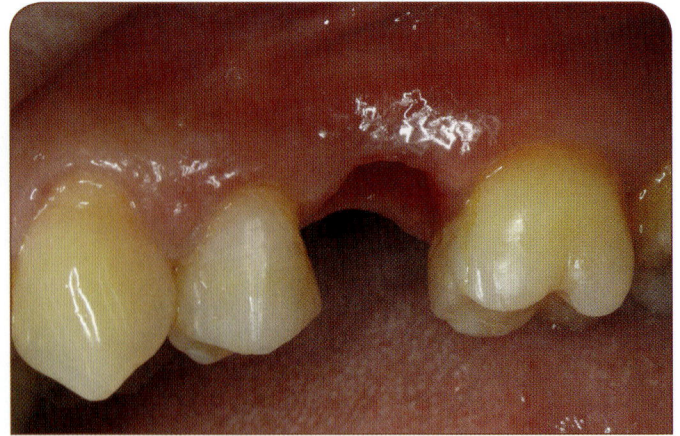

Fig. 9

Soft tissue contours at 6 months **(Fig. 9)**.

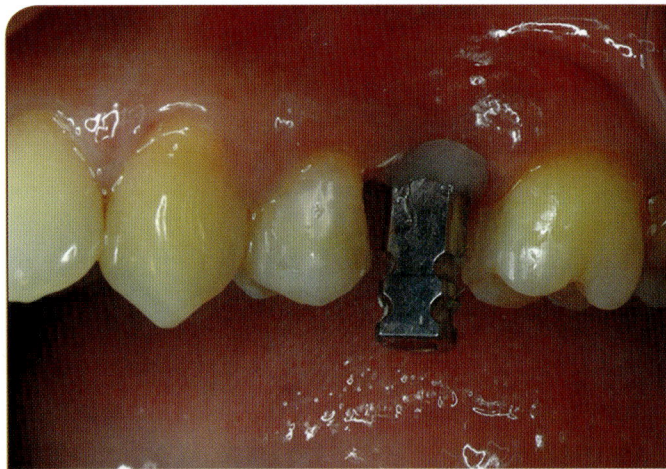

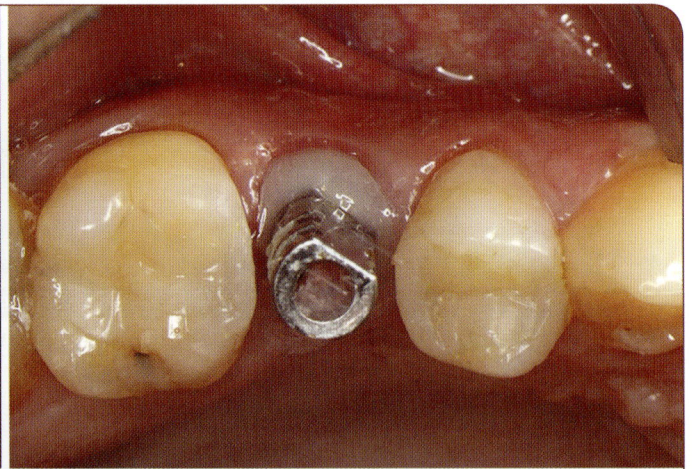

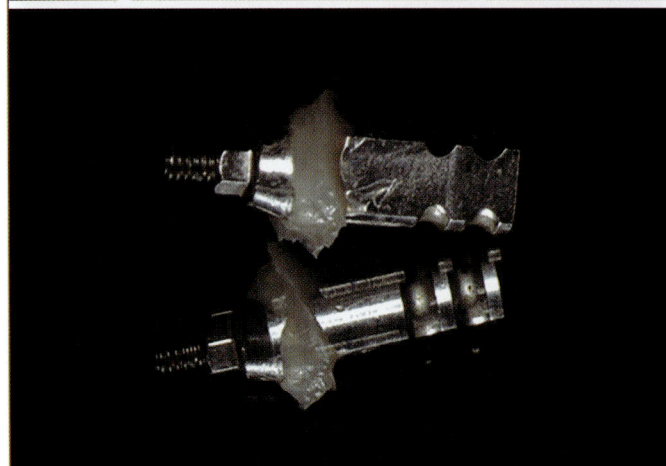

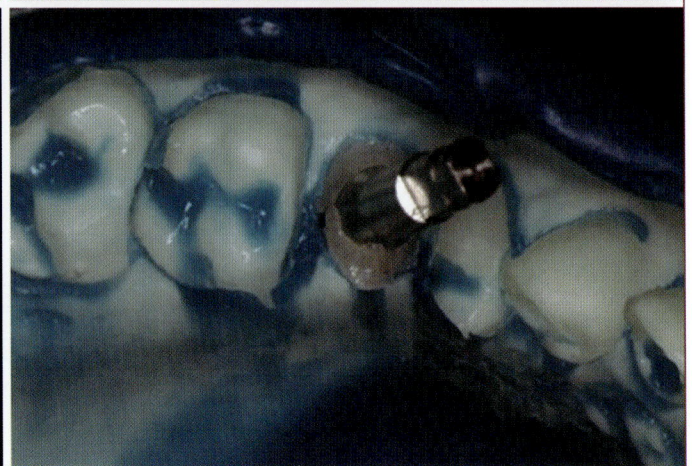

Fig. 10

Custom impression post using flowable composite to record the soft tissue contours properly **(Fig. 10)**.

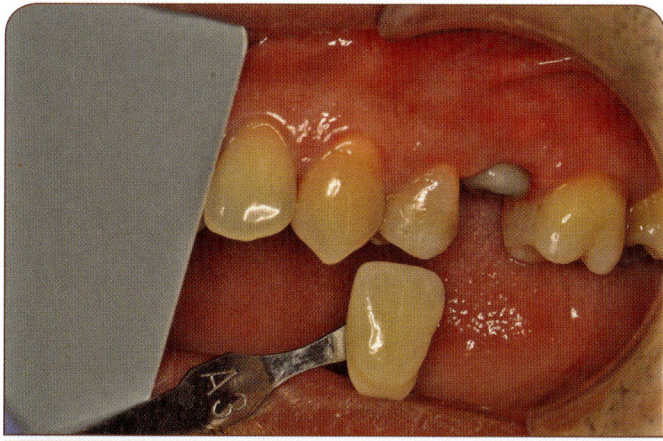

Fig. 11

Shade communication with lab, using 18% grey card **(Fig. 11)**.

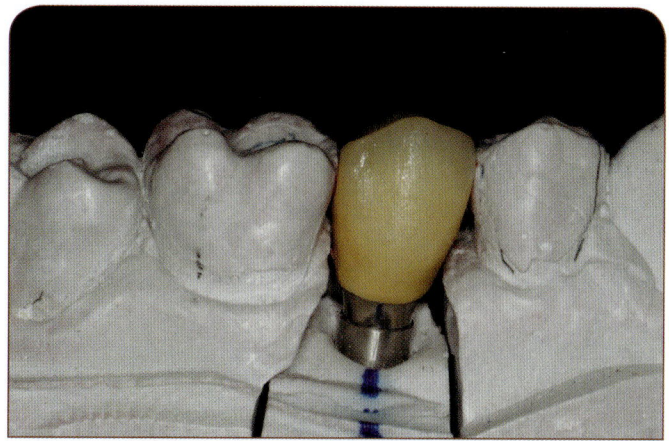

Fig. 12

Desired emergence profile created. SCR (Screw Cement Retained) crown using stock titanium abutment **(Fig. 12)**.

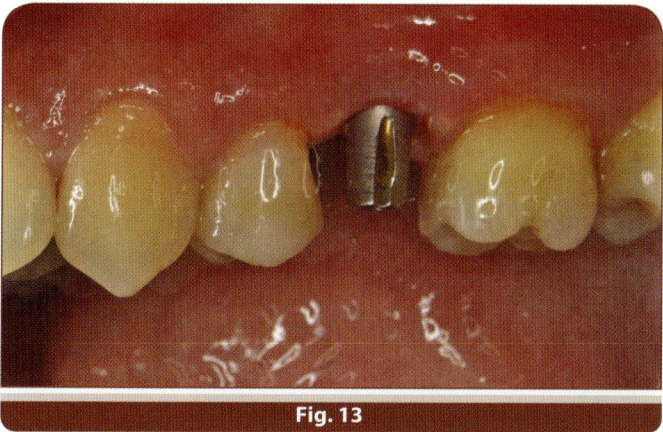

Fig. 13

Abutment in place **(Fig. 13)**.

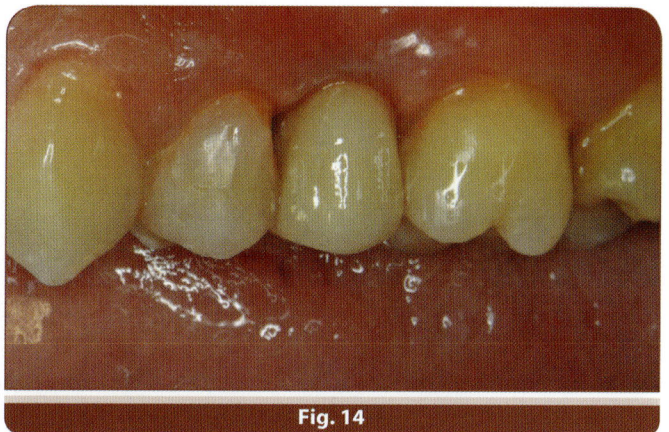

Fig. 14

Final SCR PFM prosthesis in place waiting for papillary fill to happen over time **(Fig. 14)**.

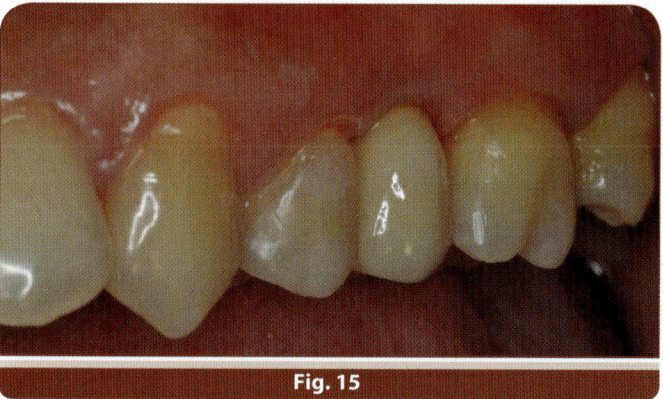

Fig. 15

Final SCR PFM prosthesis in place waiting for papillary fill to happen over time **(Fig. 15)**.

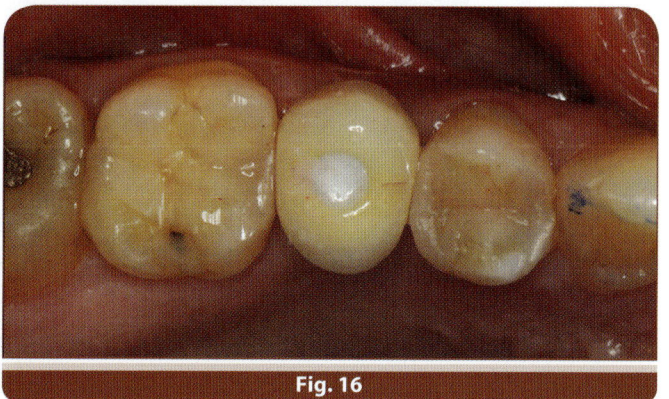

Fig. 16

Final SCR PFM prosthesis in place **(Fig. 16)**.

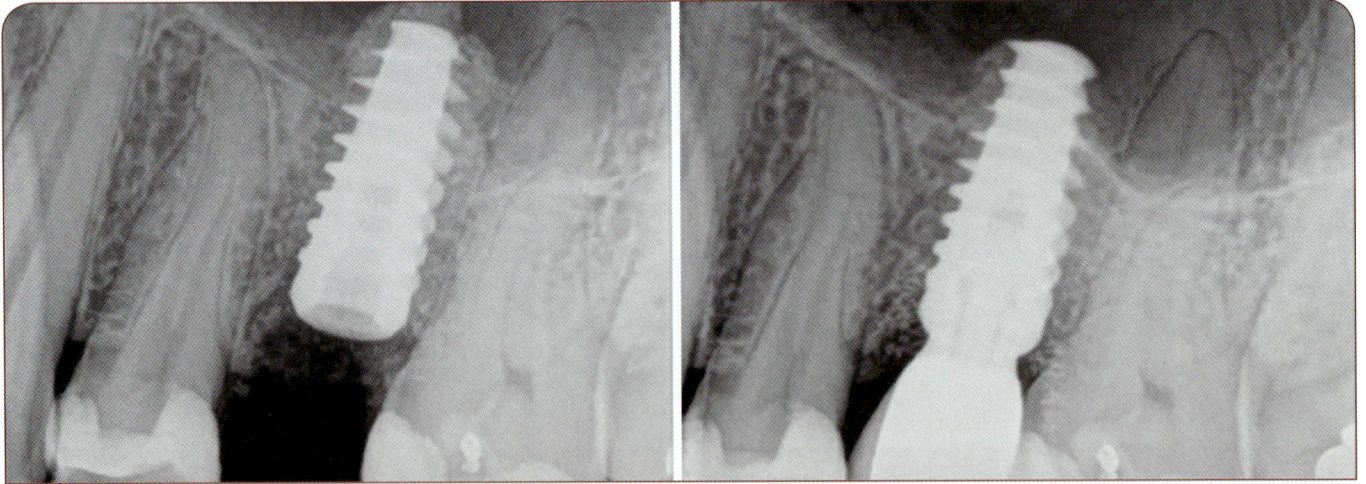

Fig. 17

After ISL and implant placement. Post prosthetic phase **(Fig. 17)**.

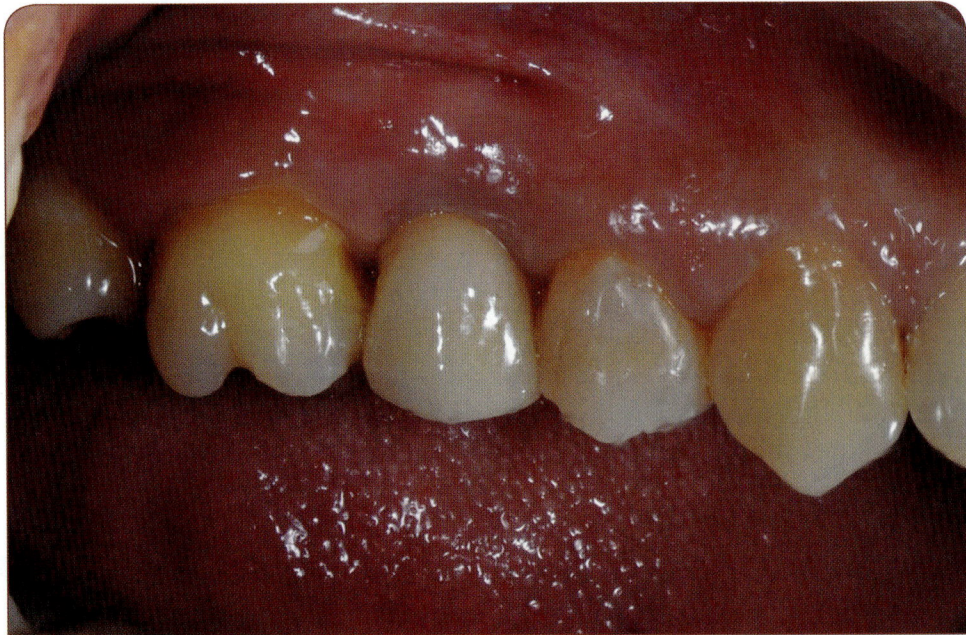

Fig. 18

Three months recall. Papillary fill in embrasures can be noticed **(Fig. 18)**.

SECTION 4

Management of Posterior Mandible

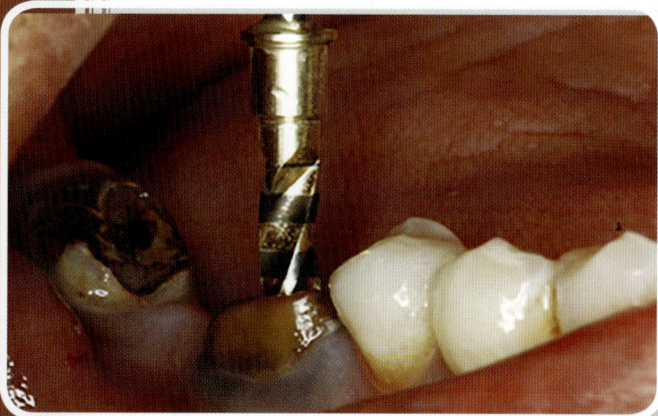

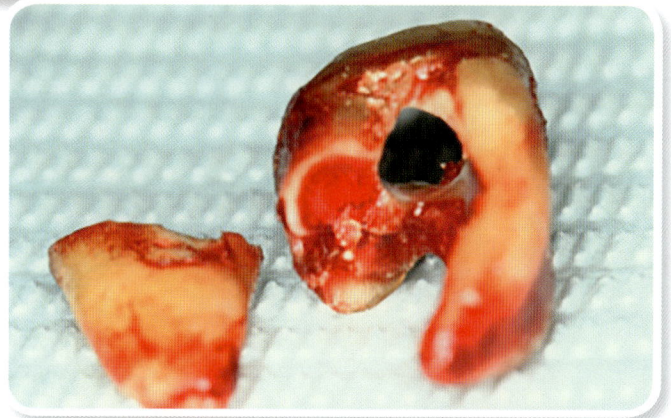

CASE STUDY 56

Lanka Mahesh

RESIDUAL ROOTS AS AN ANATOMIC GUIDE FOR IMMEDIATE IMPLANT PLACEMENT IN MANDIBULAR MOLARS

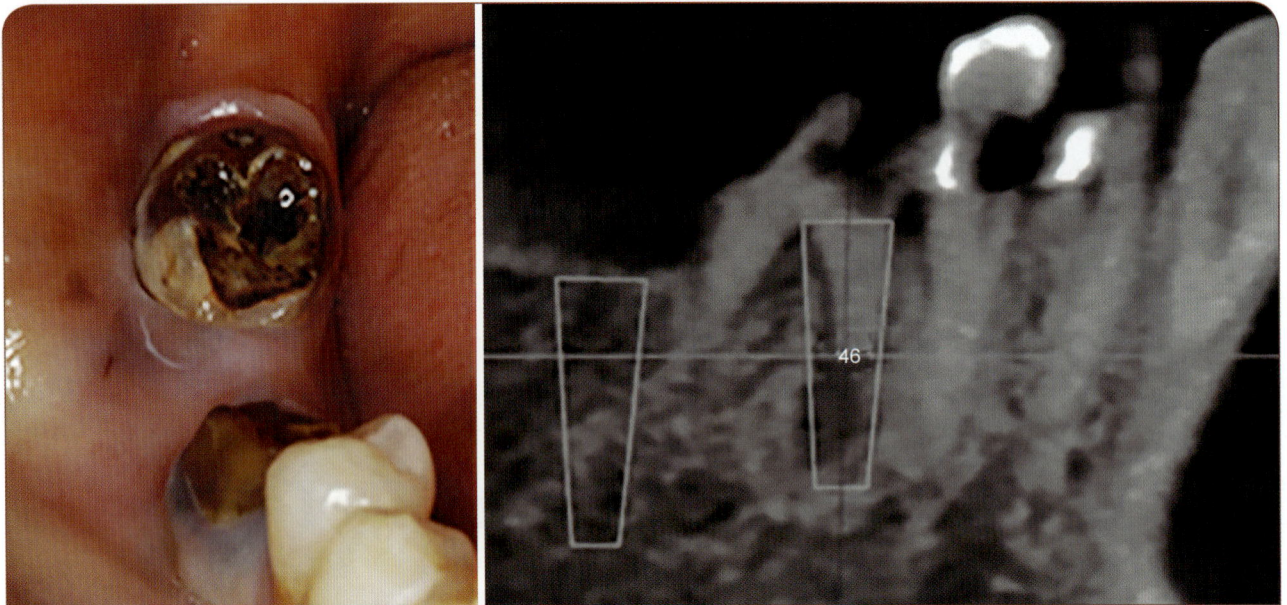

Fig. 1

A 50-year-old female patient with no relevant history.

Clinical view shows a non-restorable mandibular tooth #46, and a grossly carious #48.

The CBCT cross section shows enough bone apically to 46, and a carious 45.

Treatment plan included implant placement in 46, 47, extraction of 48 and endodontic treatment of 45.

The 46 roots were planned as an anatomic guide for implant placement for correct 3-D dimensional orientation **(Fig. 1)**.

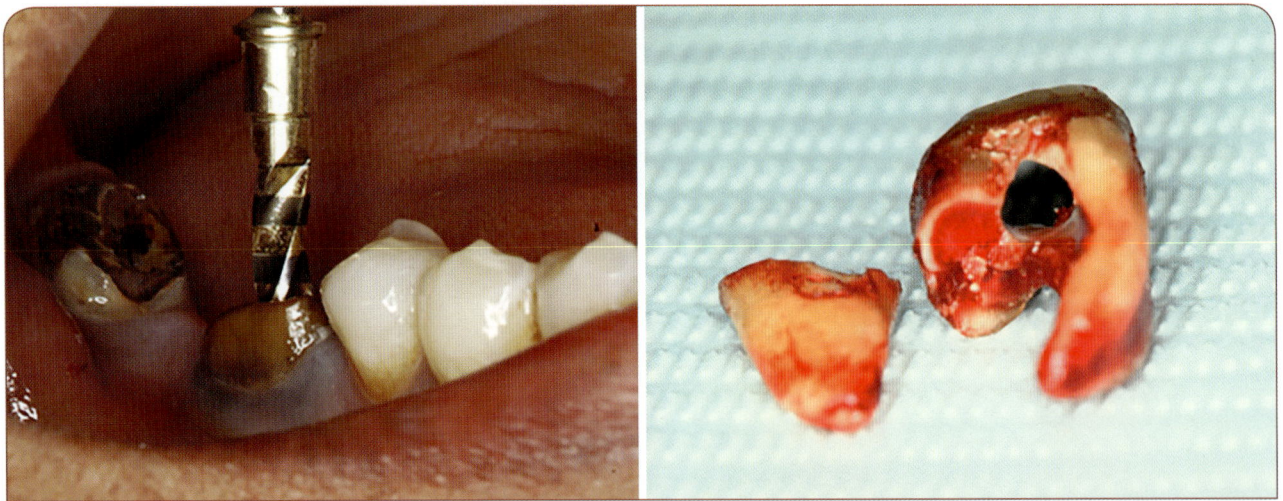

Fig. 2

Ostetomy preparation through the roots till the final drill.

The tooth is extracted at this stage.

The central location of the drills is clearly evident (the main advantage of this technique is to prevent the implant drills from slipping into the mesial or distal socket if the tooth is extracted prior and also for correct central axis fixture placement) **(Fig. 2)**.

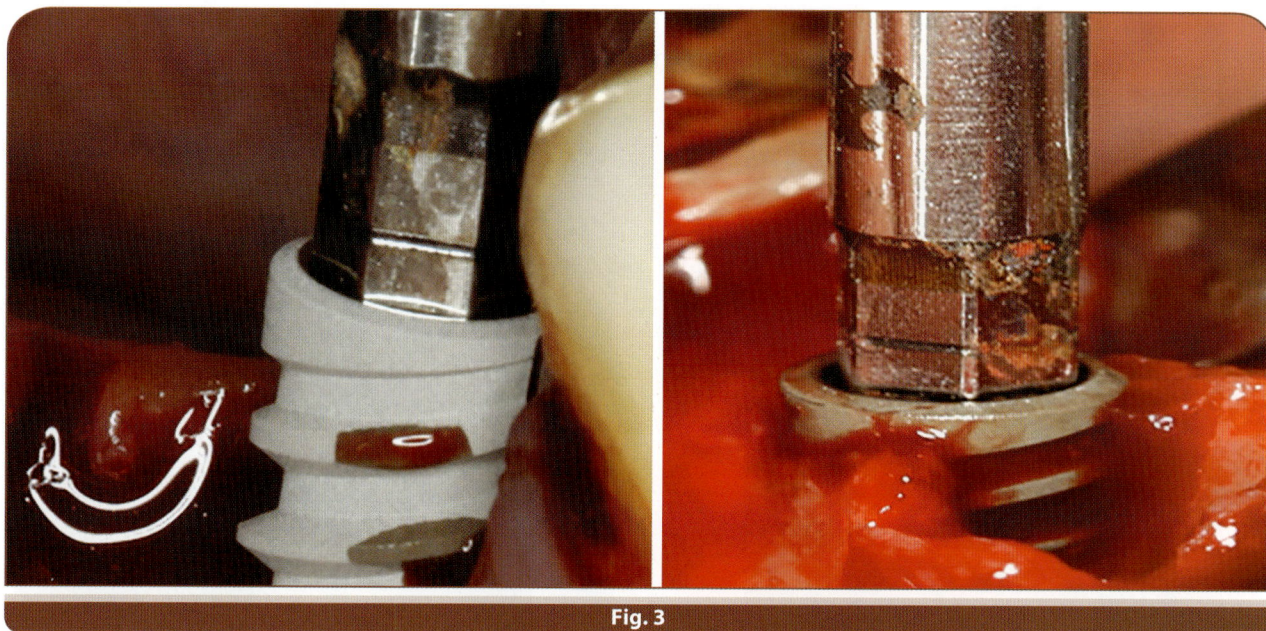

Fig. 3

2 Top DM (Bioner) implants of 4/11.5 mm are placed in the sites of 46 and 47. The 47 implant is placed in a conventional manner. Tooth number 48 is extracted in the same operative appointment **(Fig. 3)**.

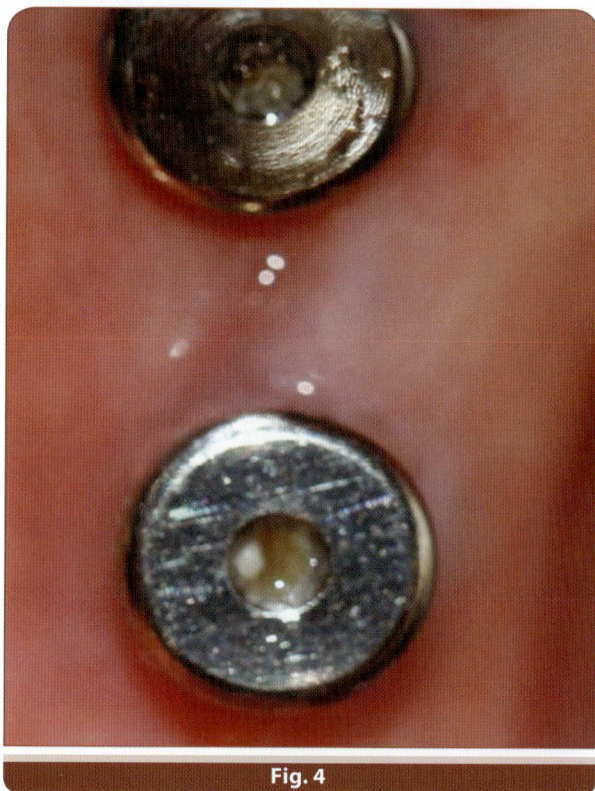

Fig. 4

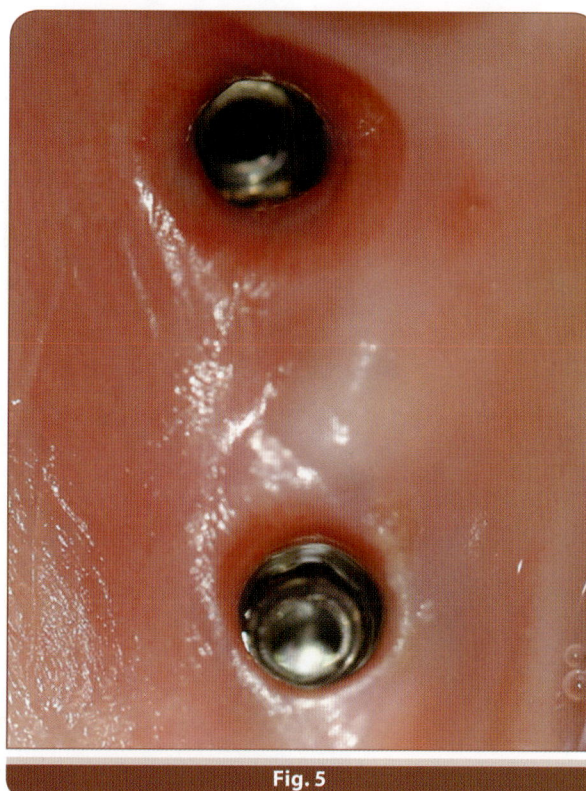

Fig. 5

Healing collars are placed at 3 months healing. Food debris tend to accumulate in the well of the collars and this picture is used most often to show the patient the importance of oral hygiene maintenance **(Fig. 4)**.

The healthy and thick peri implant tissue around the implants is clearly visible **(Fig. 5)**.

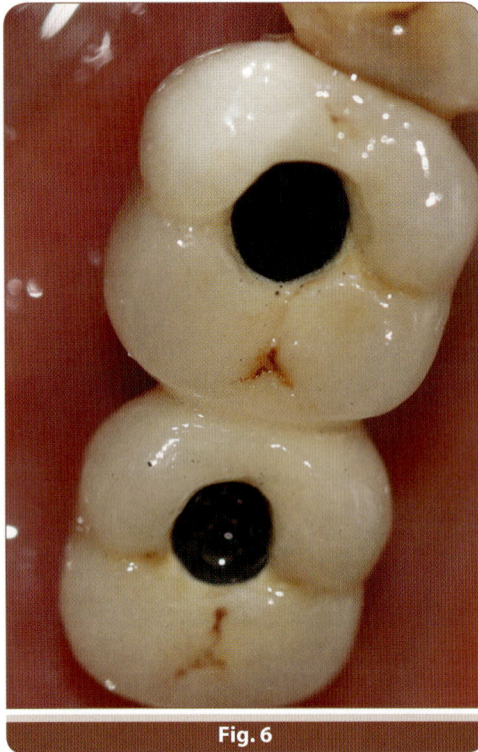

Fig. 6

The final splinted screw retained prosthesis **(Fig. 6)**.

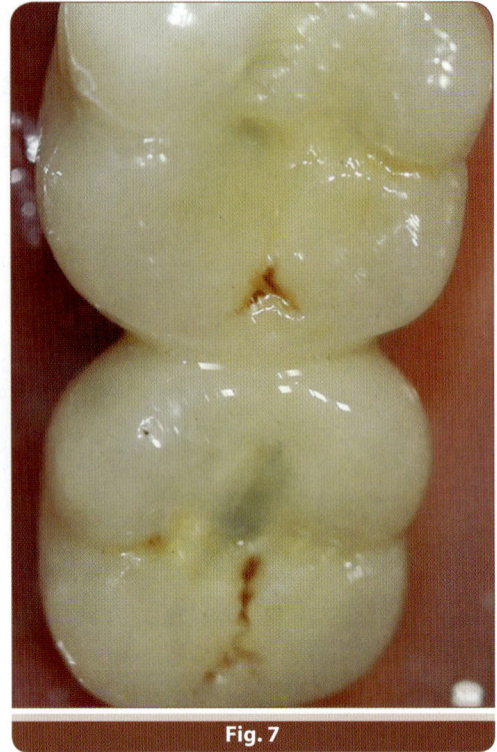

Fig. 7

After final torquing of the abutments the access holes are sealed with flowable light cure composite material (Filtek Flow, 3M) **(Fig. 7)**.

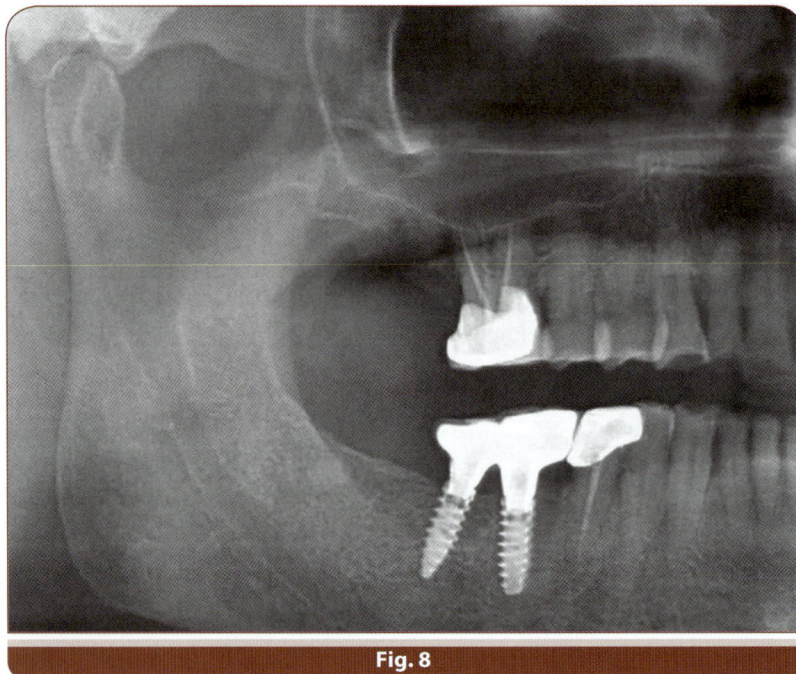

Fig. 8

Two years postoperative panorex shows extremely stable bone level maintenance. The endodontic therapy on 45 is also evident **(Fig. 8)**.

Lanka Mahesh, Nitika Poonia

RIDGE EXPANSION GBR AND IMMEDIATE IMPLANT PLACEMENT FOR MANDIBULAR MOLAR REPLACEMENT

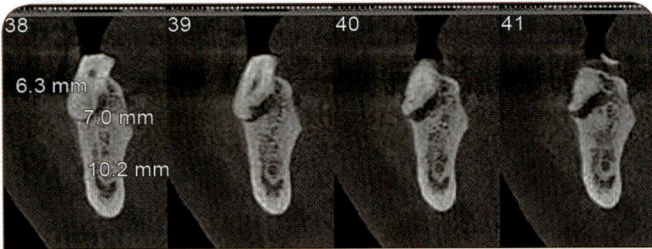

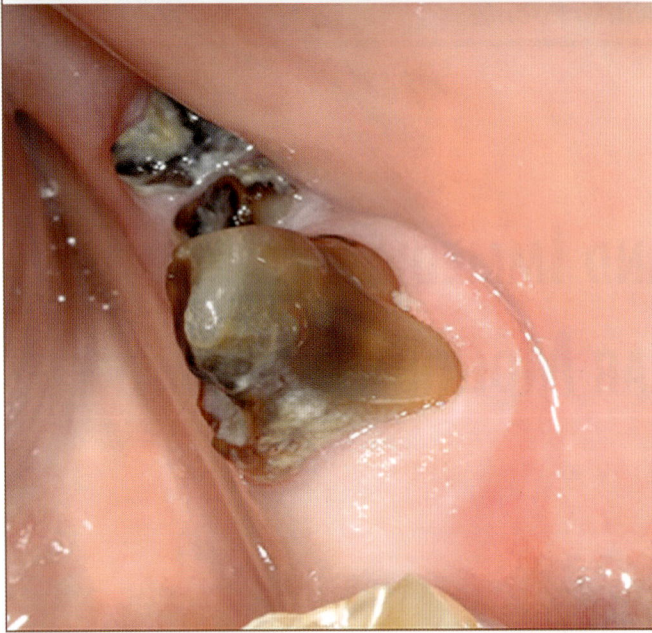

Fig. 1

Fig. 2

A large defect is clearly visible after extraction of tooth #37 (**Fig. 2**).

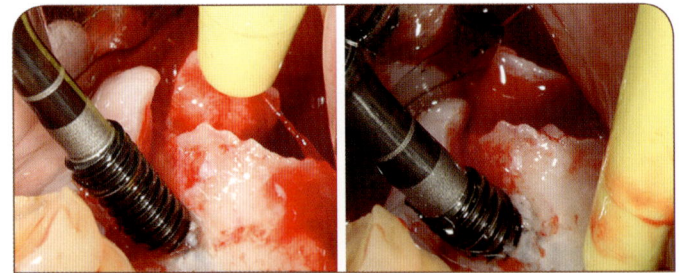

Preoperative scan and intraoral view of a 60-year-old male patient.

The defect in relation to tooth #37 is evident on the scan and narrow buccolingual with is evident in relation to tooth #36 clinically.

Treatment plan included ridge expansion in tooth 36.

Immediate implant in relation to tooth 37 as sufficient height was available GBR with DBBM (**Fig. 1**).

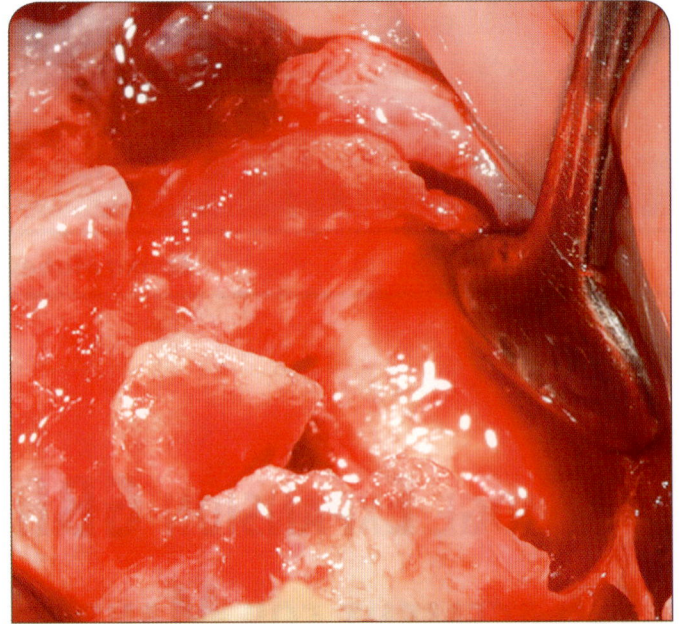

Fig. 3

The ridge is gently expanded with serial increase of the rotary expanders at 100 rpm speed.

The defect on 37 is clearly visible too (**Fig. 3**).

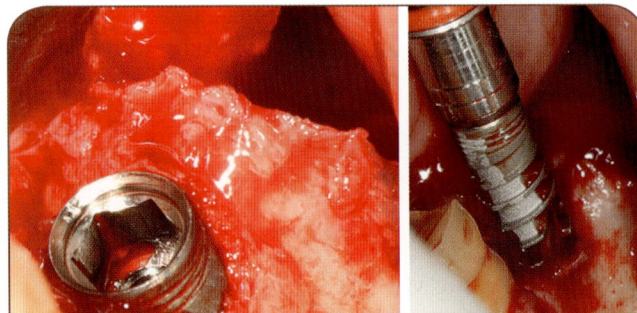

Fig. 4

A 3.75/11.5 implant is threaded into the osteotomy in relation to 36.

The coronal threads are exposed upto 2 mm (**Fig. 4**).

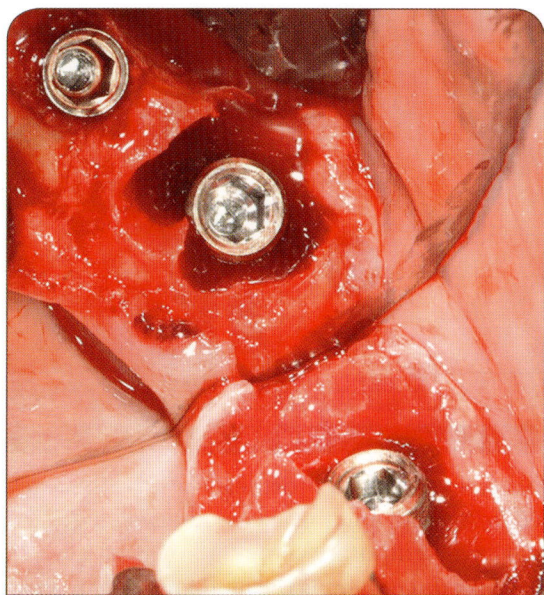

Fig. 5

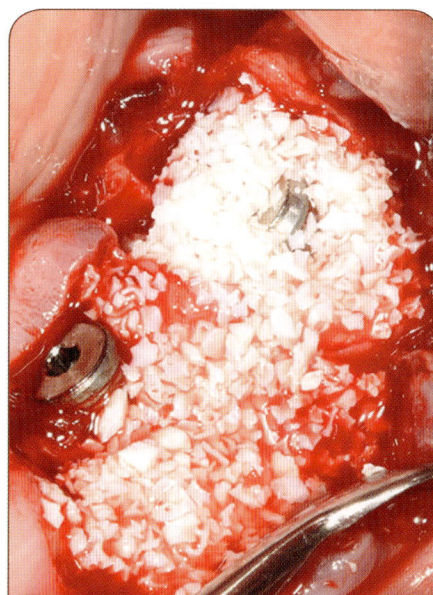

Fig. 6

A 4.2/11.5 implant, AB Dent. Is inserted into the interseptal area of the molar.

High insertion torque values are mandatory in such cases. The large circumferential defect around the implant is clearly seen **(Fig. 5)**.

Bio-Oss particles are packed all around the socket and densely packed.

It is always beneficial to over pack GBR cases to compensate graft shrinkage **(Fig. 6)**.

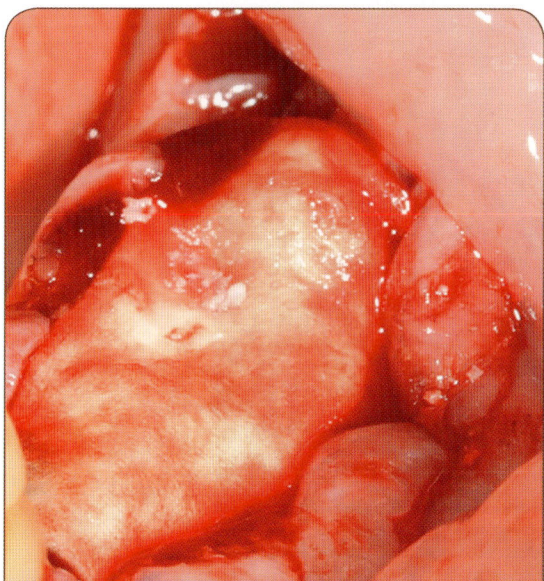

Fig. 7

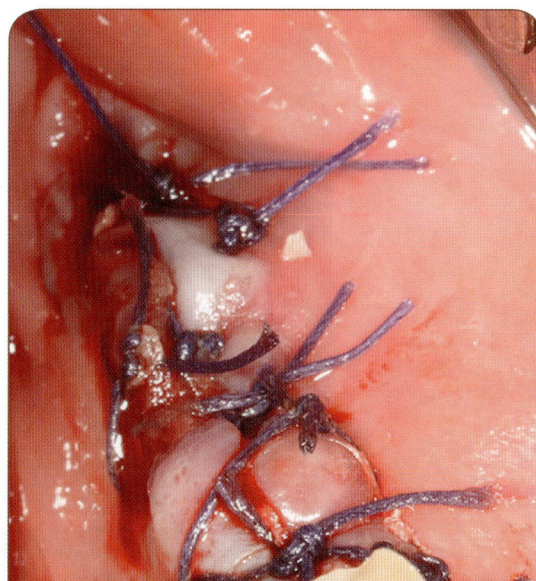

Fig. 8

The area is covered with a large size membrane RCM (ACE Surgical).

The membrane should be tacked well below the lingual/palatal flaps to ensure good wound closure **(Fig. 7)**.

After adequate periosteal release.

The flap is closed with 3-0 vicryl sutures.

Sutures (resorbable or non resorbable) should not be removed for at least 14 days to prevent premature suture line opening **(Fig. 8)**.

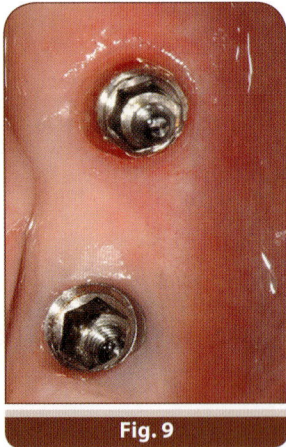

Fig. 9

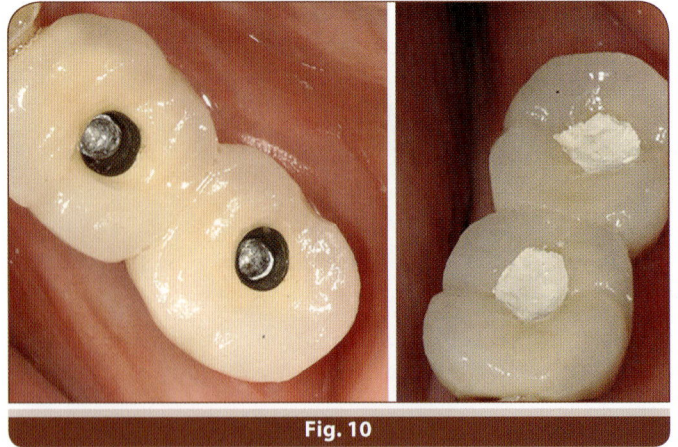

Fig. 10

The healed site at 4 months with robust tissue **(Fig. 9)**.

The final screw retained prosthesis in situ. The screws are torqued to 30 N cm and the access holes sealed with teflon tape and cavit temporary cement (3M).

After 2 weeks the patient is recalled for a check up and the temporary cement is changed to a flowable composite **(Fig. 10)**.

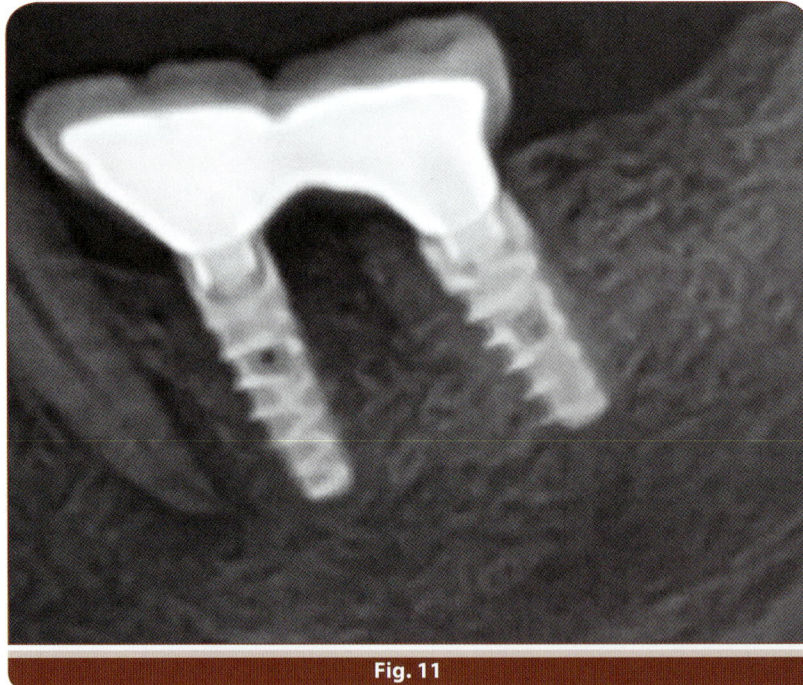

Fig. 11

Recall radiograph at 22 months. Showing excellent crestal bone maintenance and graft consolidation around tooth 37 **(Fig. 11)**.

Lanka Mahesh

SOCKET GRAFTING WITH LARGE PARTICLE DBBM AND DELAYED IMPLANT PLACEMENT

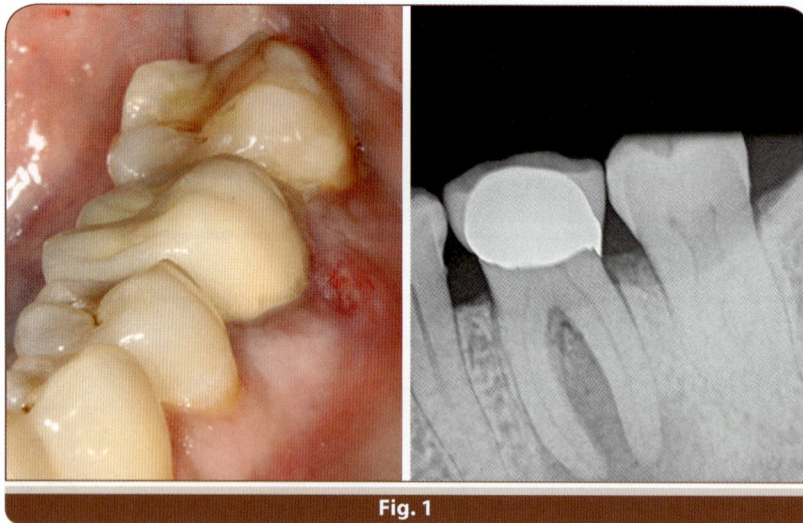

Fig. 1

A 65-year-old female patient with chief complaint of constant pain in lower left tooth crowned 4 years ago. Clinically pus exudate on palpation with tenderness and Grade 2 mobility.

IOPA X-ray reveals a large periapical pathology. Treatment plan for the case was extraction of involved tooth socket bone graft with delayed implant placement **(Fig. 1)**.

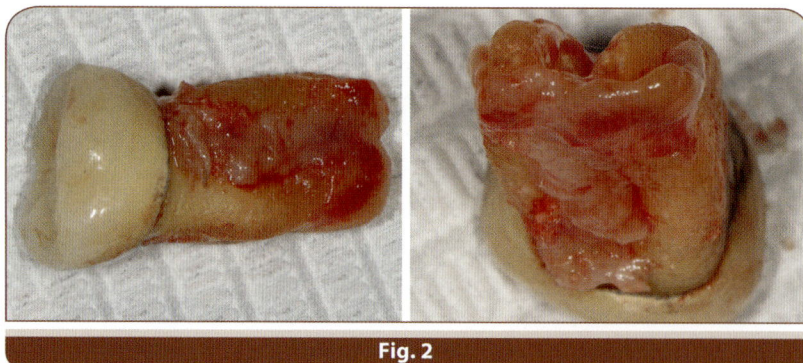

Fig. 2

Following extraction a large granuloma is clearly evident **(Fig. 2)**.

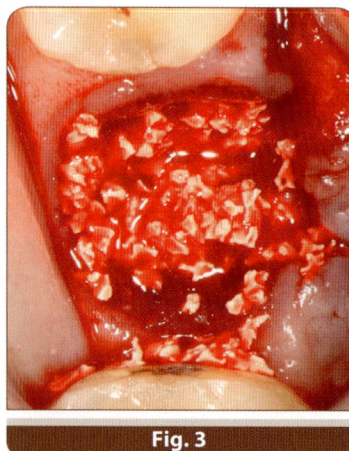

Fig. 3

Following thorough curettage and saline irrigation the socket is grafted with a 1–2 mm particle size Botis bone graft **(Fig. 3)**.

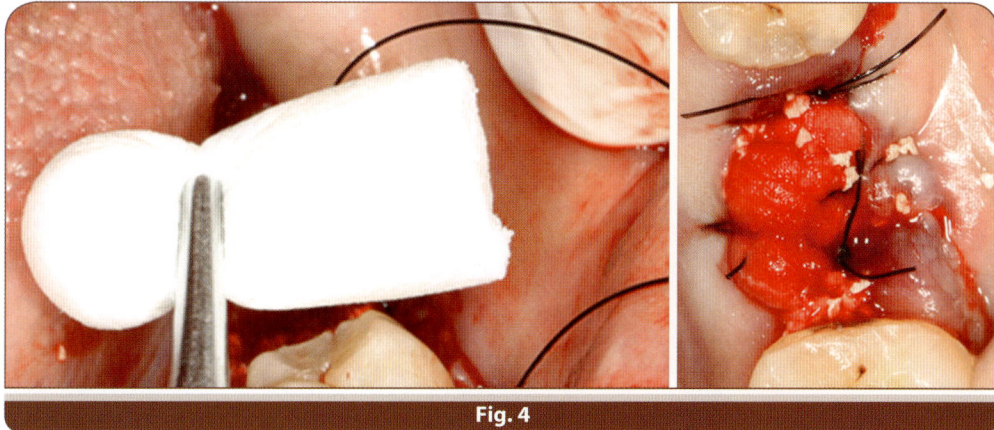

Fig. 4

The socket is sealed with a resorbable collagen plug (rcp – ace) and is stabilized with a horizontal mattress suture and interrupted sutures (3–0 polyamide sutures) **(Fig. 4)**.

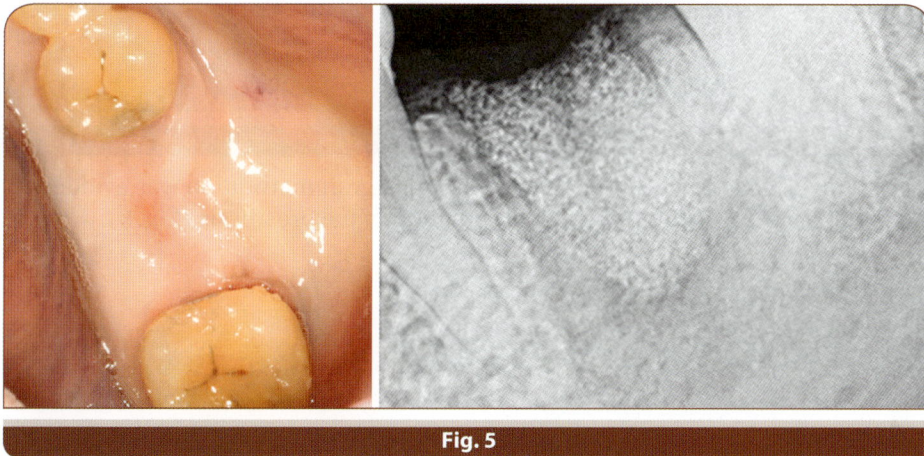

Fig. 5

Four months postoperative clinical and radiographic view demonstrates adequate healing **(Fig. 5)**.

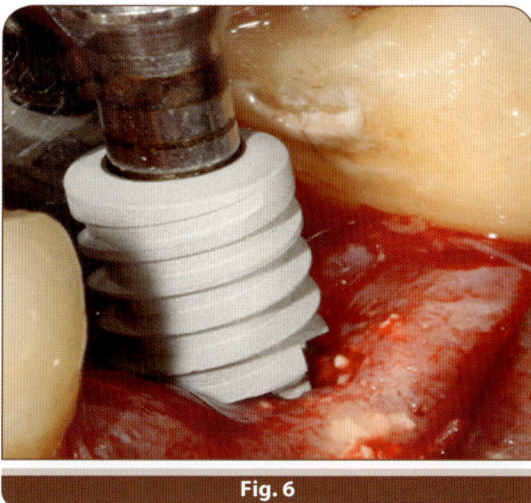

Fig. 6

A 5/10 mm bioner implant is placed at 50 N cm torque **(Fig. 6)**.

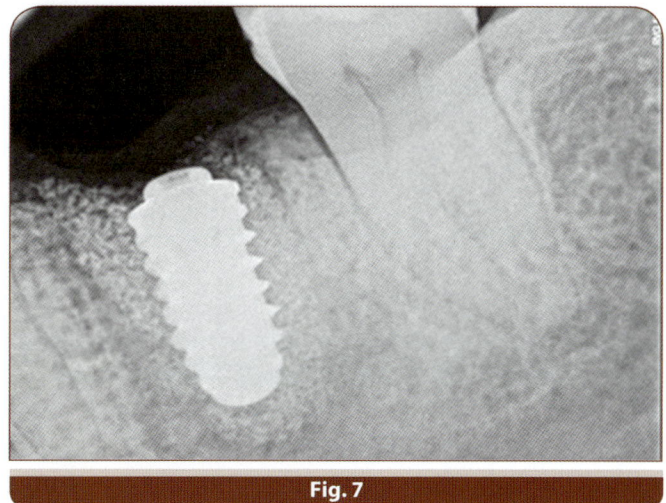

Fig. 7

Postoperative radiograph **(Fig. 7)**.

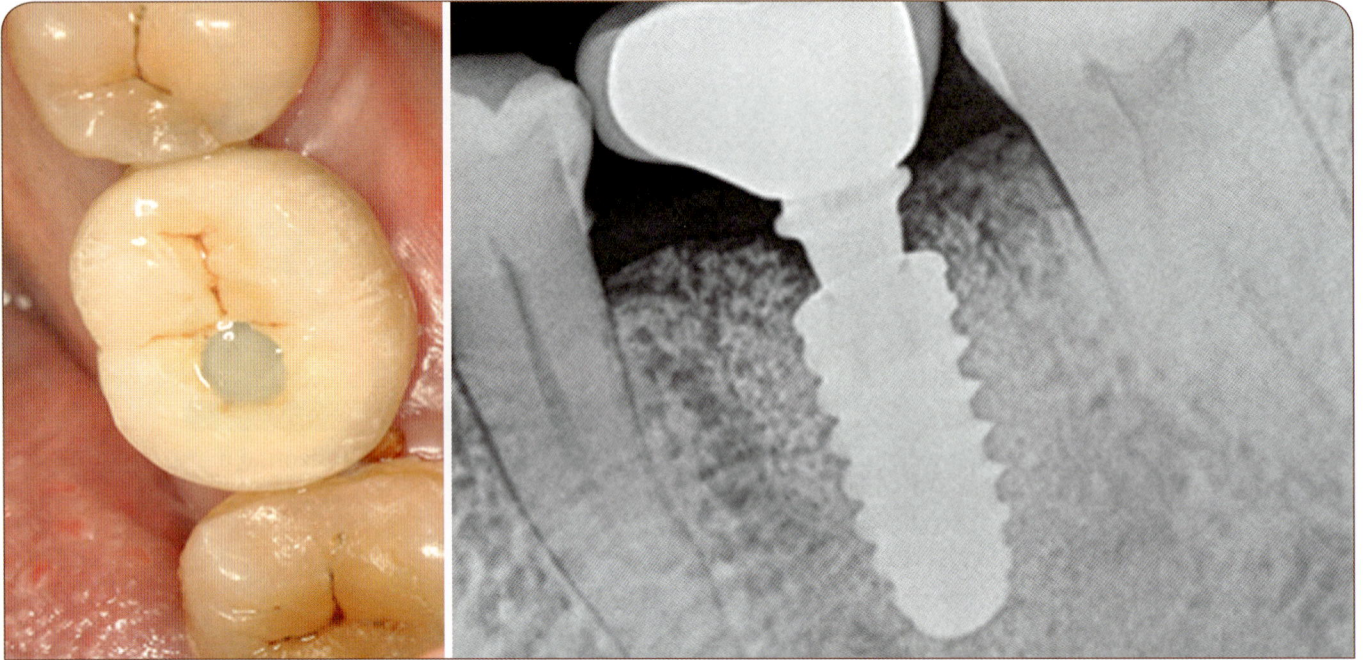

Fig. 8

One year recall. Clinical stability of soft tissue and radiographic bone graft maturation was evident. Acceptable minor remodelling at the crest is visible which is due to occlusal stimulation of the prosthesis **(Fig. 8)**.

CASE STUDY 59

Lanka Mahesh

Socket Grafting and Delayed Implant Placement with Small Particulate DBBM

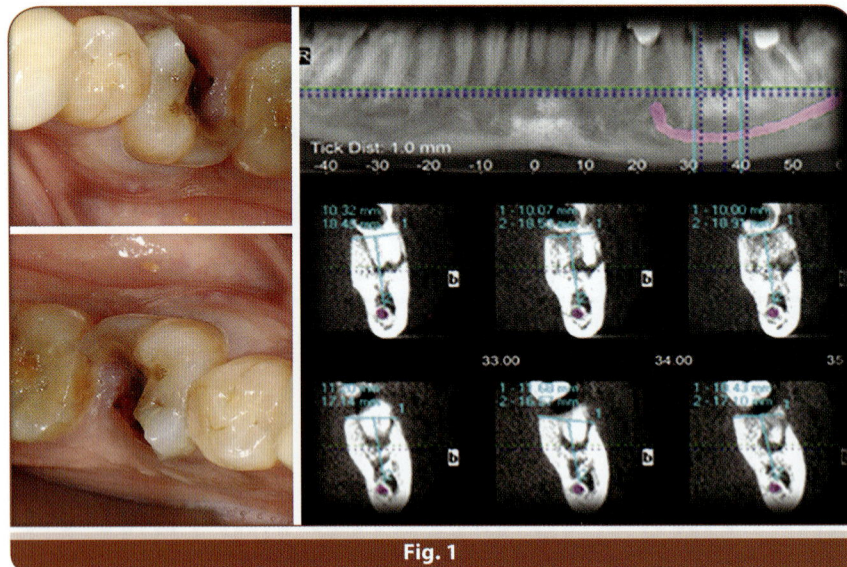

Fig. 1

A 50-year-old female patient with a non-restorable molar was advised a socket bone graft with delayed implant placement as the tooth was very wide and the periapical infection too deffered immediate implant placement **(Fig. 1)**.

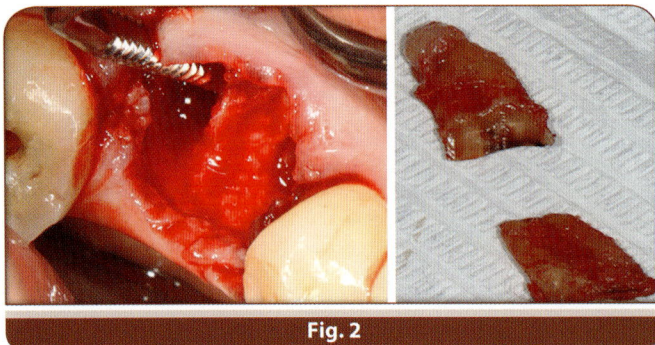

Fig. 2

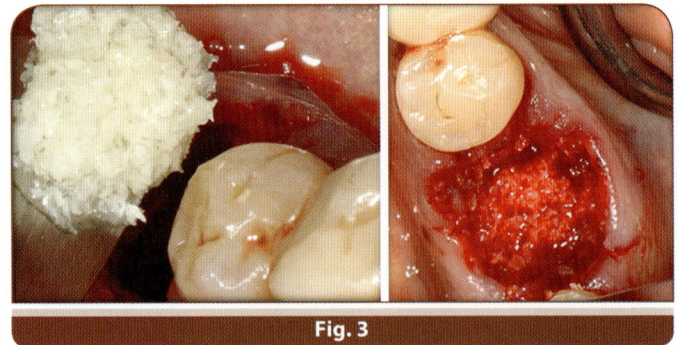

Fig. 3

The tooth was gently extracted the socket curetted thoroughly with a buck file (Hu-Friedy). The sectioned roots **(Fig. 2)**.

The socket was grafted with small bone DBBM (Smartbone). Complete fill of the socket was achieved **(Fig. 3)**.

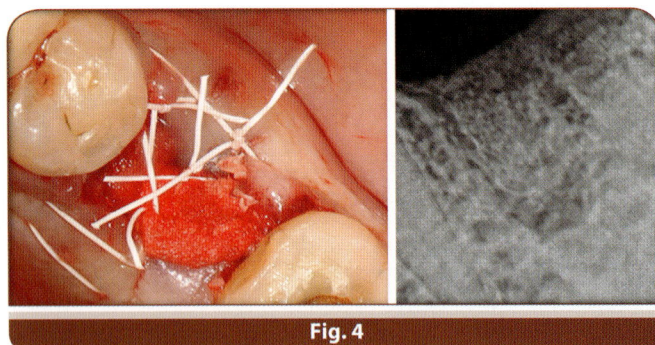

Fig. 4

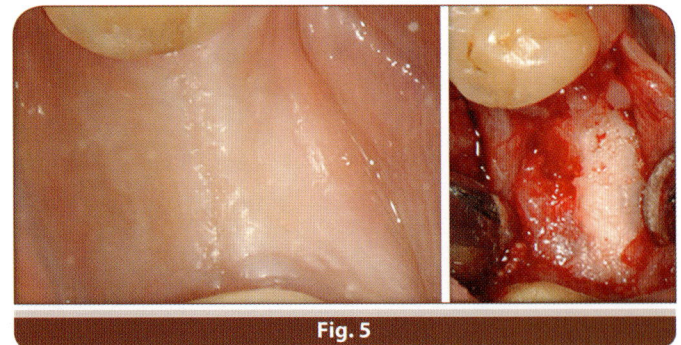

Fig. 5

The wound was closed with 3-0 cytoplast sutures (Ostegenics) and a resorbable collagen plug, RCP a (Ace surgicals) immediate postoperative radograph **(Fig. 4)**.

Five months postoperative clinical view. The site after flap reflection **(Fig. 5)**.

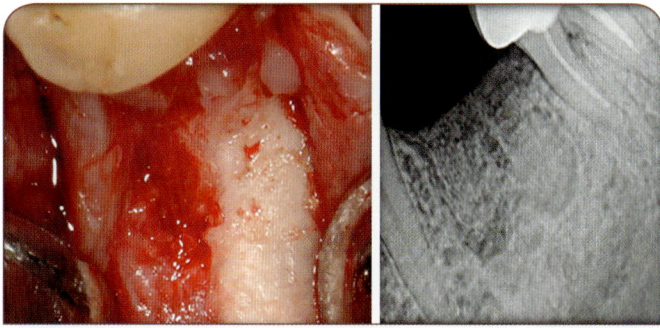

Fig. 6

The grafted site appears to be well vascularized. The X-ray reveals a graft that is integrating well with surrounding host bone **(Fig. 6)**.

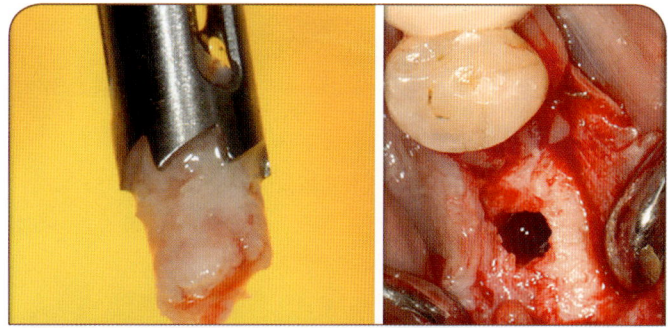

Fig. 7

A trephine of inner diameter 2.8 mm outer diameter 3 mm (Koine) was used to obtain a core for histological examination. The core should be harvested from the center of the site where the implant placement and future restoration is planned **(Fig. 7)**.

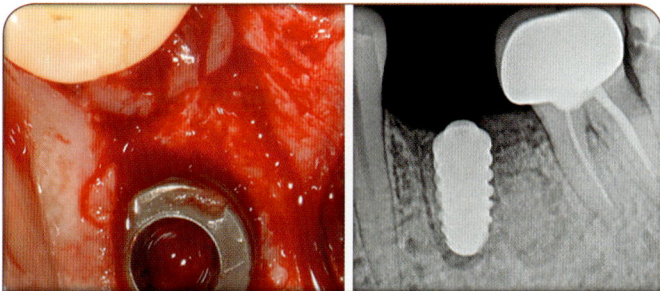

Fig. 8

A 5/11.5 top implant (Bioner) was inserted at 50 N cm. Immediate postoperative X-ray showing the implant in grafted bone **(Fig. 8)**.

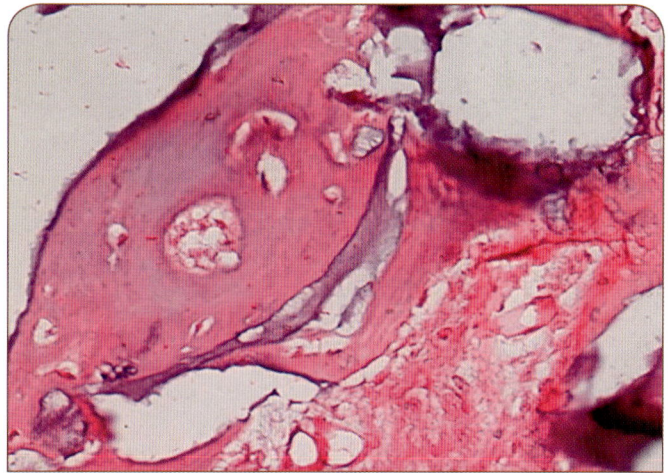

Fig. 9

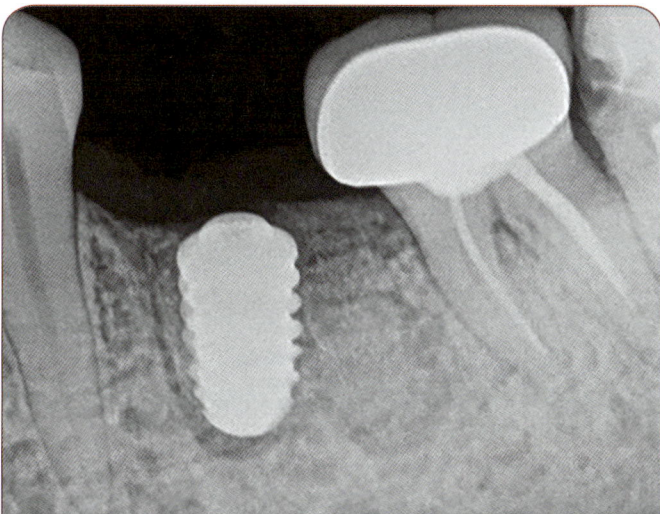

Fig. 10

Four months postoperative IOPA X-ray **(Fig. 10)**.

The biopsied cores were studied histopathologically after decalcifying in mild decalcifying agent and processing it using routine procedures. Four micron thick sections were taken and stained with hematoxylin and eosin stain and observed under the research microscope for histopathological examination.

The histopathological examination revealed areas of graft material progressively resulting in formation of new vital bone. There is coexistence of the graft material and newly formed bone. Growth lines were also seen indicating good osteoconduction. Osteoblasts are seen to be lining the bone along with presence of osteocytes within the bony lacunae indicating viable bone. The bone is seen to be in various stages of osteogenesis and presence mature surrounding connective tissue with good vascularity indicates good osteoconduction **(Fig. 9)**.

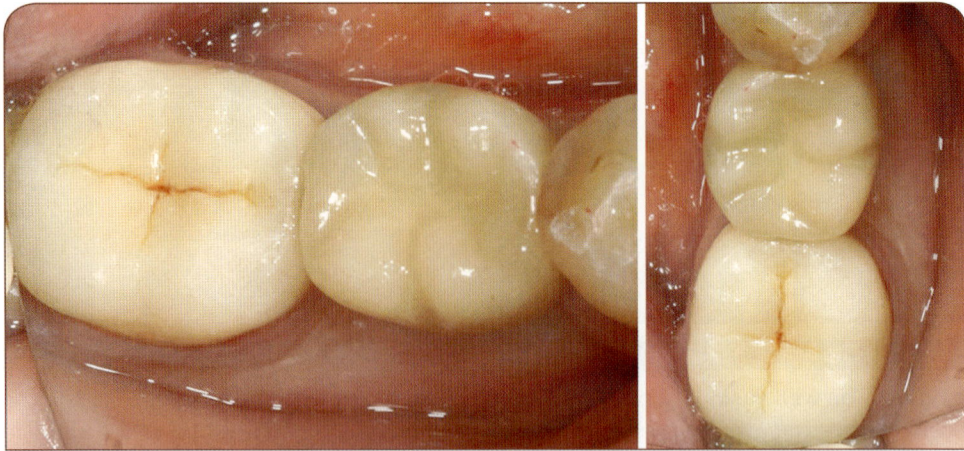

Fig. 11

Final prosthesis given after 4 months osseointegration **(Fig. 11)**.

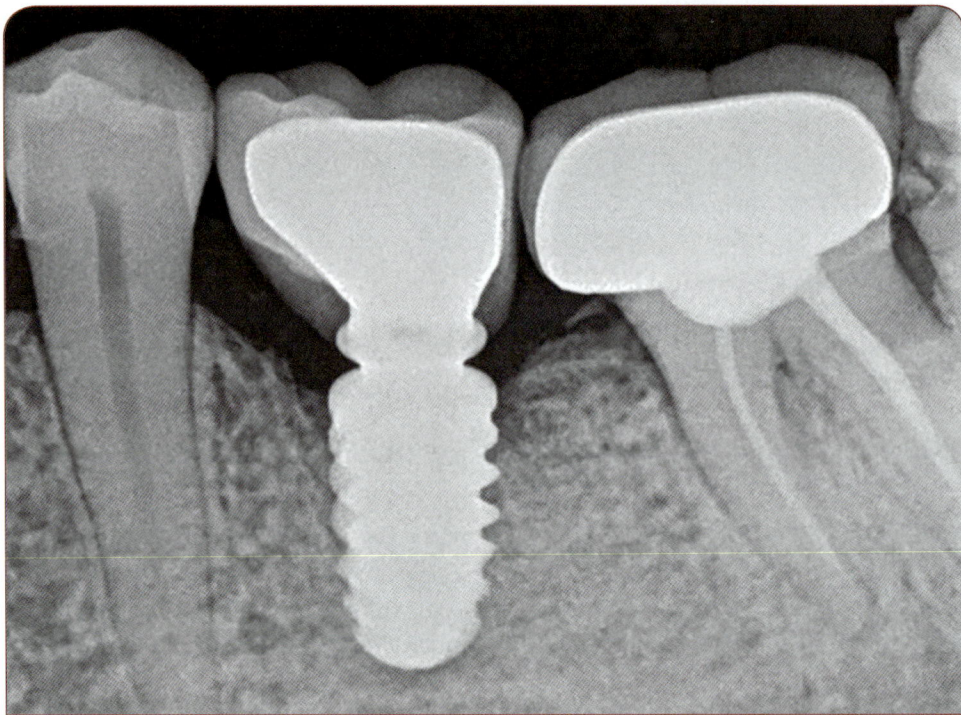

Fig. 12

Recall radiograph at 18 months showing complete maturation of the grafted socket **(Fig. 12)**.

CASE STUDY 60

David Morales Schwarz, Hilde Morales

RIDGE EXPANSION IN A LOWER POSTERIOR REGION WITH THIN RIDGE WIDTH

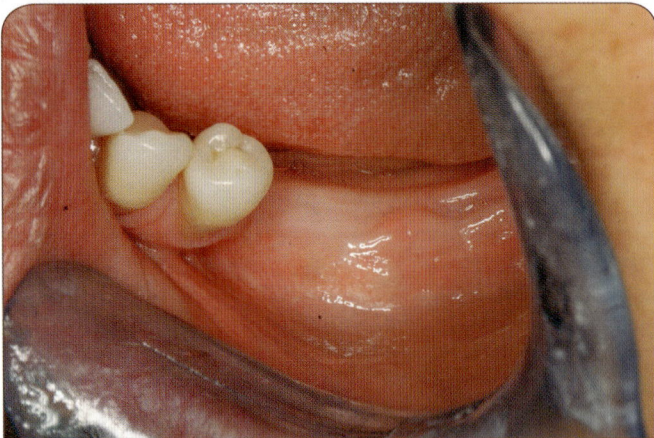

Crestal incision **(Fig. 1)**.

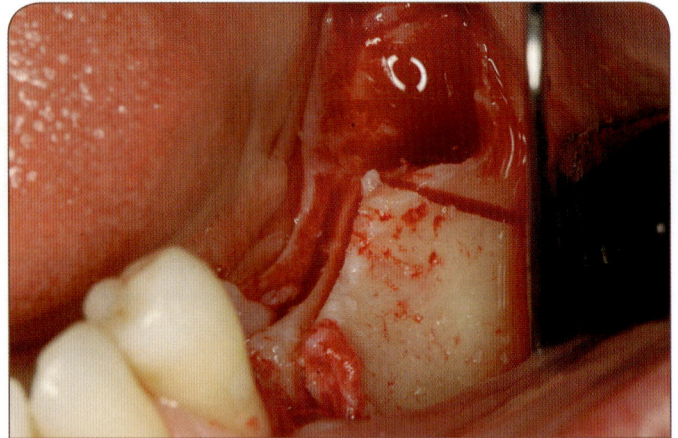

Full width flap was elevated. Piezosurgery osteotomy was made vertical and longitudinal **(Fig. 2)**.

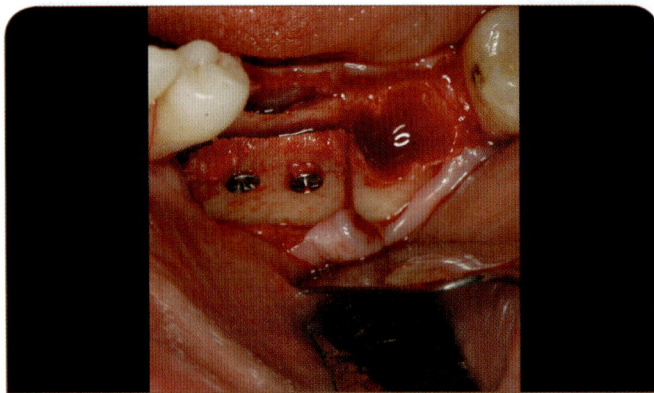

Drilling vestibular wall for dull screws placing dull screws **(Fig. 3)**.

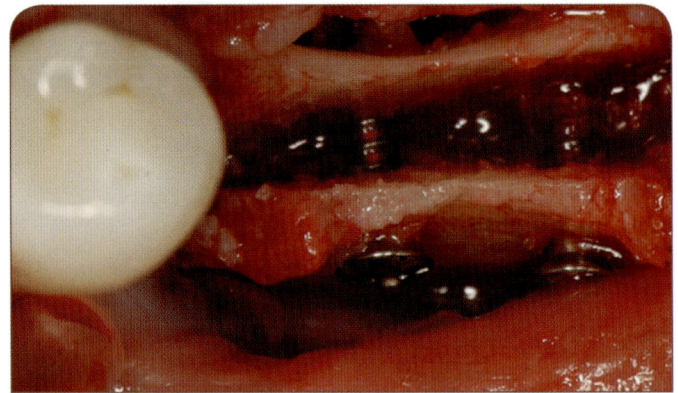

Controlled ridge augmentation **(Fig. 4)**.

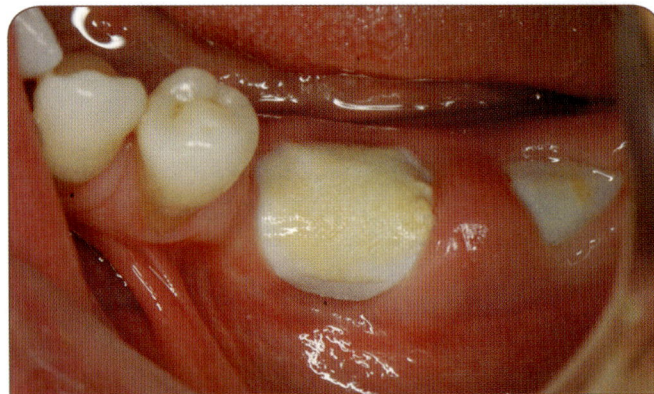

Membrane was placed **(Fig. 5)**.

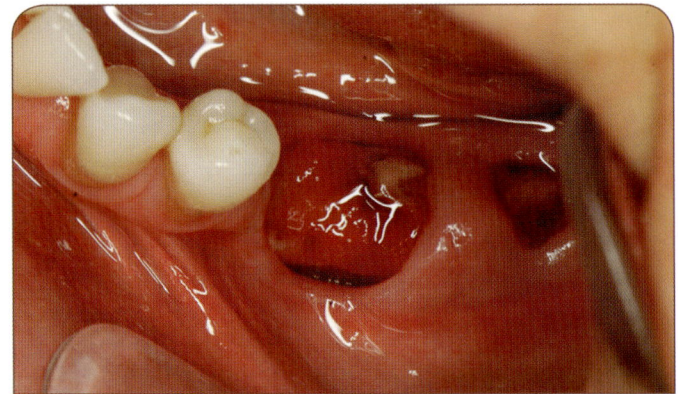

After three weeks membrane was removed **(Fig. 6)**.

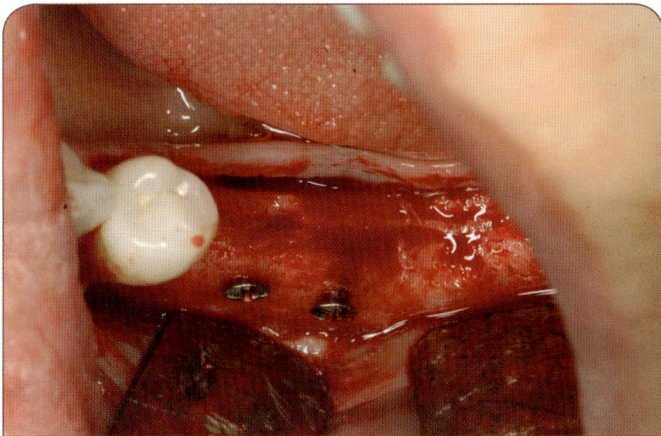
Fig. 7

Second surgery three months later **(Fig. 7)**.

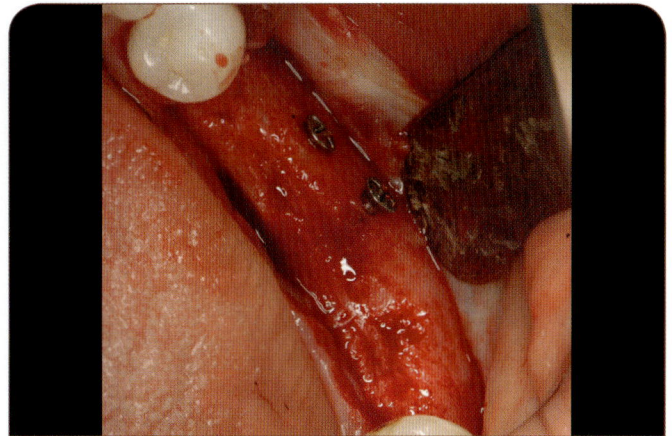
Fig. 8

Second surgery **(Fig. 8)**.

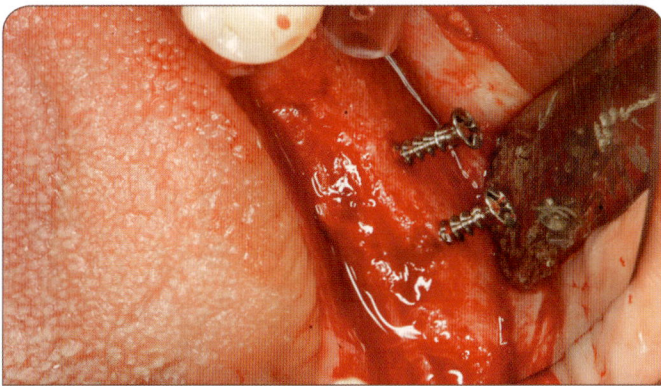
Fig. 9

Remove the screws **(Fig. 9)**.

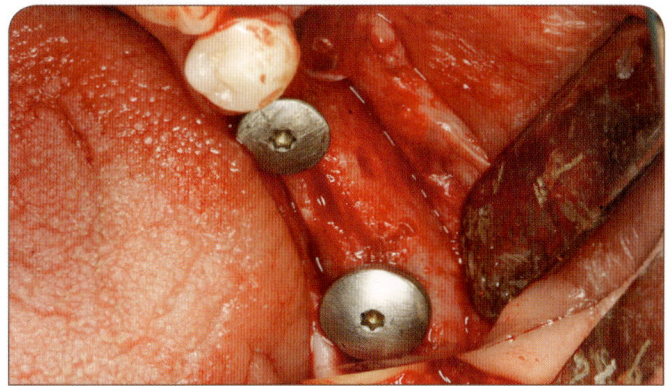
Fig. 10

Straumann implants were placed **(Fig. 10)**.

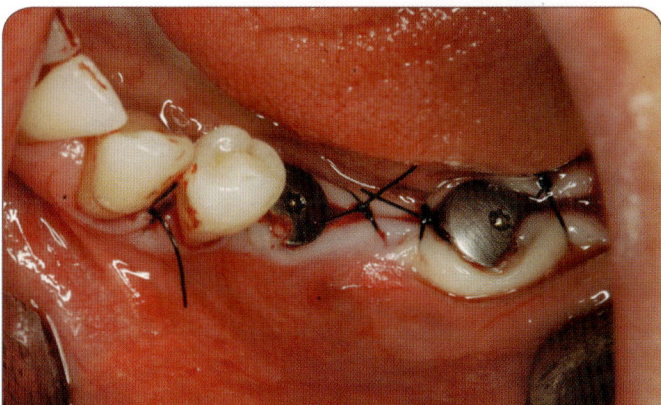
Fig. 11

Suture **(Fig. 11)**.

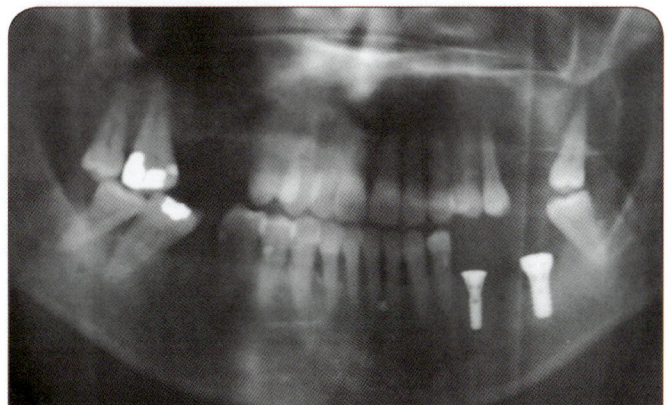
Fig. 12

Immediate postoperative orthopantomogram showing perfectly placed implants (Fig. 12).

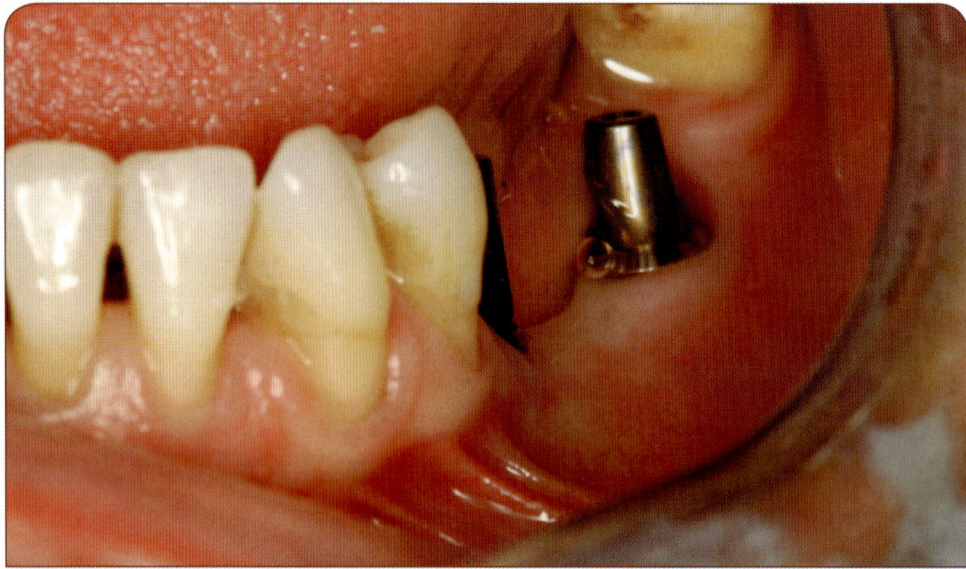

Fig. 13

Good gingival healing around the abutment **(Fig. 13)**.

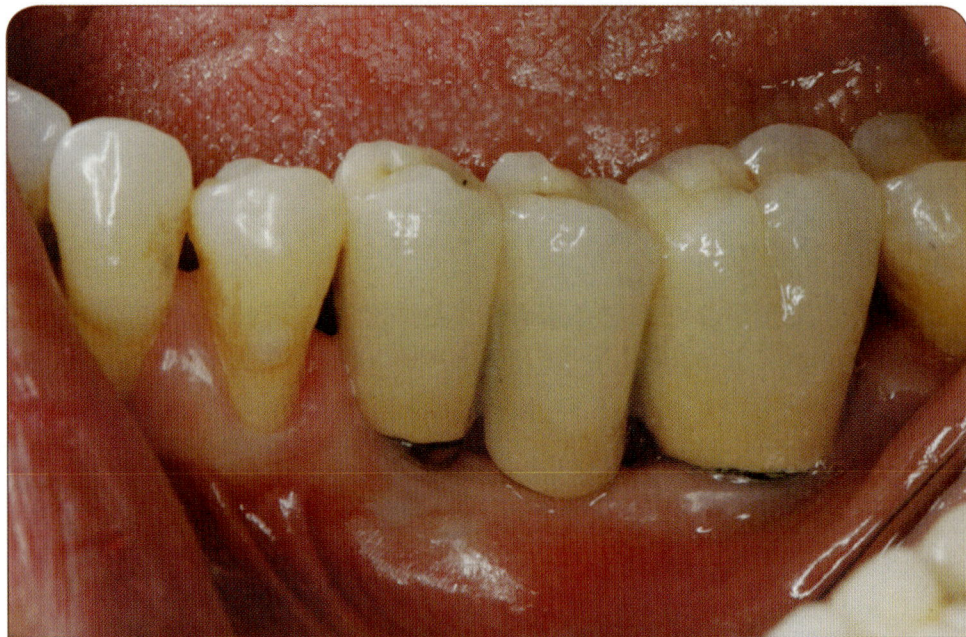

Fig. 14

Definitive restoration **(Fig. 14)**.

CASE STUDY 61

David Morales Schwarz , Hilde Morales

Ridge Split Procedure for Thin Mandibular Posterior Region; GBR done with PRP and Calcium Sulfate

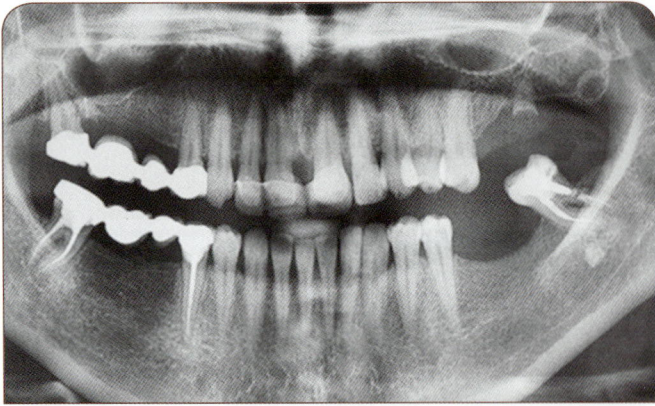

Fig. 1

A 38-year of patient complains of food lodgement with respect to right lower fixed prosthesis. Treatment plan for the case was removal of teeth # 47, 44 and 38 followed by placement of 3 implant in right mandibular side and 1 implant in left mandibular side (**Fig. 1**).

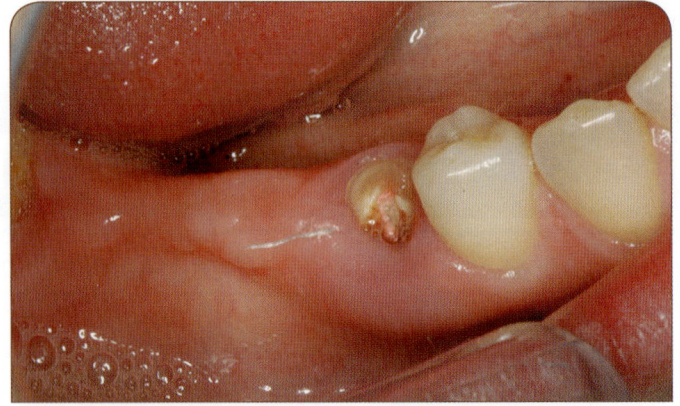

Fig. 2

Clinical view of the ridge (**Fig. 2**).

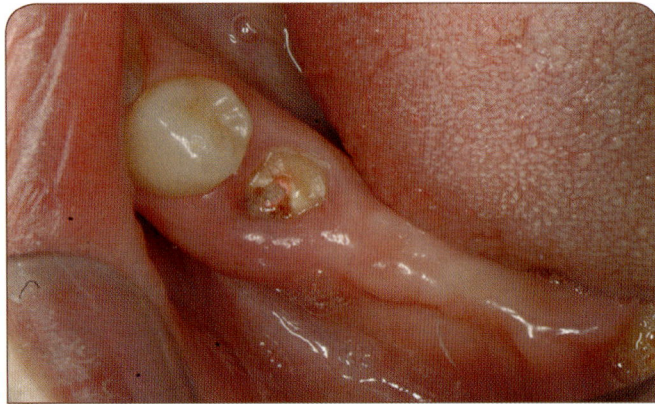

Fig. 3

Occlusal view of the ridge (**Fig. 3**).

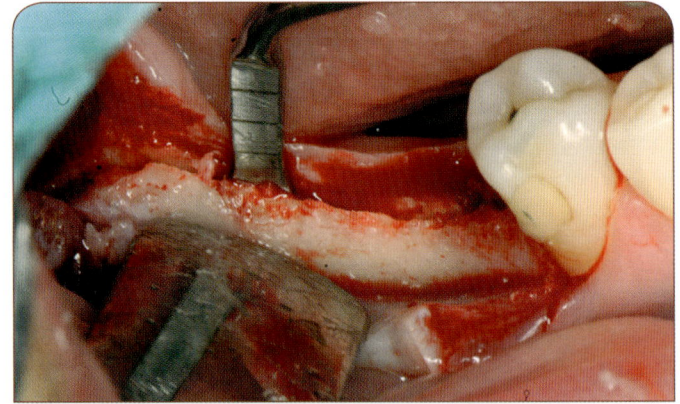

Fig. 4

Piezoelectric was used to perform crestal osteotomy (**Fig. 4**).

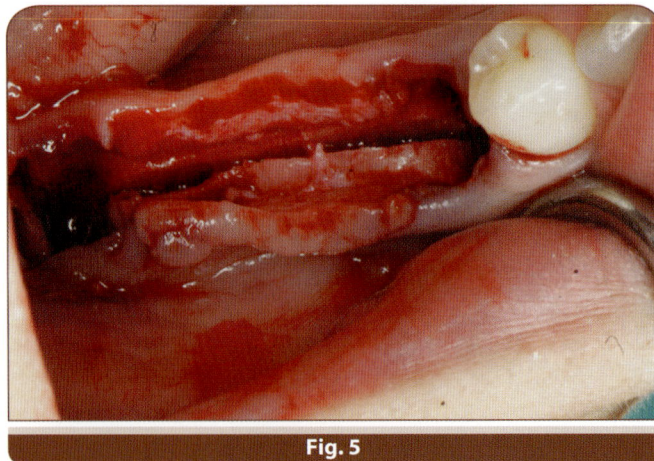

Fig. 5

A horizontal incision was made along the crestal bone (**Fig. 5**).

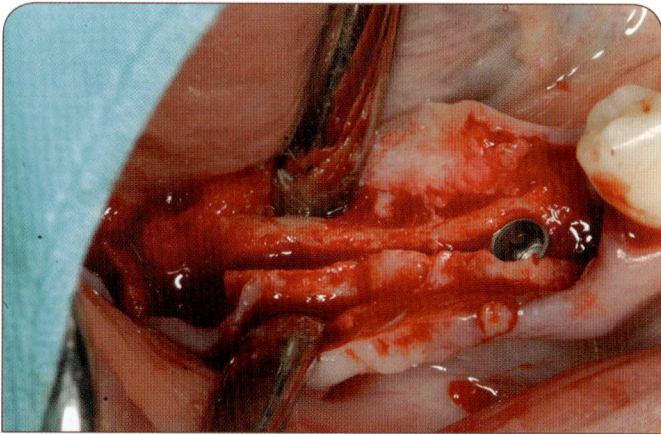

Fig. 6

Occlusal view of the osteotomy (**Fig. 6**).

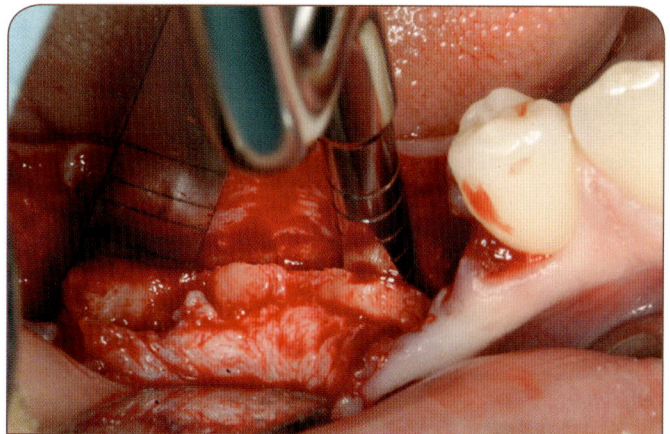

Fig. 7

Initial luxation with osteotomes (**Fig. 7**).

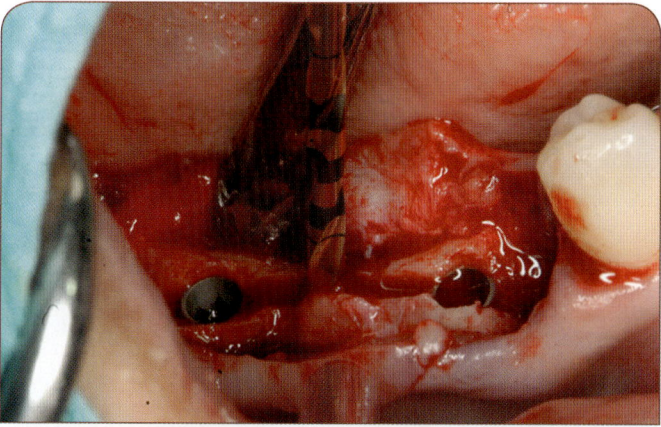

Fig. 8

Implant drilling top DM bioner (**Fig. 8**).

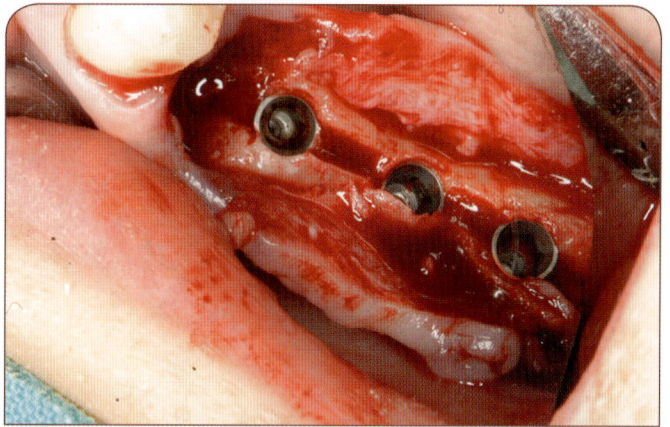

Fig. 9

The 3 top DM implants were placed (**Fig. 9**).

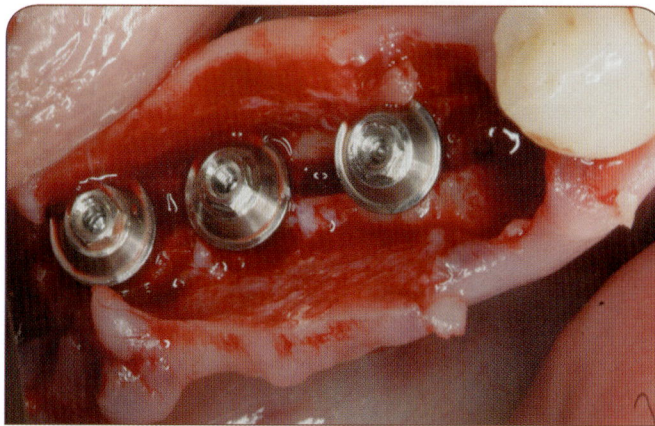

Fig. 10

Implants top DM bioner 3.5 × 13 (**Fig. 10**).

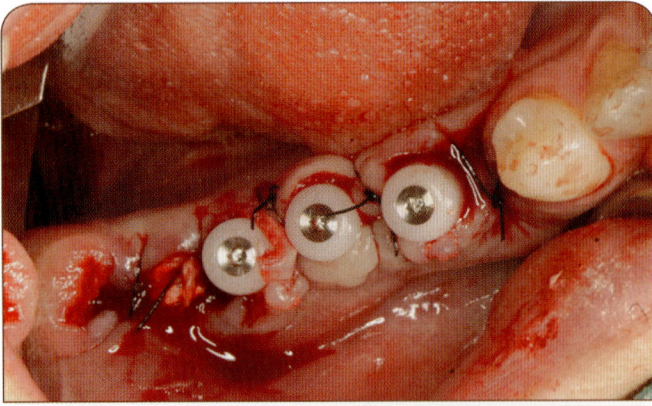

Fig. 11

Implants top DM bioner 3.5 × 13. Filled with platelet rich plasma and calcium sulfate **(Fig. 11)**.

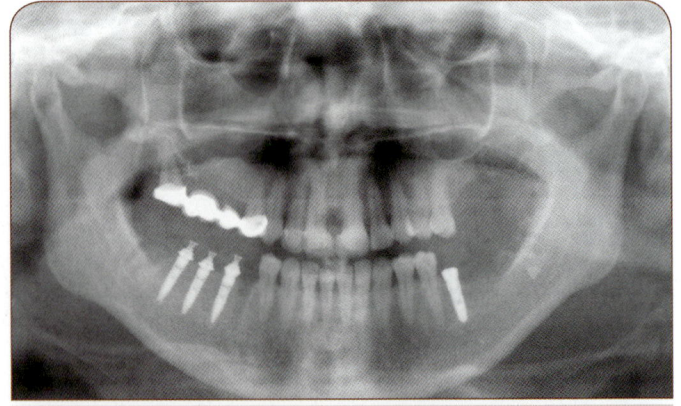

Fig. 12

Immediate postoperative orthopantomogram showing implant placed **(Fig. 12)**.

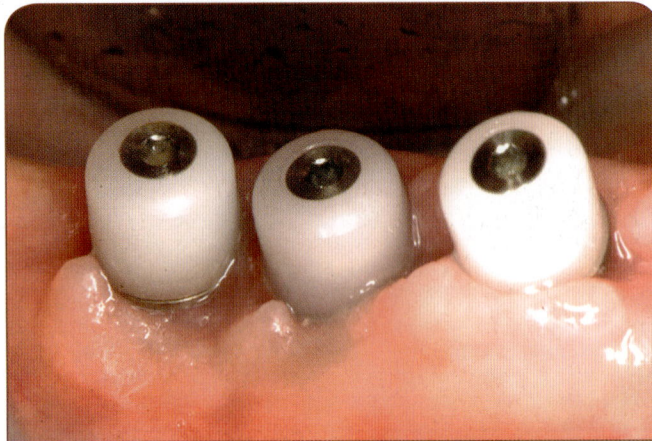

Fig. 13

One month after surgery **(Fig. 13)**.

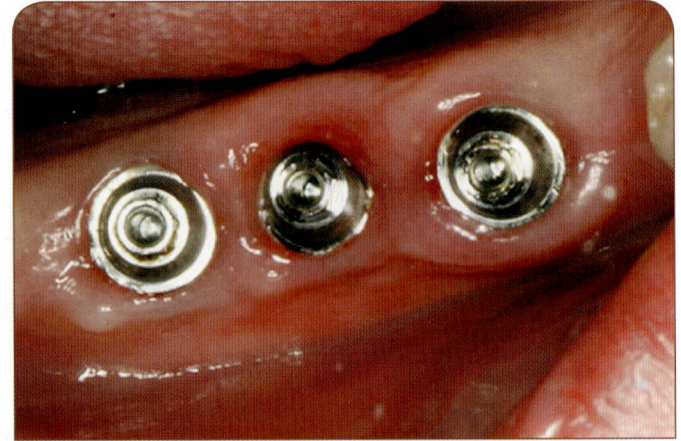

Fig. 14

Two months after surgery **(Fig. 14)**.

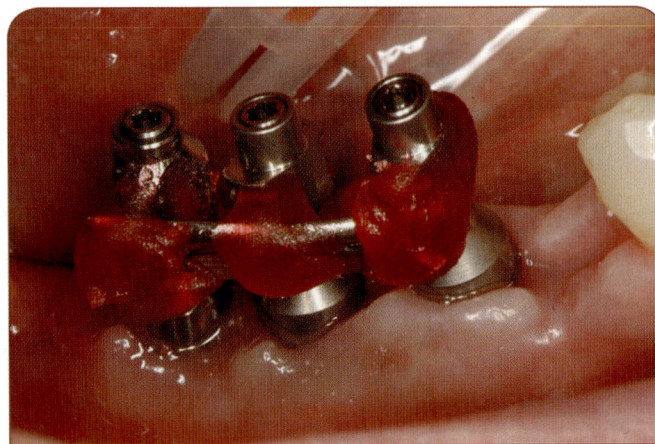

Fig. 15

Measures for definitive crowns **(Fig. 15)**.

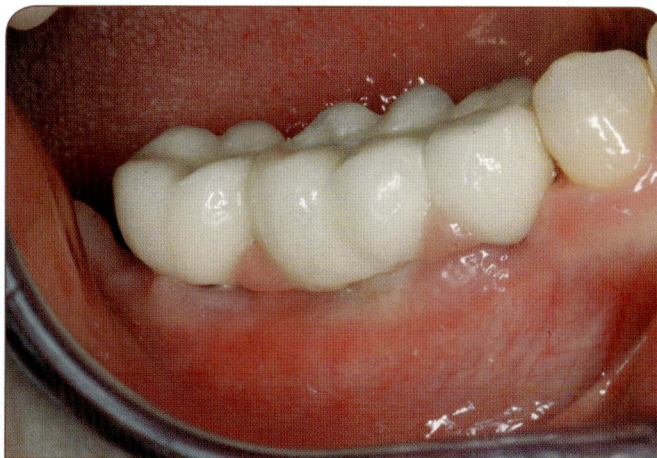

Fig. 16

Final prosthesis cemented **(Fig.16)**.

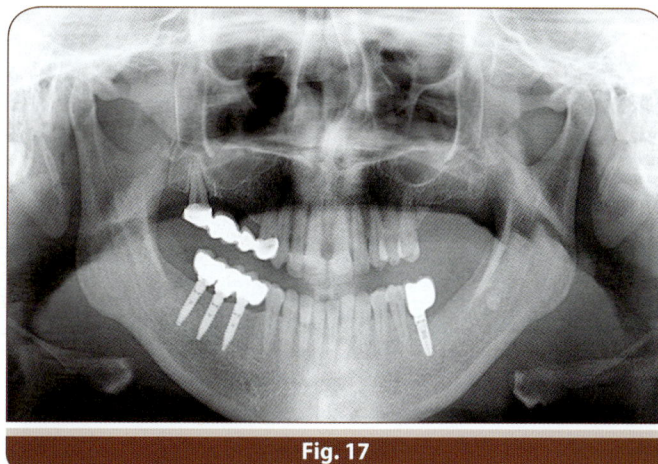

Fig. 17

Postoperative orthopantomogram with final prosthesis **(Fig. 17)**.

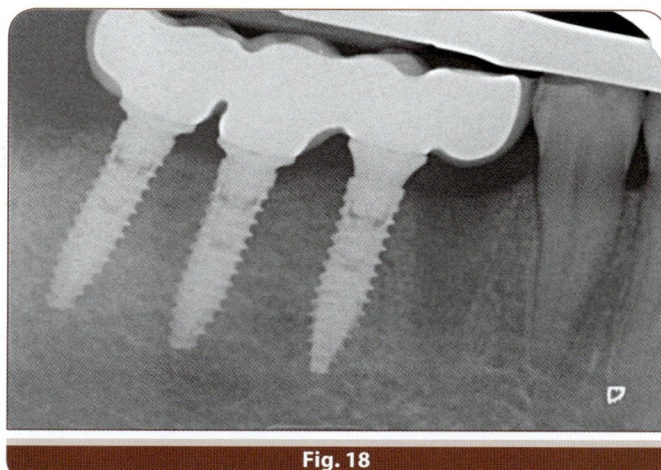

Fig. 18

intraoral periapical radiograph (IOPA) illustrating perfectly placed implants with final prosthesis **(Fig. 18)**.

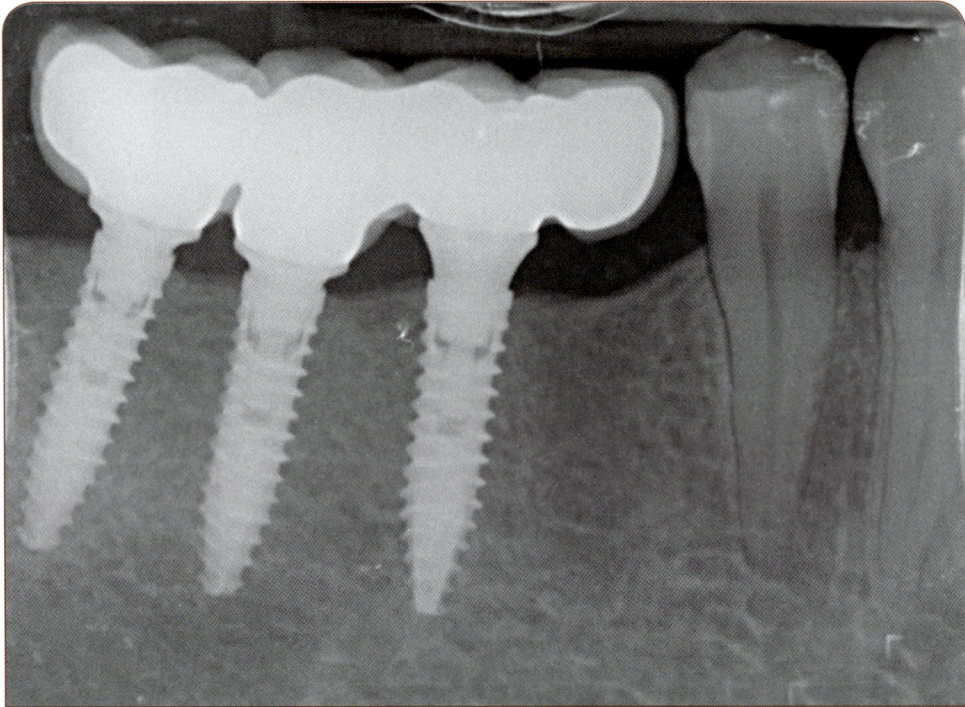

Fig. 19

Two years after implants placement **(Fig. 19)**.

Narayan TV

Ridge Expansion using Densah Burs for Implant Placement: the +1 Protocol

A 59-year-old female with history of implant failure in 36 regions after ridge split procedure about 6 months ago. The ridge width at the crest was around 3 mm and progressively wider apically. Using the +1 ™protocol of Densah burs, the ridge was expanded to >7 mm at the crest and a 4 mm × 10 mm Bioner DM implant was installed with insertion torque of 45 Ncm and a one stage healing pro-tocol was adopted. After 3 months of uneventful healing, a screw retained crown was fabricated and installed. The orthopantogram (OPG) is at 4 month recall.

'The +1 protocol' is the ability of placing an implant of diameter 1 mm greater than the pre-existing width of bone in a given location. It is facilitated by expansion of the ridge when there is an abundance of cancellous bone.

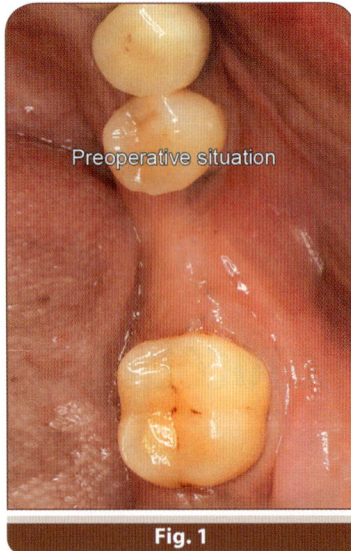
Preoperative view (Fig. 1).

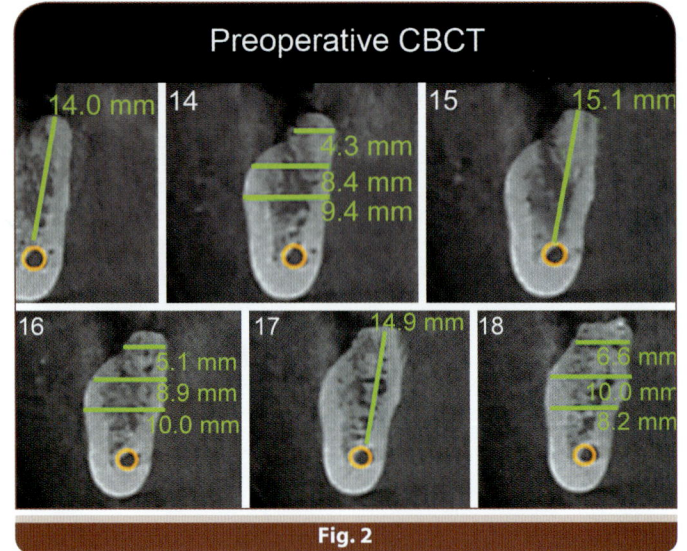
Preoperative CBCT (Fig. 2).

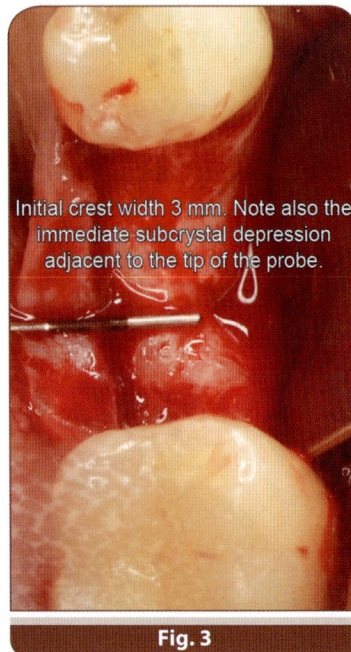
After flap reflection, with a perio-probe in place: Note the crestal width of 3 mm and the immediate subcrestal depression on the facial side (Fig. 3).

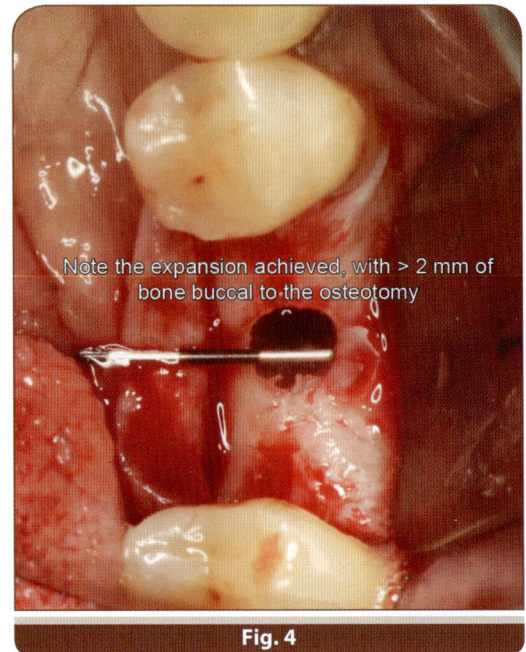
After osteotomy preparation using Densah burs, expansion achieved to 7 mm crestal width with > 2 mm bone buccal to the osteotomy (Fig. 4).

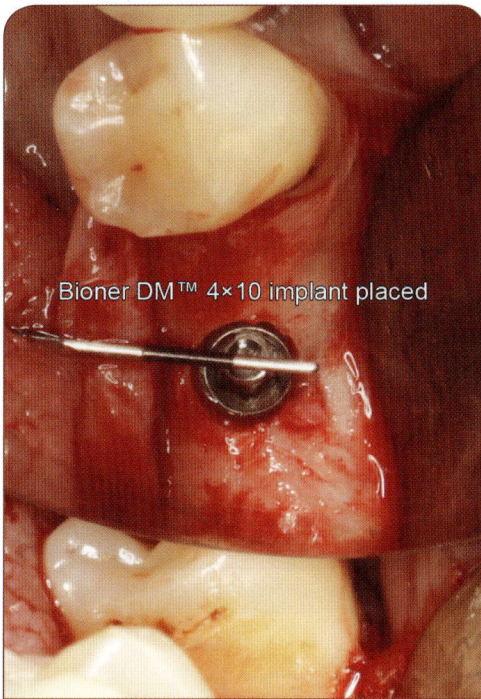

Fig. 5

Immediate postoperative photograph (**Fig. 5**).

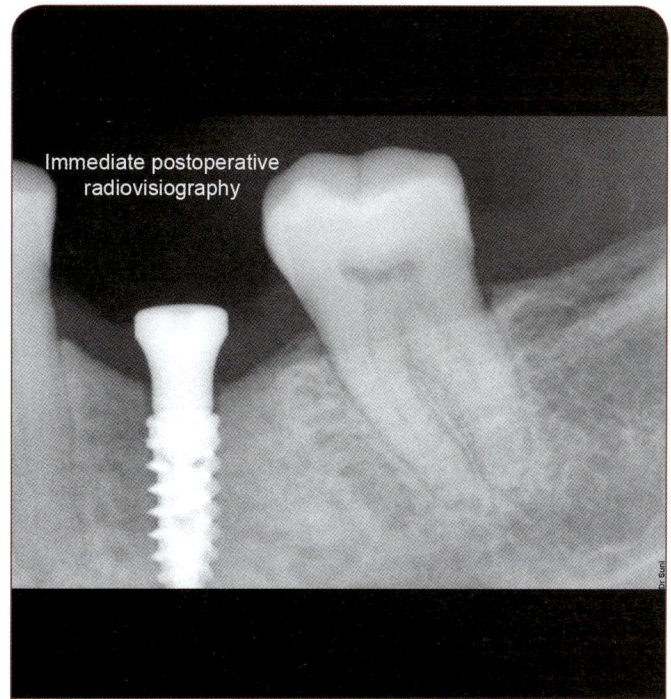

Fig. 6

Immediate postoperative radiograph (**Fig. 6**).

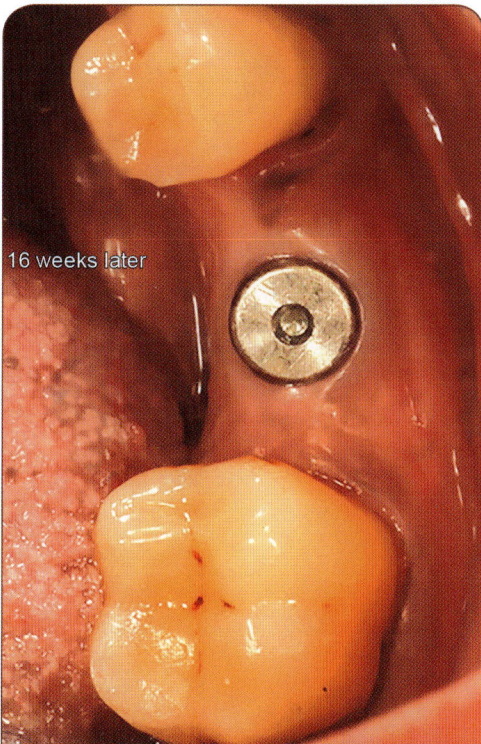

Fig. 7

16 weeks recall photo (**Fig. 7**).

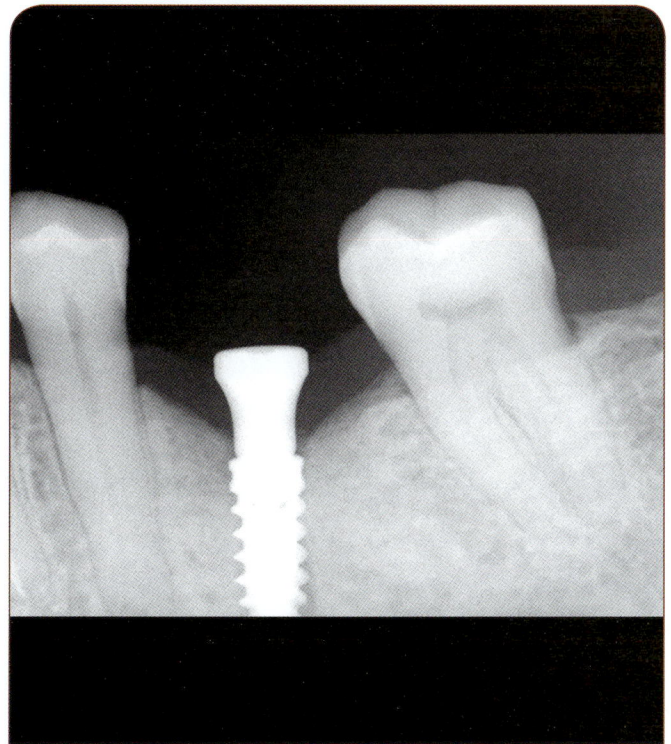

Fig. 8

16 weeks recall radiograph (**Fig. 8**).

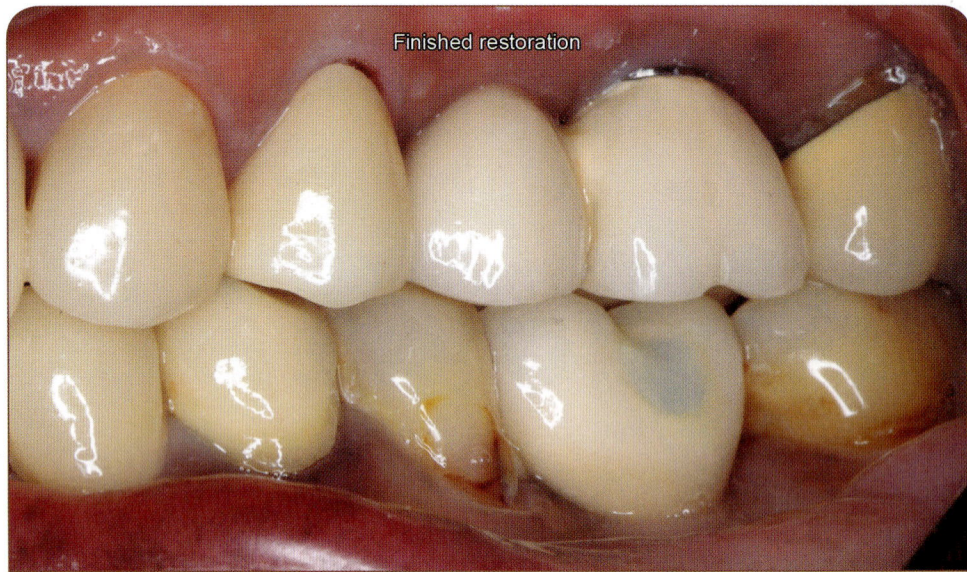

Fig. 9

Final restoration **(Fig. 9)**.

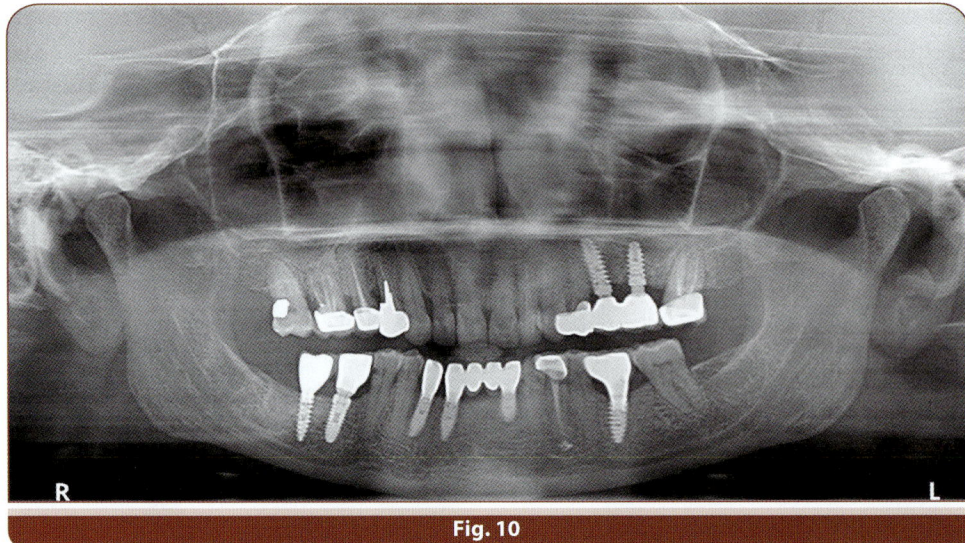

Fig. 10

Four months after final restoration radiograph **(Fig. 10)**.

CASE STUDY 63

David Morales Schwarz , Hilde Morales

Inferior Alveolar Nerve Repositioning to Manage Severely Atrophic Posterior Mandible

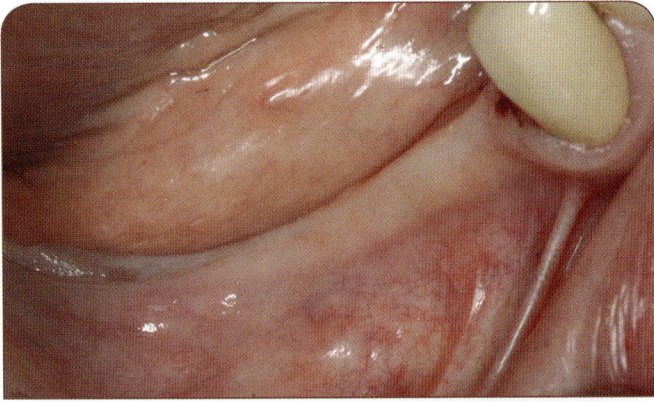

Fig. 1

A fifty three years old lady with bilateral atrophic posterior mandible. After discussing possible alternatives such as bone augmentation with guided bone regeneration or block graft, finally the decision was made a bilateral inferior alveolar nerve transposition **(Fig. 1)**.

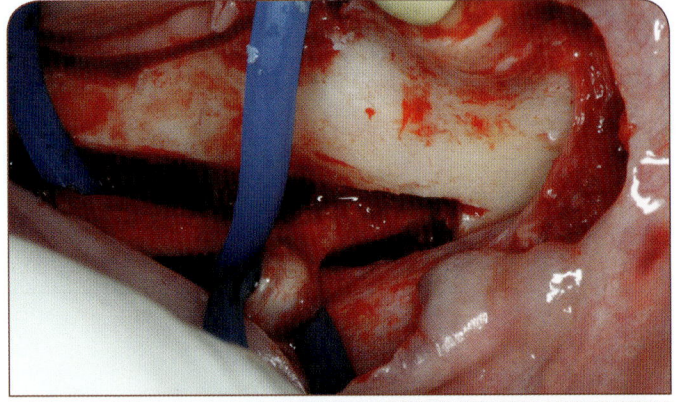

Fig. 2

After performing a rectangular osteotomy with a piezosurgery device the inferior alveolar nerve (IAN) was exposed and isolated with a silicone vessel band **(Fig. 2)**.

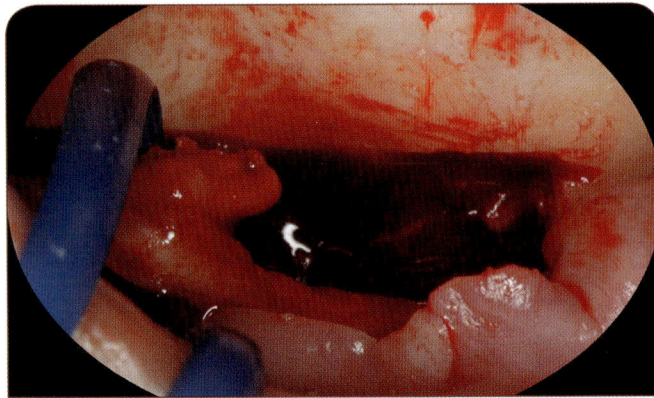

Fig. 3

The incisive branch was cut off so the entire IAN inferior alveolar nerve can be mobilized **(Fig. 3)**.

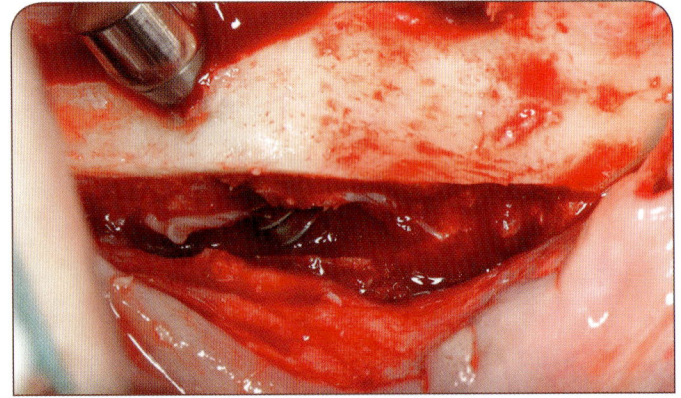

Fig. 4

Two implants were inserted and the IAN inferior alveolar nerve was mobilized distal to the last implant **(Fig. 4)**.

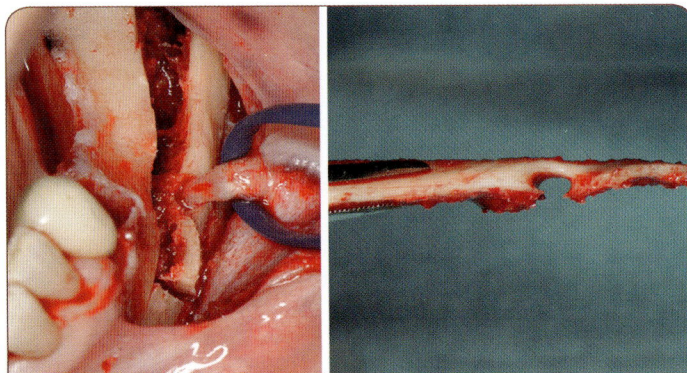

Fig. 5

Appreciate the nerve mobilization **(Fig. 5)**.

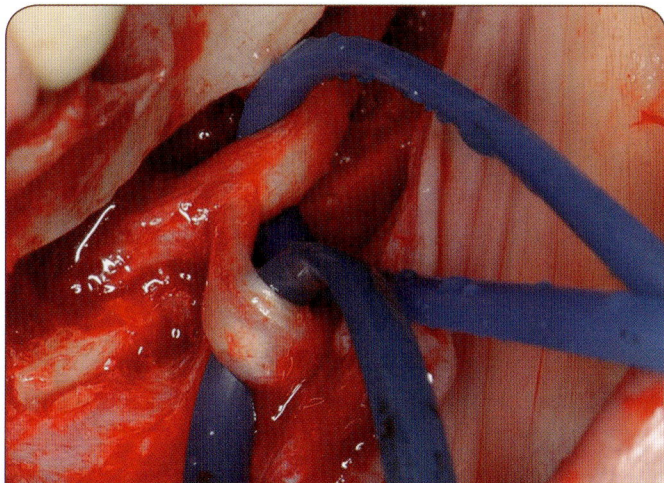

Fig. 6

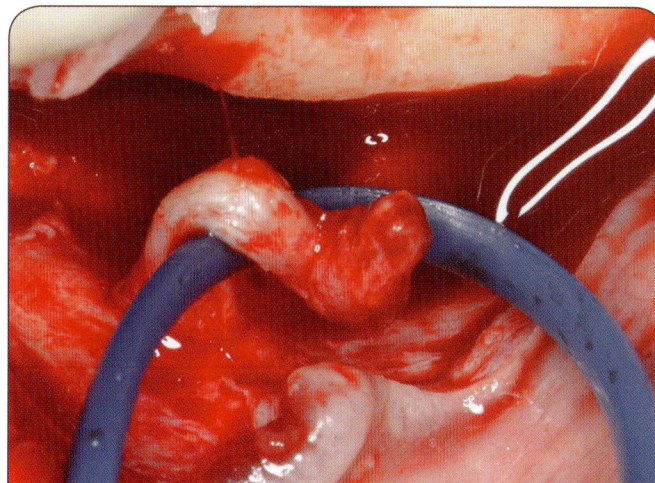

Fig. 7

Left side of the same patient in which a single rectangular osteotomy was performed including the mental foramen **(Fig. 6)**.

In this way we can avoid the vertical osteotomy next to the mental nerve. The inferior alveolar nerve (IAN) was isolated using silicone vessel band. We can observe the incisor branch and the mental branch **(Fig. 7)**.

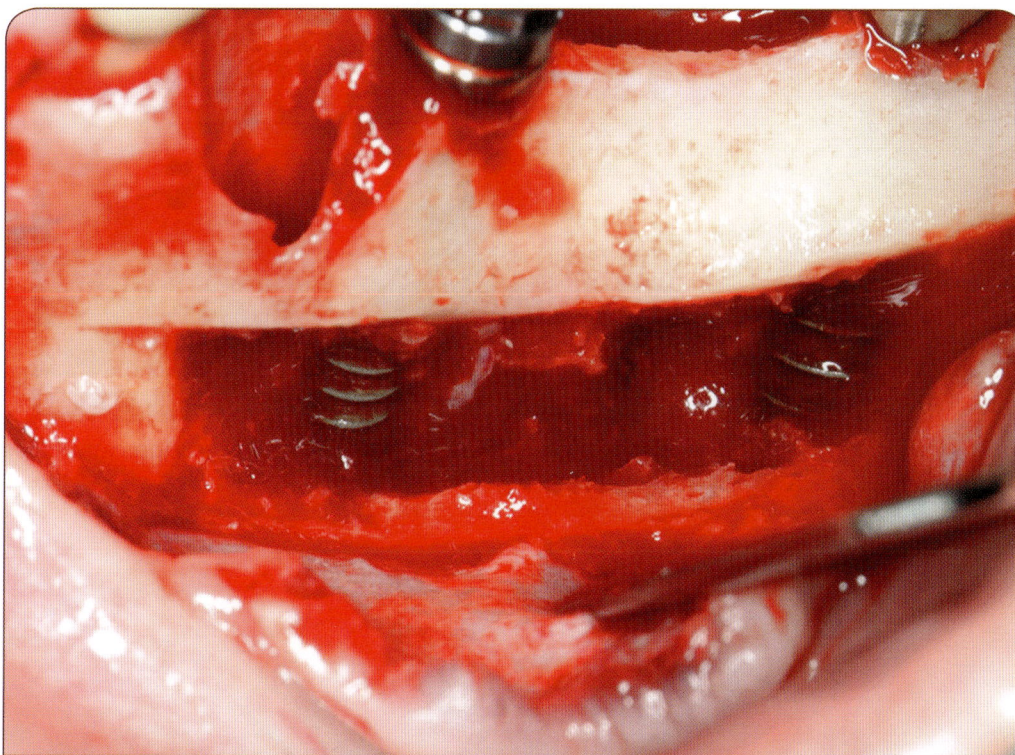

Fig. 8

The incisor branch was cut from mesial to the mental loop so the inferior alveolar nerve became loose and emerge in a distal position for the mandibular body. Two implants were inserted **(Fig. 8)**.

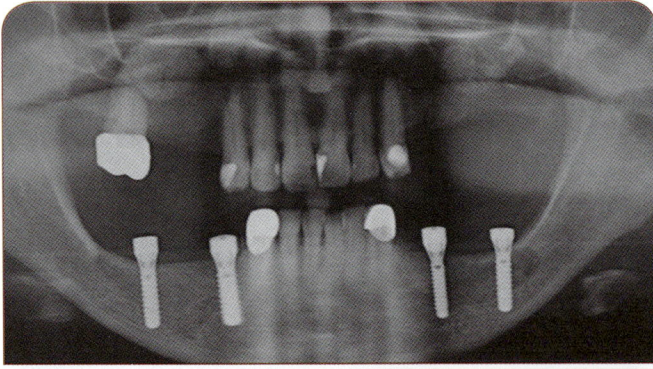

Fig. 9

Postoperative radiograph in which we can observe all the four implants and the osteotomy performed **(Fig. 9)**.

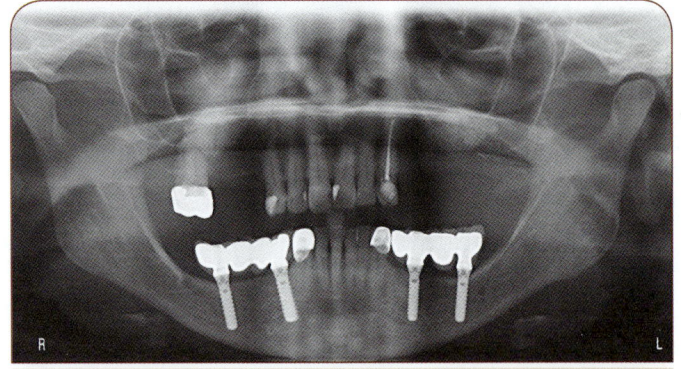

Fig. 10

Prosthesis was delivered at four months. New mental foramen can be observed distally the last implant in each side **(Fig. 10)**.

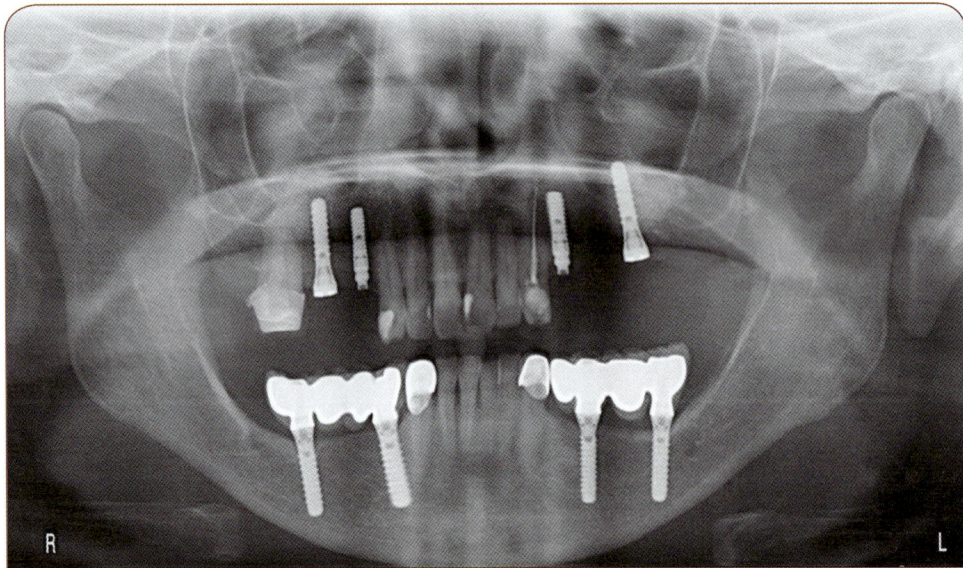

Fig. 11

One year after postoperative where the remodelation of mental foramen in a distal position can be observed on each side. Patient's report normal sensitivity on each side **(Fig. 11)**.

SECTION 5

Guided Bone Regeneration (GBR)

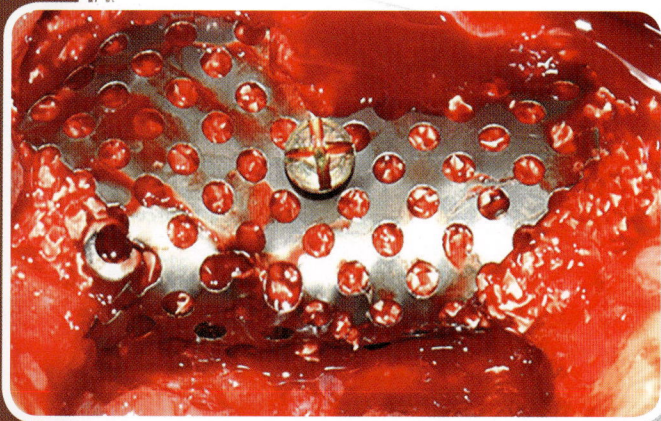

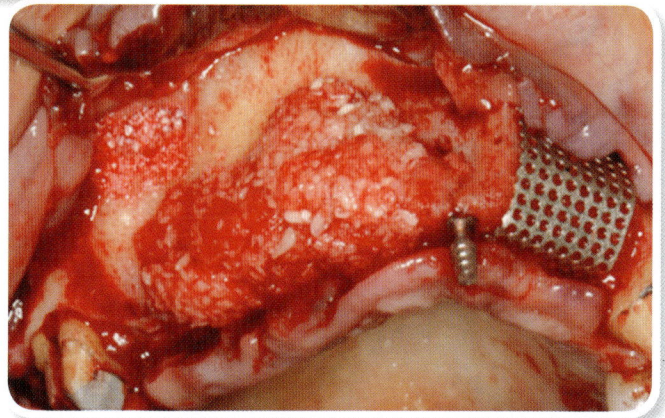

CASE STUDY 64

Lanka Mahesh

Mesh Assisted GBR in a Large Maxillary Defect Restored with a Malo Prosthesis

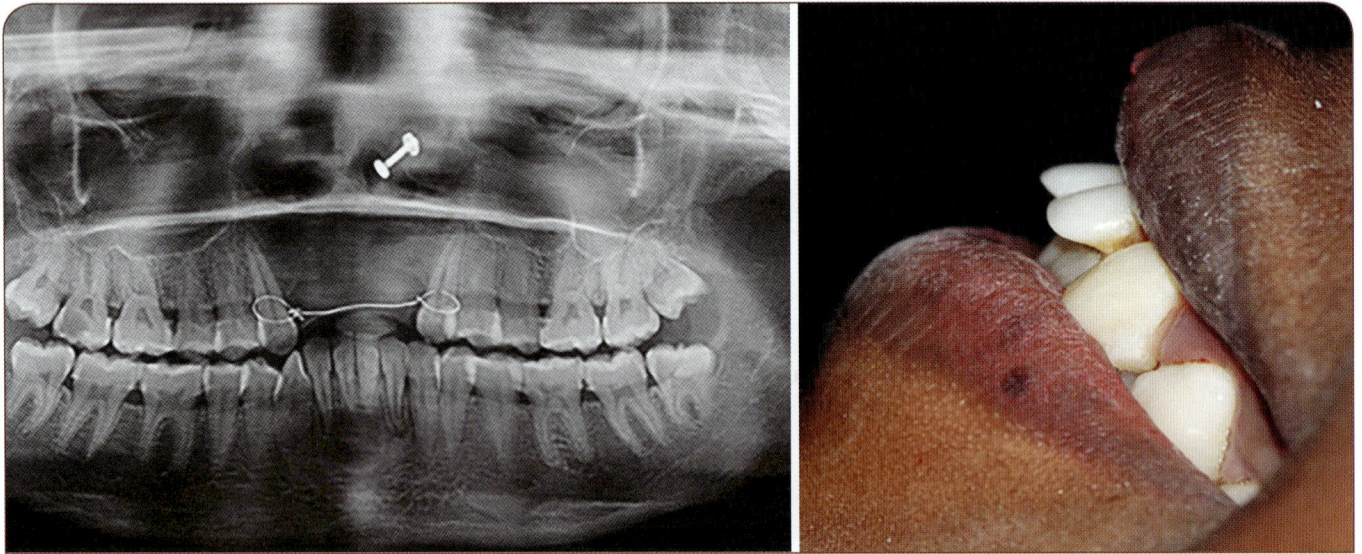

Fig. 1

Preoperative orthopantomogram and clinical presentation **(Fig. 1)**.

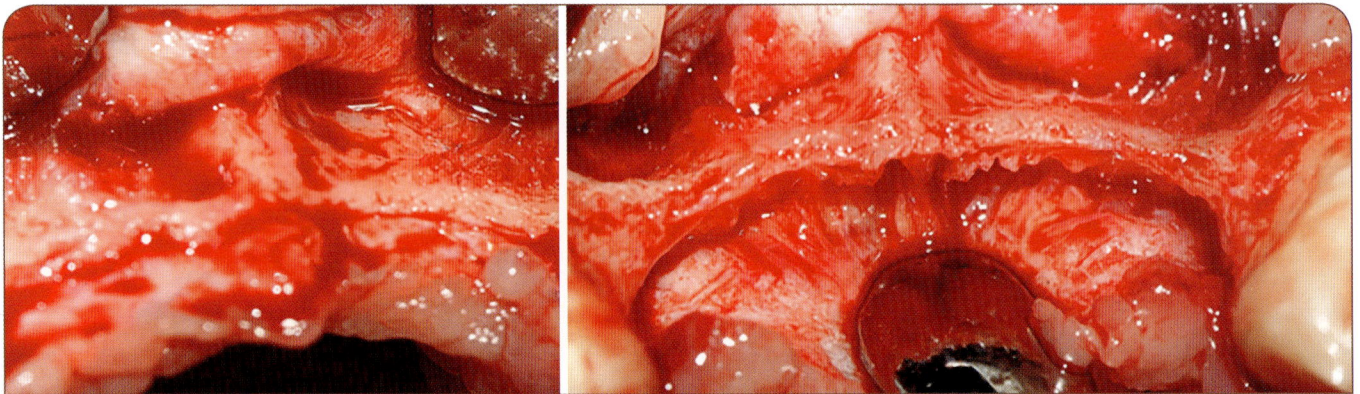

Fig. 2

After flap elevation. Atrophic Anterior Maxilla **(Fig. 2)**.

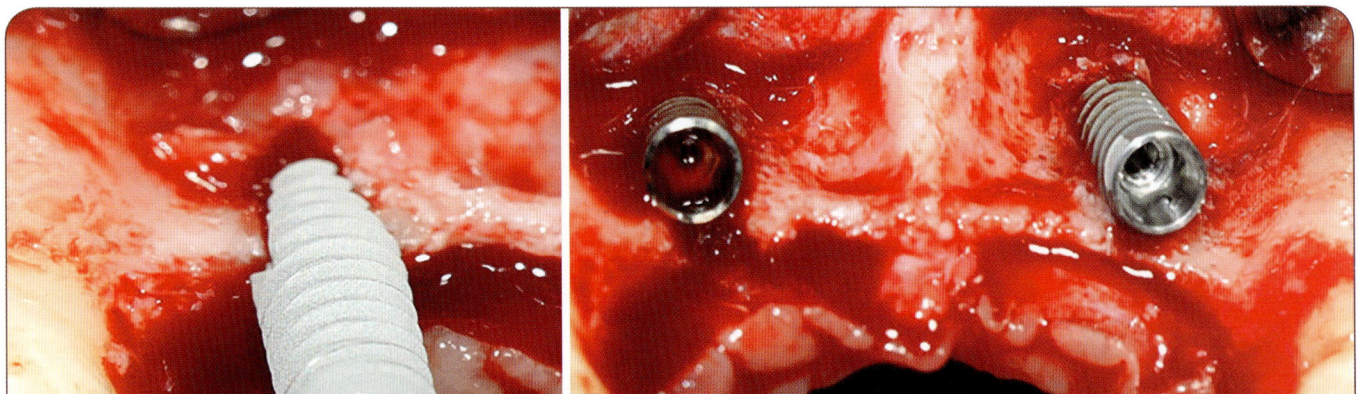

Fig. 3

Two implants placed in the upper front region **(Fig. 3)**.

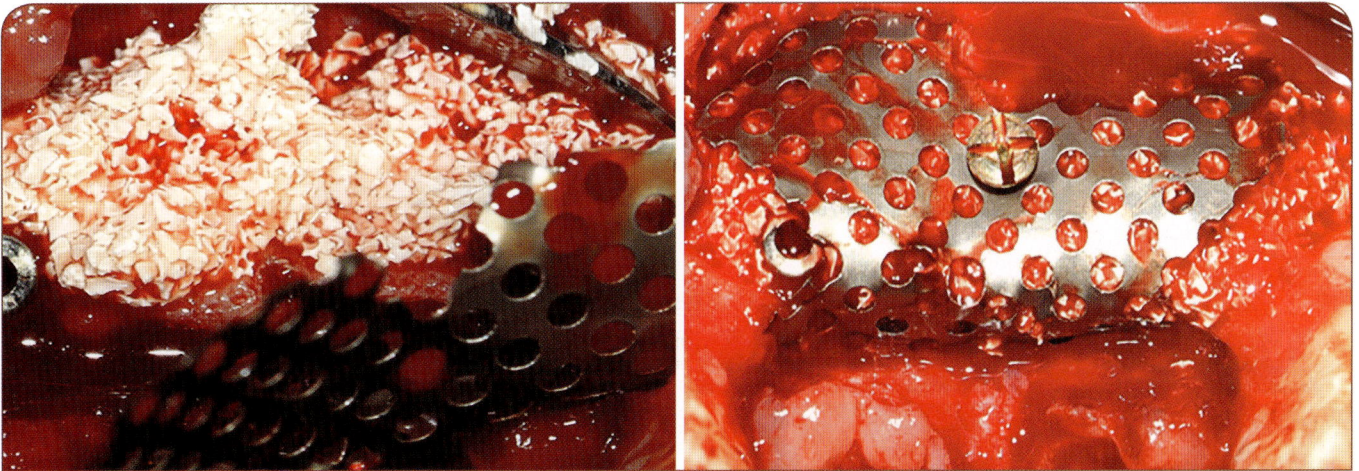

Fig. 4

Titanium mesh adapted and secured with tac after GBR done with bioass **(Fig. 4)**.

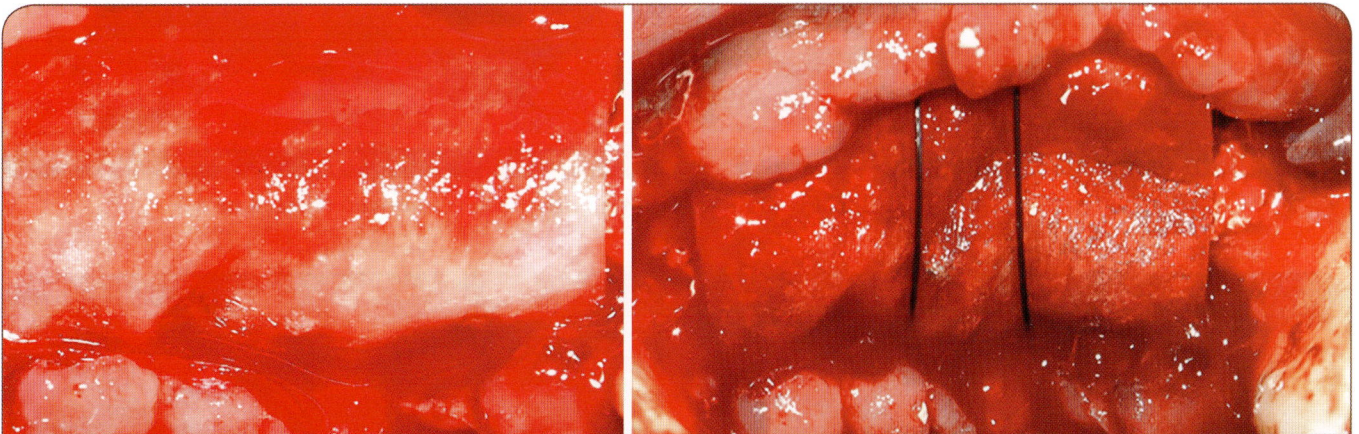

Fig. 5

Collagen membrane coverage over the Titanium mesh **(Fig. 5)**.

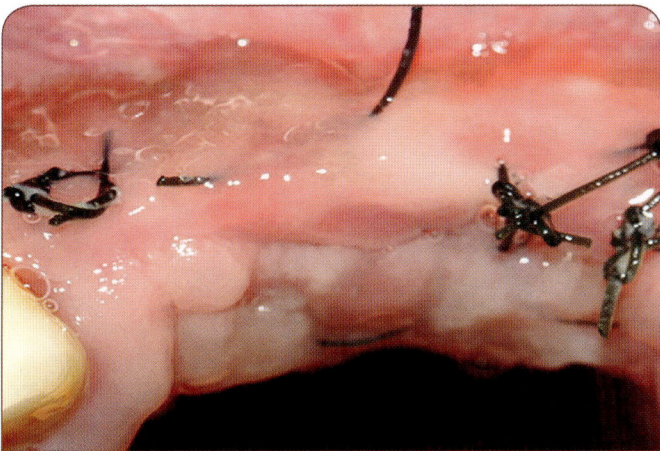

Fig. 6

Sutures placed **(Fig. 6)**.

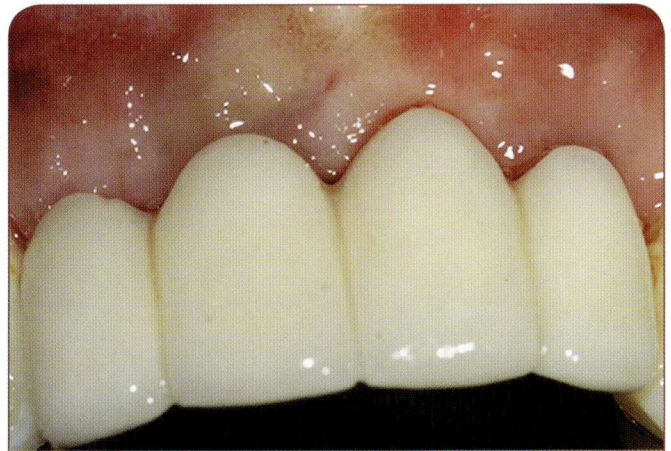

Fig. 7

Fixed temporary prosthesis given **(Fig. 7)**.

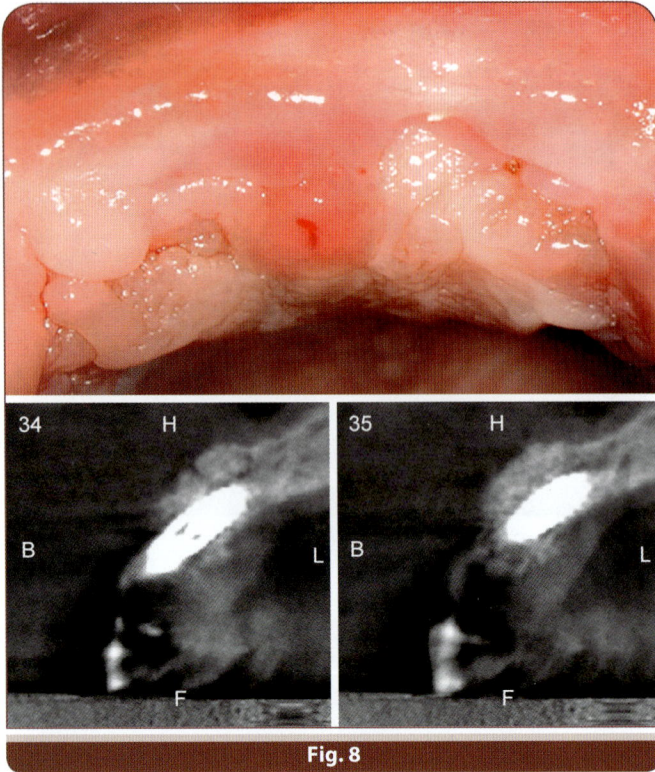
Fig. 8

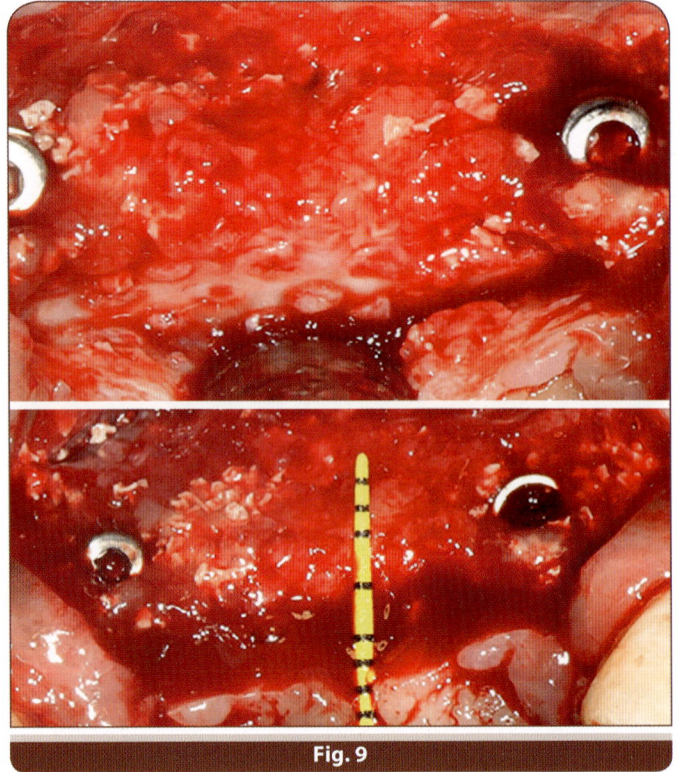
Fig. 9

Clinical representation and OBG evaluation after 3 month mesh is removed **(Figs. 8 and 9)**.

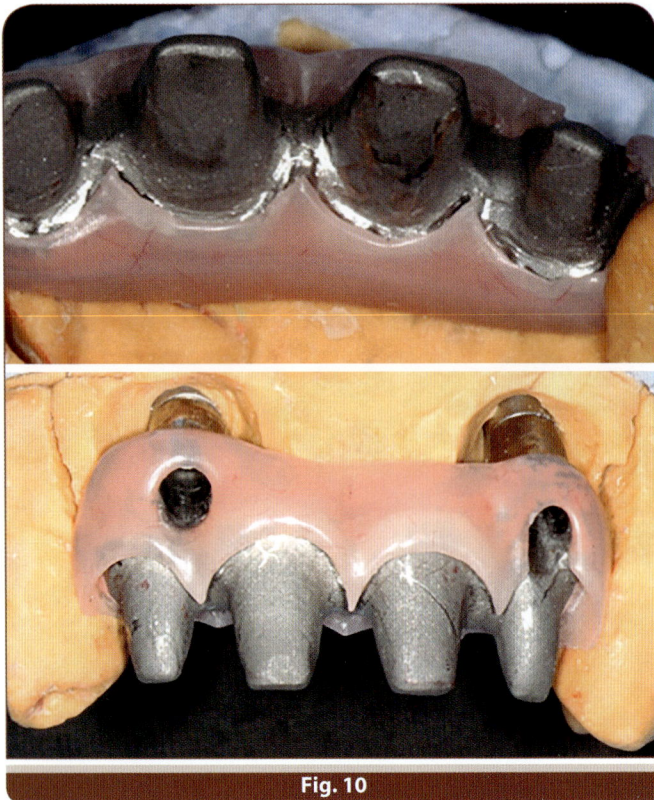
Fig. 10

Malo type prosthesis made metal trial done **(Fig. 10)**.

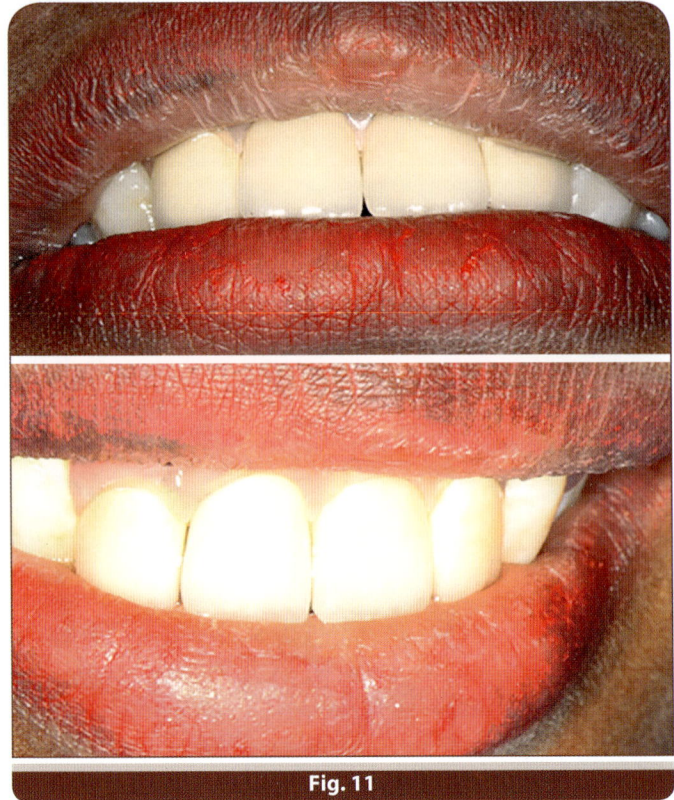
Fig. 11

Fixed prosthesis in place **(Fig. 11)**.

CASE STUDY 65

Craig M Misch

MAXILLARY AUGMENTATION WITH A rhBMP-2 BONE GRAFT FOLLOWING REMOVAL OF FAILED DENTAL IMPLANTS

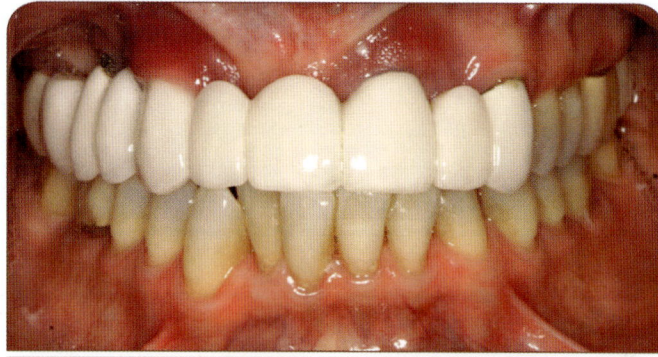

Fig. 1

A 56-year-old female patient with a history of dental implants and a fixed bridge completed two years ago.
No relevant medical history. Clinical exam found acute erythema of the maxillary gingiva around the implants **(Fig. 1)**.

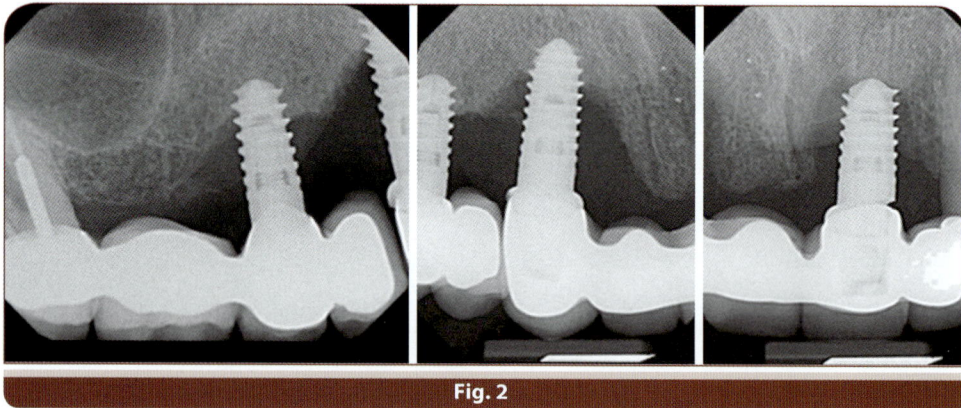

Fig. 2

Periapical radiographs of the three failing implants shows severe marginal bone loss to the apical areas **(Fig. 2)**.
Severe bone loss around the failing implants. Treatment plan included a rhBMP-2 bone graft to reconstruct the sites for new implant placement **(Fig. 2)**.

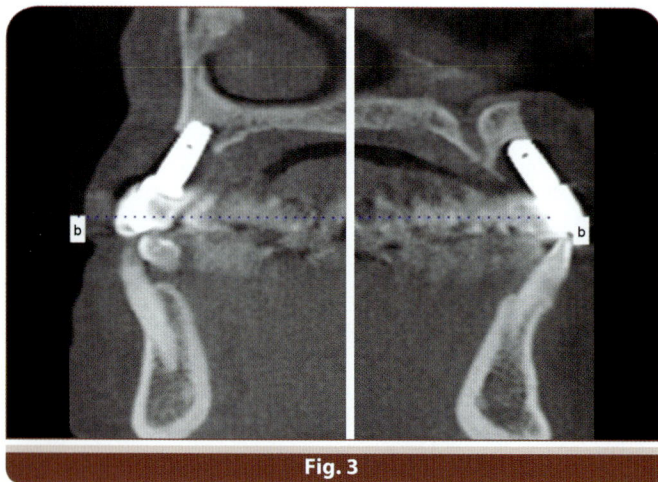

Fig. 3

A cone beam computed tomograph scan shows the bone loss extends to the apices of the implants resulting in significant vertical defects in the maxilla **(Fig. 3)**.

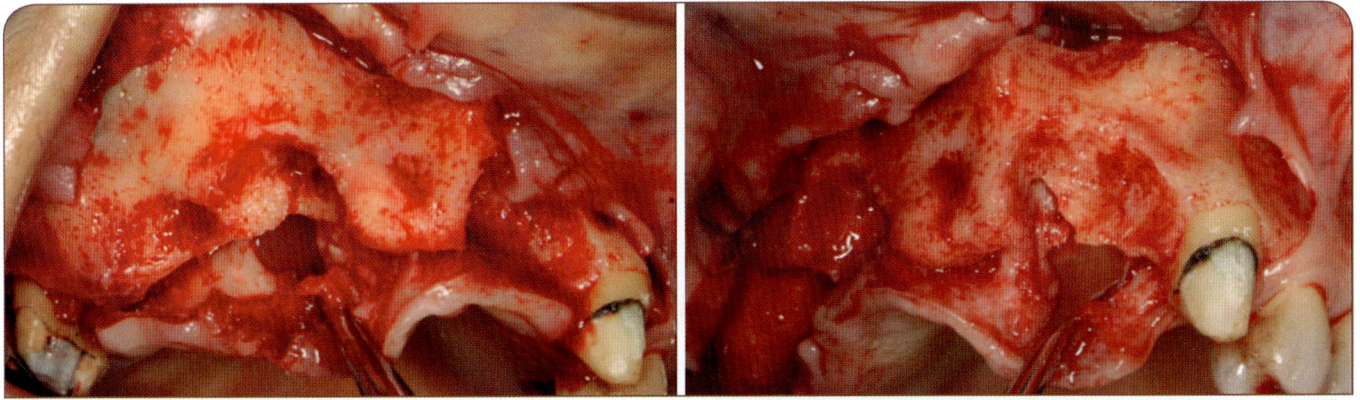

Fig. 4

The implants were removed and the defects were curetted of all soft tissue. Significant osseous defects were present requiring vertical bone augmentation **(Fig. 4)**.

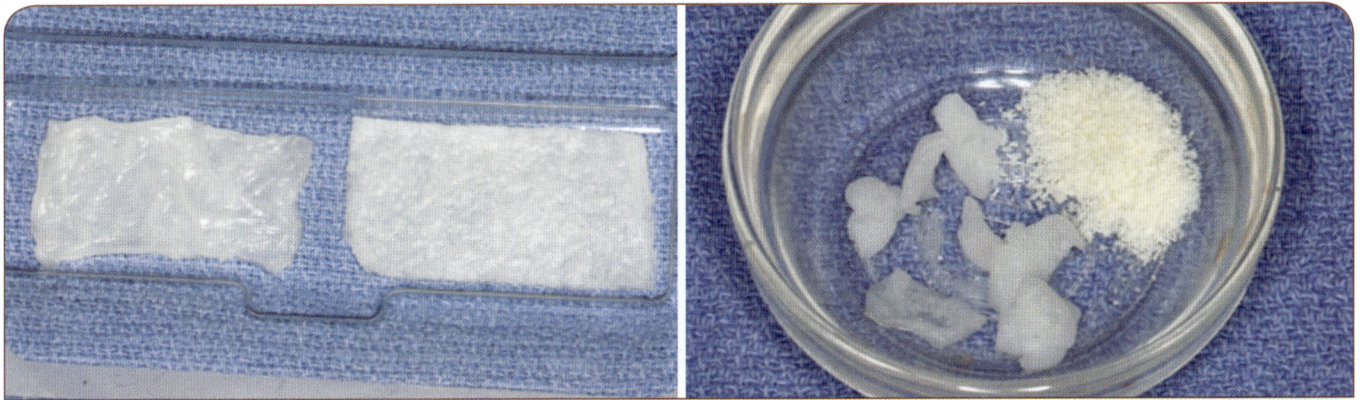

Fig. 5

rhBMP-2 is placed onto collagen sponges, as the carrier for the growth factor. The sponges were then cut into pieces and mixed to a 50:50 ratio with mineralized bone allograft **(Fig. 5)**.

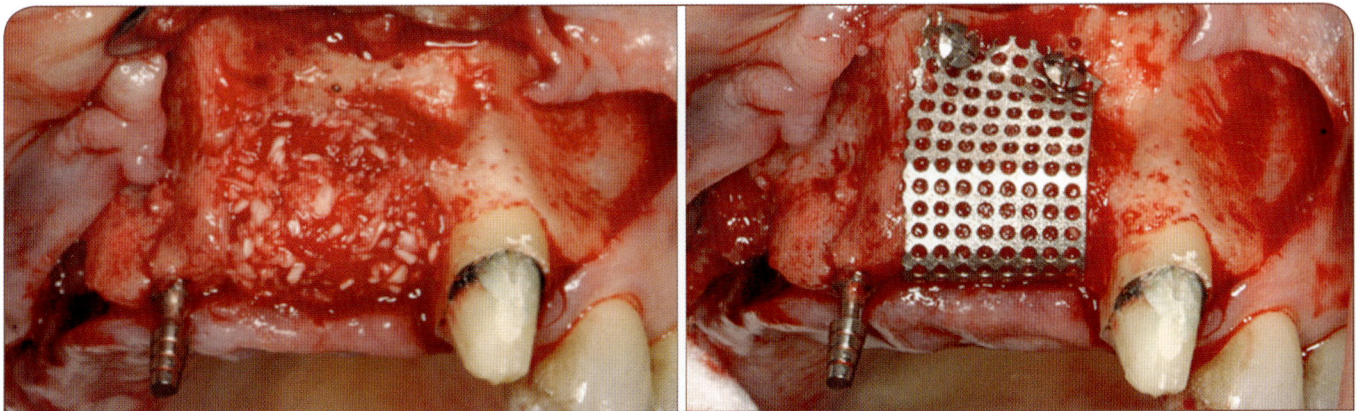

Fig. 6

The composite mixture of rhBMP-2 mixed with mineralized bone allograft and platelet rich plasma was packed into the maxillary left vertical defect. The grafted site was covered with a titanium mesh fixated with titanium screws. A provisional implant was inserted to support the fixed provisional bridge and avoid graft loading **(Fig. 6)**.

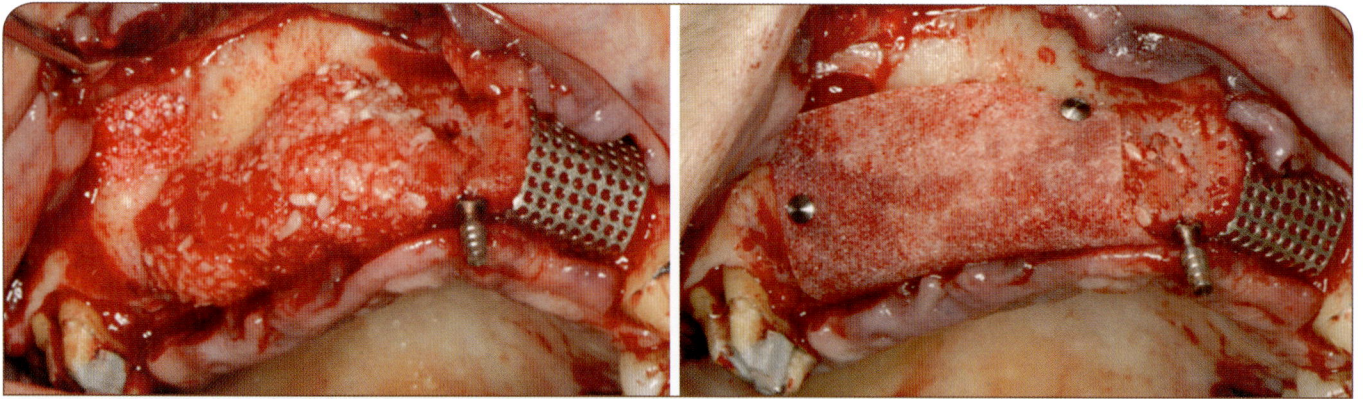

Fig. 7

The composite mixture of rhBMP-2 mixed with mineralized bone allograft and platelet rich plasma was packed into the maxillary right vertical defects. The grafted site was covered with a porous high density polyethylene membrane and secured with titanium tacks **(Fig. 7)**.

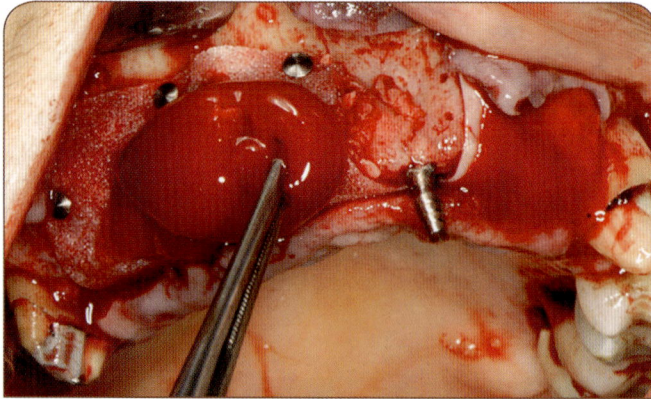

Fig. 8

The grafted sites were covered with platelet rich plasma to enhance soft tissue wound healing **(Fig. 8)**.

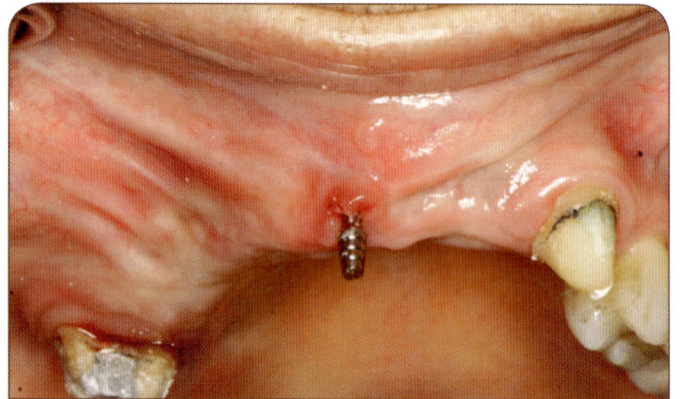

Fig. 9

The graft was allowed to heal for six months. The provisional implant remained stable and supported the provisional bridge to prevent graft loading **(Fig. 9)**.

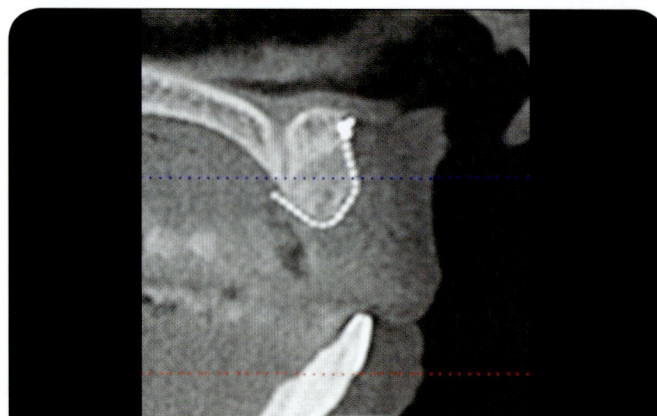

Fig. 10

A CT scan of the healed graft reveals excellent bone growth under the mesh and complete repair of the vertical defect **(Fig. 10)**.

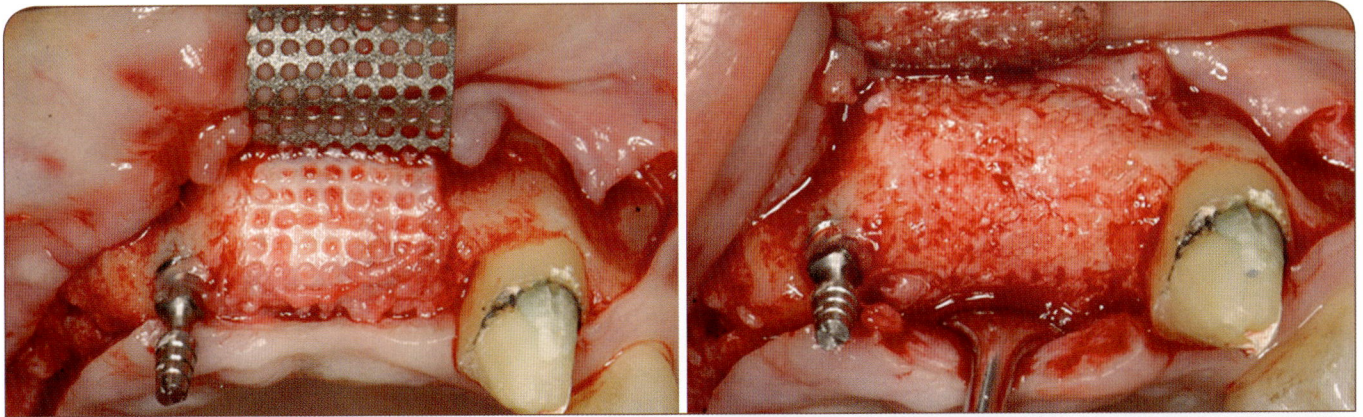

Fig. 11

Removal of the mesh reveals the pseudoperiosteum. Reflection of this layer of soft tissue exposes the reconstructed site. Note the complete bone fill and vascular appearance **(Fig. 11)**.

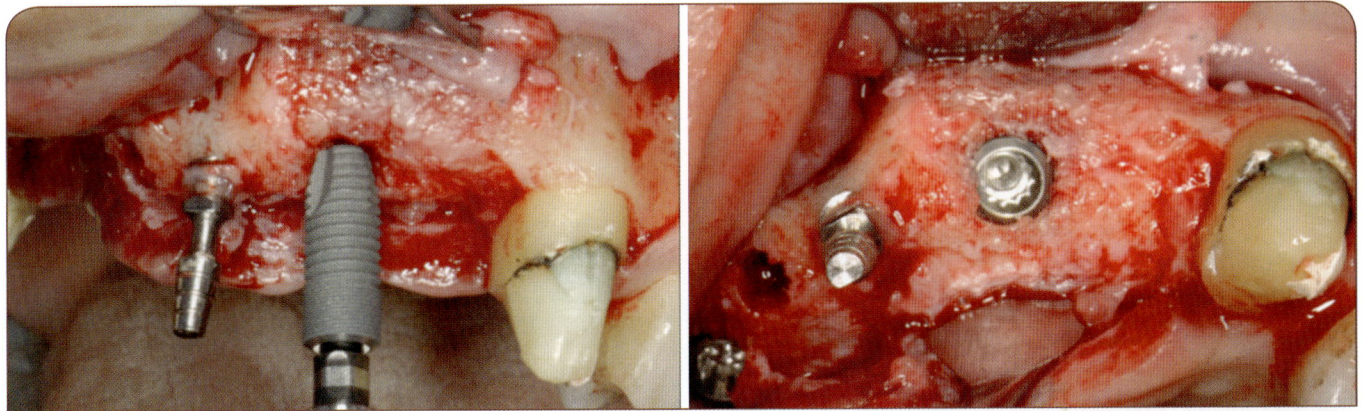

Fig. 12

A 4.0 × 11.0 mm implant is placed into the reconstructed left maxillary site. Note the significant ridge width generated by the BMP graft **(Fig. 12)**.

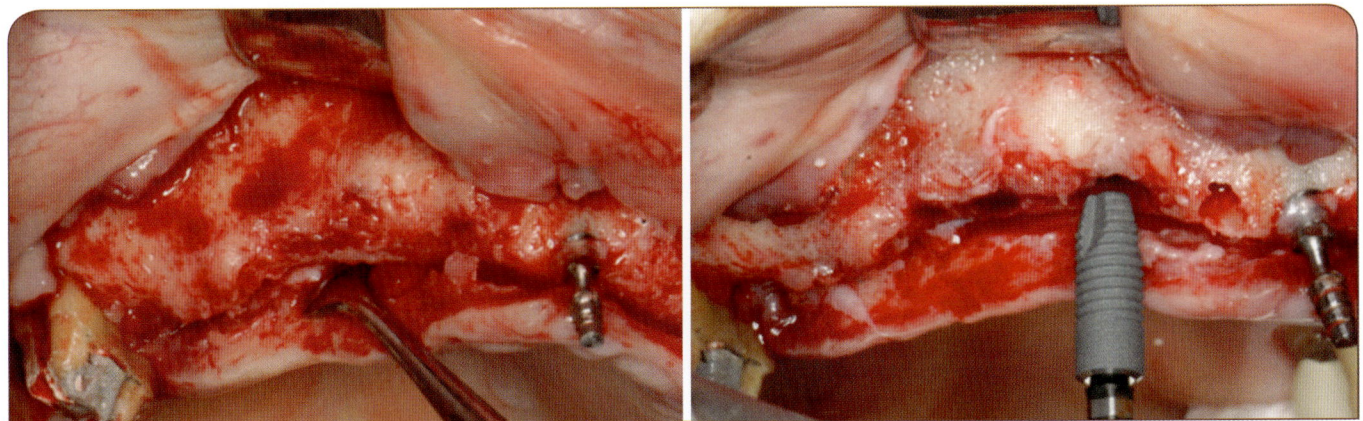

Fig. 13

The BMP graft in the right maxilla is well healed allowing the placement of new dental implants **(Fig. 13)**.

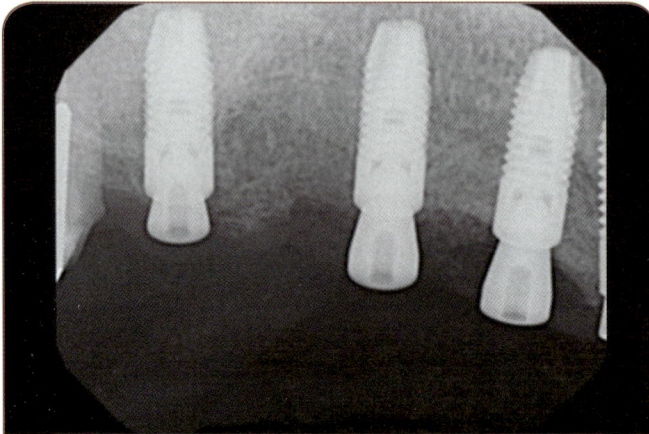

Fig. 14

Fig. 15

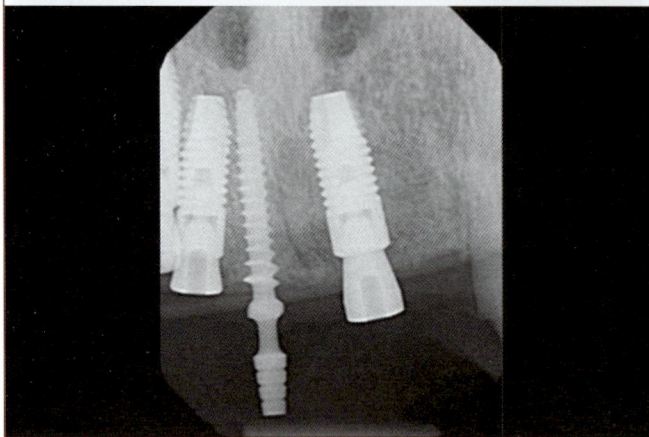

Periapical radiographs of the new implants in the reconstructed maxilla **(Fig. 14)**.

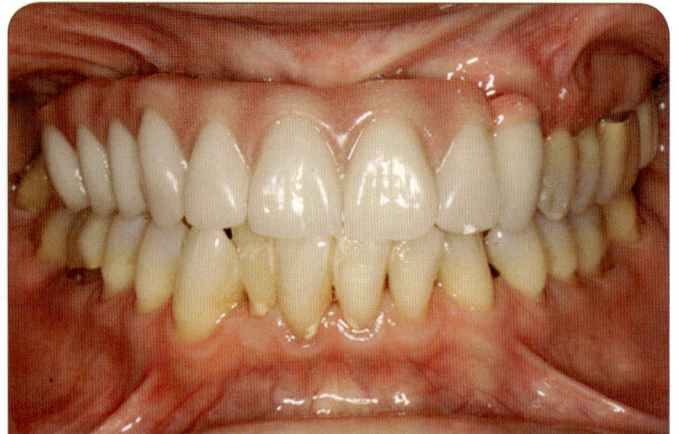

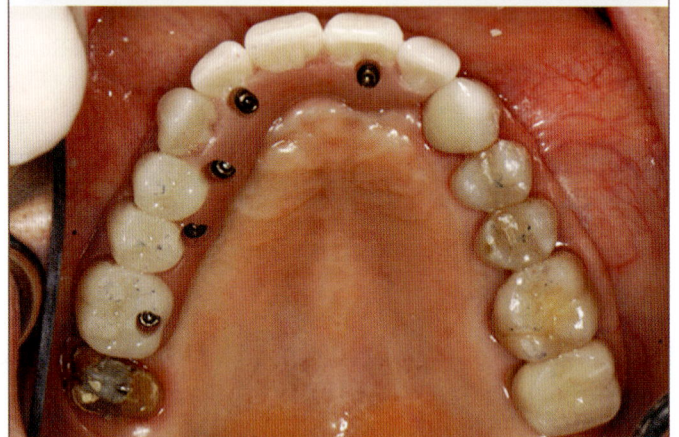

After four months of healing, the implants were restored with a screw retained fixed zirconia prosthesis **(Fig. 15)**.

Craig M Misch

RECONSTRUCTION OF A TRAUMATIC MAXILLARY DEFECT WITH AN ILIAC BLOCK BONE GRAFT

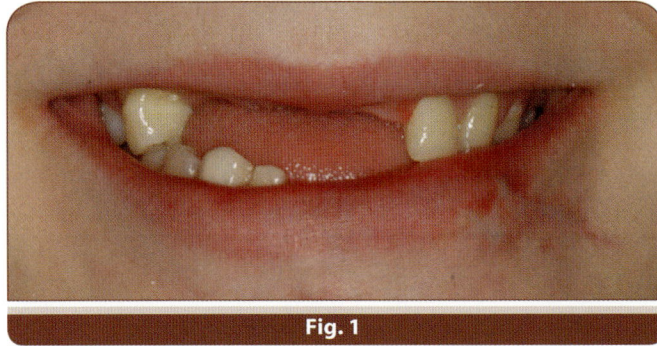

Fig. 1

A 24-year-old female patient with a history of a motor vehicle accident. She was an unrestrained passenger and ejected from the vehicle. She suffered maxillary fractures and traumatic tooth loss. No relevant medical history. Clinical exam found multiple missing teeth and a severe bone defect in the right maxilla. Treatment plan included a block bone graft harvested from the iliac crest to reconstruct the site for implant replacement (**Fig. 1**).

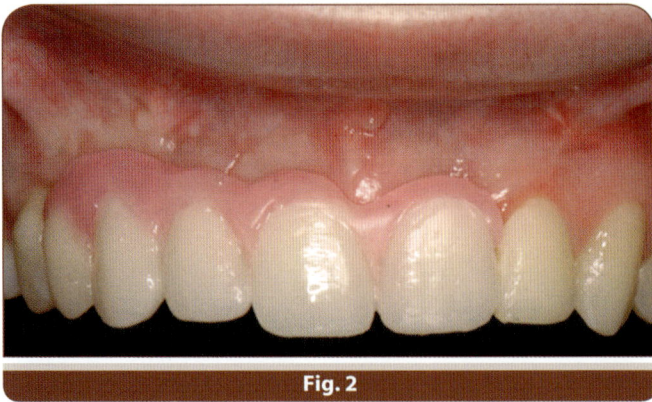

Fig. 2

A diagnostic wax up was performed for a clinical evaluation of the prosthetic requirements. The patient approved of the try-in but she did not want prosthetic gingiva (**Fig. 2**).

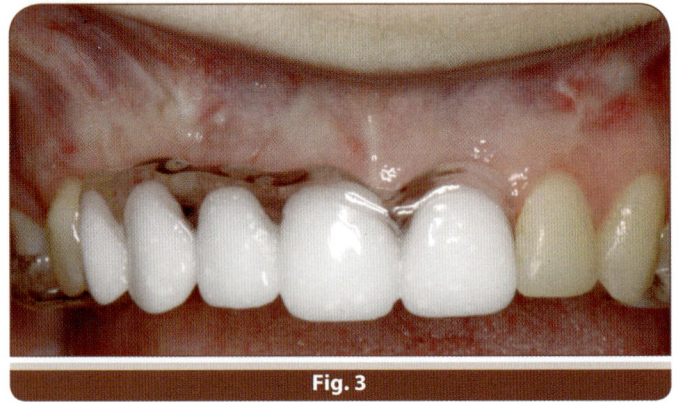

Fig. 3

A radiographic template was fabricated from the diagnostic set up. The template was worn during a cone beam computed tomography scan of the maxilla (**Fig. 3**).

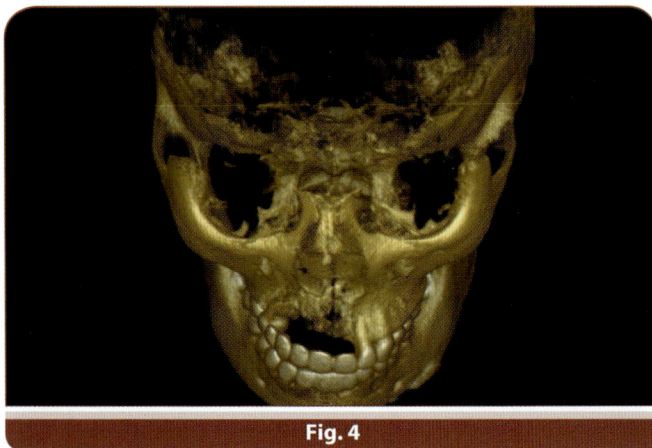

Fig. 4

A three-dimensional reconstruction of the maxilla reveals a severe horizontal and vertical defect. The prosthetic template shows the grafting requirements for future implant placement (**Fig. 4**).

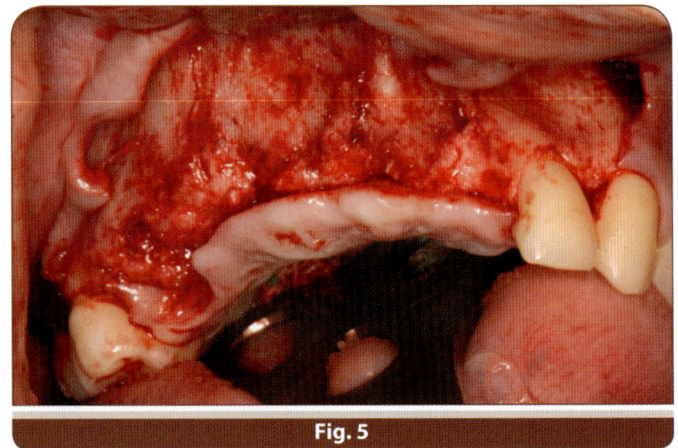

Fig. 5

Surgical exposure of the maxillary defect. Vertical releasing incisions are made remote from the defect and a large mucoperiosteal flap is elevated to allow flap advancement (**Fig. 5**).

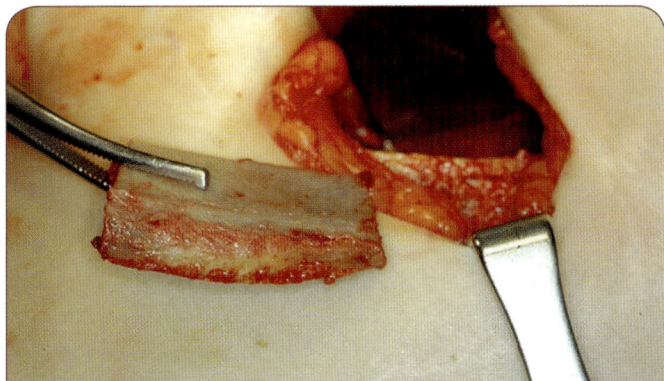

Fig. 6

The block corticocancellous bone graft was harvested from the iliac crest **(Fig. 6)**.

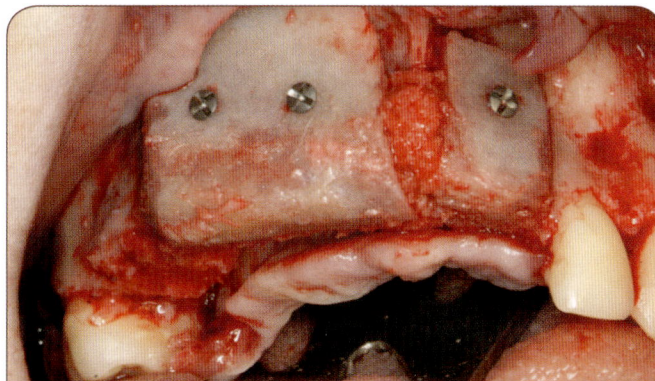

Fig. 7

The block graft is shaped and contoured to reconstruct the maxillary defect according to the prosthetic template. Cancellous bone is packed around the periphery of the bone blocks **(Fig. 7)**.

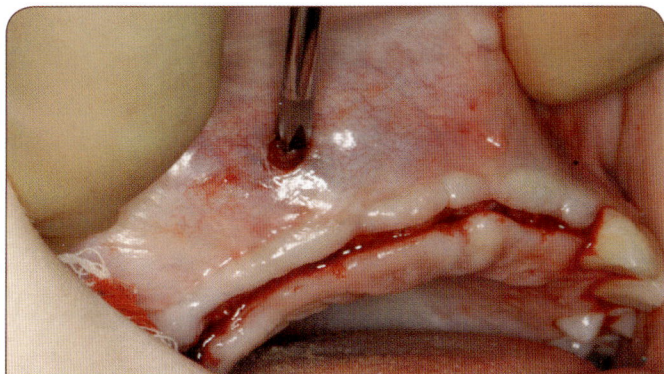

Fig. 8

After a four-month healing period the fixation screws are removed through a remote incision to maintain vascular supply to the healed bone graft **(Fig. 8)**.

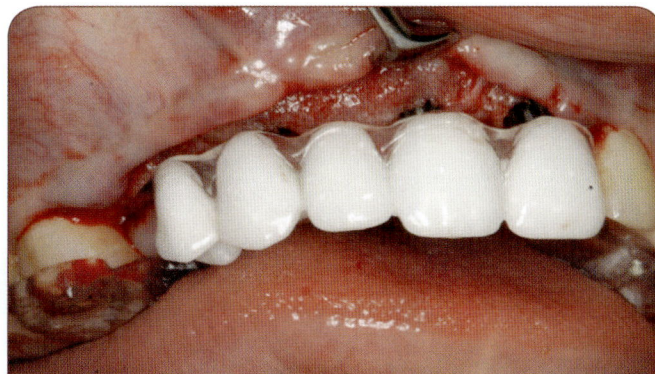

Fig. 9

The radiograph template was converted into an implant template to guide the implant positions **(Fig. 9)**.

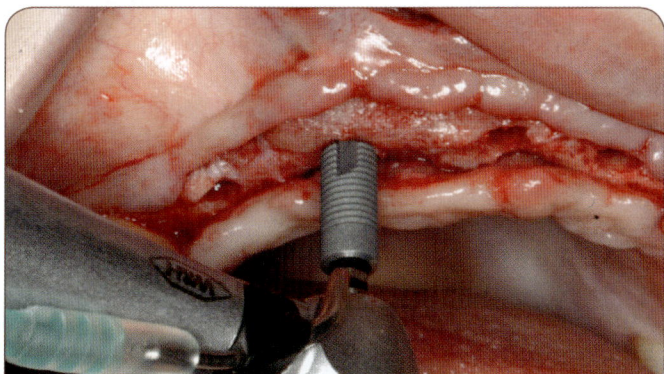

Fig. 10

Exposure of the healed graft shows good incorporation and favorable bone dimensions for implant placement **(Fig. 10)**.

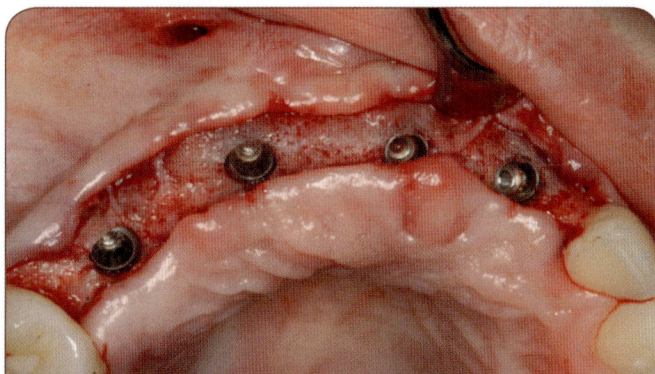

Fig. 11

Four dental implants were placed in the maxillary graft according to the implant template **(Fig. 11)**.

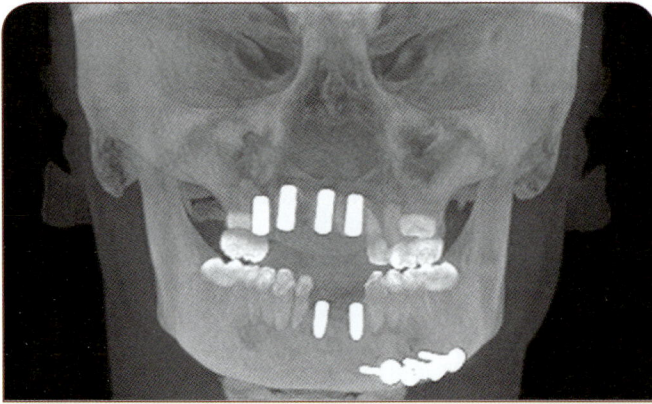

Fig. 12

A postoperative CBCT after dental implant surgery in the maxilla and mandible **(Fig. 12)**.

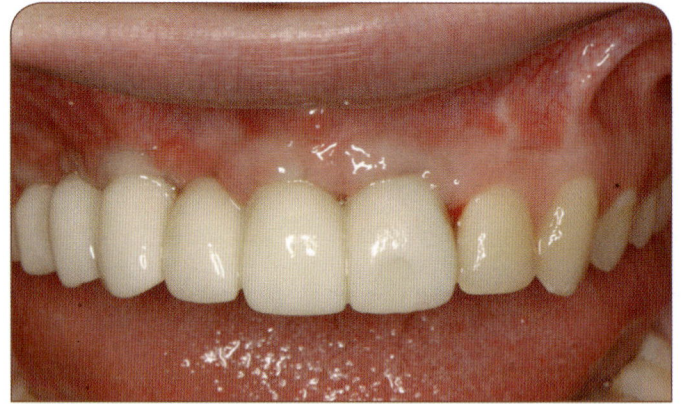

Fig. 13

The implants were uncovered after four months healing and a provisional bridge was fabricated to guide the soft tissue healing **(Fig. 13)**.

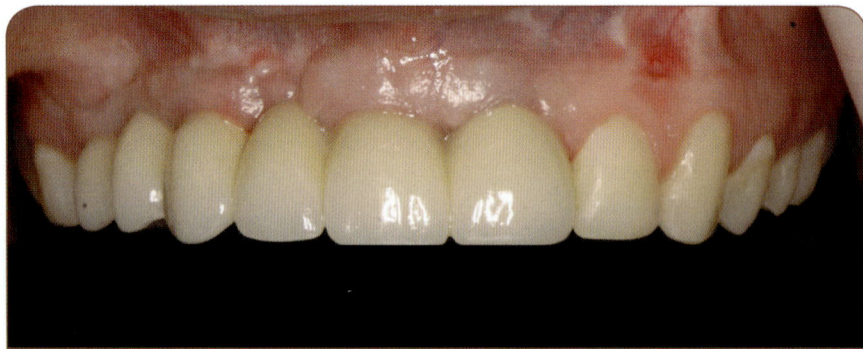

Fig. 14

The final porcelain fused to metal implant bridge was fabricated on four custom made CAD/CAM titanium abutments **(Fig. 14)**.

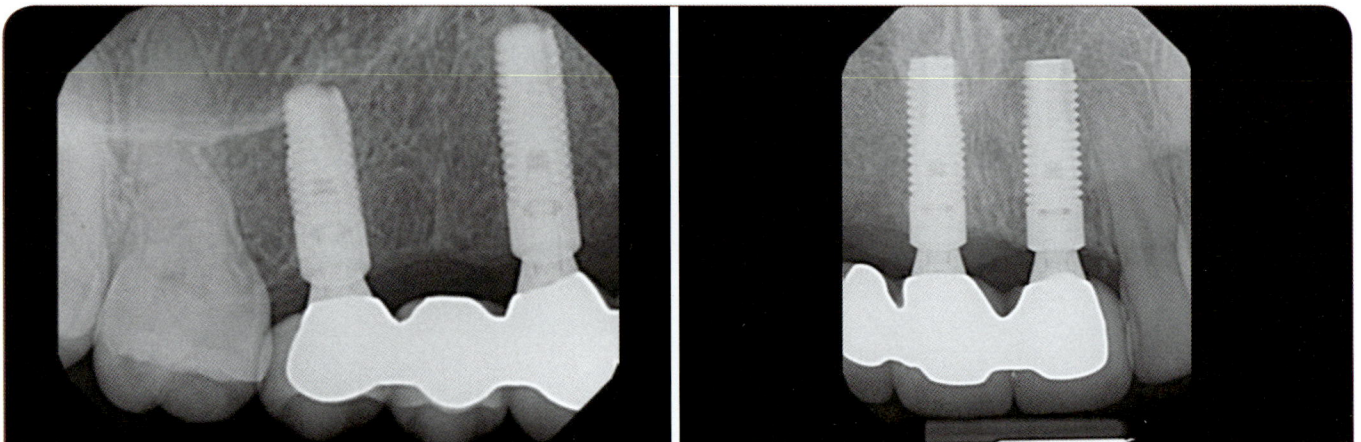

Fig. 15

Periapical radiographs at one year post-prosthetic delivery reveal the implants appear well integrated with stable marginal bone levels **(Fig. 15)**.

CASE STUDY 67

Alejandro Vivas Rojo, Jesus Gomez Perez

Maxillary Augmentation with Autogenous Bone, Allogeneic Bone RHBMP-2 Graft and Titanium Mesh

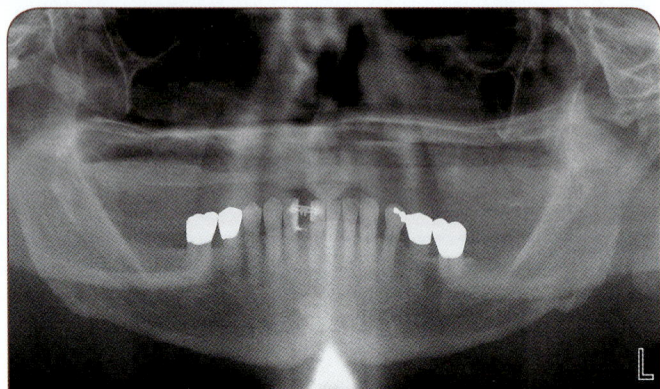

Fig. 1

Preoperative Panorex **(Fig. 1)**.

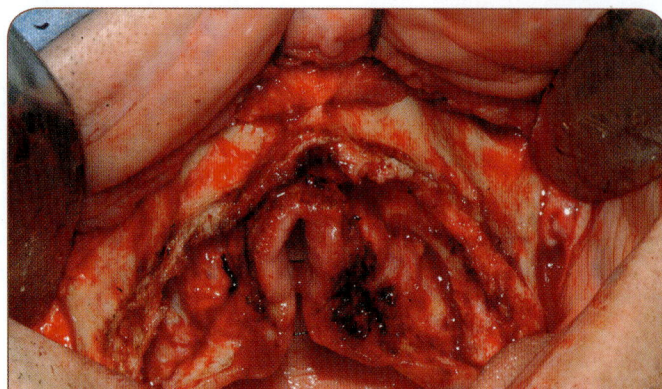

Fig. 2

Preoperative clinical, full thickness flap **(Fig. 2)**.

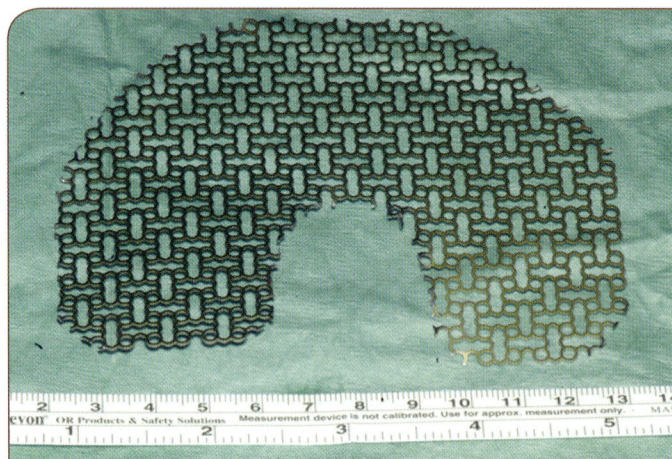

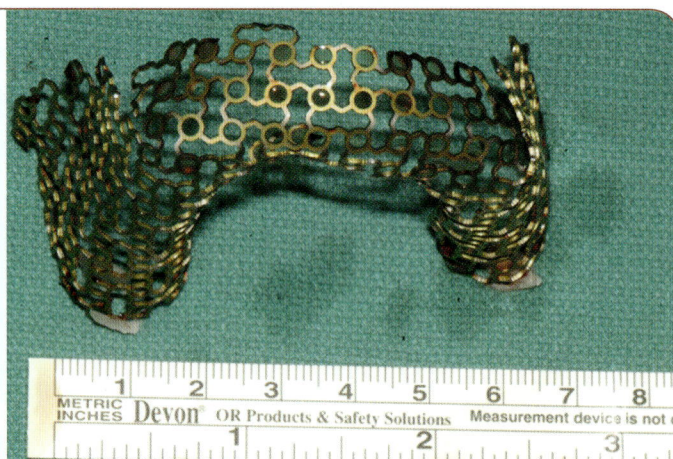

Fig. 3

Titanium mesh adapted intraoperatively **(Fig. 3)**.

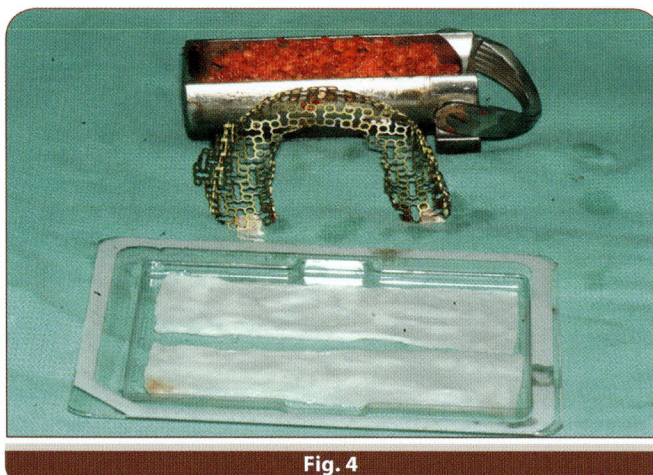

Fig. 4

Osteoinduction + Osseoconduction concept. BMP2 + FDAB + Autogenous bone. Carrier: Titanium mesh **(Fig. 4)**.

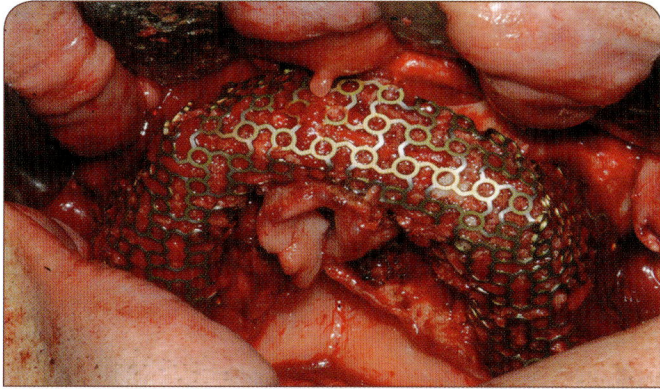

Fig. 5

Titaniun mesh adapted, with graft inside (**Fig. 5**).

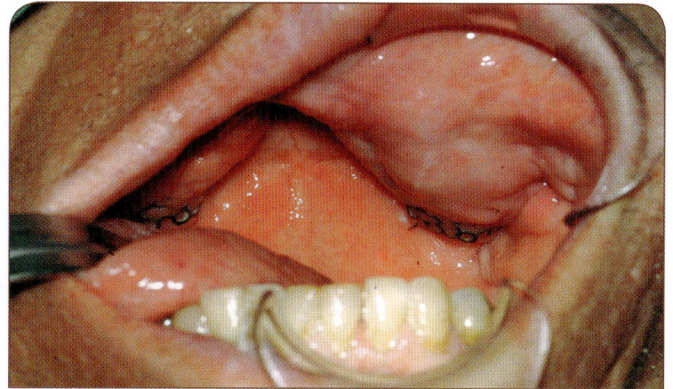

Fig. 6

After 6 months titanium mesh exposed to cavity. Notice the amount of new-formed bone (**Fig. 6**).

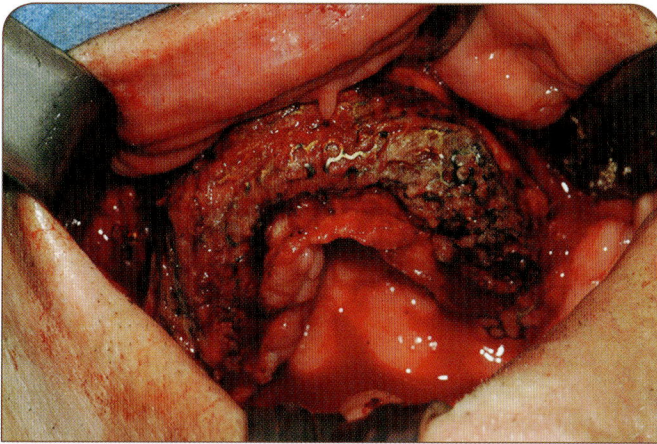

Fig. 7

Taking out the titanium mesh. Full thickness flap (**Fig. 7**).

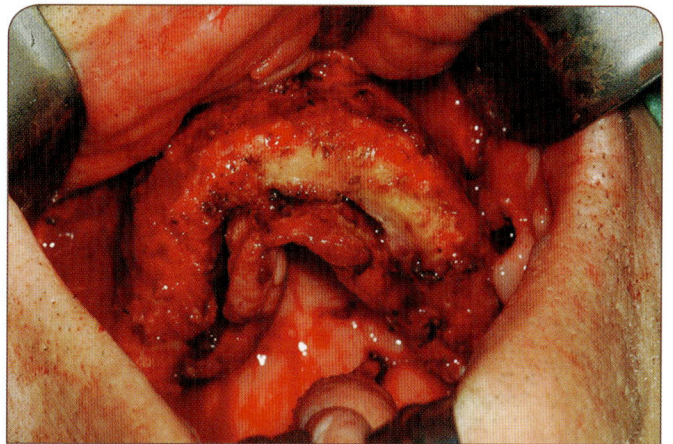

Fig. 8

New-formed bone. Density D-4 (**Fig. 8**).

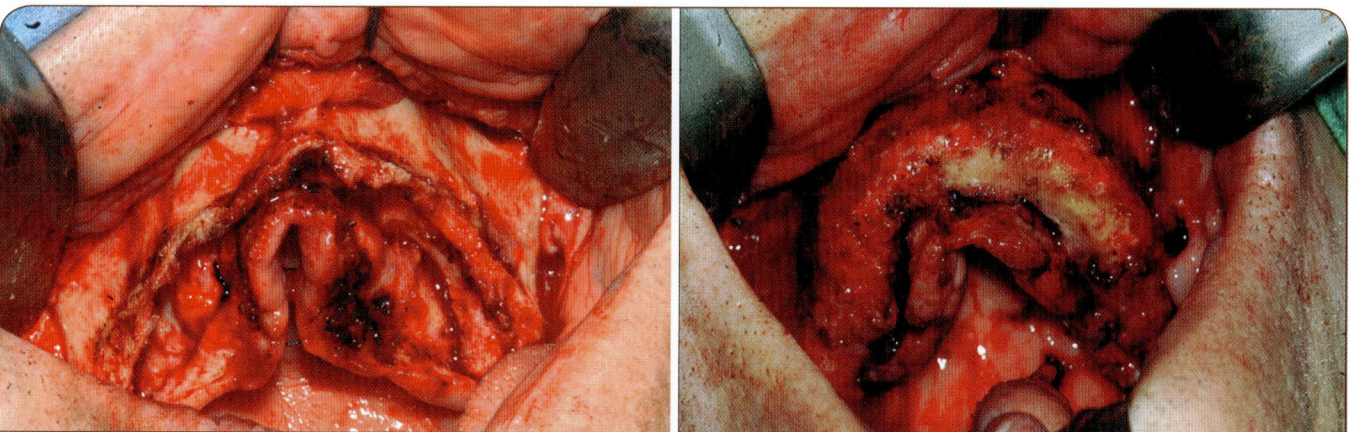

Fig. 9

Preoperative atrophied maxilla and postoperative maxilla with D-4 type bone (**Fig. 9**).

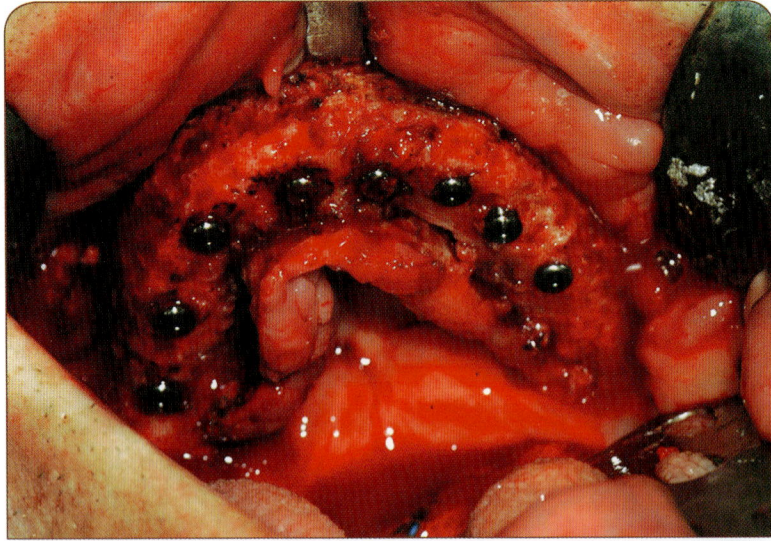

Fig. 10

Implant placed **(Fig. 10)**.

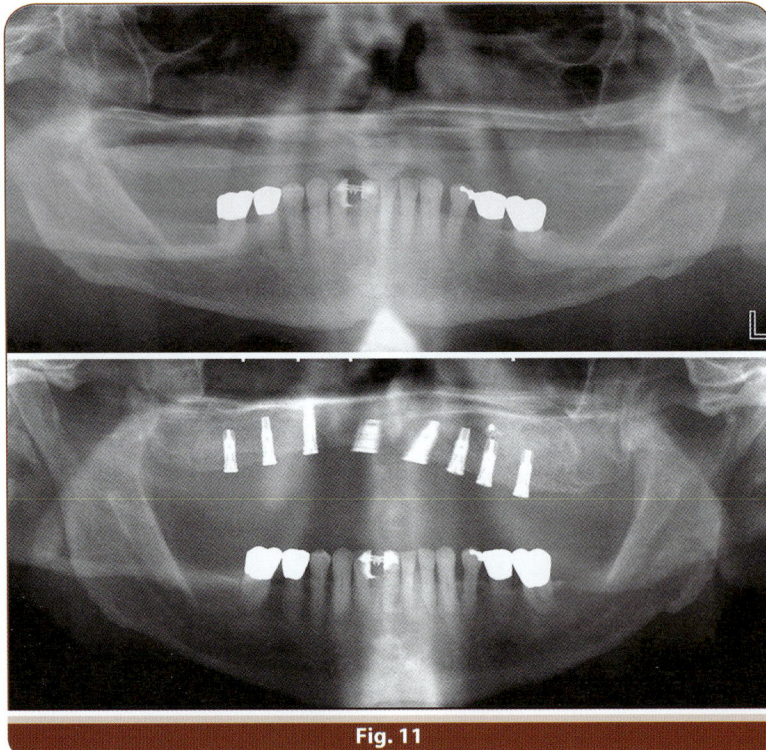

Fig. 11

Preoperative/postoperative orthopantomogram (OPG) **(Fig. 11)**.

Lanka Mahesh

MAXILLARY CORTICAL SPLIT WITH GBR

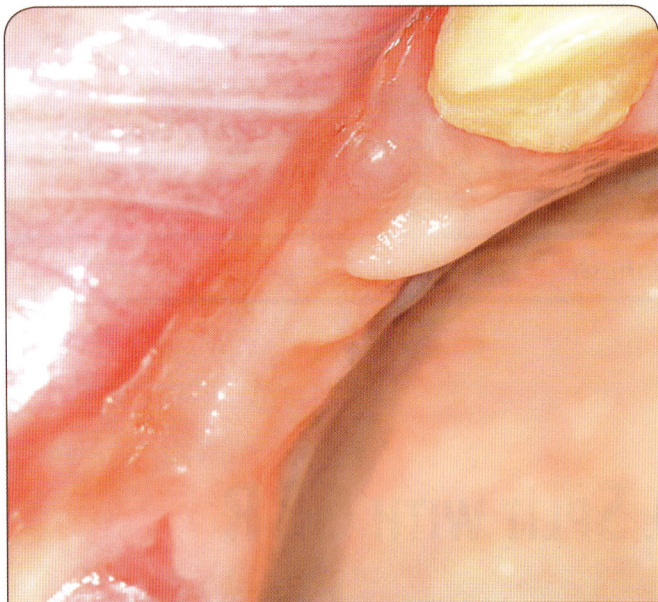

Fig. 1

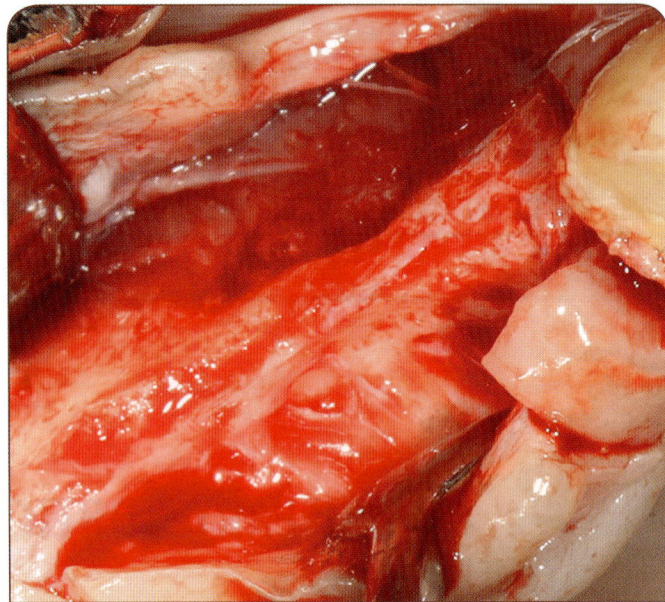

Fig. 2

Preoperative clinical view of a female patient. Aged 60 years. Patient had undergone prior fixture placements in other regions of the maxilla. It is evident from the clinical view and the soft tissue collapse that the bone below would be resorbed to a great extent **(Fig. 1)**.

Options in such cases include:
- A block graft
- Staged GBR
- The above two options involve delayed implant placement after 4–6 months after bone graft maturation
- Split and simultaneous implant placement with GBR which was planned here **(Fig. 2)**.

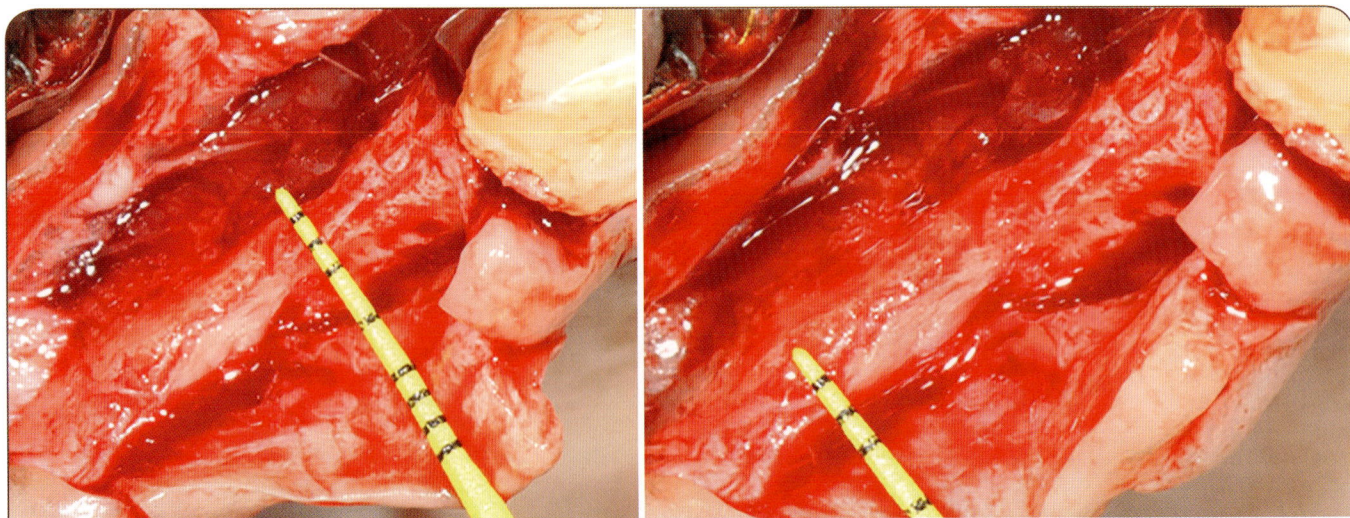

Fig. 3

The width at the crest in both regions of planned implant placement is 2 mm **(Fig. 3)**.

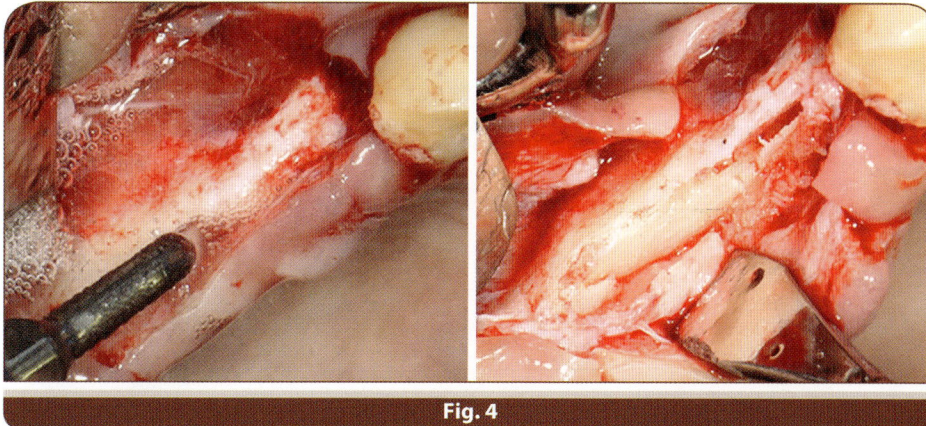

Fig. 4

A saw tip of the piezosurgery unit is used to create the split. (Piezo art—Dowell Dental). The completed split (the main criteria for a cortical split is available height which should at least be 10 mm) **(Fig. 4)**.

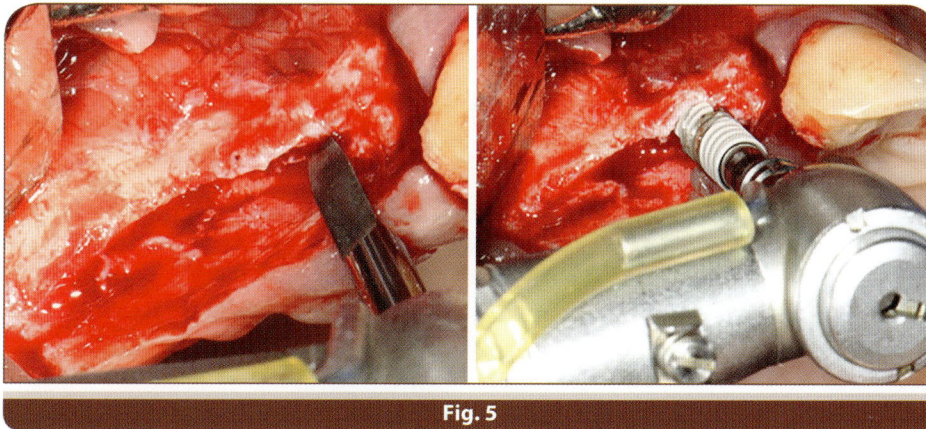

Fig. 5

Lancet/pilot drilling for the mesial implant. This step should have the drill at high speed upto 2500 rpm to prevent 'walkng' of the drill and creating fractures of the facial plate. A Bioner Top DM (Bioner) is inserted at 30 rpm and 50 Ncm torque **(Fig. 5)**.

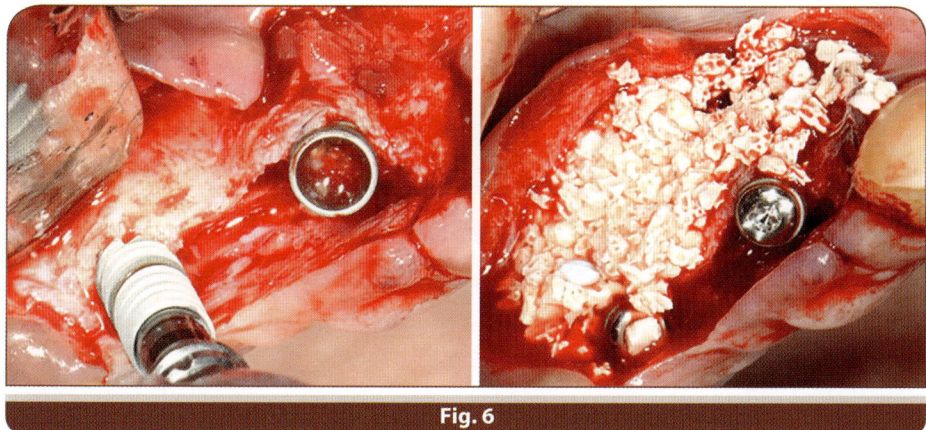

Fig. 6

The design of the implant facilitates the bony cortices to expand without the use of any additional expansion screws or chisels. The area is covered with a DBBM (cerabone-botiss) **(Fig. 6)**.

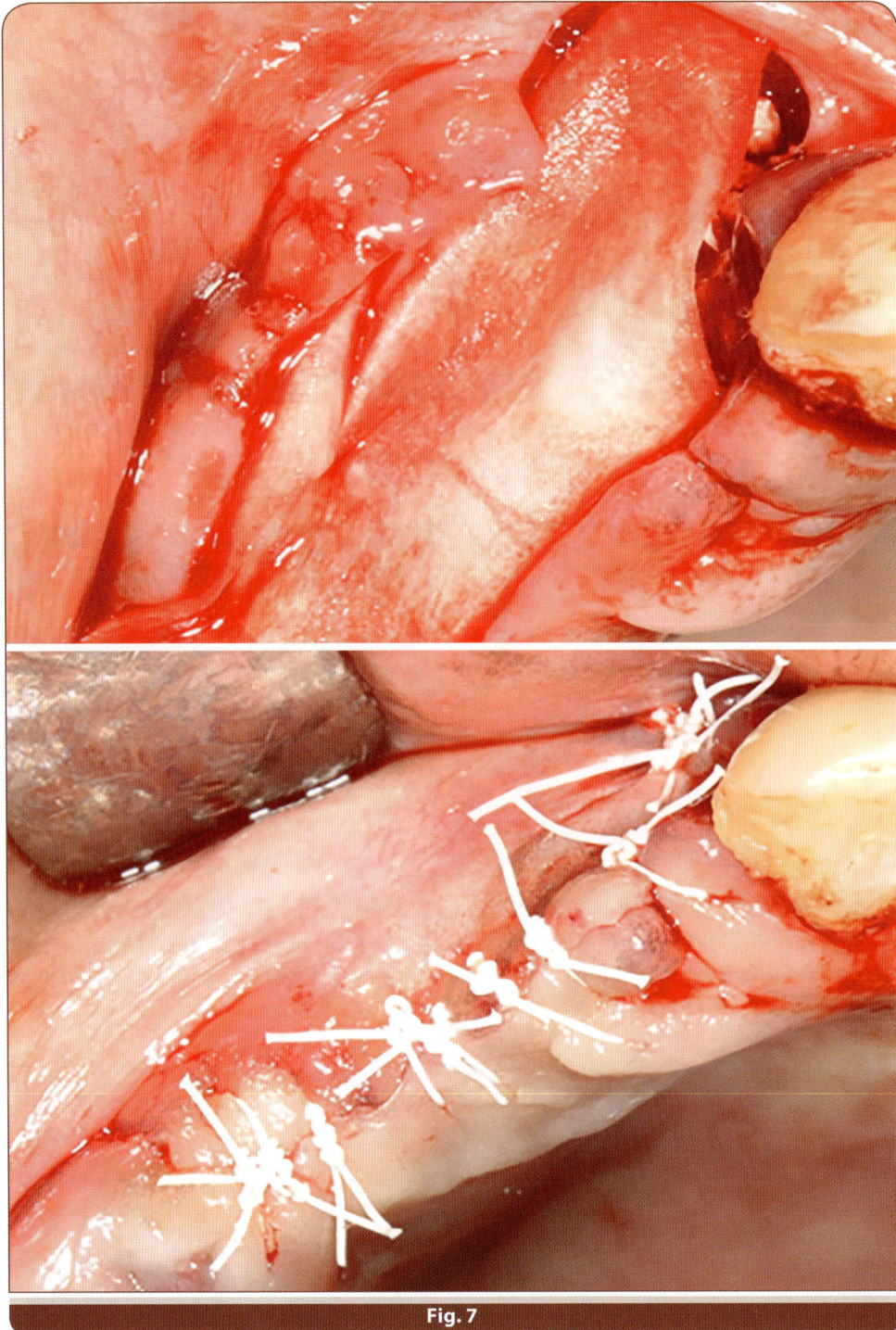

Fig. 7

The operated site is covered with a resorbable collagen membrane (Jason pericardium membrane-botiss). Closure is attained with 3–0 cytoplast sutures **(Fig. 7)**.

Praful Bali

BONE AUGMENTATION WITH AUTOGENOUS BONE SCRAPINGS FOR ABSENCE OF BUCCAL BONE IN THE CENTRAL INCISOR AREA

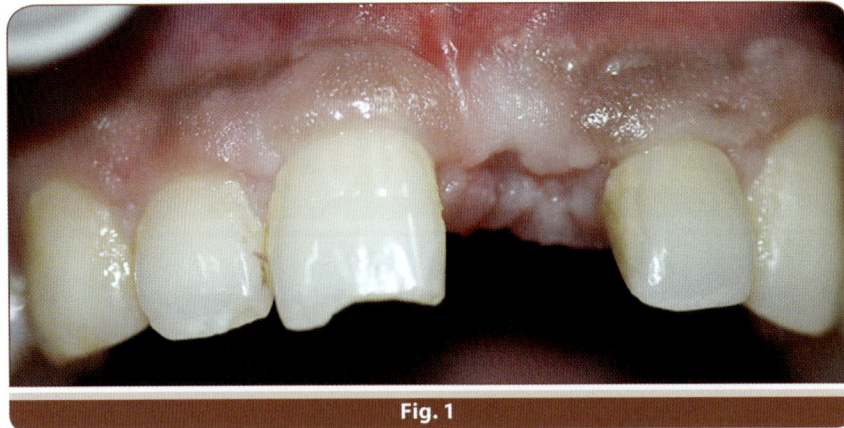

Fig. 1

A clinical surmisation of gingivo-osseous alterations for an indefectible upshot. Patient's smile disported a missing central incisor accompanied with flexous gingival tissue. A closer look revealed defalcated cortical plates, that had to be amended for an optimal rehabilitation **(Fig. 1)**.

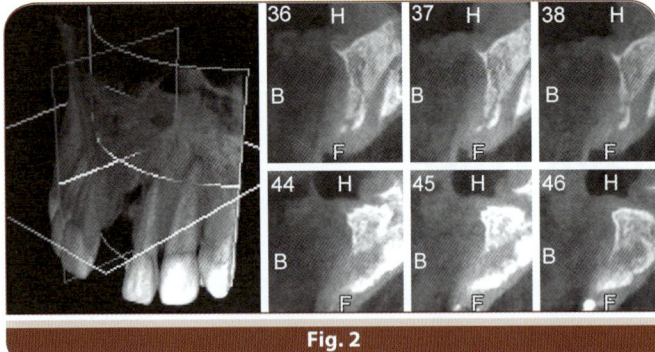

Fig. 2

CBCT images were wielded for an accurate diagnosis **(Fig. 2)**.

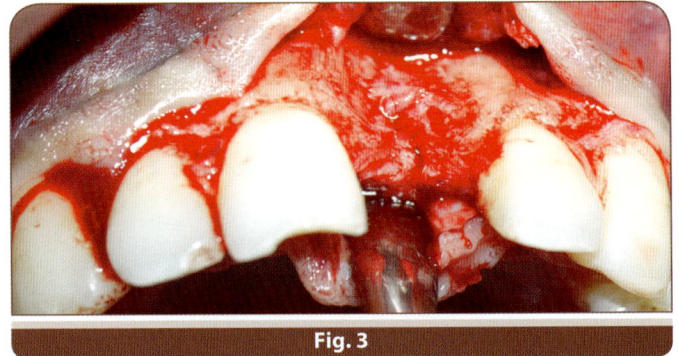

Fig. 3

A full thickness mucoperiosteal flap was raised, the underlying bony architecture was evaluated and the surgical osteotomy was prepared **(Fig. 3)**.

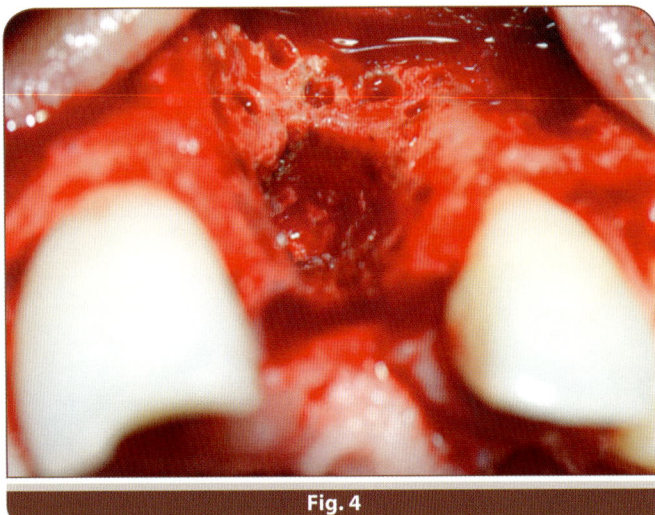

Fig. 4

The labial cortical plate superior to the osteotomy was honeycombed for hybridization with the bone graft burst **(Fig. 4)**.

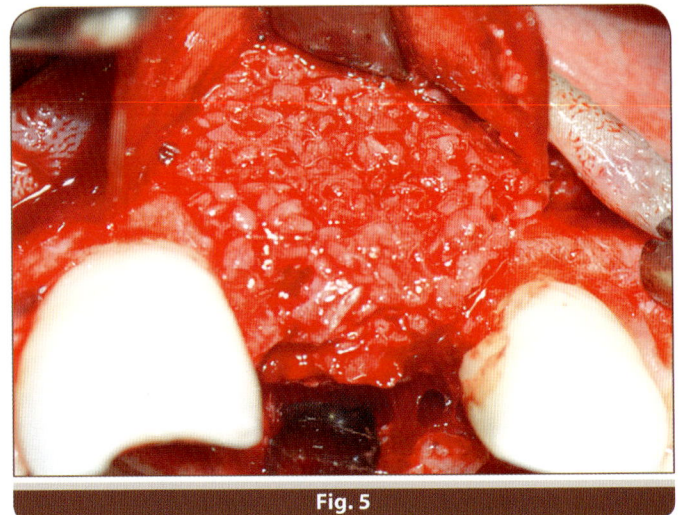

Fig. 5

Cortical bone scrapings were augmented to the host bed and GBR was completed using a resorbable membrane **(Fig. 5)**.

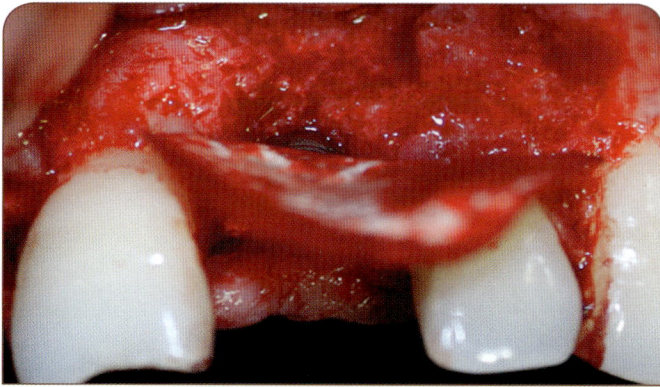

Fig. 6

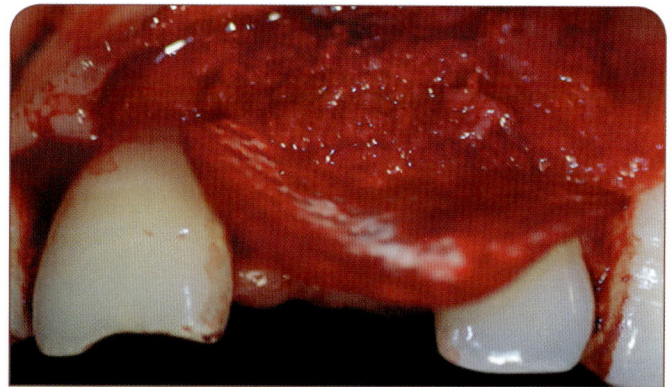

Fig. 7

The site was revisited after 4 months of healing and 3.5/ 13 mm implant was placed in the 3D position vertically and horizontally. Slight augmentation was performed again and regain the bone esthetics to the fullest (**Fig. 6**).

Cortical bone scrapings were augmented again and GBR completed (**Fig. 7**).

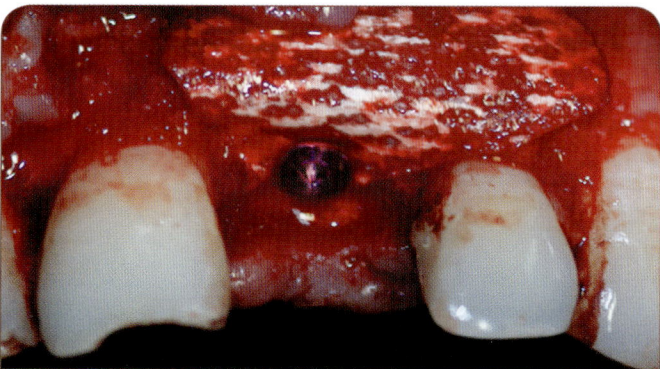

Fig. 8

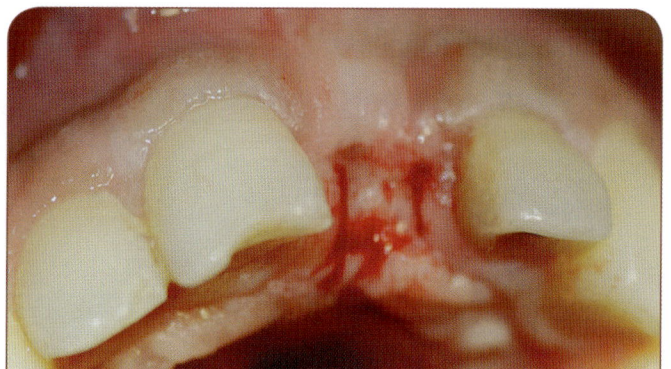

Fig. 9

The endosteal implant was immured, taking cognisance of the final prosthesis (**Fig. 8**).

After 4 months of osseointegration soft tissue—'Roll in Tissue' Graft was done to enhance the soft tissue esthetics (**Fig. 9**).

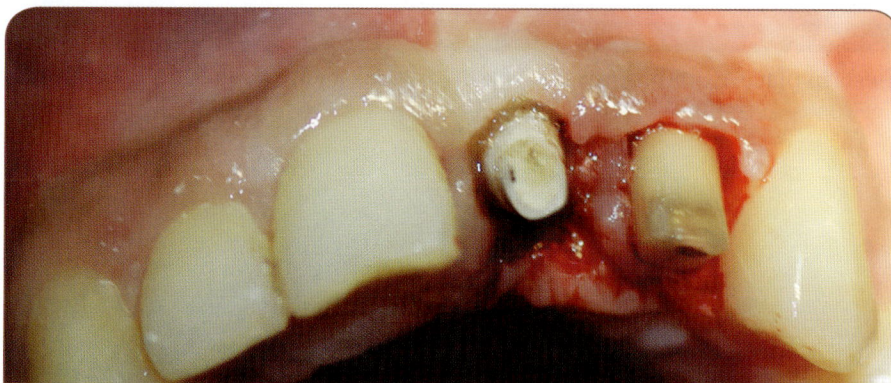

Fig. 10

Post-soft tissue integration, the site was uncloaked, a procera temporary abutment annexed, and as visualized in the picture, the adjacent incisor was prepared (**Fig. 10**).

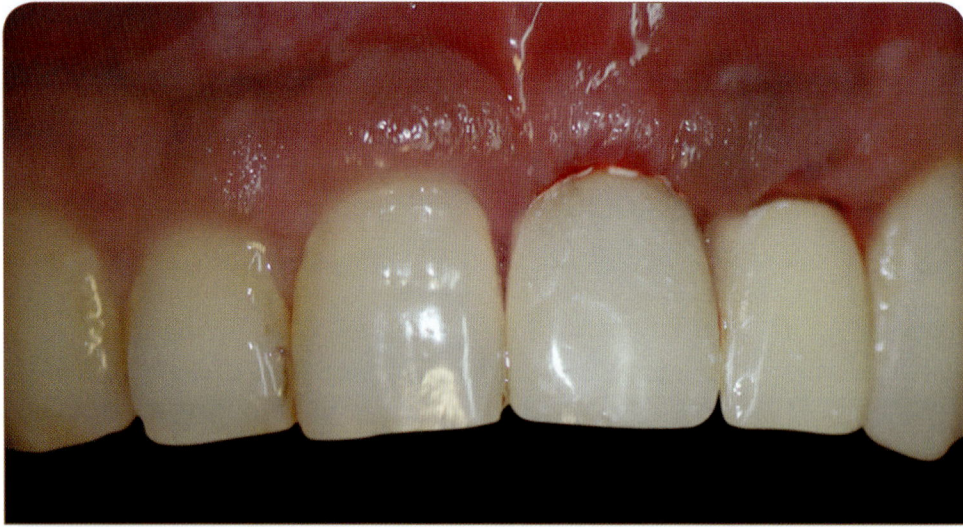

Fig. 11

Interim crowns were appended for an amiable gingival fringe **(Fig. 11)**.

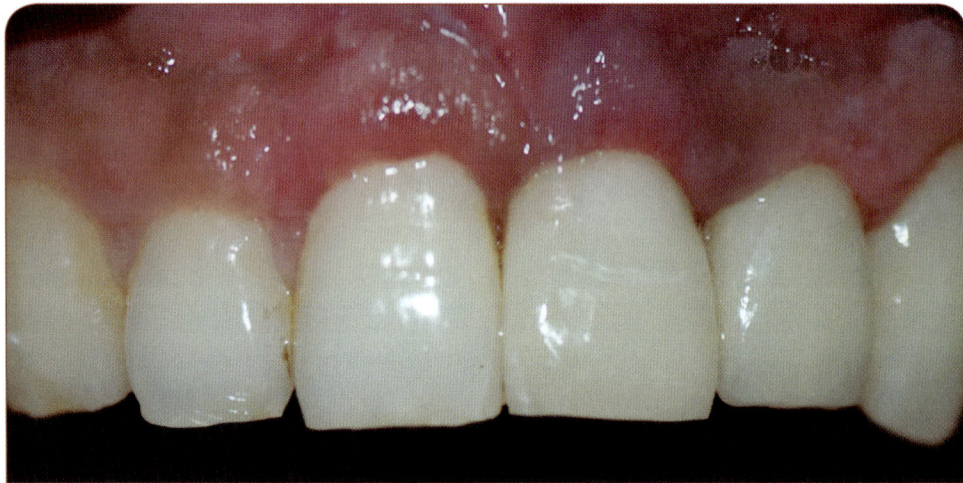

Fig. 12

The final prosthesis in place, exhibiting an ideal osseogingival set off, congruent to our intention **(Fig. 12)**.

Lanka Mahesh, Nitika Poonia

GBR AND SIMULTANEOUS IMPLANT PLACEMENT WITH OSSEODENSIFICATION IN A COMBINED VERTICAL AND HORIZONTAL MAXILLARY DEFECT

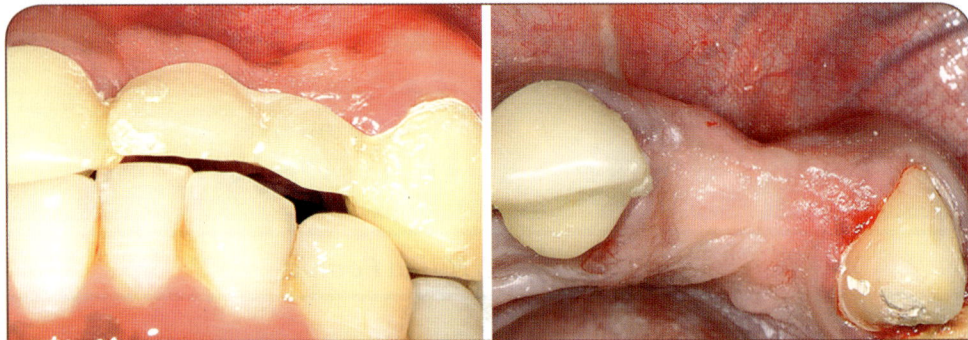

Fig. 1

Preoperative clinical view of a 28-year-old male patient wearing a fixed acrylic resin prosthesis. After removal of the prosthesis the soft tissue defect is evident **(Fig. 1)**.

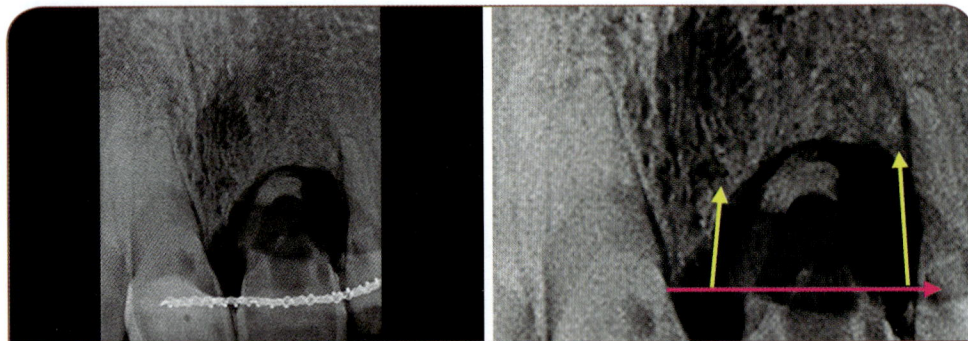

Fig. 2

Radiographs revealed a splinted prosthesis with marked root resorption. The yellow and pink arrows depict the vertical and horizontal defect present (the vertical component is close to 5 mm) **(Fig. 2)**.

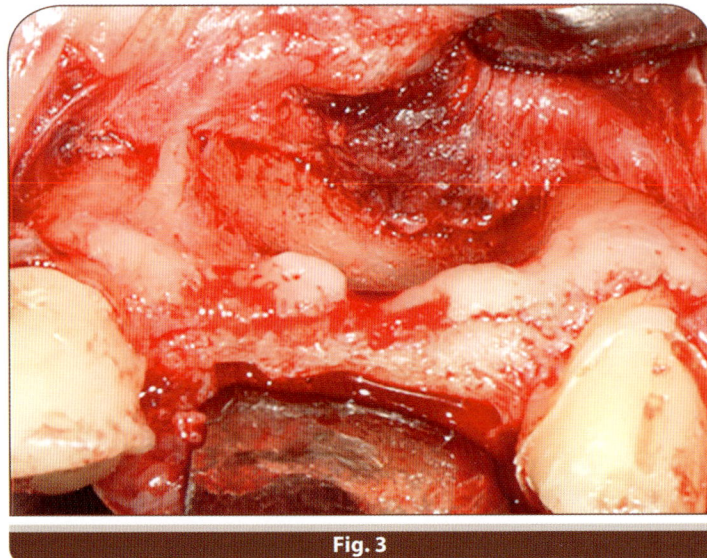

Fig. 3

After a full mucoperiosteal flap is reflected the large defect is clearly seen. An intraoperative decision was made to place simultaneous implants with GBR with a titanium re-enforced EPTFE membrane using Densah osseodensification burs. The burs used in this case **(Fig. 3)**.

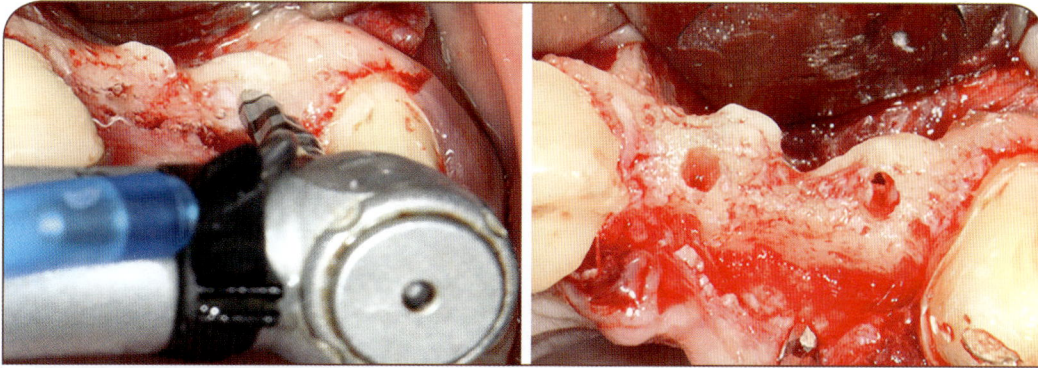

Fig. 4

After pilot bur osteotomy the Densah burs are used in reverse/counter clockwise motion thereby not cutting the bone rather expanding it by osseodensification. Clinical view after the 2.5 mm bur is used **(Fig. 4)**.

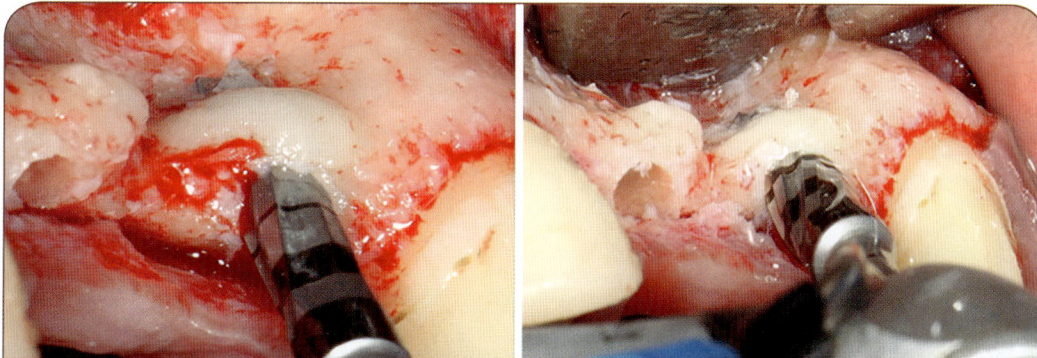

Fig. 5

A 3 mm drill is the last bur used for osteotomy preparation. The bur is clearly visible on the facial wall elucidating a very thin cortical wall **(Fig. 5)**.

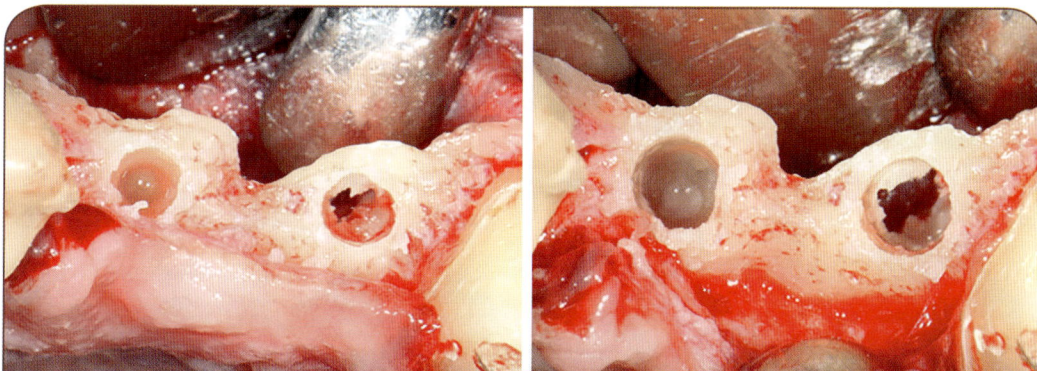

Fig. 6

The osteotomies are enlarged to accommodate a 3.75 mm implant in 21 and 3/11.5 mm implant in 22 (AB). The defect is clearly visible from an occlusal view **(Fig. 6)**.

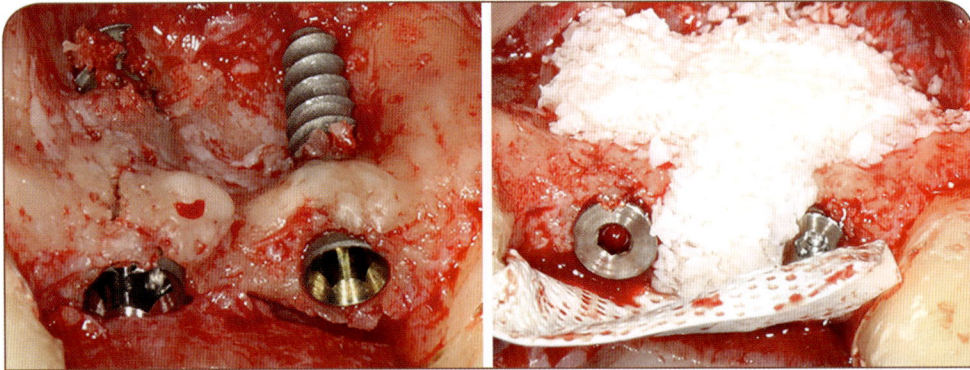

Fig. 7

The implants are inserted at 30 Ncm , a fracture of the facial wall over 21 is evident and a nearly complete exposure of the implant in 22 can be seen. Medium particle DBBM, bio oss (Geistlisch, Sui) is gently packed over the defect in a horizontal and vertical placement **(Fig. 7)**.

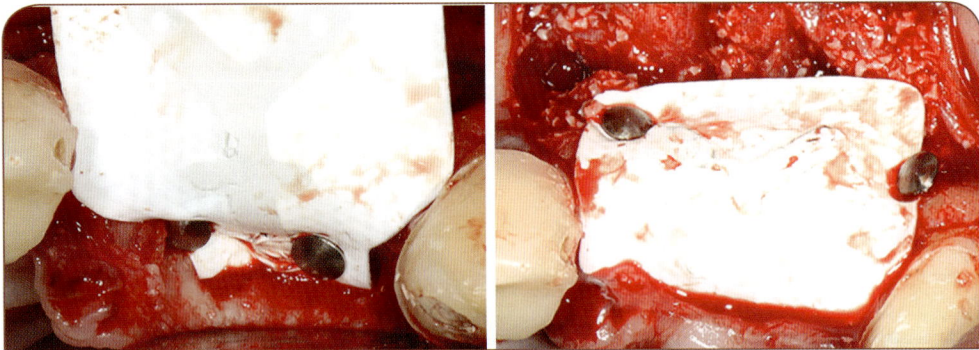

Fig. 8

The membrane is prebent to conform to the defect site. The membrane used in this case. Two membrane tacs (Bioner) are placed palatally to stabilize the membrane prior to graft placement. Two tacs are placed after graft packing to have a completely stable enviornment for the graft to mature **(Fig. 9)**.

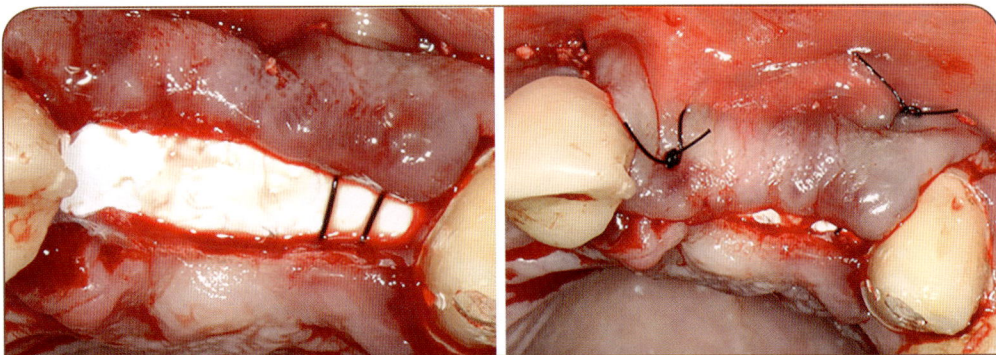

Fig. 9

After a periosteal release incision the flap is approximated with a stabilizing suture at the distal end. Both ends of such flaps are best treated with a horizontal mattress suture to maintain flap passivity and creating a stable suture line **(Fig. 9)**.

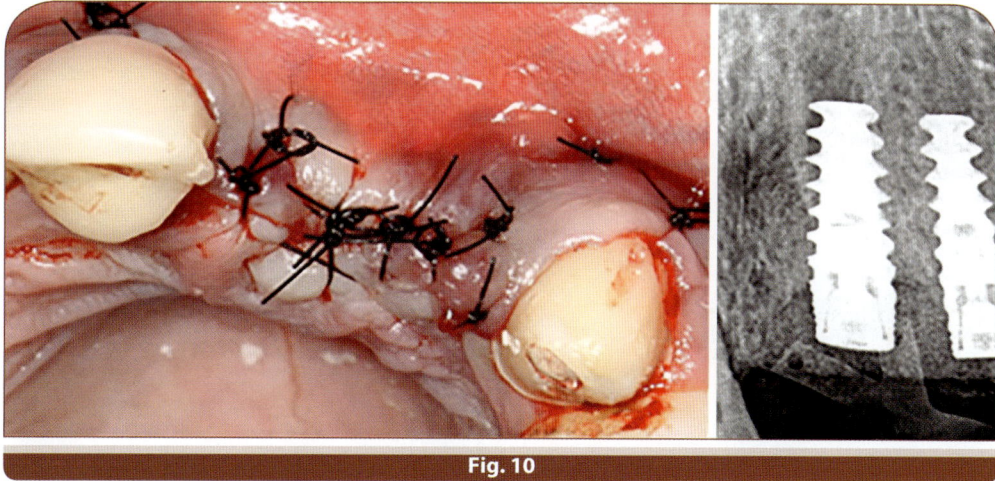

Fig. 10

The wound closure is completed with interuppted sutures. Immediate postoperative radiograph shows implants in correct position and adequate vertical fill of the bone graft **(Fig. 10)**.

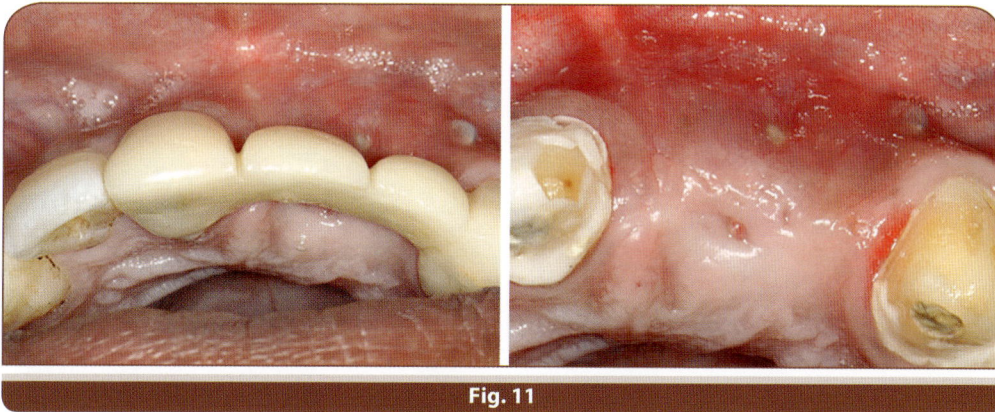

Fig. 11

Five months postoperative view shows good bulk achieved. A tissue tac is visible subgingival (if this happens in the early stages of wound healing it is better to make a minor incision and removing it rather than it causing a tissue dehiscence) **(Fig. 11)**.

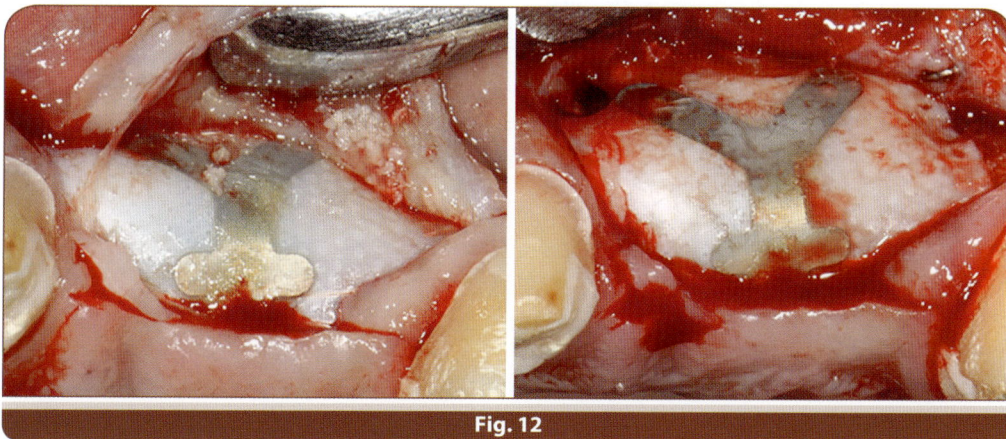

Fig. 12

A papilla preserving incision is made to expose the membrane. A stable membrane is visible which is the most important criteria in a GBR procedure especially with a nonresorbable membrane (The tac visible subgingival can be seen on the inner aspect of the flap) **(Fig. 12)**.

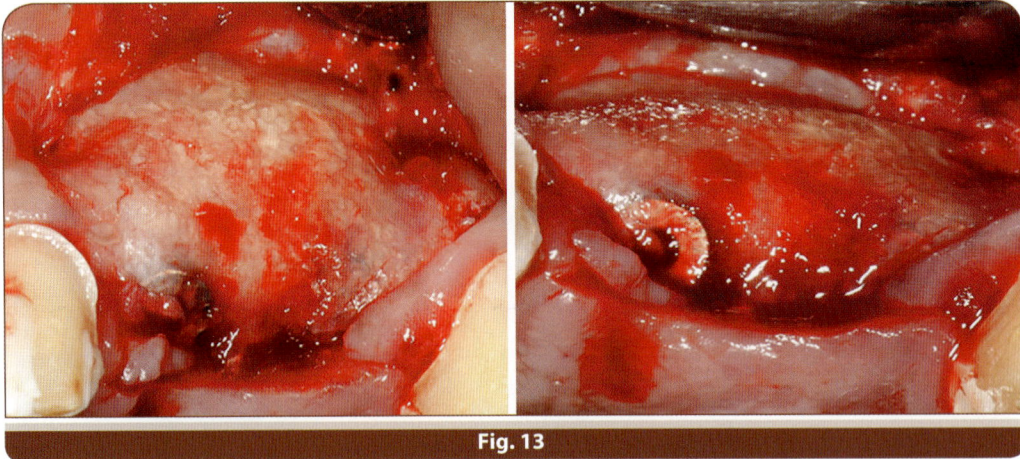

Fig. 13

Excellent healing and a robust graft uptake are evident, the implants are buried within new bone illustrating excellent vertical bone gained (new blood vessels are also seen in the grafted bone). Occlusal view also depicts good volume of bone regeneration **(Fig. 13)**.

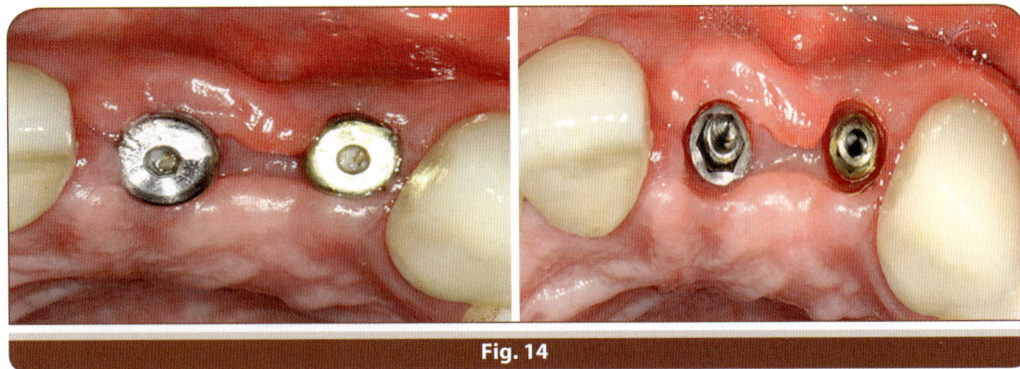

Fig. 14

Two weeks post second stage surgery the tissue is healing well. The 11 and 23 have been restored with individual zirconia crowns and impressions are recorded for the implant fixtures **(Fig. 14)**.

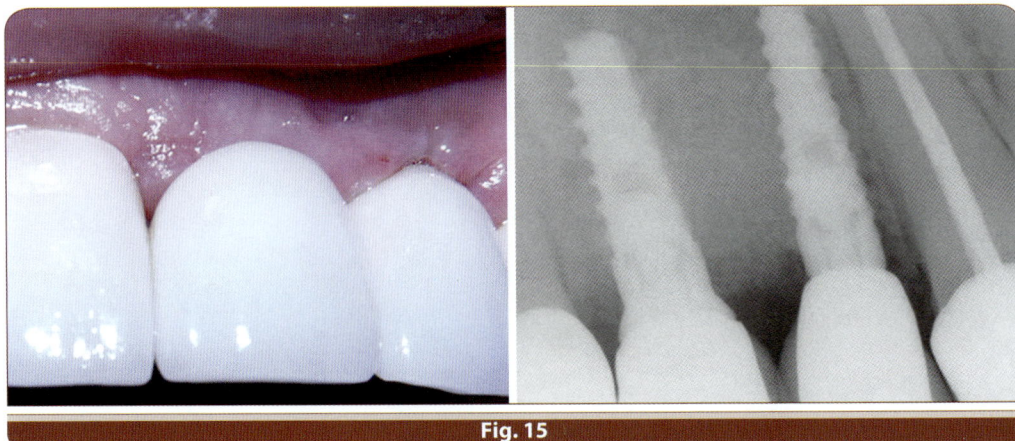

Fig. 15

The prosthesis at insertion (four individual zirconia crowns were fabricated). The final radiograph demonstrates complete vertical bone fill and excellent stability of the regenerated osseous tissue **(Fig. 15)**.

Cary Bopiah

RECONSTRUCTION OF THE ANTERIOR MAXILLA WITH AN AUTOGENOUS BLOCK GRAFT FROM THE RAMUS

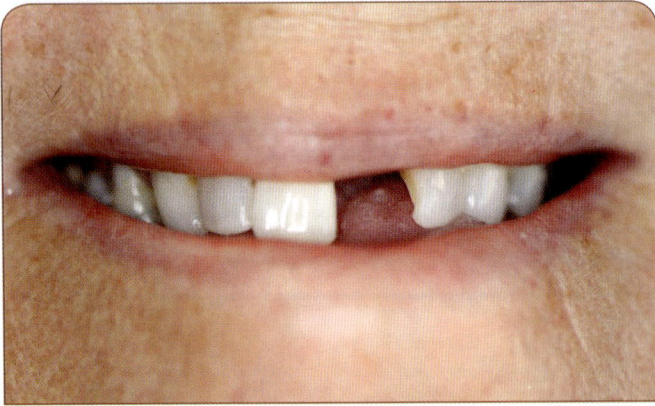

Fig. 1

Preoperative view of patient smiling showing a low lip line **(Fig. 1)**.

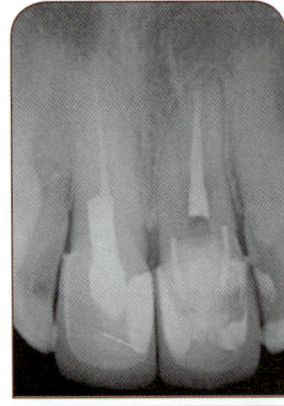

Fig. 2

Routine radiograph taken of the tooth#11 and tooth #21 region. The tooth #21 shows not canal treatment and a composite coronal restoration supported by dentine pins **(Fig. 2)**.

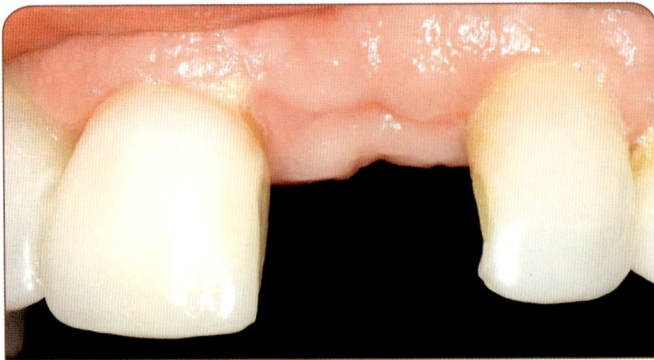

Fig. 3

Intraoral view of the upper left central incisor region **(Fig. 3)**.

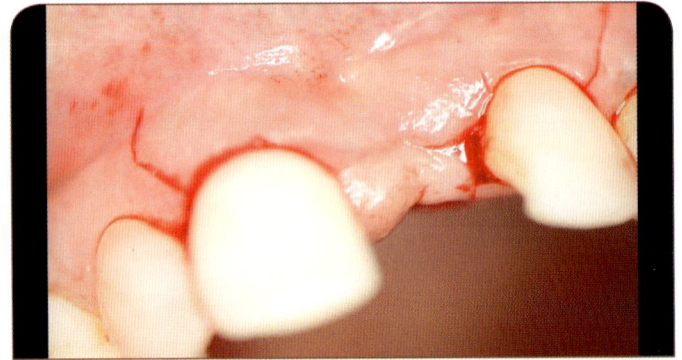

Fig. 4

Outline of the remote palatal incision with vertical relieving incisions made opposite the upper right central incisor and upper left lateral incisor **(Fig. 4)**.

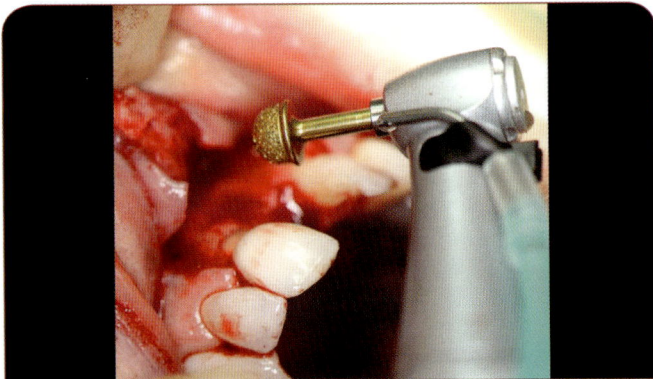

Fig. 5

Site exposure and smoothening of bony irregularities with a DASK bur (Implantium) **(Fig. 5)**.

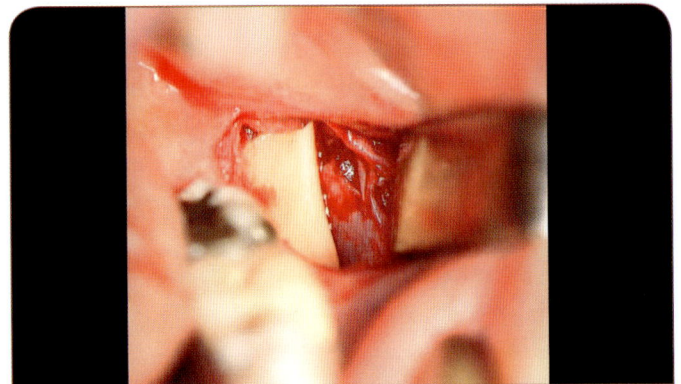

Fig. 6

Exposure of the donor site (left ramus) **(Fig. 6)**.

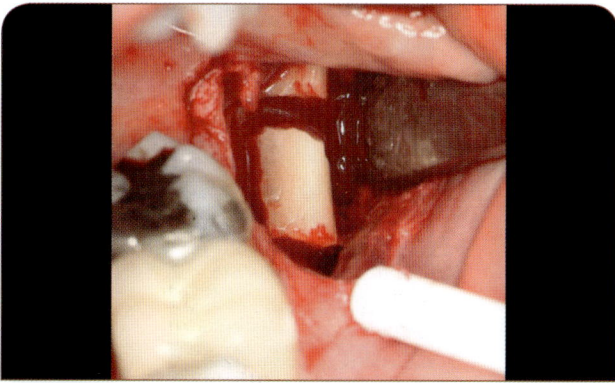

Fig. 7

Completed osteotomy for the left ramus J-shaped block graft **(Fig. 7)**.

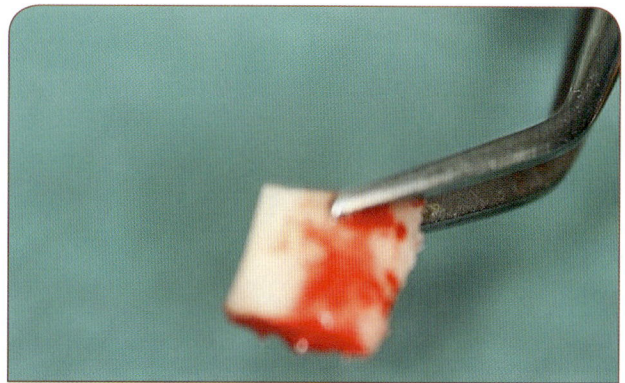

Fig. 8

Harvested ramus graft **(Fig. 8)**.

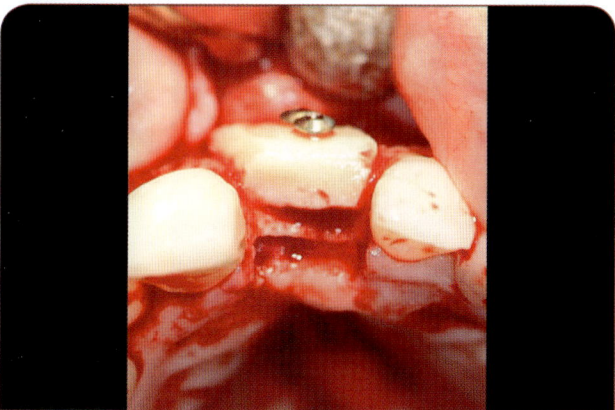

Fig. 9

Ramus graft secured to the recipient site and held with bone screws. **(Fig. 9)**.

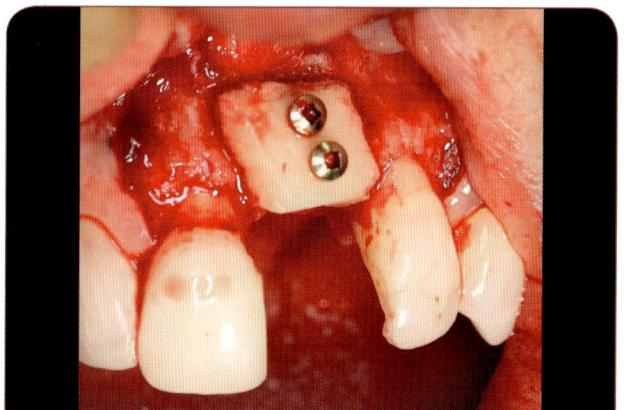

Fig. 10

Labial view of the ramus graft secured to the recipient site **(Fig. 10)**.

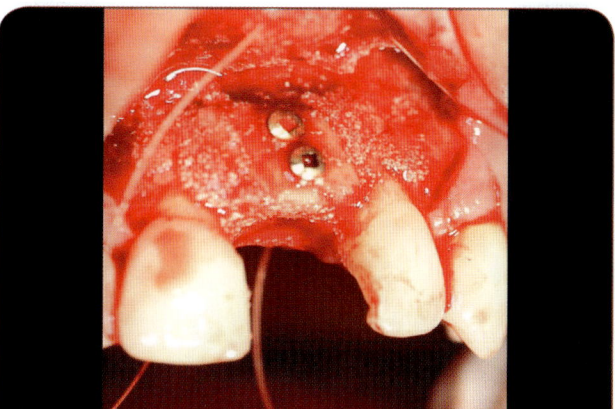

Fig. 11

Voids filled with particles of synthetic bone (SynthoGraft, Bicon) **(Fig. 11)**.

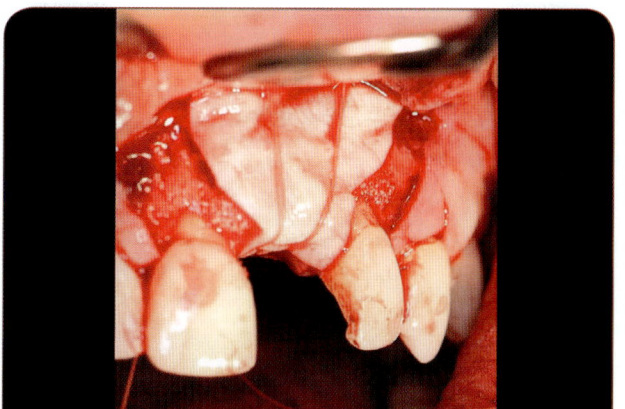

Fig. 12

Grafted site covered with a membrane (Bio-Gide, Geistlich) **(Fig. 12)**.

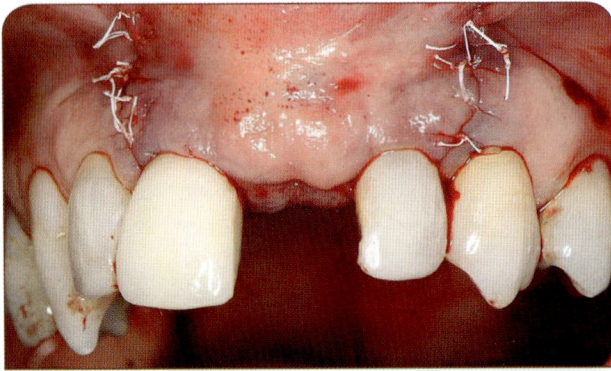

Fig. 13

Grafted site closed with 5-0 polytetrafluoroethylene sutures **(Fig. 13)**.

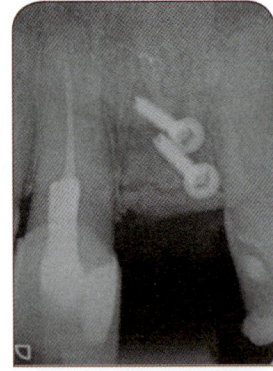

Fig. 14

Radiograph on the day of ramus grafting graft held in place with bone pins **(Fig. 14)**.

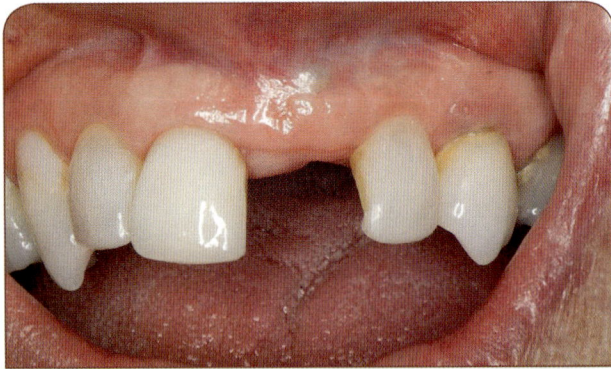

Fig. 15

Healed site 5 months after grafting, the shadow of the bone screws are visible **(Fig. 15)**.

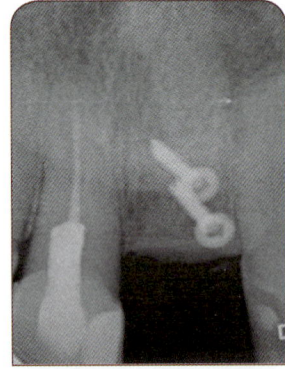

Fig. 16

Five month postoperative radiographic view, notice a more homogeneous appearance of the graft with the recipient site **(Fig. 16)**.

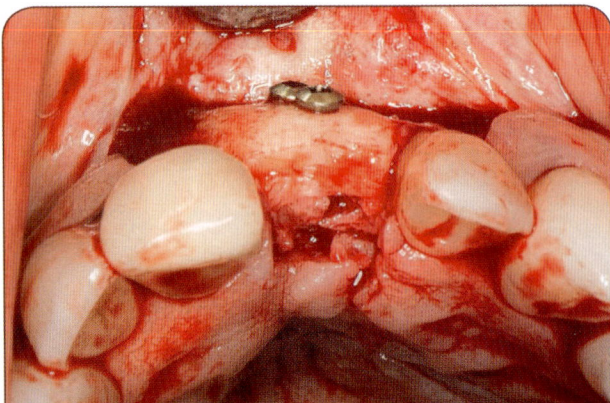

Fig. 17

Occlusal view of the exposed tooth 21 region **(Fig. 17)**.

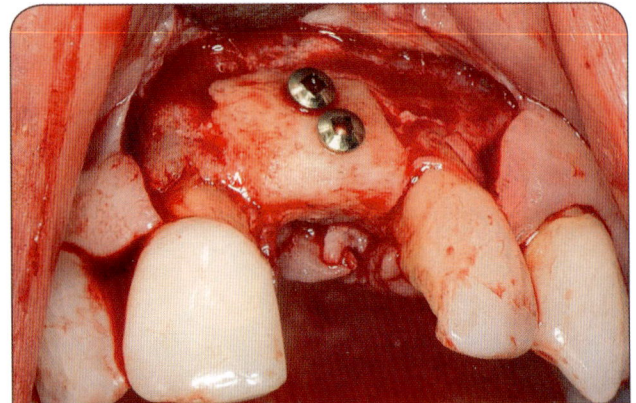

Fig. 18

Osteotomy made 2/3rds in the ramus graft and 1/3rd on the recipient bone **(Fig. 18)**.

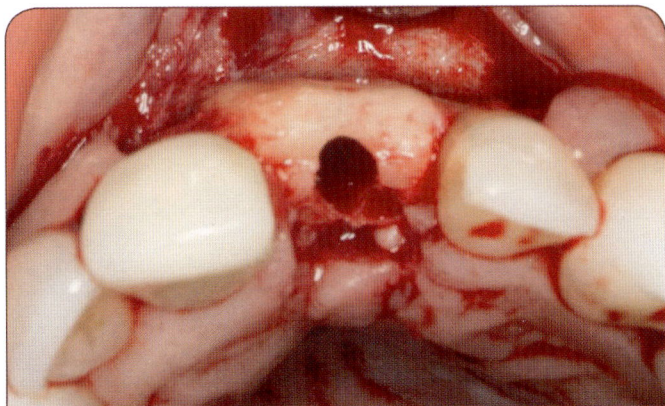

Fig. 19

Labial view of the grafted site **(Fig. 19)**.

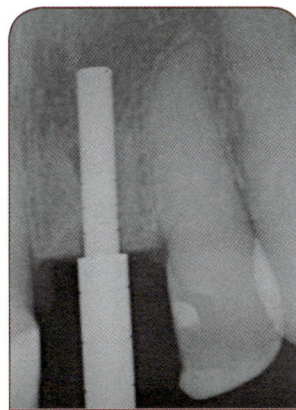

Fig. 20

Periapical radiograph of a guide pin in the tooth#21 region **(Fig. 20)**.

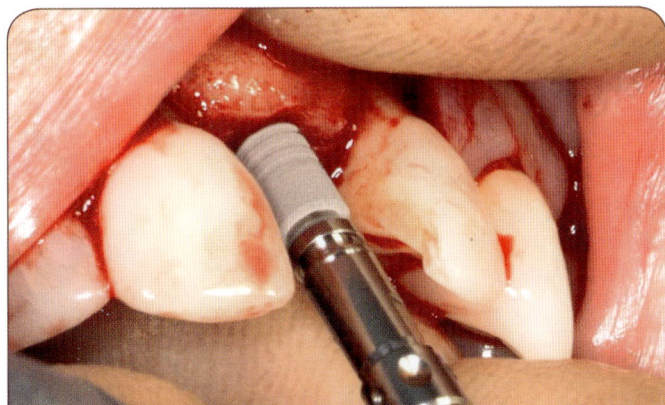

Fig. 21

Insertion of an Ankylos (Dentsply) Implant **(Fig. 21)**.

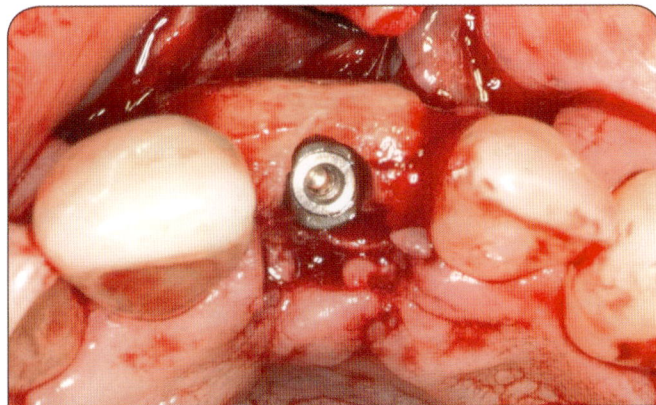

Fig. 22

Implant placed 1 mm subcrestal, in line with the cingulum of the adjacent upper right central incisor **(Fig. 22)**.

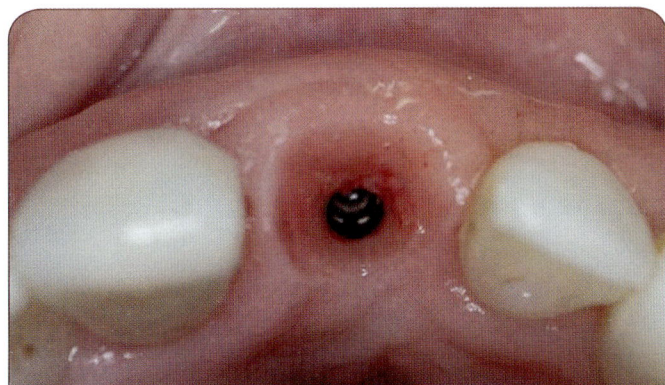

Fig. 23

Occlusal view of the 21 region after site development the labial profile of the site shows a healthy common curvature **(Fig. 23)**

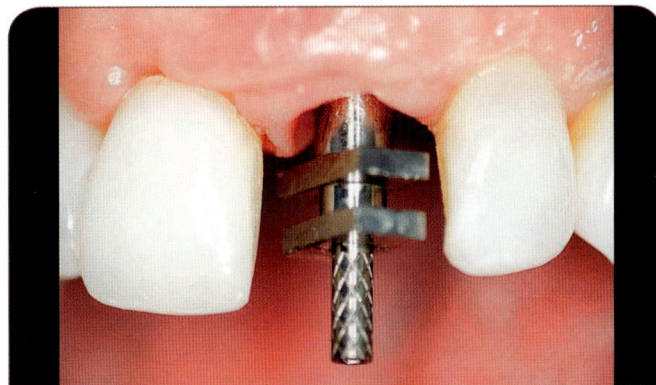

Fig. 24

Transfer post secured to the body of the implant for final impressions after site development was completed with temporary abutment and temporary acrylic crown **(Fig. 24)**.

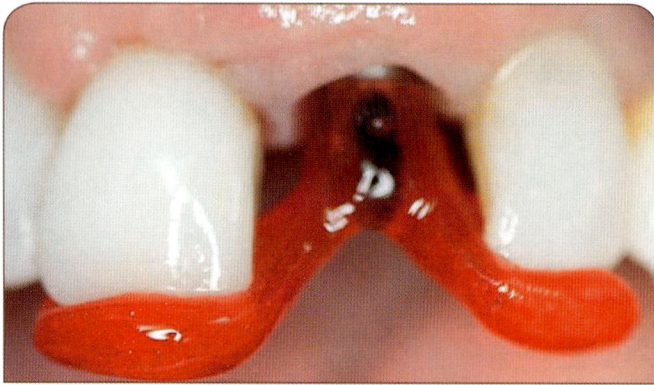

Fig. 25

Duralay jig used to index the abutment (**Fig. 25**).

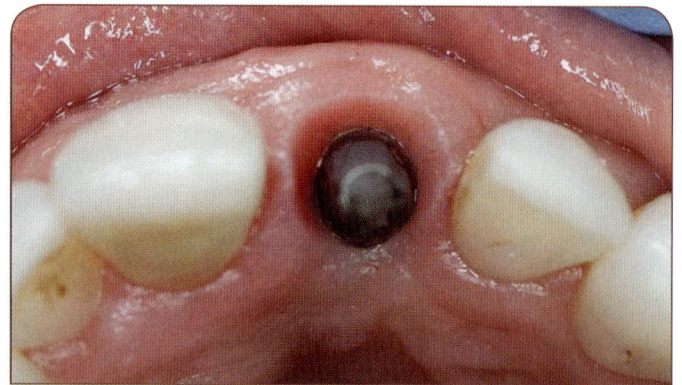

Fig. 26

Occlusal view of the abutment with emergence in line with the ingulum of the adjacent upper right central incisor (**Fig. 26**).

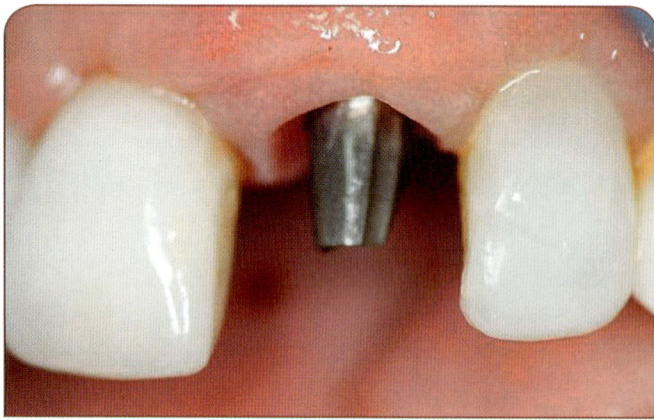

Fig. 27

Implant abutment in position (**Fig. 27**).

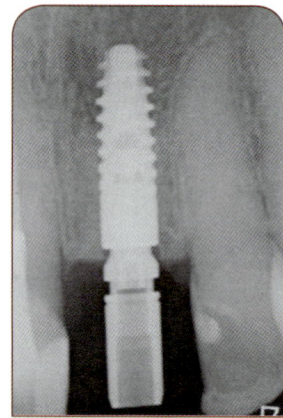

Fig. 28

Implant abutment in position (**Fig. 28**).

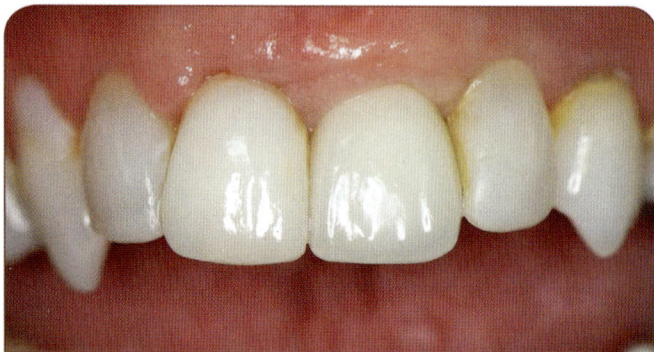

Fig. 29

Intraoral view of porcelain bonded crown on the implant in the tooth #21 region (**Fig. 29**).

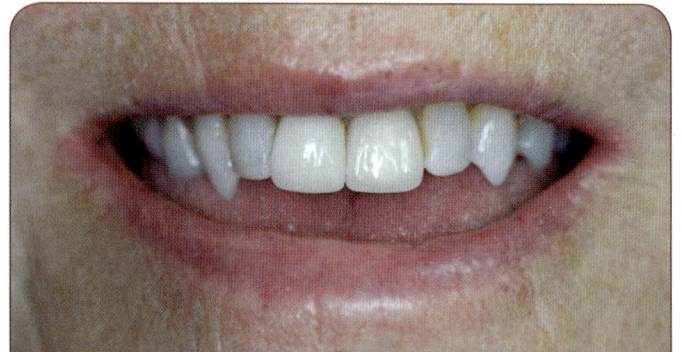

Fig. 30

Extraoral view of patient smiling (**Fig. 30**).

Lanka Mahesh, Vishal Gupta

Horizontal and Vertical Ridge Augmentation with Simultaneous Implant Placement

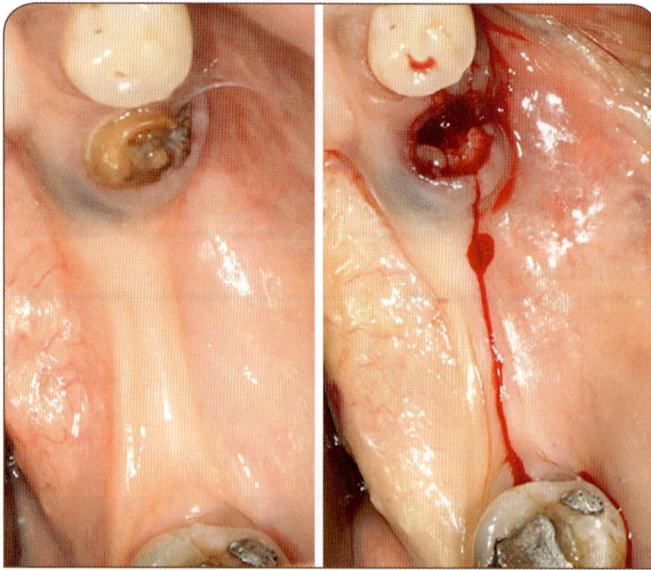

Fig. 1

Baseline situation. Root stump extracted. Mid crestal incision extending one tooth mesial and one tooth distal to operating site **(Fig. 1)**.

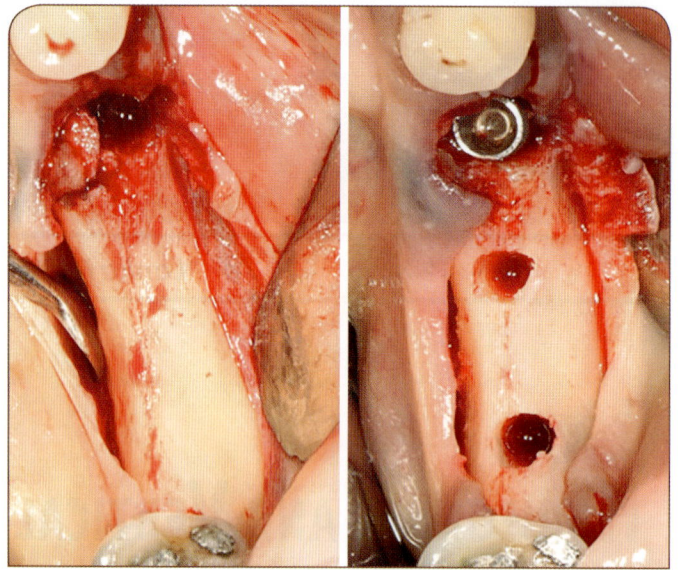

Fig. 2

Buccal and lingual flap reflected. Nobel Active (Nobel Biocare) 4.3/11.5 placed in extraction socket. Osteotomy prepared for implant in teeth #36 and 37 **(Fig. 2)**.

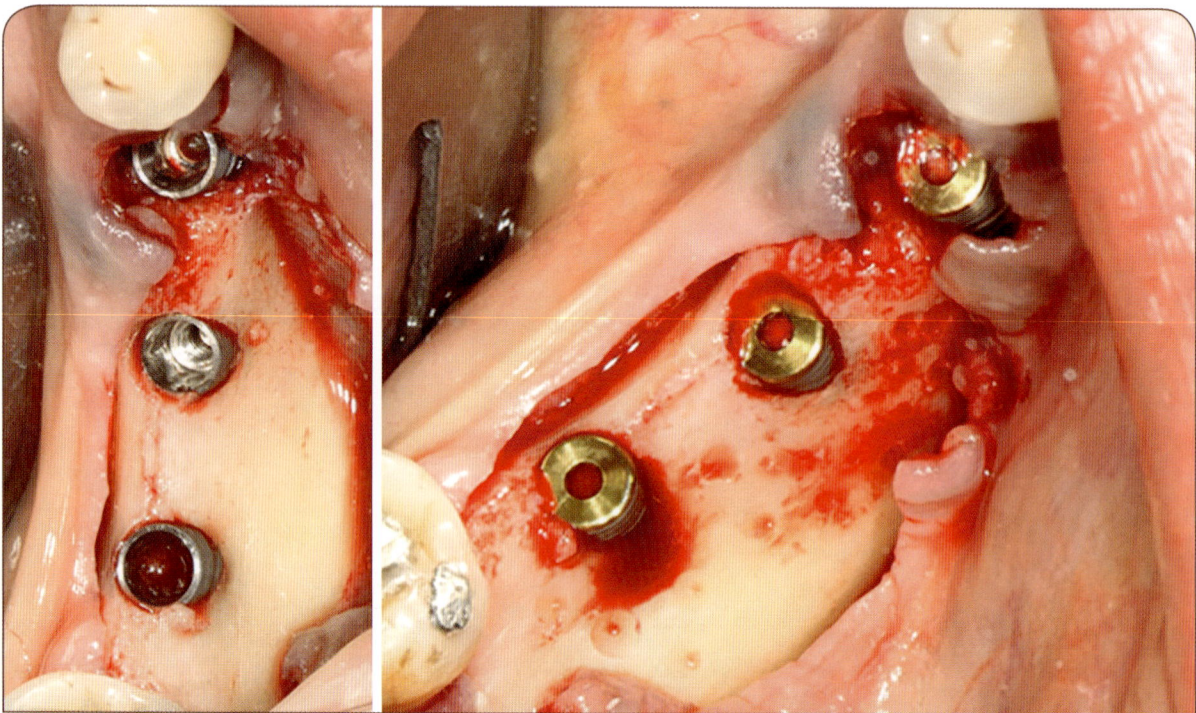

Fig. 3

Nobel Active (Nobel bio care) 4.3/10 placed at 36 and 37 area. Horizontal and vertical bone defect evident **(Fig. 3)**.

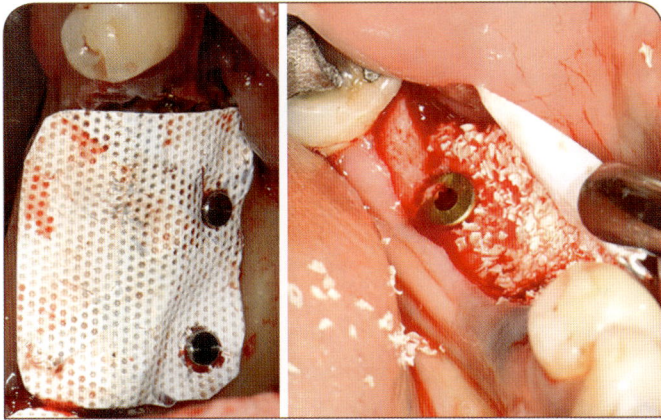

Fig. 4

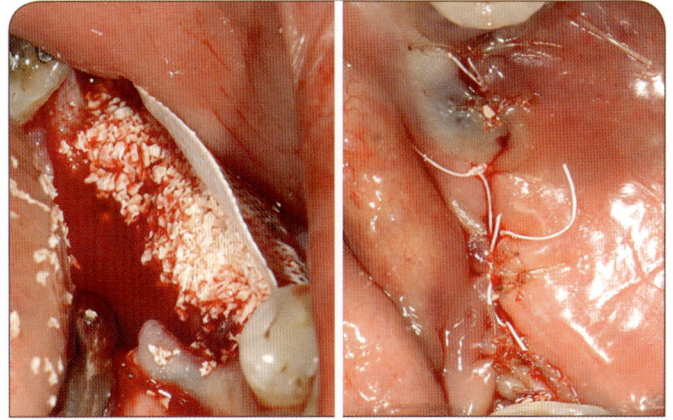

Fig. 5

Cytoplast XL (Osteogenics) stabilized with tacs (Bioner). Cerabone (Botiss) graft placed after decortication to fill the defect **(Fig. 4)**.

Complete filling of the area with graft is noted. Water tight sutures Cytoplast 3–0 (Osteogenics) **(Fig. 5)**.

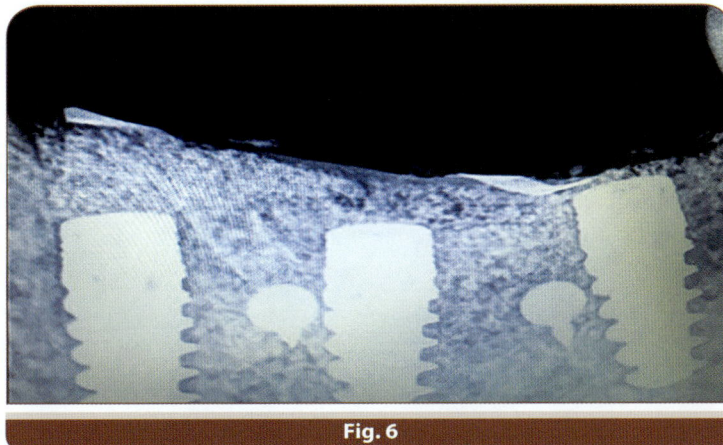

Fig. 6

Immediate postoperative RVG shows complete fill of defects and tacs can also be seen **(Fig. 6)**.

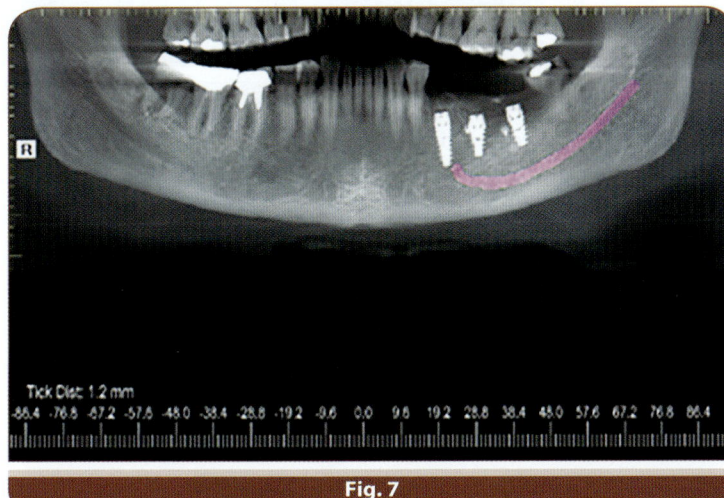

Fig. 7

6 months post of CBCT **(Fig. 7)**.

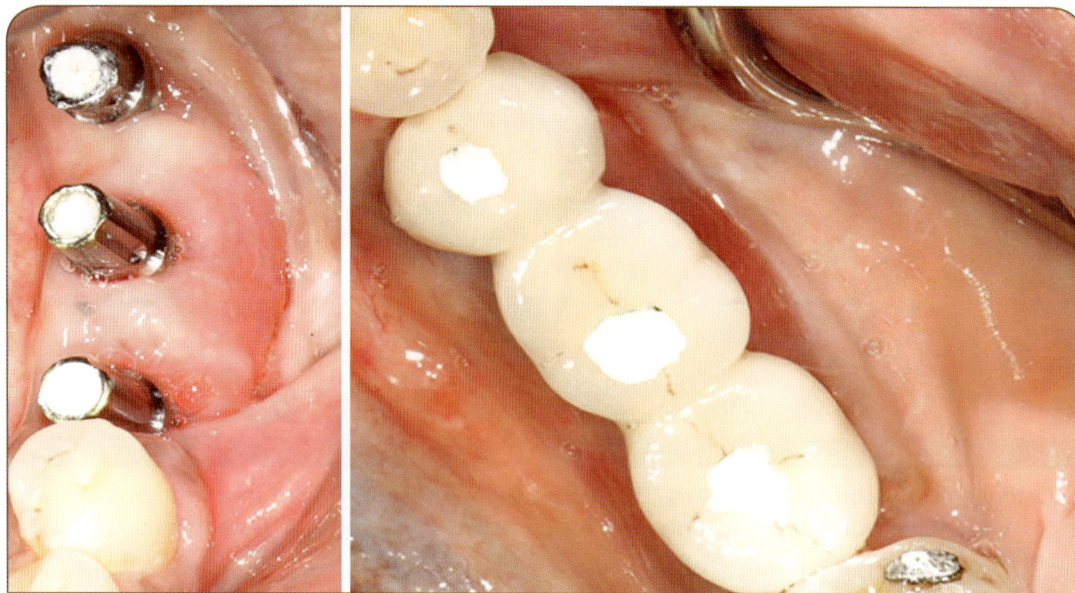

Fig. 8

Abutment placed and torqued to 30 N cm. Cemented crowns with Implant cement (Premier), occlusal vents closed with cavit (3M) for 3 weeks and eventually changed to light cure compost (3M) **(Fig. 8)**.

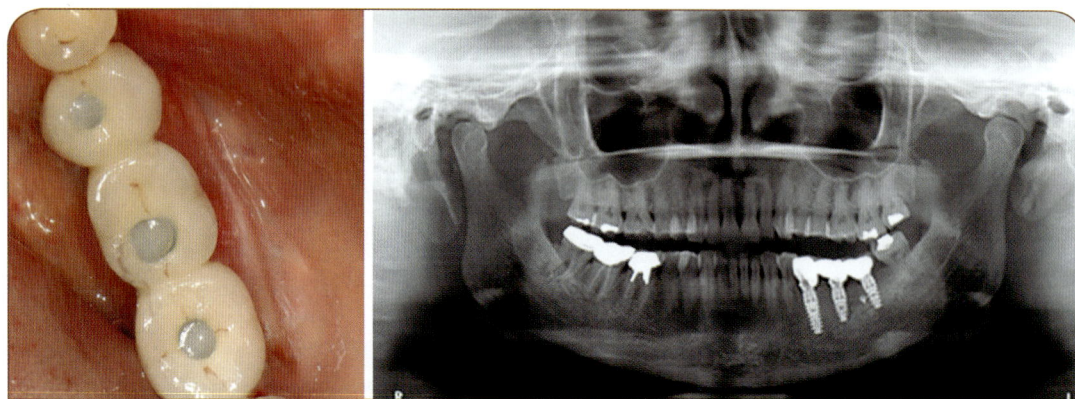

Fig. 9

Two years postoperative clinical view and X-ray **(Fig. 9)**.

Tarun Kumar

Horizontal Ridge Augmentation using Autogeneous Block Bone Graft Followed by Implant Placement

Female patient, 22 years of age reported with the chief complaint of missing upper right front tooth and wanted replacement for the same. There was no contributory past medical and dental history.

The treatment plan included ridge augmentation using autogenous block graft harvested from the chin, followed by placement of implant after 4 months of grafting post.

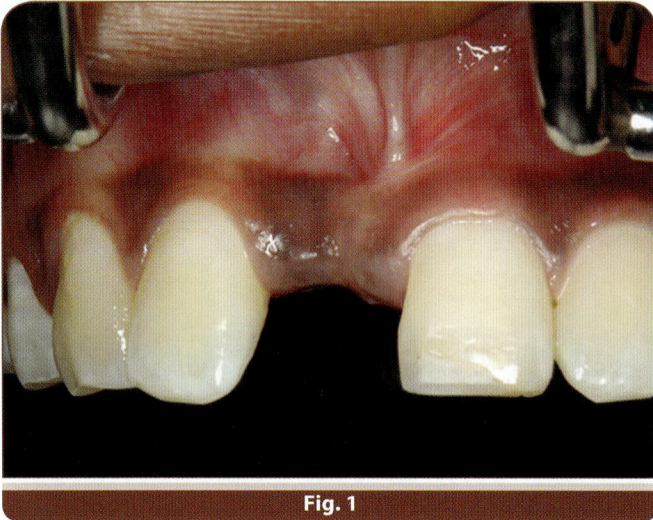

Fig. 1

Preoperative labial view of the surgical site—view of the edentulous gap and the soft tissue condition **(Fig. 1)**.

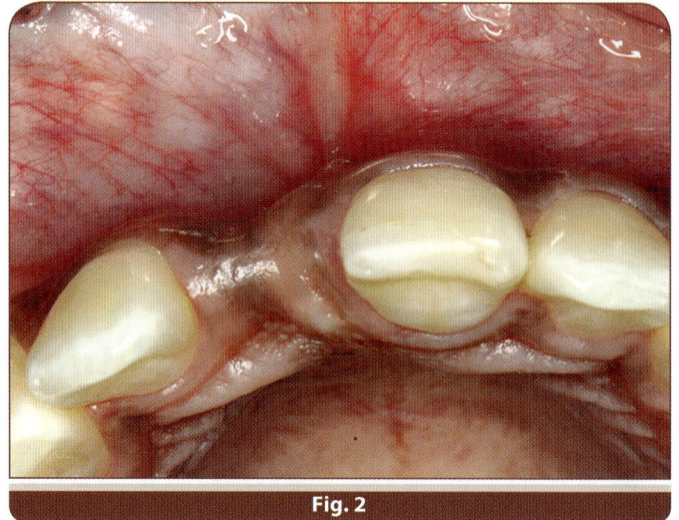

Fig. 2

Preoperative occlusal view of the surgical site tooth #11 **(Fig. 2)**.

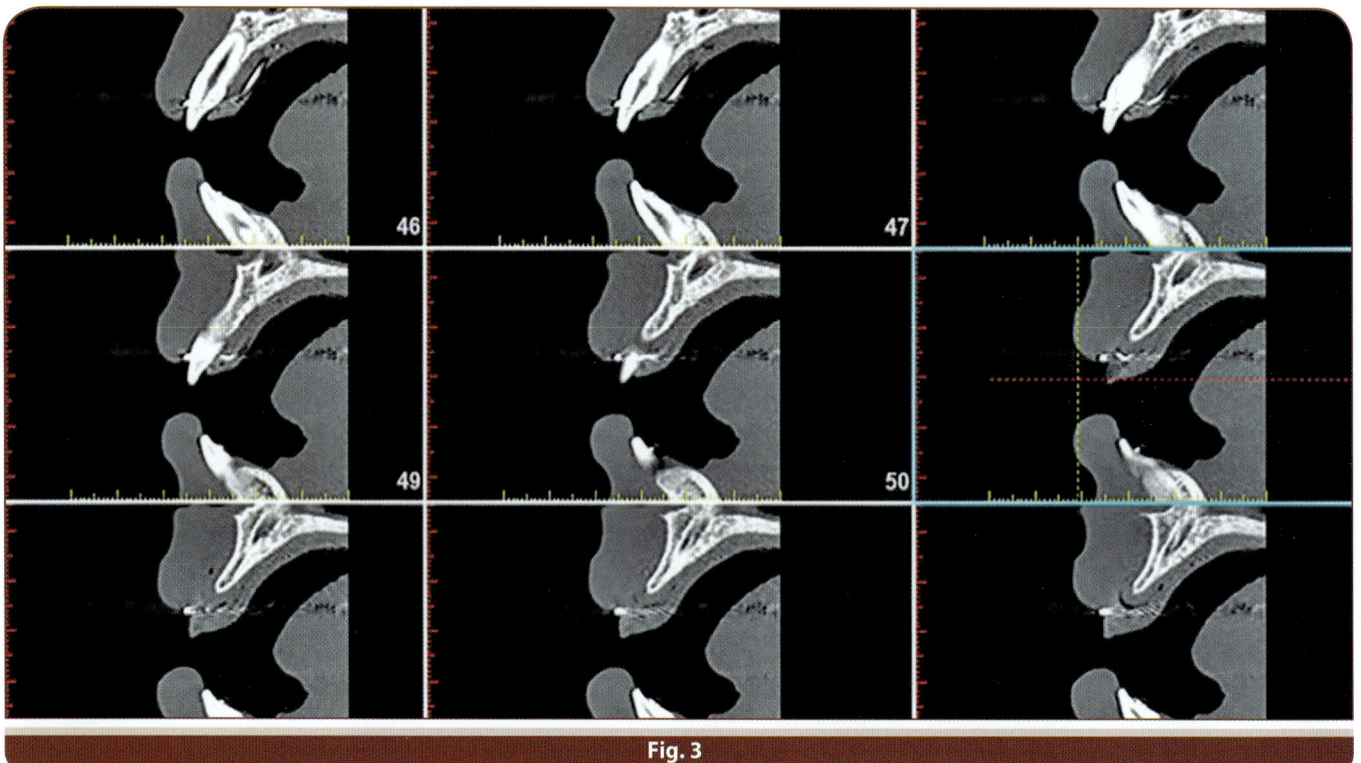

Fig. 3

CBCT showing Seibert's class I deficiency **(Fig. 3)**.

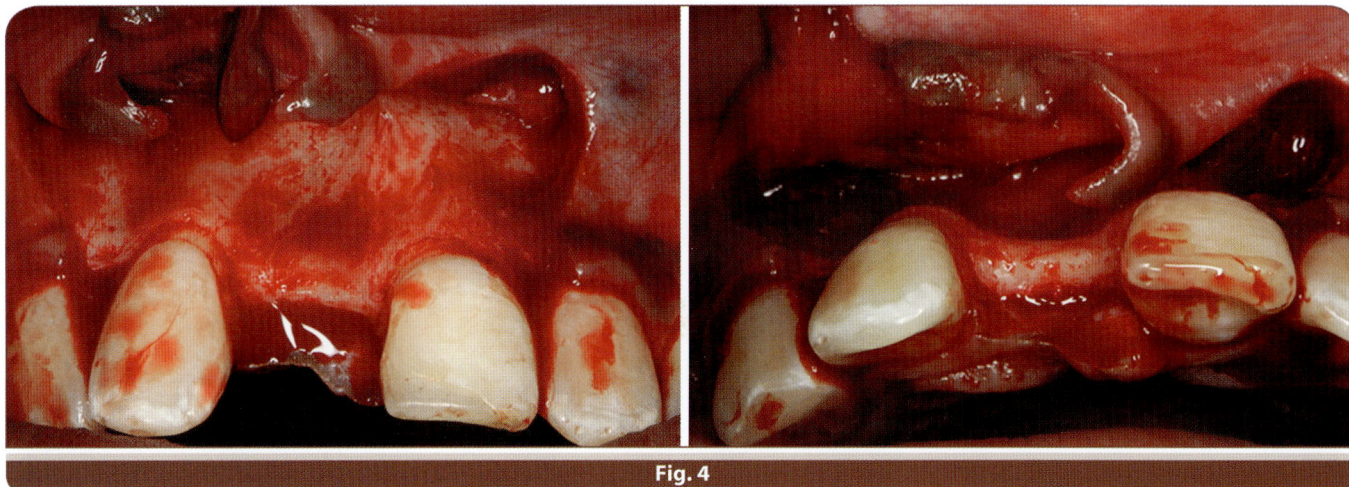

Fig. 4

Intraoperative labial and occlusal view of ridge width depicting the Seibert's class I ridge deficiency after full thickness flap reflection utilizing mid Crestal and vertical releasing incision **(Fig. 4)**.

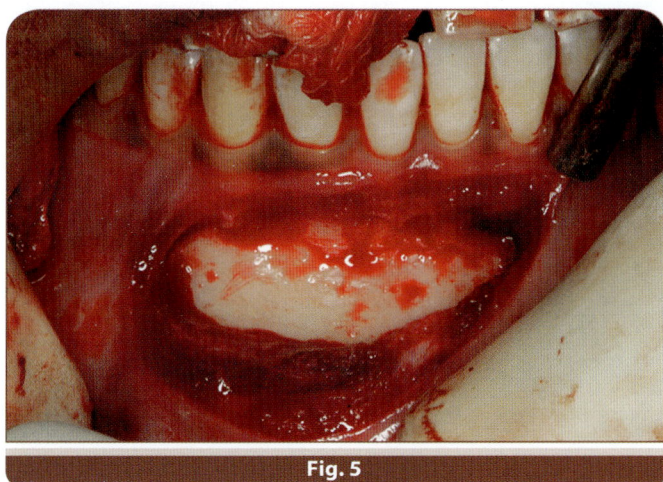

Fig. 5

Intraoperative view of the donor site (chin) **(Fig. 5)**.

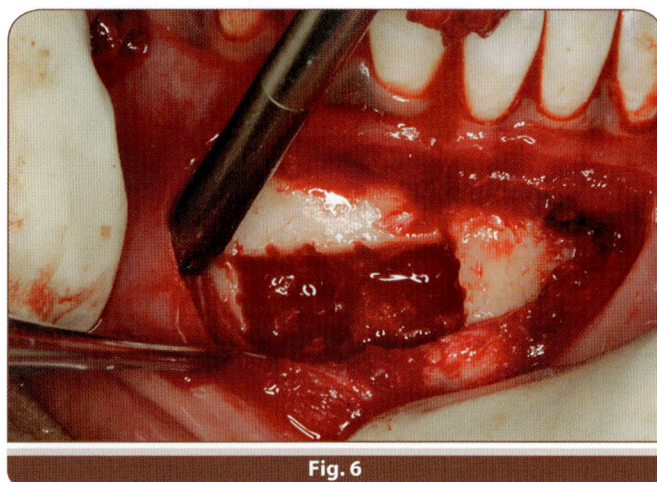

Fig. 6

Harvesting of the chin block graft from the donor site **(Fig. 6)**.

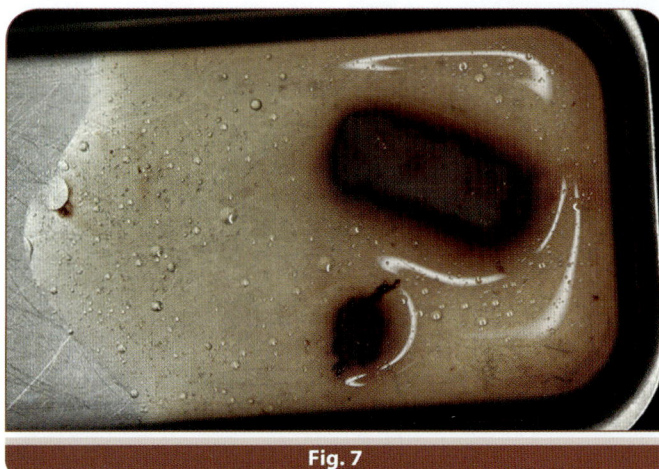

Fig. 7

Block graft harvested **(Fig. 7)**.

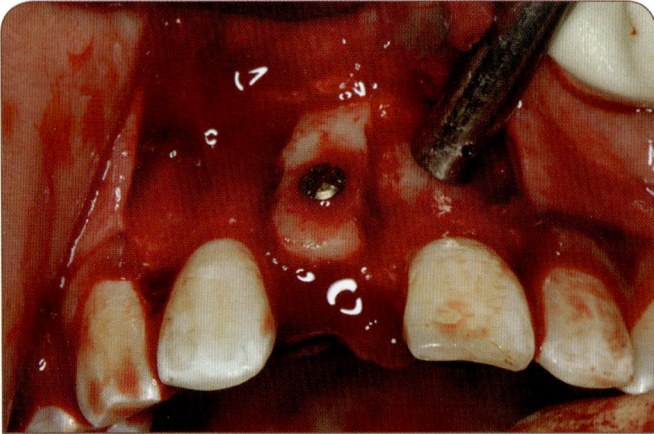
Fig. 8

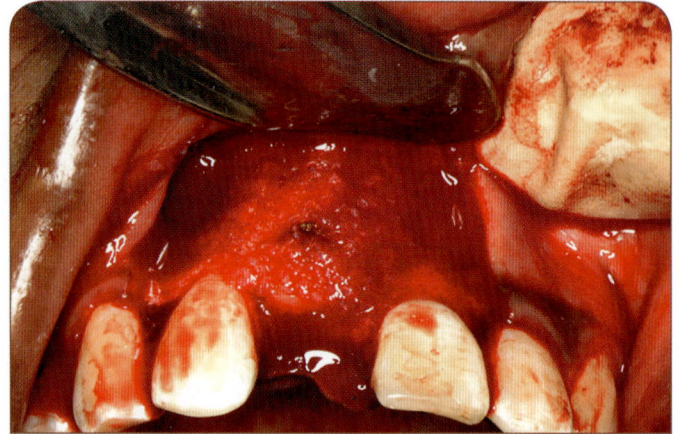
Fig. 9

Fixation of the block graft at the recipient site with 1.5 × 10 mm micro screws **(Fig. 8)**.

Mineralized particulate allograft placed over the fixed block graft **(Fig. 9)**.

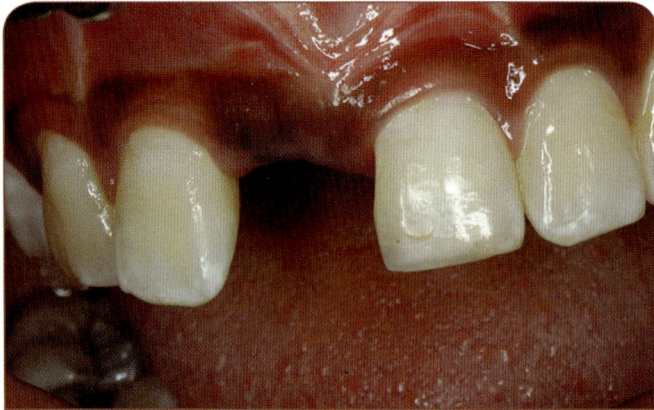
Fig. 10

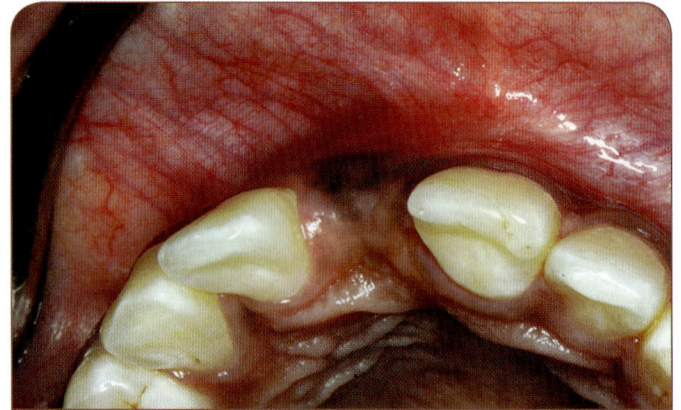
Fig. 11

Four months postoperative labial view of the grafted site **(Fig. 10)**.

Four months postoperative occlusal view of the grafted site **(Fig. 11)**.

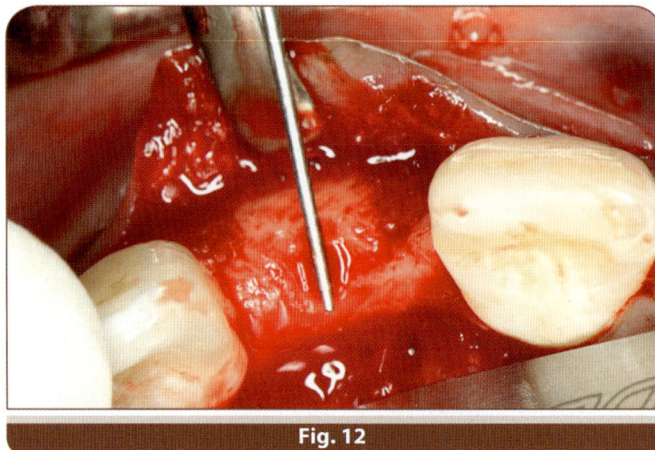
Fig. 12

Intraoperative view of the ridge width 4 months after block grafting. This view shows a well integrated block graft with gain in the ridge width **(Fig. 12)**.

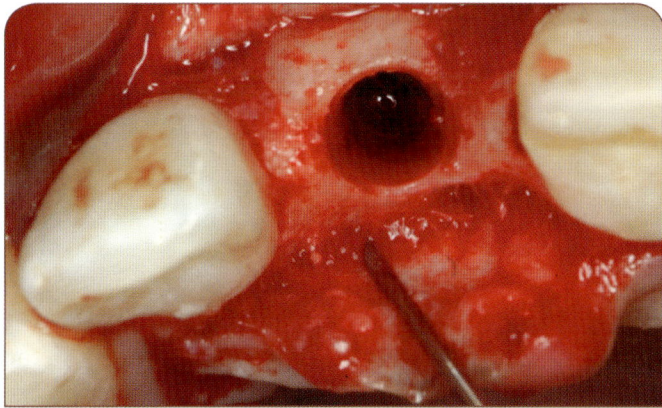

Fig. 13

Osteotomy site prepared for the placement of the implant (**Fig. 13**).

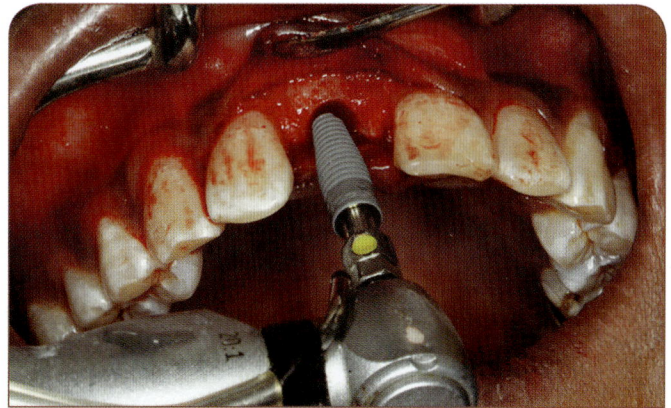

Fig. 14

Implant placement (4.3 × 11.5 mm) in the prepared osteotomy site tooth #11 (**Fig. 14**).

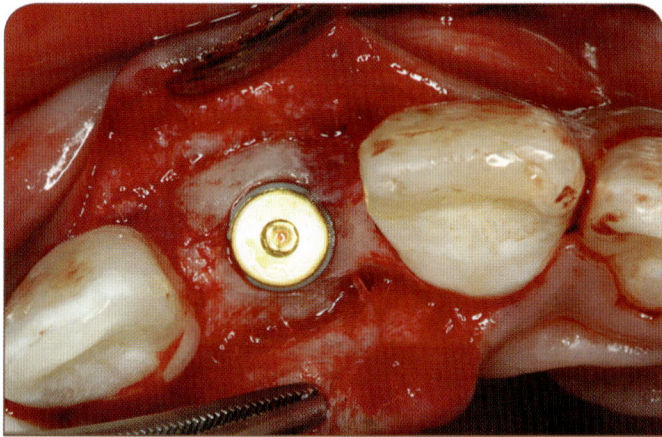

Fig. 15

Fixation of healing cap on the implant placed in relation to tooth #11 (**Fig. 15**).

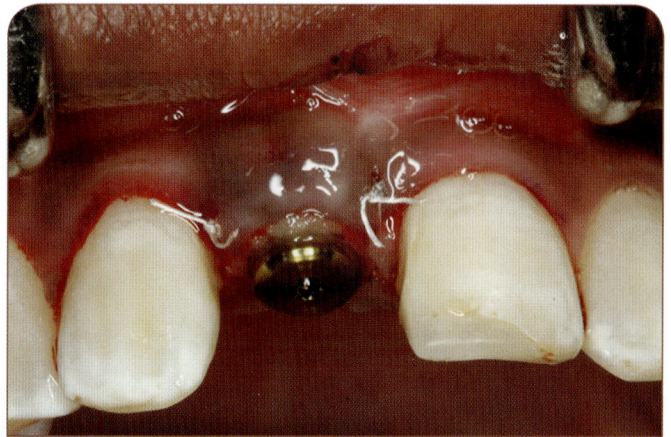

Fig. 16

Closure of the surgical site achieved by suturing using 4–0 polytetrafluoroethylene (cytoplastic) suture material (**Fig. 16**).

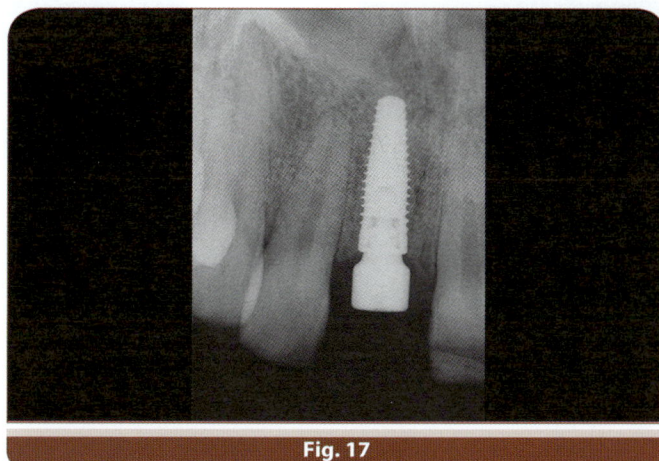

Fig. 17

Immediate postoperative intraoral periapical radiograph after placement of implant (**Fig. 17**).

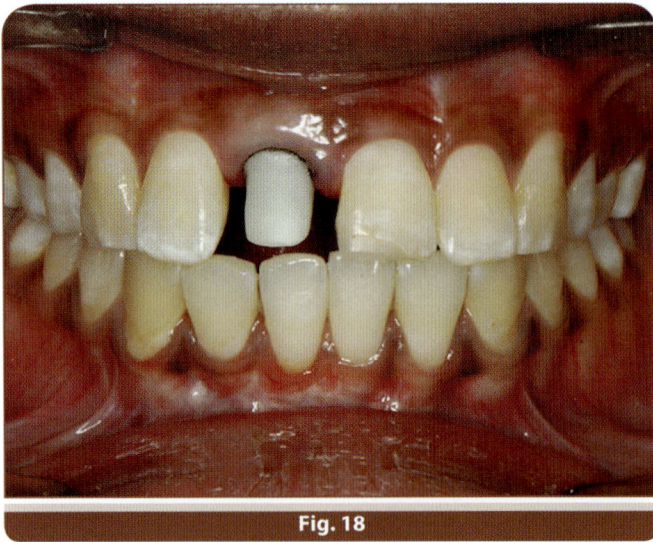
Fig. 18

Customized zirconia abutment placed in relation to tooth #11 (Fig. 18).

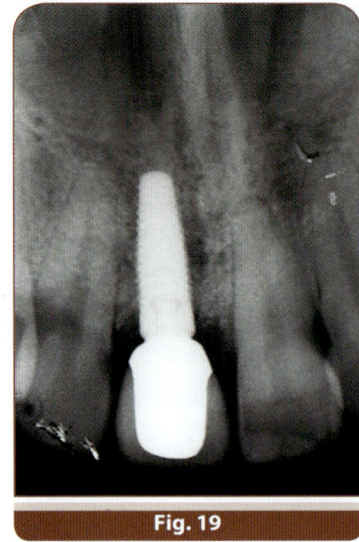
Fig. 19

Intraoral periapical radiograph after loading the implant (Fig. 19).

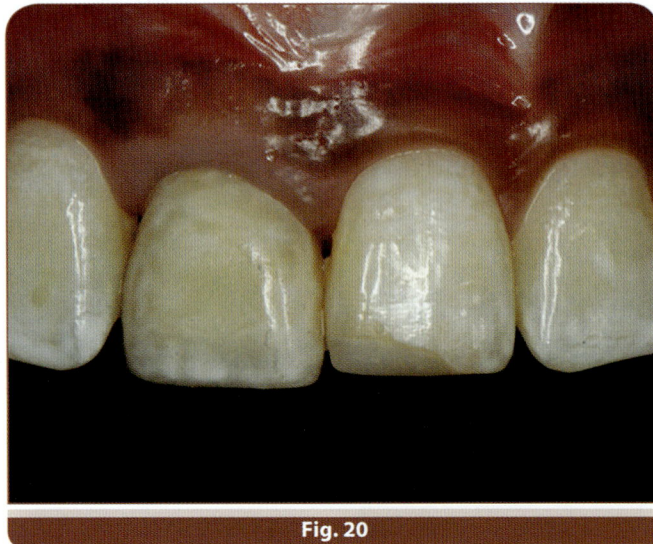
Fig. 20

Prosthesis (Emax Lithium disilicate crown) delivered in relation to tooth #11 (Fig. 20).

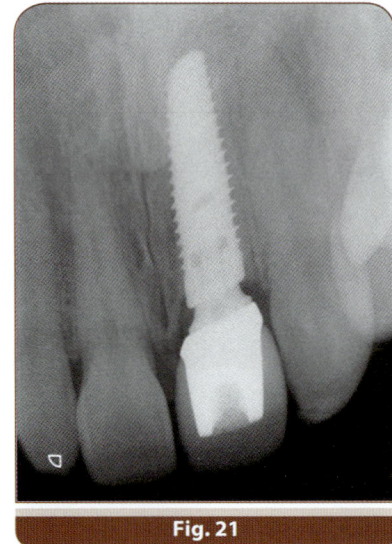
Fig. 21

Follow-up intraoral periapical radiograph after 1 year of the implant placement (Fig. 21).

Lanka Mahesh, Vishal Gupta

MESH ASSISTED GBR FOR A SINGLE MAXILLARY ANTERIOR TOOTH REPLACEMENT

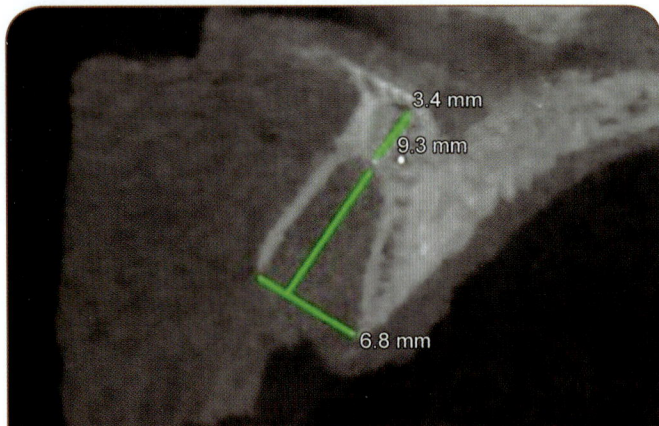

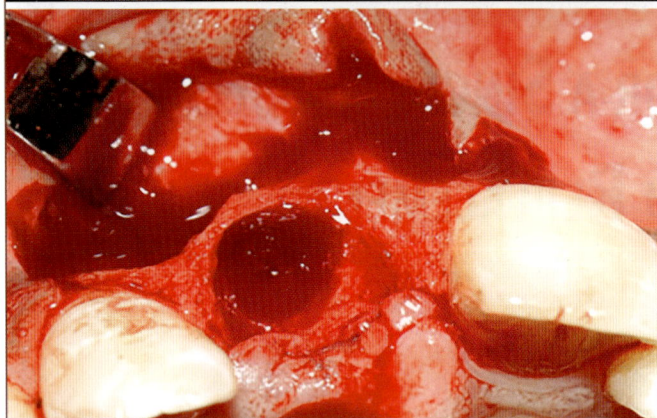

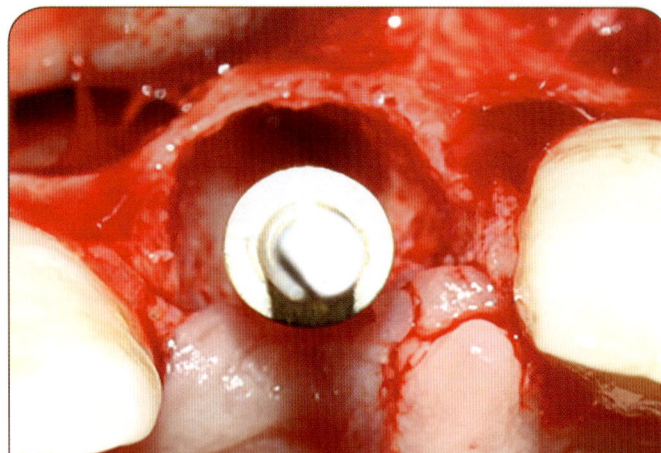

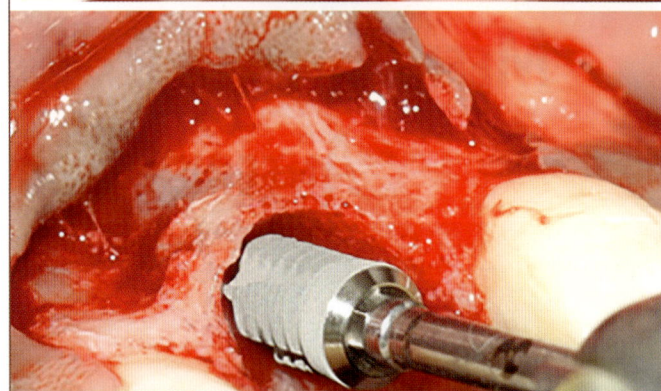

Fig. 1

Fig. 2

A 24-year-old male patient with tooth #11 avulsed in a trauma event. Preoperative CBCT view exhibits an extremely thin facial plate. Flap reflection confirms the scan findings. Treatment plan included immediate implant placement with mesh assisted GBR to bulk the implant site **(Fig. 1)**.

Palatal drilling to obtain correct implant position. A 4.7/11.5 kelt implant (Bioner) is placed at 30 Ncm **(Fig. 2)**.

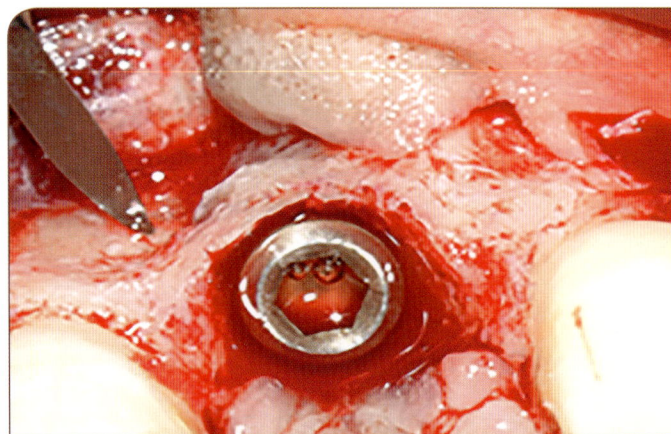

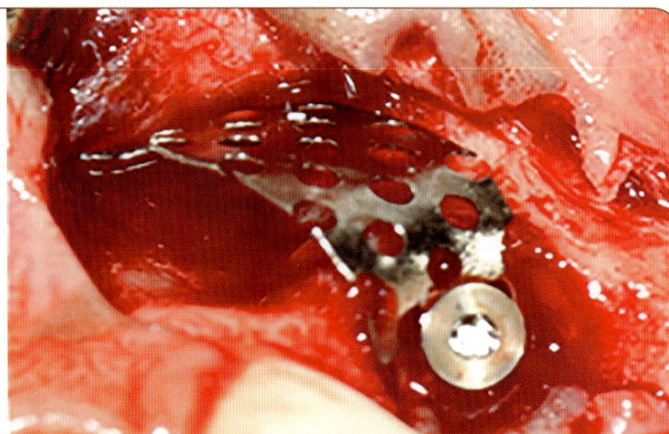

Fig. 3

Decortication with a lancet drill to get fresh BMP into the wound. A mesh (Salvin) is adapted and secured with the implant cover screw **(Fig. 3)**.

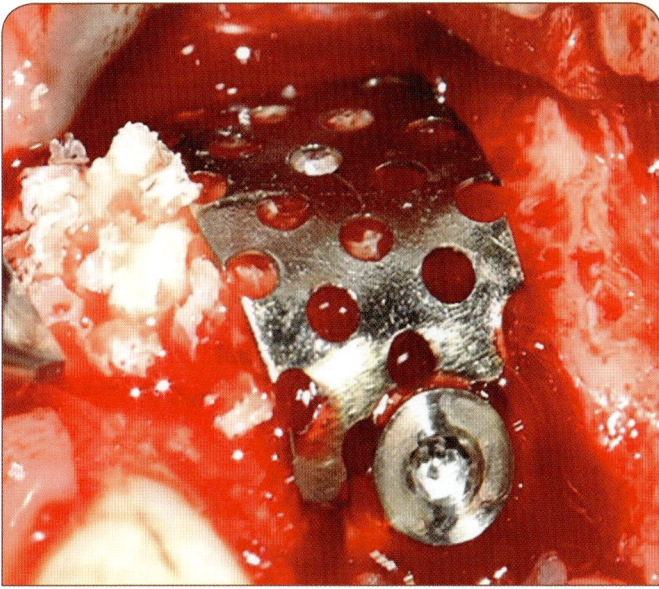

Fig. 4

Fig. 5

Bio-Oss® (geistlisch) particles along with NovaBone Morsels (NovaBone) are packed into the space created by the mesh.

The advantage of using a mesh in such cases is sustained space maintenance lasting over a long period unlike collagen membranes which collapse over the wound (Fig. 4).

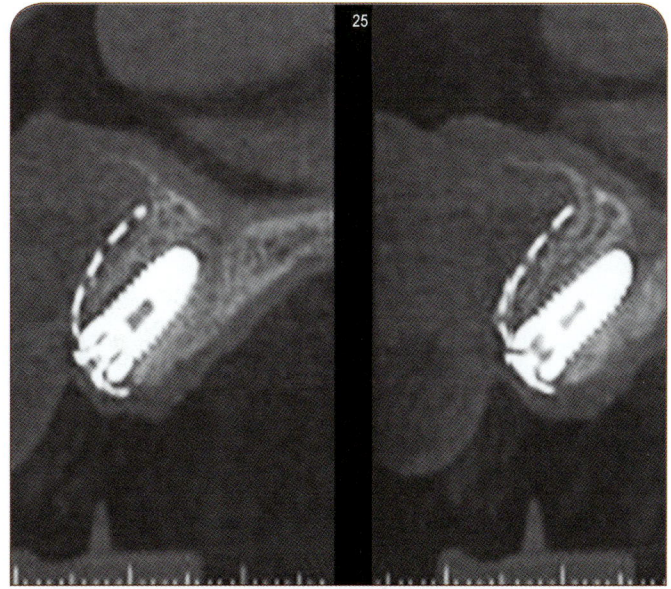

Postoperative scan views at 5 months show adequate bone volume regeneration over the facial wall over the implant. Every case in the anterior segment should be augmented to maintain long-term stability of the prosthesis (Fig. 5).

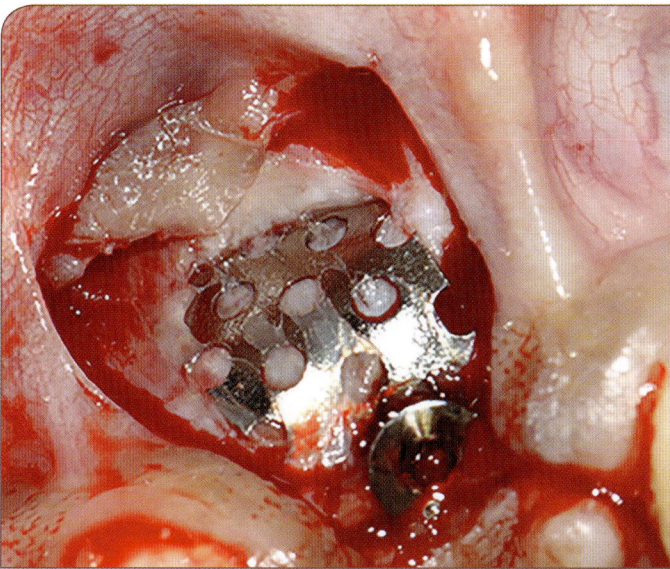

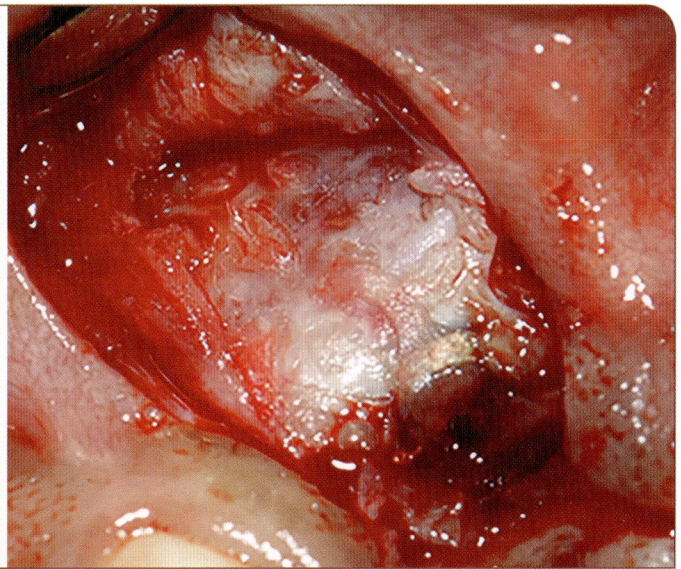

Fig. 6

At second stage surgery the mesh is seen adhering tightly to underlying bone, the cover screw is removed and the mesh is gently pried away without disturbing the regenerated bone bed. After mesh removal robust bone growth is clearly evident (Fig. 6).

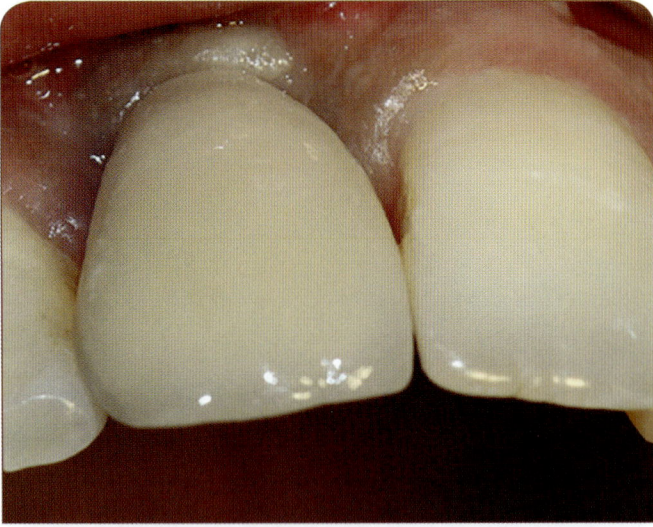

Fig. 7

The final PFM prosthesis inserted **(Fig. 7)**.

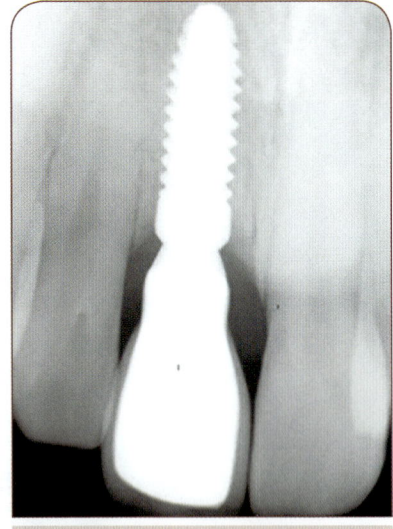

Fig. 8

Control X-ray at after 18 months **(Fig. 8)**.

Robert A Horowitz

SOCKET GRAFTING FOR PREPARATION OF IMPLANT BONE

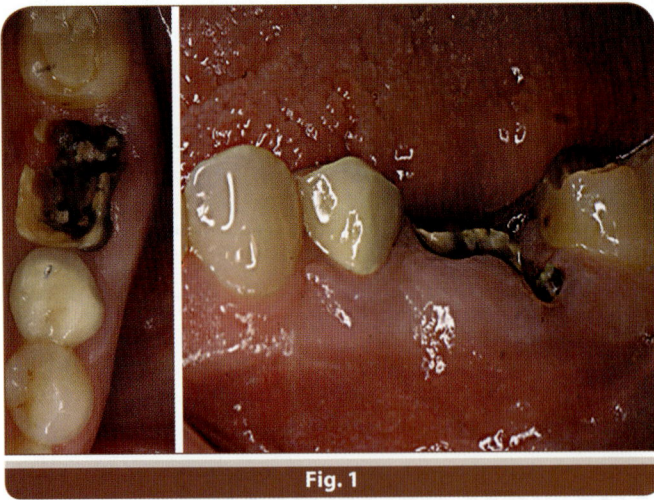

Fig. 1

The patient presents with a severely decayed, infected lower left first molar tooth **(Fig. 1)**.

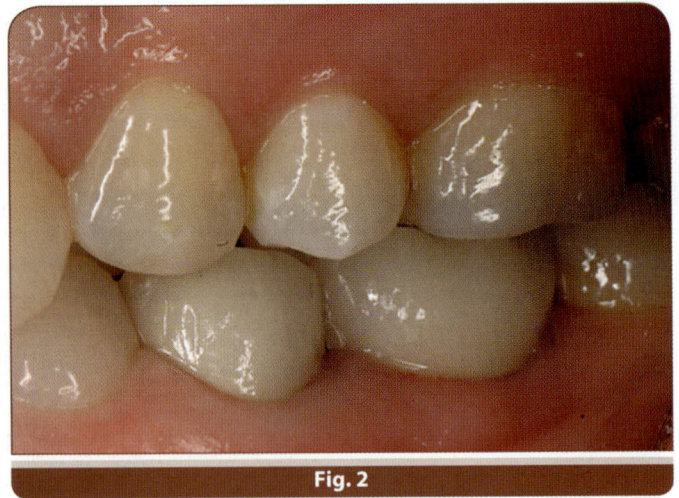

Fig. 2

This is all the patient wants— aesthetic, functional "teeth" that require little to no maintenance on her part **(Fig. 2)**.

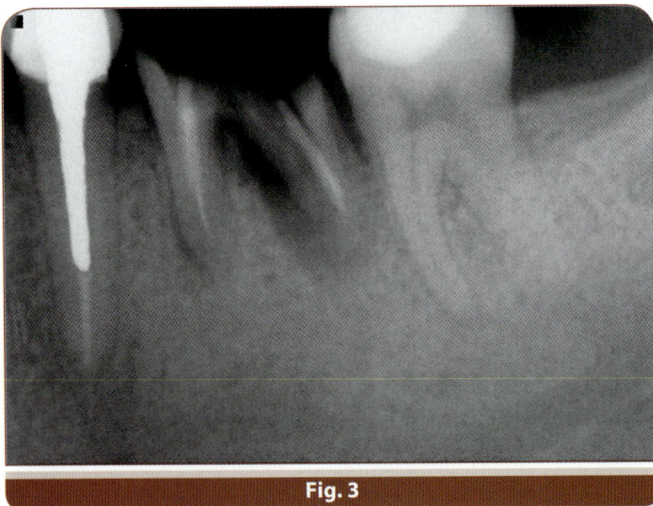

Fig. 3

Minimal number of visits: Surgical, Restorative. Maximal volume preservation/augmentation: Bone, Keratinized tissue. Maximum VITAL bone. Longevity of aesthetic and functional outcome. Minimal—morbidity, financial

The initial periapical radiograph demonstrated the severe decay, poor endodontic therapy and fractured distal root— a hopeless tooth **(Fig. 3)**.

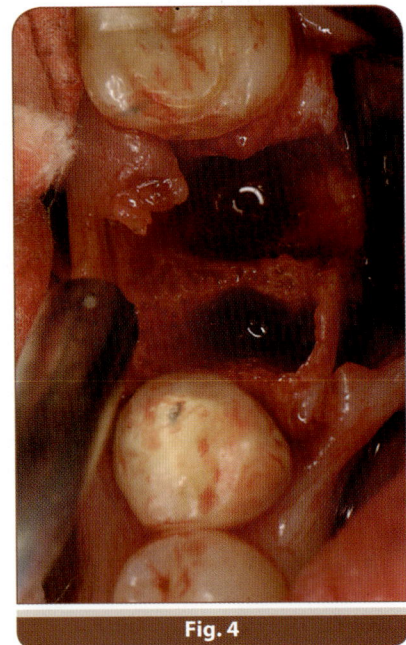

Fig. 4

Failed endodontic therapy. Missing buccal plate on the distal root. Sufficient proximal bone on adjacent teeth. Failing restoration on the adjacent premolar.

Minimal flap elevation is performed just past the crest of the ridge demonstrating thin residual bone and significant loss of the distobuccal plate **(Fig. 4)**.

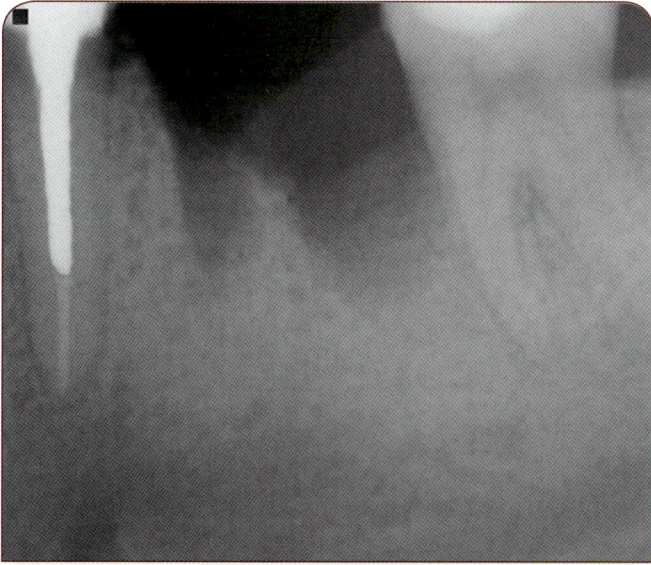

Fig. 5

Periapical X-ray verifies bone loss. Radiograph shows missing height of bone and area where the buccal plate is missing in the area of the distal root **(Fig. 5)**.

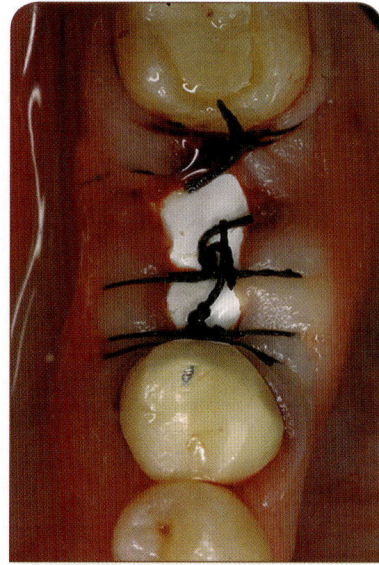

Fig. 6

Five months later, minimal flap elevation reveals a healed ridge with bleeding bone and sufficient width to enable placement of a wide diameter implant **(Fig. 6)**.

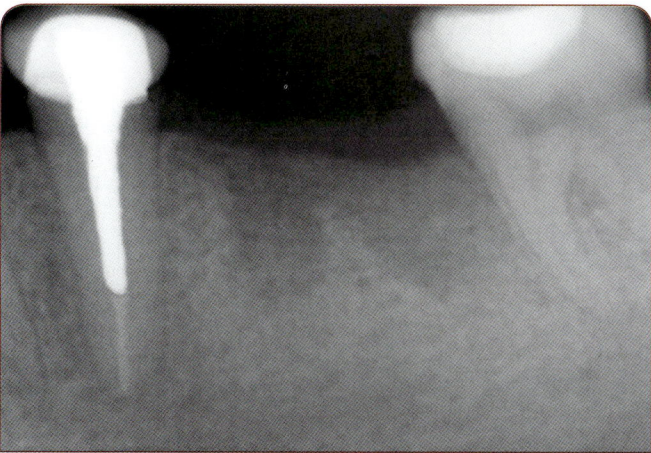

Fig. 7

Mineralized bone at 5 months. The periapical radiograph at the time of implant placement shows no graft remnants and mineralized bone in the entire area of the extraction **(Fig. 7)**.

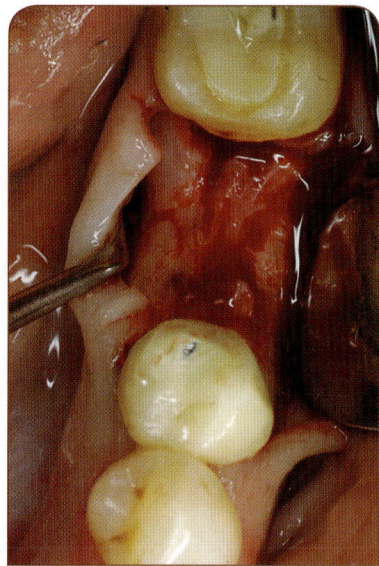

Fig. 8

Cytoplast over a blood clot. In site—3 weeks. Implant planned after healing period. This quick regeneration of alveolar bone and preservation of the ridge width were accomplished by placement of a Cytoplast (Osteogenics, Lubbock, TX) dense PTFE barrier over a blood clot. No attempt for primary closure was made as this barrier is designed to remain in an exposed manner for 3–4 weeks after insertion **(Fig. 8)**.

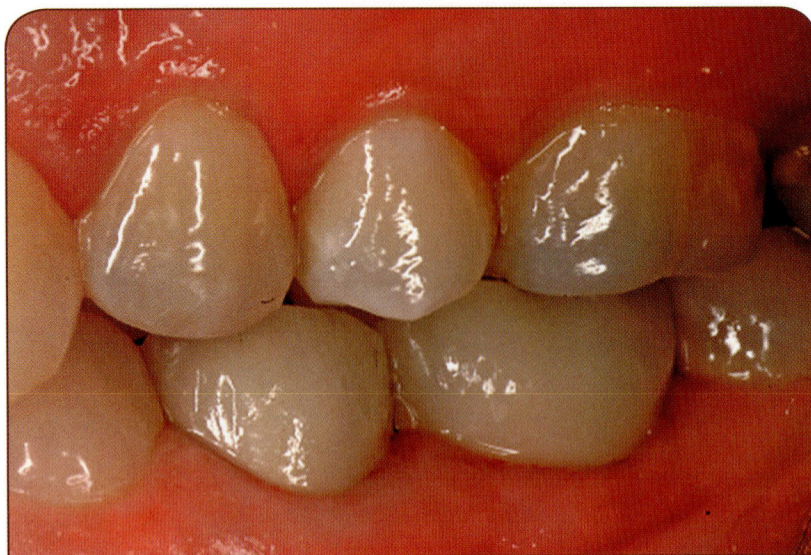

Fig. 9

Six months after insertion of the final prosthesis on the retained premolar and the implant-supported molar, the tooth shapes are ideal and they are surrounded by adequate bands of thick, healthy keratinized tissue **(Fig. 9)**.

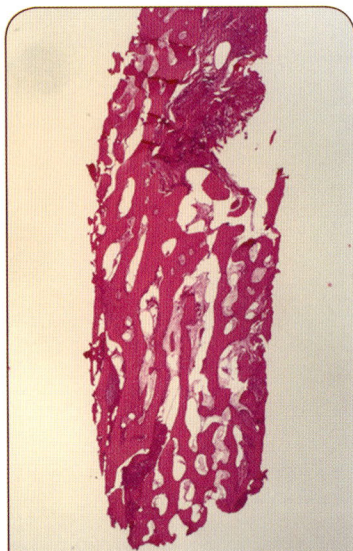

Fig. 10

Core taken at implant insertion is kept in 10% formalin. Successively dehydrated and demineralized. Embedded in wax. Stained with H&E. Viewed through traditional microscope.

Ideal results: Vital bone, No residual graft. Quick healing, Followed on X-ray. Hematoxylin and eosin staining of the core (Gloria Turner, NYU College of Dentistry) taken at the time of implant placement demonstrates 70% bone, all vital. This is a significant accomplishment as "normal" alveolar bone in this region demonstrates approximately 35% vital bone. At 70% there is excellent vital bone—to implant contact at placement and the ability to immediately provisionalize with a restoration **(Fig. 10)**.

Robert A Horowitz

SOCKET GRAFTING

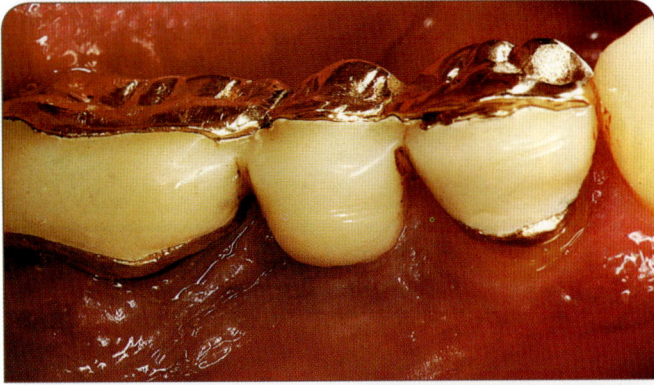

Fig. 1

This 70-year-old male has smoked 1–2 packs of cigarettes per day for over 40 years. Clinically poor gingival tone and a narrow edentulous ridge are noted **(Fig. 1)**.

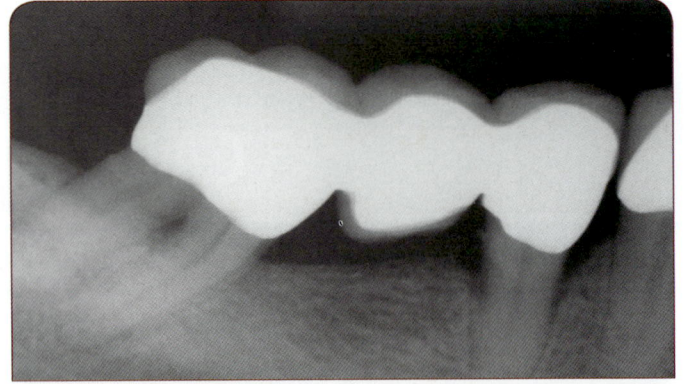

Fig. 2

Radiographically, there is furcation involvement on the non-vital molar, 30–50% bone loss on the premolar and subgingival calculus present around both teeth **(Fig. 2)**.

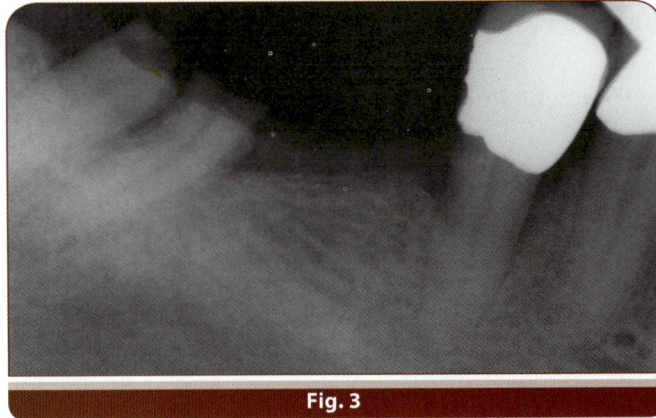

Fig. 3

Tooth #45: Questionable prognosis, save or extract? Tooth #47: Hopeless—Decay, CI III furcation involvement, extract, graft, replace. Site lower right back after sectioning - tooth #47 had deep decay and furcation involvement. As the first step of atraumatic extraction, the molar tooth is sectioned **(Fig. 3)**.

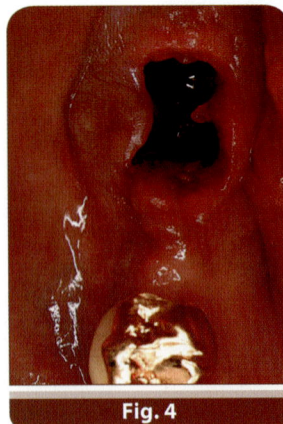

Fig. 4

Minimal flap elevation: Not flapless—placing implant, minimal trauma to bone: Piezosurgery, Periotomes, Elevators. Both roots of the molar can be removed after sectioning with no flap elevation, no damage to the alveolar bone and no trauma to the gingival tissues **(Fig. 4)**.

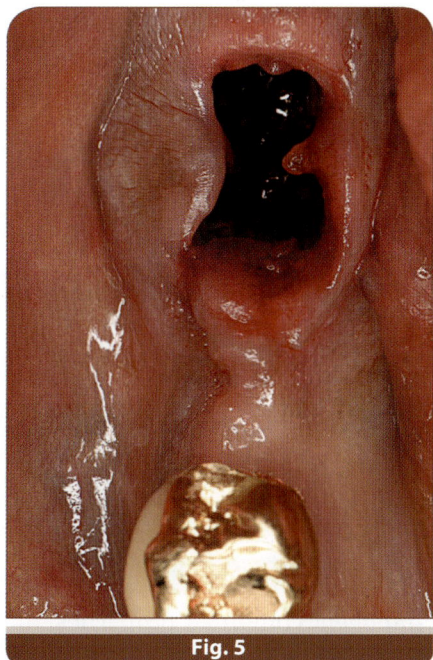

Fig. 5

Loss of keratinized tissue, loss of bone, bloodless surgery. Occlusally, the site collapse in the region of the first molar tooth shows decreased alveolar width and loss of keratinized tissue. There is no bony support for the facial keratinized tissue in the second molar site, as determined on X-ray **(Fig. 5)**.

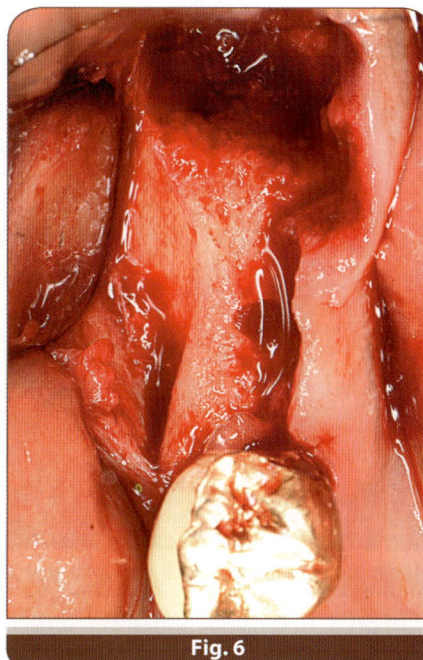

Fig. 6

No buccal plate tooth #47 confirmed! Flap elevation (to place the first molar implant) confirms significant horizontal ridge collapse in the edentulous ridge and lack of buccal bone in the extraction socket **(Fig. 6)**.

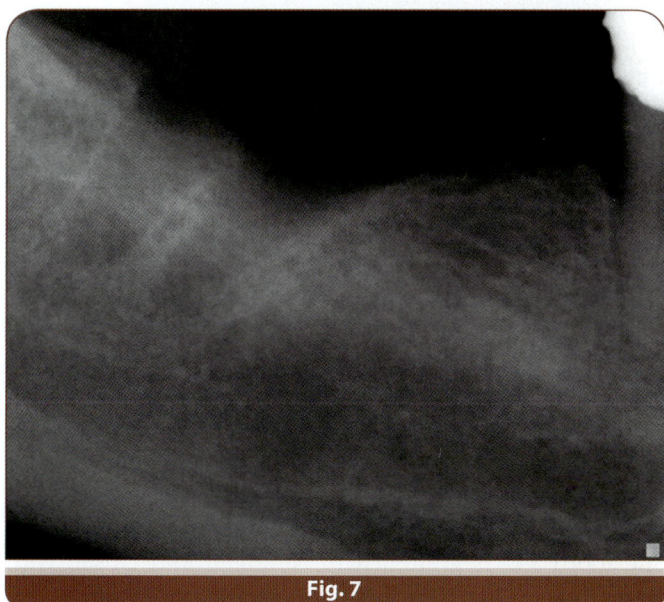

Fig. 7

Site tooth #46 and 47 after extraction. Radiographic confirmation of the loss of alveolar height and buccal plate after extraction **(Fig. 7)**.

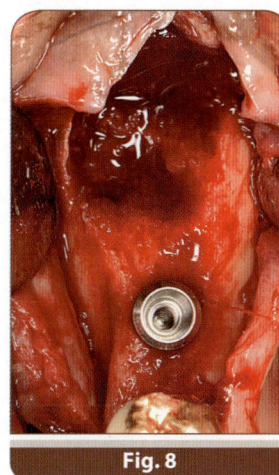

Fig. 8

Narrow ridge, slight lingual location, can still work fine, not as aesthetic, not as hygienic. Though the ridge width in the second molar site is 12 mm, it is only 6.5 mm in the first molar site. Without appropriate bone regenerative grafting there would be similar bone loss in this site as seen clinically and reinforced in the dental literature **(Fig. 8)**.

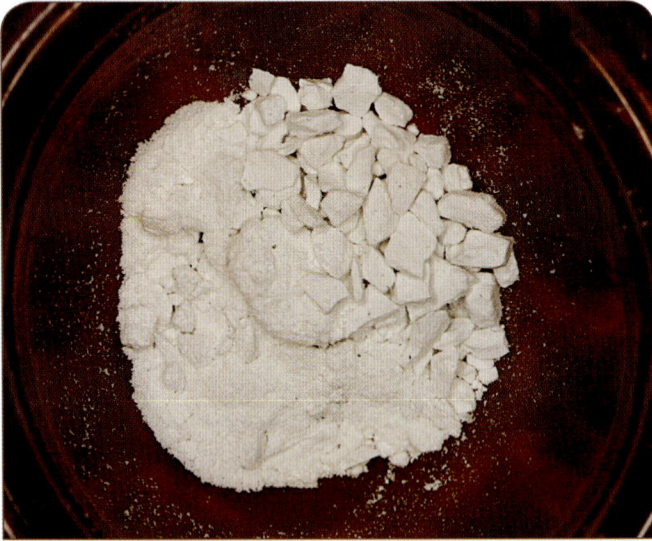
Fig. 9

With the patient's history of smoking and bone loss, an osteogenic mixture of calcium sulfate hemihydrate and dihydrate (Dentogen, Orthogen, NJ, USA) was used **(Fig. 9)**.

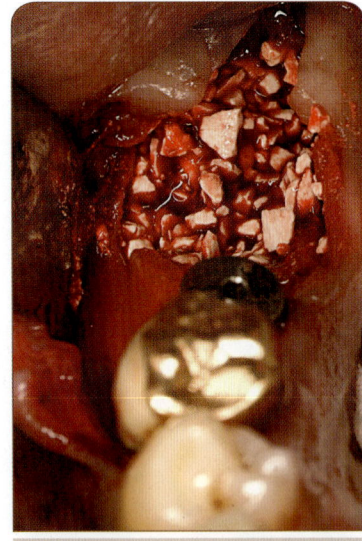
Fig. 10

Dentogen, nanogen, combined properties, alter resorption, better volume preservation, still fully resorbable.

This was hydrated with sterile saline and inserted into the defect. Combination of the 2 phases of Calcium Sulfate enables improved handing properties and setting of the material to maintain shape and prevent washout **(Fig. 10)**.

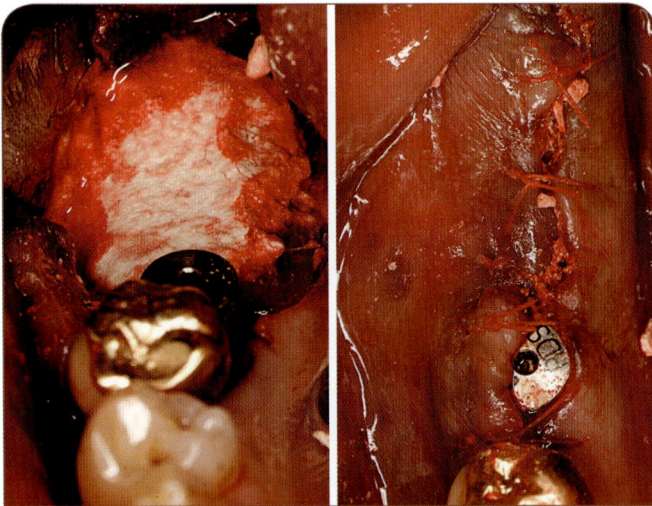
Fig. 11

Minimally invasive surgery, setting graft—support shape, healing followed on X-ray, no barrier removal needed, good for an apprehensive patient. A calcium sulfate barrier (Dentogen, Orthogen) was placed and allow to set over the graft and then covered completely with mobilized facial and lingual flaps **(Fig. 11)**.

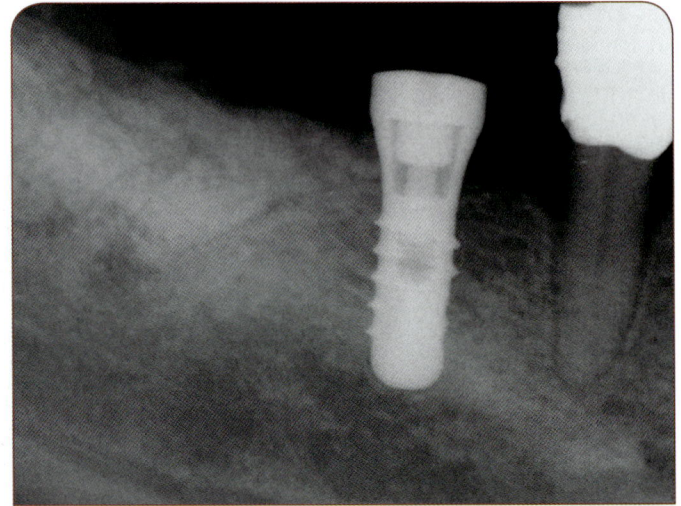
Fig. 12

Site tooth #46 had adequate bone and is now implanted. Site tooth #47 is grafted with Nanogen and closed with Dentogen—calcium sulfate barrier.

The socket is completely filled to ideal contour with the graft material, first molar implant placed and the infrabony defect fully debrided after root planning of the premolar tooth **(Fig. 12)**.

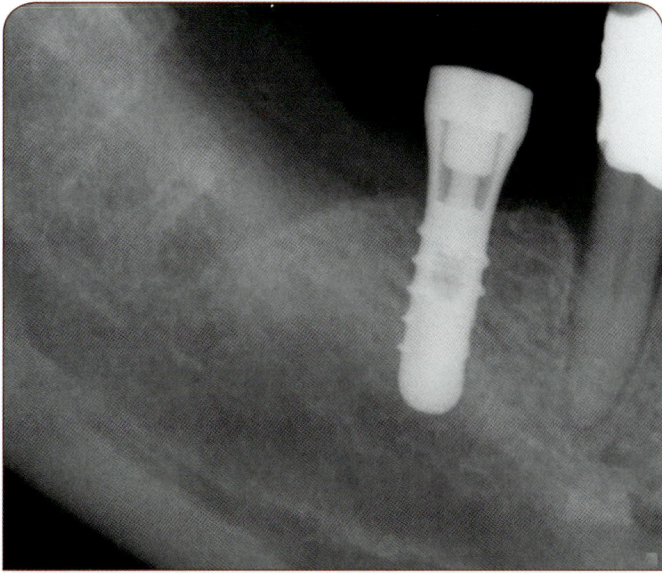

Fig. 13

Nanogen pellets are degrading and bone is forming apically in the site tooth # 47 at 1 month post grafting. One month postoperatively, the graft particles have not dislodged. They are dissolving at the appropriate time frame and at the same rate as vital bone is beginning to enter the osteoid forming after extraction **(Fig. 13)**.

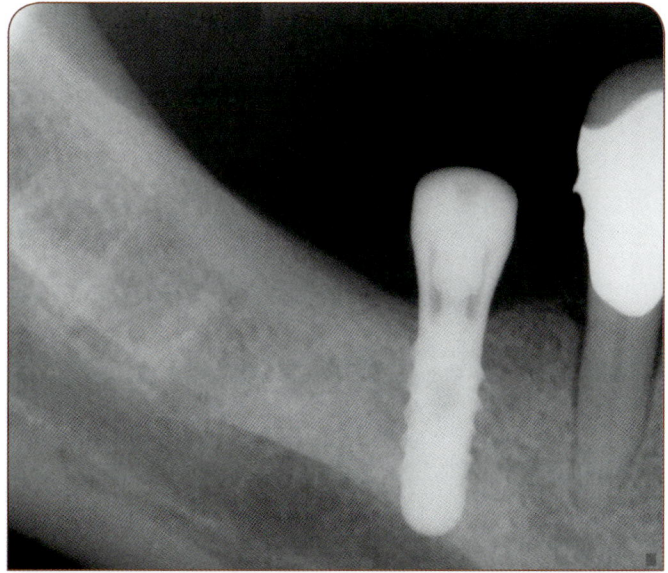

Fig. 14

More bone growth up to the alveolar crest in site tooth #47 at 2 months post grafting. Two months postoperatively, mineralized tissue has filled the socket to the level of the lingual plate of bone **(Fig. 14)**.

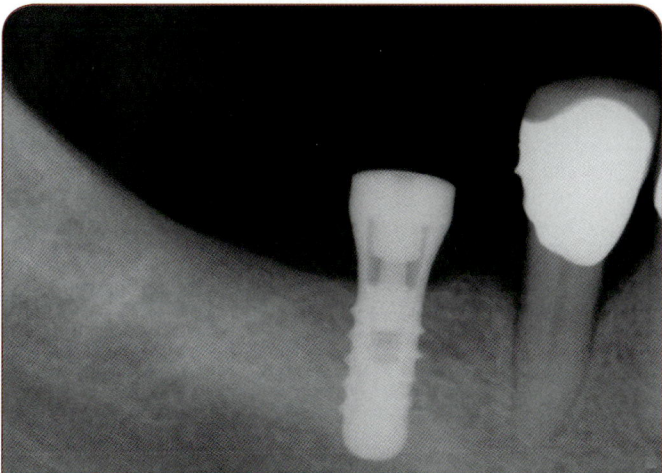

Fig. 15

Robust bone growth in site tooth # 47 at 5 months post grafting—site is as dense radiographically as the rest of the alveolar bone. At five months the new bone appears to have the same radio-opacity as the adjacent, native bone **(Fig. 15)**.

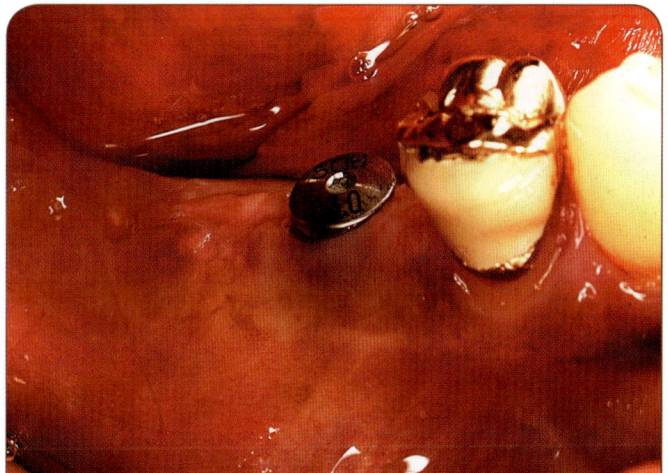

Fig. 16

Ideal gingival healing is shown at the same time point **(Fig. 16)**.

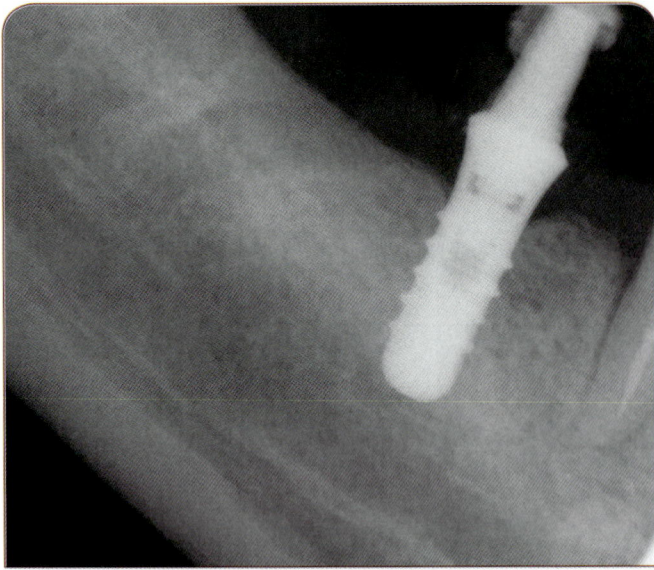

Fig. 17

Site tooth #47 healed fully with bone at 6 months post grafting—no vertical collapse. Plenty of keratinized tissue. Radiographically the bone has fully healed at 6 months when an abutment is temporarily placed on the first molar implant to enable laboratory fabrication of a surgical guide and transitional restoration **(Fig. 17)**.

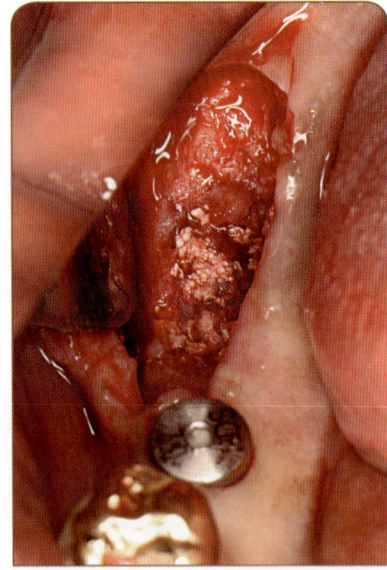

Fig. 18

Ridge width full, some particles: new Nanogen smaller particles, resorb fully in 3–4 months. A full thickness, papilla sparing incision shows full preservation of the alveolar ridge width with some graft not completely resorbed **(Fig. 18)**.

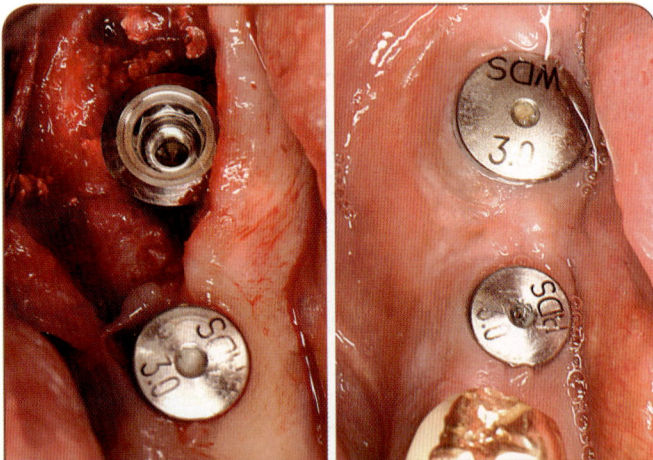

Fig. 19

A wide body, wide platform tissue level implant is placed in the 11 mm ridge. The gingiva matures quickly showing thick and healthy keratinized tissue **(Fig. 19)**.

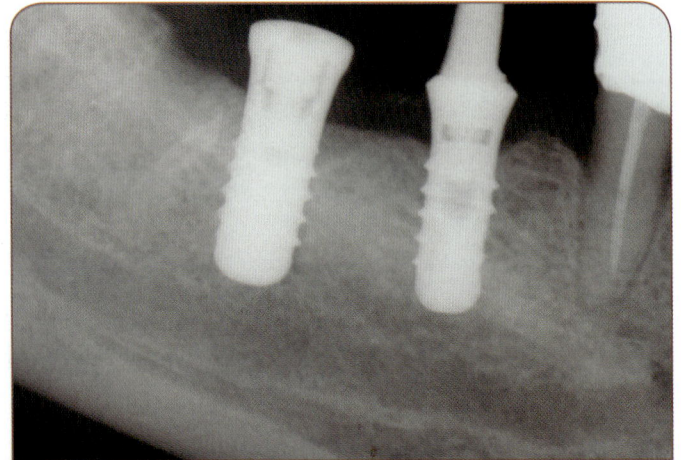

Fig. 20

Implant placed in site tooth #47 at 6 months post grafting. The two implants have a 2.7 mm machined collar to enable biologic width to reform coronally. In a patient like this with compromised healing, this could lessen the osseous severity of peri-implant disease **(Fig. 20)**.

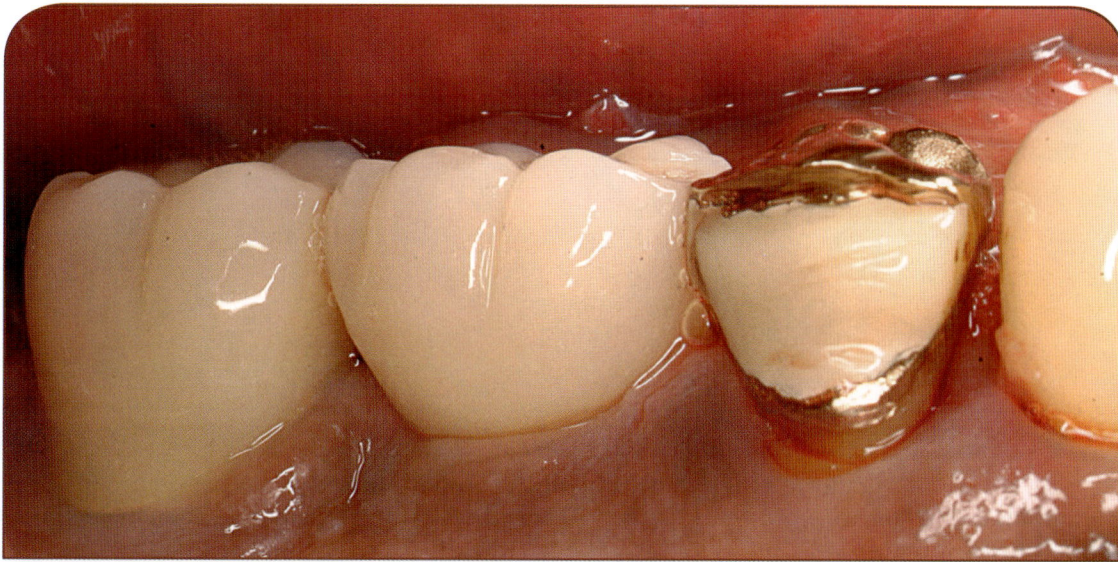

Fig. 21

One year after final restoration on the implants, more inflammation is noted proximal to the adjacent tooth than the healthy keratinized tissue around the implant-supported crowns **(Fig. 21)**.

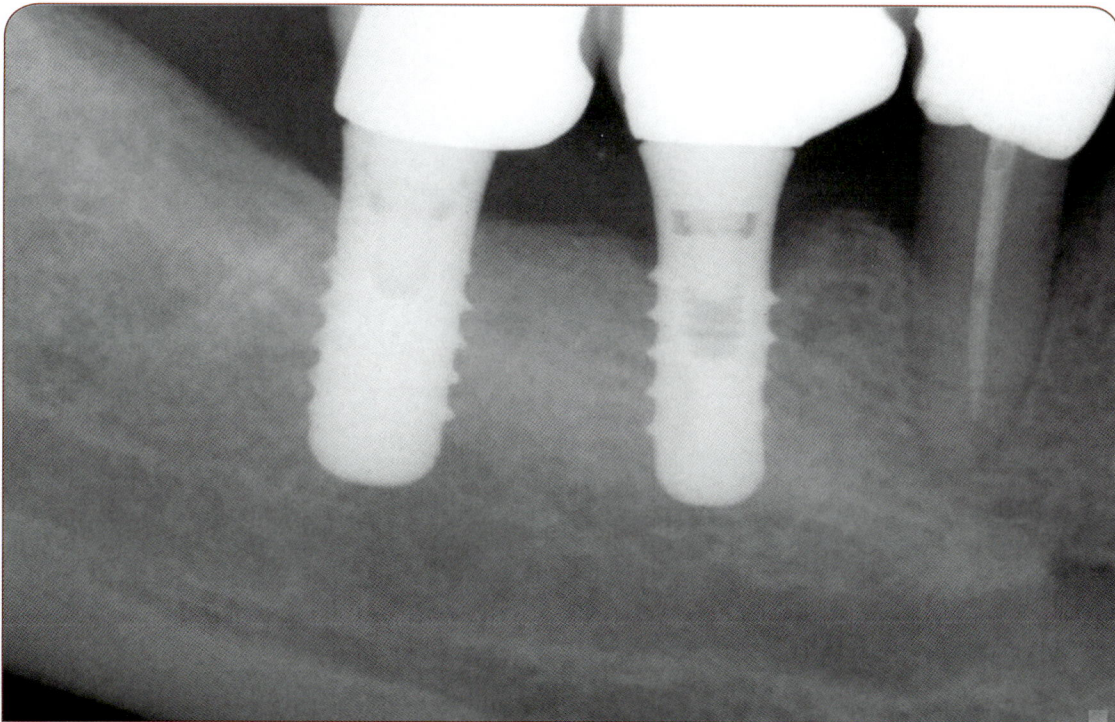

Fig. 22

Bone grew in site implanted with pure calcium sulfate pellets well. Implant was placed easily 6 months after grafting. The site was supported well by bone, surrounded by keratinized tissue. Implant is doing well 8 years after placement in this site. Crestal bone has been better preserved around the implant placed in the extracted and grafted site than where prior site collapse had occurred. Peri-implant disease can be affected by placement of an implant in too narrow a ridge, smoking and improper restoration, all seen in this site **(Fig. 22)**.

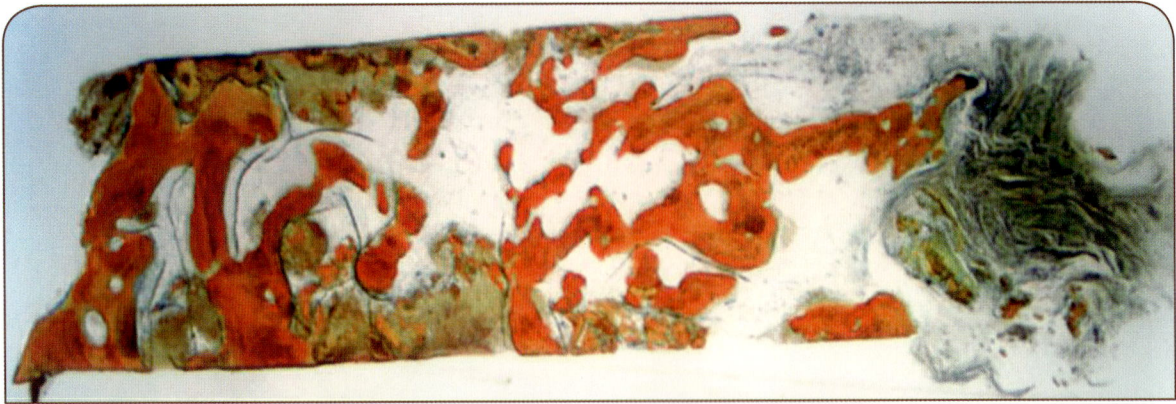

Fig. 23

64% bone, all vital, No residual graft. Histologically, the bone regenerative response was excellent. There is 65% bone, all vital in the socket itself. Near the crest, where the facial plate was absent, some dense, inflamed keratinized tissue was present **(Fig. 23)**.

Lanka Mahesh, Maurice A Salama

Extraction of an Impacted Maxillary Canine and Simultaneous Implant Placement with GBR

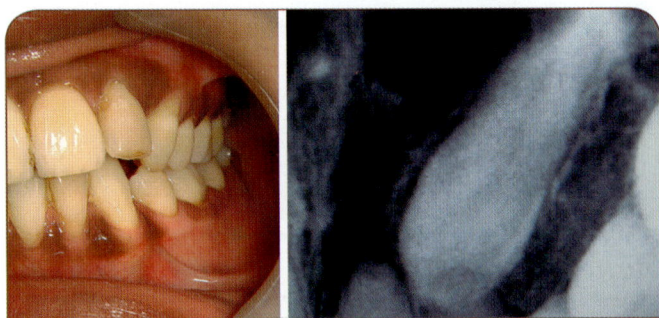

Fig. 1

A 32-year-old female patient with a retained deciduous lateral incisor which was mobile. The radiograph showed an impacted canine in relation to teeth #23. Treatment plan included extraction of teeth #23 and 25 and simultaneous placement of an implant with GBR **(Fig. 1)**.

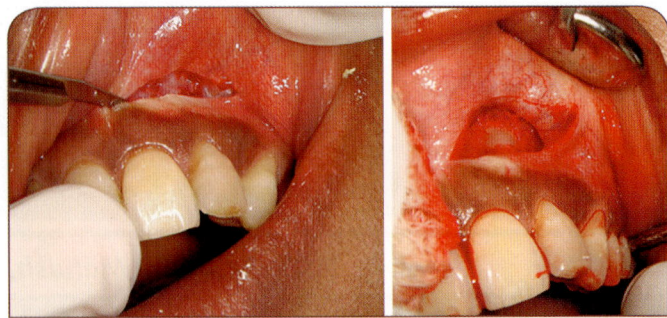

Fig. 2

A crevicular incision is made in the attached gingiva at the exact location of the canine with a 15 C blade, not raising a full mucoperiosteal flap is essential whenever feasible to prevent marginally tissue recession and prevent papilla loss. The canine is exposed after gentle dissection of the flap **(Fig. 2)**.

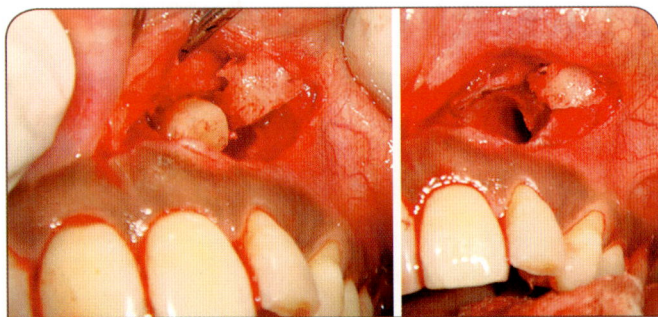

Fig. 3

A round tip of a UBS (Resista) is used to make the bony cuts around the canine to completely expose the tooth from all directions. The canine is gently luxated and removed in toto **(Fig. 3)**.

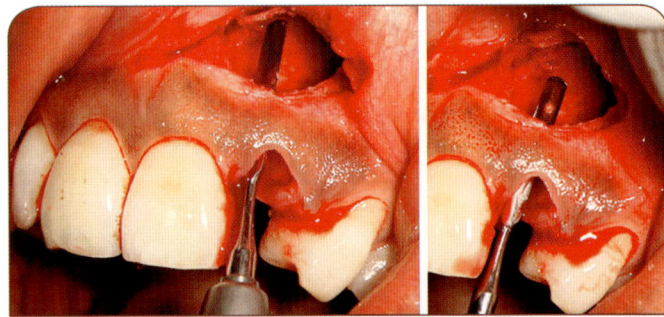

Fig. 4

A periotome has been used to show the extent of the bony defect following the impacted tooth removal.

Such large defects are usually best treated with staged GBR, in cases where primary stability is achieved simultaneous implant placement and GBR may be performed **(Fig. 4)**.

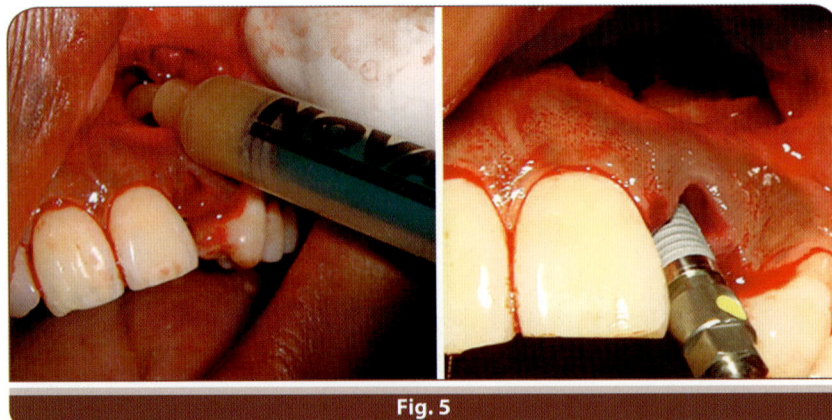

Fig. 5

1 cc of calcium phosphosilicate putty (novabone) is injected into the defect and packed with a flat ended instrument. A 4.3/13 mm Nobel replace (Nobel Biocare) implant is gently threaded into the ostetomy at 30 N cm **(Fig. 5)**.

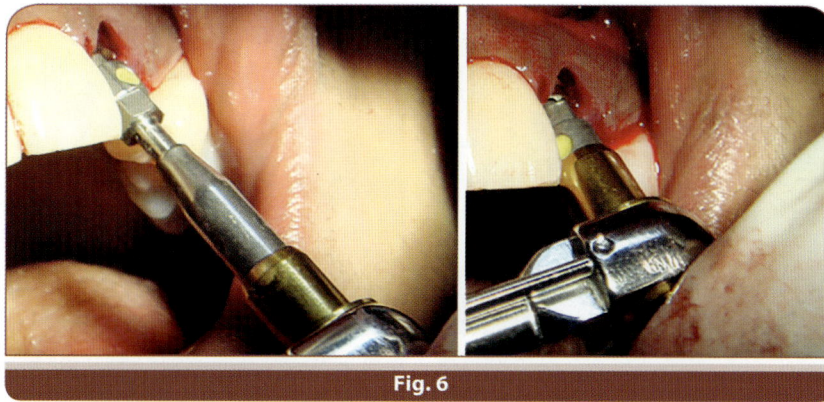

Fig. 6

An extender is best utilized in such cases in the anterior segment to prevent interference from the neighboring teeth incisal edges. A manual ratchet is used for final seating of the implant (positive finger pressure on the ratchet is very essential to prevent the implant from wobbling, as the only point of implant stability is the coronal 2 mm of bone) **(Fig. 6)**.

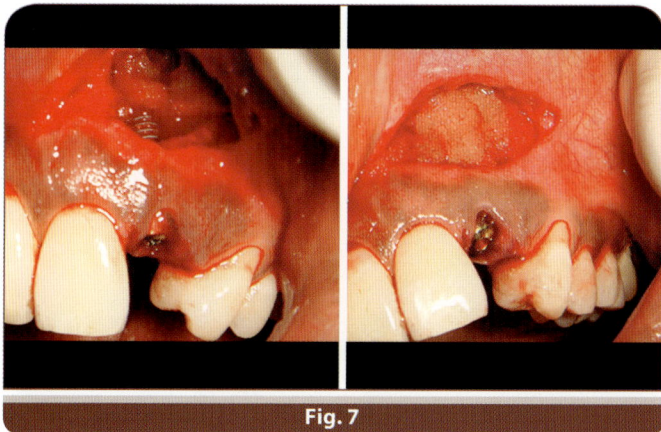

Fig. 7

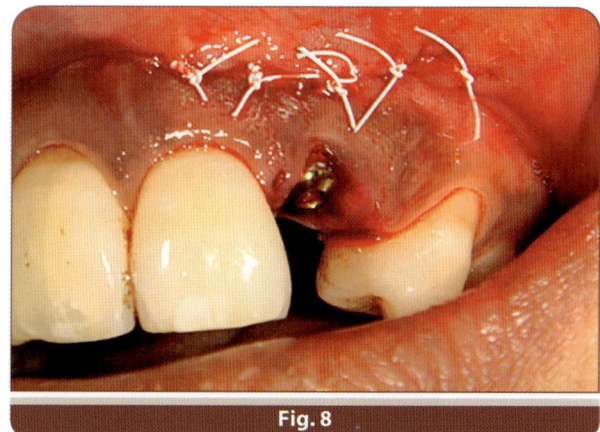

Fig. 8

The implant body is clearly visible within the osteotomy . 1 cc of NovaBone putty is placed over the implant surface to achieve a 'sandwich' effect **(Fig. 7)**.

The wound is closed with biomend collagen membrane (Zimmer Dental) and 3-0 simple interuppted EPTFE sutures (Osteogenics) **(Fig. 8)**.

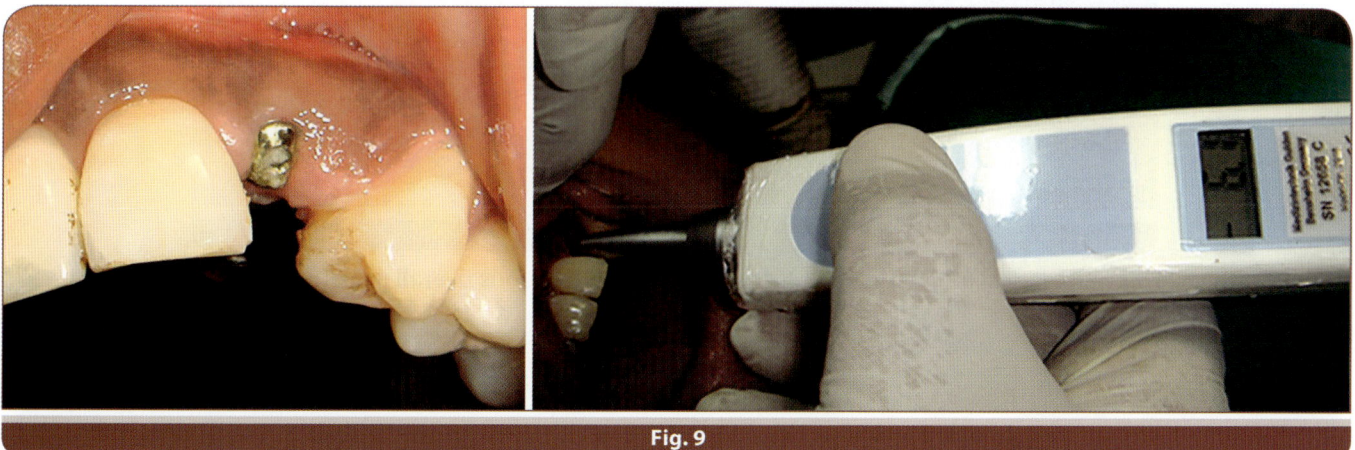

Fig. 9

At 5 months postoperative visit,the bulk of tissue can be appreciated. After removal of the temporary bonded prosthesis. A periotest (is utilised giving a reading of –6.1 suggesting the implant has achieved adequate osseointegration **(Fig. 9)**.

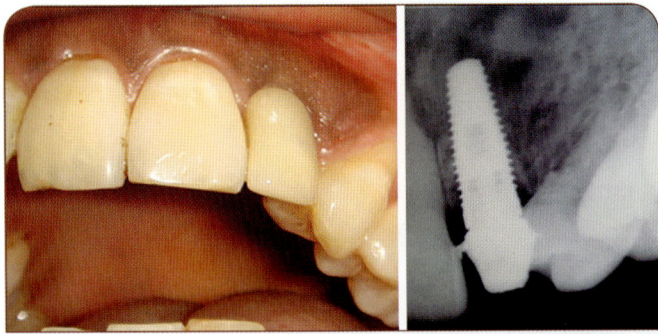

Fig. 10

A temporary composite crown is fabricated and kept in place for 4 months. An X-ray at this stage clearly shows initial graft maturation (the outline of the impacted canine is still visible) **(Fig. 10)**.

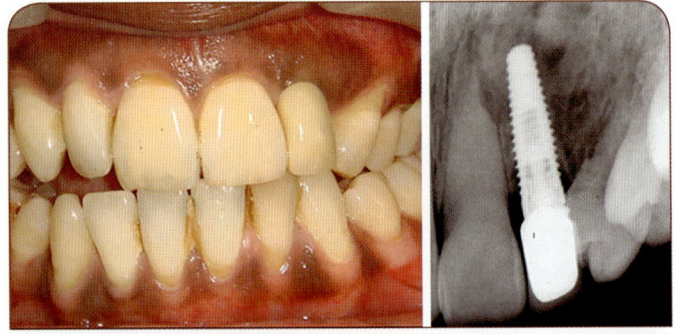

Fig. 11

The final zirconia crown in place. X-ray at insertion showing nearly complete graft maturation **(Fig. 11)**.

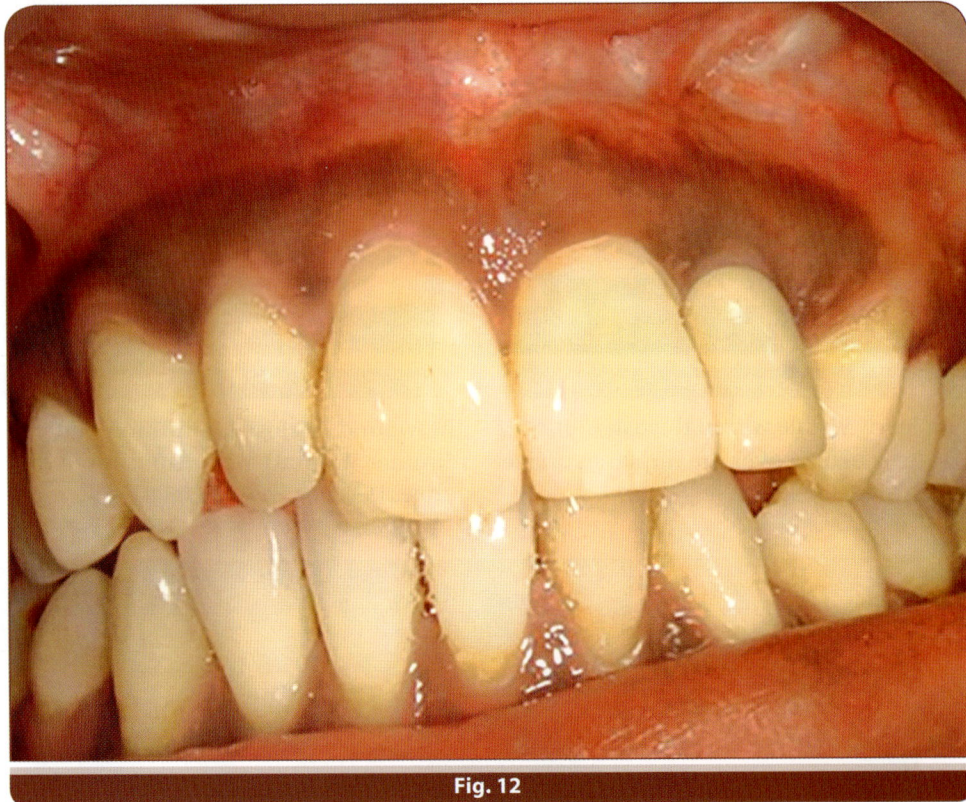

Fig. 12

Seven year clinical follow-up exhibits a stable and harmonious overall prosthesis **(Fig. 12)**.

CASE STUDY 78

Bassam F Rabie

One Stage Hard and Soft Tissue Grafting Around Immediate Post Extraction Implant

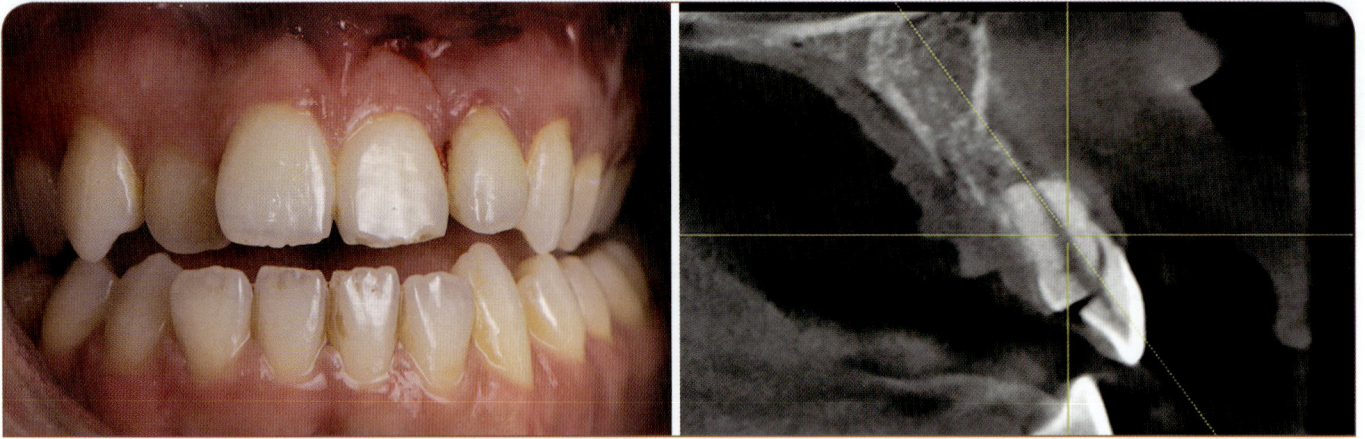

Severe resorption of the apex of the root. Confirmed with a CBCT **(Fig. 1)**.

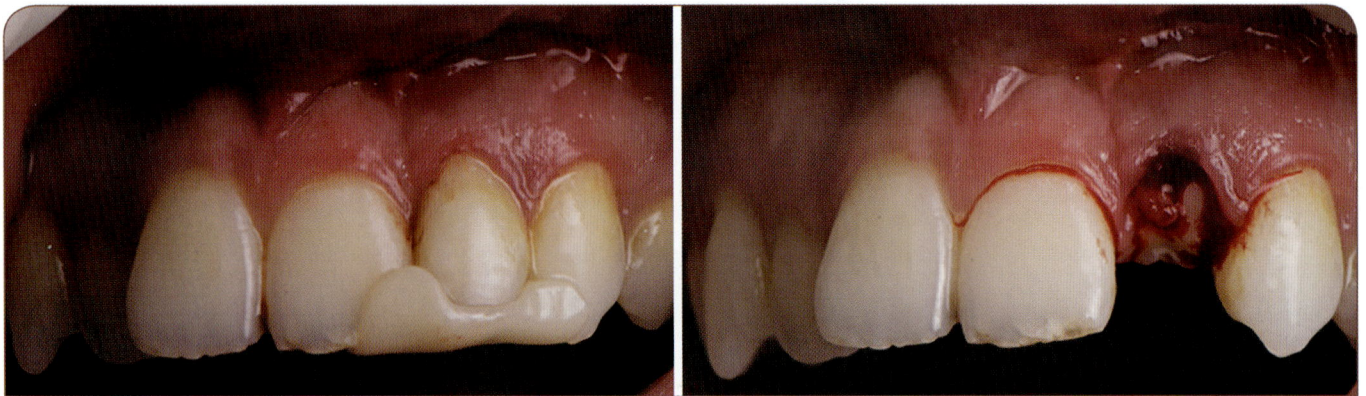

Fabrication of incisal resin guide before extraction of the lateral incisor. Extraction and flap elevation **(Fig. 2)**.

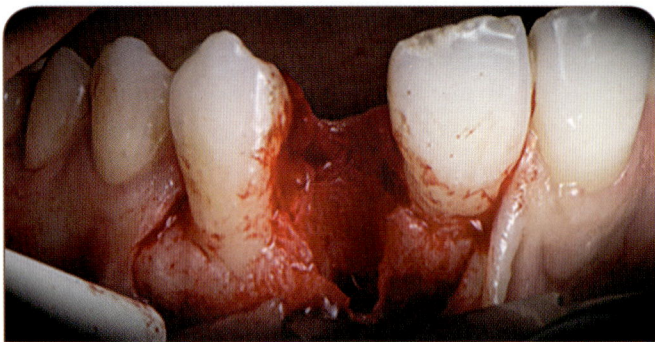

Absence of labial plate after extraction **(Fig. 3)**.

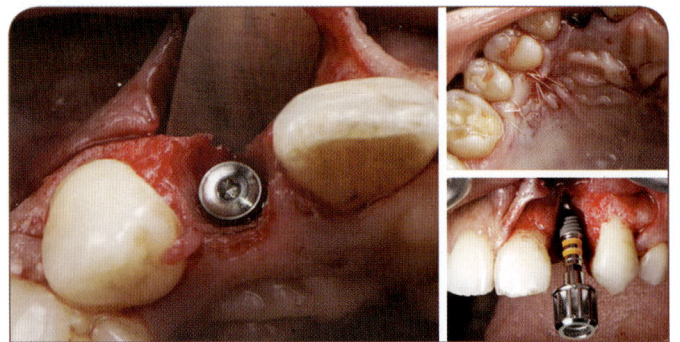

Connective tissue harvested, and implant placed. Loss of the labial plate, but intact interproximal heights of bone **(Fig. 4)**.

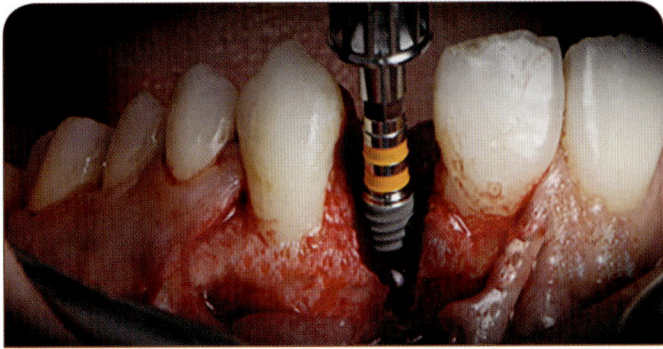

Fig. 5

Implant placement **(Fig. 5)**.

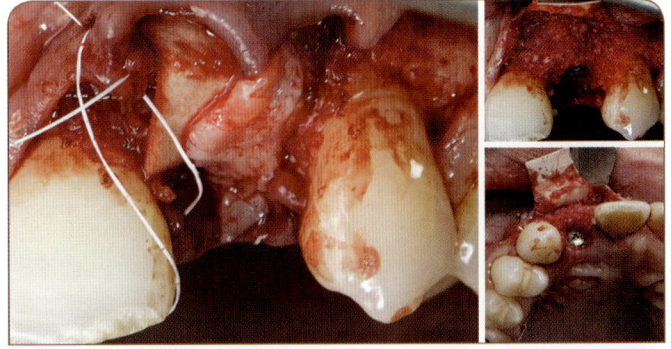

Fig. 6

Grafting with cortical cancellous allograft and slow resorbing collagen membrane and placement of the soft tissue CT graft **(Fig. 6)**.

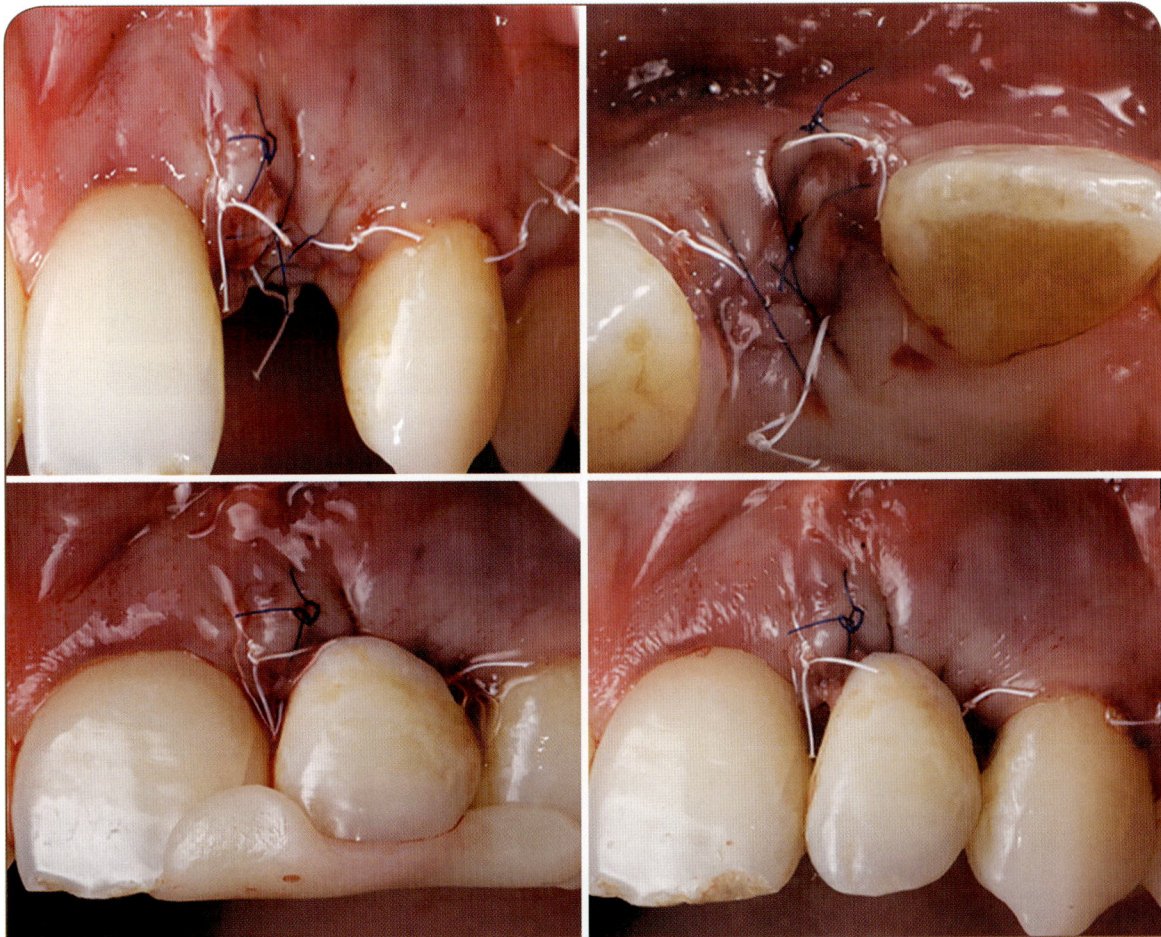

Fig. 7

Suturing, and use of the same natural crown of the extracted lateral, guided by the resin incisal guide to bond it palatally on both adjacent natural teeth as a temporary since no immediate nonfunctional loading was done **(Fig. 7)**.

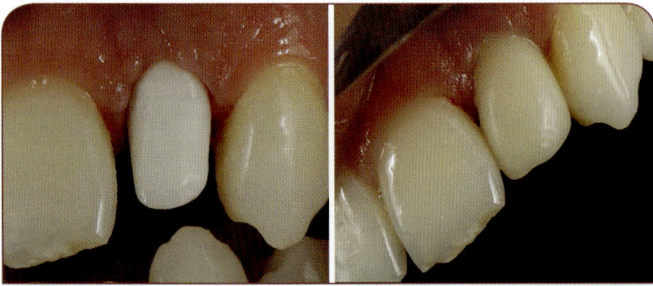

Fig. 8

After 4 months, temporization and then Zirconia try in **(Fig. 8)**.

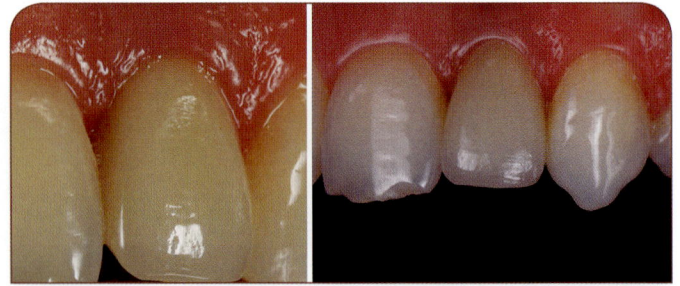

Fig. 9

Final crown in place. Note the soft tissue integration around the implant crown **(Fig. 9)**.

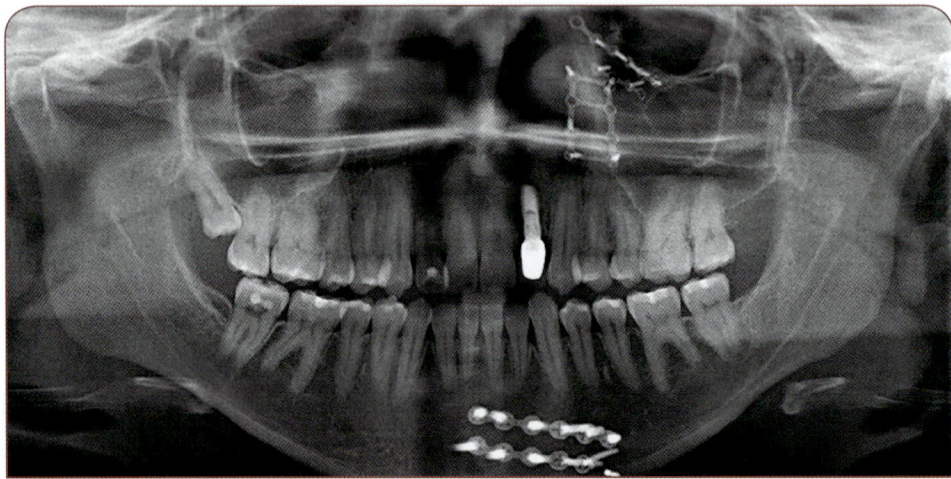

Fig. 10

Postoperative radiograph (OPG) of final prosthesis **(Fig. 10)**.

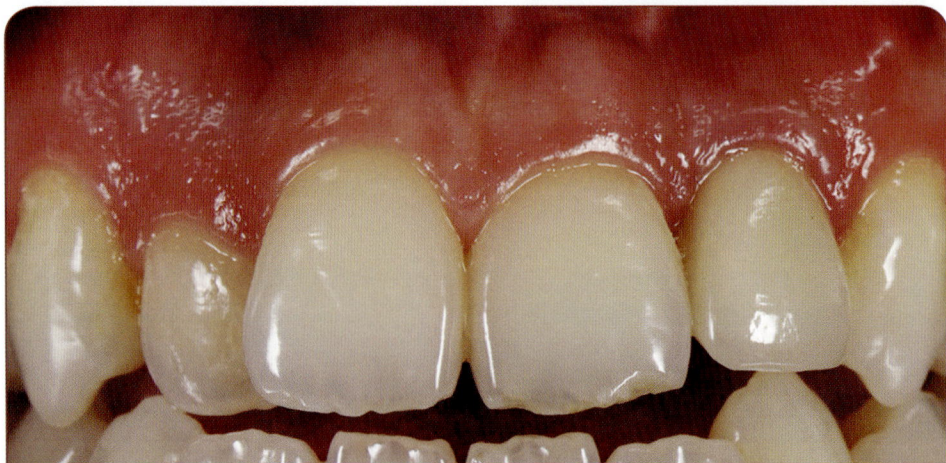

Fig. 11

Five years follow up. Note continued improvement in soft tissue architecture and papilla fill **(Fig. 11)**.

CASE STUDY 79

Alejandro Vivas Rojo, Jesus Gomez Perez

MAXILLARY AUGMENTATION WITH AUTOGENOUS BONE

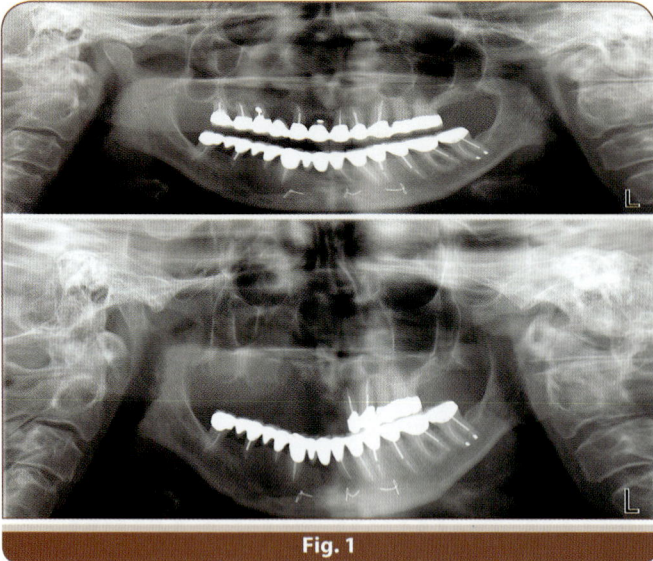

Fig. 1

Radiographic evaluation, preoperative **(Fig. 1)**.

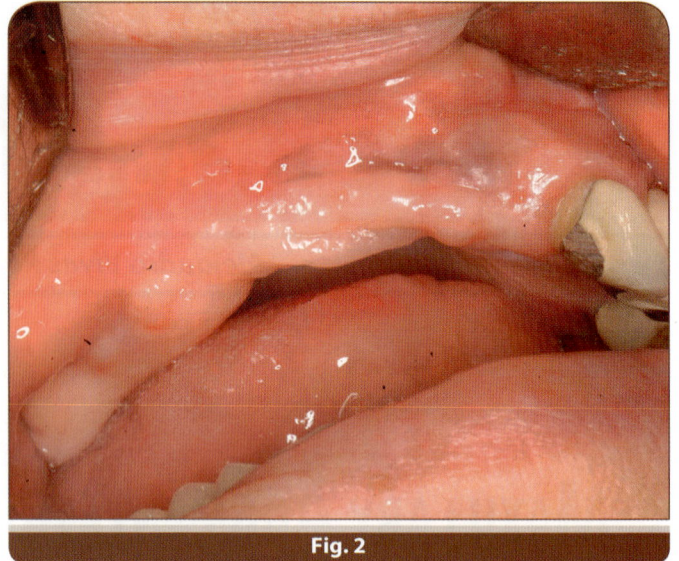

Fig. 2

Clinical evaluation, preoperative **(Fig. 2)**.

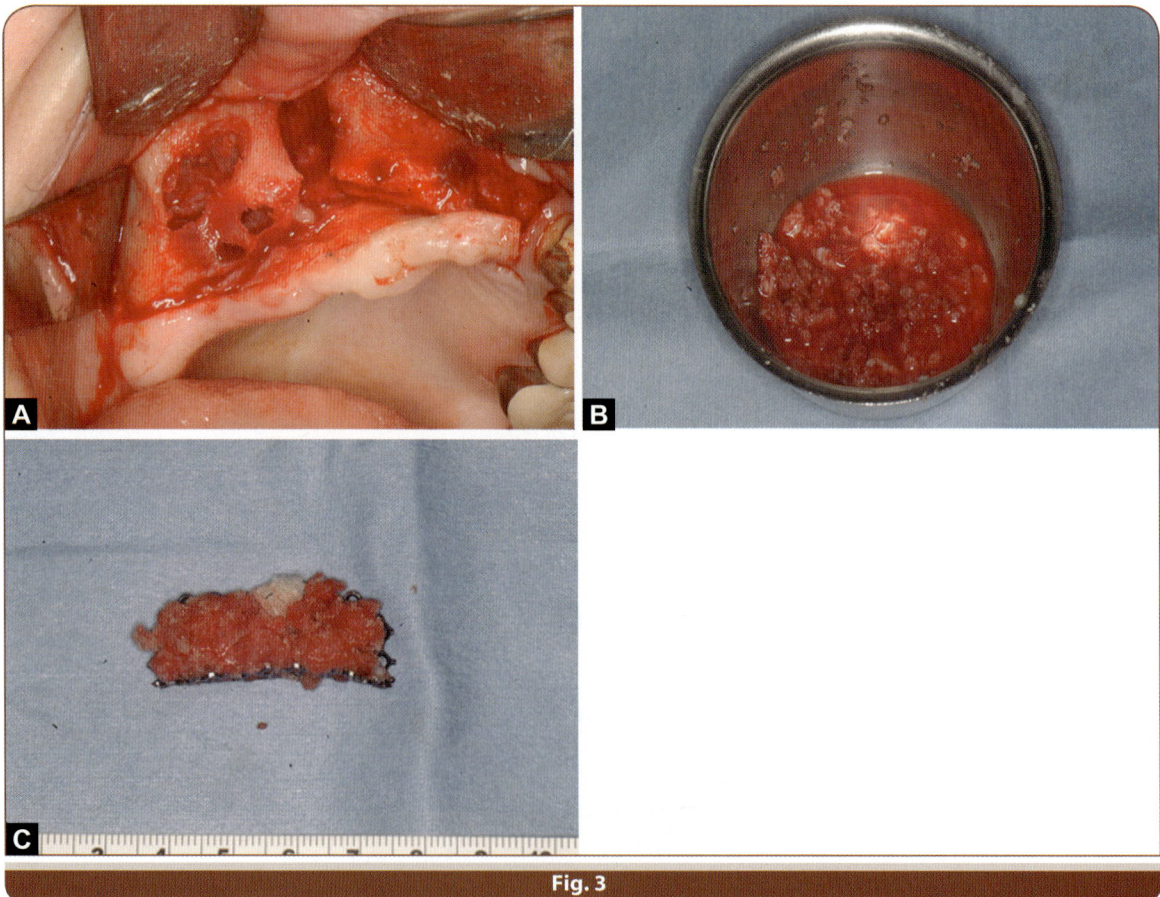

Fig. 3

(A) Design and release of flap, sinus graft procedure (B) BMP2 + autogenous bone, (C) Graft inside the titanium mesh **(Fig. 3)**.

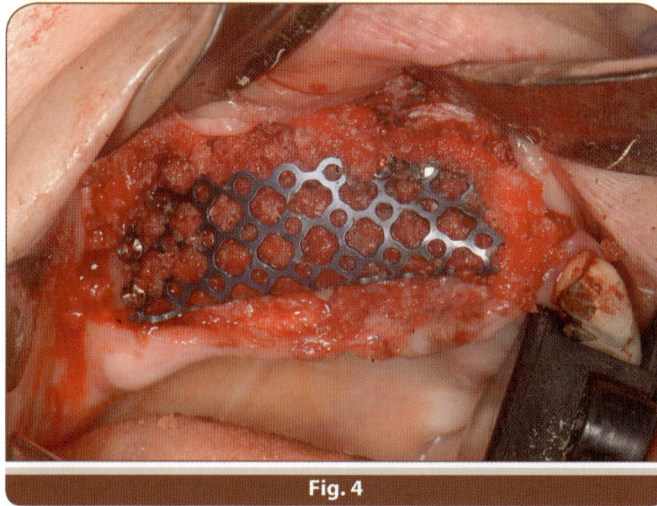

Fig. 4

Titanium mesh + osseoconduction (BMP 2 + autogeous bone) **(Fig. 4)**.

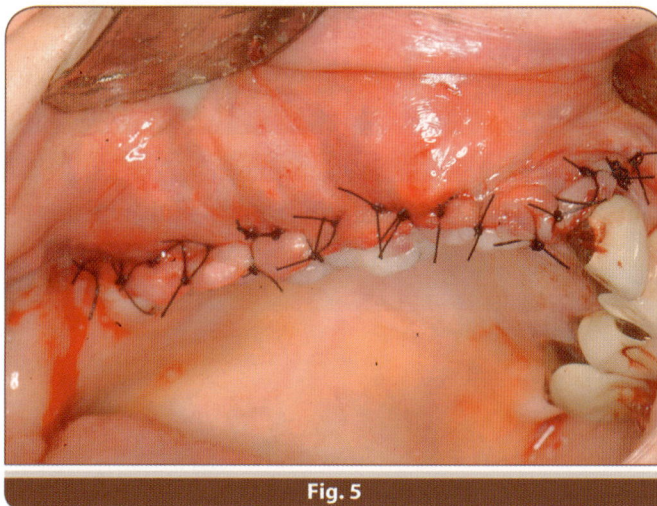

Fig. 5

Tension free closure **(Fig. 5)**.

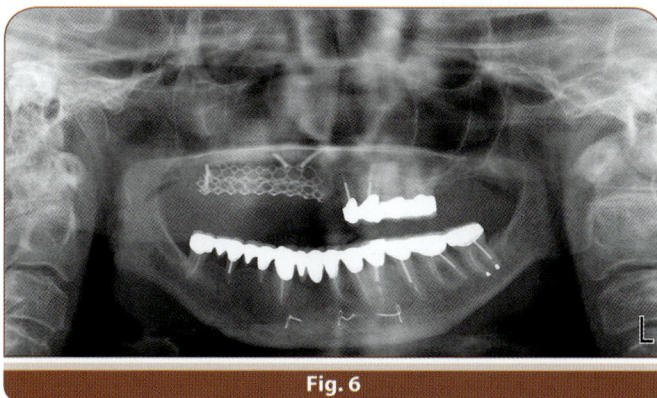

Fig. 6

Orthopantomogram after ridge augmentation **(Fig. 6)**.

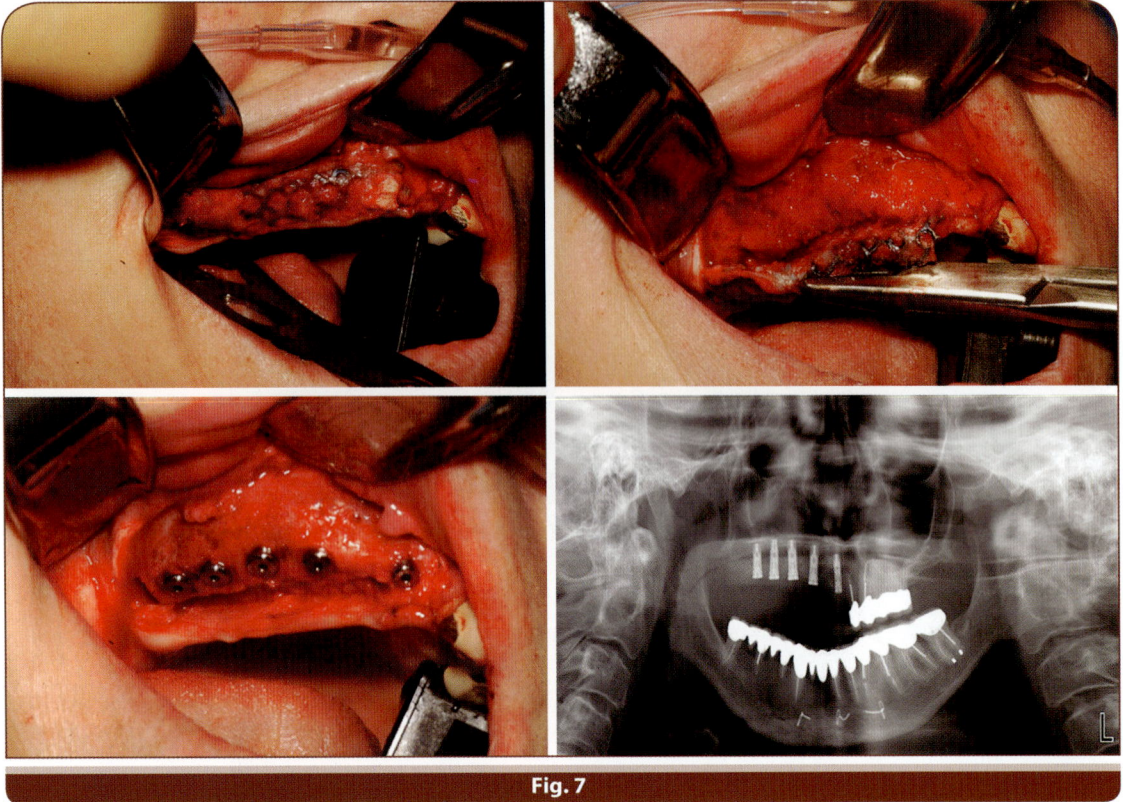

Fig. 7

After 6 months, titanium mesh removal and evident D4 type bone seen. Fine implants placed and checked radiographically **(Fig. 7)**.

Cary Bopiah

RECONSTRUCTION OF THE ANTERIOR MAXILLA WITH AN AUTOGENOUS BLOCK GRAFT FROM THE MANDIBULAR SYMPHYSIS

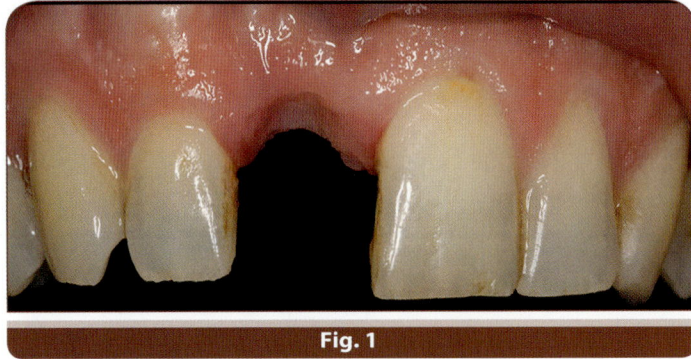

Fig. 1

A view of the upper right central incisor region 6 months after extraction. A 47-year-old Caucasian man was referred for an implant to replace the upper right central incisor. The tooth #11 had historically undergone a root canal treatment and restored with a post core crown approximately 20 years ago. The patient developed an abscess with the tooth which was subsequently extracted by his dentist **(Fig. 1)**.

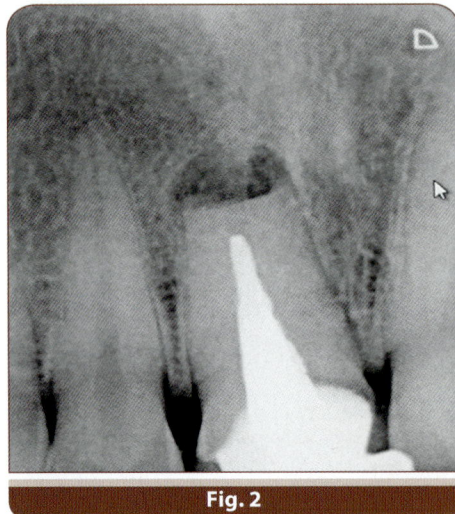

Fig. 2

Periapical radiograph of the upper right central incisor showing the evidence of root resection, a root canal treatment with a large post in the root canal. Evidence of periapical pathology can also be seen **(Fig. 2)**.

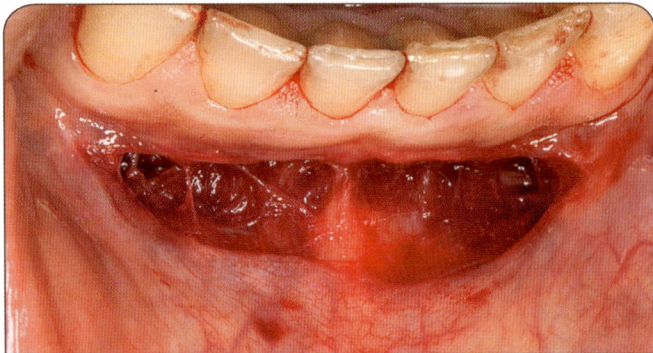

Fig. 3

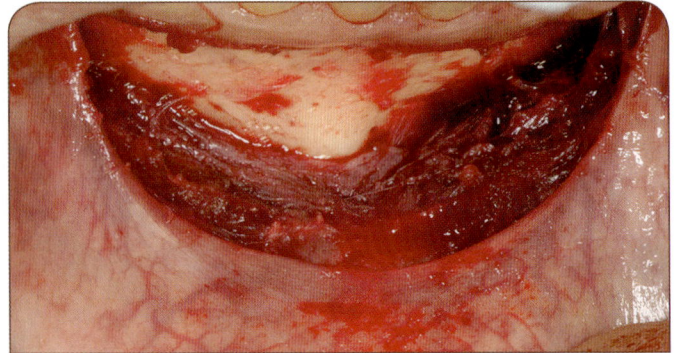

Fig. 4

Circumvestibular incision for exposure of the donor site (mandibular symphysis) **(Fig. 3)**.

Postage stamp outline for a symphysis graft **(Fig. 4)**.

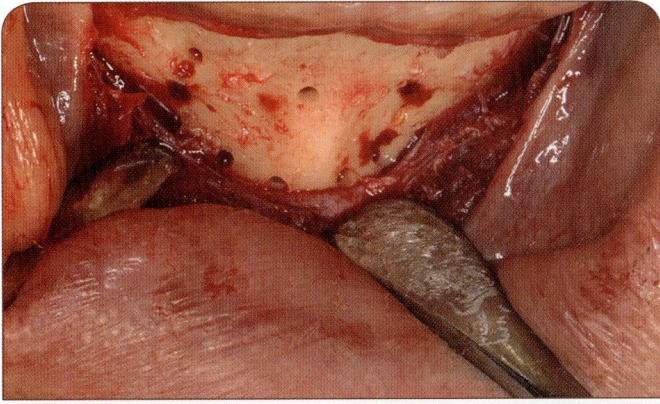
Fig. 5

Osteotomy outlined and completed through the labial cortex and into the spongiosa. The superior cut was made 5 mm below the root apices of the mandibular anteriors (**Fig. 5**).

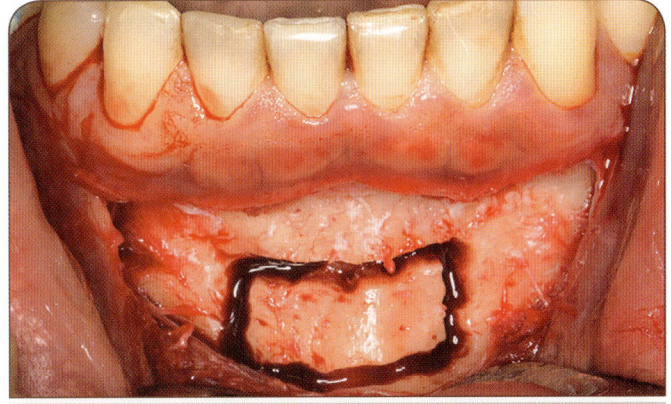
Fig. 6

Osteotomy outlined and completed (**Fig. 6**).

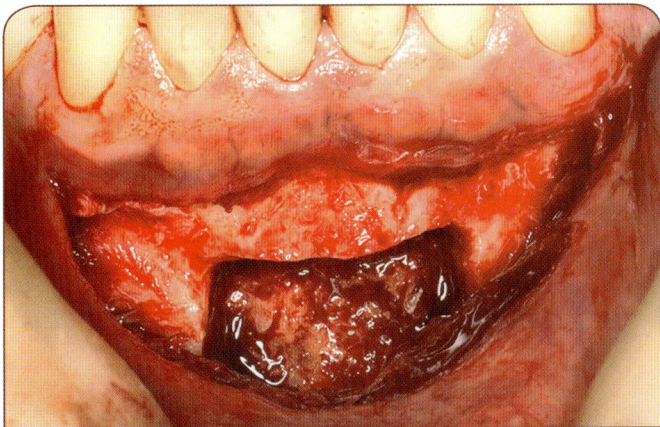
Fig. 7

Donor site after harvesting (**Fig. 7**).

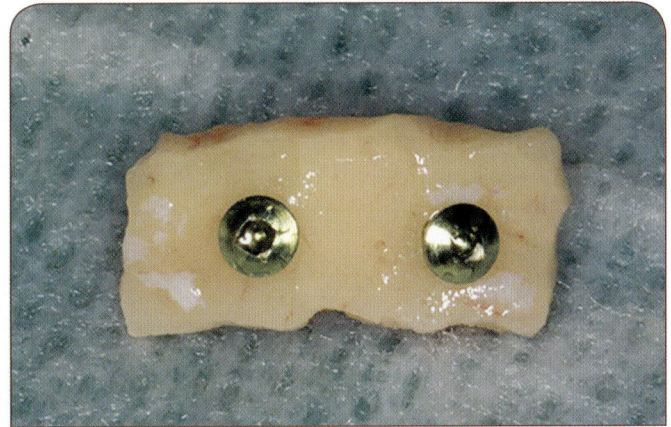
Fig. 8

Symphysis graft prepared with bone screws in situ (**Fig. 8**).

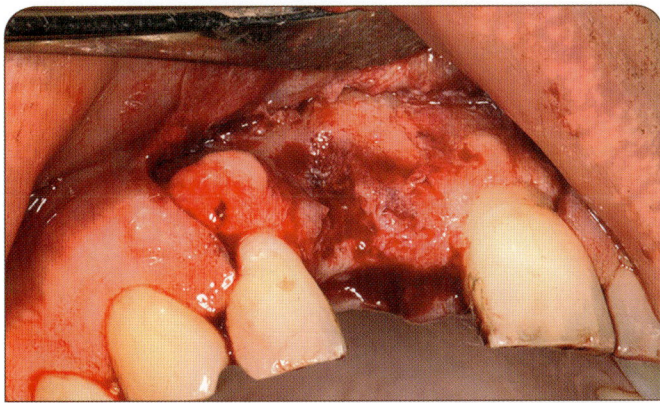
Fig. 9

Recipient site (upper right central incisor) showing horizontal deficiency of the site (**Fig. 9**).

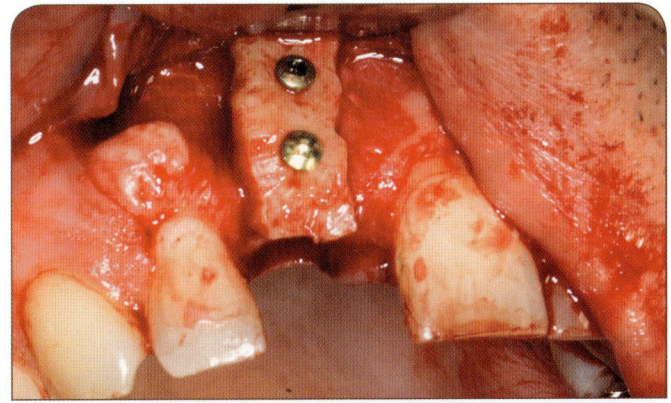
Fig. 10

The symphysis graft secured to the recipient site with two bone screws (**Fig. 10**).

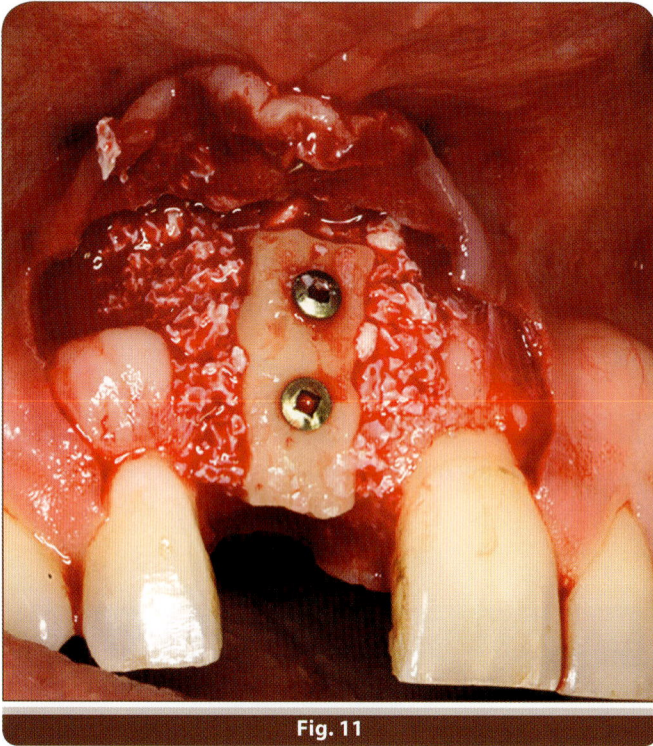

Fig. 11

Bio-oss® packed alongside the cortical graft to fill voids (site overbuilt and overfilled) **(Fig. 11)**.

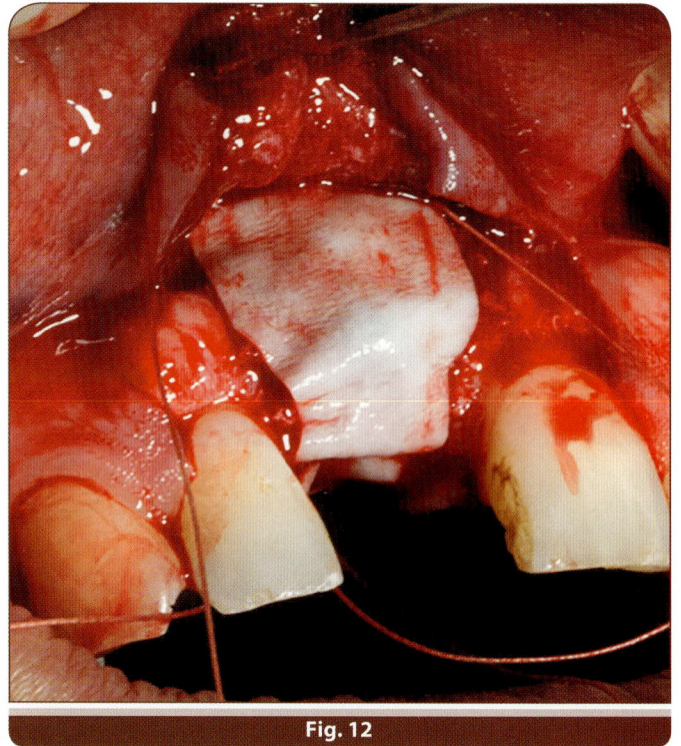

Fig. 12

Biogide membrane to be held with a sling suture **(Fig. 12)**.

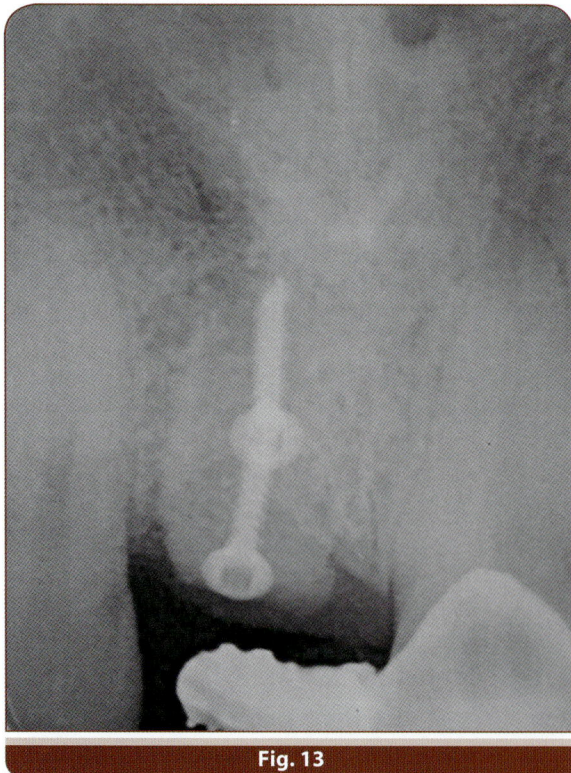

Fig. 13

Postoperative radiograph of bone graft in situ **(Fig. 13)**.

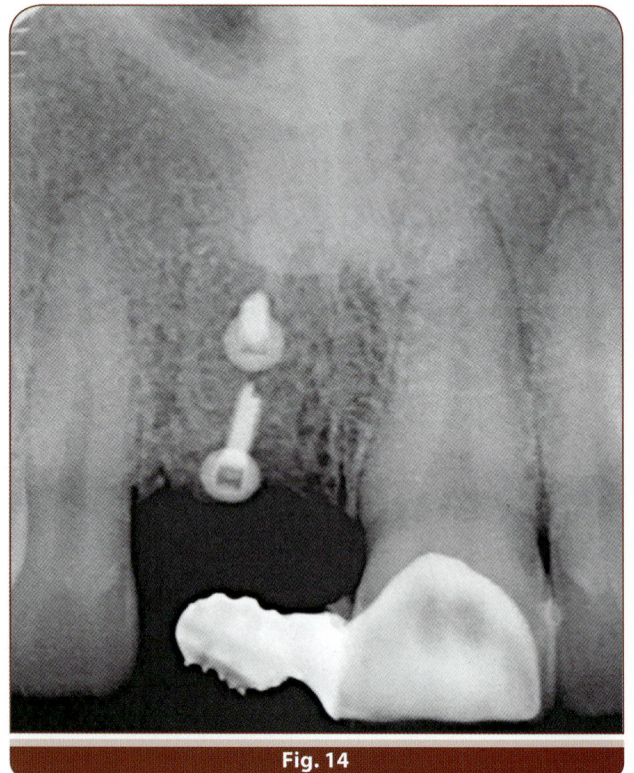

Fig. 14

Bone graft healed after 5 months **(Fig. 14)**.

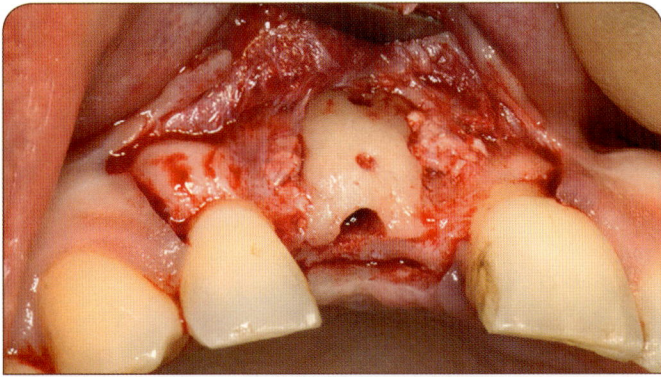

Fig. 15

Healed grated site, reopened after 6 months and implant osteotomy prepared **(Fig. 15)**.

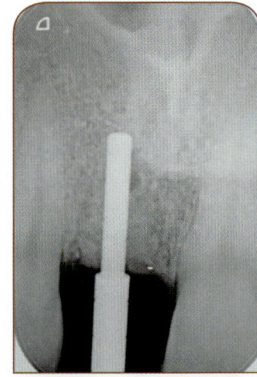

Fig. 16

Periapical of a guide pin in the initial osteotomy **(Fig. 16)**.

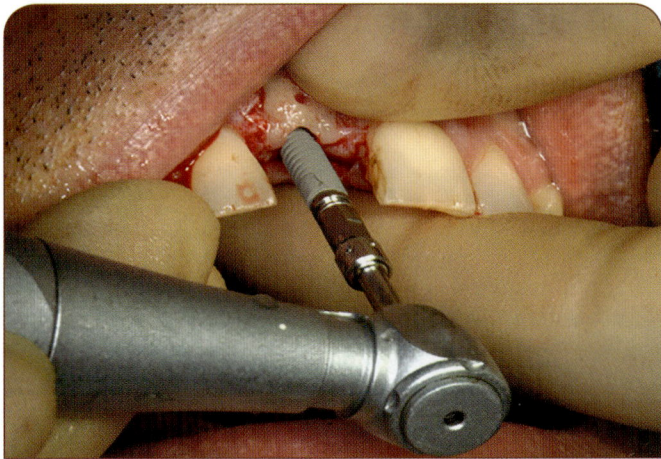

Fig. 17

An ankylos 3.5 × 11 mm (DENTSPLY) implant being placed into the osteotomy **(Fig. 17)**.

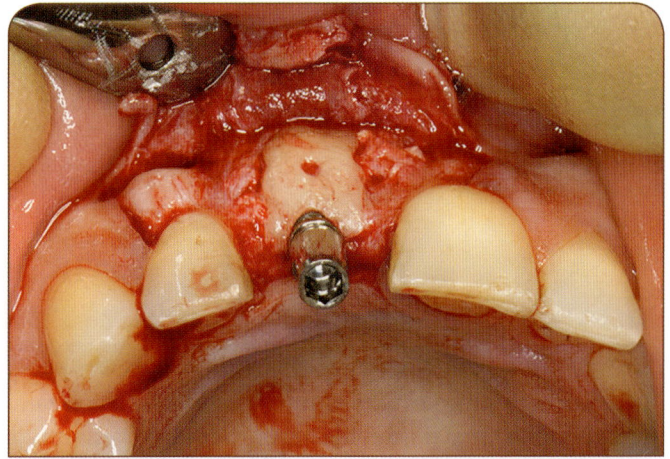

Fig. 18

Implant in situ emergence in line with the cingulum of the tooth #21 **(Fig. 18)**.

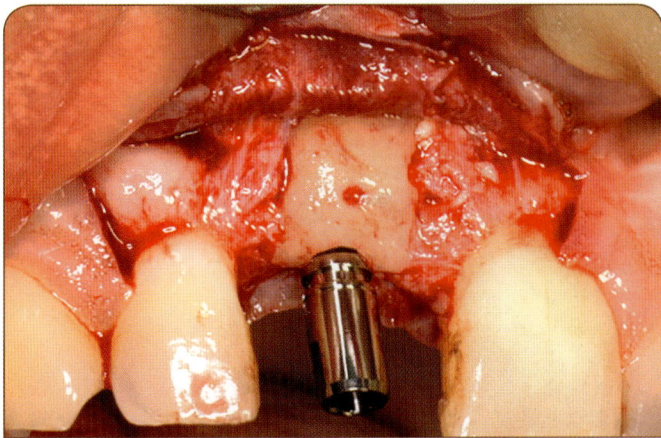

Fig. 19

Implant in situ **(Fig. 19)**.

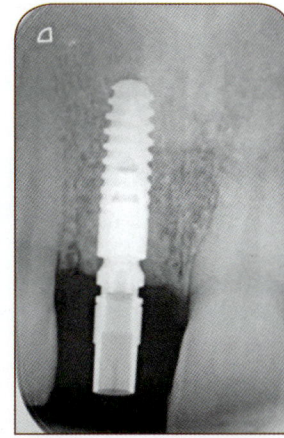

Fig. 20

Ankylos (DENTSPLY) implant in situ **(Fig. 20)**.

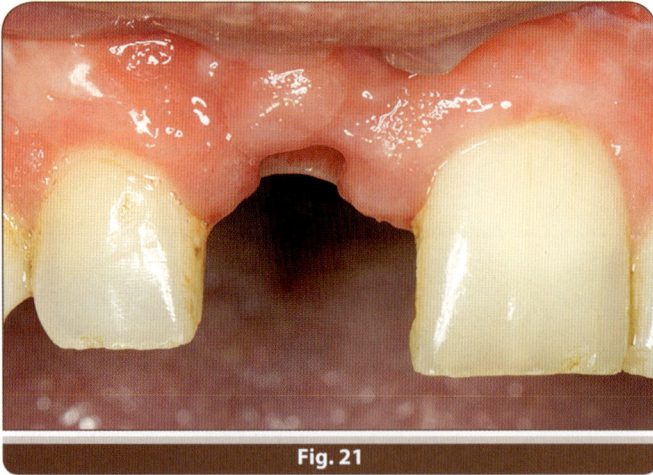

Healed site 2 weeks after uncovery **(Fig. 21)**.

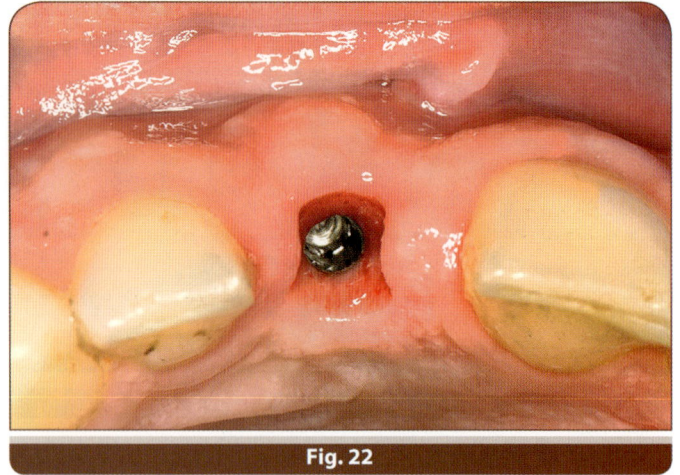

Two weeks after uncovery **(Fig. 22)**.

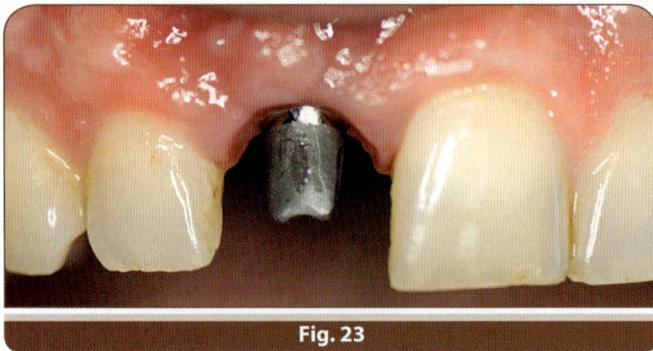

After site development with temporary abutment and temporary crown, final impressions were taken and a titanium post was secured into the body of the implant **(Fig. 23)**.

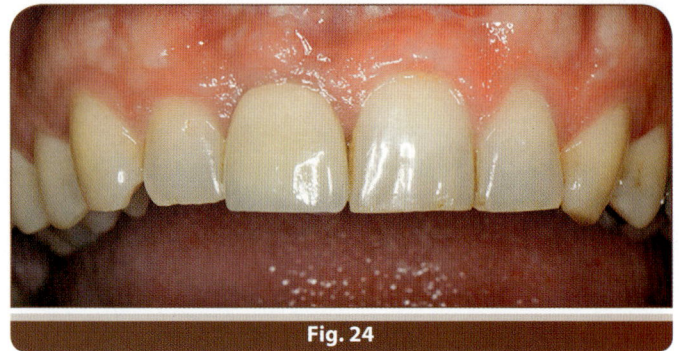

Intraoral view of the final crown on the titanium abutment in the tooth #11 region **(Fig. 24)**.

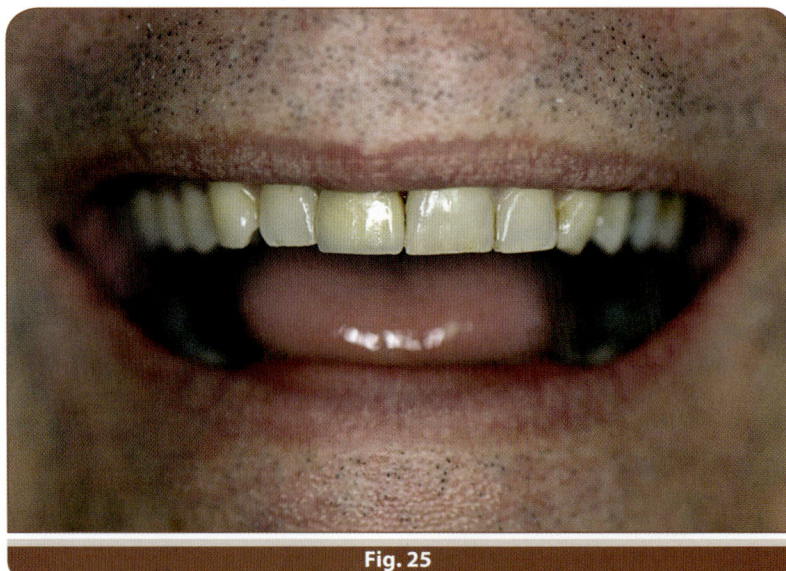

An extraoral view of the patient smiling **(Fig. 25)**.

CASE STUDY 81

Tarun Kumar

LATERAL RIDGE SPLIT FOLLOWED BY IMMEDIATE IMPLANT PLACEMENT

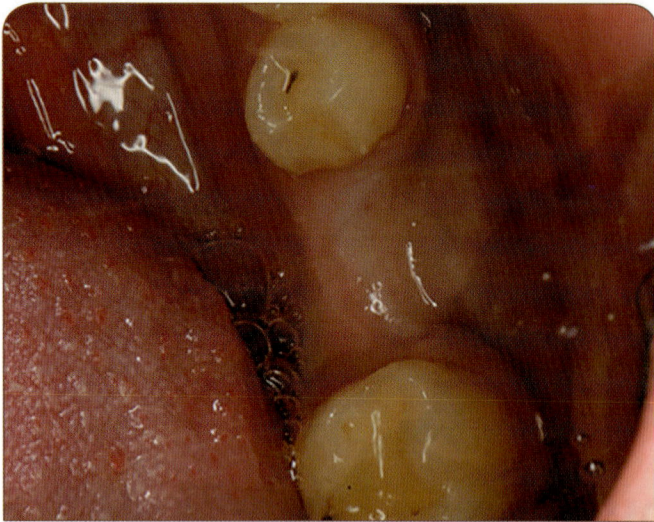

Fig. 1

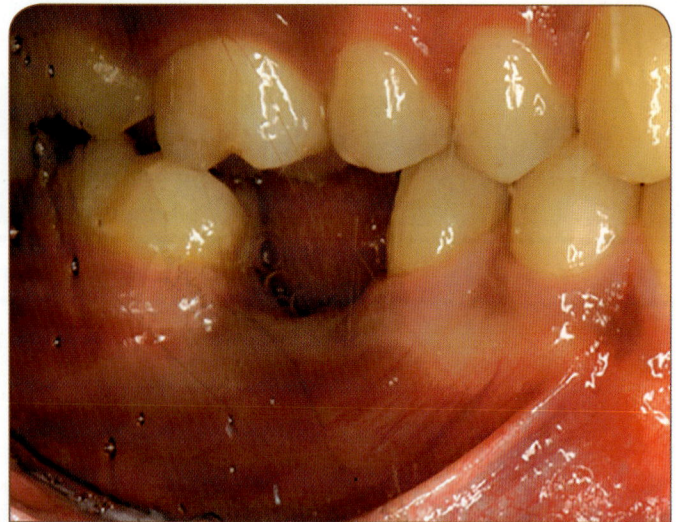

Fig. 2

A 20-year-old healthy male patient came with the chief complaint of missing left lower back tooth with inability to chew in the same area. His medical history was non-contributory. His past dental history revealed that he had got his tooth extracted due to caries 2 years back **(Figs. 1 and 2)**.

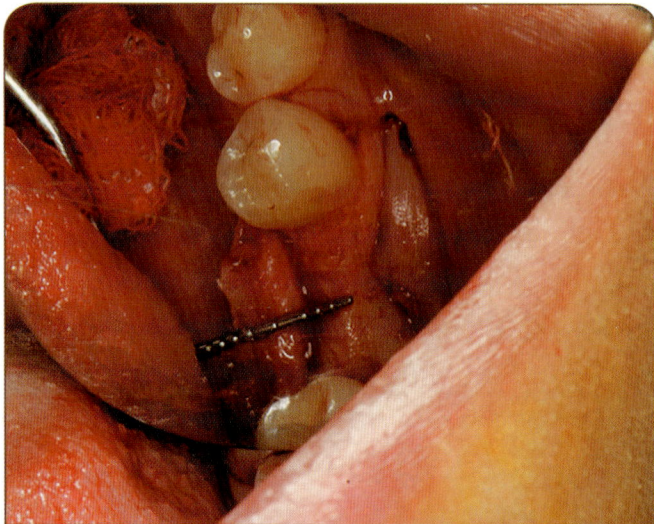

Fig. 3

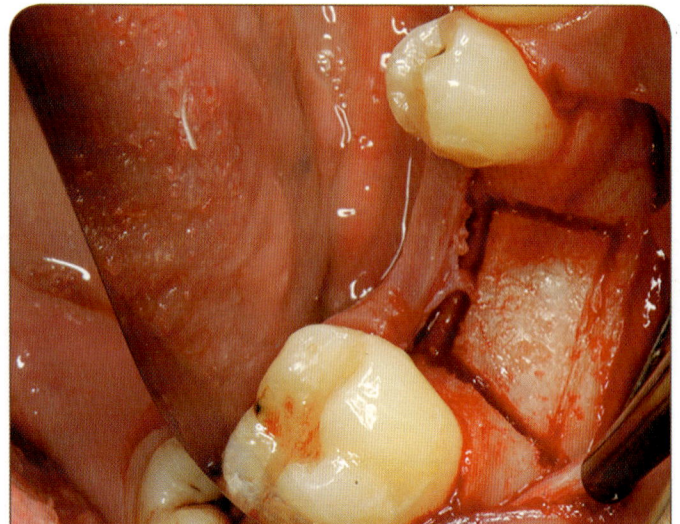

Fig. 4

Perioperatively a deficient horizontal ridge width of about 2.5 mm was seen **(Fig. 3)**.

Horizontal bone osteotomy was then performed in the middle of the ridge using an ultrasonic bone surgery unit, to a depth of 8 mm, starting 2 mm distal to the premolar, and extending 2 mm posterior to the planned distal implant site, after which two vertical relaxing osteotomies in the buccal bone plate was given which extended from the cortical into the cancellous bone. The two vertical cuts were then joined at the base by another horizontal cut called the "hinge cut" which does not breach the labial cortical plate **(Fig. 4)**.

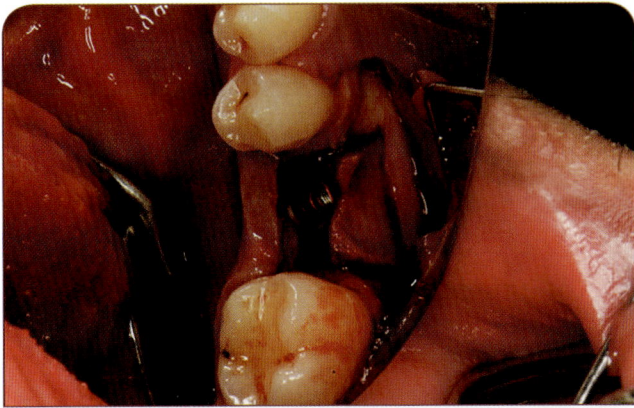
Fig. 5

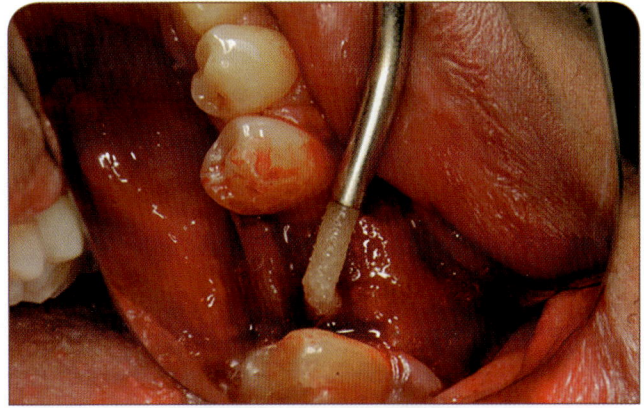
Fig. 6

Implant placement was done at the prepared osteotomy site at the expanded ridge. The osteotomy site was prepared starting with the pilot drill and the ridge was expanded further using compression screws till the final ridge expansion was achieved (**Fig. 5**).

A collagen membrane was adapted over the osteotomy site and the expanded ridge which was grafted using novabone putty under the membrane (**Fig. 6**).

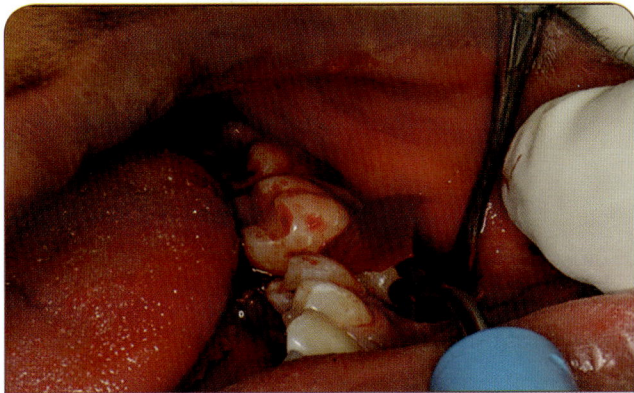
Fig. 7

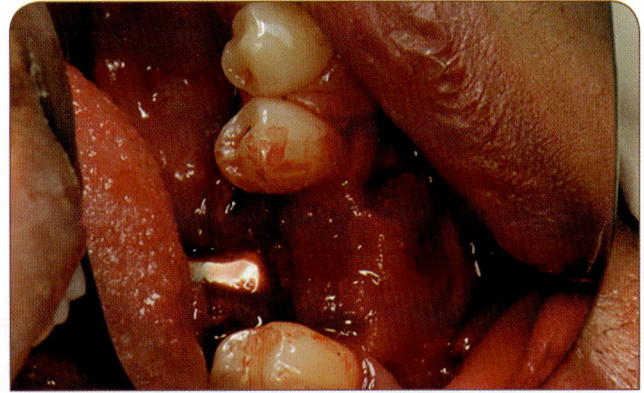
Fig. 8

Collagen membrane adapted (**Fig. 7**).

Bone graft filled to cover osteotomy site (**Fig. 8**).

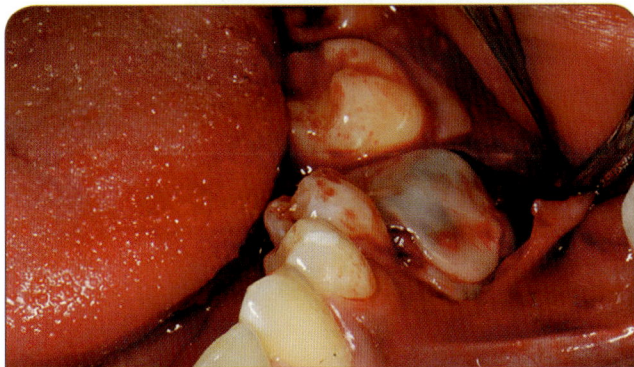
Fig. 9

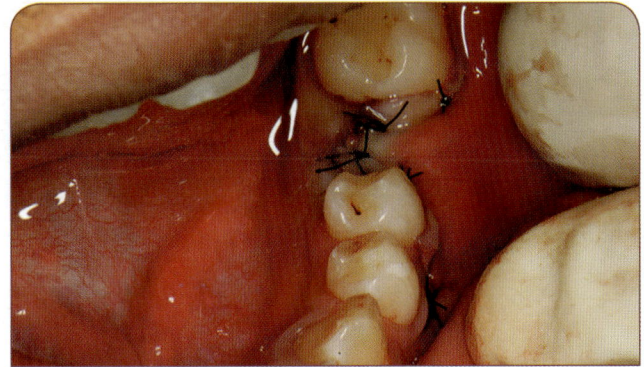
Fig. 10

A PRF membrane was obtained and adapted over the implant site that was grafted (**Fig. 9**).

A tension free closure of the flap was achieved (**Fig. 10**).

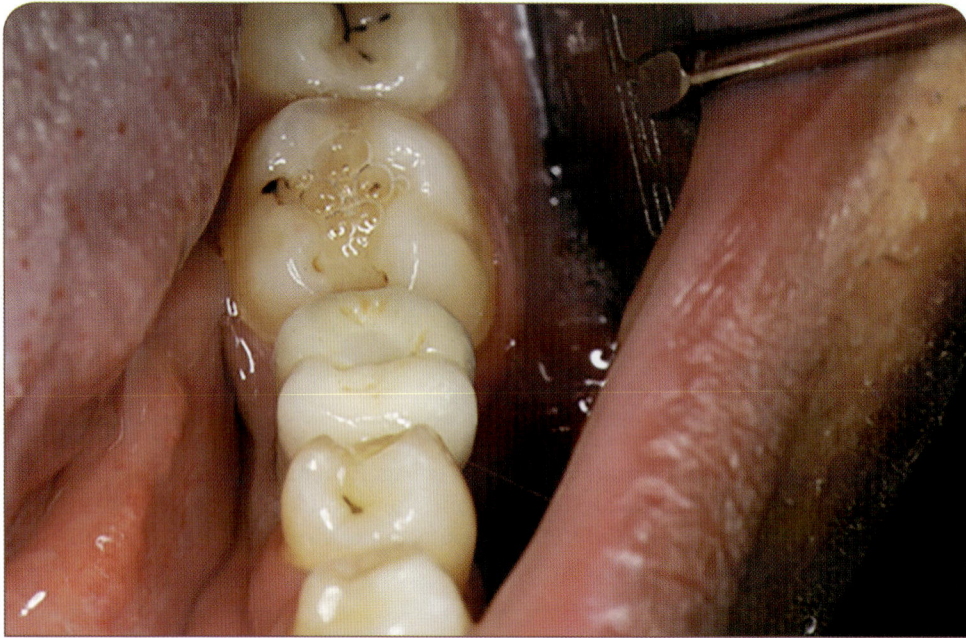

Fig. 11

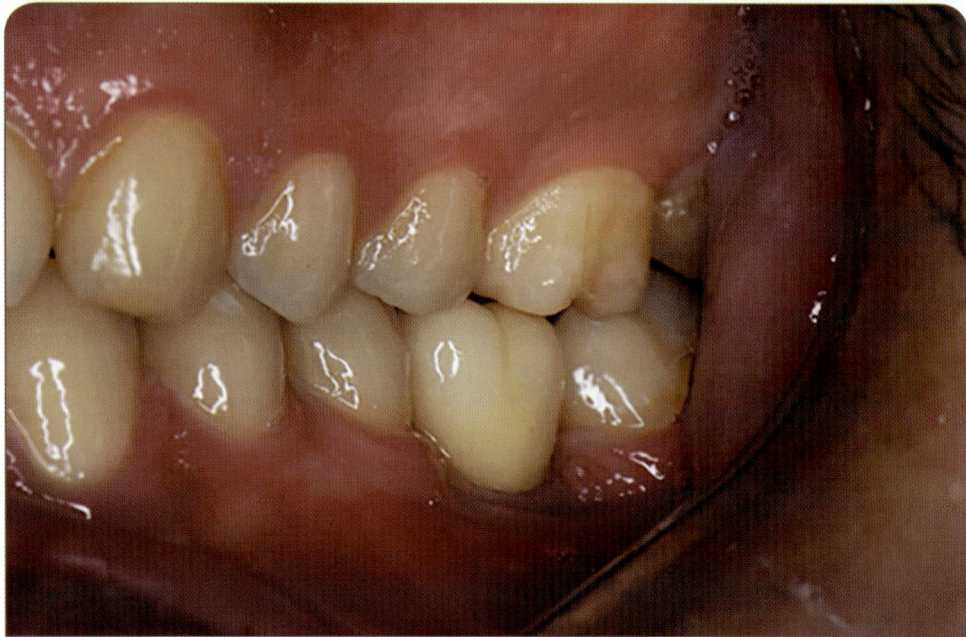

Fig. 12

Prosthesis was delivered 6 months after the implant placement and adequate occlusion was achieved **(Figs. 11 and 12)**.

Robert A Horowitz

Piezosurgery: An Important Tool to Harness Bone for Immediate Implant Placement

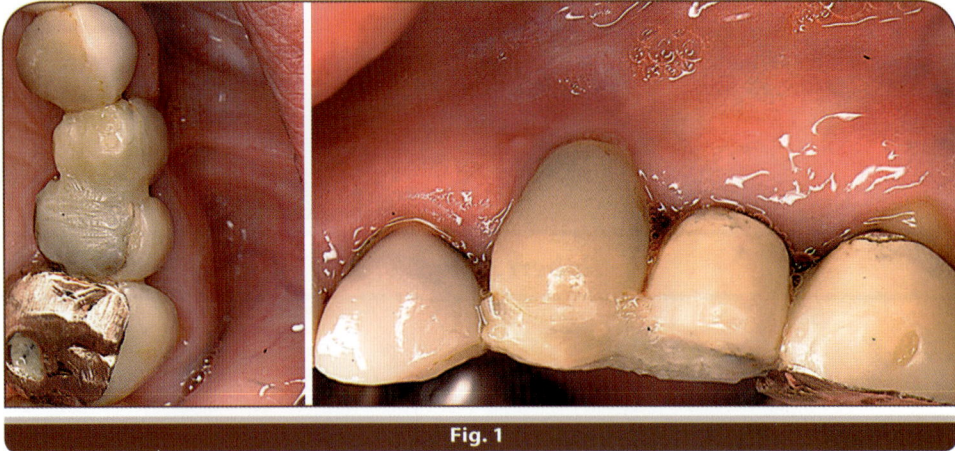

Fig. 1

This patient presented with a failing fixed prosthesis—decay under the anterior abutment and site collapse in the pontic area **(Fig. 1)**.

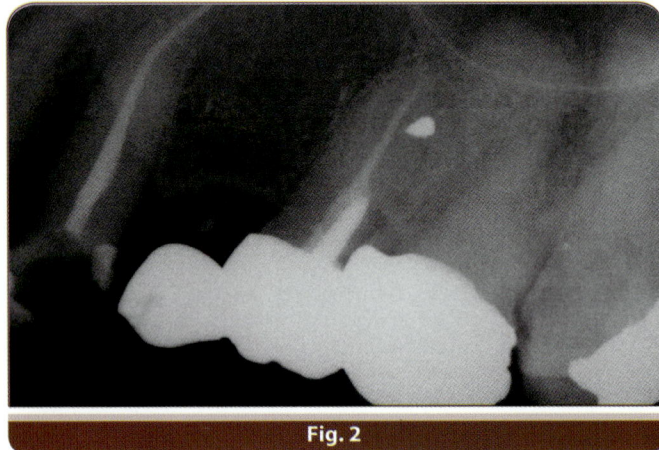

Fig. 2

The radiograph shows significant decay in the maxillary left canine and decreased radio-opacity in the edentulous site **(Fig. 2)**.

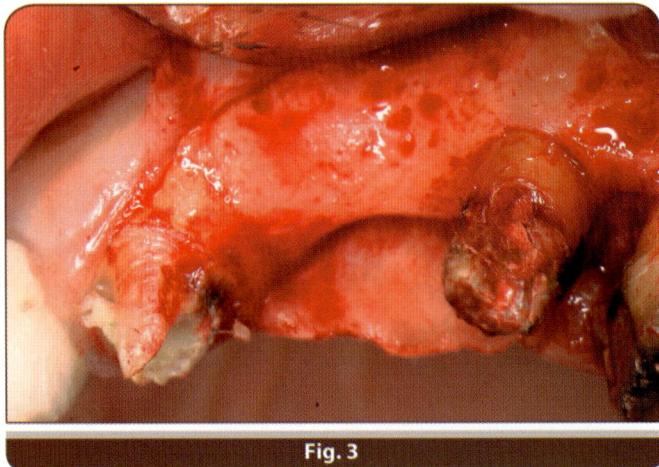

Fig. 3

- Patient desires
  - Individual teeth
  - Minimal number of procedures

Insufficient crown length to restore. After flap elevation, inadequate crown length is noted **(Fig. 3)**.

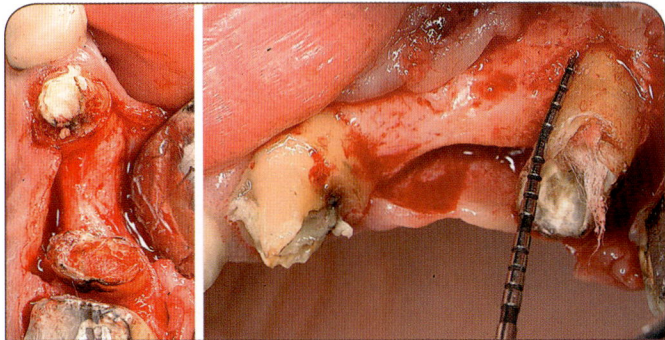

Fig. 4

Sufficient crown length has been achieved using Piezosurgery; horizontal and vertical ridge collapse are noted in the edentulous area **(Fig. 4)**.

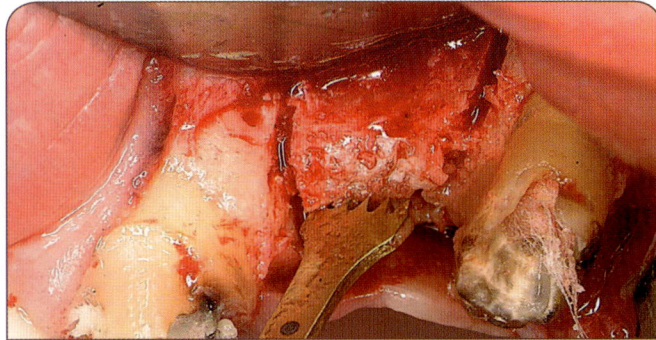

Fig. 5

Saw cuts to free buccal segment. Utilizing micro-oscillating piezosurgery saws, absolute precision enables vertical and horizontal osseous cuts to be made **(Fig. 5)**.

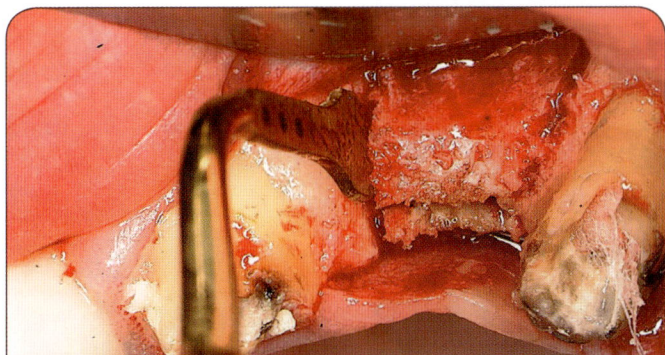

Fig. 6

Ensure potency between cuts. The facial cuts are reinforced to ensure they meet with the apico-coronal cut close to the palatal bone **(Fig. 6)**.

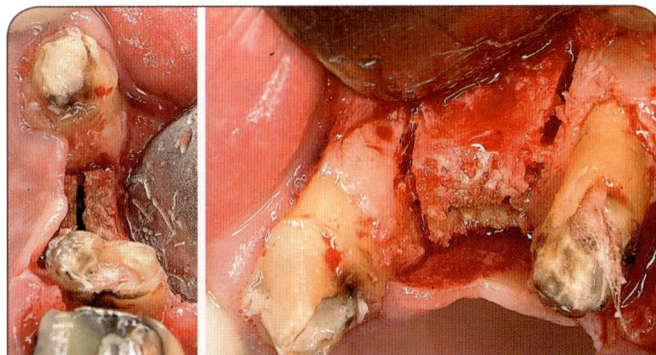

Fig. 7

Occlusal and facial view of completed cuts through the alveolar bone show proximity to adjacent tooth, palatal bone and remaining periosteum on the segment to be mobilized **(Fig. 7)**.

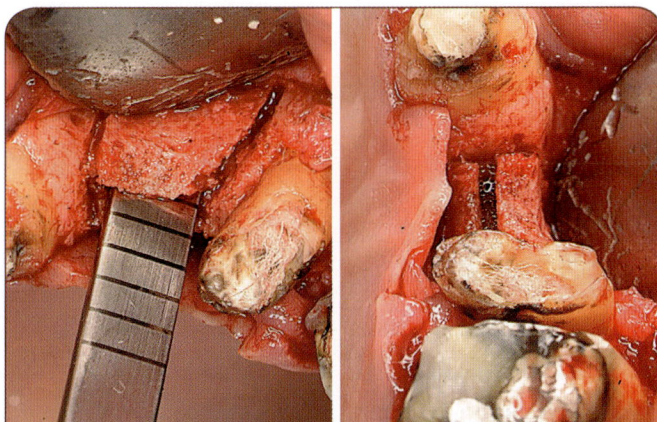

Fig. 8

Narrow chisel to mobilize. Thin bladed chisels are gently malleted to begin spreading the facial bone **(Fig. 8)**.

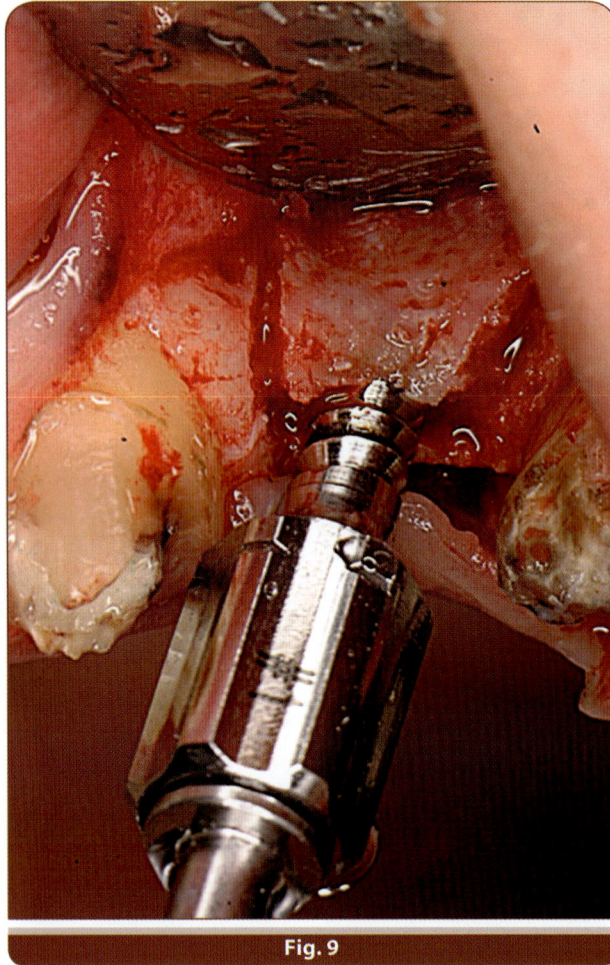

Fig. 9

Non-cutting rotary bone spreaders (MIS) follow the apical path the implant will track along to continue spreading the facial plate of bone **(Fig. 9)**.

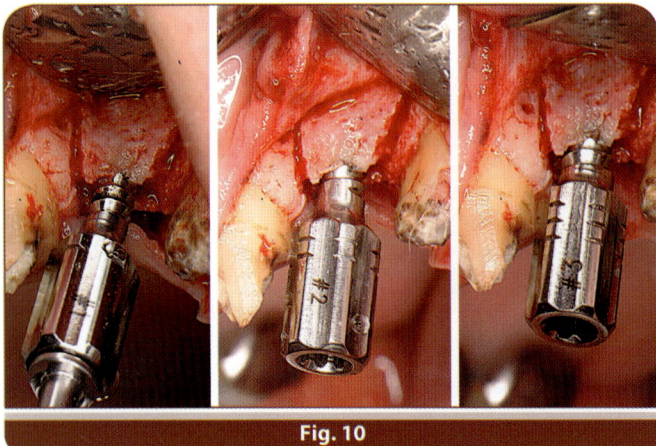

Fig. 10

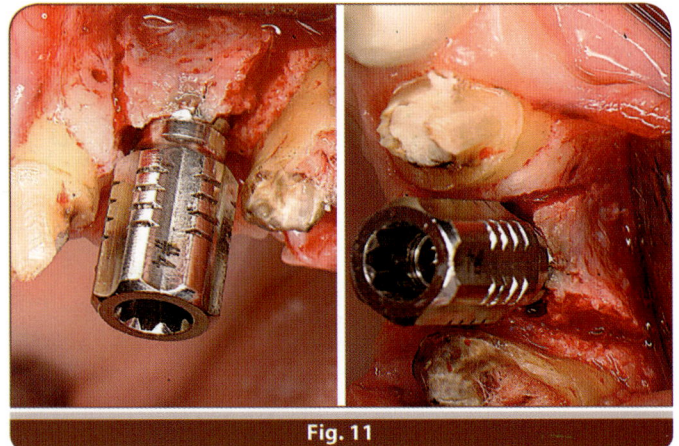

Fig. 11

Sequential widening of "gap". Wider spreaders facilitate gentle movement of the mobilized segment **(Fig. 10)**.

Long cuts so segment bends. Facial and occlusal view with the final spreader demonstrate lack of trauma to the facial bone **(Fig. 11)**.

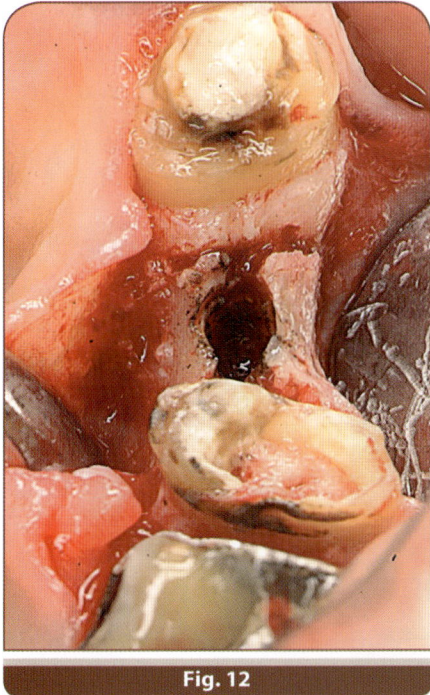

Fig. 12

The site is now 3 mm wider. The rotary devices do not cut but gently compress some of the less dense facial bone **(Fig. 12)**.

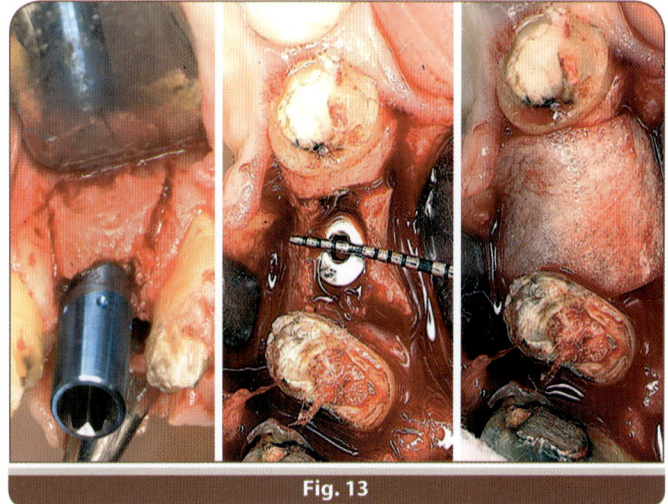

Fig. 13

Graft over crest and gap. Ideal implant position is noted. Additional graft material is placed on the buccal surface of the bone and covered with a resorbable (Cytoplast RTM) barrier. Initial placement, graft, barrier.

Initial implant placement and site after grafting with DFDBA and Calcium Sulfate (Dentogen) with a calcium sulfate barrier prior to placing the collagen **(Fig. 13)**.

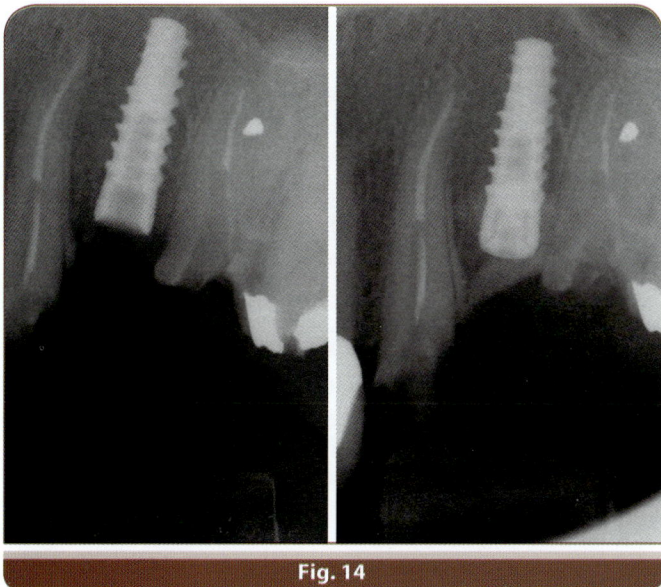

Fig. 14

Postoperative IOPA **(Fig. 14)**.

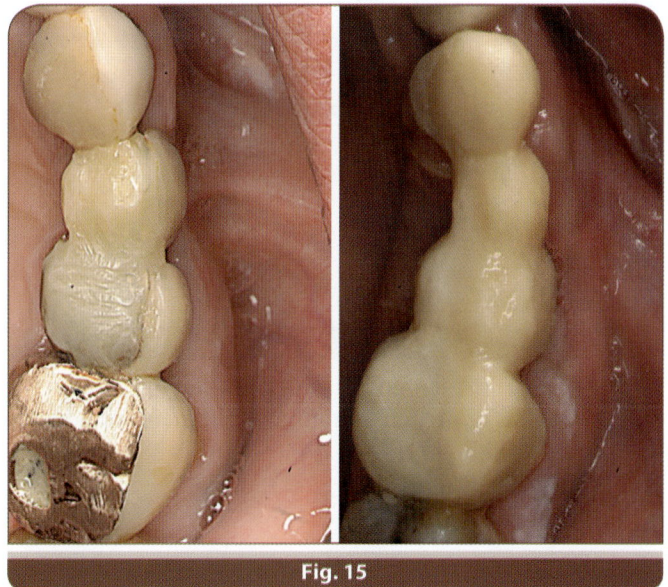

Fig. 15

Two weeks postoperative—wider ridge. The occlusal views preoperatively and 2 weeks postoperatively show the increased alveolar ridge width obtained with this procedure **(Fig. 15)**.

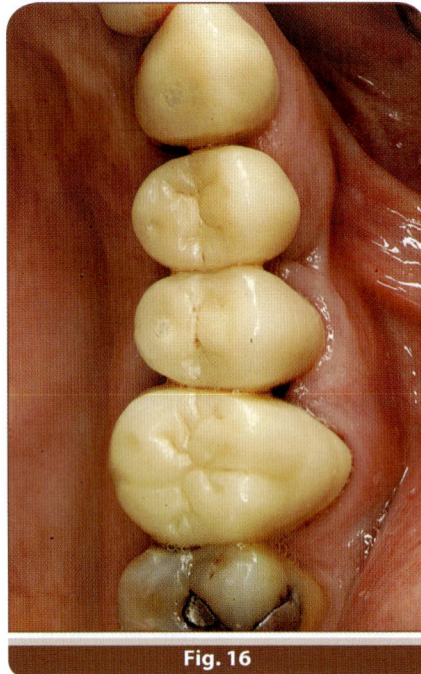

Fig. 16

Six years postoperatively: the ridge width has been maintained, crowns are of an appropriate size and shape **(Fig. 16)**.

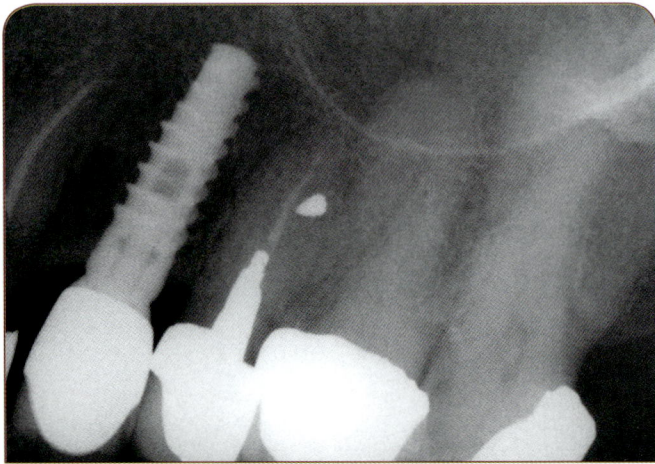

Fig. 17

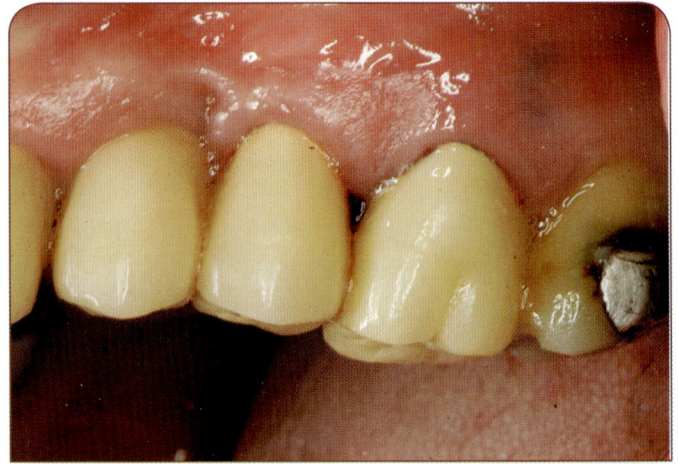

Fig. 18

Crestal bone preserved all sites. Radiographically the crestal bone is quite dense and has been maintained at an ideal height **(Fig. 17)**.

Final restoration 6 year postoperative. Facially, sufficient and healthy keratinized tissue is shown. The patient is maintaining the restorations free from inflammation **(Fig. 18)**.

Tarun Kumar

Simultaneous Implant Placement with Titanium Mesh Assisted Guided Bone Regeneration

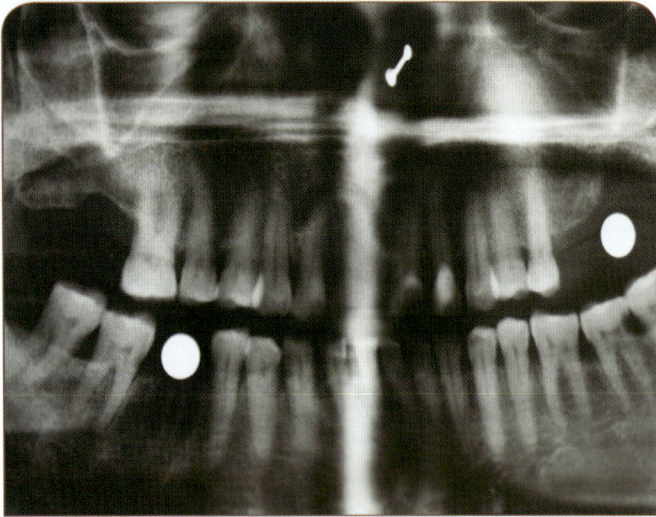

Fig. 1

A 58-year-old female patient with a chief complaint of missing teeth in the upper anterior region. History of road traffic accident and extraction of right central incisors. No relevant medical history. Radiological and clinical examination of the area revealed. Seibert's Class I ridge deficiency. Treatment plan included simultaneous implant placement titanium mesh assisted guided bone regeneration using sandwich augmentation protocol **(Fig. 1)**.

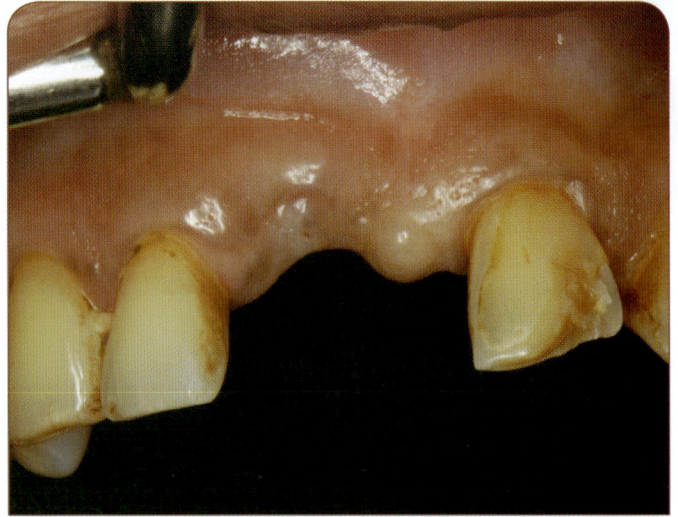

Fig. 2

Preoperative labial view of the edentulous area **(Fig. 2)**.

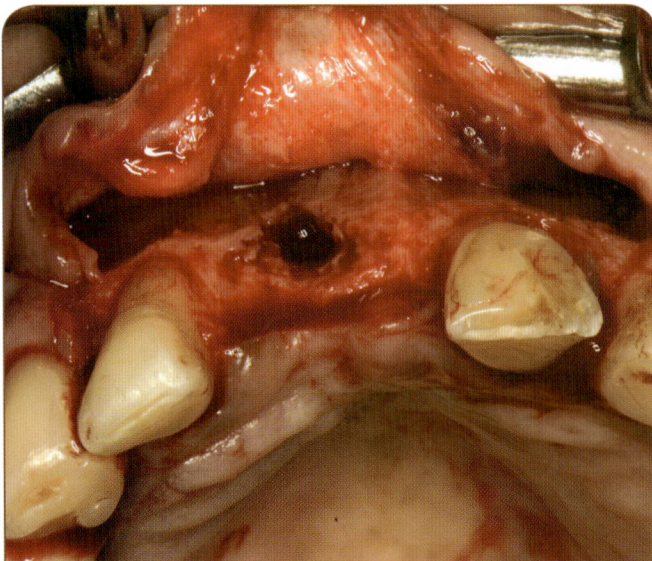

Fig. 3

A full thickness flap reflection utilizing mid crestal and two vertical release incisions **(Fig. 3)**.

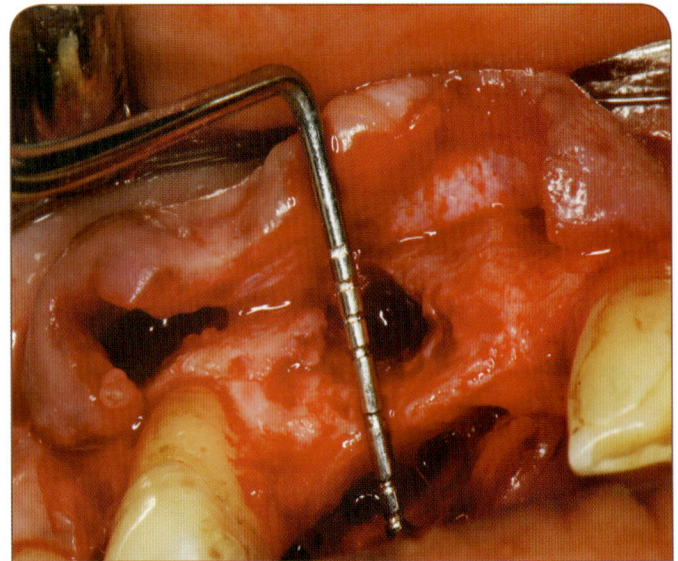

Fig. 4

Occlusal view showing the horizontal deficiency of the ridge **(Fig. 4)**.

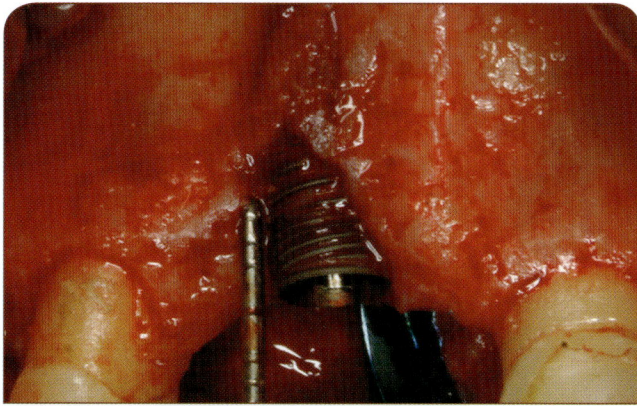
Fig. 5

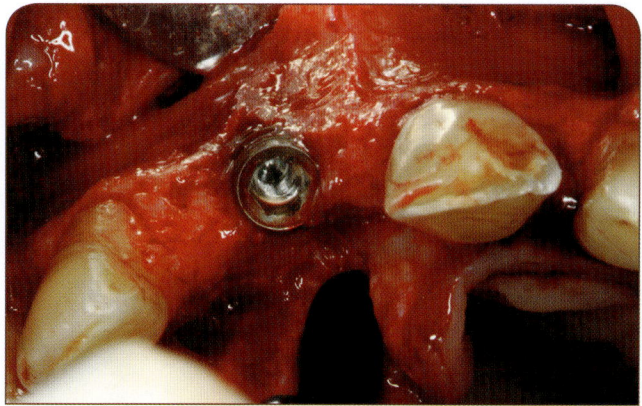
Fig. 6

Implant placement 4.2 × 13 mm. 7 mm dehiscence on the buccal aspect of the implant **(Figs. 5 and 6)**.

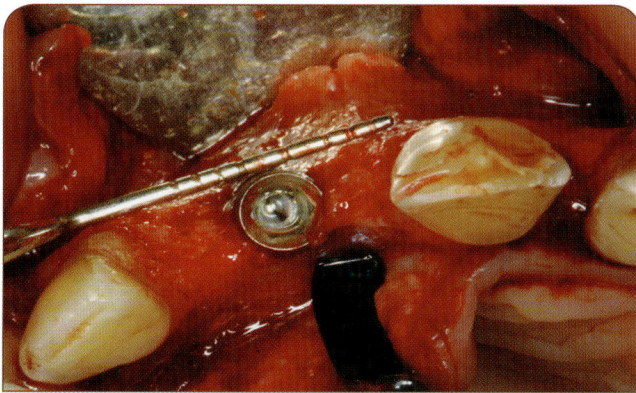
Fig. 7

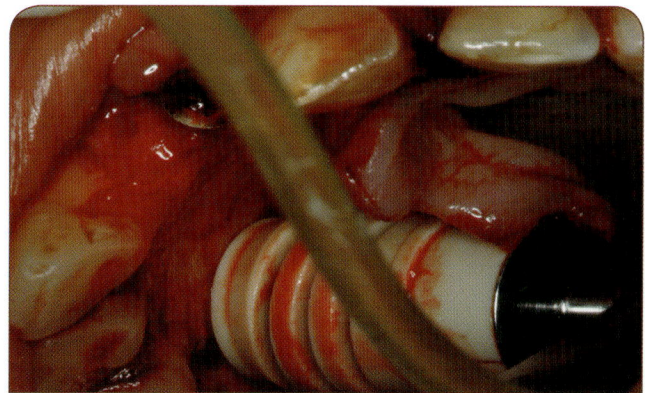
Fig. 8

Occlusal view.
Note: Class II dehiscence **(Fig. 7)**.

Harvesting of autogenous bone using auto chip maker (ACM) Neo Biotech **(Fig. 8)**.

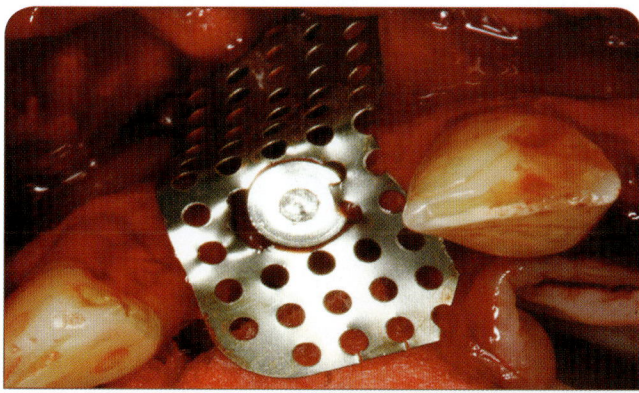
Fig. 9

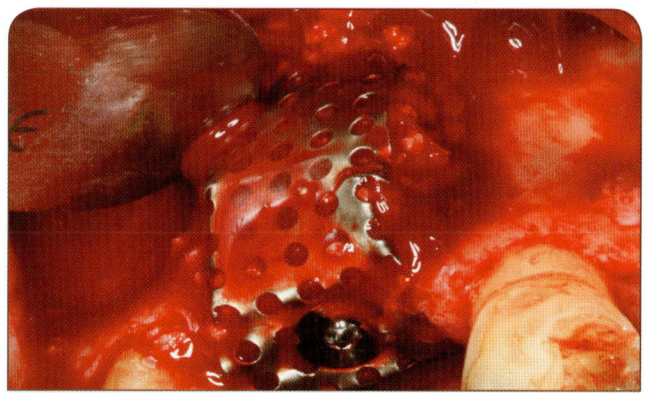
Fig. 10

Titanium mesh contoured and adapted **(Fig. 9)**.

Sandwich bone augmentation protocol with autogenous bone layered over the exposed threads layered by calcium phosphosilicate (CPS) morsels. Mesh adapted over the graft **(Fig. 10)**.

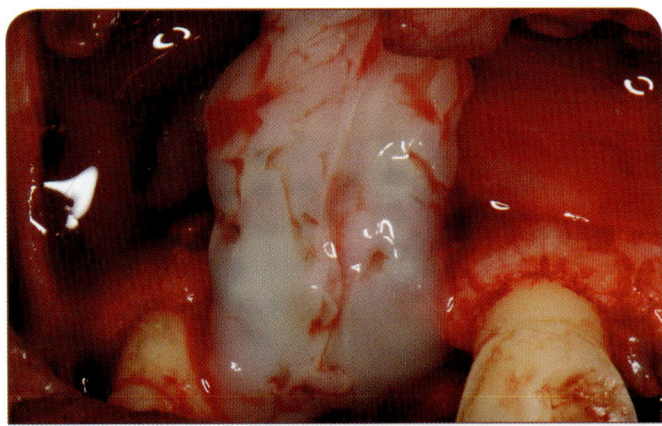

Fig. 11

Platelet rich fibrin (PRF) membrane placed over the mesh **(Fig. 11)**.

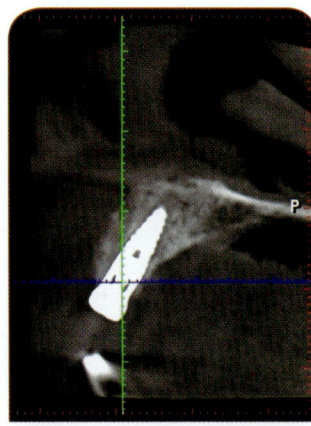

Fig. 12

Four months postoperative CBCT showing regenerated bone **(Fig. 12)**.

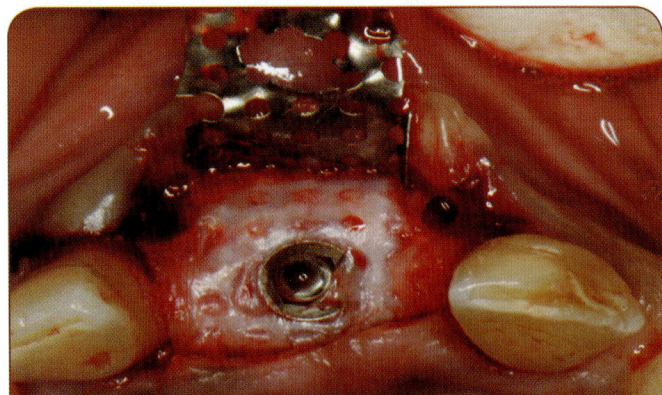

Fig. 13

Five months postoperative mesh removal. Note the full volume of regenerated bone **(Fig. 13)**.

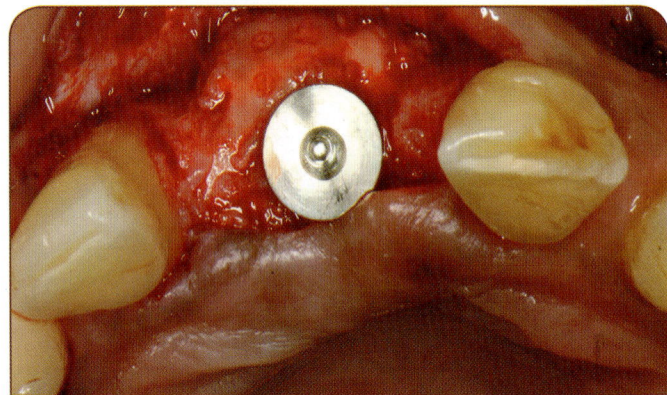

Fig. 14

Healing cap placed. This view shows minimum 3 mm thick buccal bone regenerated over the previously dehiscence **(Fig. 14)**.

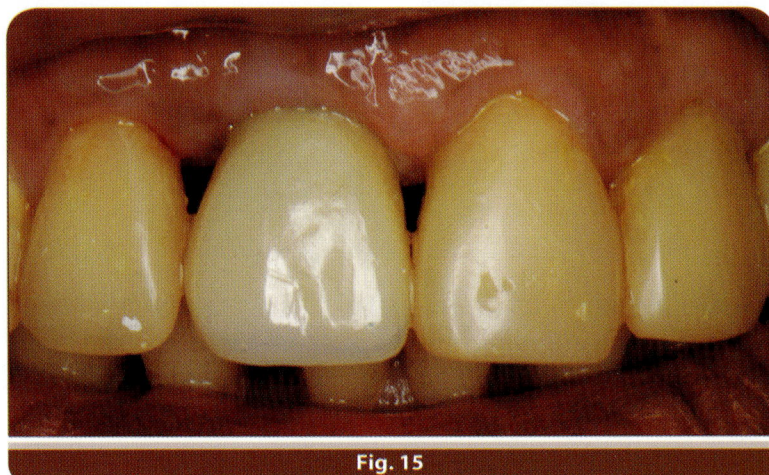

Fig. 15

Final cement retained PFM **(Fig. 15)**.

CASE STUDY 84

Robert A Horowitz

SCREW RETAINED ZIRCONIA CROWN: TREATMENT CHOICE TO MINIMIZE PERI-IMPLANT DISEASE

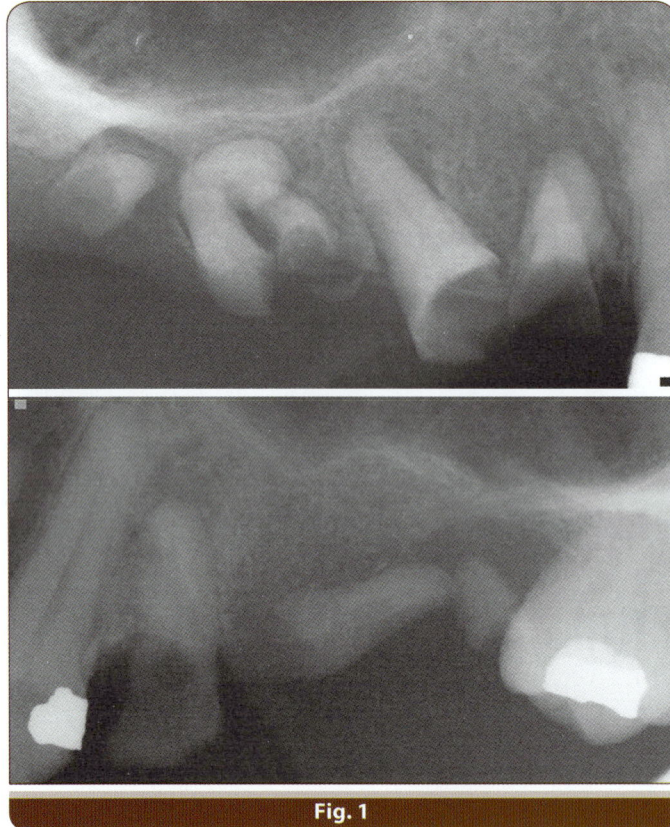

Fig. 1

Extraction socket therapy goals: Whether to presence socket or to augment. Diagnosis—extremely fearful patient. Extraction alone would lead to further bone loss, need for sinus augmentation and poor aesthetics from high crown-to-implant ratio **(Fig. 1)**.

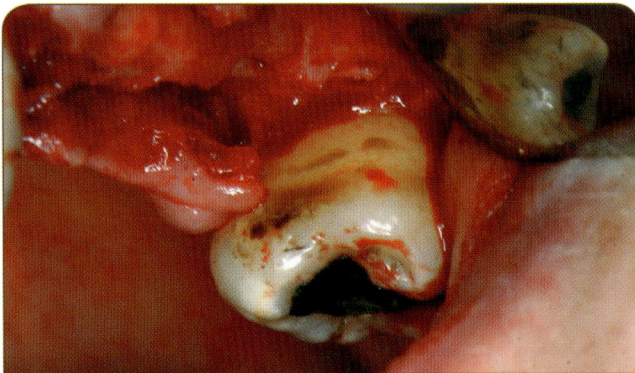

Fig. 2

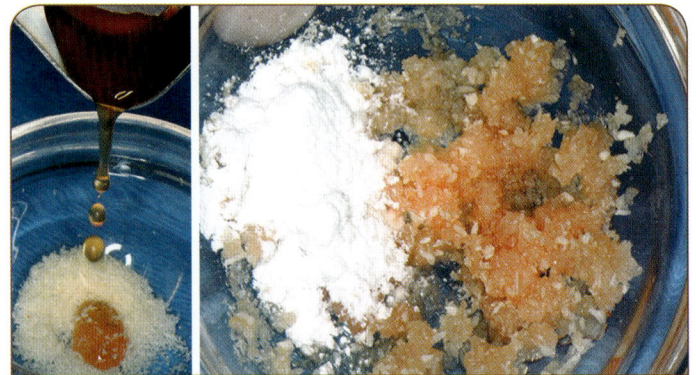

Fig. 3

Highest percentage of vital bone. Minimal residual graft, approach through biology, literature, appropriate diagnosis and treatment. Significant calculus deposits and bone loss are noted at the time of flap elevation for socket debridement **(Fig. 2)**.

Mineralized cancellous allograft: Slowly resorbing, good scaffold. Hydrate in L-PRF (Leucocyte and platelet rich fibrin): Growth enhancing autologous compounds. Mix calcium sulfate (3D Bond, Dentogen): Increase osteogenesis, angiogenesis and improve handling. To enhance the biologic activity of mineralized cancellous allograft, it was hydrated in L-PRF and mixed with calcium sulfate hemihydrate (Dentogen, Orthogen Corp,. NJ) **(Fig. 3)**.

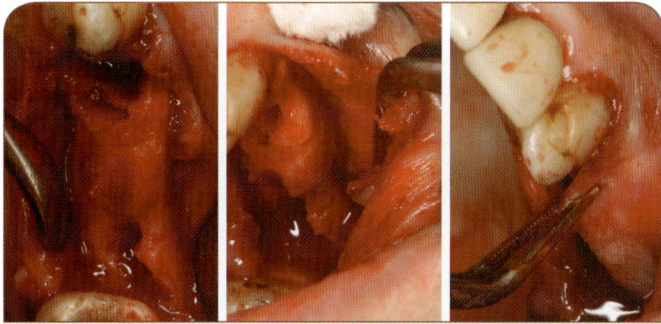

Fig. 4

Thorough debridement enables full visualization of the amount of bone loss and thinness of the residual plates of bone. Periosteal releasing incisions will enable primary closure over the grafted sites **(Fig. 4)**.

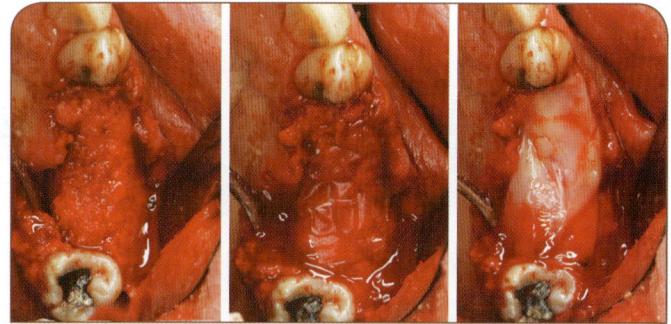

Fig. 5

Barriers: BioXclude, L-PRF. Full contour particulate grafting is covered by a bioactive amnion-chorion barrier (BioXclude, Snoasis Medical, Denver, CO) and membranes from L-PRF to enhance biologic activity and decrease the chance of flap retraction and graft loss **(Fig. 5)**.

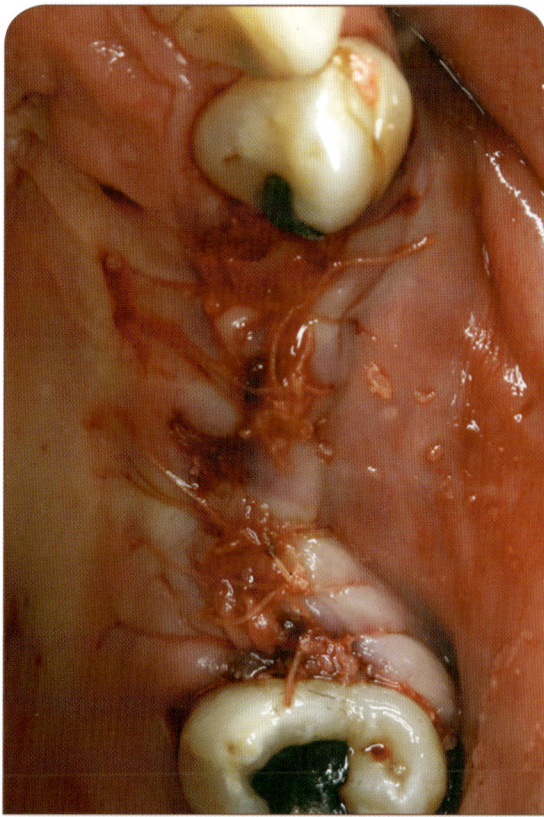

Fig. 6

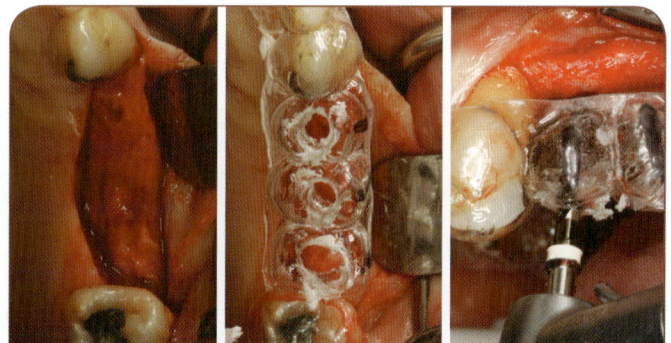

Fig. 7

Surgical guide from prosthetic setup. A surgical guide made from articulated casts and a prosthetic wax-up is used for implant placement in the fully healed ridge six months after extraction and grafting **(Fig. 7)**.

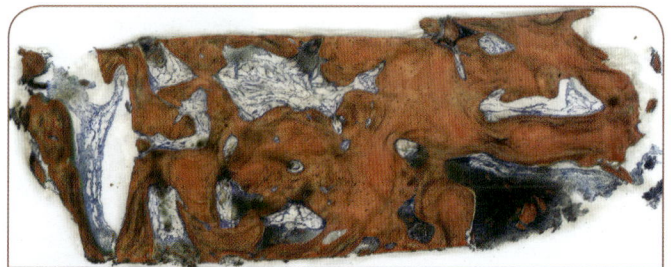

Fig. 8

Bioactive barriers: Hold shape, speed healing, decrease risk of flap exposure of graft. Ensure primary closure obtained, maintained, wait for healing: Follow on X-ray. Reenter after radiographic evidence of new bone: Calcium sulfate dissolves—radiolucent, Bone forms, mineralizes- radiopaque. Primary closure is obtained to assist in healing following the principles of Guided Bone Regeneration **(Fig. 6)**.

Ideal result: Vital bone shown on non-demerarized histo with Von Gieson's Picric Acid Fuchsin Stain.

Non-demineralized processing of a core of regenerated material shows 73% bone, 65% vital (Hard Tissue Research Lab, U. of Minnesota Dental School, Minneapolis, MN) **(Fig. 8)**.

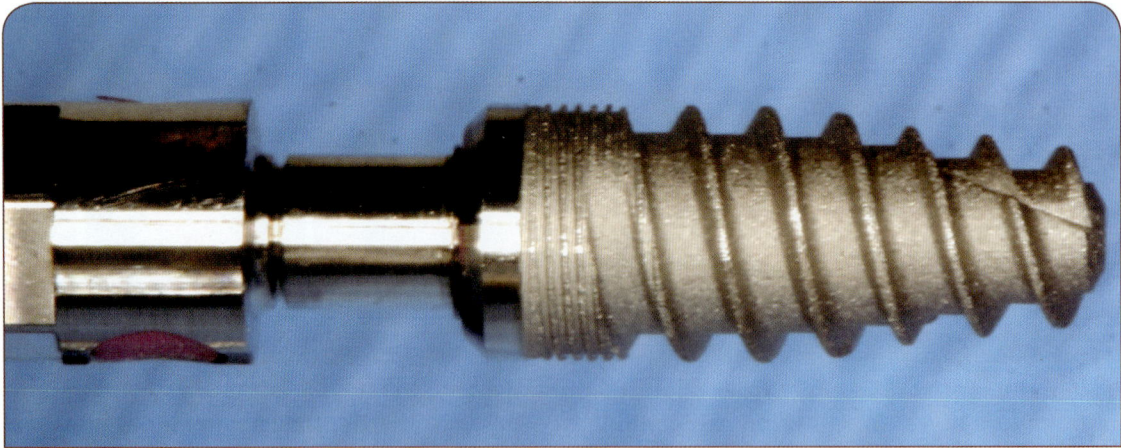

Fig. 9

Preserve bone—Glidewell (Hahn) implant with machined collar. Choosing an appropriate implant (J Hahn Implant, Glidewell Dental) with both a polished shoulder and platform shifting should decrease the chance of peri-implant disease **(Fig. 9)**.

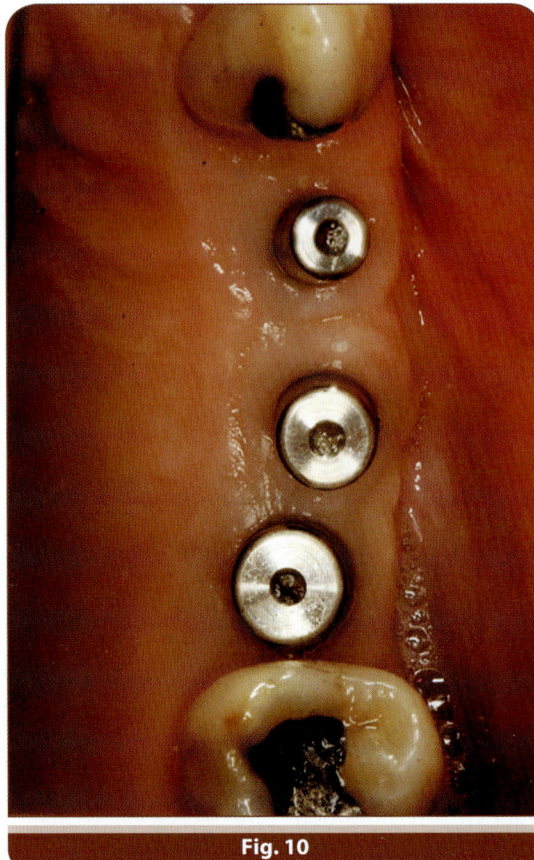

Fig. 10

Bone and gingiva healed: Thick keratinized tissue Buccal, Palatal. Implants ready to restore at 3 months. Ideal restoration: Screw retained, Zirconia on Ti base, CAD-CAM designed, fabricated. The occlusal view 3 months after implant placement shows ideal ridge width and mature keratinized tissue **(Fig. 10)**.

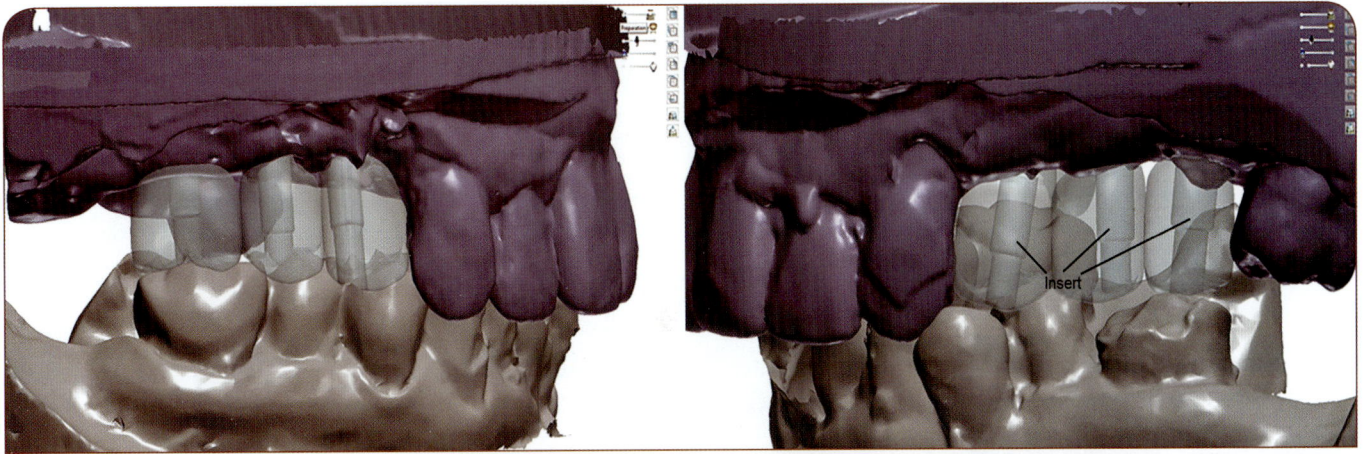

Fig. 11

CAD CAM designed restorations. Digital design of CAD/CAM restorations enables proper contour, contacts and aesthetics (Glidewell Dental) to be designed and approved or modified by the dentist prior to fabrication **(Fig. 11)**.

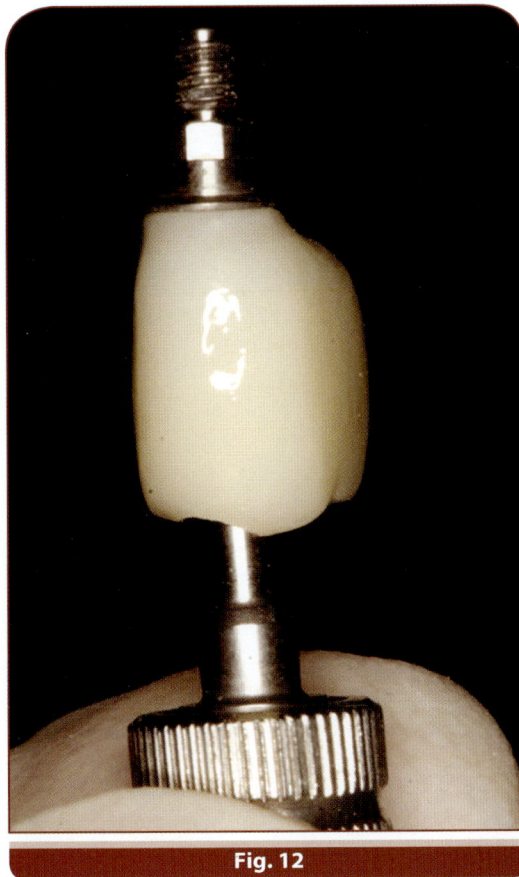

Fig. 12

Less plaque accumulation than Titanium, Gold. Easy to get: Aesthetics, contour, contact, emergence profile. Retrievable, inexpensive titanium base: No abrasion inside implant, machined fit of parts and a screw-retained Brux Zir crown on a titanium base (Glidewell Dental) has complete retrievability with no residual subgingival cement. Contours designed to facilitate ideal home and to reduce the risk of peri-implant disease **(Fig. 12)**.

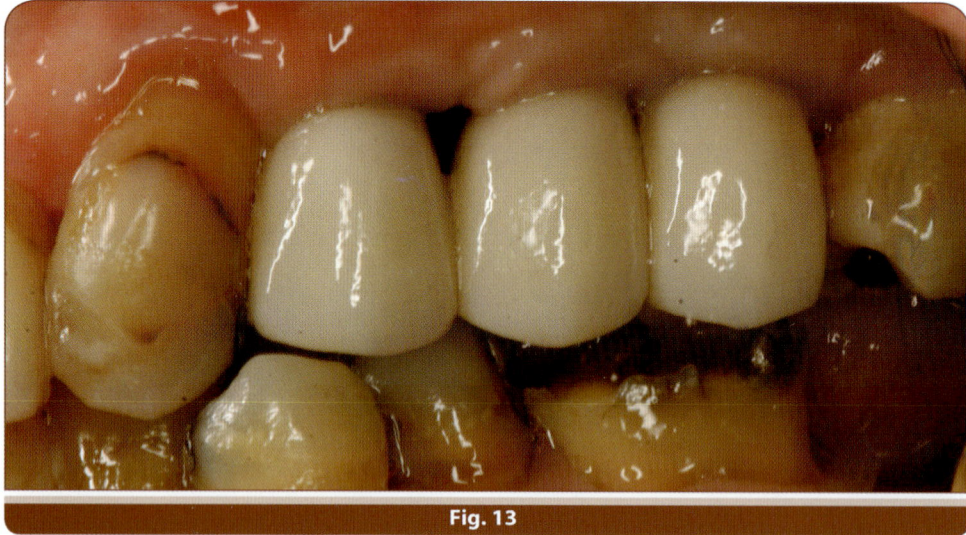

Fig. 13

Final screw-retained restorations. Embrasure spaces are designed into the final restorations to minimize food impaction where possible, facilitate cleaning and deliver aesthetic, functional, maintainable restorations to the patient **(Fig. 13)**.

SECTION 6

Soft Tissue Grafting

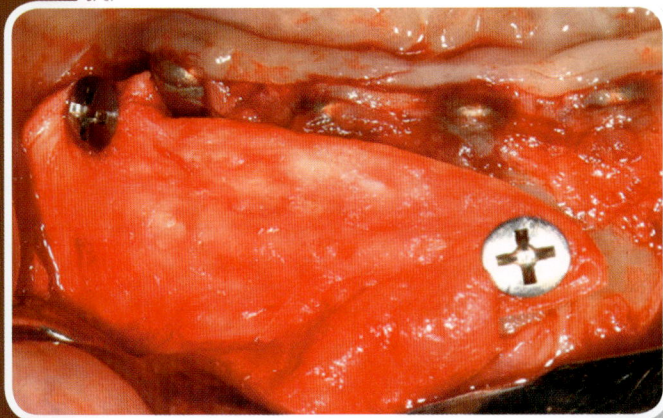

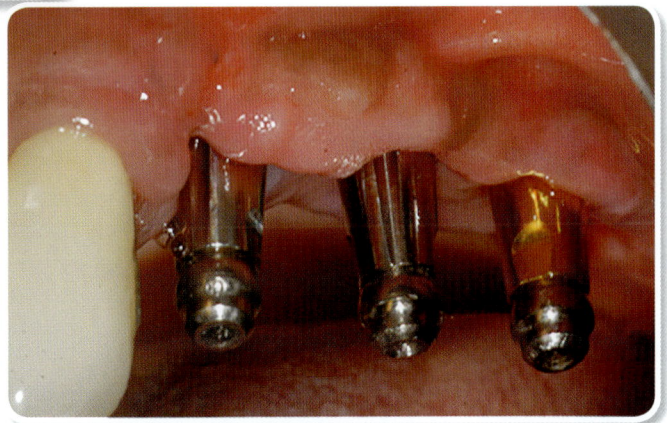

Praful Bali

Soft Tissue Grafting as a Tool to Improve Gingival Esthetics of a Malpositioned Implant with Absence of Buccal Bone

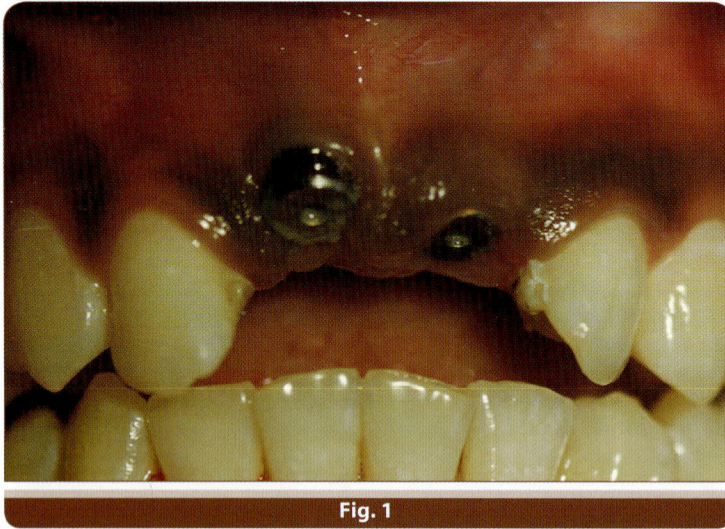

Fig. 1

Preoperative—facial view, after removing temporary Maryland type prosthesis–gingival formers in place **(Fig. 1)**.

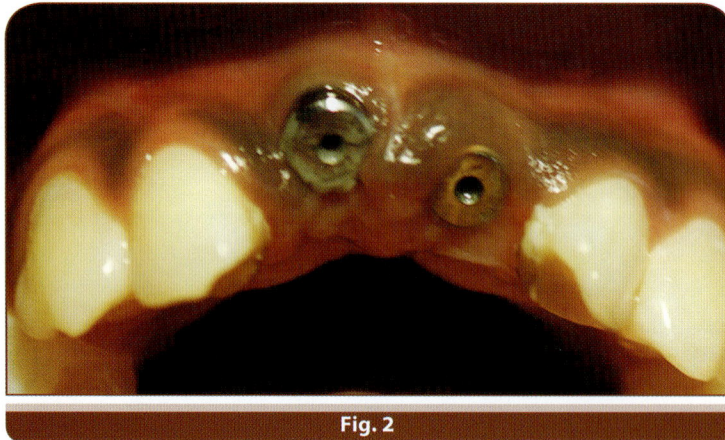

Fig. 2

Preoperative—occlusal view, note buccal placement of implant no#11. Also a wide implant placed in that area **(Fig. 2)**.

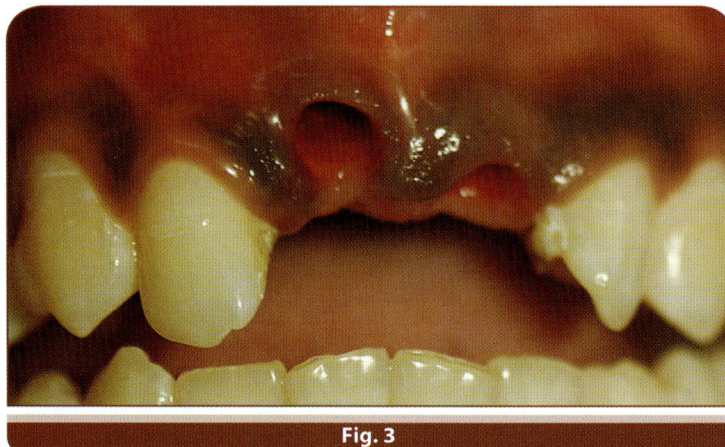

Fig. 3

Preoperative—facial view, after removing gingival formers. Note the emergence level of implant no#11 **(Fig. 3)**.

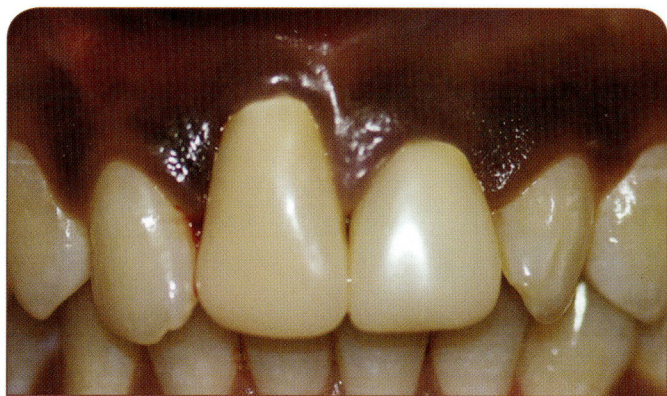

Fig. 4

Temporary crown once made after shaping permanent abutments after removing gingival formers. Note the emergence level of implant #11 **(Fig. 4)**.

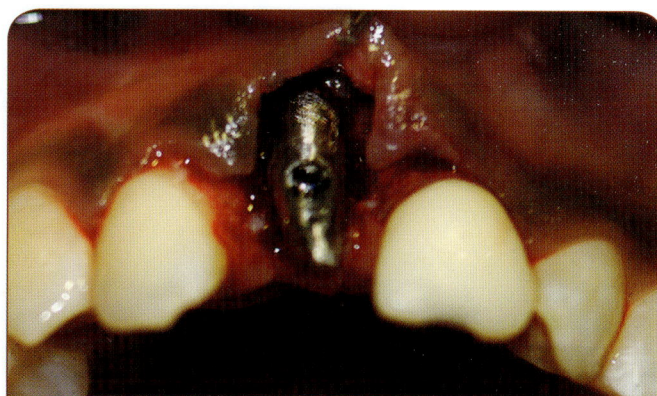

Fig. 5

Reflexion of conservative flap exposing complete exposed buccal surface of the implant **(Fig. 5)**.

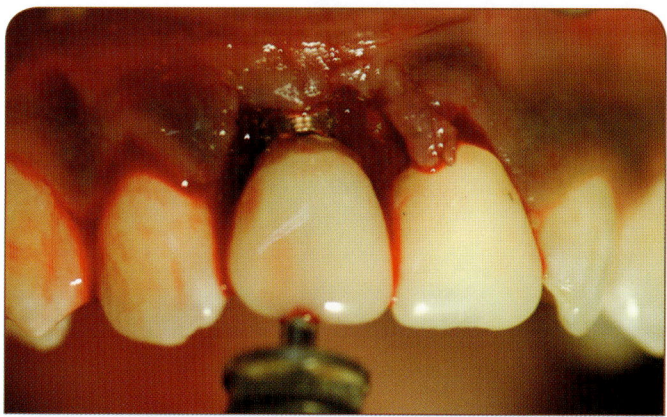

Fig. 6

Screw retained temporary crowns on both the implants and mobilization of flap **(Fig. 6)**.

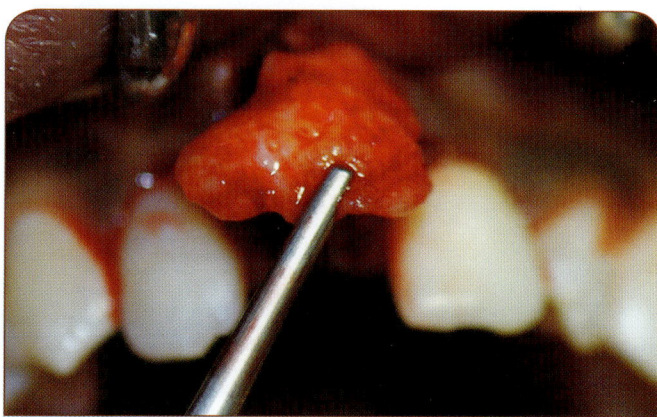

Fig. 7

Pedicle connective tissue graft taken from palate **(Fig. 7)**.

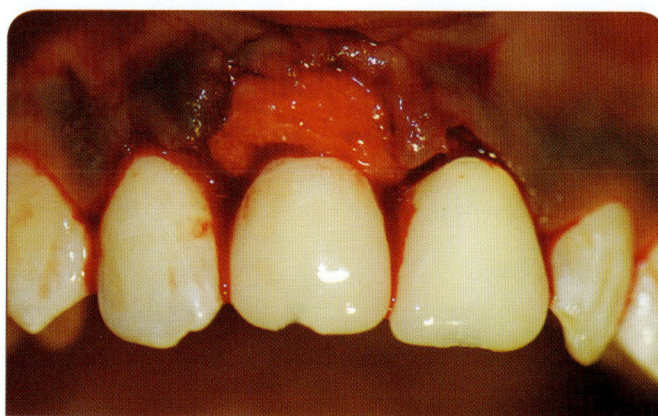

Fig. 8

Connective tissue graft in place stabilized by 6-0 internal sutures **(Fig. 8)**.

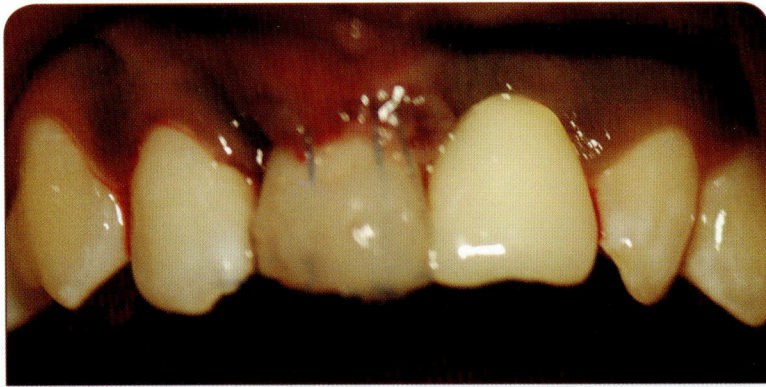

Fig. 9

Non-resorbable 6-0 sutures secured with composite on the temporary tooth **(Fig. 9)**.

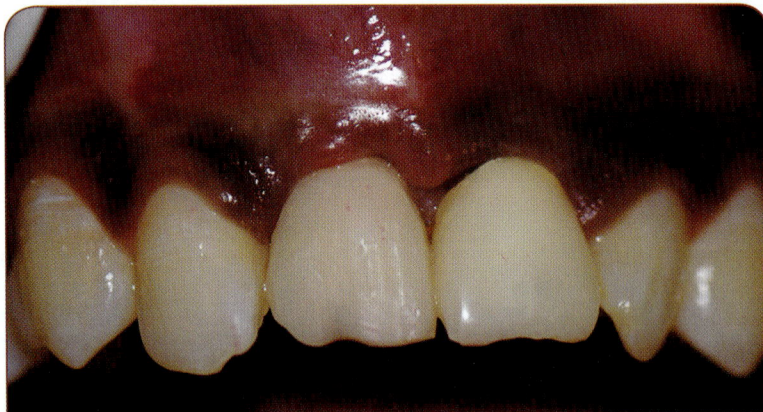

Fig. 10

Two months post healing **(Fig. 10)**.

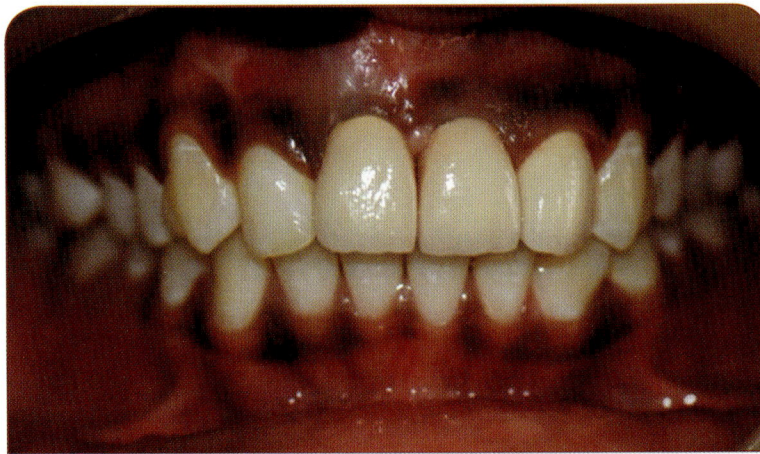

Fig. 11

Final all ceramic restorations on 11, 21, 22. Tooth #22 is endotreated before the crown is given **(Fig. 11)**.

CASE STUDY 86

Sudhindra Kulkarni

FREE CONNECTIVE TISSUE GRAFT

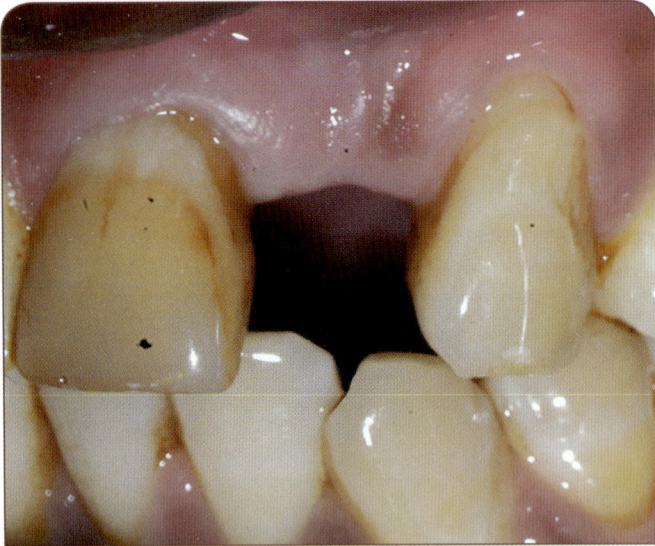

Fig. 1

Deficient ridge contour in relation to tooth #22 **(Fig. 1)**.

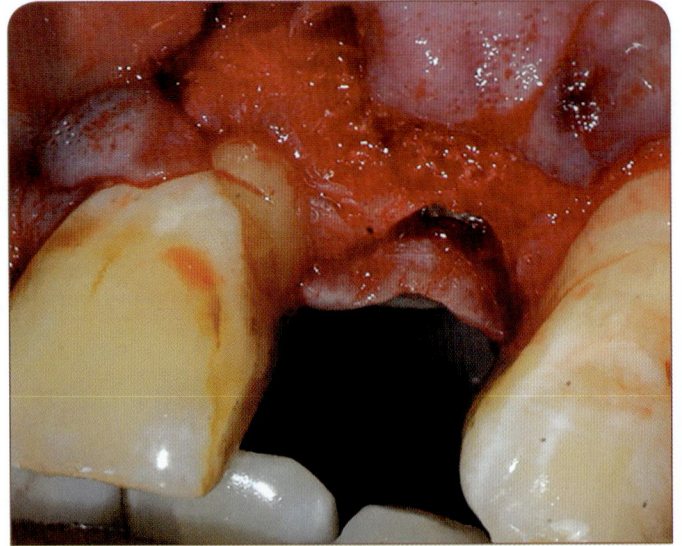

Fig. 2

Tear on the mid buccal flap. Inadvertent flap tear in relation to the mid buccal area of tooth #21 **(Fig. 2)**.

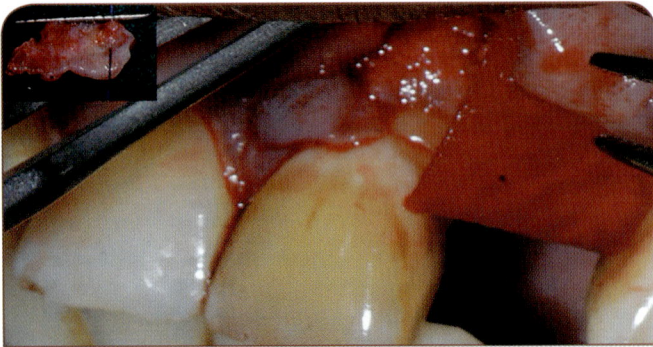

Fig. 3

Use of connective tissue graft (CTG) to cover the tear, the membrane was used to cover the bone graft. Guided bone regeneration done with tooth #22. Connective tissue harvested from the palate the cover the tear **(Fig. 3)**.

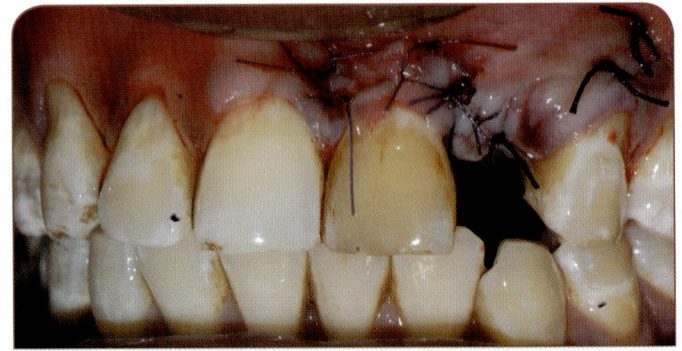

Fig. 4

Connective tissue placed on the exposed root of tooth #21 and secured by sutures to the adjacent tissues. The buccal flap is then advanced and sutured to achieve primary closure **(Fig. 4)**.

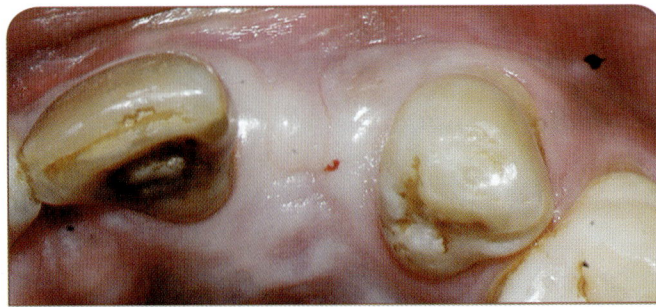

Fig. 5

Four months after implant placement, note the lack of buccal contour **(Fig. 5)**.

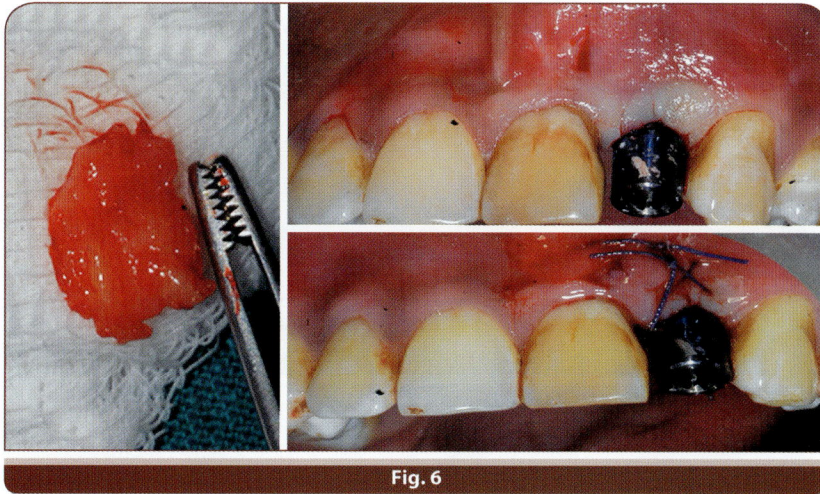

Fig. 6

Connective tissue harvested from palate. Remote incision to create a pouch to place the graft. Graft secured. Remote incision made mesial and apical to tooth #22 to create tunnel to pass the CTG. The CTG is secured in place **(Fig. 6)**.

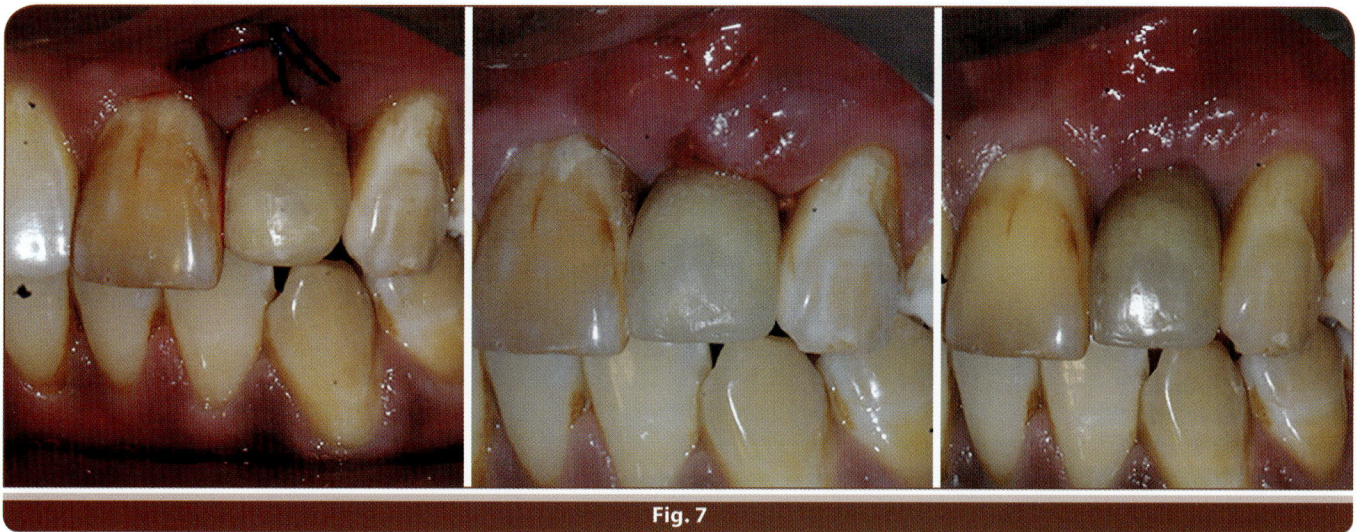

Fig. 7

Graft secured. Temporary restoration is placed on the implant in #22 site. After 1 month: well settled tissues. At 1-week after the CTG. The tissue appears inflamed. At 15 days after CTG placement. 15 days later, the tissue is well-matured **(Fig. 7)**.

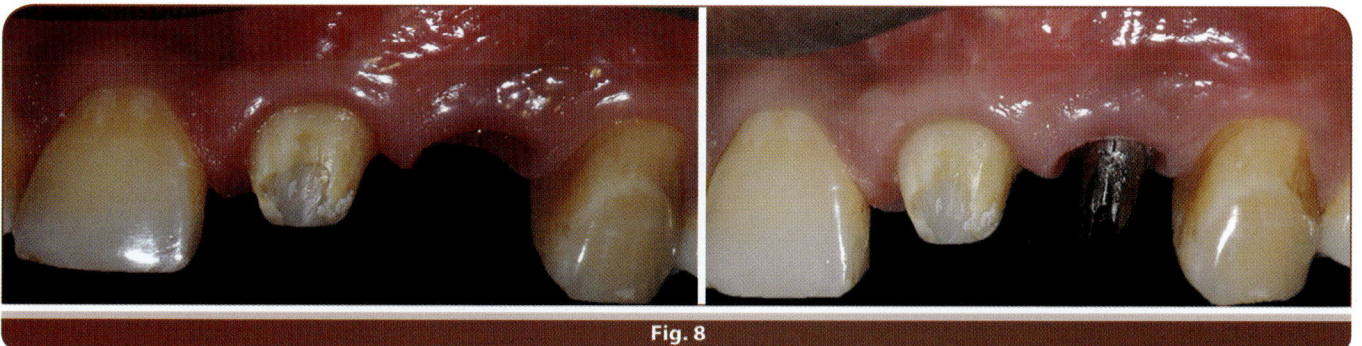

Fig. 8

At final cementation. Note the tissue health and contour **(Fig. 8)**.

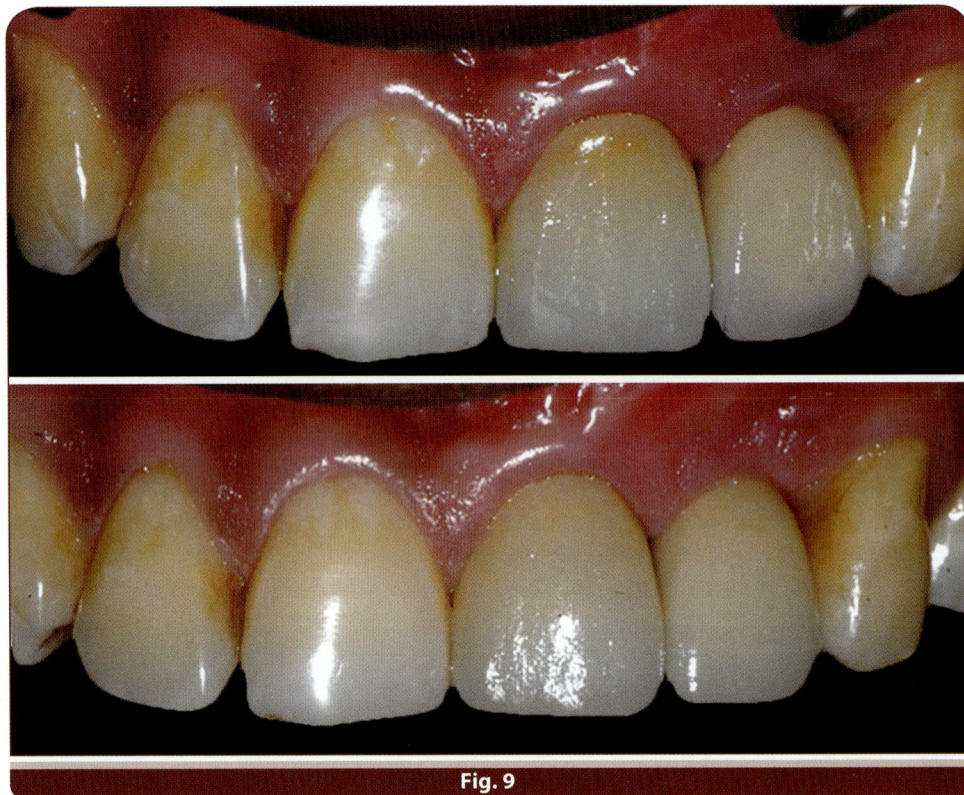

Fig. 9

At 3 months post cementation. Note the soft tissue health and contour. The restorations have an ideal emergence from the underlying tissue **(Fig. 9)**.

Lanka Mahesh

Soft Tissue Augmentation with ADM at Second Stage Surgery

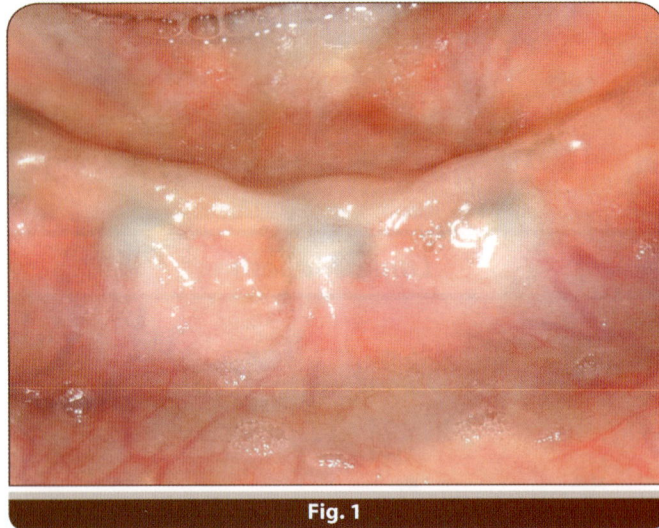

Fig. 1

Preoperative view of the mandibular arch. With 4 implants (Bioner) inserted for an over denture 4 months prior to second stage surgery. Lack of kertatinized tissue is clearly evident. Also the lack of vestibular depth is noted. The goal of treatment in such cases is to have healthy thick tissue with adequate vestibular depth to ensure long term stability of the implant restoration. Treatment plan included placement of an acellular dermal matrix with locators at the same appointment **(Fig. 1)**.

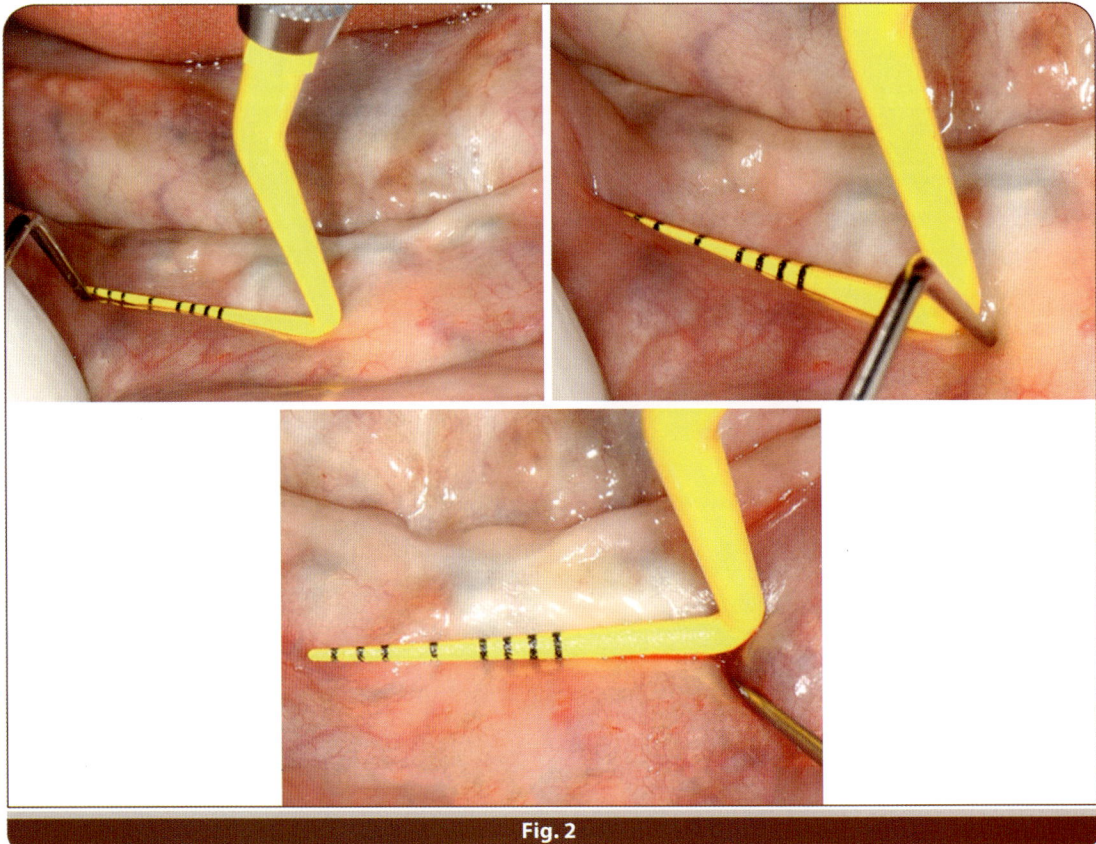

Fig. 2

The areas of the incision are clearly marked to know the correct size of the graft to be used with an Colorvue probe (Hu-Friedy) **(Fig. 2)**.

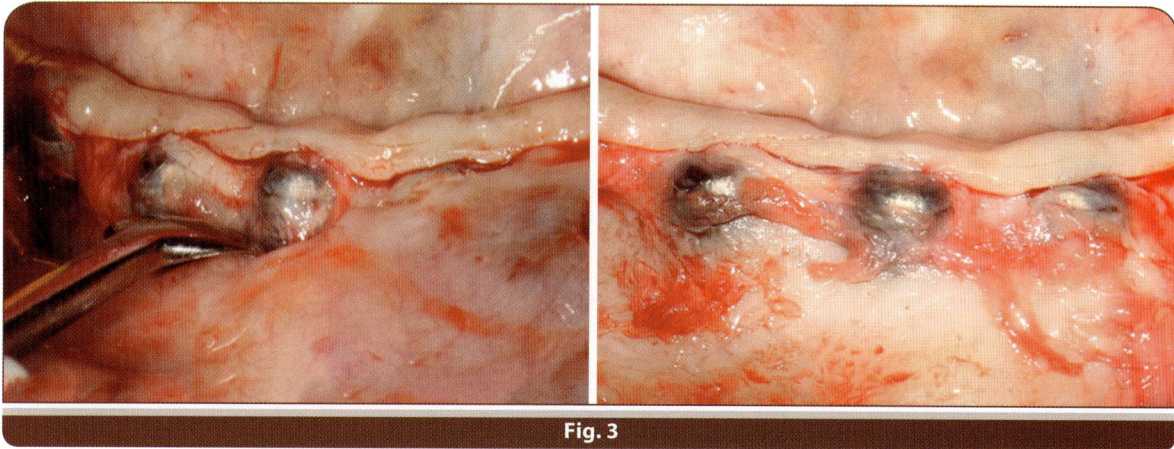

Fig. 3

The incision in such cases is para-crestal keeping a 2 mm border of attached crestal soft tissue, which helps in preventing tissue loss and tearing of the flap and also in getting a good seal with the prosthetic component attached **(Fig. 3)**.

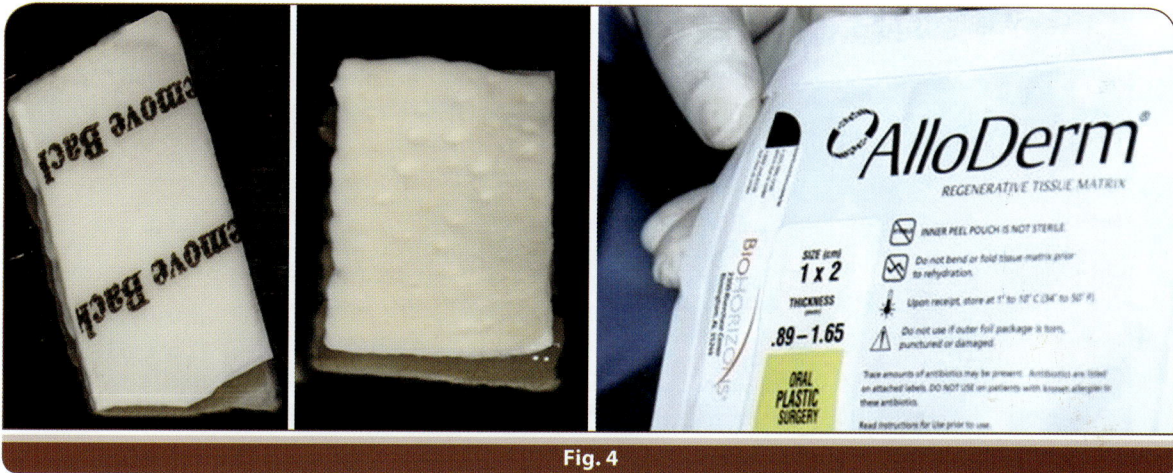

Fig. 4

A 1 × 2 cm graft is used here. The graft is soaked in saline for 20 minutes prior to use to allow rehydration thereby making it more pliable to adapt **(Fig. 4)**.

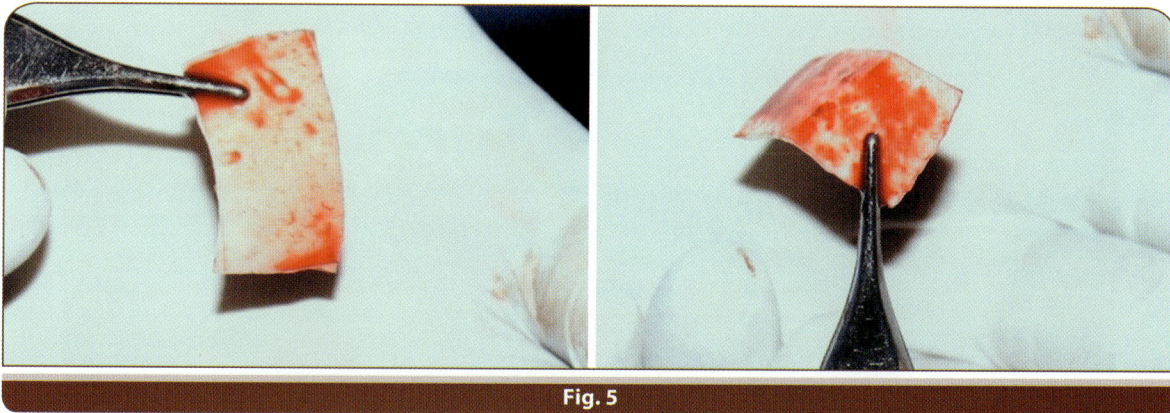

Fig. 5

The graft is soaked in blood for a few minutes to identify the basement membrane and the epithelium side. The basement membrane side absorbs blood and should be placed on the host site **(Fig. 5)**.

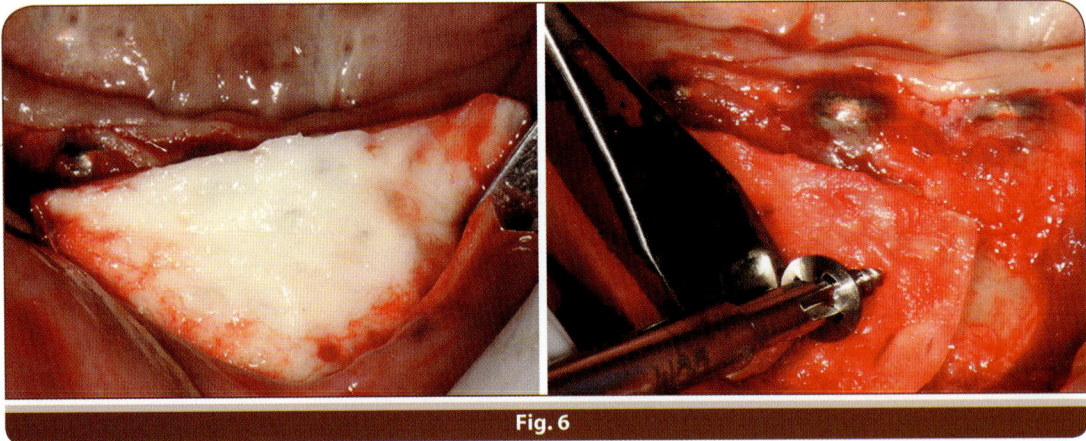

Fig. 6

Alloderm is placed on the operative site and fixed with soft tissue screws. A three point fixation is preferably desired for graft fixation **(Fig. 6)**.

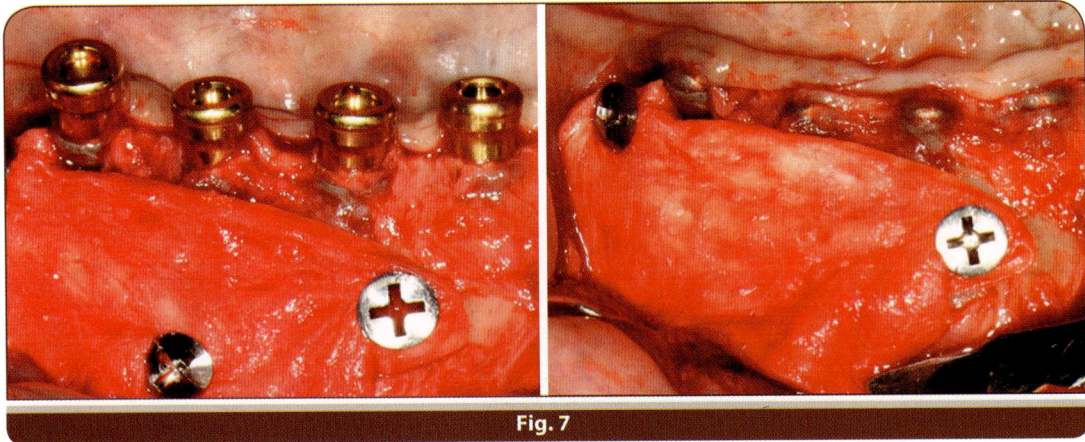

Fig. 7

After the graft is fixated with 3 screws locator attachments (Zest Anchors) are placed instead of healing collars to prevent disruption of the tissue seal achieved post surgery, also because it was decided to do a chair side relining of the final denture **(Fig. 7)**.

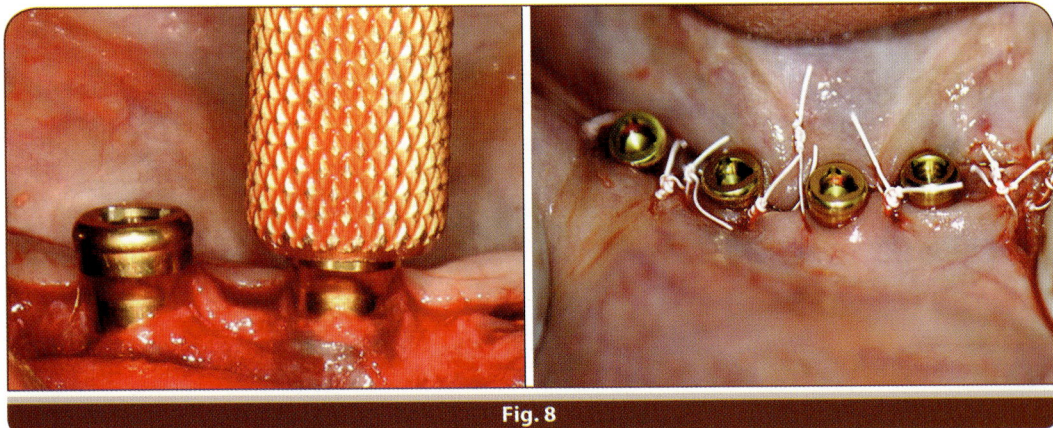

Fig. 8

The locator core tool is used to place the locator abutment and torqued to 30 Ncm. The surgical site is closed with 3-0 cytoplast interrupted sutures (Osteogenics) **(Fig. 8)**.

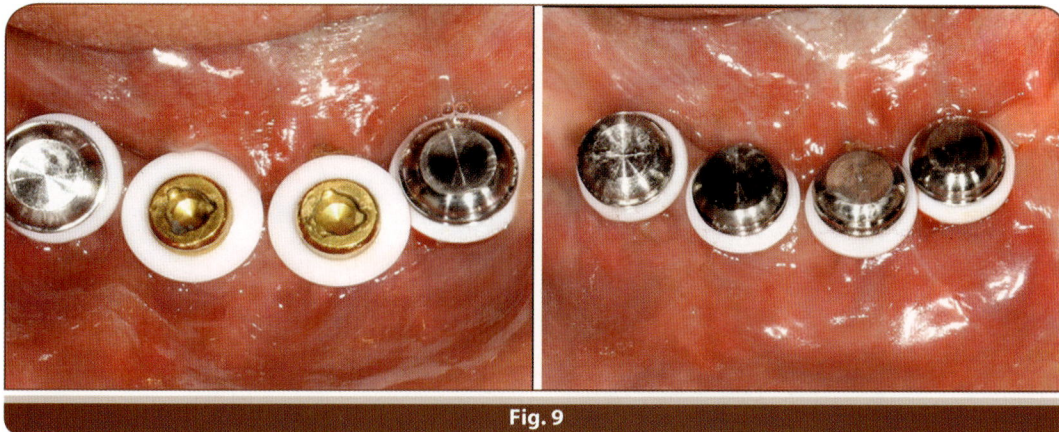

Fig. 9

After 3 weeks thick healed tissue with good vestibular depth is clearly visible. At this appointment the male processing units are placed over the locator abutments with a block out ring to prevent resin from flowing into any undercuts. The denture is relined chairside, polished and delivered to the patient **(Fig. 9)**.

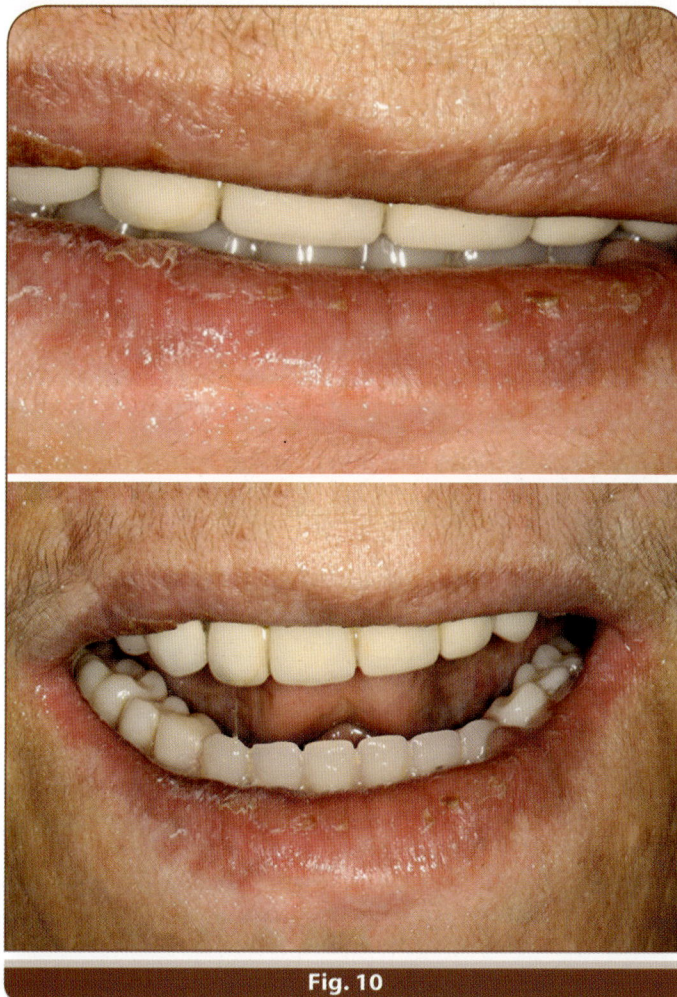

Fig. 10

All movements are checked to achieve complete harmony in centric, protrusive and lateral movements also to check the phonetics and over all facial symmetry of the prosthesis **(Fig. 10)**.

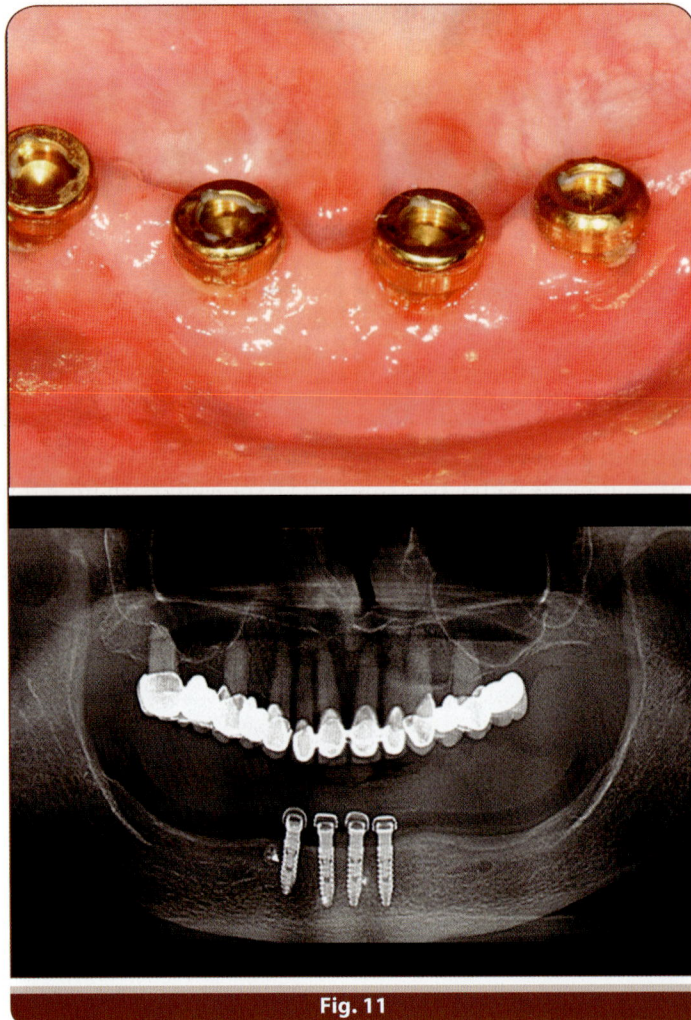

Fig. 11

Two years follow-up shows a thick band of tissue and a very stable soft tissue environment around the implants. Two years follow-up panorex shows good maintenance of crestal bone levels. The soft tissue screws can also be seen **(Fig. 11)**.

Sudhindra Kulkarni

CORRECTION OF FACIAL TISSUE DEFICIT AND LACK OF VESTIBULAR DEPTH

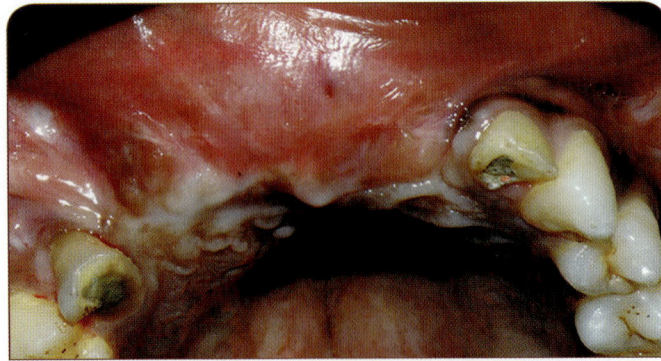

Fig. 1

Lack of keratinized tissue after buccal flap advancement to cover the augmented area. Lack of vestibular depth as well as keratinized tissue. This condition is observed in situations wherein the flap is advanced to achieve primary closure and cover the augmented areas **(Fig. 1)**.

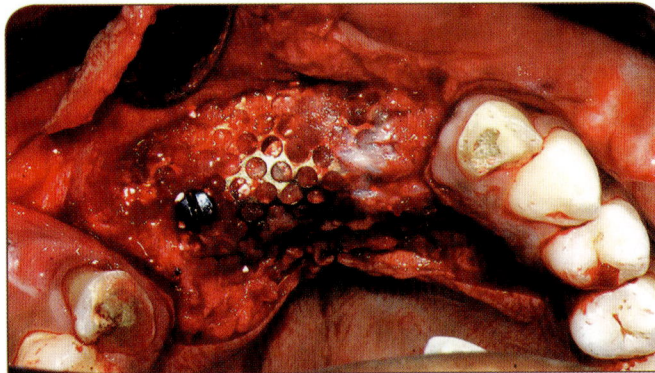

Fig. 2

After reflecting the flap and displacing the palatal flap: A split thickness flap from the palate to the ridge, then a full thickness flap on the ridge and again a split thickness till the muccogingival junction (MGJ). A split-full-split incision flap is reflected and the palatal tissue is displaced buccally **(Fig. 2)**.

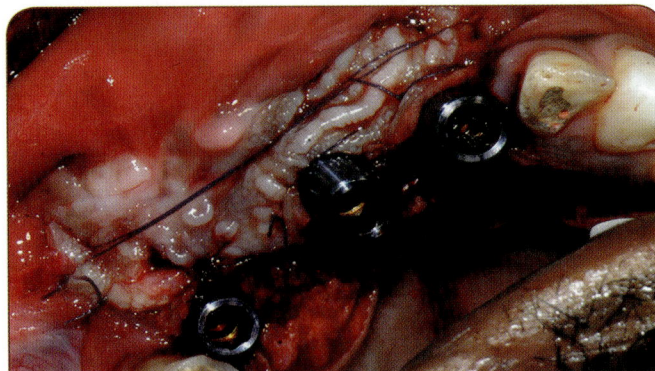

Fig. 3

Flap secured on the buccal. The flap is positioned and secured on the buccal side. The de-epithelialized area on the palate is allowed to heal by secondary intention **(Fig. 3)**.

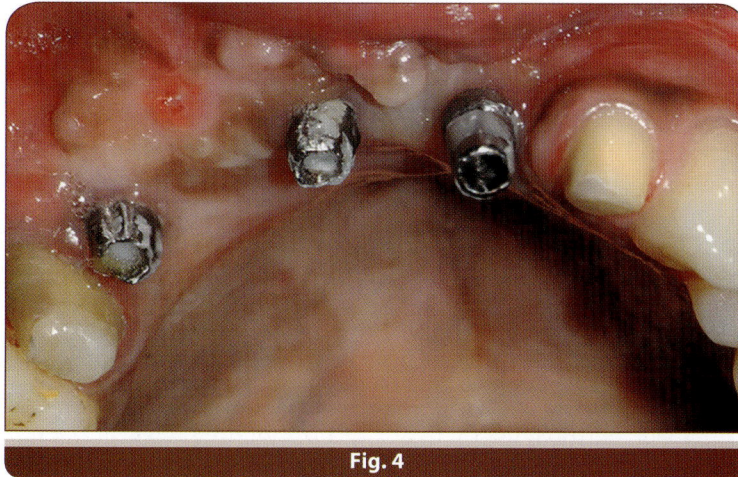

Fig. 4

Lack of vestibule. Well-formed keratinized tissue around all the implants **(Fig. 4)**.

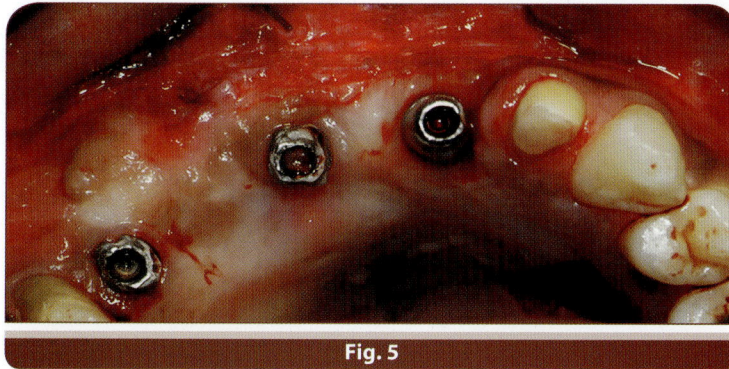

Fig. 5

Tissue surface prepared by shifting the buccal tissues apically. To gain adequate vestibular depth that facilitates oral hygiene measures, it was decided to do a free gingival graft. The buccal tissue including the frenii were dissected exposing the connective tissue bed **(Fig. 5)**.

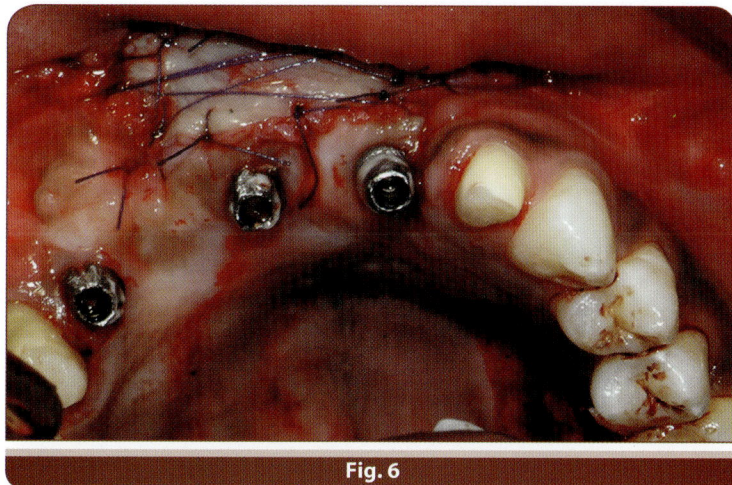

Fig. 6

Free gingival graft (FGG) harvested from the palate and secured. FGG harvested from the palated and secured on the de-epithelialized areas on the buccal side. The buccal flap is now secured at the base of the incision **(Fig. 6)**.

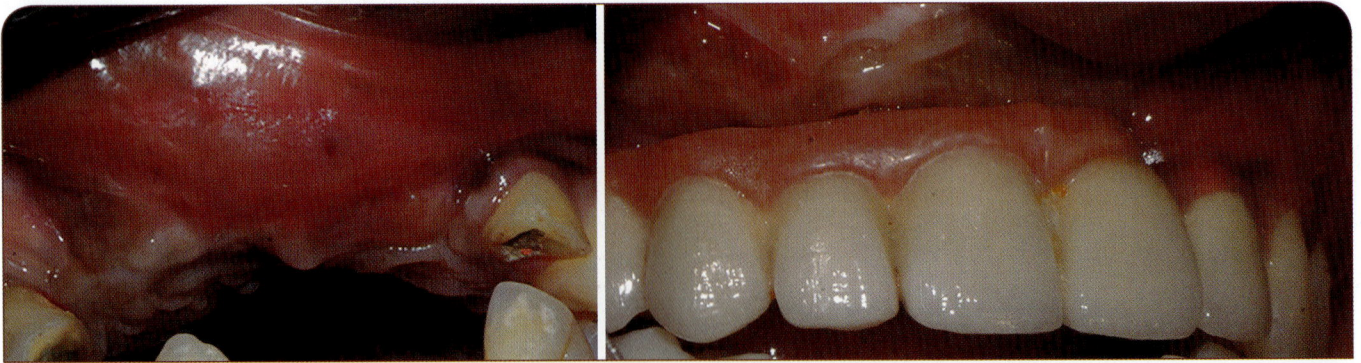

Fig. 7

Tissue and sulcus depth gained. Comparison of the pre- and postoperative soft tissue level and the buccal vestibule **(Fig. 7)**.

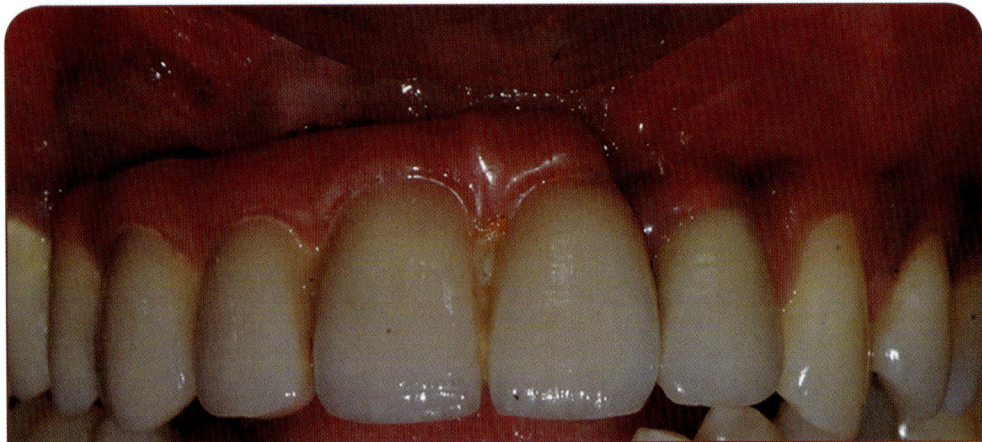

Fig. 8

Buccal view showing the gained vestibular depth **(Fig. 8)**.

CASE STUDY 89

Sudhindra Kulkarni

Palatal Rotated Flap Technique and Free Gingival Graft & Facially Displaced Palatal Graft

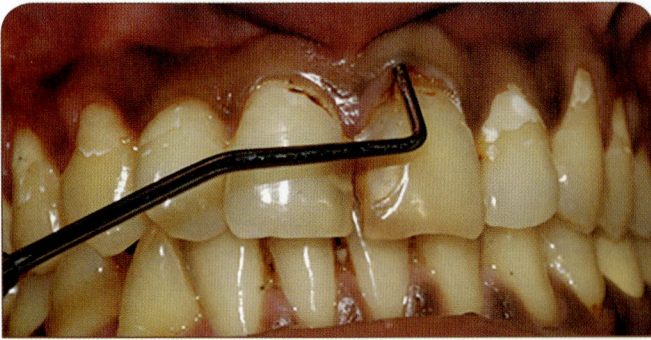

Fig. 1

Labial tissue deficit in relation to tooth #21. Probing-checking for pocket depth and evaluating whether the buccal bone can be felt **(Fig. 1)**.

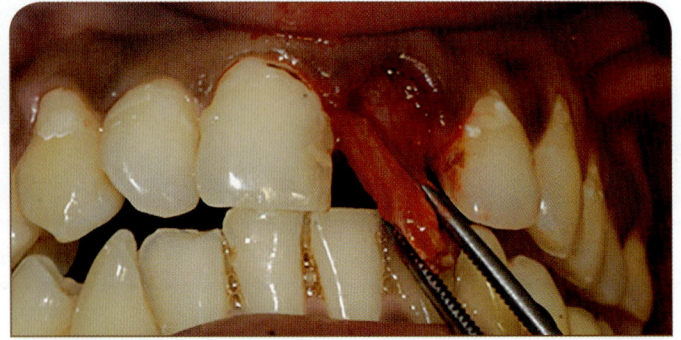

Fig. 2

Left maxillary central incisor removed. Removal of the cystic lining from the socket **(Fig. 2)**.

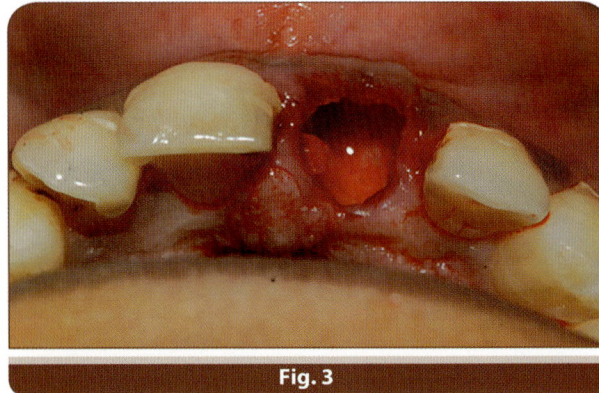

Fig. 3

Socket cleaned. The buccal wall is missing **(Fig. 3)**.

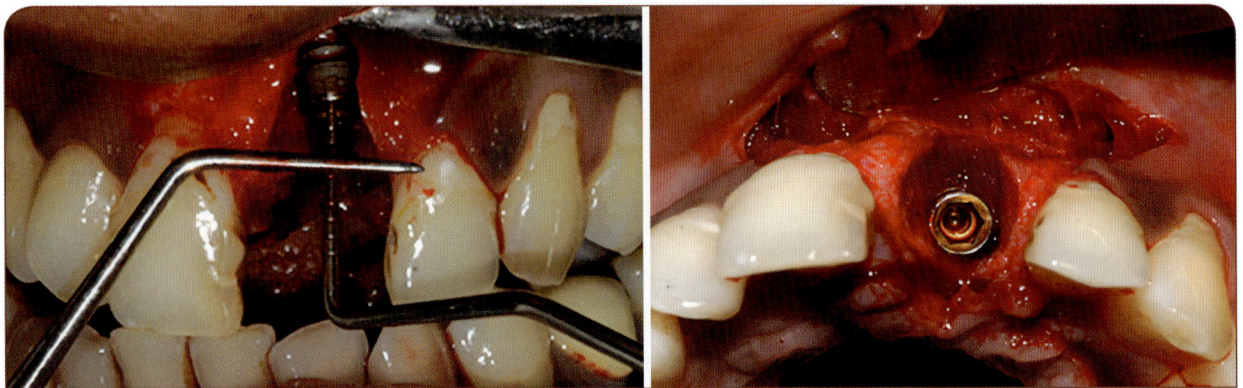

Fig. 4

Implant placed in the site. The graduated probe is used to check the depth of the seating of the implant in relation to the imaginary line joining the two adjacent CEJ's. Buccolingual positioning of the implant. Implant is placed within the envelop of the maxilla **(Fig. 4)**.

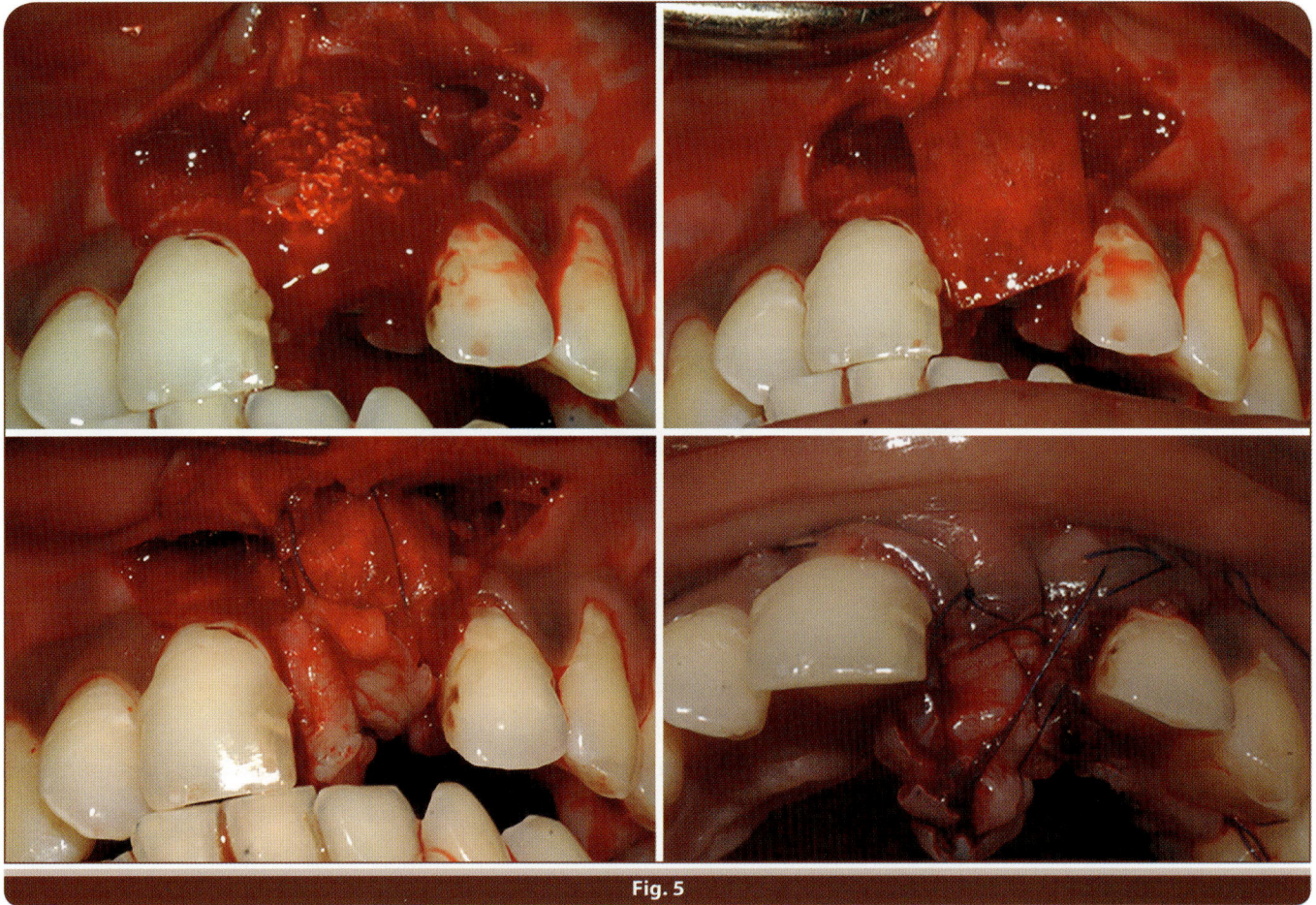

Fig. 5

Guided bone regeneration (GBR) done. Bone graft placed at the site. A combination of autogenous and xenograft is placed. The autogenous bone is placed in contact with the implant and the xenogenic bone is layered on top of the ABG (Autogenous bone graft).

Bilayered collagen membrane placed on top of the bone graft. The membrane is shaped to the site. The palatal flap is rotated and secured to the periosteum of the buccal side to get primary closure. The buccal flap is secured in position without advancing it **(Fig. 5)**.

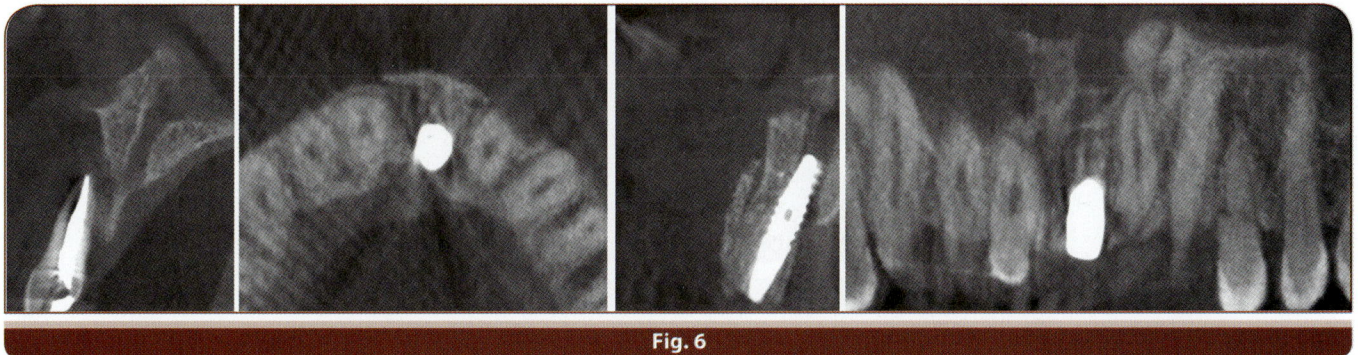

Fig. 6

Radiograph showing the bone and the implant in the site **(Fig. 6)**.

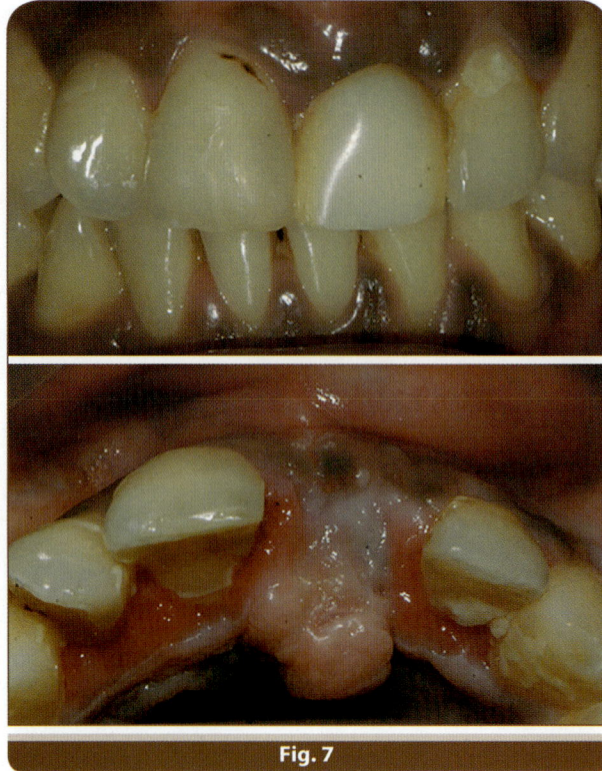

Fig. 7

The site at 4 months postoperative. The tissue health looks good. Excess palatal tissue is visible. The buccal contour looks adequate **(Fig. 7)**.

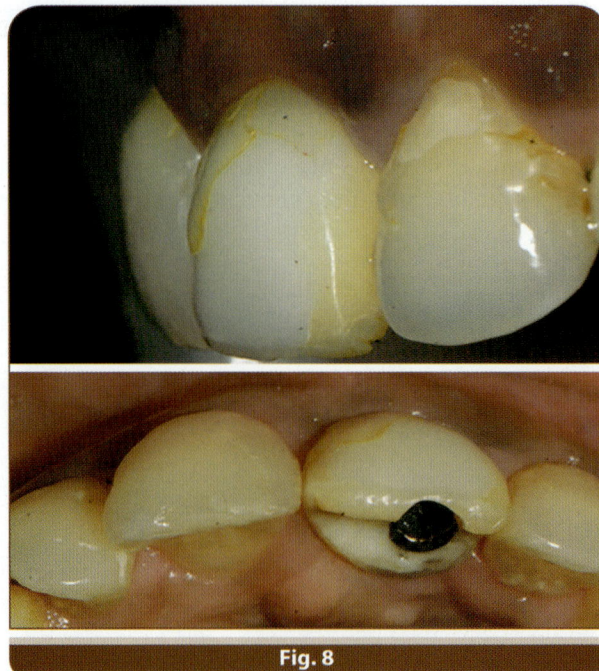

Fig. 8

Guided bone regenaration/Palatal rotation/dual zone. Proximal view showing the buccal contour. The implant was uncovered and restored with a screw retained temporary prosthesis **(Fig. 8)**.

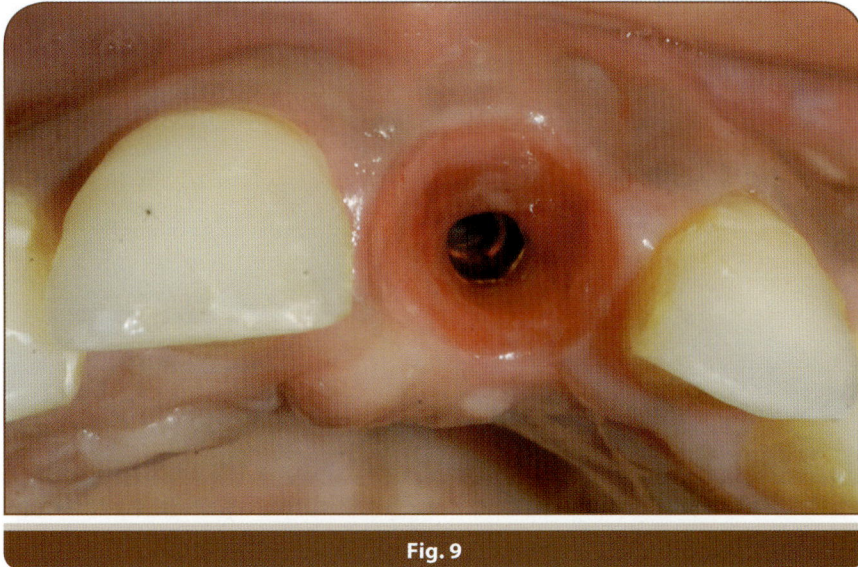

Fig. 9

Guided bone regeneration/Palatal rotation/dual zone. Final contour. Well-formed tissue cuff around the implant **(Fig. 9)**.

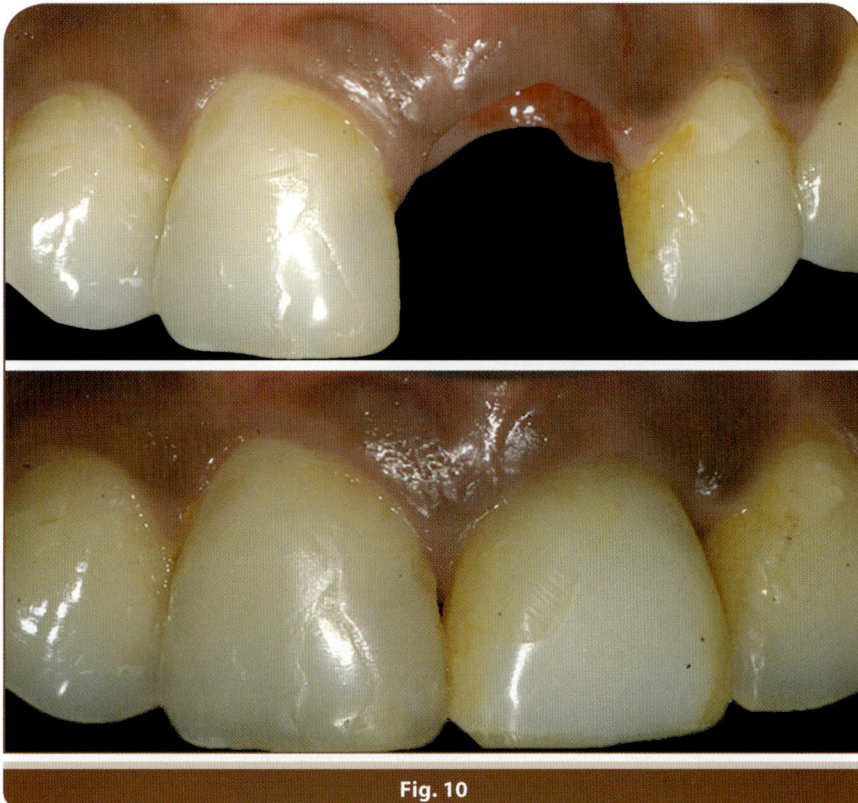

Fig. 10

Tissue contours. Buccal scallop and zenith is perceptible. The modification of the temporary prosthesis is key to achieve ideal tissue contours **(Fig. 10)**.

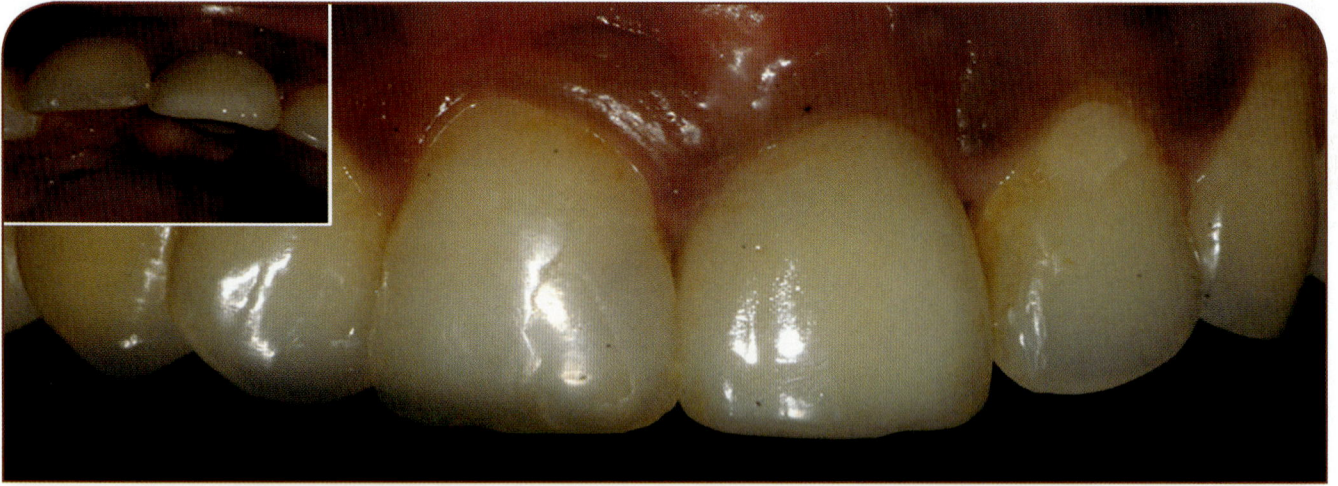

Fig. 11

Palatal flap displacement as facial gingival graft. Final restorations, merging into and emerging from the soft tissue **(Fig. 11)**.

Tarun Kumar

Reconstruction of Attached Gingiva around an Implant by Free Gingival Graft

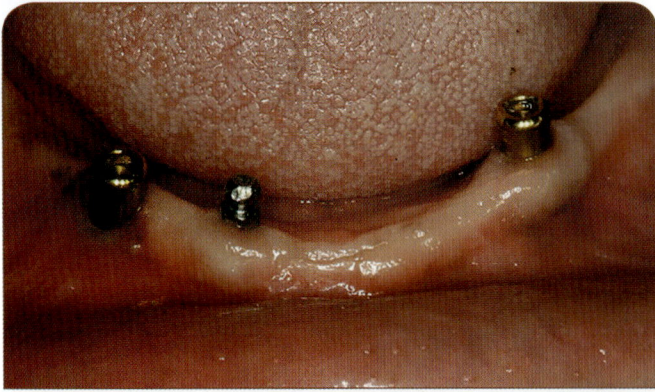

Fig. 1

Inadequate width of attached gingiva **(Fig. 1)**.

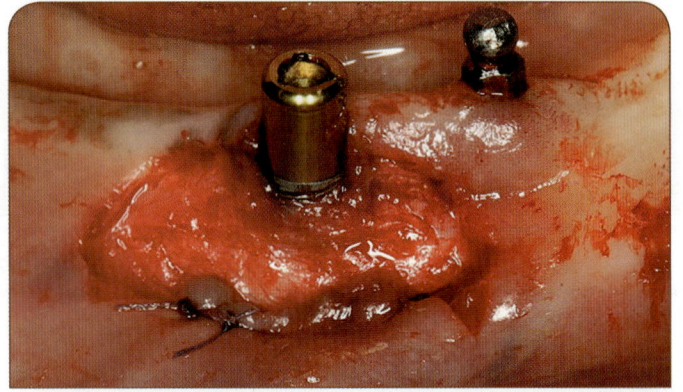

Fig. 2

Apical repositioning of flap **(Fig. 2)**.

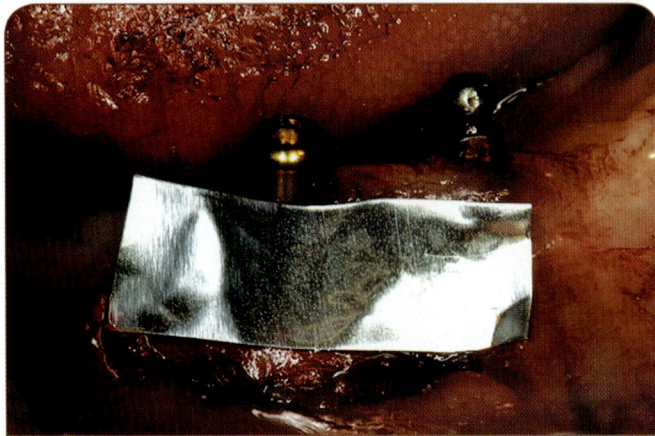

Fig. 3

Placement of aluminum foil as template in the recipient site **(Fig. 3)**.

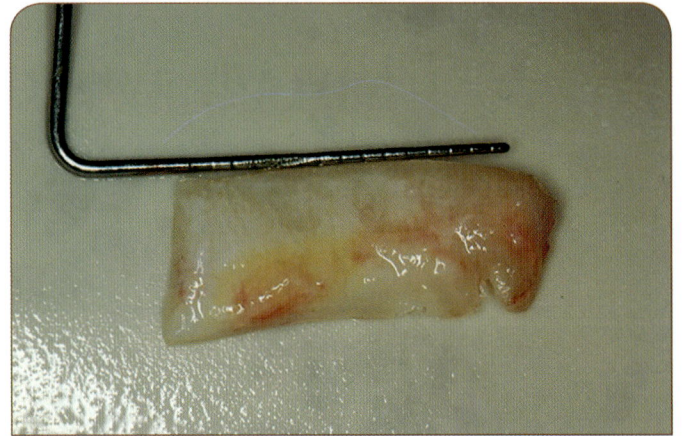

Fig. 4

Dimensions of the free gingival graft retrieved from the patient's palate **(Fig. 4)**.

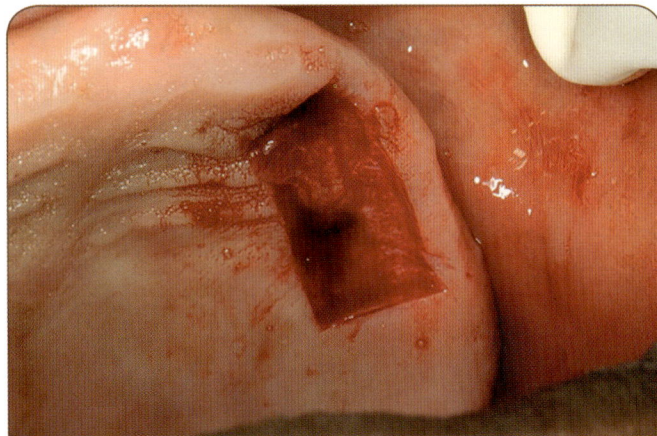

Fig. 5

Donor site after graft harvestation **(Fig. 5)**.

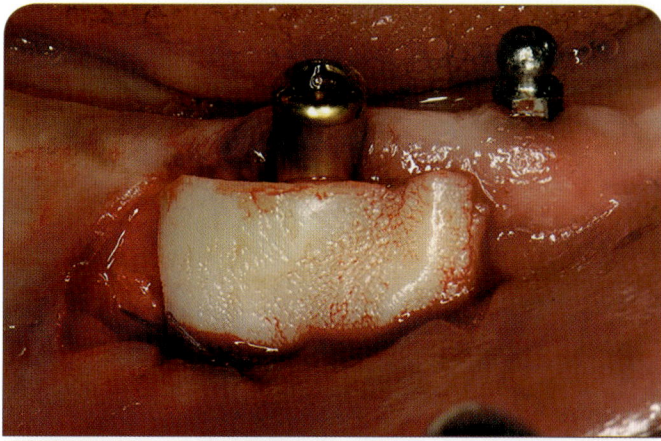
Fig. 6

Placement of the graft at recipient site **(Fig. 6)**.

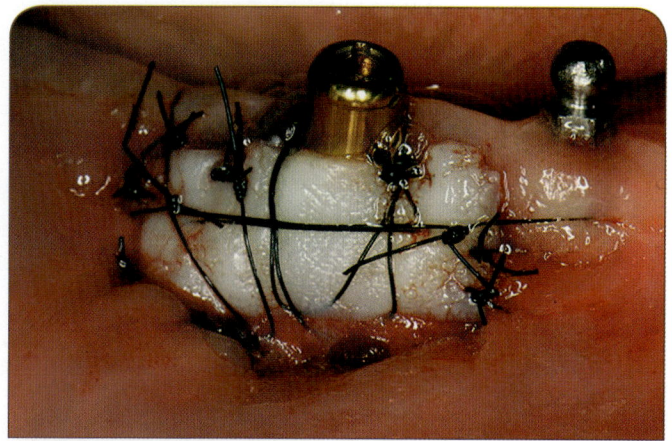
Fig. 7

Free gingival graft sutured at recipient site **(Fig. 7)**.

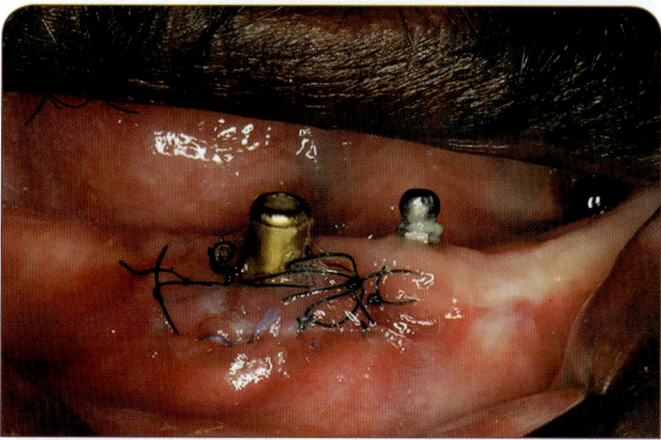
Fig. 8

Postoperative view after 7 days **(Fig. 8)**.

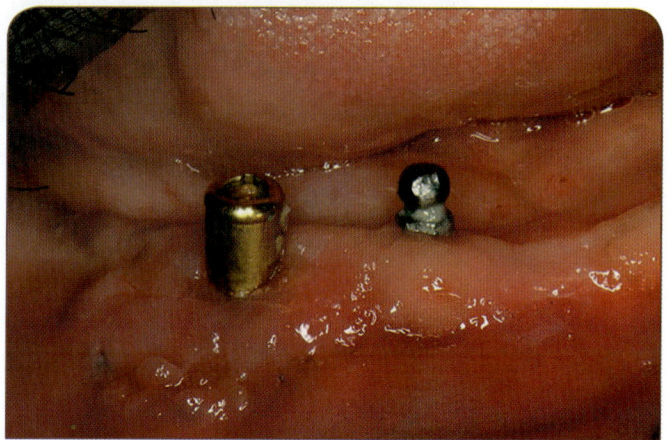
Fig. 9

Postoperative view after 15 days **(Fig. 9)**.

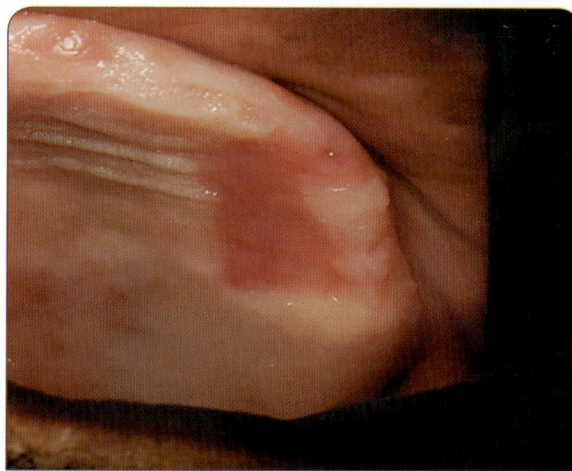
Fig. 10

Postoperative donor site view after 15 days **(Fig. 10)**.

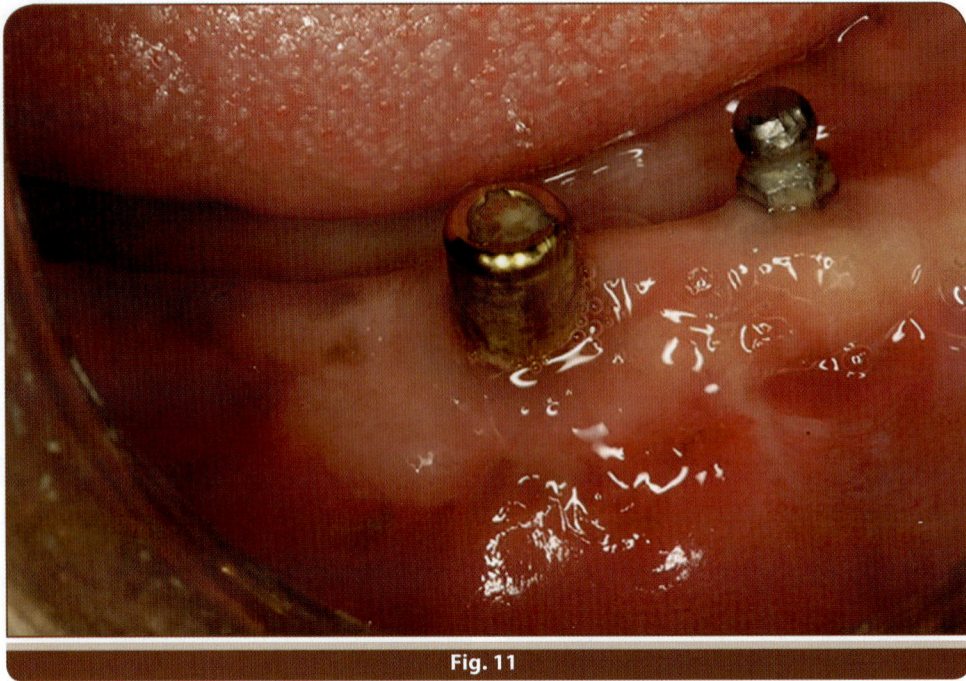

Fig. 11

Postoperative recipient site after 1 month showing increase in the width of attached gingiva **(Fig. 11)**.

Lanka Mahesh

Soft Tissue Augmentation in a Full Arch Rehabilitation with a Hybrid Prosthesis in the Maxilla

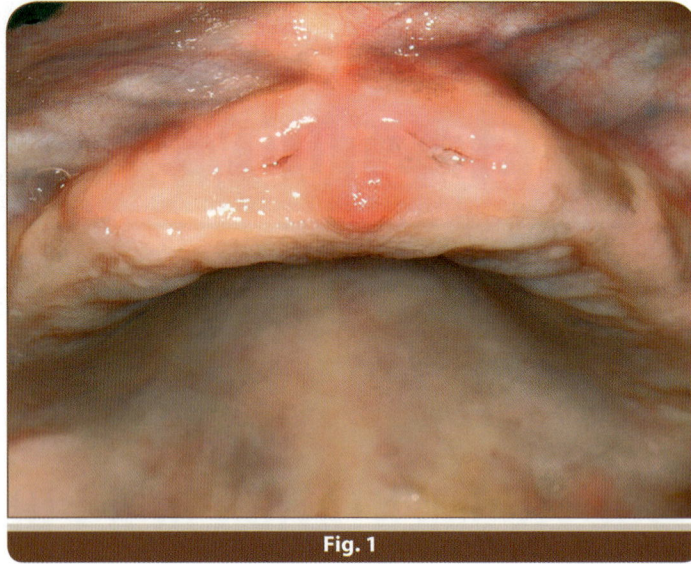

Fig. 1

Intraoral view. Treatment plan included placement of six implants followed by a soft tissue augmentation at second stage to bulk the tissue **(Fig. 1)**.

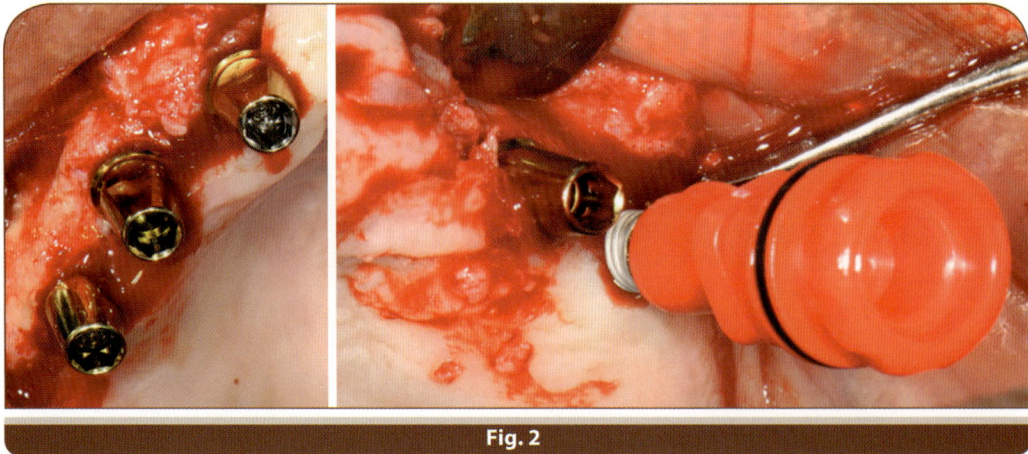

Fig. 2

Six 3.8/11.5 mm Cortex Dynamix implants were placed and left for submerged healing protocol for 5 months **(Fig. 2)**.

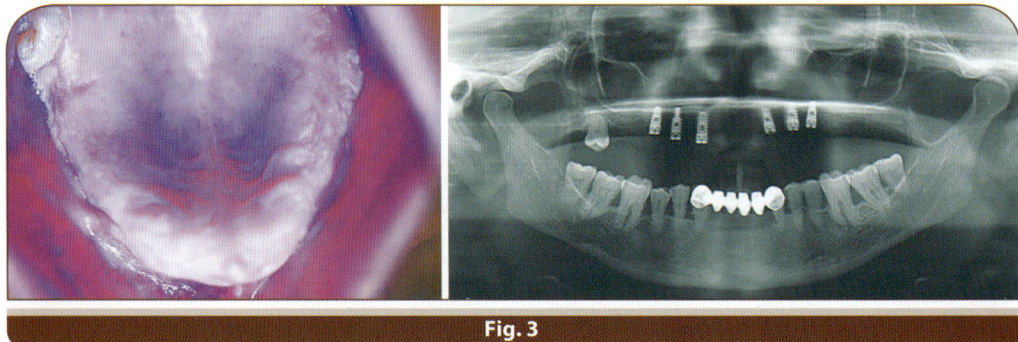

Fig. 3

Five months postoperative clinical view shows the lack of thick tissue that is desired around implant fixtures. Radiographic view shows well integrated implants **(Fig. 3)**.

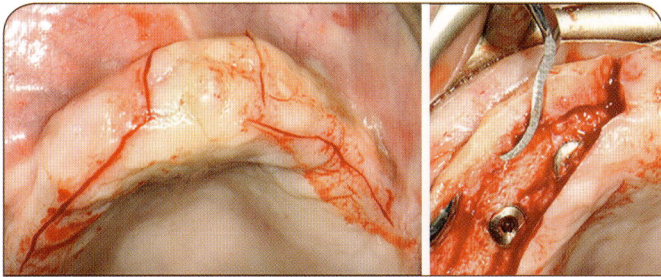

Fig. 4

The incision at second stage is 3 mm paracrestal thereby allowing palatal tissue to be displaced facially. The implants are exposed using a back action chisel **(Fig. 4)**.

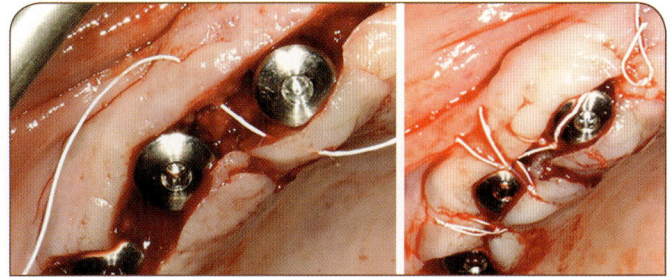

Fig. 5

Pedicles are created with a 15c blade and rotated between the healing collars and wound closure is done with 4-0 cytoplast (osteogenics). The sutures should not be placed too tight which would cause tissue necrosis **(Fig. 5)**.

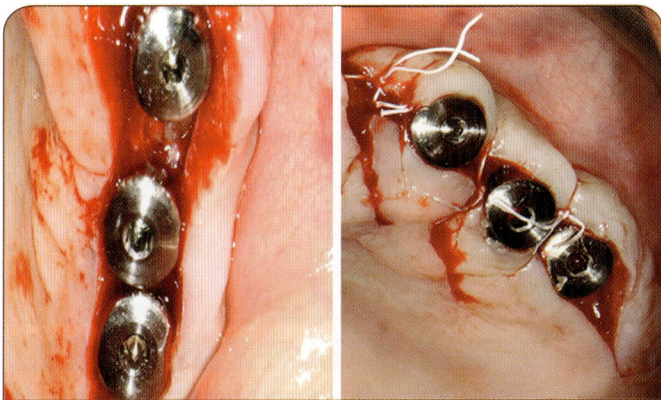

Fig. 6

The same procedure is done of the left side **(Fig. 6)**.

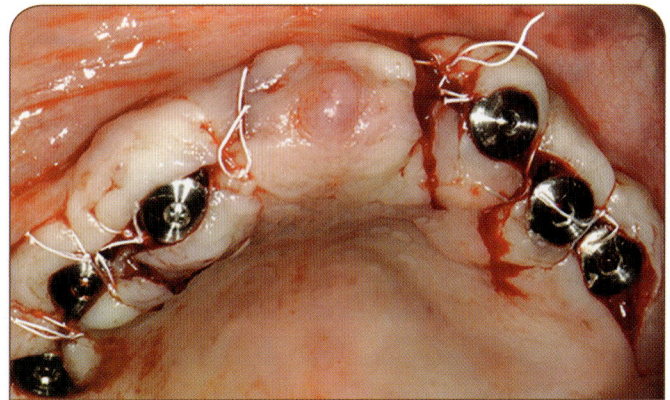

Fig. 7

The operated sites are left to heal undisturbed with no interim prosthesis **(Fig. 7)**.

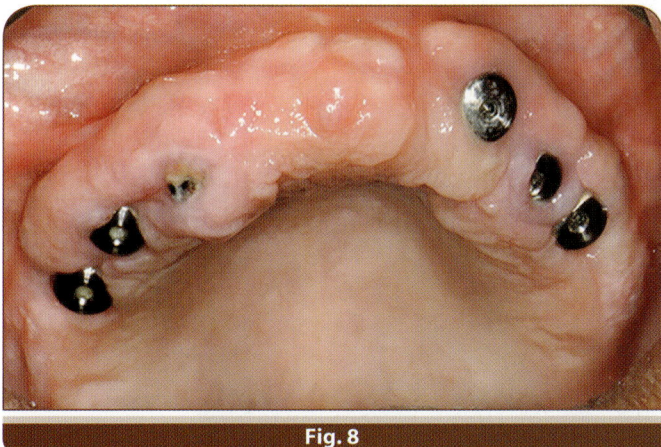

Fig. 8

Three weeks postoperative the healing tissue appears normal and tissue thickness has been clearly achieved **(Fig. 8)**.

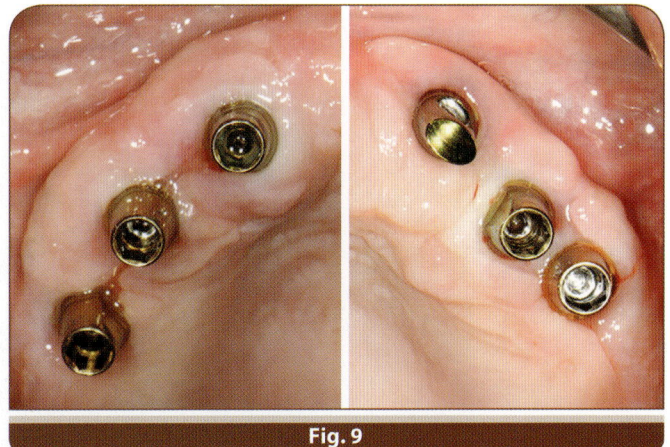

Fig. 9

Eight weeks from second stage surgery a healthy thick band of tissue around the implants can be seen **(Fig. 9)**.

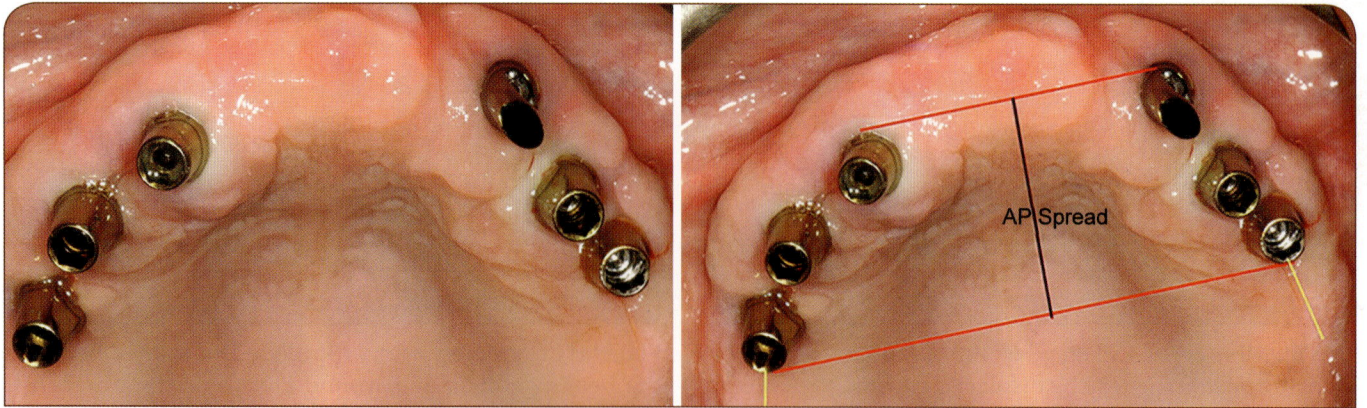

Fig. 10

The cantilever extension (yellow line) should never be more than 1-1/2 times the AP spread (purple line) **(Fig. 10)**.

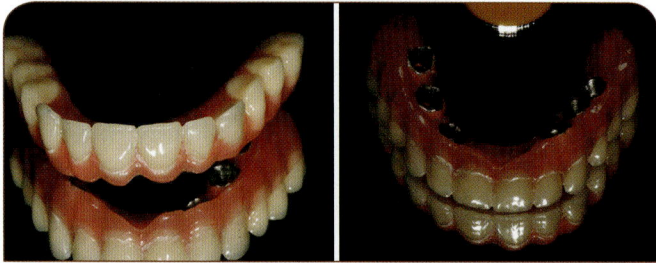

Fig. 11

The hybrid prosthesis which will be cemented onto the implants **(Fig. 11)**.

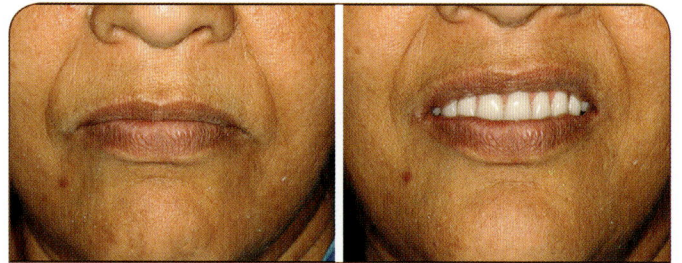

Fig. 12

Adequate lip support leading to an overall pleasing facial appearance is noted **(Fig. 12)**.

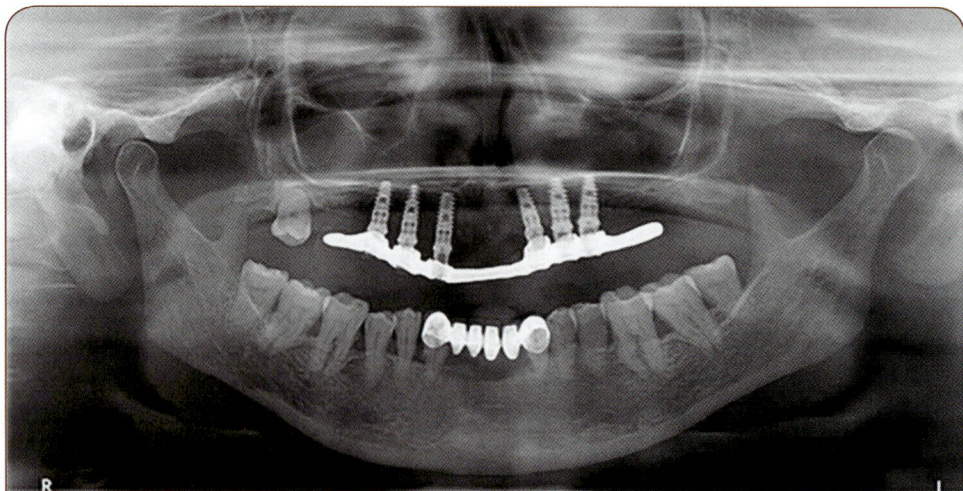

Fig. 13

Control panorex four years postoperatively shows overall harmony of the entire prosthetic rehabilitation **(Fig. 13)**.

CASE STUDY 92

Bach Le

Treatment of Labial Soft Tissue Recession around a Dental Implant in the Esthetic Zone using the Screw Tent-Pole Technique with Mineralized Allograft

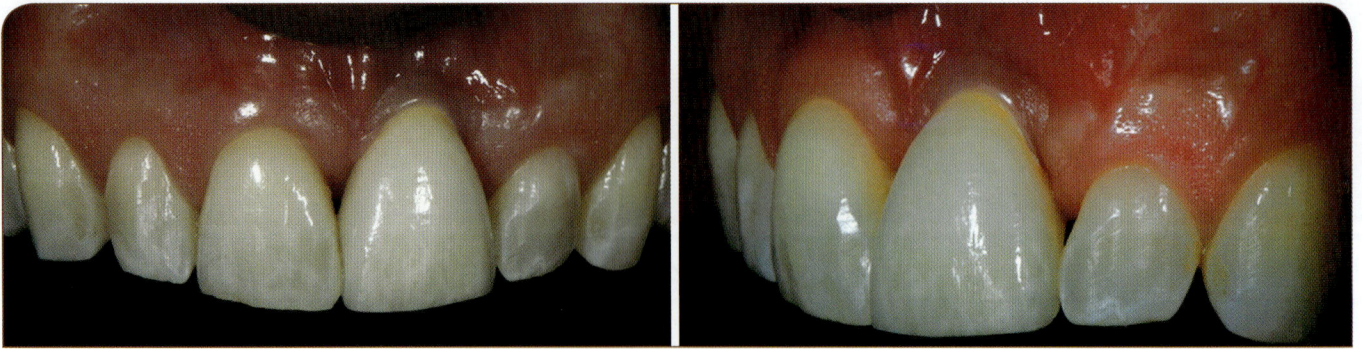

Fig. 1

Preoperative clinical view shows maxillary left central incisor with gingival recession and discoloration caused by exposure of the underlying dental implant. Note that there are no signs of infection or inflammation (peri-implant disease) **(Fig. 1)**.

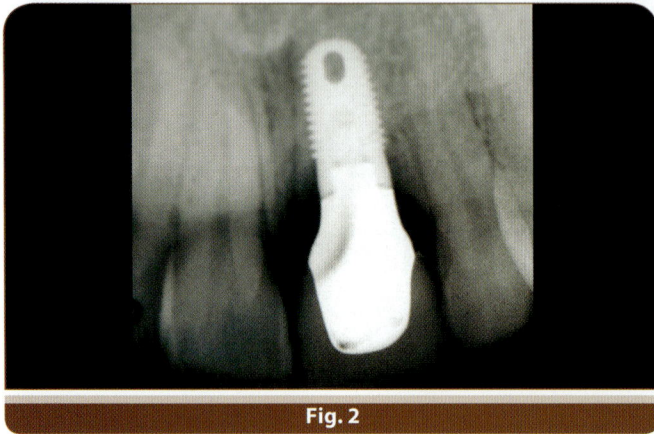

Fig. 2

Radiograph showing healthy crestal bone level **(Fig. 2)**.

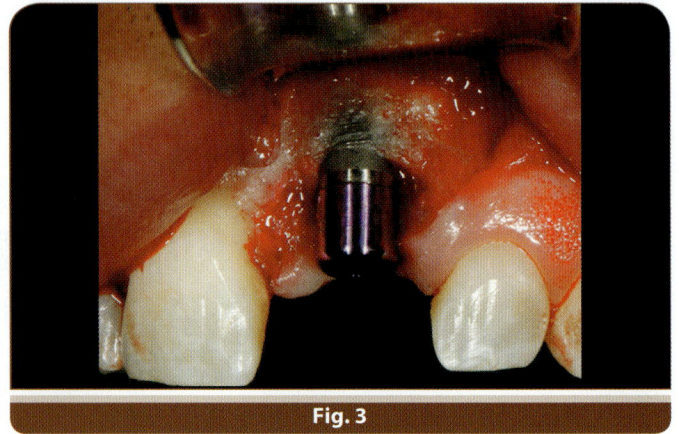

Fig. 3

Surgical exposure showing dehiscenced labial bone and exposed implant surface **(Fig. 3)**.

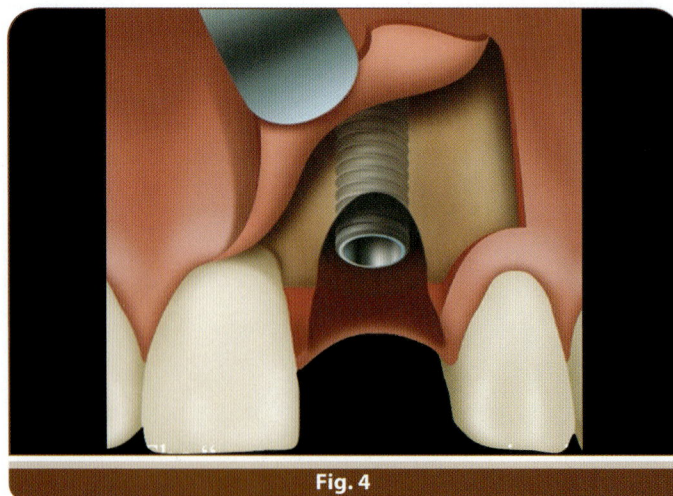

Fig. 4

Incision design: The 'open book flap design is utilized for better graft containment and allow for coronal advancement of the gingival margin. The flap is developed with a distal, curvilinear, vertical incision that follows the gingival margin of the distal tooth. A wide subperiosteal reflection is made up to the level of the nasal spine to expose 2 to 3 times the treatment area, and then the papilla is reflected on the mesial side of the edentulous site **(Fig. 4)**.

Treatment of Labial Soft Tissue Recession Around a Dental Implant in the Esthetic....

475

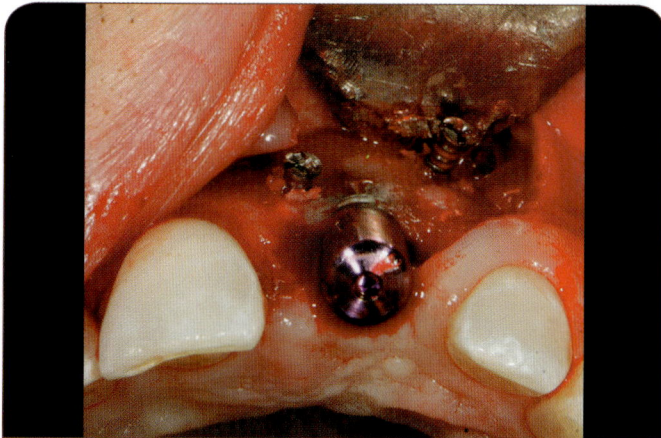
Fig. 5

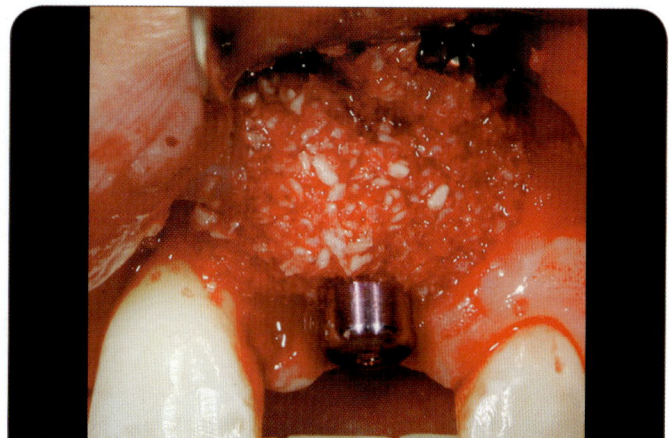
Fig. 6

Two tenting screws are strategically placed near the exposed textured implant surface. It is important to note that this technique has the best prognosis for success when the implant is not severely malpositioned and there is only a small (< 3 mm) amount of implant exposure **(Fig. 5)**.

A mineralized allograft (MinerOss Cortical Cancellous mix or Puros Cancellous) material mixed with the patient's blood placed on the labial surface of the implant and covered with a resorbable membrane (CopiOs Pericardium) **(Fig. 6)**.

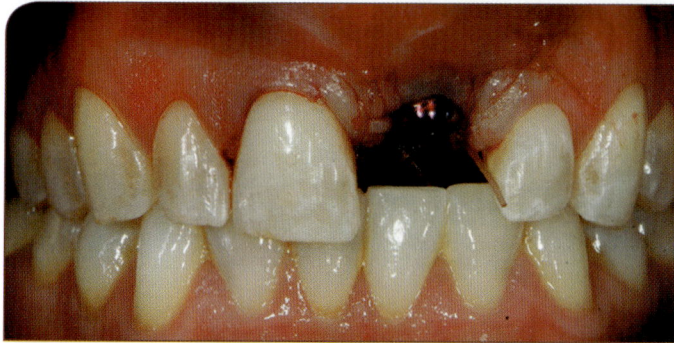
Fig. 7

A wide healing abutment was connected to the implant to create an additional tenting effect over the graft site and help to contour the overlying soft tissue **(Fig. 7)**.

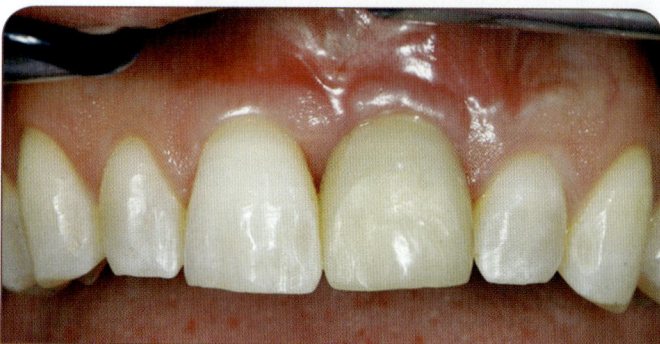
Fig. 8

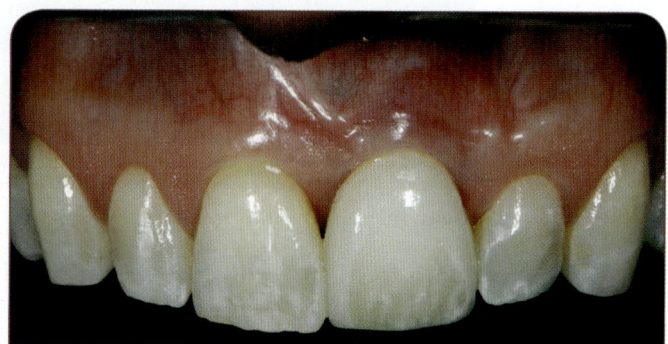
Fig. 9

Screw-retained provisional restoration delivered after 4 months of healing **(Fig. 8)**.

Follow-up clinical view shows significant improvement in soft tissue parameters with a corresponding decrease in crown length at 1 year **(Fig. 9)**.

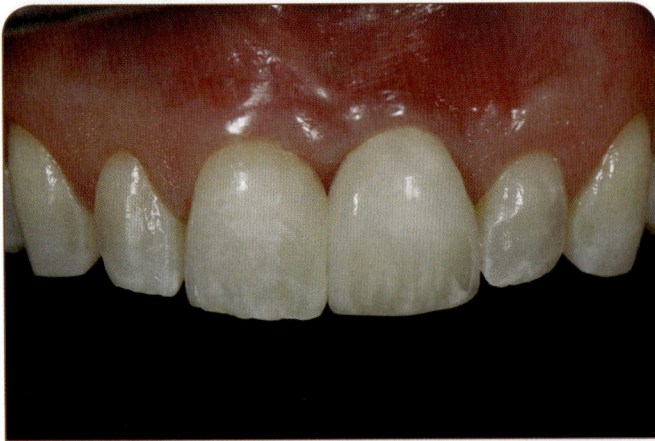

Fig. 10

Follow-up clinical view shows stable gingival margin level at 3 years. Composite bonding was performed on the right central incisor to improve symmetry between the two incisors **(Fig. 10)**.

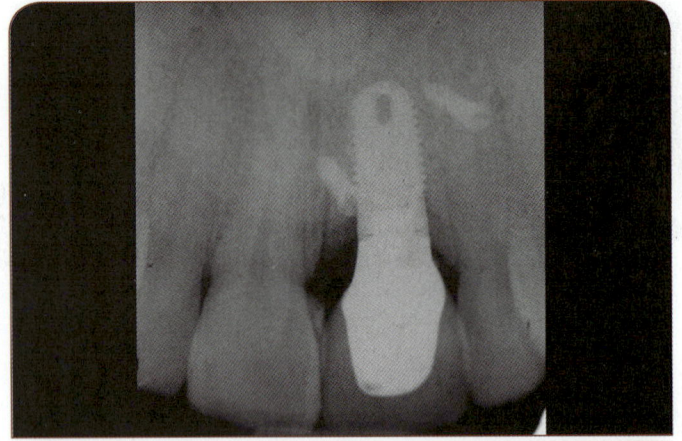

Fig. 11

Postoperative radiograph taken 2 years after GBR procedure shows stable peri-implant bone level. Tenting screws are not removed unless they become exposed **(Fig. 11)**.

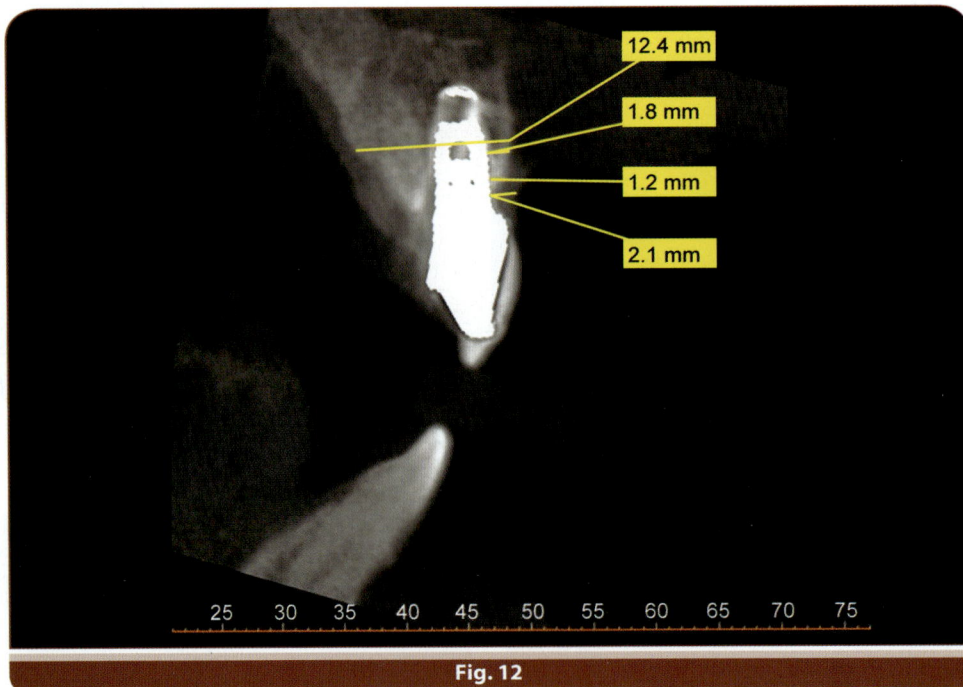

12.4 mm

1.8 mm

1.2 mm

2.1 mm

Fig. 12

Postoperative CT scan taken 2 years after GBR procedure shows restoration of hard and soft tissue dimensions **(Fig. 12)**.

CASE STUDY 93

Sudhindra Kulkarni

LATERAL DISPLACEMENT OF THE PALATAL TISSUE

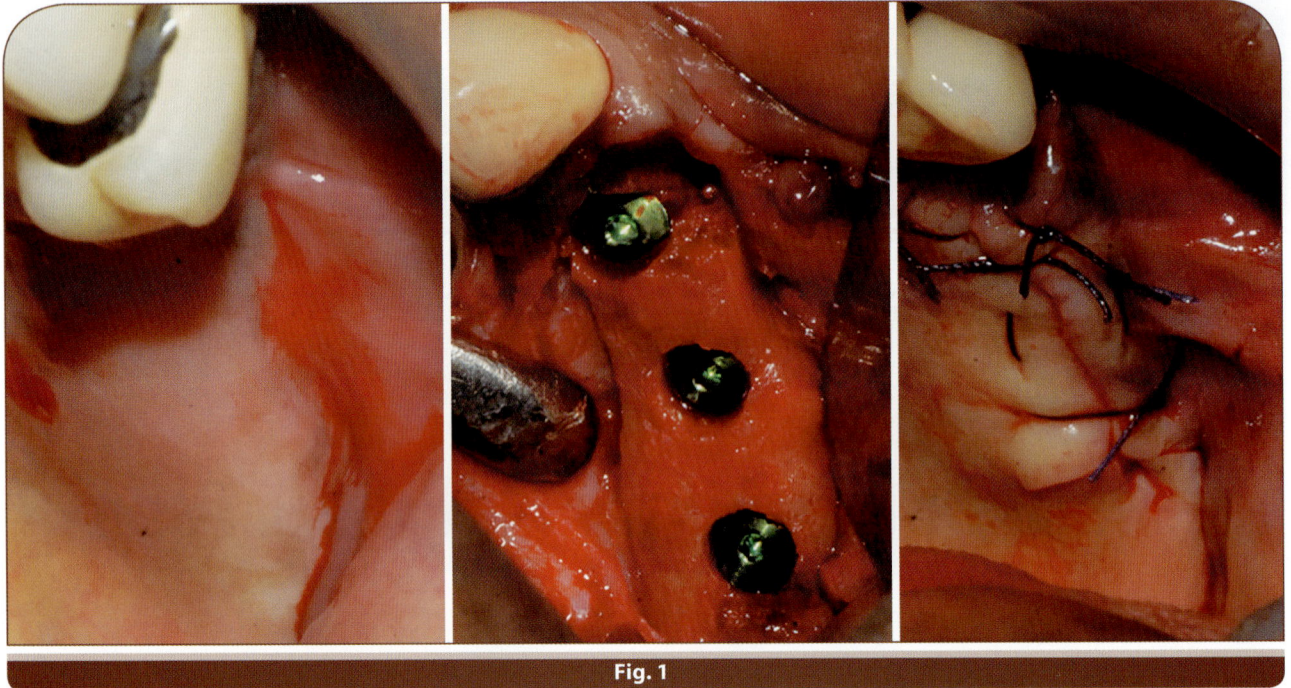

Fig. 1

Palatal tissue displacement. Implant placed and primary closure attained **(Fig. 1)**.

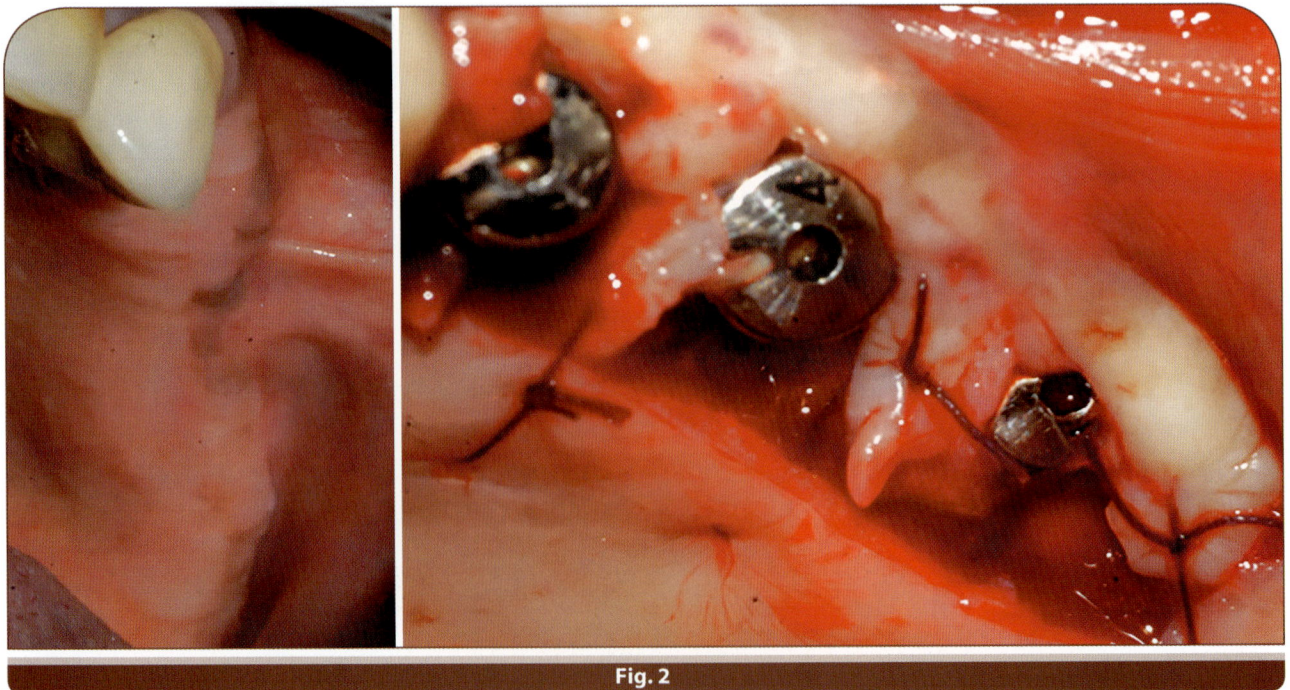

Fig. 2

Palatal tissue displacement. At 3 months, re-entry time: Paracrestal incision made to displace the flap on to the buccal side. The flap is then incised in a 'C' shape, staring from distal to the mesial, around each implant/healing abutment creating 'fingers', which are then passed in the inter-implant area and secured with 5-0 sutures **(Fig. 2)**.

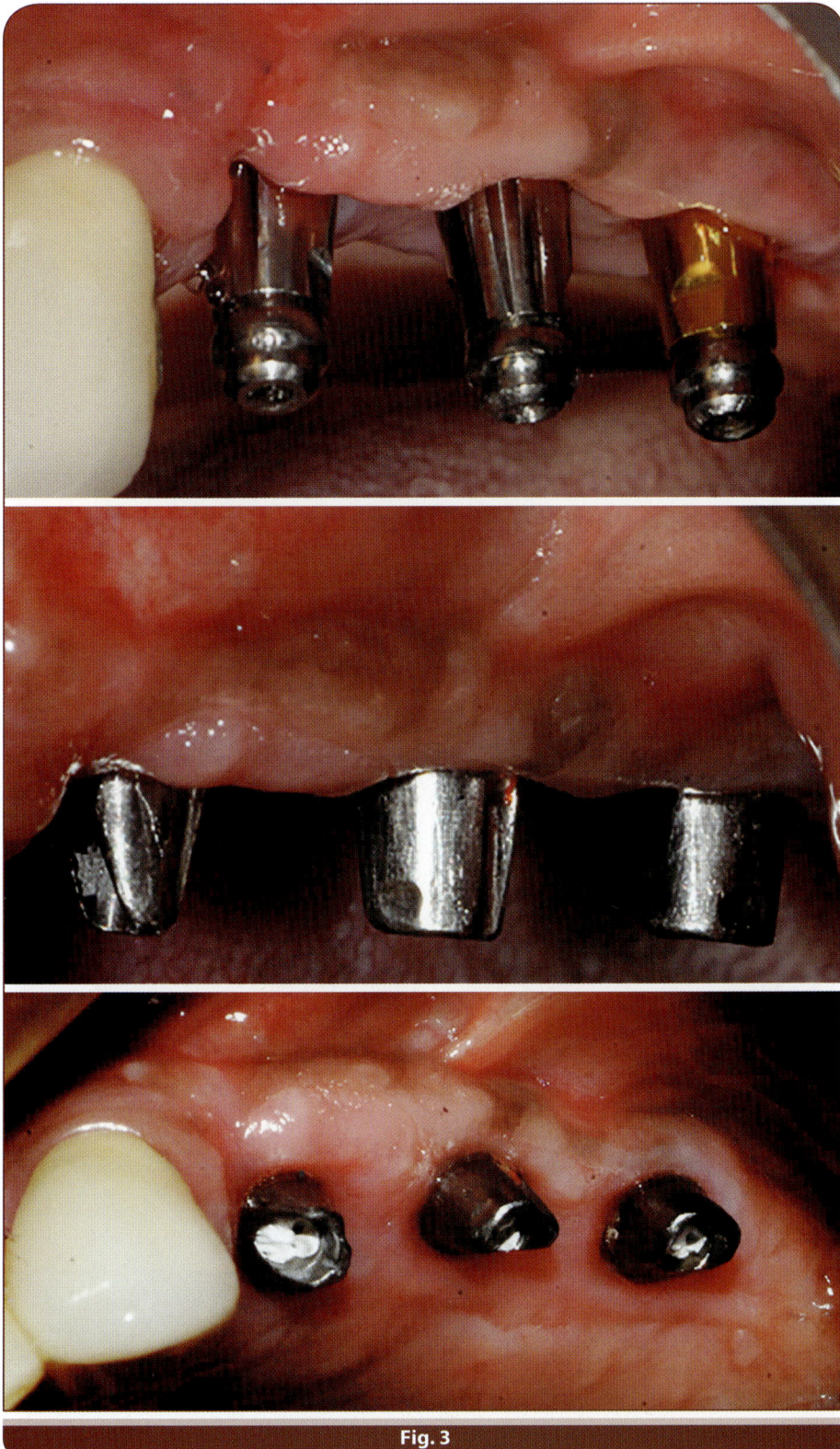

Fig. 3

Palatal tissue displacement. Well-healed tissue healing at impression. Final abutments for cemented prosthesis. Palatal view—note the scar line on the palatal side **(Fig. 3)**.

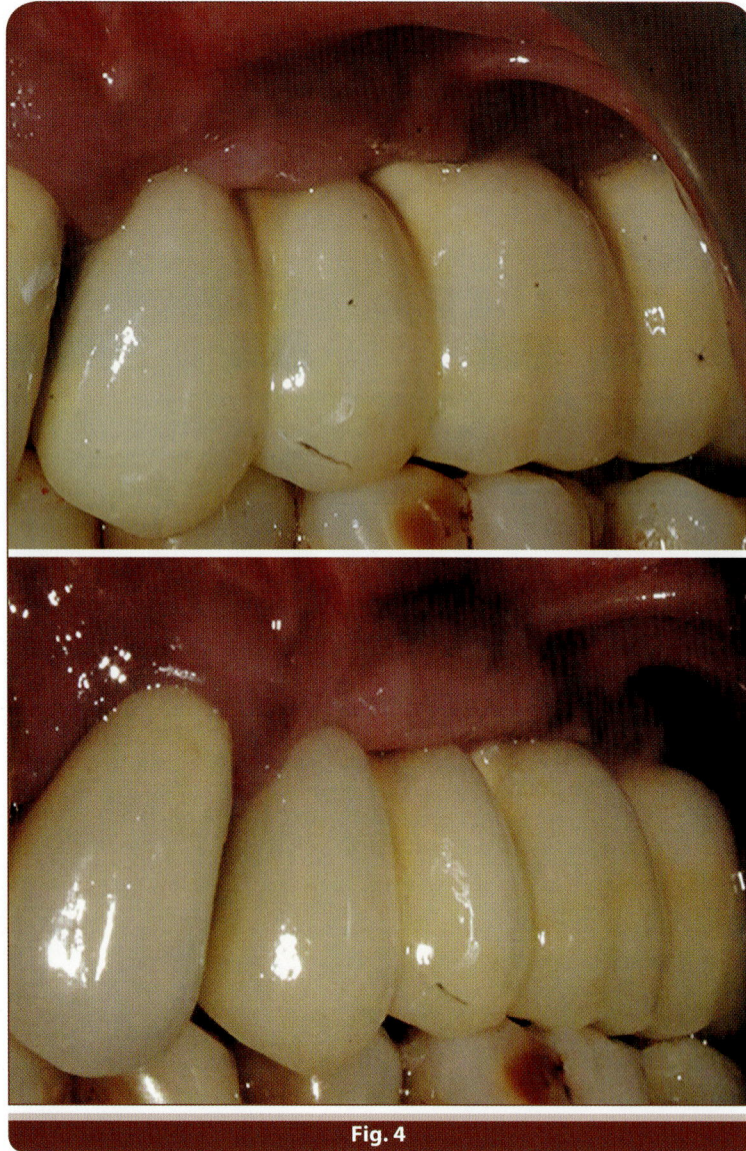

Fig. 4

Palatal tissue displacement. At final cementation. Pouch and tunnel technique **(Fig. 4)**.

CASE STUDY 94

Sudhindra Kulkarni

LATERAL DISPLACEMENT OF THE PALATAL TISSUE—PART 2

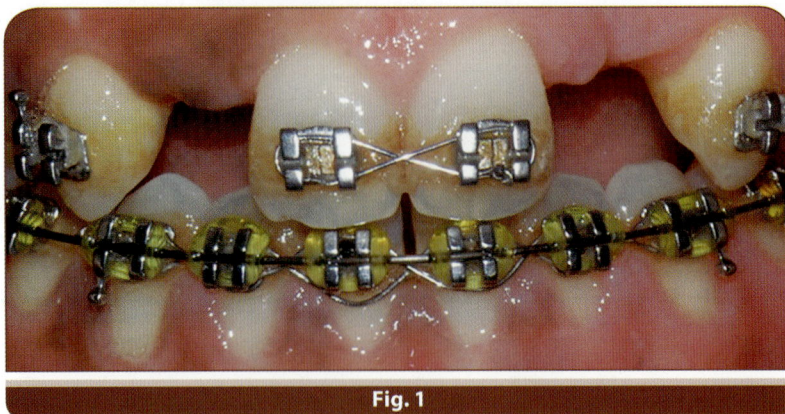

Fig. 1

Palatal roll and finger split. Preoperative **(Fig. 1)**.

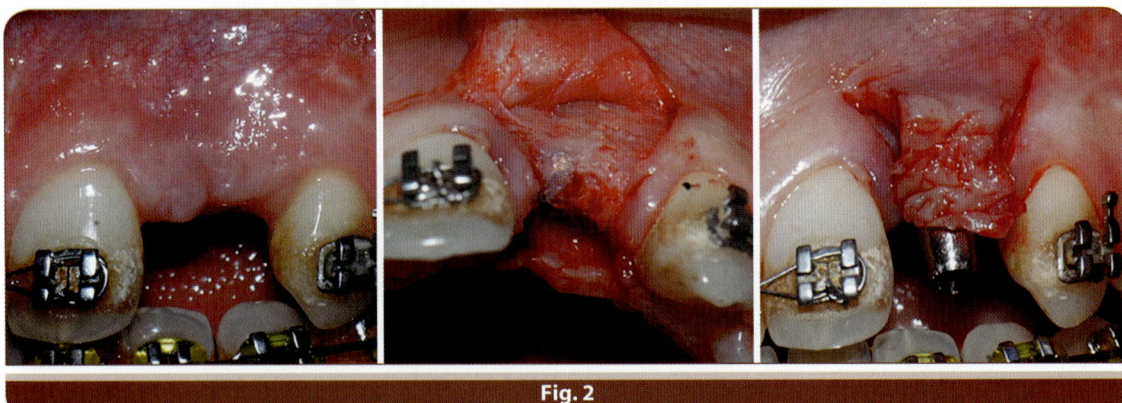

Fig. 2

Lack of contour. Note the buccal contour deficiency with tooth #22 area. Deep palatal flap elevated and de-epithelialized. Flap reflected, with a split-full-split incision. The buccal periosteum is left intact. The palatal tissue is now de-epithelialized and rolled under the buccal flap **(Fig. 2)**.

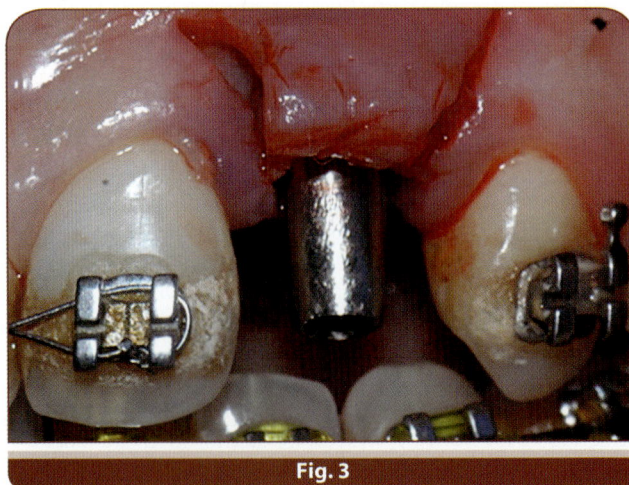

Fig. 3

Flap rolled into the pouch. The de-epithelialized part is tucked underneath the buccal flap. Abutment is placed to temporize the site **(Fig. 3)**.

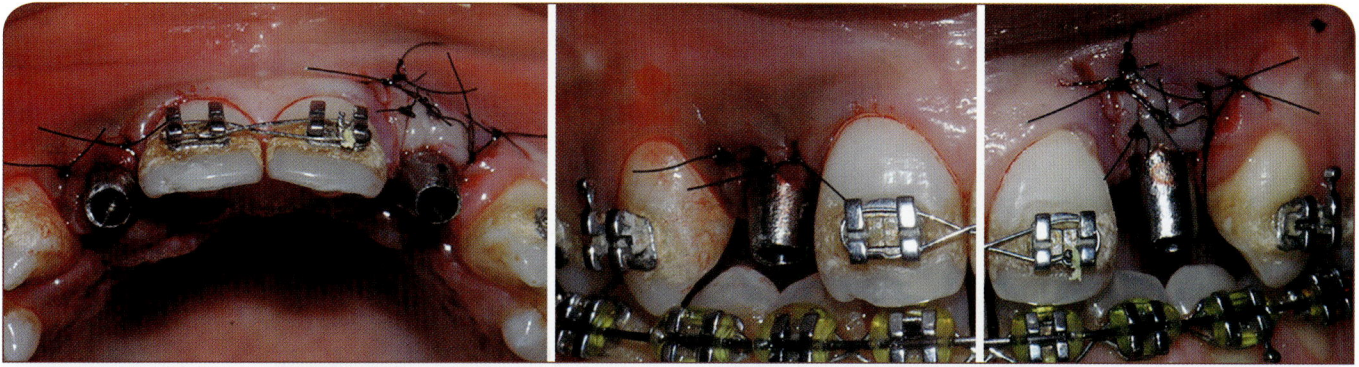

Fig. 4

In the tooth #12 site, the implant site is uncovered and abutment is placed to temporize the area. Buccal view of the tooth #22 site. Flap secured. Occlusal view—the flaps are closed with 5-0 polyamide monofilament sutures **(Fig. 4)**.

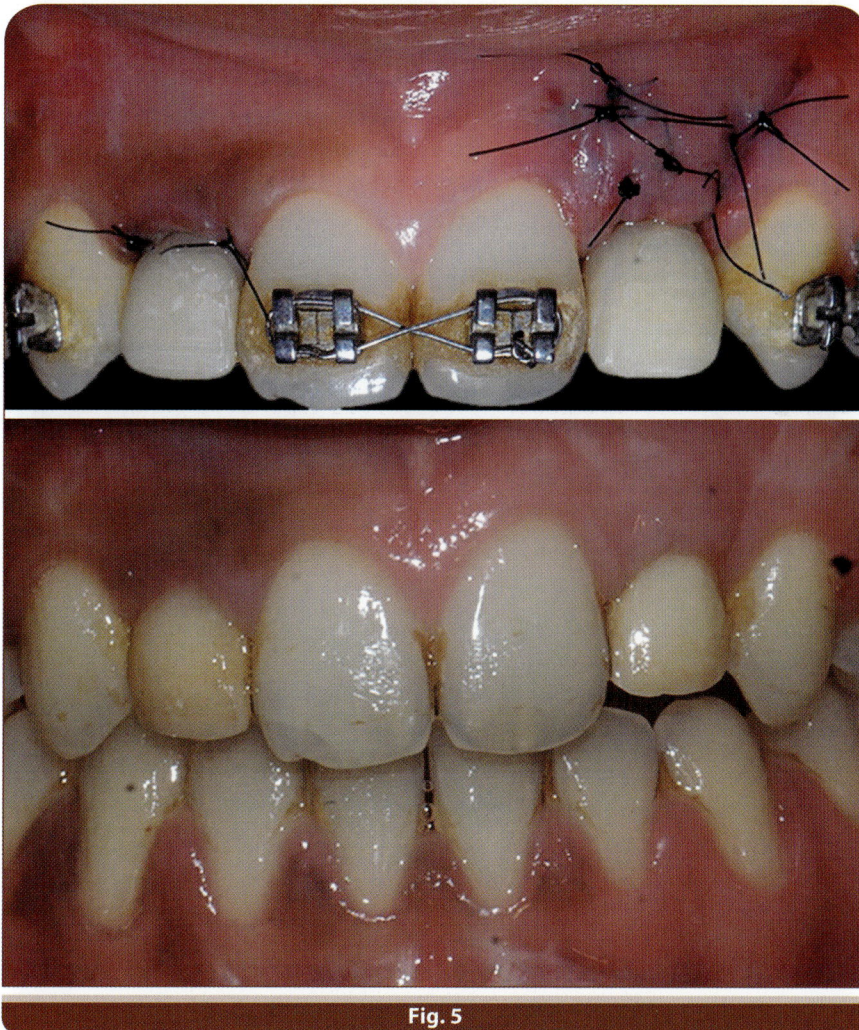

Fig. 5

Temporary placed. One week postoperative site. Note the tissue contour. Four weeks after removal of the sutures and soft tissue maturation. The site is now ready for final restorations **(Fig. 5)**.

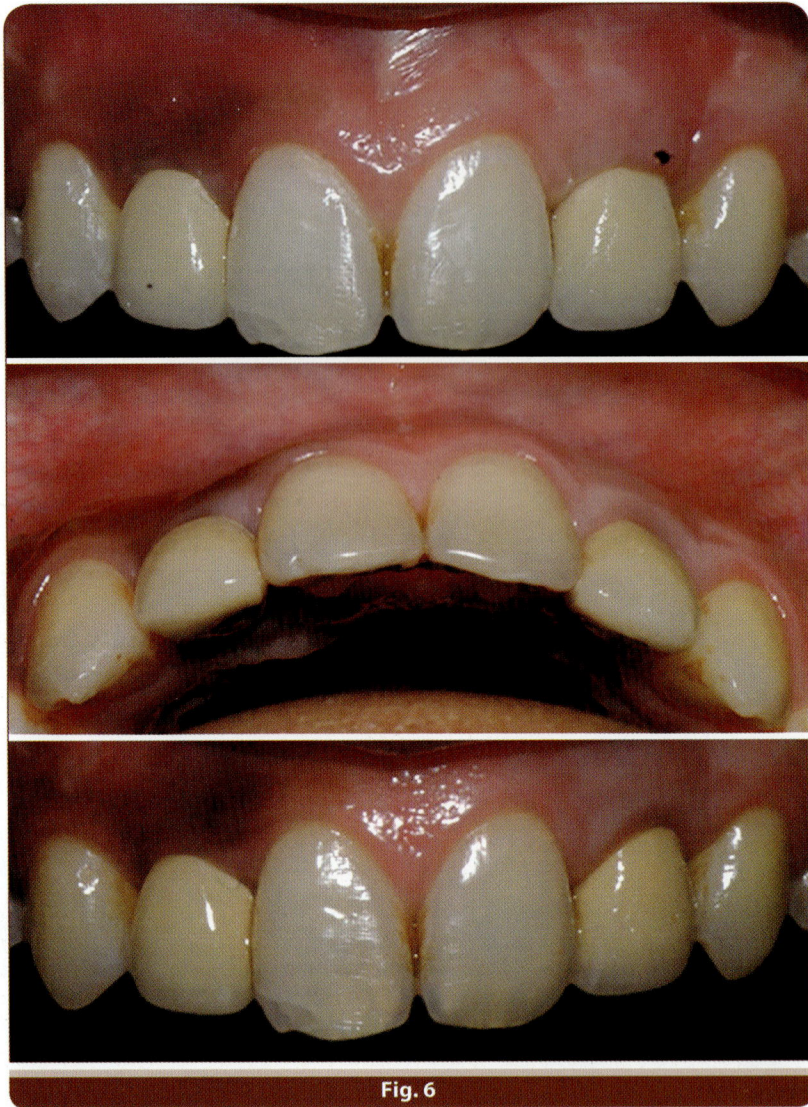

Fig. 6

At final restorations. Final cemented restorations on tooth #12 and tooth #22. At 2-year, postoperative follow-up. Note the ideal tissue contours on both the sites **(Fig. 6)**.

Cary Bopiah

Inverted Pedicled Connective Tissue Palatal Graft for the Correction of an Anterior Soft Tissue Defect

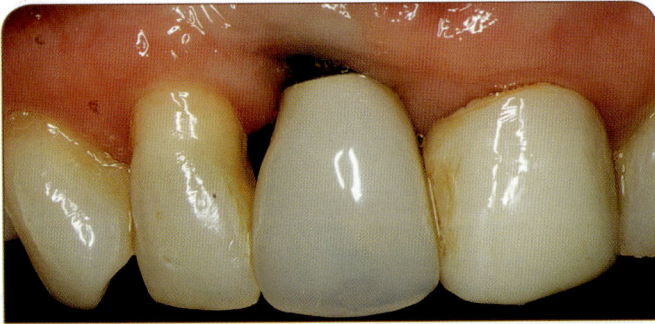

Fig. 1

Intraoral view showing the degree of gingival recession and exposure of the implant abutment and shoulder **(Fig. 1)**.

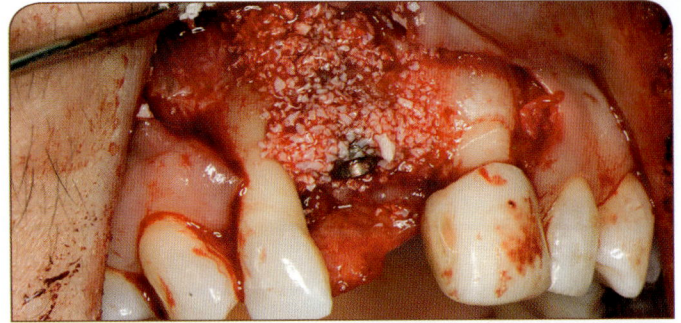

Fig. 2

Crown and abutment removed and the site exposed. The threads of the implant cleant and the site grafted with a mix of an allograft (SynthoGraft™) and locally harvested bone chips **(Fig. 2)**.

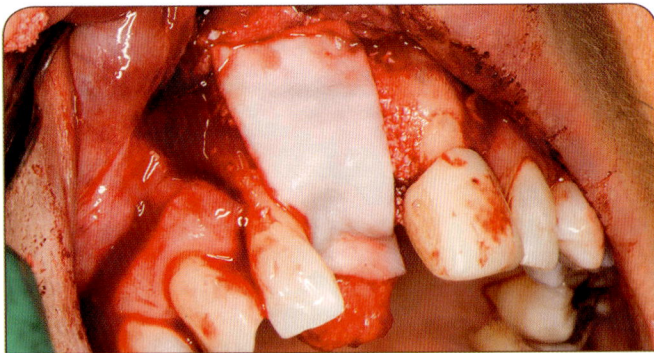

Fig. 3

A collagen membrane (Bio-Guide®, Geistlich) was used to cover the bone graft **(Fig. 3)**.

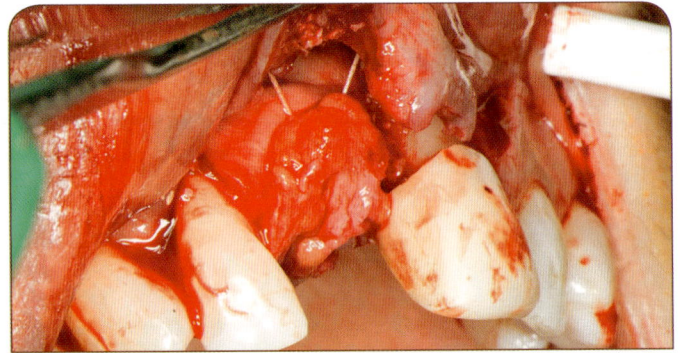

Fig. 4

The palatal connective tissue graft folded on its belly and inverted onto the labial side. The graft was held by a horizontal mattress sling suture and the end of the graft was secured into a pouch made in the labial gingiva **(Fig. 4)**.

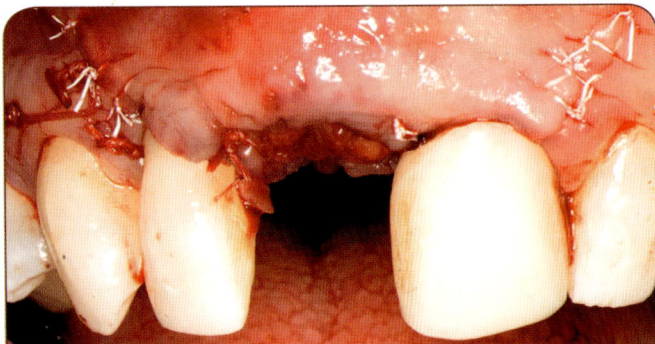

Fig. 5

Site closure with 5-0 PTFE sutures. **(Fig. 5)**

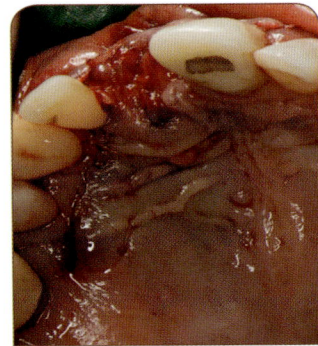

Fig. 6

Occlusal view of the palate after closure of the wound **(Fig. 6)**.

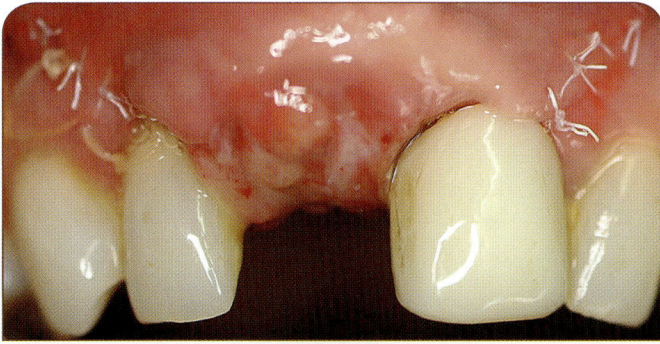

Fig. 7

Intraoral labial view after 2 weeks of healing **(Fig. 7)**.

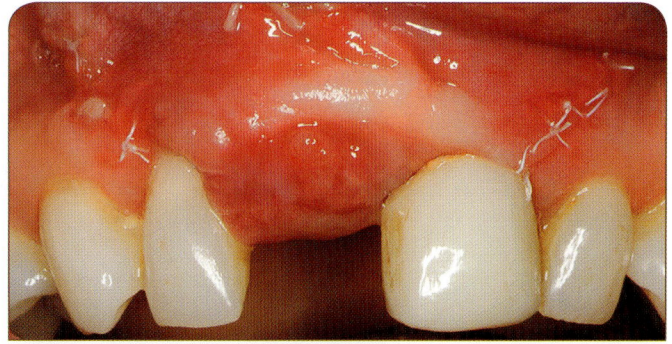

Fig. 8

Intraoral labial view after 6 weeks of healing **(Fig. 8)**.

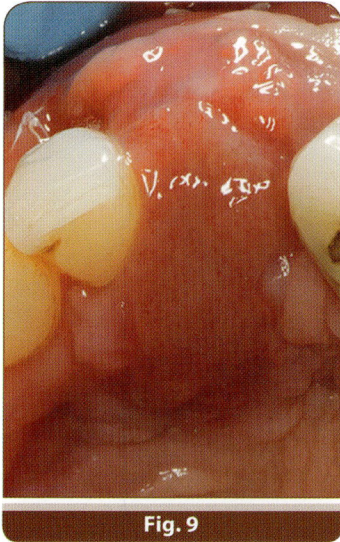

Fig. 9

Occlusal view of the palate 6 weeks after healing **(Fig. 9)**.

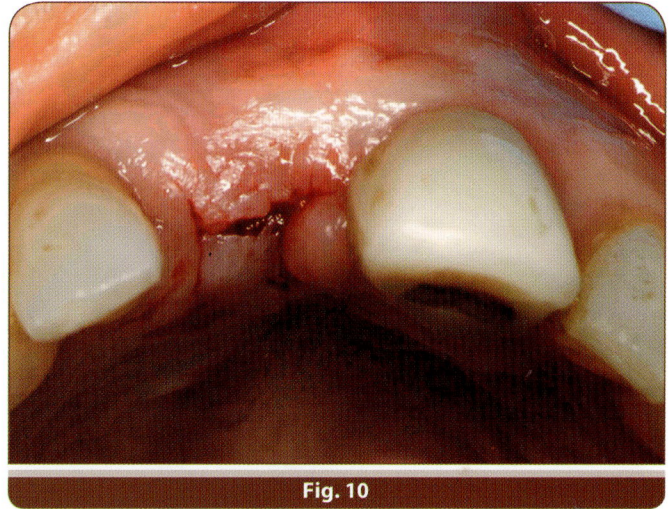

Fig. 10

H-shaped uncovery incision made after a 3-month healing period **(Fig. 10)**.

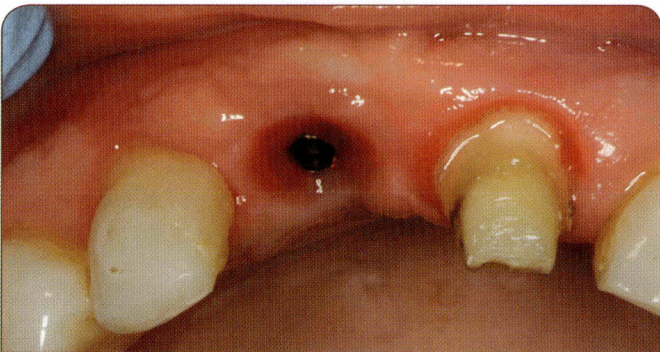

Fig. 11

Occlusal view for the grafted upper right central incisor area 2 weeks after uncovery. The crown on the upper left central incisor was removed and the tooth re-prepared for a new crown **(Fig. 11)**.

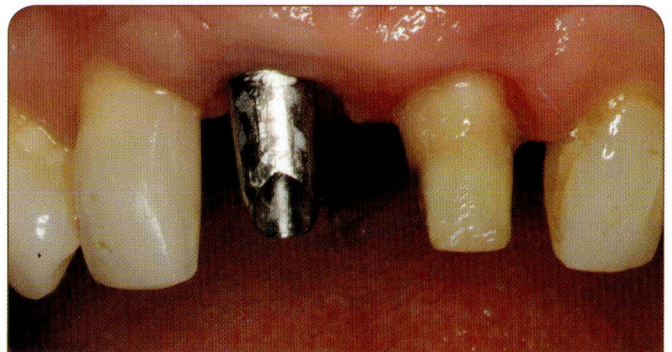

Fig. 12

Labial view of the upper right and left central incisors. Note the equitable gingival heights for the upper two central incisors **(Fig. 12)**.

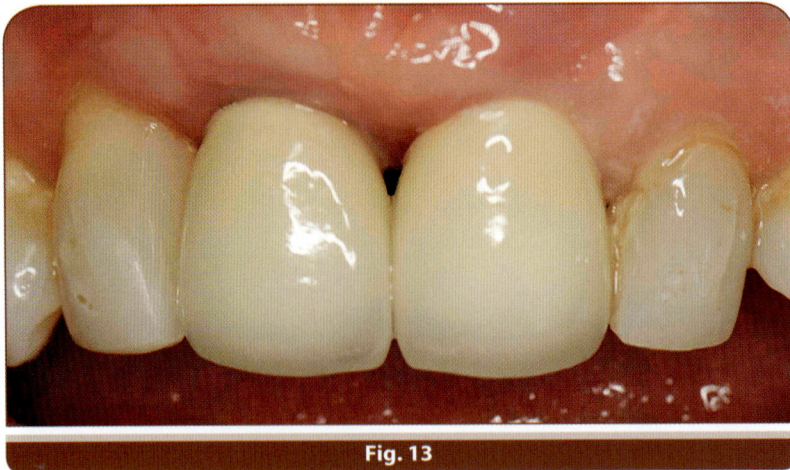

Fig. 13

Porcelain bonded crowns for the upper centrals incisors in place **(Fig. 13)**.

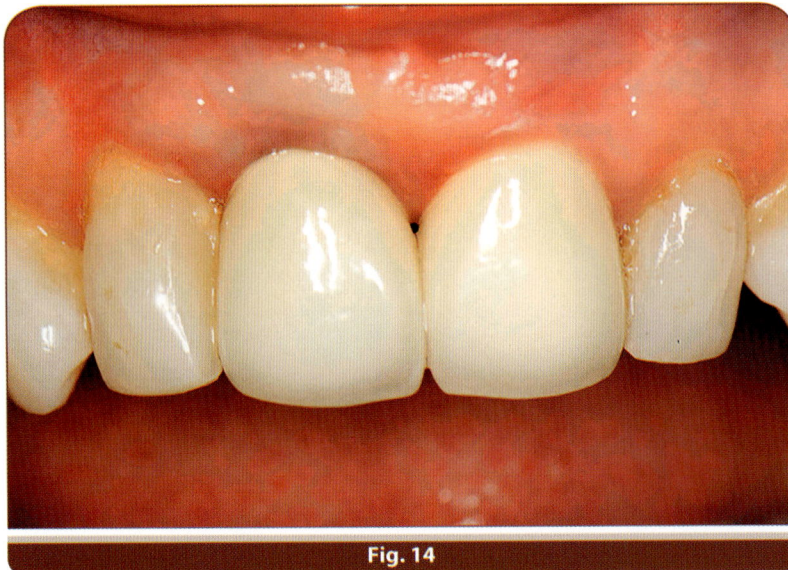

Fig. 14

Labial view five years after placement of crowns. Note the healthy and stable height of the surrounding gingival tissue **(Fig. 14)**.

CASE STUDY 96

Sudhindra Kulkarni

FREE SOFT TISSUE GRAFT

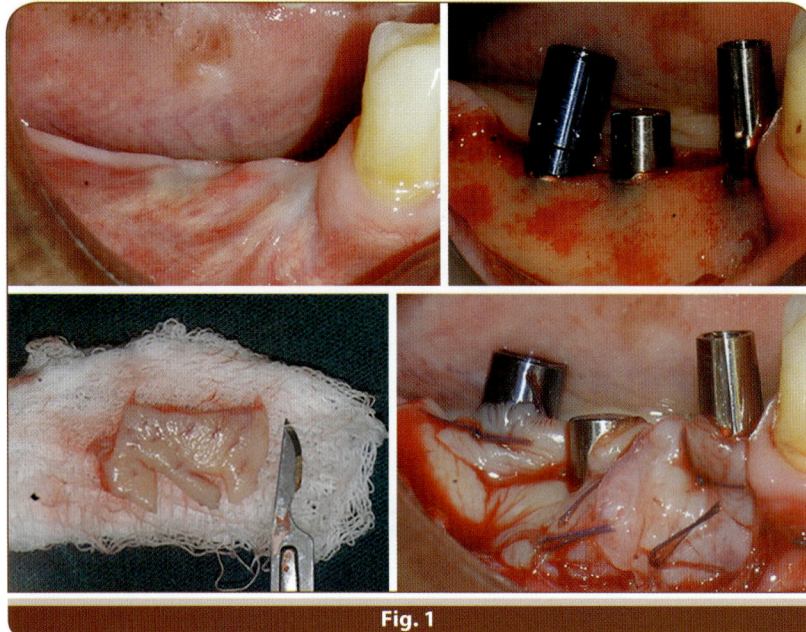

Fig. 1

Lack of Keratinized tissue in the implant site from tooth #44-46. Full Thickness flap reflected to expose the site. Free gingival graft harvested from the palate. Cuts made to facilitate placement in the implant area **(Fig. 1)**.

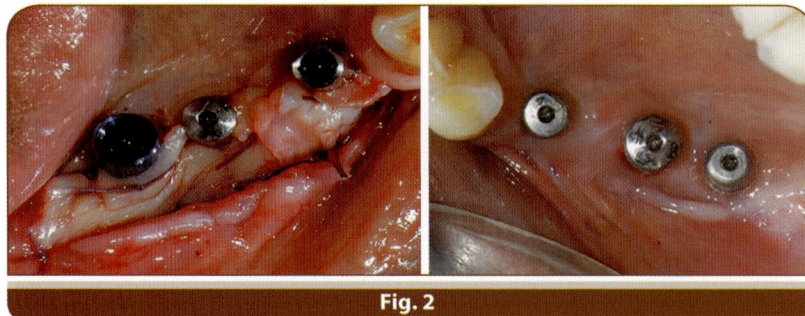

Fig. 2

Occlusal view showing the adaptation of the soft tissue to the recepient site. Well healed soft tissue around the implants at 3 weeks postoperative **(Fig. 2)**.

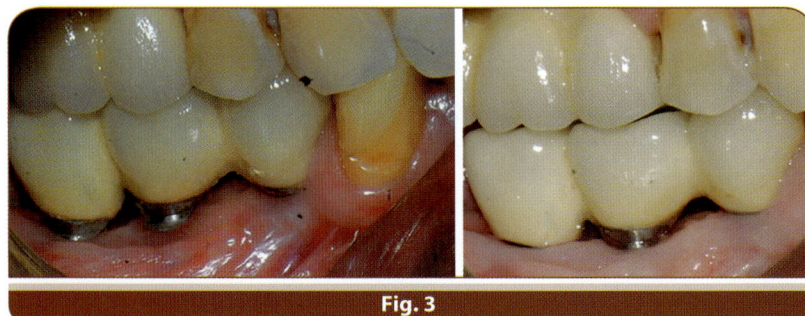

Fig. 3

At final restoration. Note the tissue levels and presence of keratinized tissue around the 3 implants. At 1 year follow-up. Note the creeping of the soft tissue over the abutments as compared to the time of cementation of the prosthesis. The tissue appears thicker and healthier. This also shows that the presence of keratinized tissue also facilitates oral hygiene **(Fig. 3)**.

Prosthetic Options: Single Tooth to Full Arch

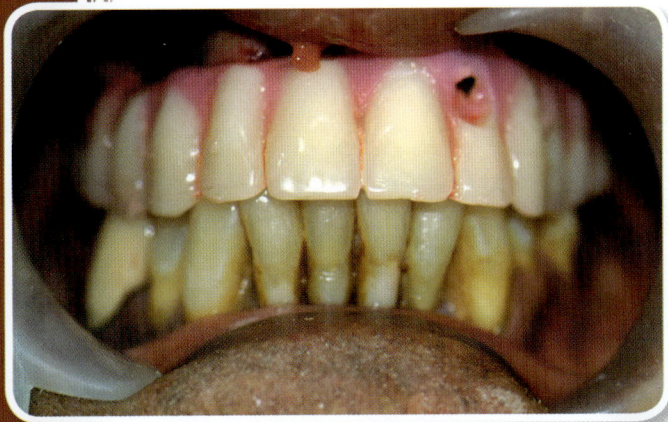

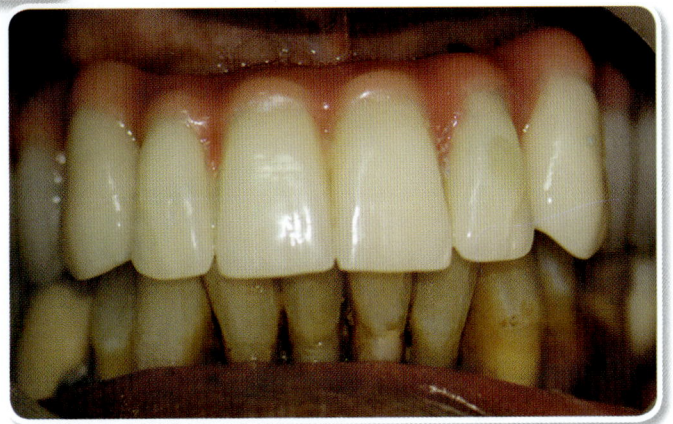

Praful Bali

Maxillary "All on 4" to avoid Sinus Augmentation

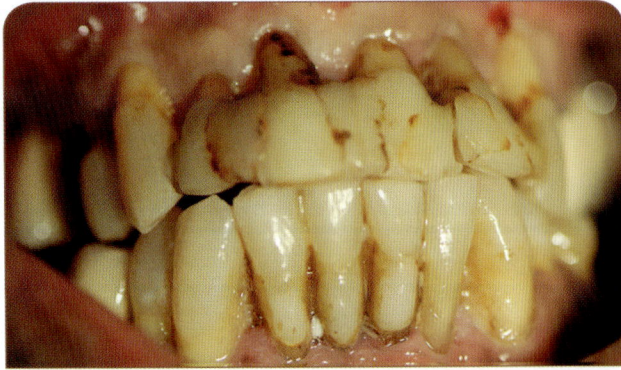

Fig. 1

A 58-year-old patient presents with hopeless upper dentition with the aim to replace all teeth with implants. Patient is afraid of being without teeth and hence has been postponing the definitive treatment for a long time (**Fig. 1**).

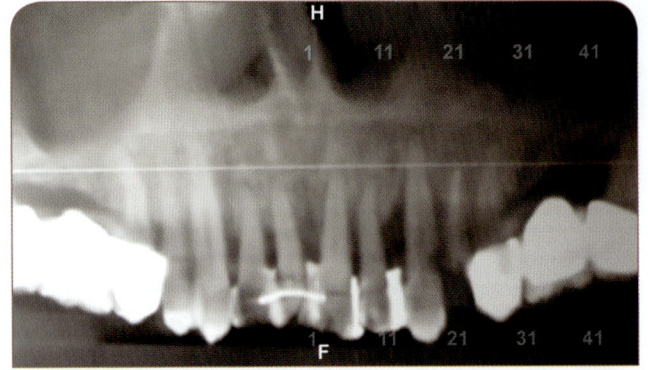

Fig. 2

On clinical and radiographic examination a decision is taken to do a full arch rehabilitation for the patient with the "All on 4" treatment concept as the patient is not ready for sinus lifts. An immediate temporary prosthesis is also planned so that the patient is not edentulous for any time (**Fig. 2**).

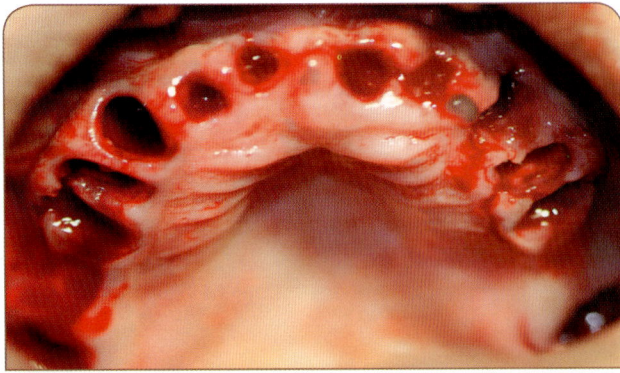

Fig. 3

Total extraction done before raising the flap (**Fig. 3**).

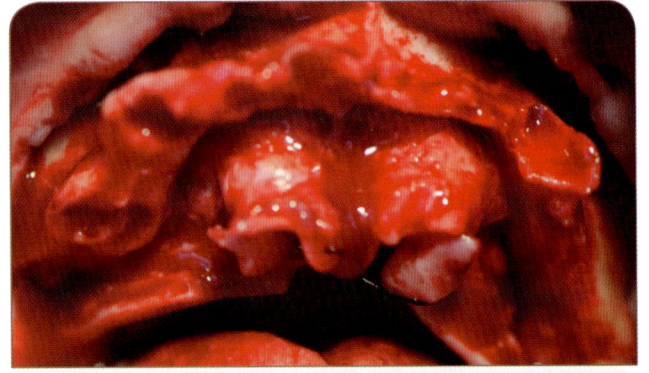

Fig. 4

The ridge is flattened and prepared for osteotomy (**Fig. 4**).

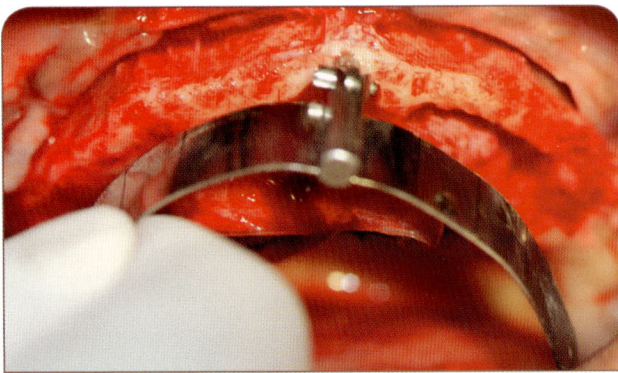

Fig. 5

The Malo clinic guide is placed after a 2 mm/10 mm drilling is done in the center of the ridge (**Fig. 5**).

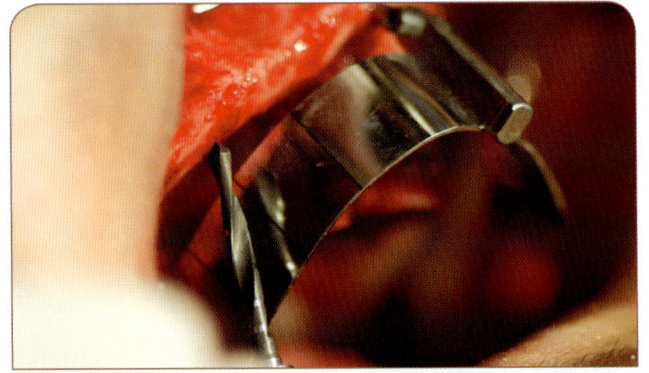

Fig. 6

The pilot drill is oriented bisecting the parallel lines on the Malo clinic guide. This gives the orientation for the tilted posterior implants to be placed at 45 degrees angle (**Fig. 6**).

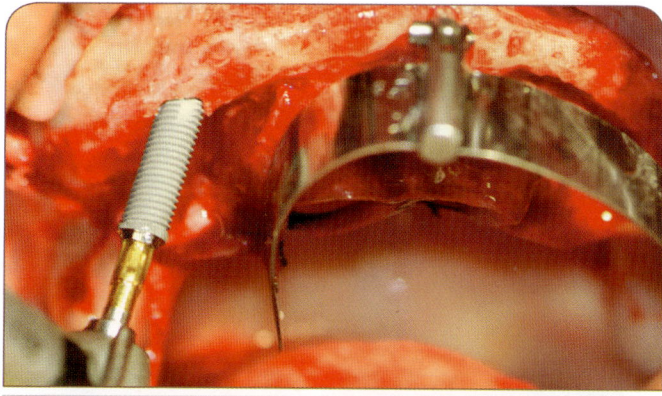

Fig. 7

The posterior implants are placed at an angle of 45 degrees. The implants are torqued at 50 N/cm (**Fig. 7**).

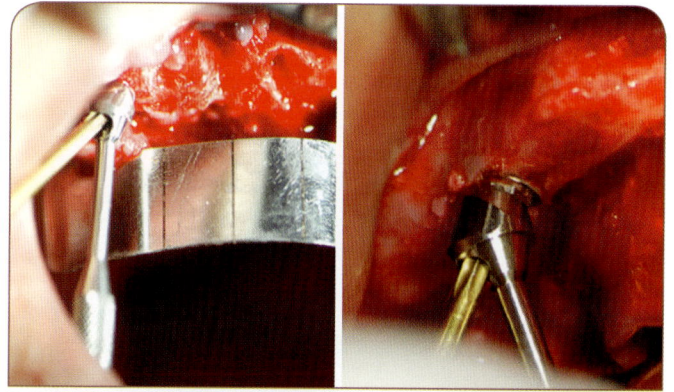

Fig. 8

A 35 degree abutment is torqued at 30 N/cm (**Fig. 8**).

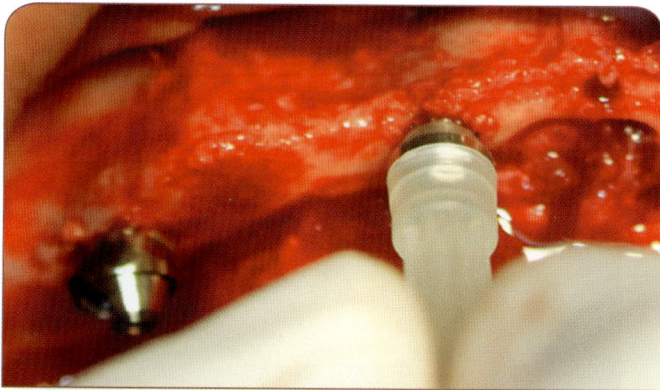

Fig. 9

Anterior implants are placed at 0 degree angulation at the same torque and a straight abutment is placed over them at the prescribed torque (**Fig. 9**).

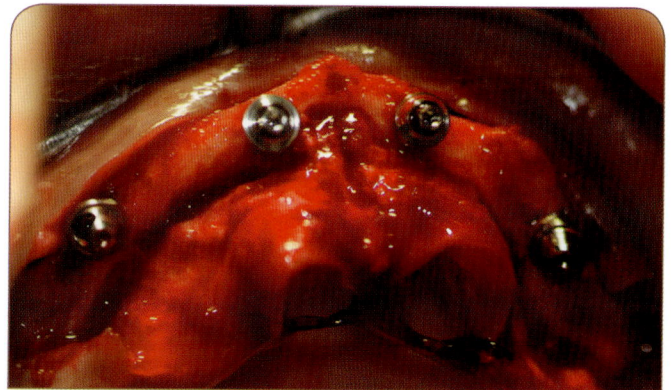

Fig. 10

Occlusal view of the 4 implants with 4 multi-unit abutments (**Fig. 10**).

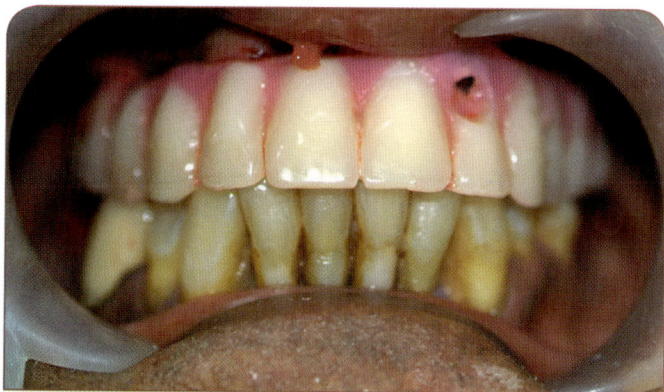

Fig. 11

An immediate fixed prosthesis is given on the same day— Teeth in a day concept (**Fig. 11**).

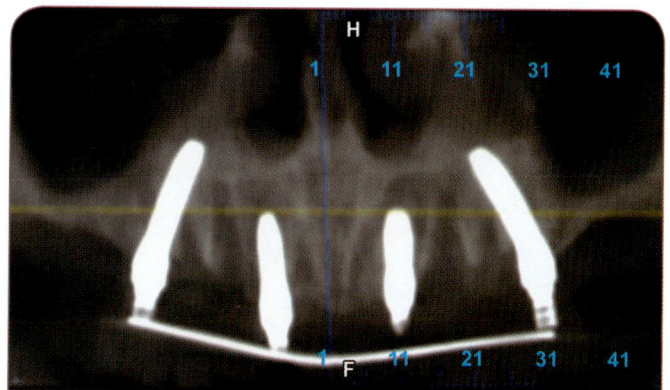

Fig. 12

Final X-ray of the All on 4. Note the 45 degree tilted posterior implants and the 0 degree anterior implants (**Fig. 12**).

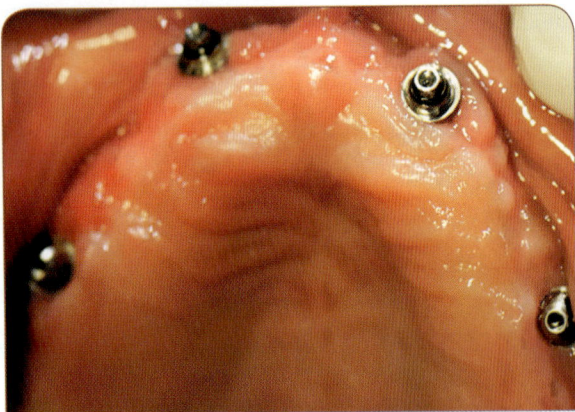
Fig. 13

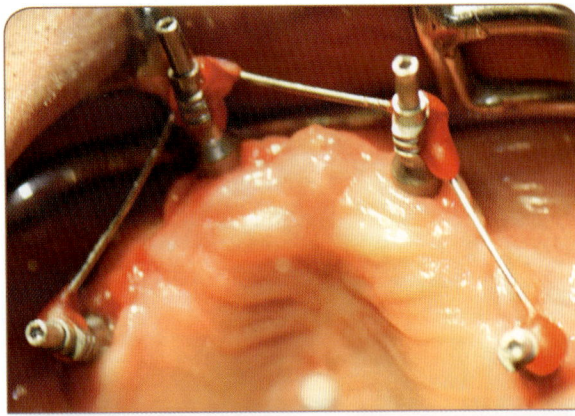
Fig. 14

Clinical situation after 3 months of healing (**Fig. 13**).

Open tray impression posts—abutment level, are placed over the multi-unit abutments and the posts are splinted together with wire and pattern resin (**Fig. 14**).

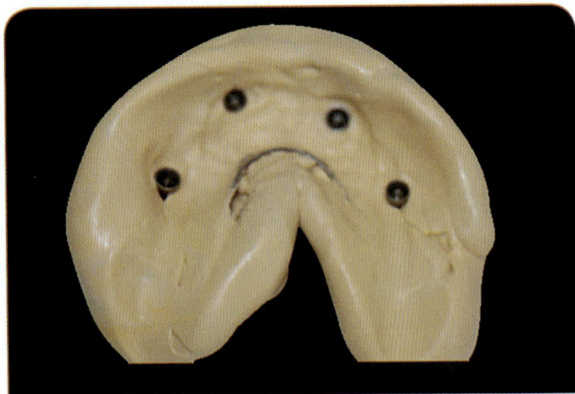
Fig. 15

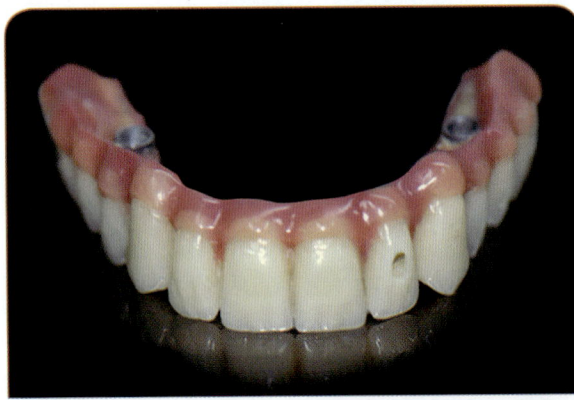
Fig. 16

The open tray impression taken. A model is poured in this and a framework is fabricated over which the final prosthesis is constructed (**Fig. 15**).

The final prosthesis made in visio.lign (**Fig. 16**).

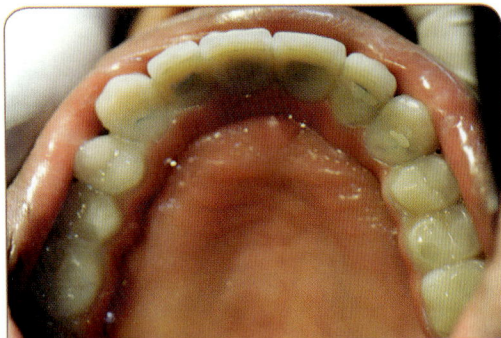
Fig. 17

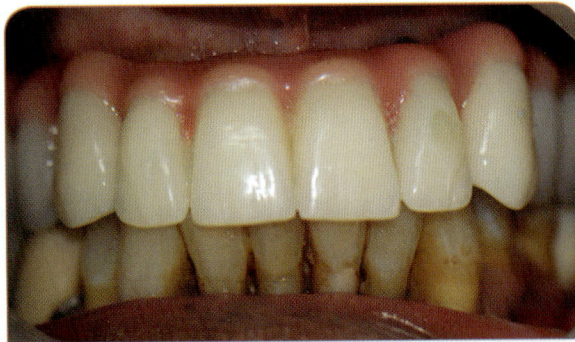
Fig. 18

Occlusal view if the final prosthesis. The screw holes filled with composite. The design made so that the patient can clean with a floss, water pick (**Fig. 17**).

Visio.lign final prosthesis is torqued at 15 N/cm and the screw holes filled with composite (**Fig. 18**).

Praful Bali

Full Mouth Rehabilitation with Tilted Implants, Immediate Loading and Temporization of a Case of Failed Dentition with Collapsed Occlusion

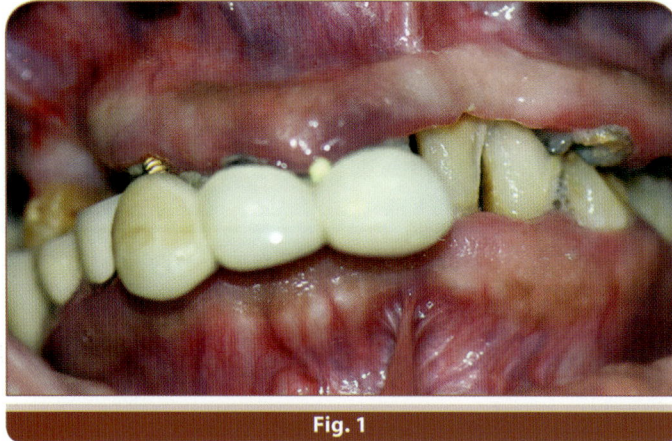

Fig. 1

A patient presents with failed dentition and collapsed occlusion. Needs immediate care and implant supported rehabilitation **(Fig. 1)**.

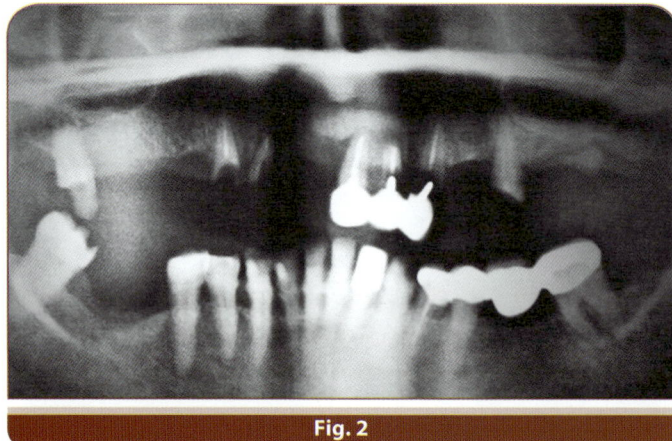

Fig. 2

Preoperative X-ray showing failed prosthesis with root stumps **(Fig. 2)**.

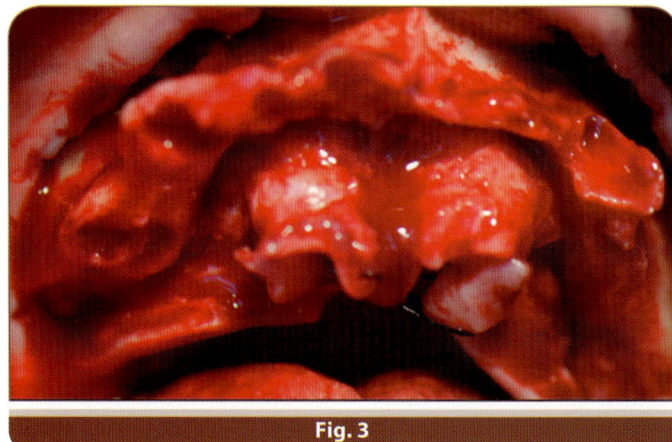

Fig. 3

Incision and flap reflection done to expose the underlying bone. Extraction of all mutilated teeth done, sockets cleaned and bone leveled **(Fig. 3)**.

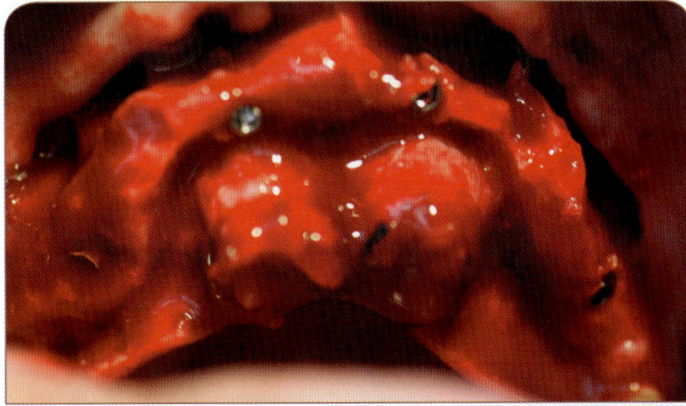

Fig. 4

All on Four Procedure done : 4 Implants placed – 2 posterior tilted implants and 2 anterior straight implants **(Fig. 4)**.

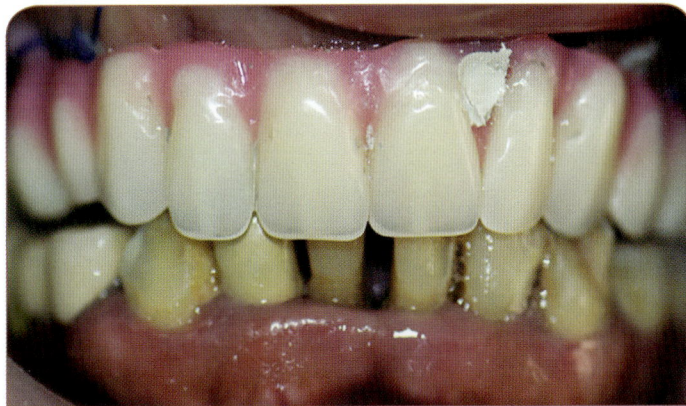

Fig. 5

Temporization done with an acrylic screw retained prosthesis. Note the establishment of the vertical dimension and occlusion. A mutually protected occlusion is generated. Patient is restored to function and esthetics within 4 hours— Teeth in a day **(Fig. 5)**.

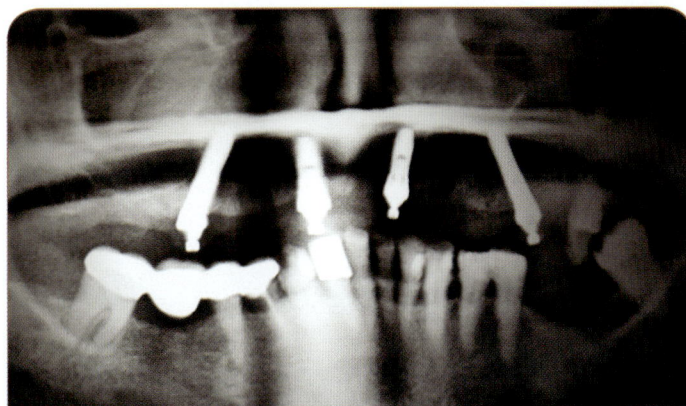

Fig. 6

X-ray showing placement of implants—All on Four **(Fig. 6)**.

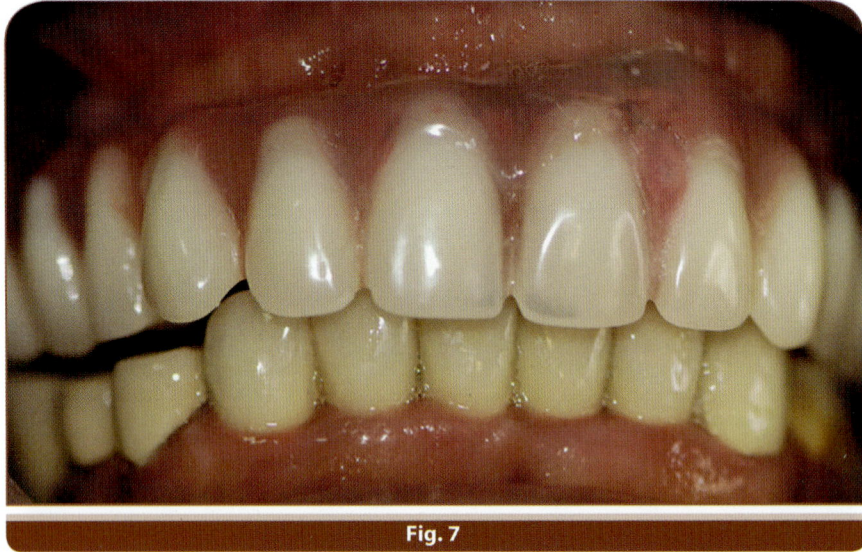

Fig. 7

The definitive prosthesis is an acrylic hybrid prosthesis. Over all health is achieved **(Fig. 7)**.

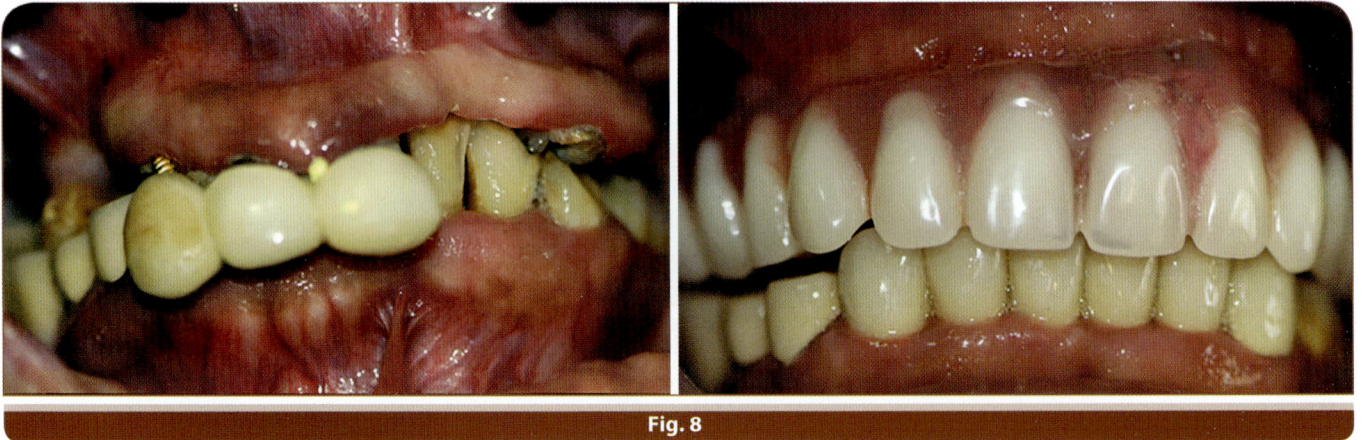

Fig. 8

Pre- and Post-comparison **(Fig. 8)**.

Amit Gulati

A Journey Spanning 6 Years
Surgical-Prosthetic-Recall

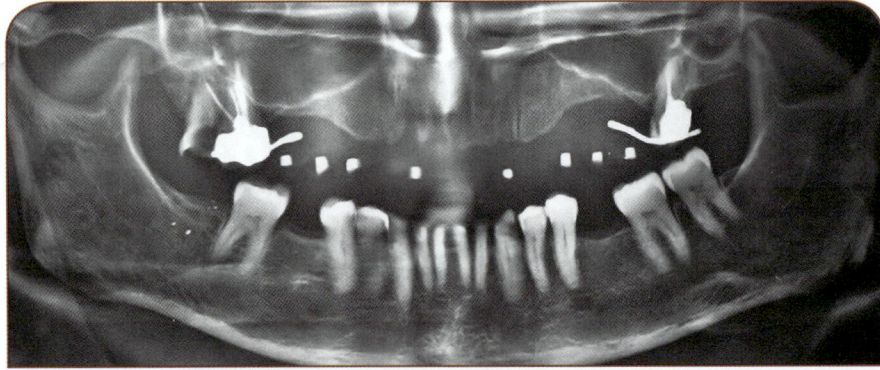

Fig. 1

Preoperative orthopantogram showing missing upper teeth **(Fig. 1)**.

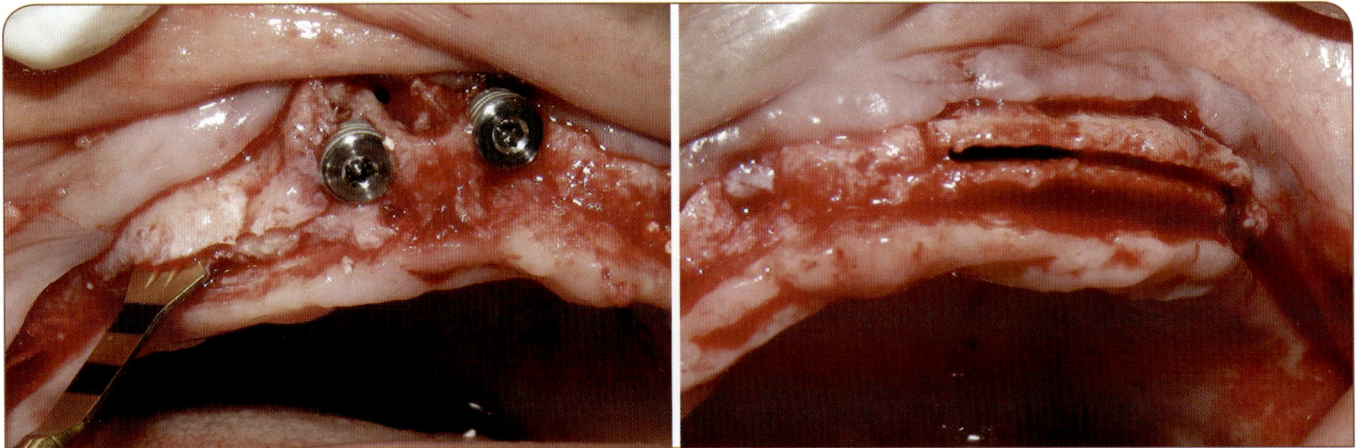

Fig. 2

Ridge split with piezo and chisels followed by expansion **(Fig. 2)**.

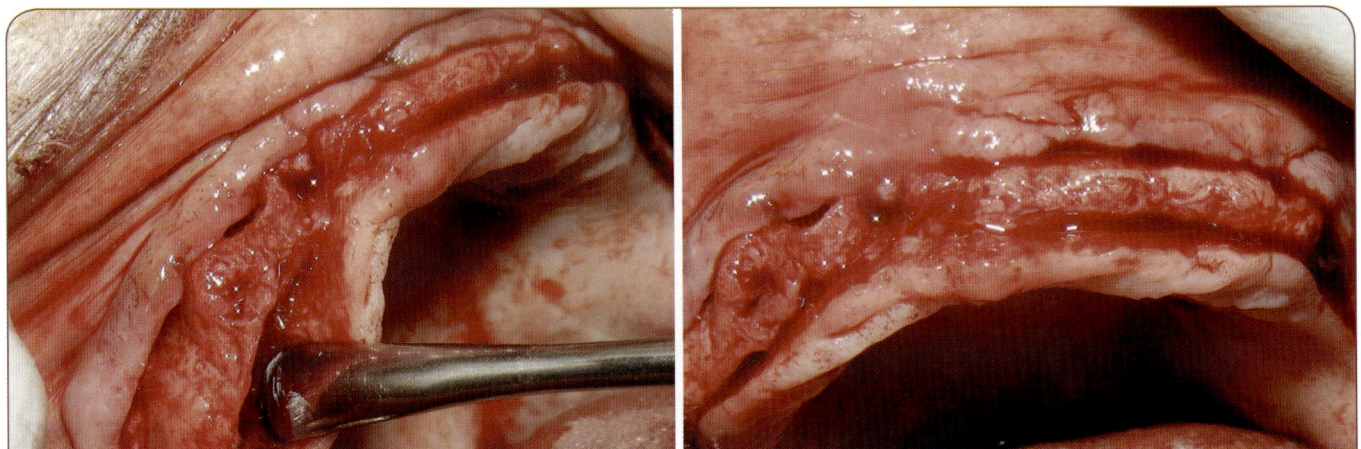

Fig. 3

Compromised width, 2–3 mm **(Fig. 3)**.

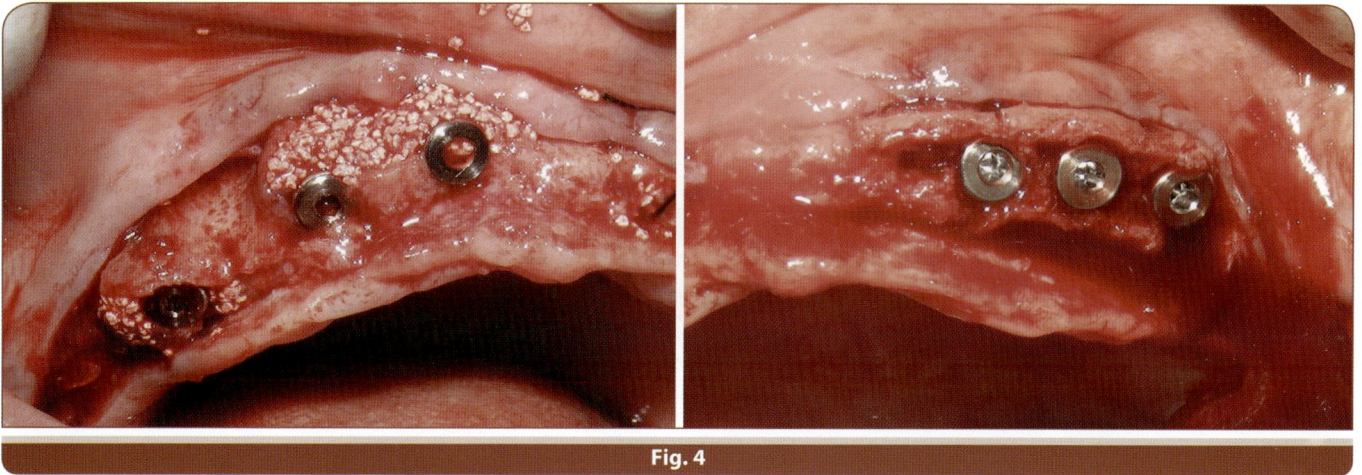

Fig. 4

Composite grafting, bTCP + autogenous, collagen membrane (Fig. 4).

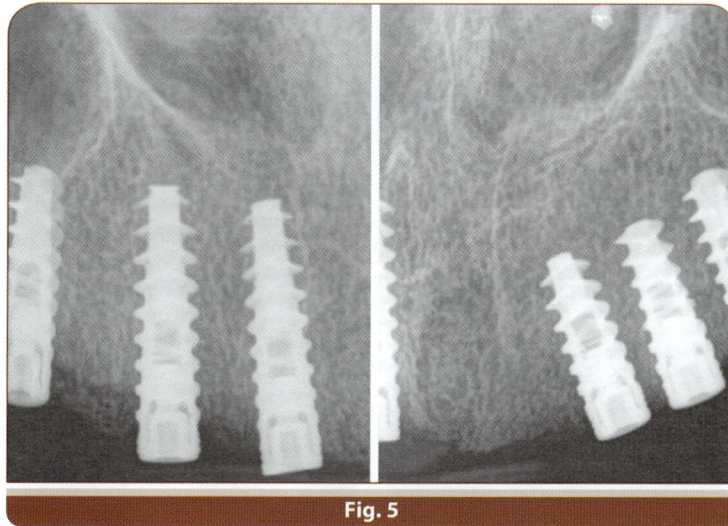

Fig. 5

Intraoral radiographs showing implants placement (Fig. 5).

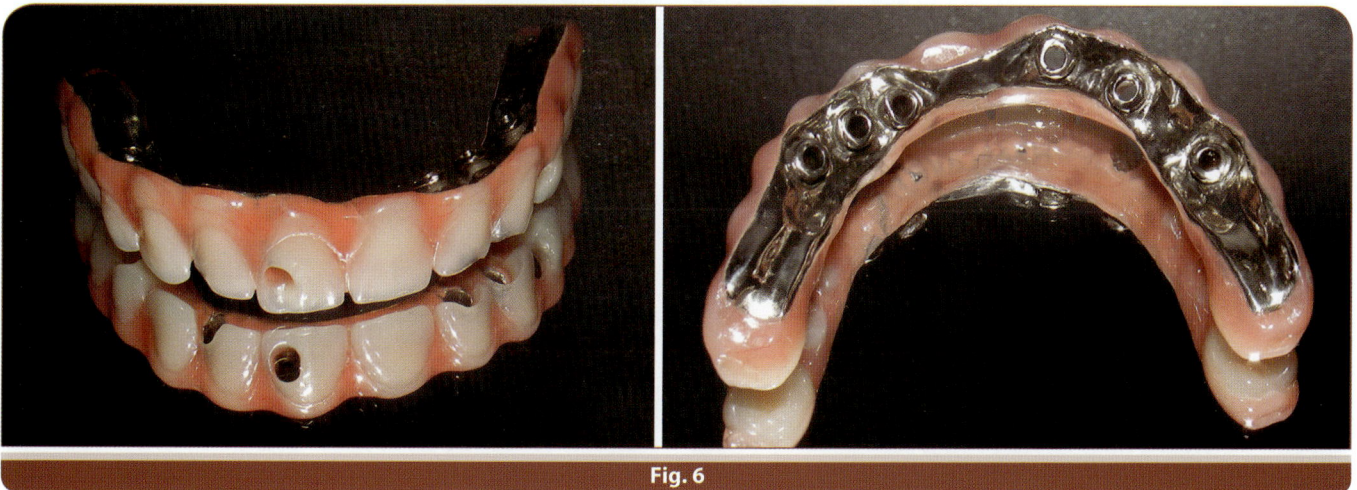

Fig. 6

Hybrid prosthesis (Fig. 6).

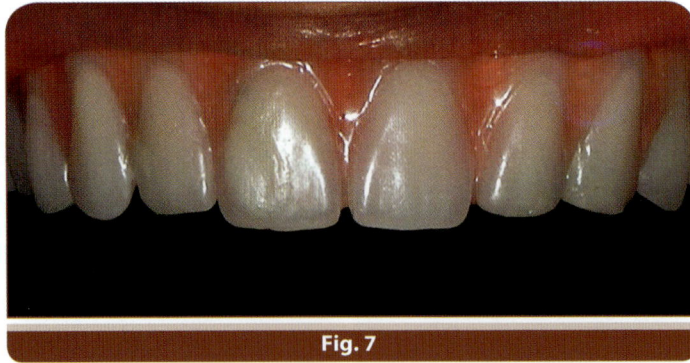

Fig. 7

Screw access holes sealed with composite **(Fig. 7)**.

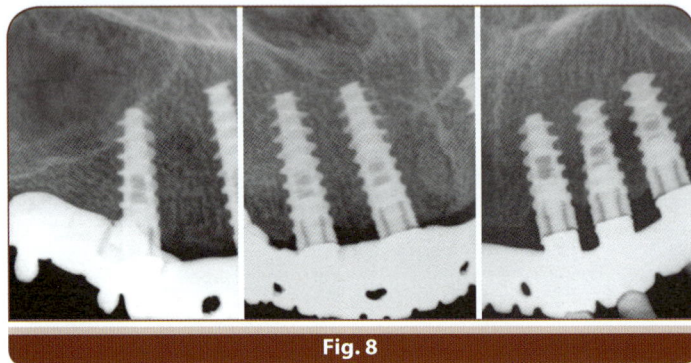

Fig. 8

Immediate postoperative **(Fig. 8)**.

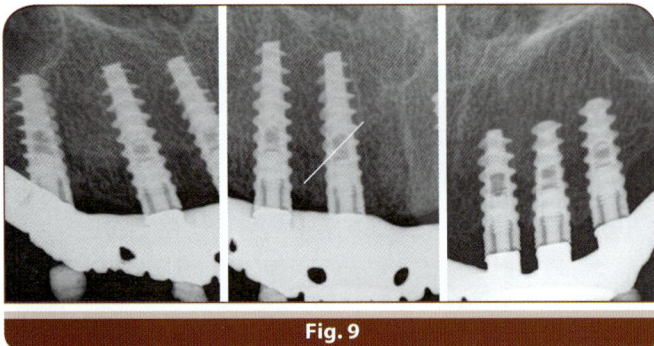

Fig. 9

Five months recall **(Fig. 9)**.

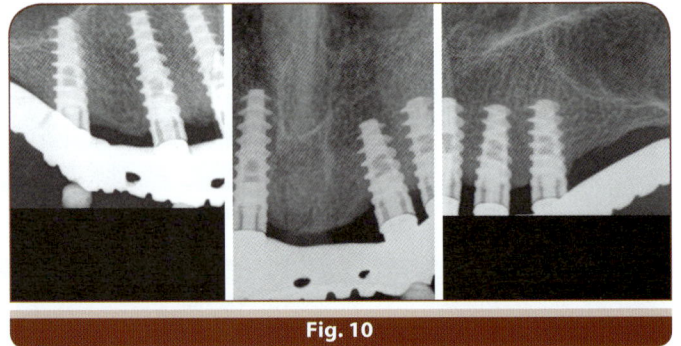

Fig. 10

Two years recall **(Fig. 10)**.

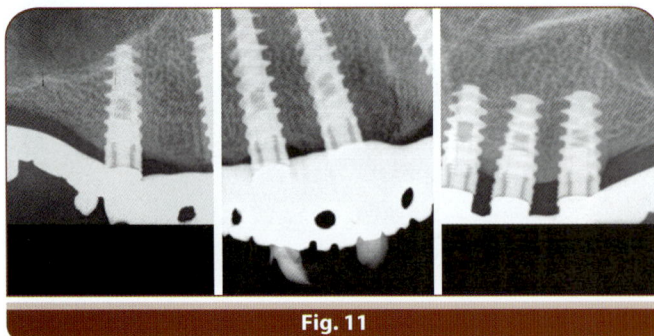

Fig. 11

Three years recall **(Fig. 11)**.

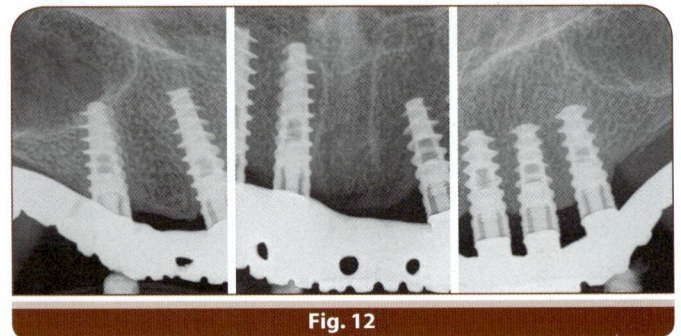

Fig. 12

Four years recall **(Fig. 12)**.

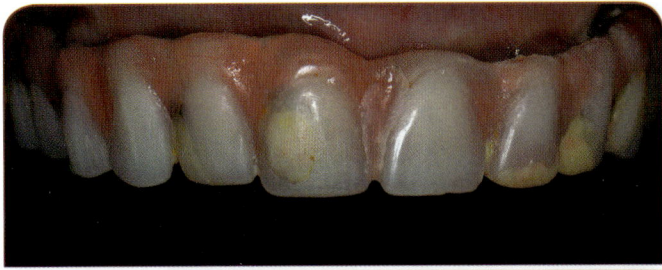

Fig. 13

State of hybrid prosthesis in 5 years **(Fig. 13)**.

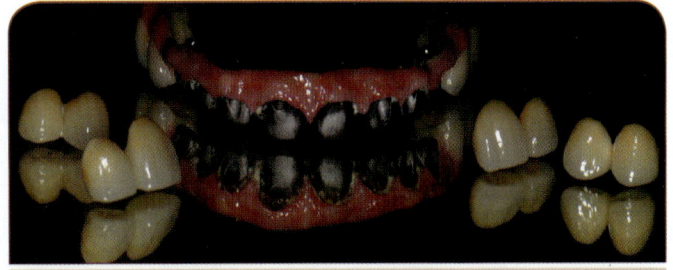

Fig. 14

New prosthesis—Malo type— crowns on primary framework **(Fig. 14)**.

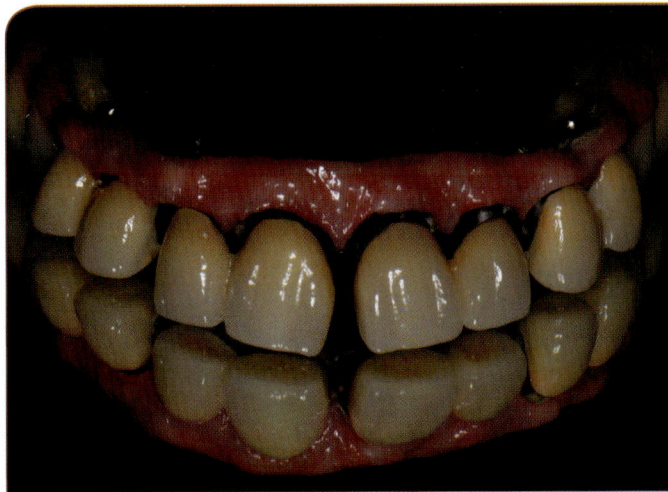

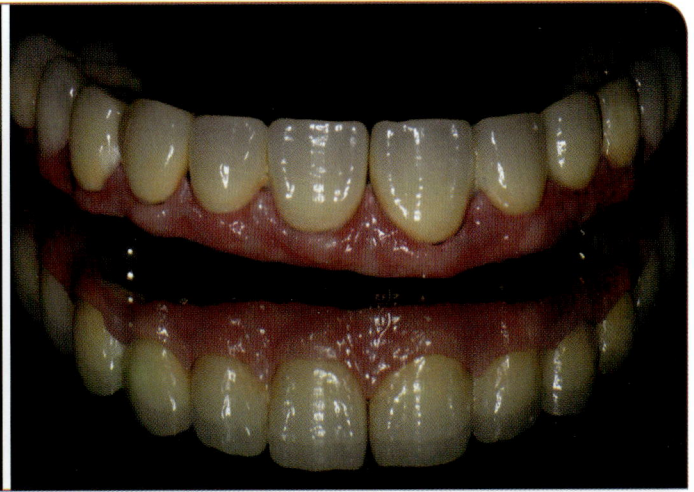

Fig. 15

New prosthesis—Malo type— crowns on primary framework **(Fig. 15)**.

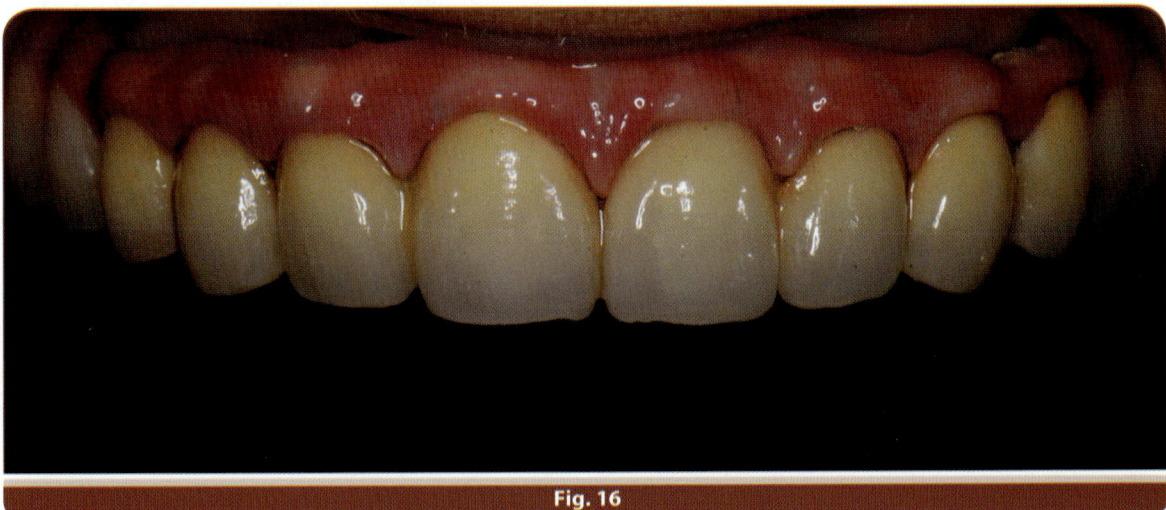

Fig. 16

New prosthesis—Malo type— crowns on primary framework in patient's mouth **(Fig. 16)**.

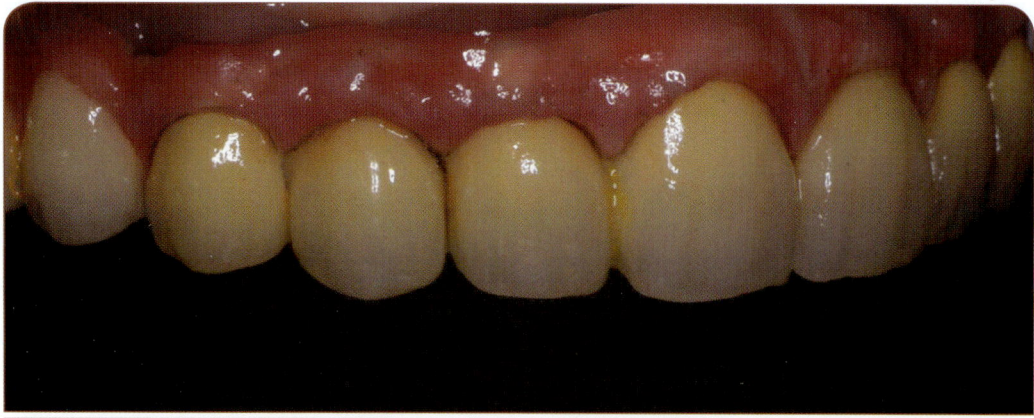

Fig. 17

New prosthesis—Malo type— crowns on primary framework lateral view **(Fig. 17)**.

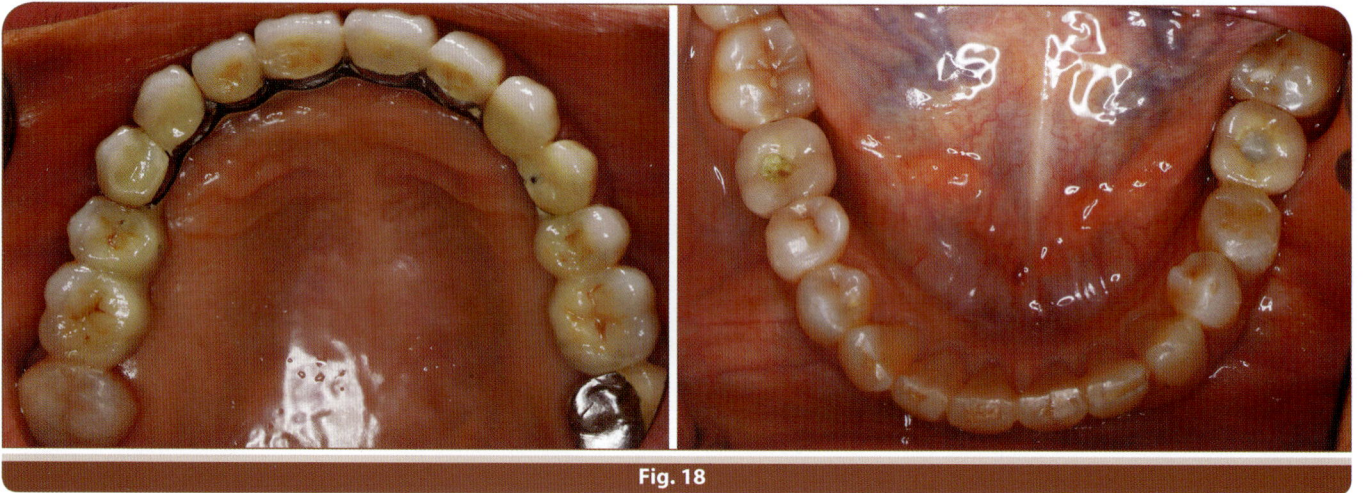

Fig. 18

New prosthesis—Malo type— crowns on primary framework occlusal view **(Fig. 18)**.

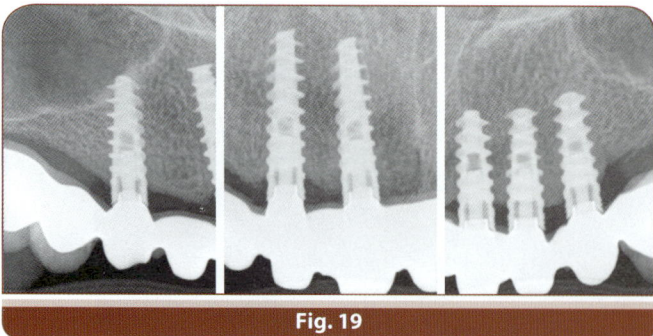

Fig. 19

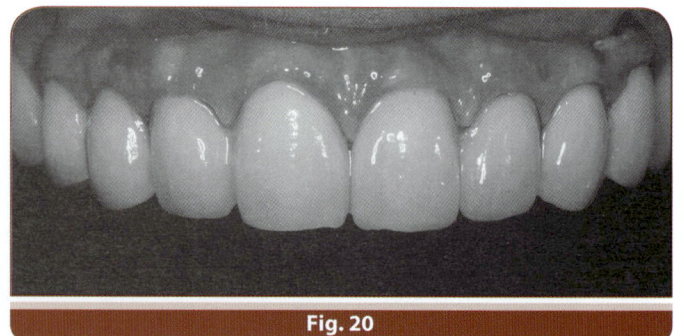

Fig. 20

Six years recall **(Figs. 19 and 20)**.

CASE STUDY 100

Praful Bali, Sourabh Nagpal

MALO TYPE BRIDGE WORK: A STATE OF ART

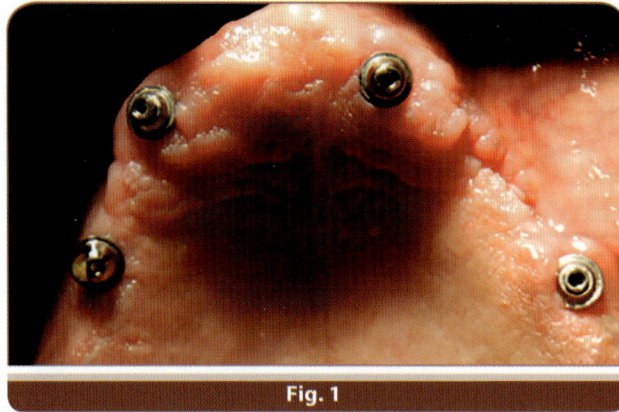

Fig. 1

"All on 4" procedure was performed in the maxilla and mandible and a Malo type prosthesis was planned **(Fig. 1)**.

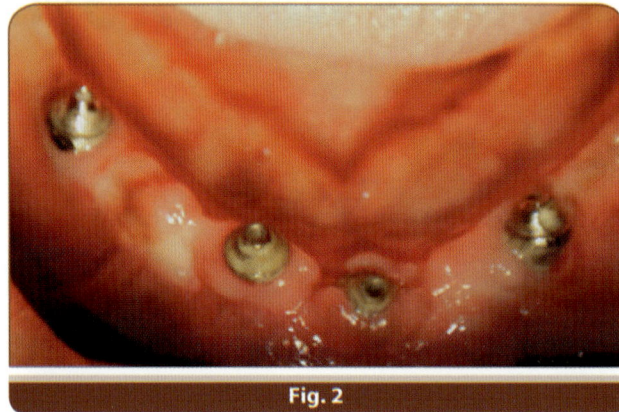

Fig. 2

The Malo Bridge—A separate framework is casted and retained on the "all on 4" MU abutments and individual crowns are made and cemented on to the framework **(Fig. 2)**.

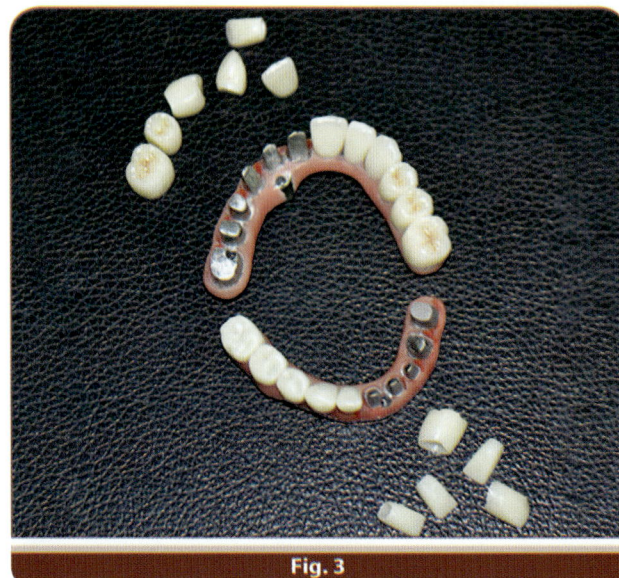

Fig. 3

Malo bridge—Separate screw retained framework and individual cementable zirconia crowns **(Fig. 3)**.

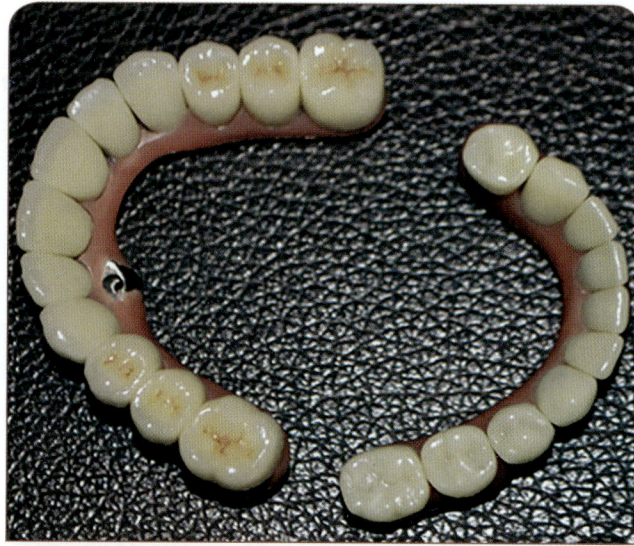

Fig. 4

The Malo Bridge assembled **(Fig. 4)**.

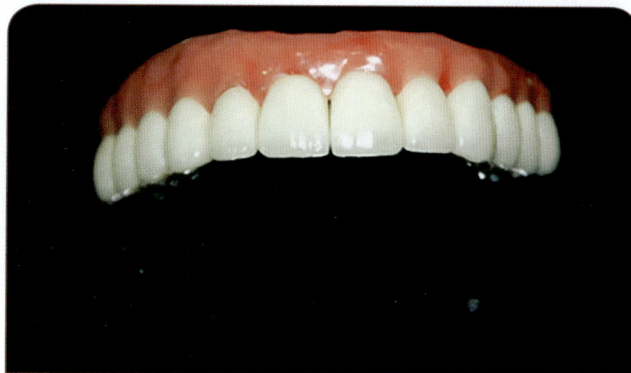

Fig. 5

The Malo Bridge facial view **(Fig. 5)**.

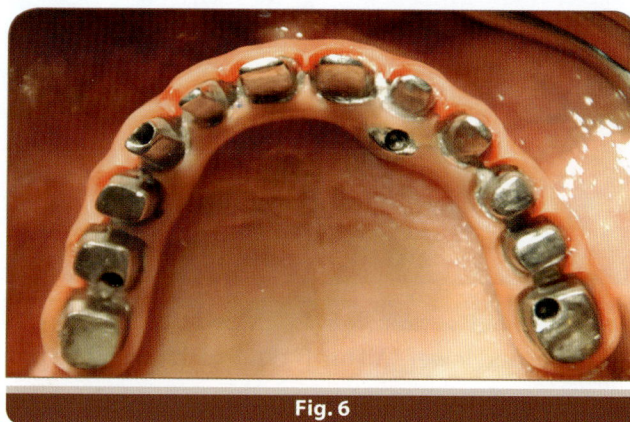

Fig. 6

The maxillary framework is torqued onto the MU abutments at 15 N cm **(Fig. 6)**.

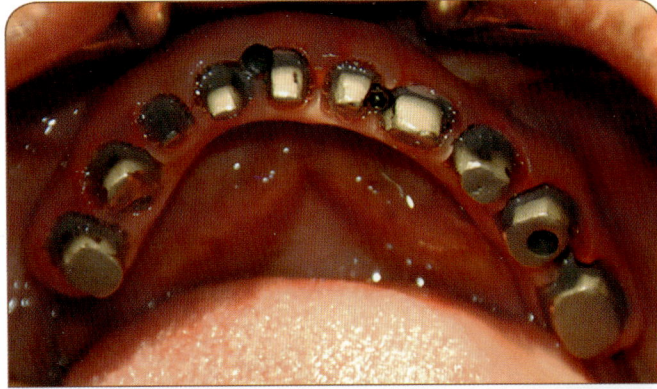

Fig. 7

The madibular framework is also torqued onto the MU abutments at 15 Ncm **(Fig. 7)**.

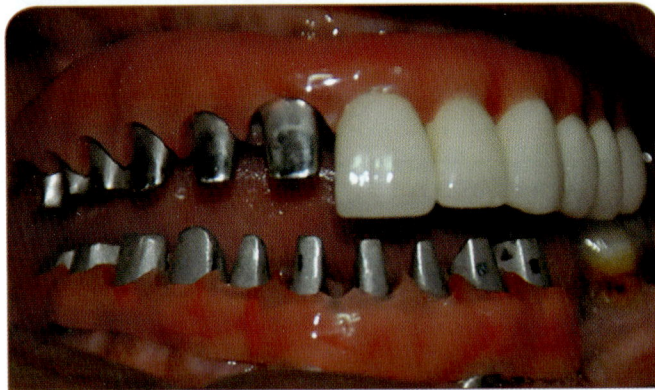

Fig. 8

Every zirconia crown is then cemented one crown at one time and the extra cement is cleaned before cementing the next crown **(Fig. 8)**.

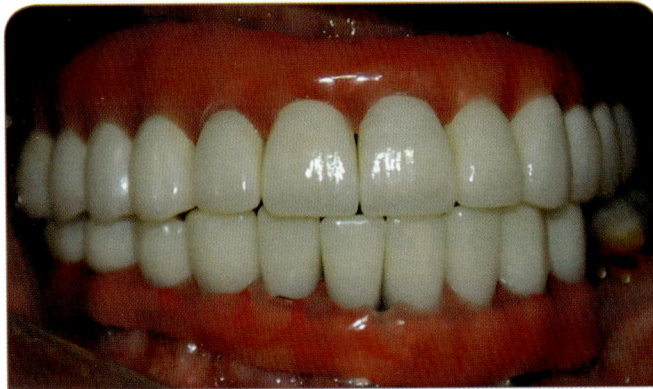

Fig. 9

Final image of the upper and lower "All on 4" done with Malo type prosthesis **(Fig. 9)**.

Amit Gulati

COMPLICATION MANAGEMENT OF IMMEDIATE EXTRACTION IMPLANT IN ESTHETIC ZONE

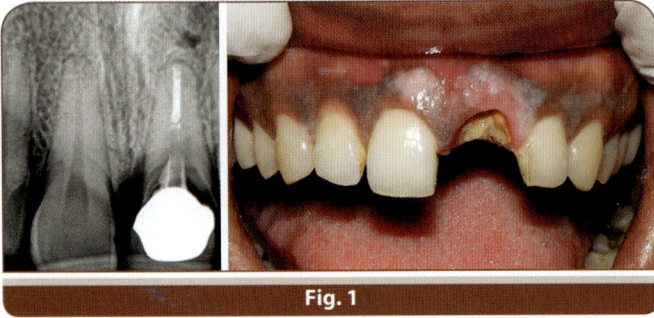

Fig. 1

Baseline: Post and Core treated tooth #21. Fractured for over 8 months resulting in some loss of facial bone. Presence of diastema. Patient's non-acceptance for a removable provisional **(Fig. 1)**.

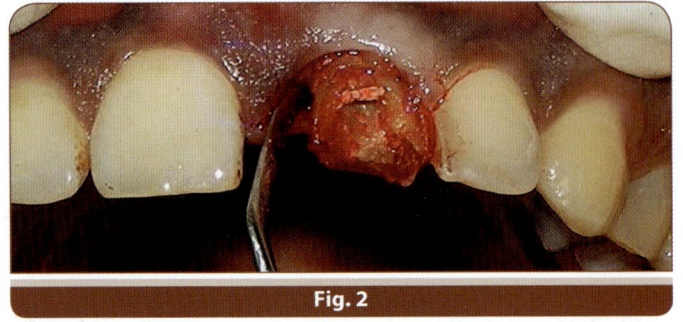

Fig. 2

Treated with extreme caution. Atraumatic extraction using periotomes **(Fig. 2)**.

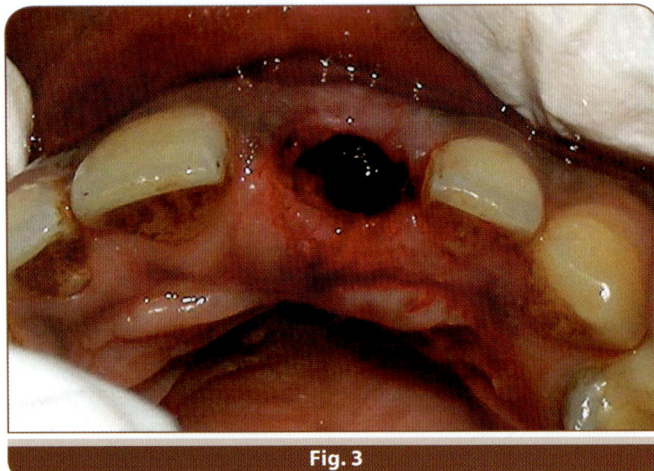

Fig. 3

Extraction socket **(Fig. 3)**.

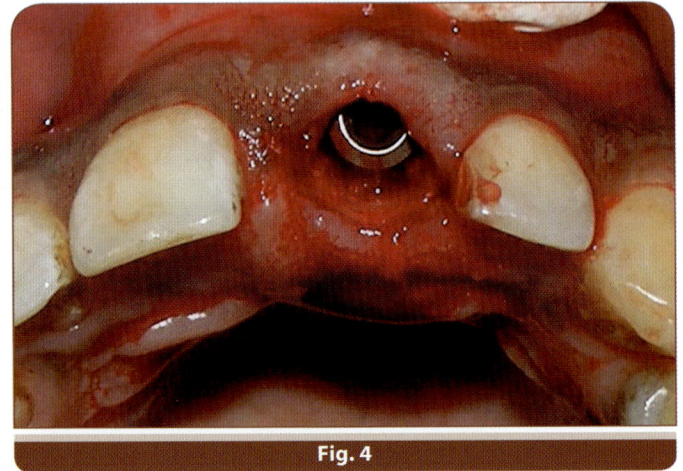

Fig. 4

Mistakes: Missing coronal part of facial bone, delayed protocol after augmentation should have been preferred. Implant pushed facially by dense palatal bone while insertion. Smaller implant diameter should have been used **(Fig. 4)**.

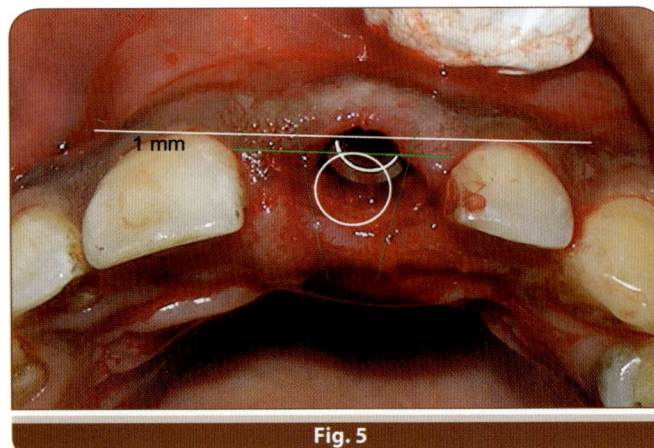

Fig. 5

Missed ideal 3D implant position in immediate extraction situations. Large diameter implant pressing on delicate and deficient facial socket wall **(Fig. 5)**.

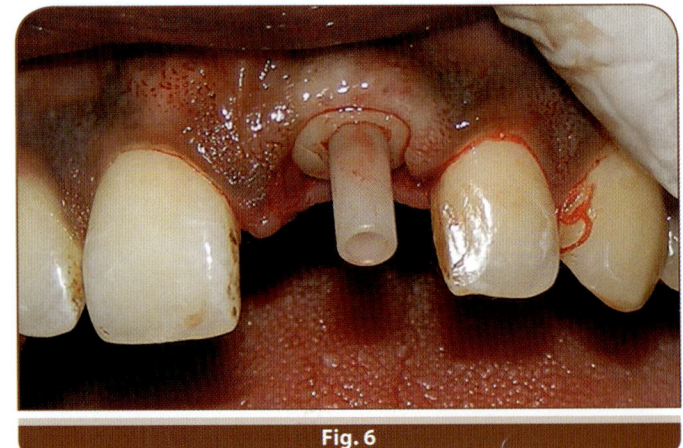

Fig. 6

Composite lined on temporary abutment cylinder to support soft tissue **(Fig. 6)**.

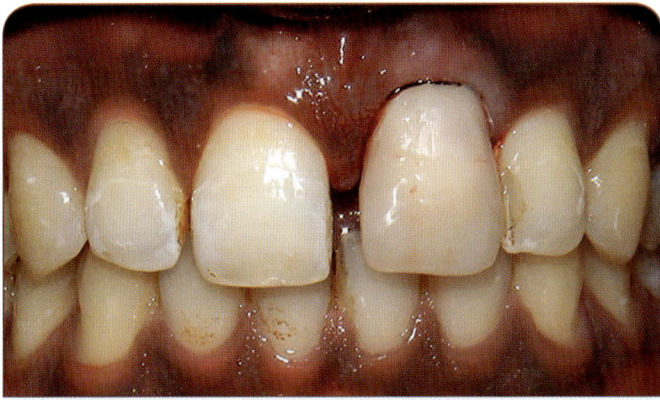

Provisional crown in place (**Fig. 7**).

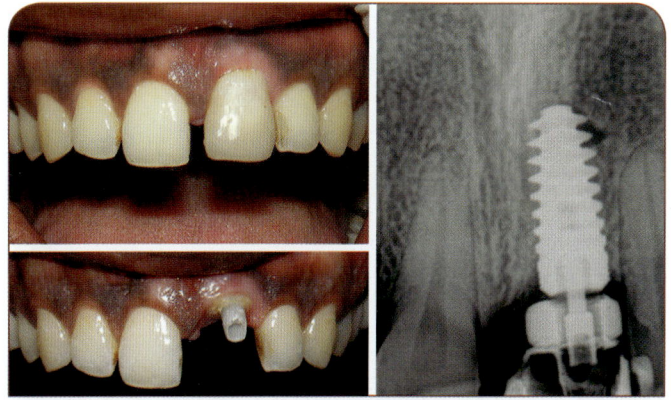

Clinical situation at 4 months (**Fig. 8**).

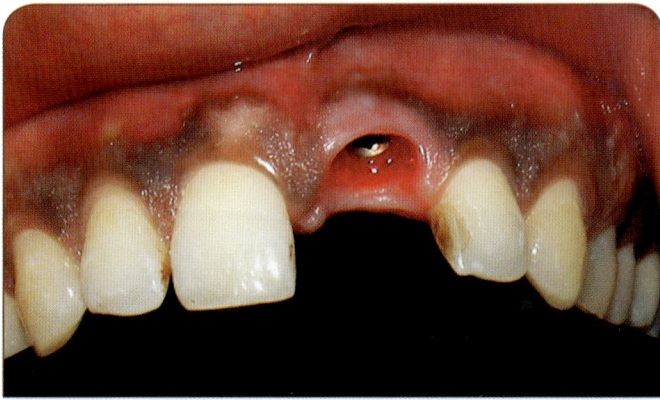

Clinical situation at 4 months (**Fig. 9**).

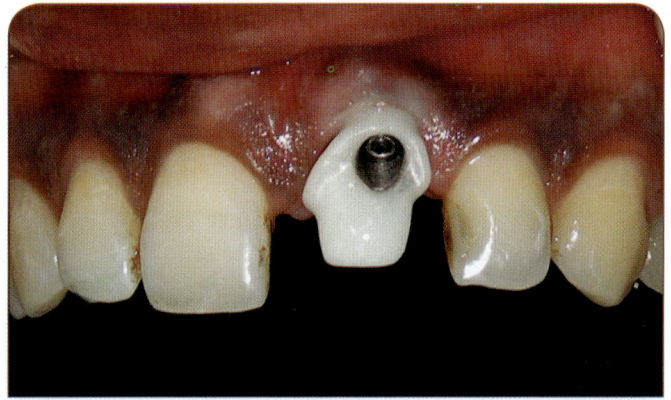

Custom hybrid abutment. E-Max pressed on stock abutment (**Fig. 10**).

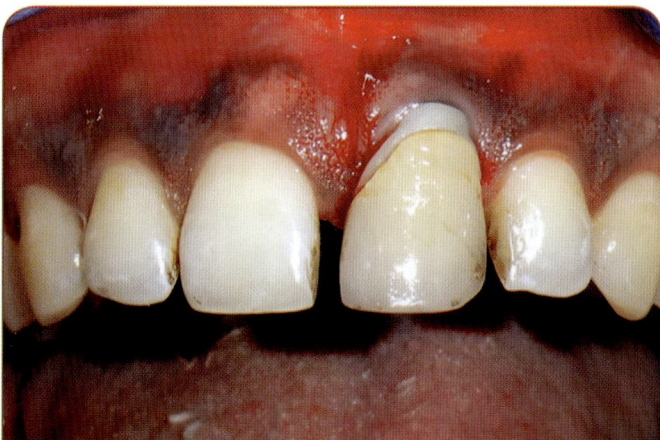

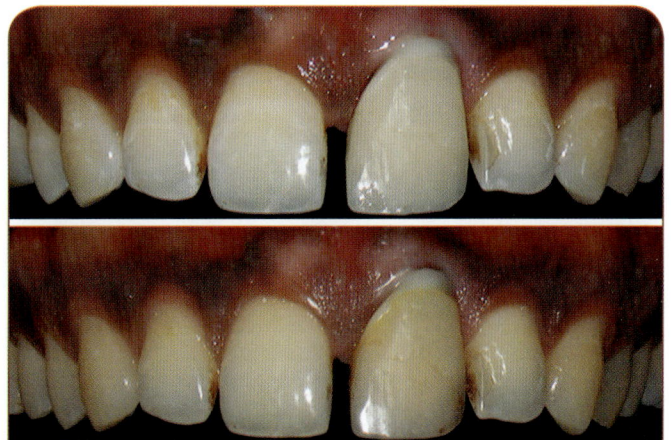

Connective tissue graft with coronally advanced flap did not work (**Figs. 11 and 12**).

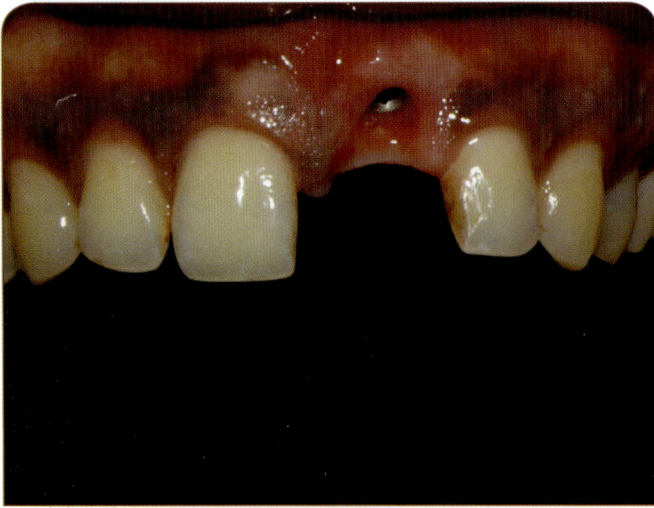

Fig. 13

New custom made abutments will be fabricated **(Fig. 13)**.

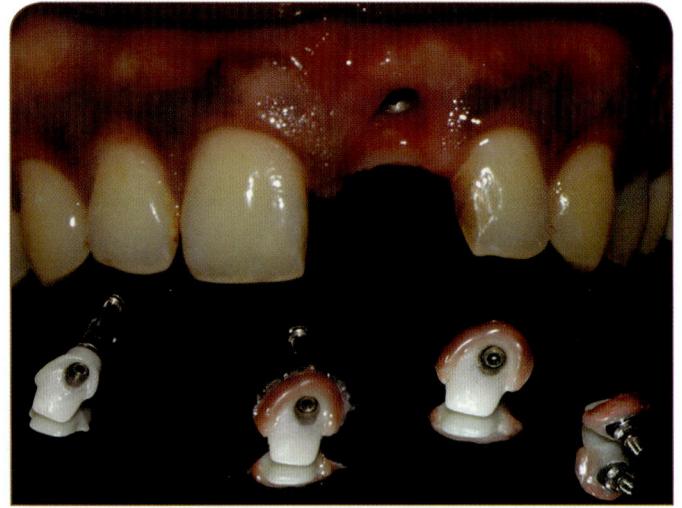

Fig. 14

E-Max abutment collar prepared with HF etch and silane for direct layering with pink composites. Layered intra-orally and characterized to match with pigmented gum tissue. Finished and polished **(Fig. 14)**.

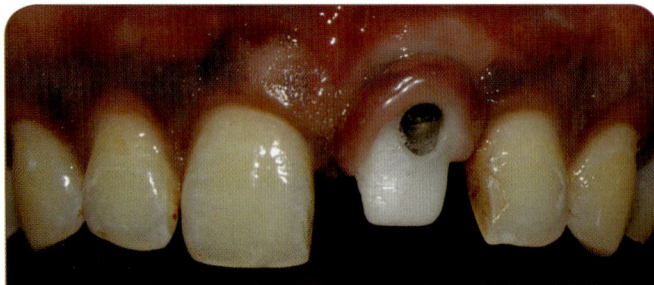

Fig. 15

Abutment placed **(Fig. 15)**.

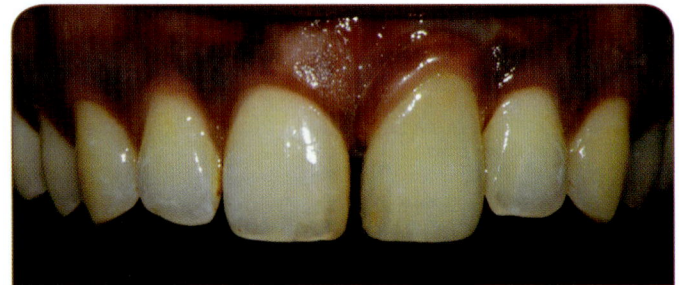

Fig. 16

Abutment level impression for an E-Max crown **(Fig. 16)**.

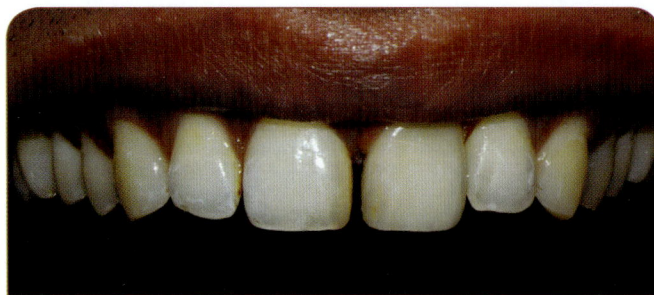

Fig. 17

Smile view **(Fig. 17)**.

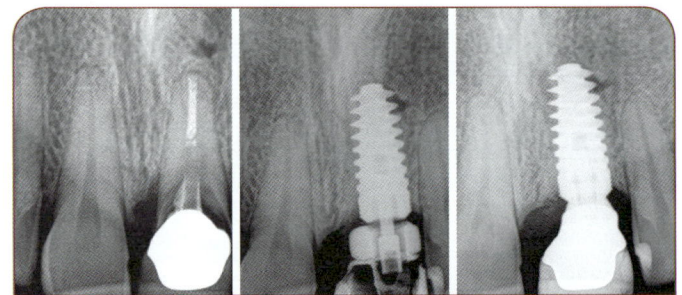

Fig. 18

Baseline, 4 months postsurgery, 6 months post-restoration **(Fig. 18)**.

CASE STUDY 102

Sujit Bopardikar

Full Mouth Rehabilitation with Fixed Implant Solution in a Failing Dentition

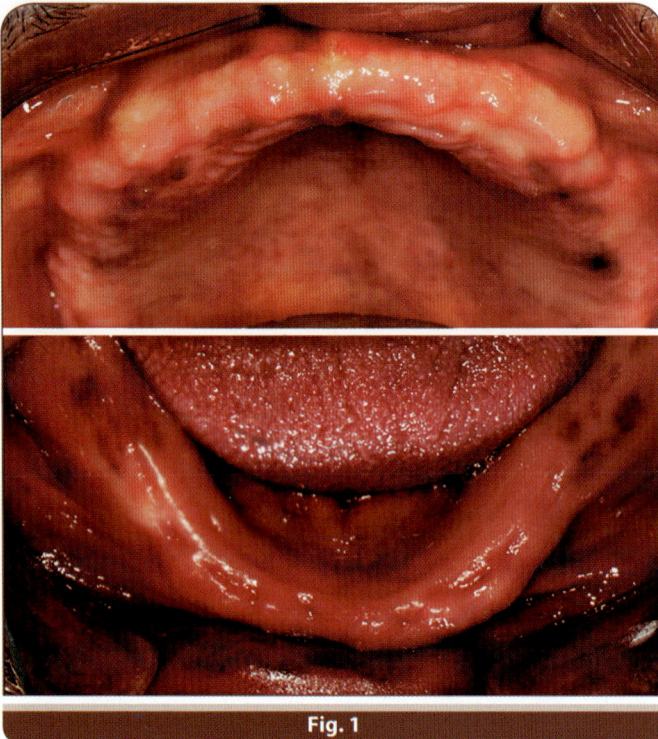

Fig. 1

A patient with 12 weeks post extraction. A well healed maxillary as well as mandibular ridges luckily a well rounded ridge with adequate bone to give a fixed solution as the patient wished. 12 weeks post extraction maxillary and mandibular arch **(Fig. 1)**.

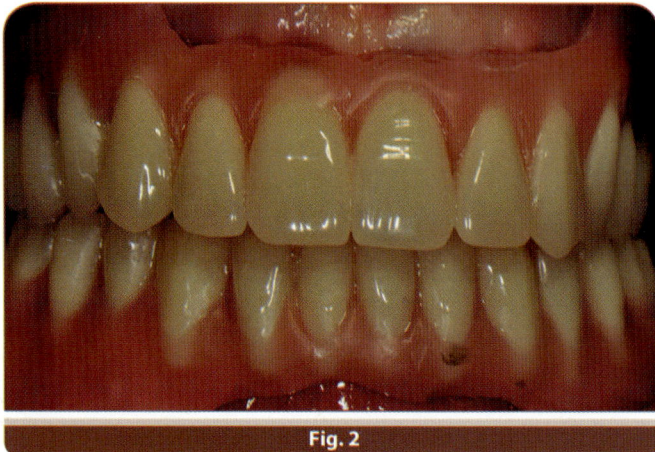

Fig. 2

A complete denture was fabricated to get a fair idea of the ridge relation, the vertical space available to fabricate the prosthesis. The occlusion that can be achieved, the esthetics, phonetics and finally to determine the implant positions. Wax up of the trial denture checked for occlusion esthetics and vertical dimension **(Fig. 2)**.

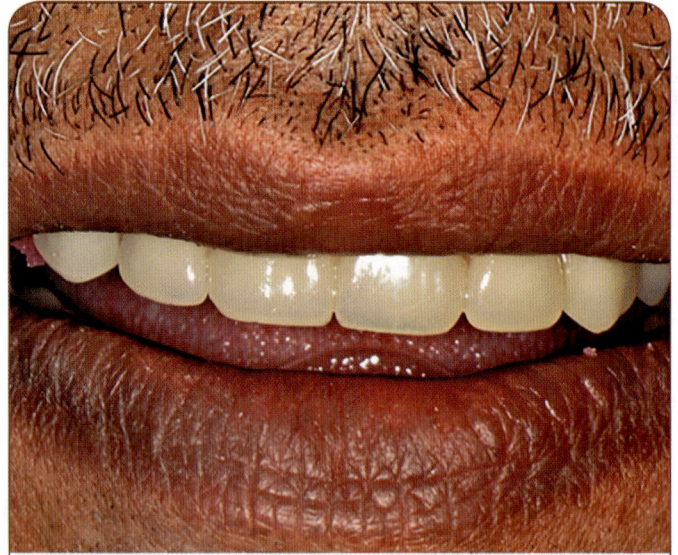

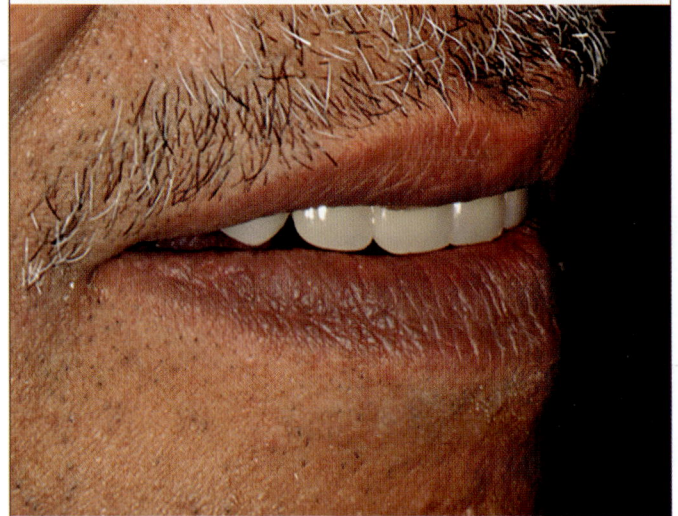

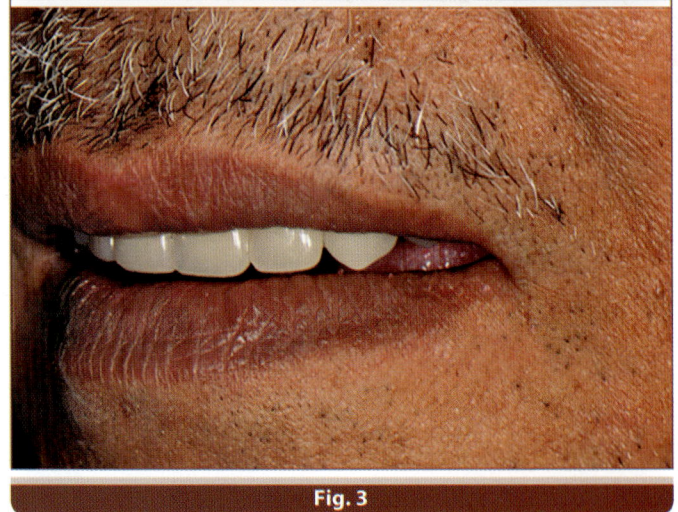

Fig. 3

Esthetics phonetics and Lip support of the trial denture checked **(Fig. 3)**.

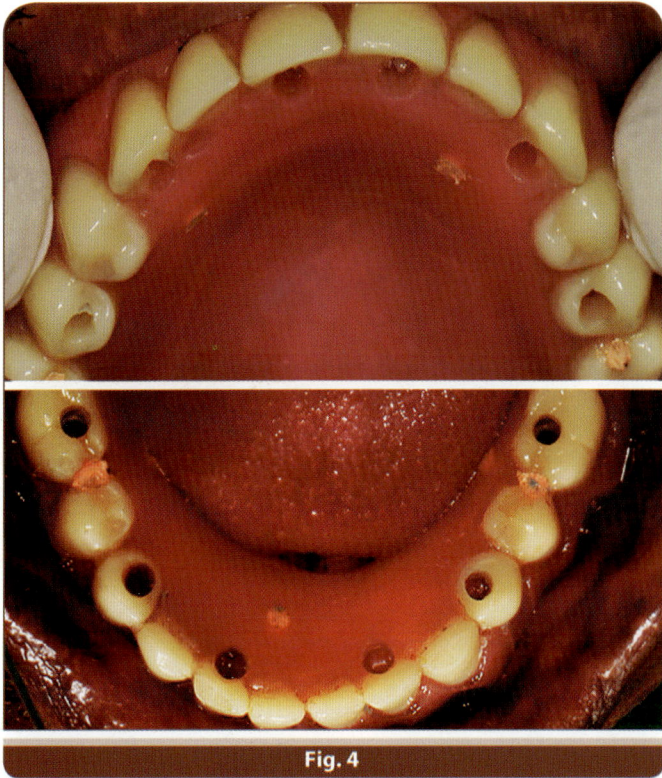
Fig. 4

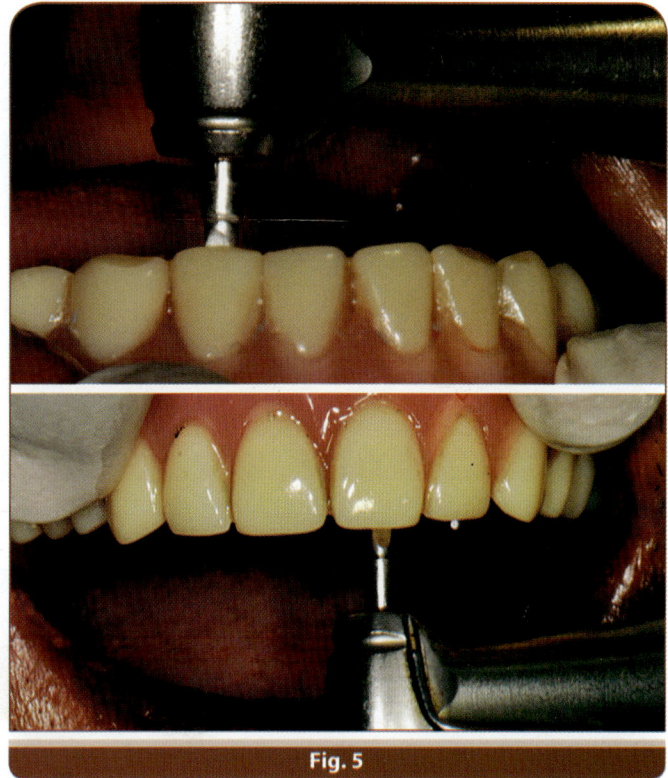
Fig. 5

Guiding holes 2 mm in diameter were made in the denture in the positions of the implants that were to be placed so that the implants could be placed in the best prosthodontically suitable position. Maxillary and mandibular denture in place with holes to serve as surgical guide **(Fig. 4)**.

With the dentures firmly in place the initial drill was used to make the osteotomy through the guiding holes made in the denture to make sure that the position of the implants are as planned to get the best prosthetic result. Osteotomy performed through the surgical guide **(Fig. 5)**.

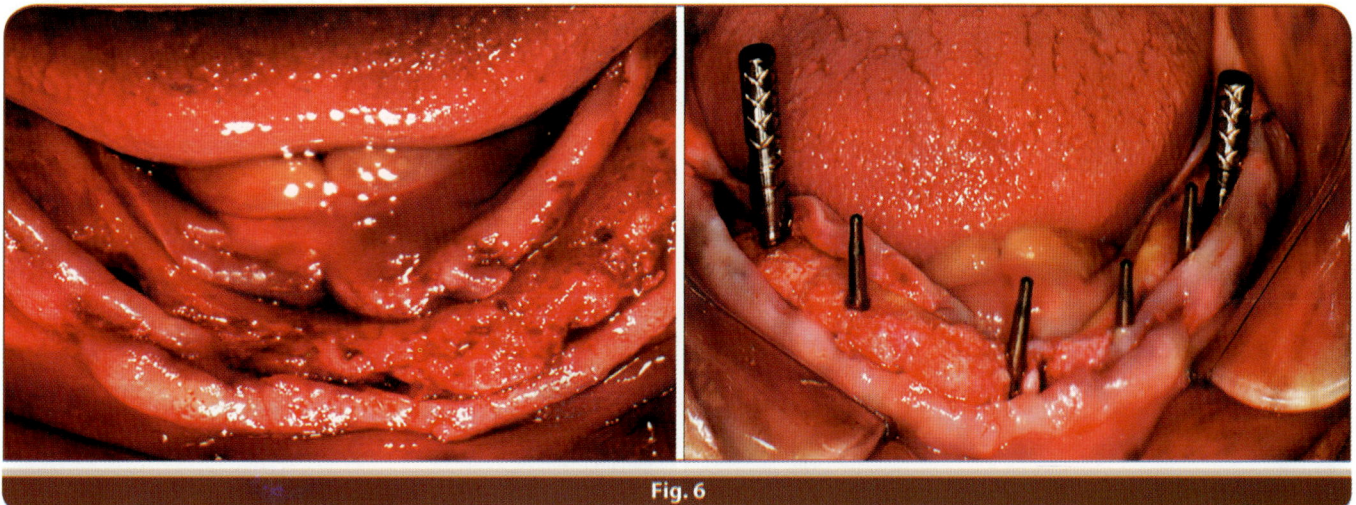
Fig. 6

Alloderm is placed on the operative site and fixed with soft tissue screws, a three point fixation is preferrably desired for graft fixation. Mandibular ridge full thickness flap reflected osteotomies completed parallelism checked **(Fig. 6)**.

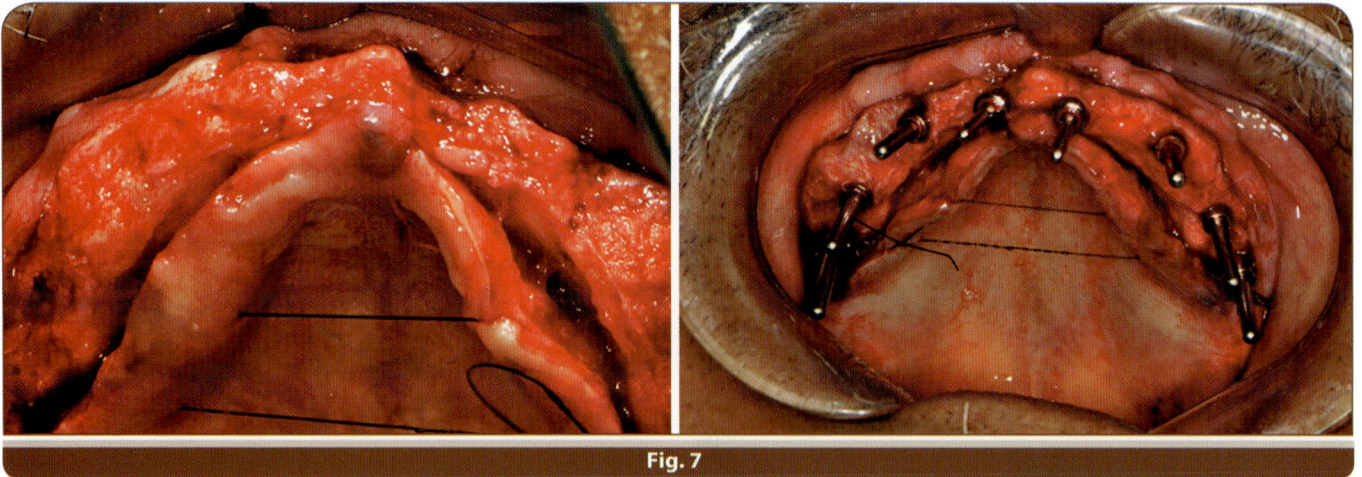

Maxillary full thickness flap reflected. Maxillary osteotomies completed with parallel pins (**Fig. 7**).

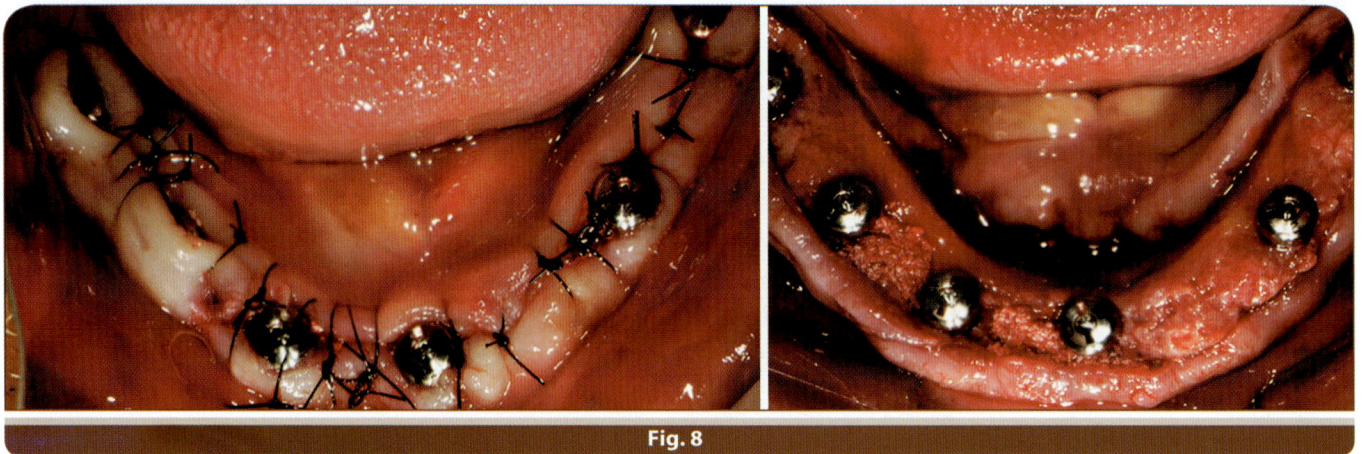

The insertion torque of the implants were between 25 Ncm to 30 Ncm hence it was decided not to load them immediately. Also this torque allowed to place transmucosal abutments in the first stage itself avoiding a second surgery to the patient. Mandibular implants with transmucosal attachment in place sutures given (**Fig. 8**).

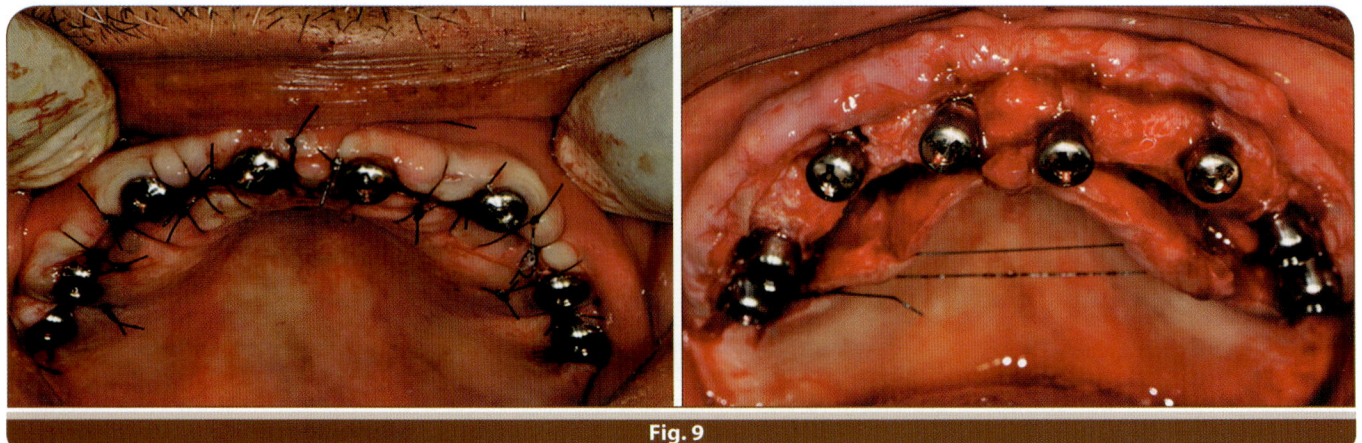

Maxillary implants with transmucosal abutments in place sutures given (**Fig. 9**).

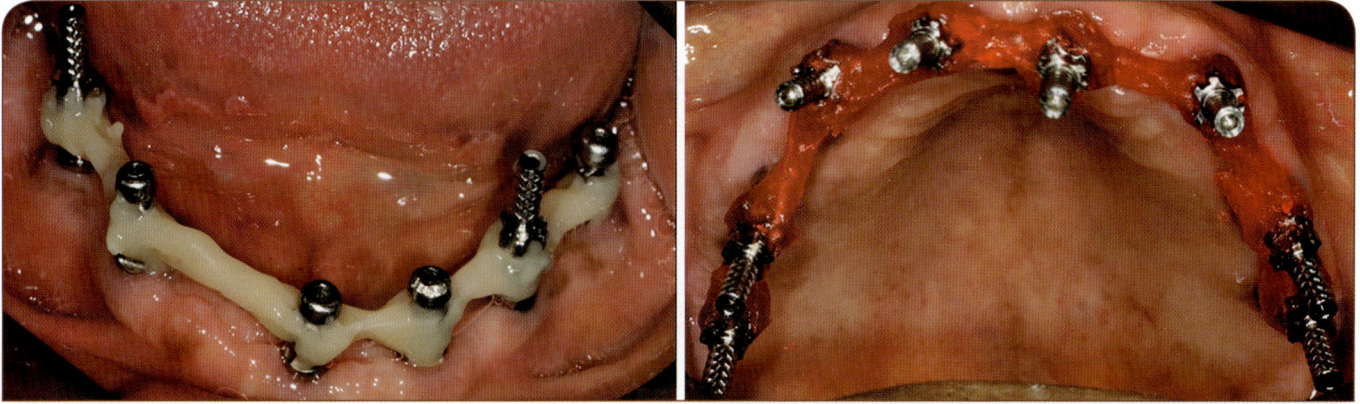

Fig. 10

16 weeks post surgery the prosthetic phase began with the impression procedures. Open tray impression with splinting of the impression posts to decrease any chances of distortion and to ensure passive fit of the prosthesis. Maxillary and mandibular implants with open tray impression posts splinted and ready for impression **(Fig. 10)**.

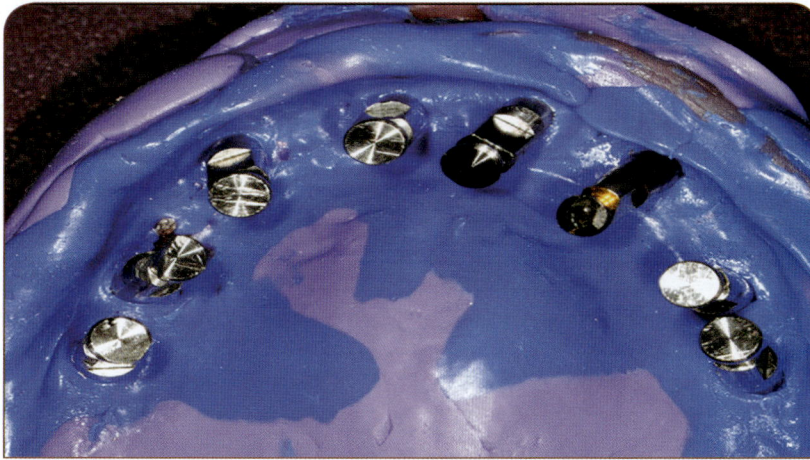

Fig. 11

Impression was poured and models prepared. Maxillary impression with Analogs in place **(Fig. 11)**.

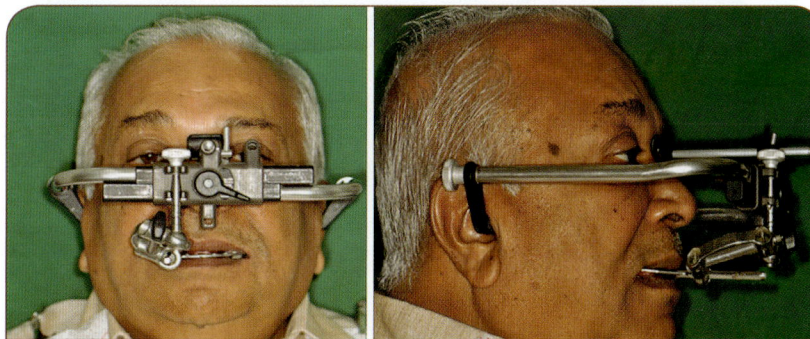

Fig. 12

Fresh jaw relation was made and a face bow record made to make sure that the framework would be best made keeping in mind the vertical and horizontal relation of the jaws. Face bow record for a perfect occlusion **(Fig. 12)**.

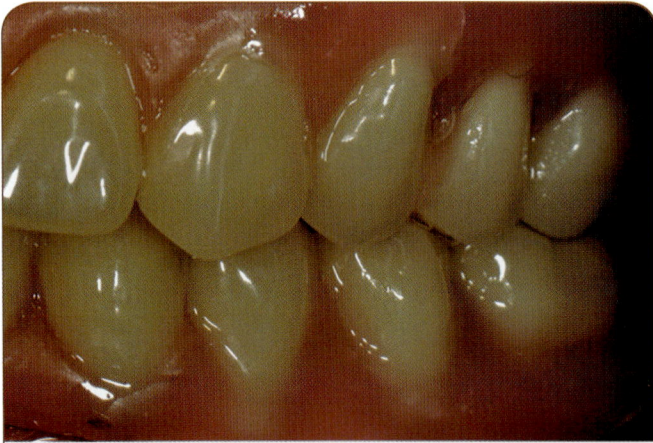

Fig. 14

Metal trial was carried out and the position of the teeth, the length of the teeth and the jaw relation were reverified. Emphasis on a passive fit of the castings. Maxillary and mandibular metal framework trial (**Fig. 14**).

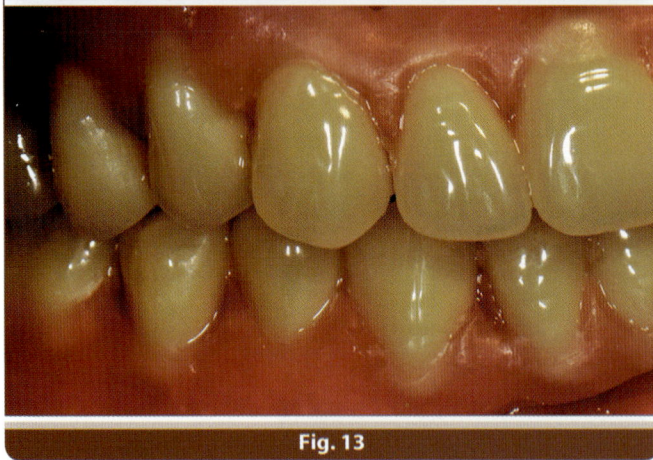

Fig. 13

Fig. 15

The setting trial was made and the jaw relation ascertained. A silicon index of the same was made to now help in the milling of the abutments and for the prosthesis. Patient desired a cement retained prosthesis without screw vents. Trial denture checked for occlusion vertical dimensions and esthetics (**Fig. 13**).

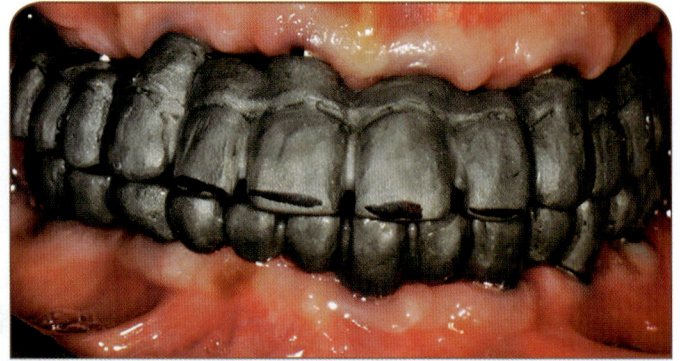

Final prosthesis made of Porcelain fused to metal with gingiva colored porcelain and separate bridges to avoid cross arch stresses and a self-cleansing design. The patient's age was taken into consideration while choosing the color and texture of teeth. Dentogenic additions like cracks and stains were incorporated. PFM prosthesis in occlusion (**Fig. 15**).

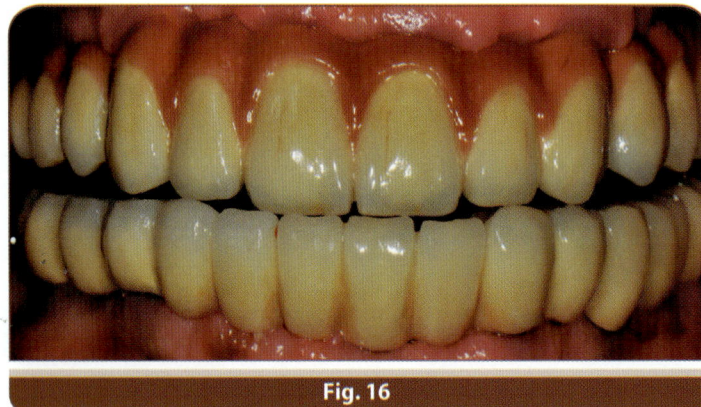

Fig. 16

Mutually protected occlusion was given during the protrusive movement of the mandible, where the posterior teeth were out of occlusion during the protrusive movement. Protrussive movement and posterior disocclusion (**Fig. 16**).

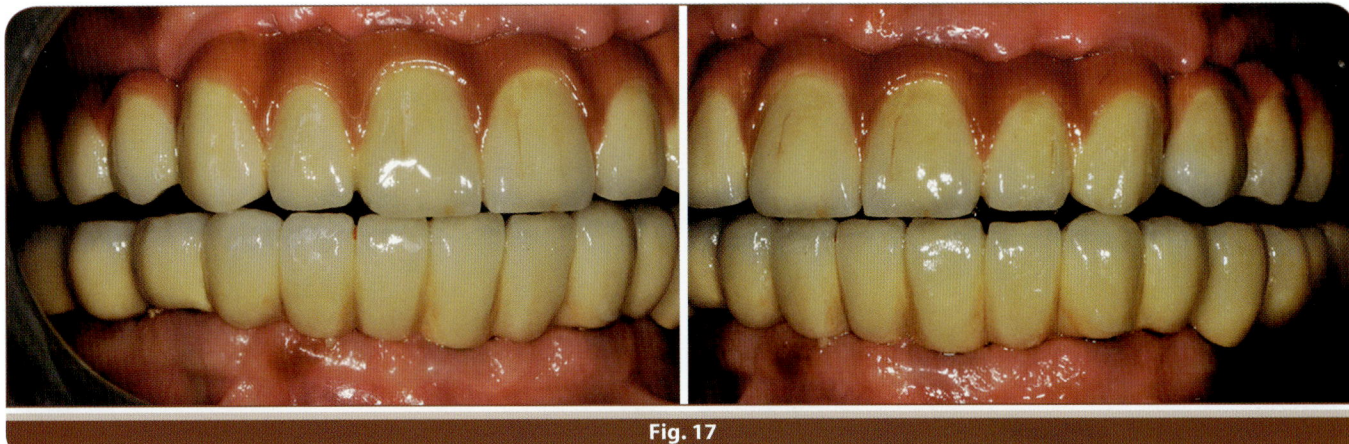

Fig. 17

Canine guided occlusion was planned during all lateral movements as the implants were splinted and any contact in the posterior teeth would result in unwanted interference. Canine guided occlusion on lateral movement **(Fig. 17)**.

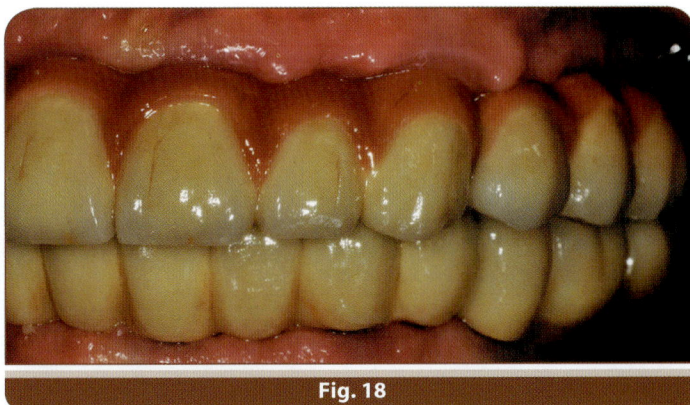

Fig. 18

Maximum intercuspation position and centric relation position were synchronized and a tripodal point contact between all maxillary and mandibular teeth were established. Lateral view in centric relation **(Fig. 18)**.

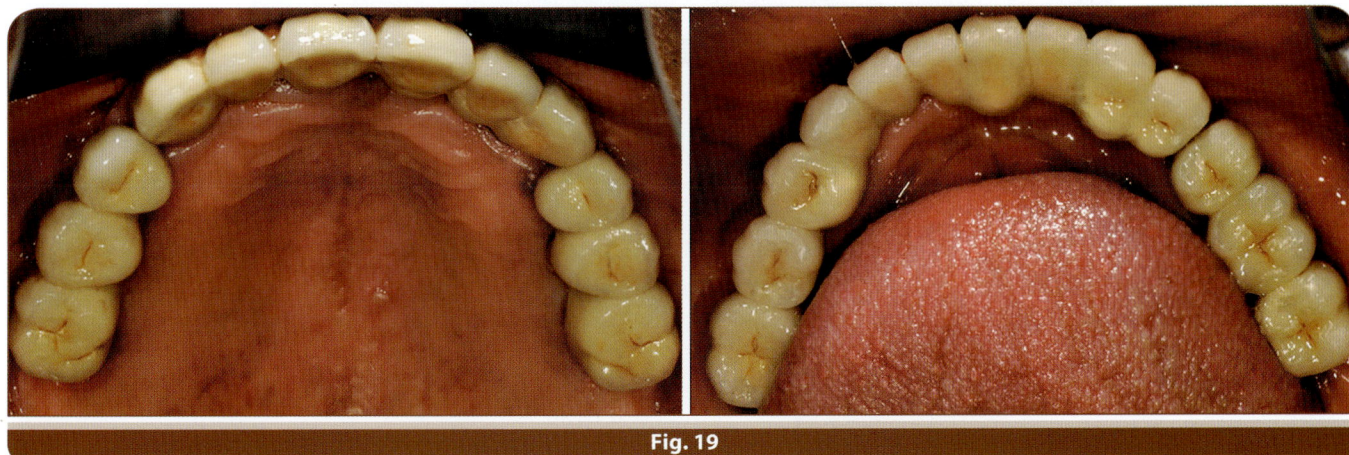

Fig. 19

Maxillary and mandibular occlusal view **(Fig. 19)**.

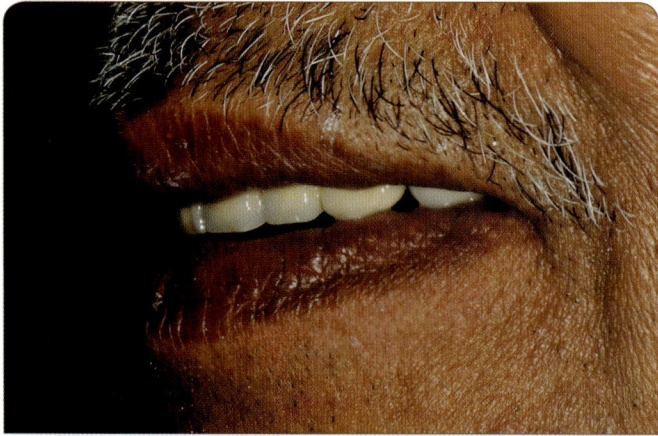

Fig. 20

Left profile **(Fig. 20)**.

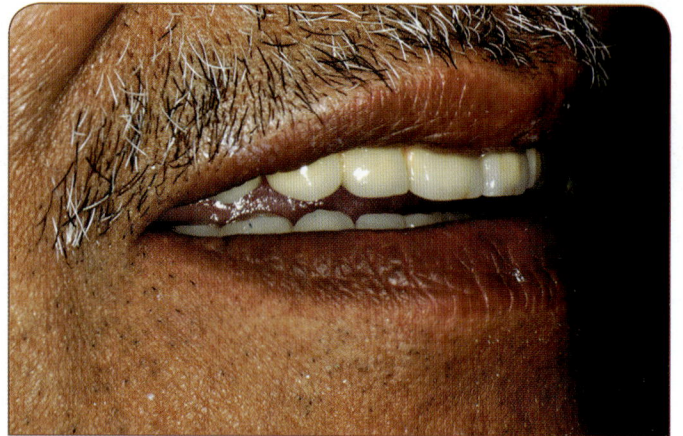

Fig. 21

Right profile view to check esthetics and vertical dimension **(Fig. 21)**.

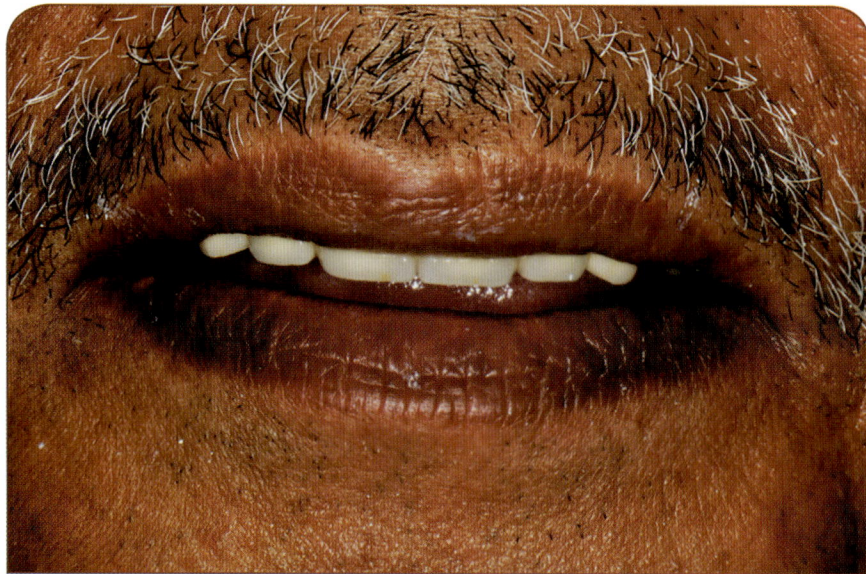

Fig. 22

Smile esthetic evaluation and lip support **(Fig. 22)**.

CASE STUDY 103

Mónica Restrepo

Computer-guided Surgery Case Series

CASE 1

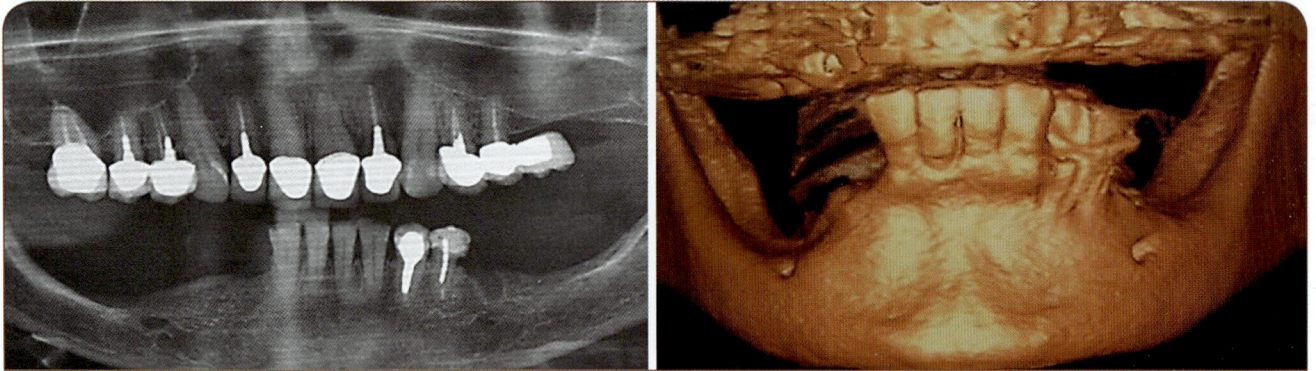

Fig. 1

Computer-guided implant surgery is a valuable treatment option in a partially edentulous patient. A panoramic visual model and a digital system are used as a diagnostic tool for surgical planning. The 3-D models data are carefully analyzed for bone topography and subjacent anatomical structures to allow favorable guided implant positioning. Presurgical visual models. Panoramic X-ray for general evaluation. CBCT volumetric data for guided surgery **(Fig. 1)**.

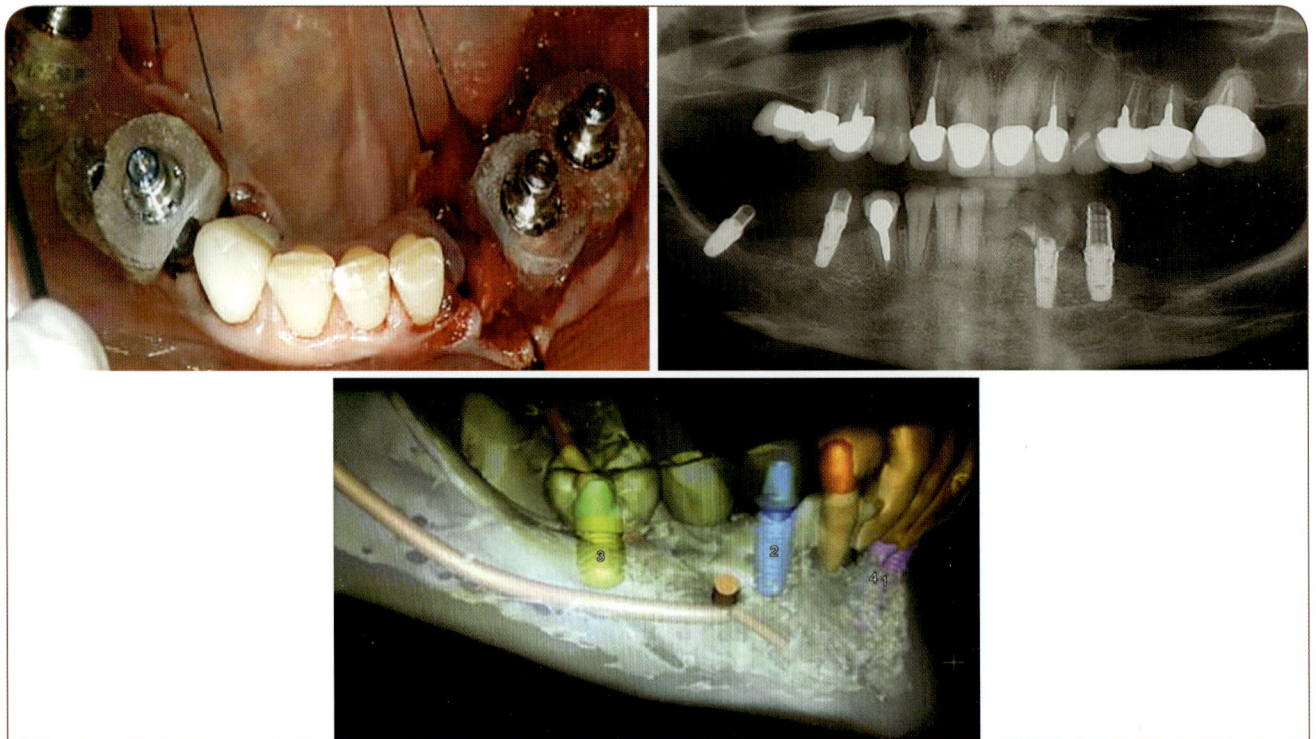

Fig. 2

A stereo-lithographic template is fabricated on previous 3-D models analyses. The surgical guide is stabilized and, the full thickness flap secure by means of sliding sutures. Virtual dental implant planning let on a prosthetically driven approach, resulting in a well designed prosthesis, better esthetics and optimizing the immediate loading procedure. Surgical procedure. Stereo lithographic surgical guide is stabilized to allow implant placement. Panoramic X-ray of 4 immediate loading implants inserted in the edentulous mandible. Dental implant and restoratively driven digital planning is assessed before treatment **(Fig. 2)**.

CASE 2

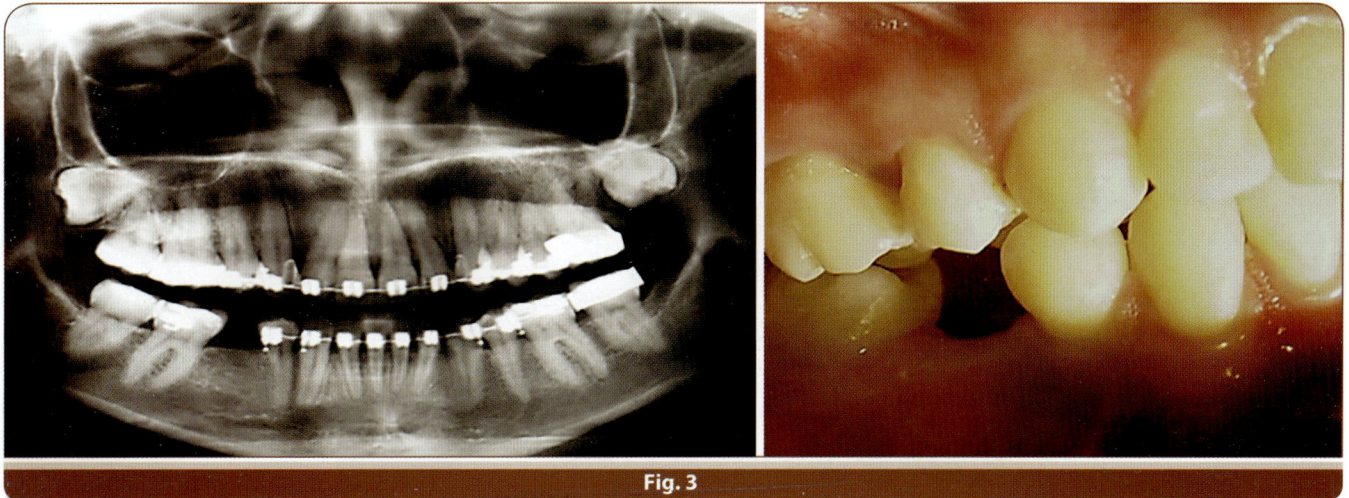

Fig. 3

"Flapless simplified approach" for implant placement. A partially edentulous patient is clinically evaluated for a single-tooth placement in post extraction site. Prior implant surgical procedure, bone quality and quantity as well as tissue width and high are evaluated. Presurgical radiographic 2-D evaluation of patient's edentulous area. Intraoral soft and hard tissue relationships for guided surgery. Intraoral soft and hard tissue relationships for guided surgery **(Fig. 3)**.

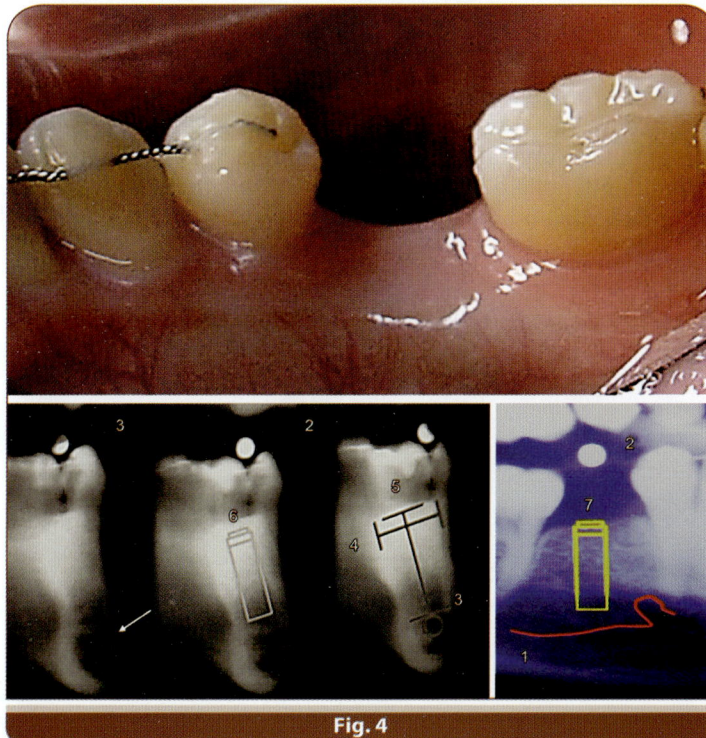

Fig. 4

A fully healed socket is observed. The 3D guidance is a driving factor during implant treatment. An adequate knowledge of hard and soft tissues are obtained from visual models to meet the biologic and functional goals. Initial clinical intraoral view of gingival soft tissue appearance is imperative for surgical decision making. 3-D volumetric tissue measurements and anatomical consideration are considered for implant selection. Hard tissue virtual volumetric data is analyzed previous implant placement **(Fig. 4)**.

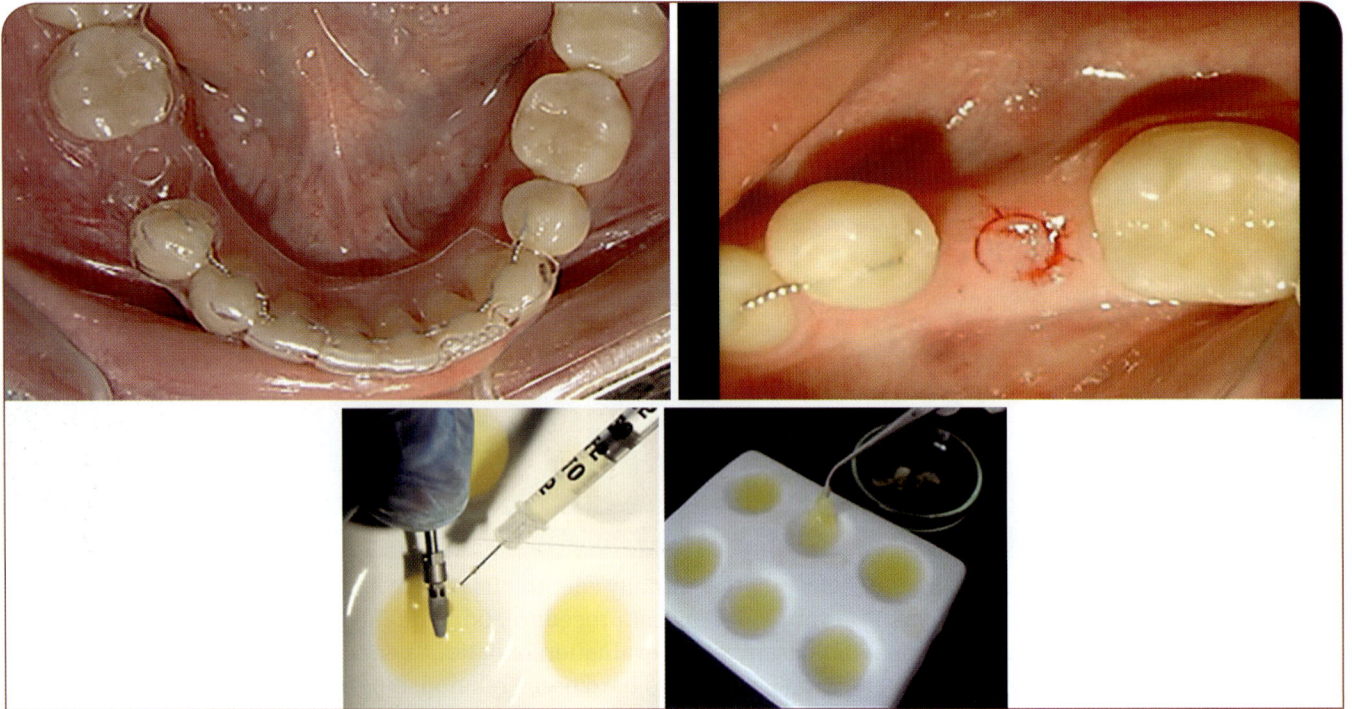

Fig. 5

A rigid, clear surgical template (1.0 mm) is fabricated over the duplicated cast using a vacuum former device. The alveolar crest is exposed by a punch—"flapless simplified approach"—to reduce post-surgical discomfort and to good will the time required for implant placement and immediate loading. A hydrogel-release growth factors is incorporated to the implant surface providing a pore network to support cell attachment, migration and tissue formation when simultaneous bone augmentation is not intended. Surgical procedure. Customized surgical template is designed to ensure transfer precision of the implant to the operative field. Flapless surgery through a connective punch technique is performed. Implant surface is embedded with fibrin and growth factors before implant insertion. Cell based kit, fibrin and growth factors hydrogels are used to improve tissue healing **(Fig. 5)**.

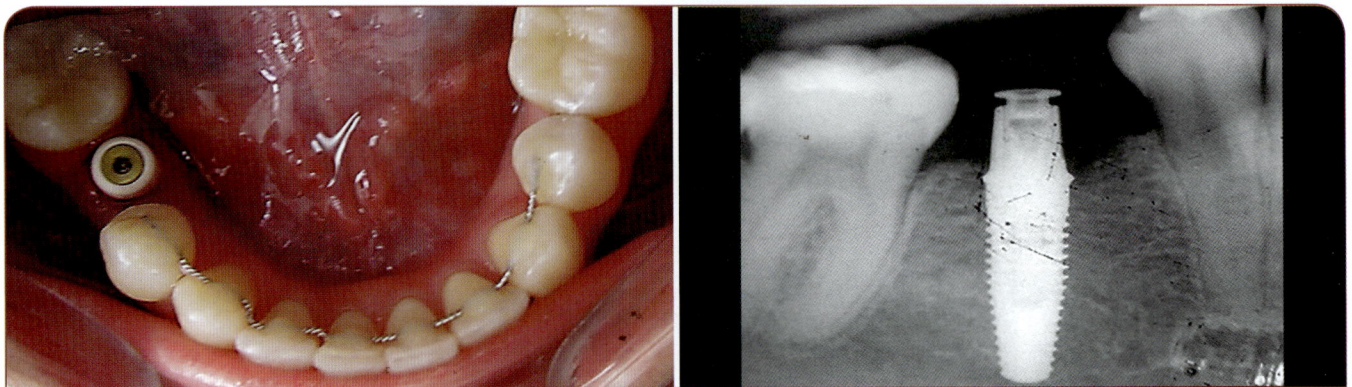

Fig. 6

The one-stage surgical procedure helps to maintain the integrity of the peri-implant soft tissues and successfully replace single posterior molars. The single implant (4.3 × 13 mm) is functionally loaded immediately after placement. One-stage surgical procedure. Uneventful peri-implant tissue healing is observed after immediate implant. Postsurgical radiographic evaluation determines vertical bone gain and stable bone levels in a single dental implant using the punch approach **(Fig. 6)**.

CASE 3

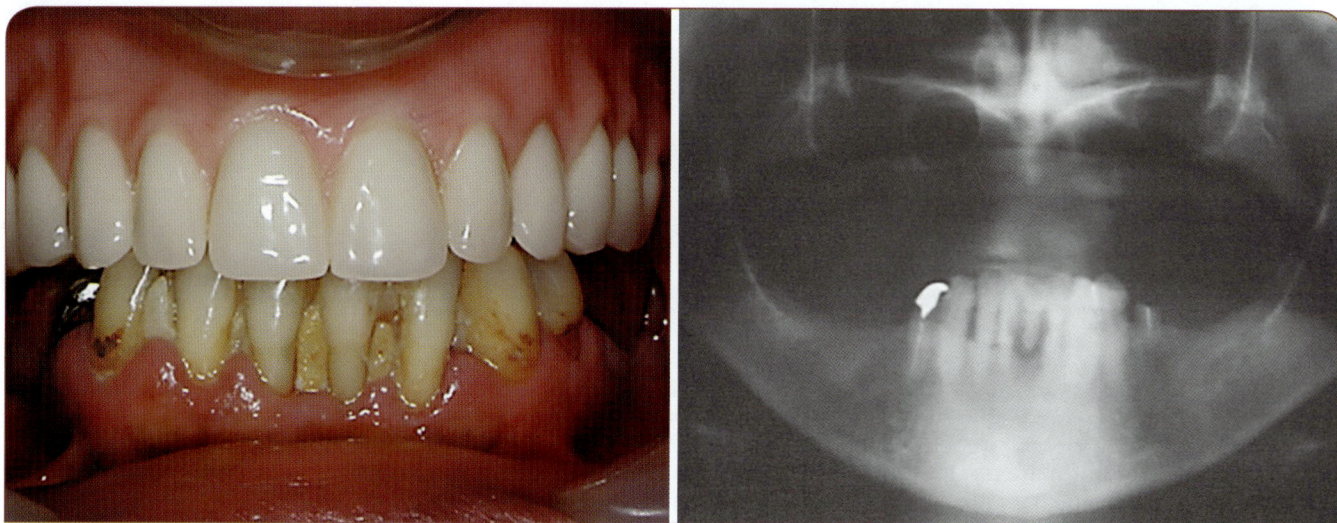

Fig. 7

Growth factor delivery-based tissue engineering for immediate implant placement and loading. Preoperatively visual models shown a partially edentulous patient with chronic periodontal disease. Clinical parameters as supragingival calculus, clinical attachment loss >3, bone loss and missing teeth can be evidentiated. Presurgical general overview of the clinical case. Generalized gingival inflammation can be seen; the chief complaint was "missing teeth". At initial radiographic evaluation, moderate to severe periodontitis, caries, missing teeth and severely deficient maxilla are evident (**Fig. 7**).

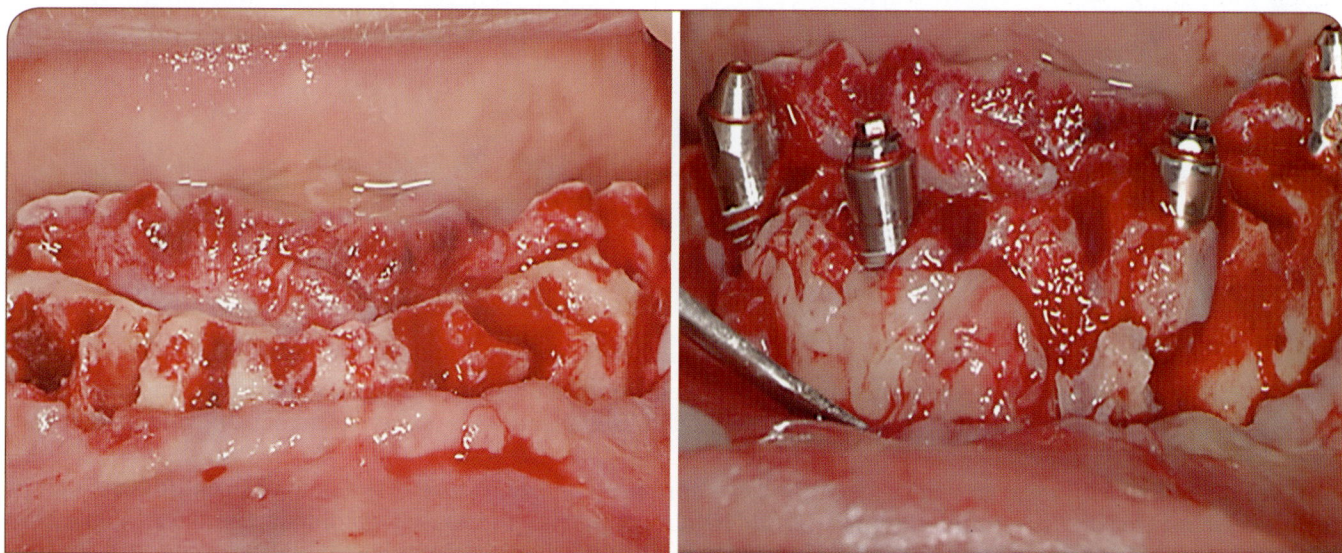

Fig. 8

After tooth extraction, the patient is rehabilitated with a provisional fixed dental prosthesis and 4 implants (4.3 × 13 mm). Final abutments are attached to the implants achieving immediate function. Surgical procedure. Full thickness flap is reflected and tooth extraction performed. Residual mandibular ridge irregularities are corrected by means of osteotomy. Four mandibular dental implants are inserted and immediately loaded. Fibrin hydrogel growth factor models are placed over to fill up osseous defects and to predict surgical outcomes (**Fig. 8**).

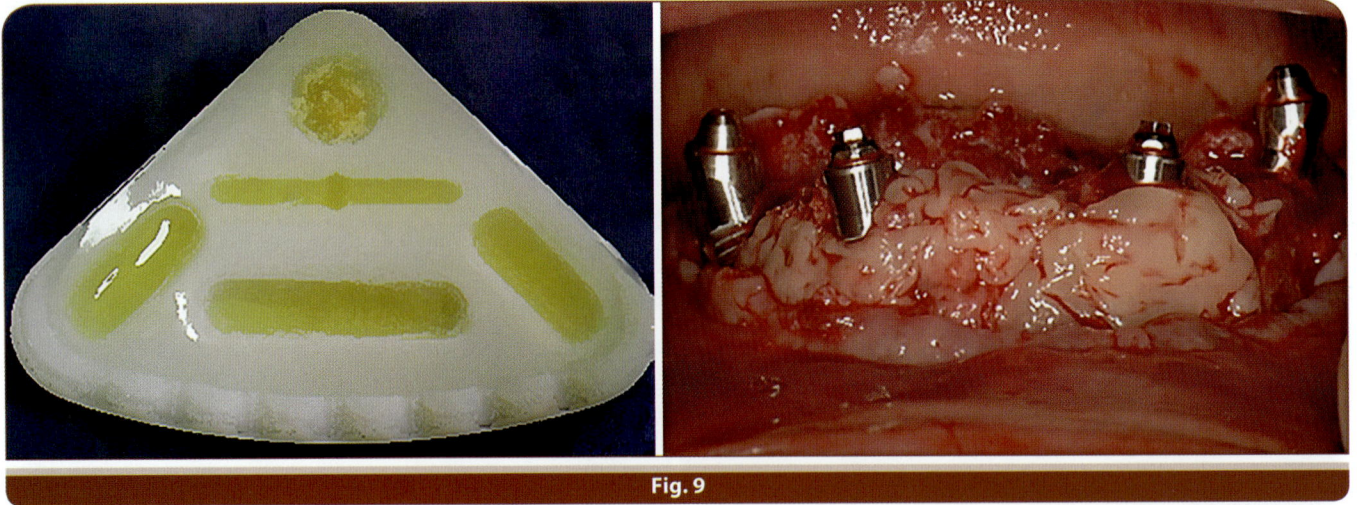

Fig. 9

Hydrogels based on fibrin are obtain from autologous blood and used to fill the appropriate spaces whenever bone volume is lacking. Clinically, DFDBA particles (1000 microns) as scaffolds retain greater concentrations of growth factors promoting bone regeneration at the implant sites The 3D structure allows fixation into the surgical site, and deliver growth factors during tissue healing. The regenerative medicine therapy kit composed of fibrin, growth factors and demineralized bone matrix are applied after implant placement. The hydrogels models are utilized to treat bony defects **(Fig. 9)**.

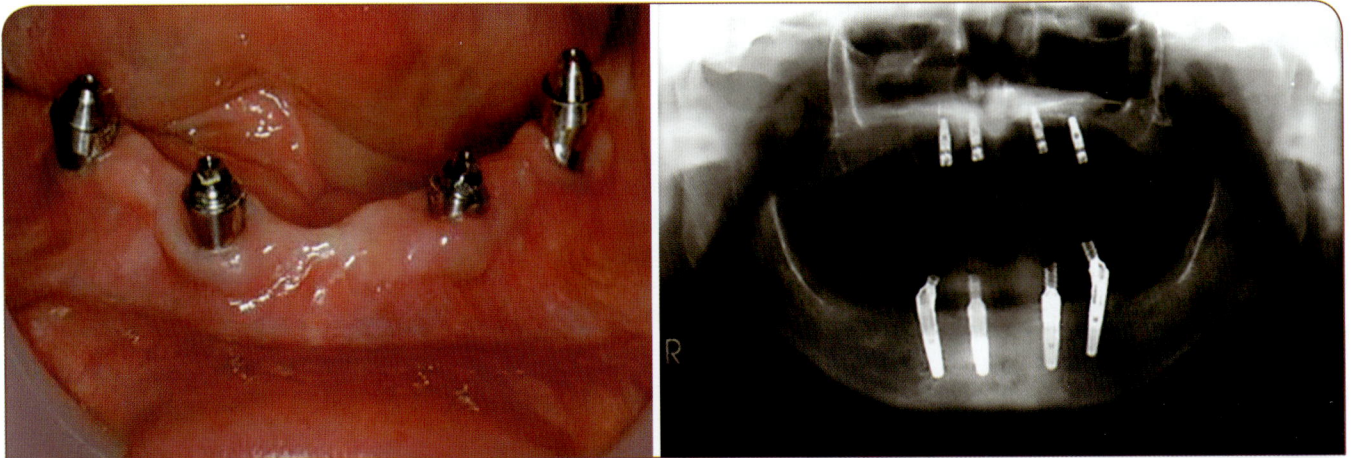

Fig. 10

Postsurgical healing after tooth extraction is uneventful. Delivery-based tissue engineering constructs improve soft tissue thickness (1–3 mm) and implants stability. Successful clinical integration is observed. No bone defects are detected by probing around all implants.

Wound healing. Fibrin and growth factors hydrogels improve color and texture of the gingiva. As a physical barrier, hydrogels moisture soft tissues and minimize wound healing time. Panoramic radiographic image shows stable bone levels after implant placement and immediate loading **(Fig. 10)**.

David Morales Schwarz, Hilde Morales

Full Mouth rehabilitation with Autologous Dentin Graft Platelet Rich Plasma (PRP) and Calcium Sulfate

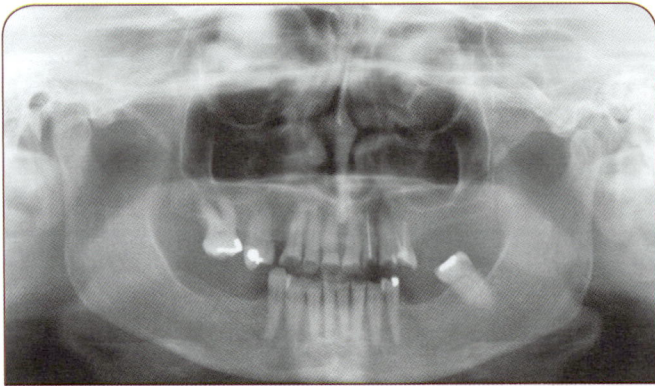

Fig. 1

A 72-year-old female patient. No relevant medical history. 6 maxillary implants and 6 mandibular implants were planned. Two short implants were planned **(Fig. 1)**.

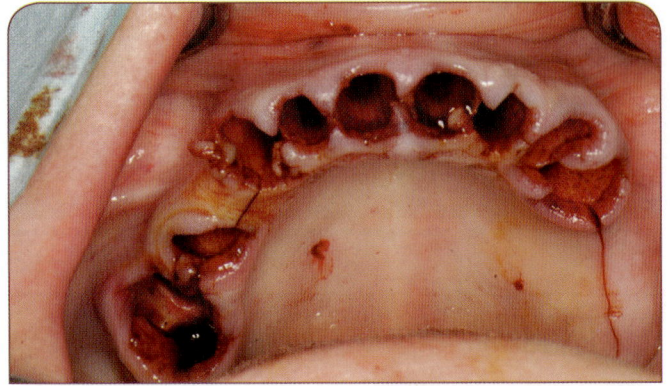

Fig. 2

Tooth extraction and crestal incision **(Fig. 2)**.

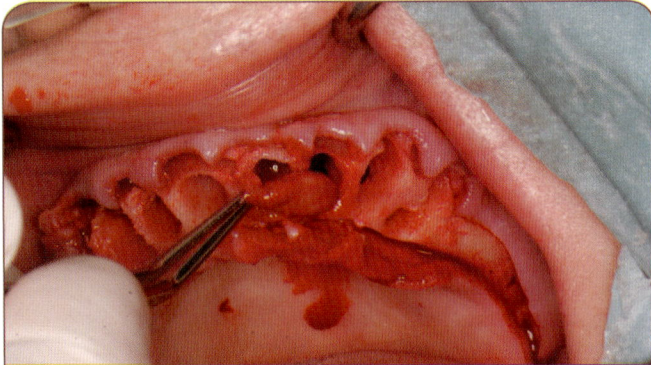

Fig. 3

Quistectomy 2.2, 2.3, 2.4 which was perforating nasal floor. Sinus communication **(Fig. 3)**.

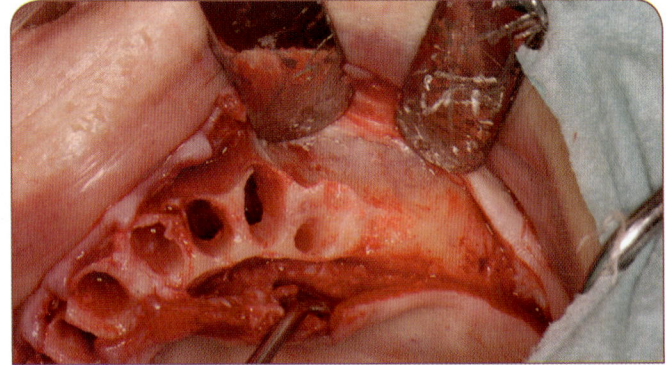

Fig. 4

Full thickness flap was elevated to expose the alveolar crest and the lateral wall of the maxillary sinus **(Fig. 4)**.

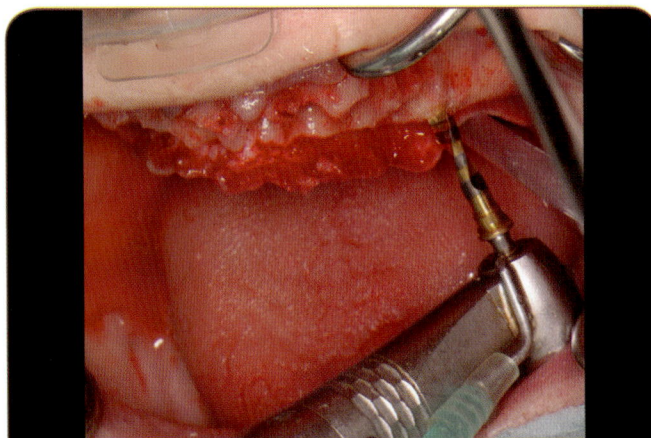

Fig. 5

Left side angulated implant drilling following the bioner top DM sequence **(Fig. 5)**.

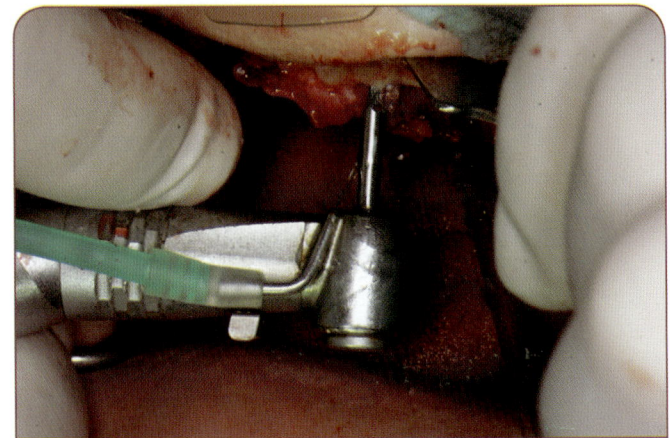

Fig. 6

2.1 drilling bioner top DM implant following bioner top DM sequence **(Fig. 6)**.

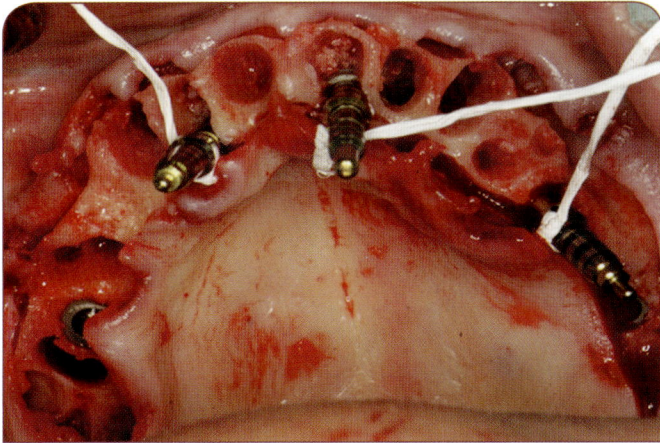
Fig. 7

One maxillary bioner top DM implants. Diameter 4 mm (**Fig. 7**).

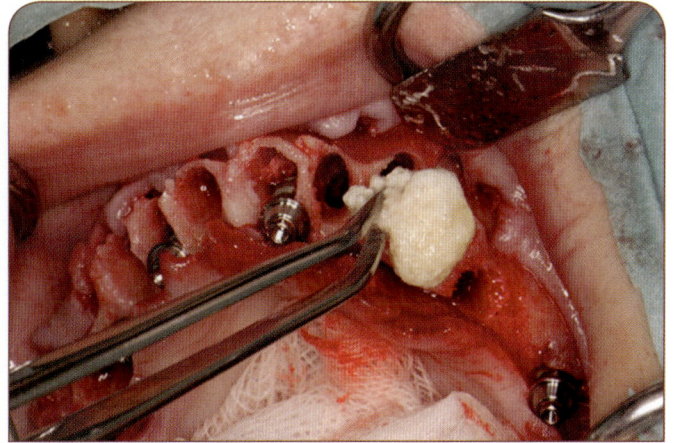
Fig. 8

Dental alveoli filled with autologous dentin graft (**Fig. 8**).

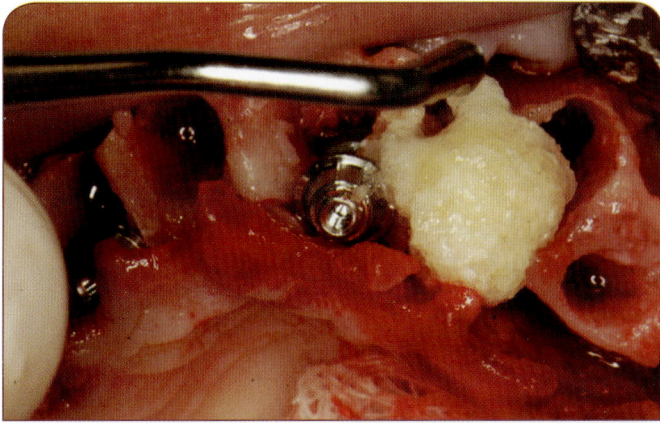
Fig. 9

Filled with autologous dentin graft + PRP + calcium sulfate (**Fig. 9**).

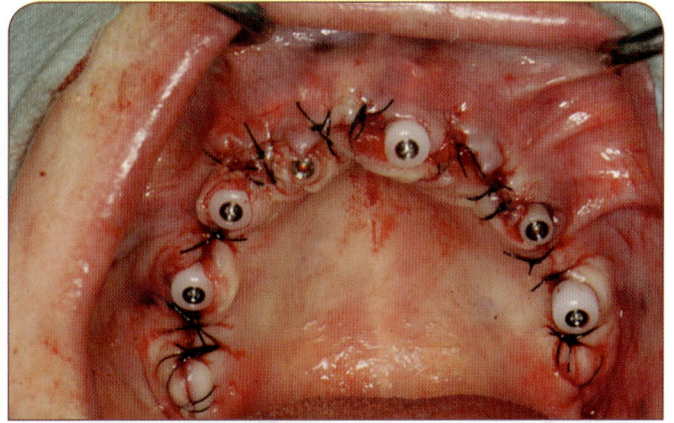
Fig. 10

6 maxillary dental implants bioner top DM (**Fig. 10**).

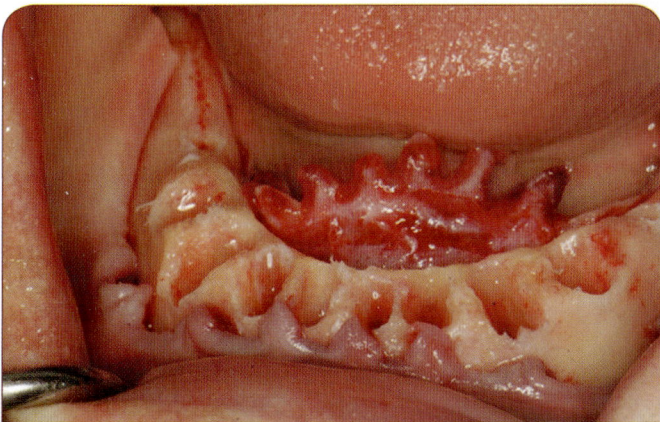
Fig. 11

Crestal mandibular incision (**Fig. 11**).

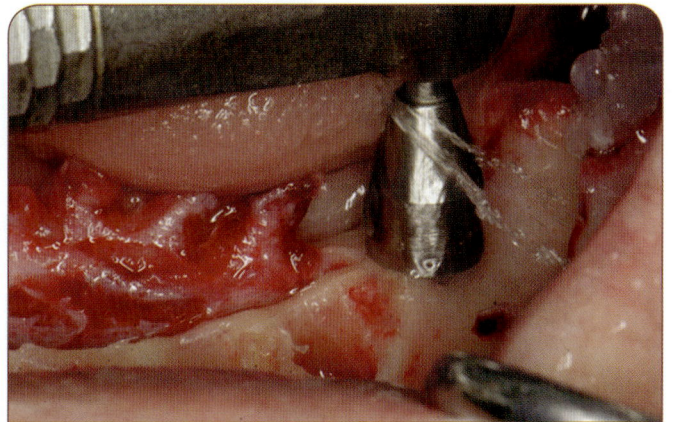
Fig. 12

Initial osteotomy with bioner FP. 1200 rpm (**Fig. 12**).

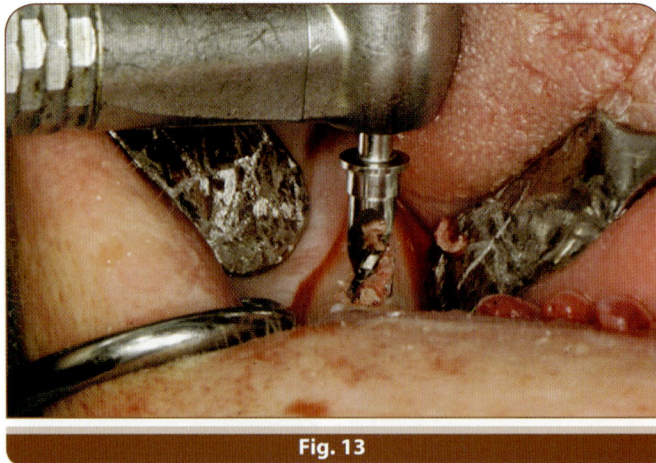

Drilling with FS 2 short DM bioner **(Fig. 13)**.

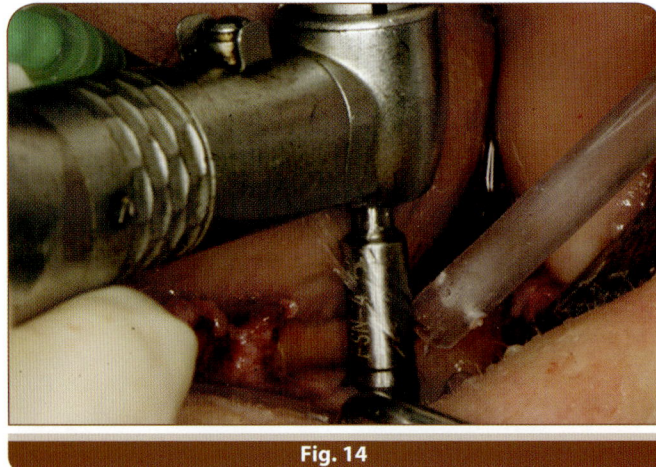

Secure milling system, composed of rotatory diamond bur that enable to work to the limit without damage important structures. 1200 rpm **(Fig. 14)**.

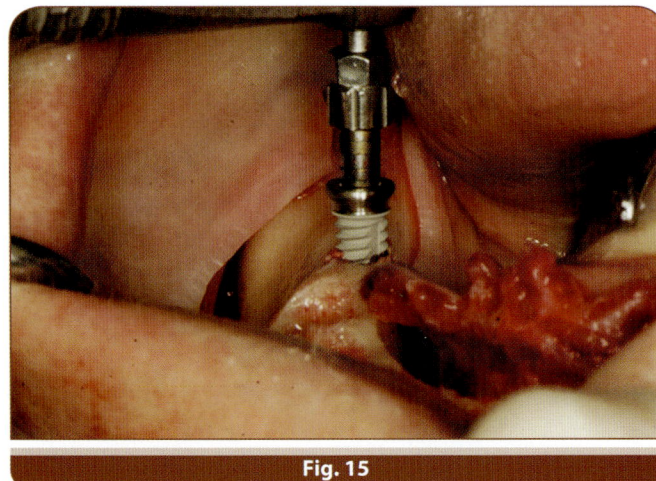

Placing short DM bioner 4 × 6 **(Fig. 15)**.

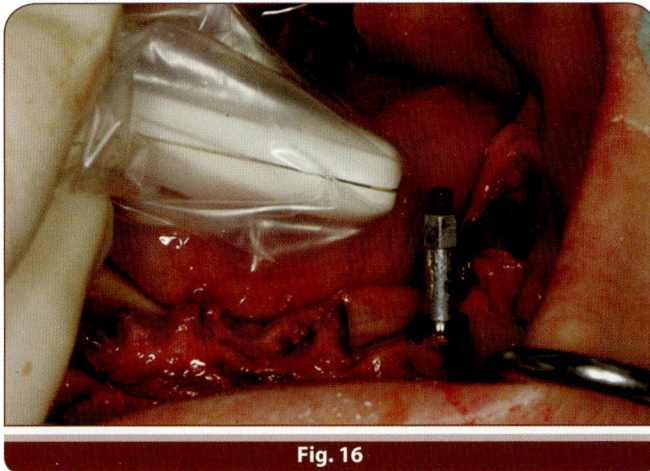

Ostell check (74) short DM 5 × 6 mm **(Fig. 16)**.

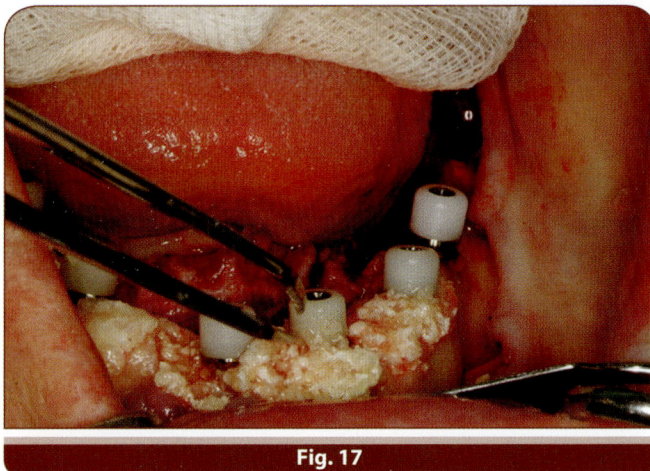

Autologous dentin graft + PRP + calcium sulfate **(Fig. 17)**.

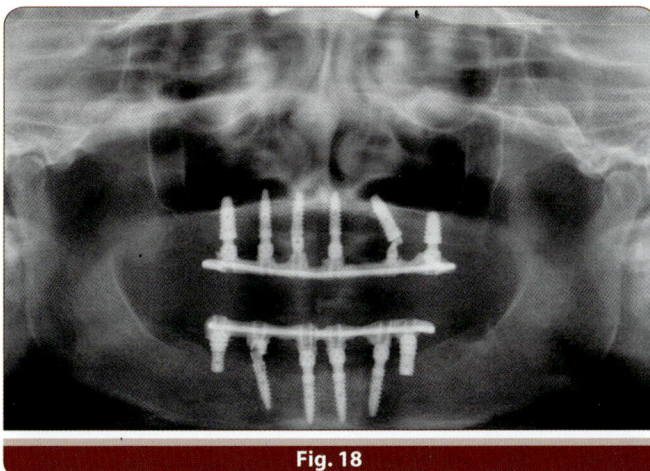

X-ray of the final prosthesis **(Fig. 18)**.

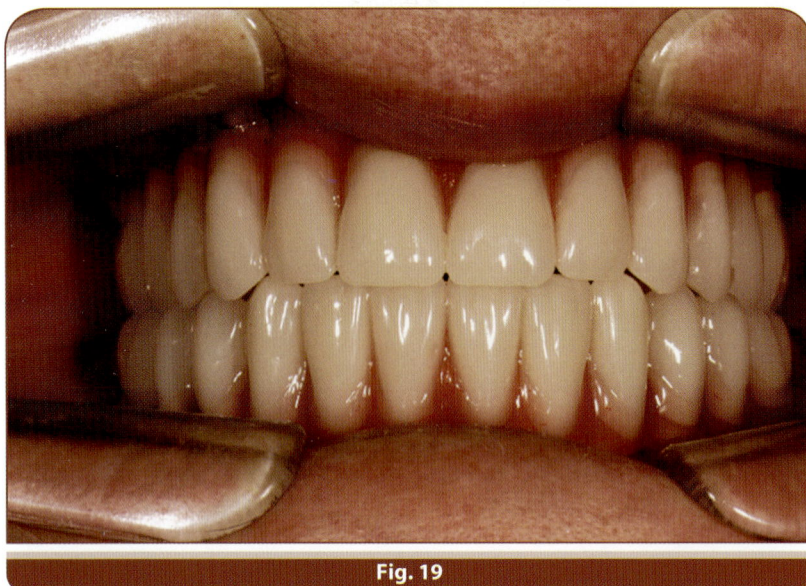

Fig. 19

Final prostheses fixed 10 days after surgery **(Fig. 19)**.

David Morales Schwarz , Hilde Morales

ZYGOMATIC IMPLANT: TREATMENT OPTION FOR ATROPHIC MAXILLA

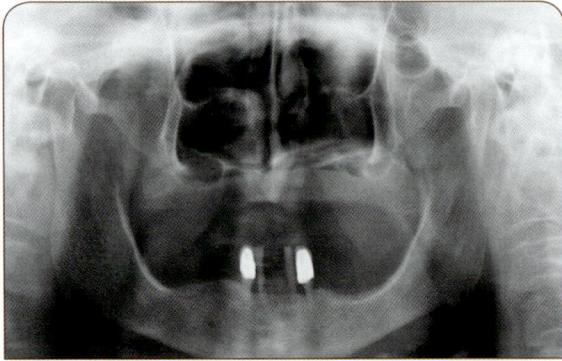

Fig. 1

Female new patient 67 years old, no relevant medical history. We plan right zygomatic implant for maxillary complete oral rehabilitation in a patient with bone atrophy in the posterior regions of the maxilla with the goal of developing and increasing posterior occlusal stability during immediate loading (**Fig. 1**).

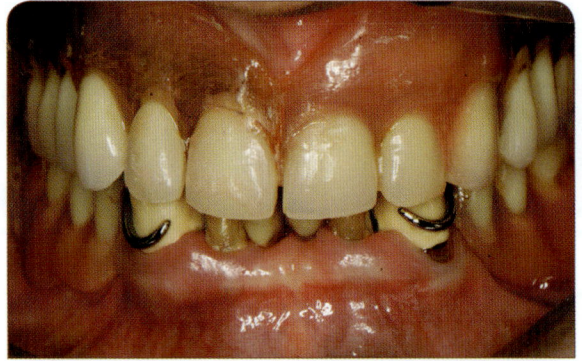

Fig. 2

She wears denture since 20 years (**Fig. 2**).

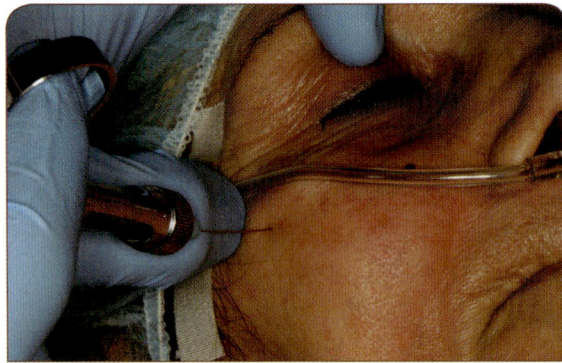

Fig. 3

The procedure was performed under local anesthesia and sedation (**Fig. 3**).

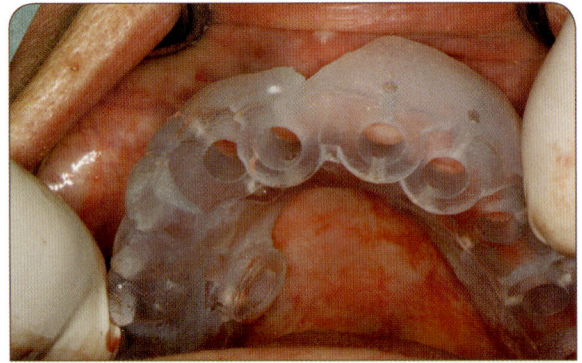

Fig. 4

Surgical guide was placed to identify prosthetically favorable position for the conventional and zygomatic implants (**Fig. 4**).

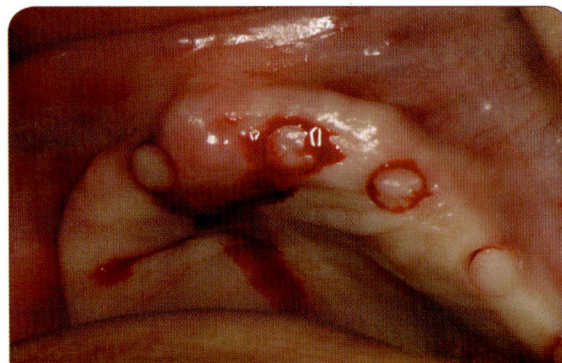

Fig. 5

Implants places were marked with circular scalpel (**Fig. 5**).

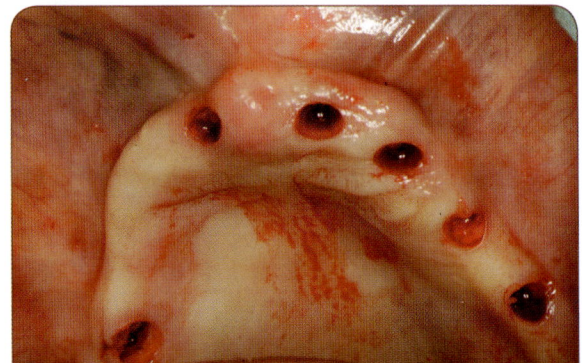

Fig. 6

Tissue removed from the future site of implant placement (**Fig. 6**).

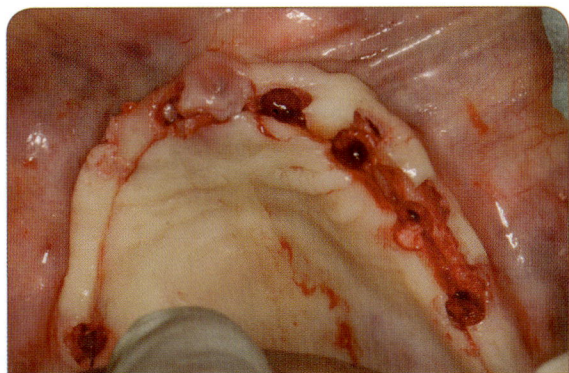
Fig. 7

A crestal incision was made **(Fig. 7)**.

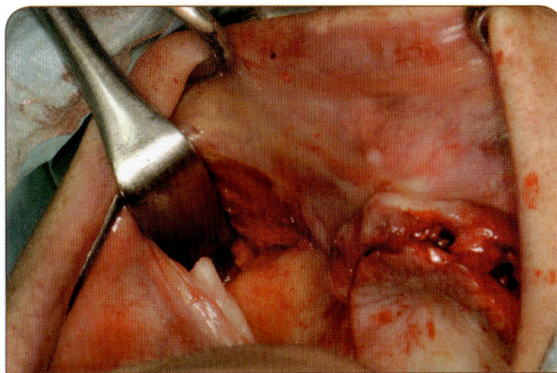
Fig. 8

Mucoperiosteal flap was elevated to expose the alveolar crest, the lateral wall of the maxillary sinus and the inferior rim of the zygomatic arch. A retractor was used to ensure good visibility of the zygomatic bone **(Fig. 8)**.

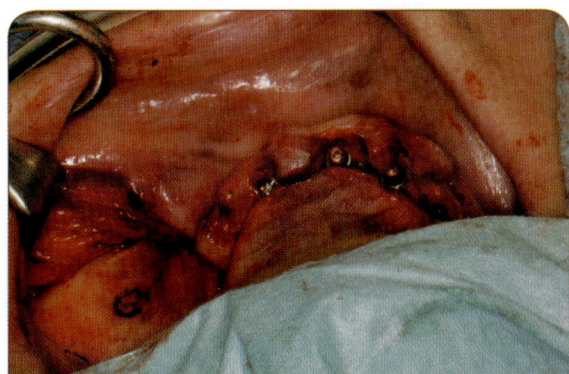
Fig. 9

Zygomatic implant's position was drawn with a pencil **(Fig. 9)**.

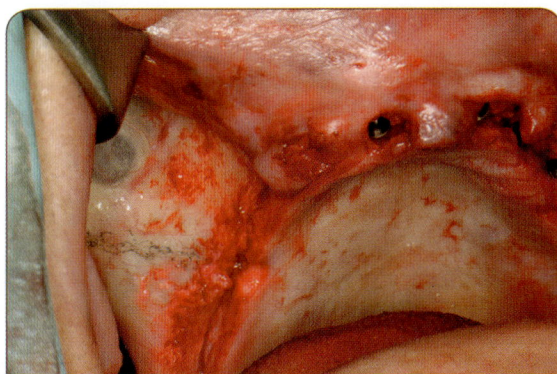
Fig. 10

We draw the path of the zygomatic implant with a pencil **(Fig. 10)**.

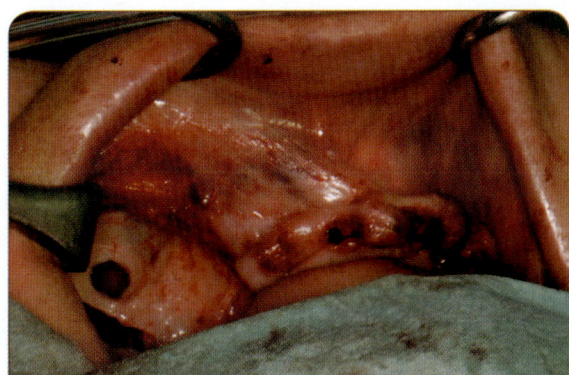
Fig. 11

Initial osteotomy preparation for sinus graft **(Fig. 11)**.

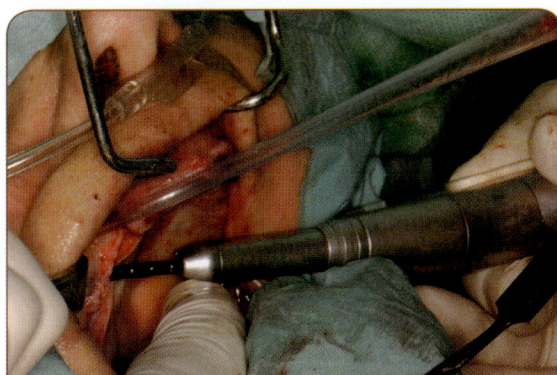
Fig. 12

Estándar drilling protocol by nobel zygoma. 1200 rpm **(Fig. 12)**.

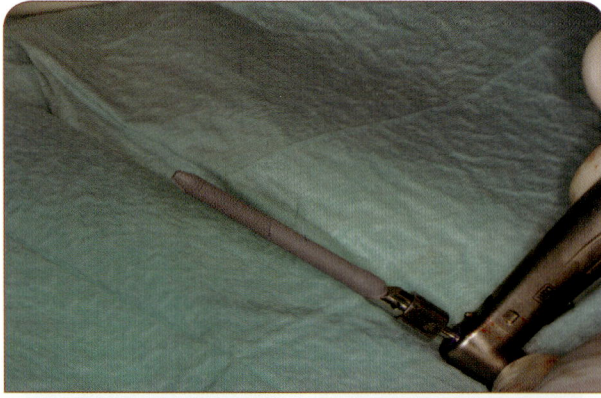

Fig. 13

37.5 mm nobel zygoma implant **(Fig. 13)**.

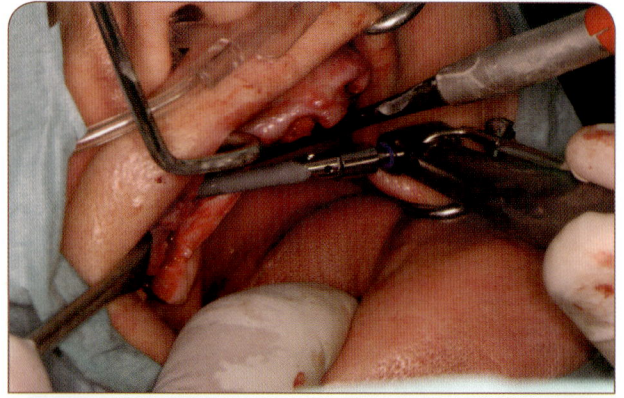

Fig. 14

We place nobel zygoma implant on zygomatic bone. 40 rpm **(Fig. 14)**.

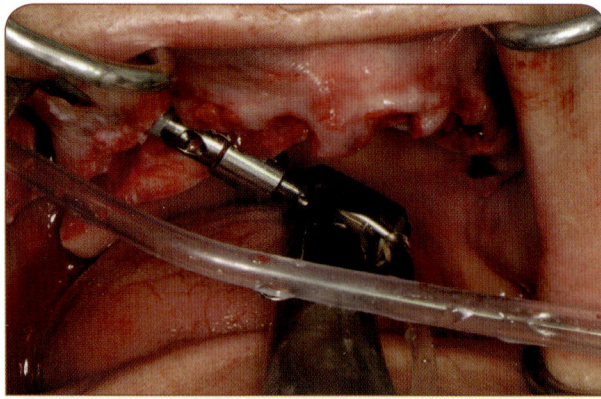

Fig. 15

Trusion of marking followed for proper implant placement **(Fig. 15)**.

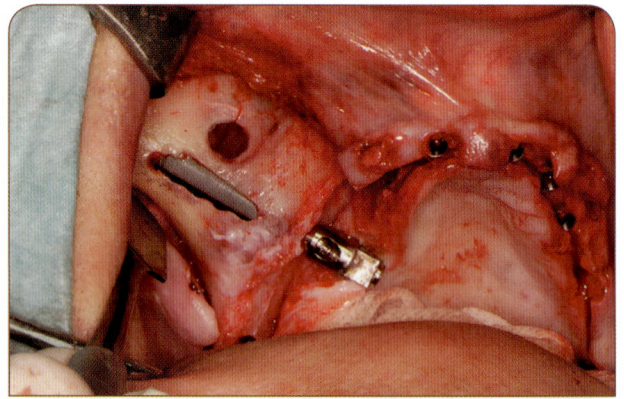

Fig. 16

Implant seated on zygomatic apophysis of maxillary bone **(Fig. 16)**.

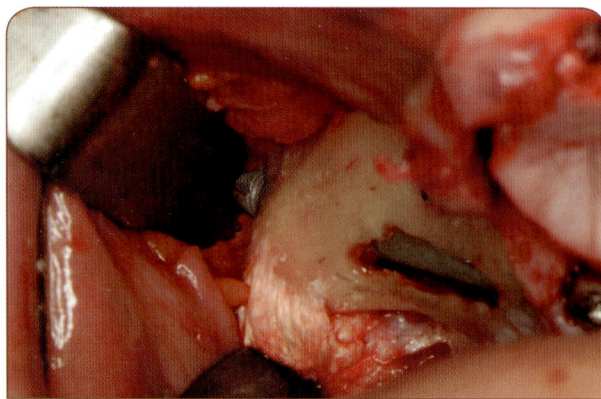

Fig. 17

Zygoma implant apex **(Fig. 17)**.

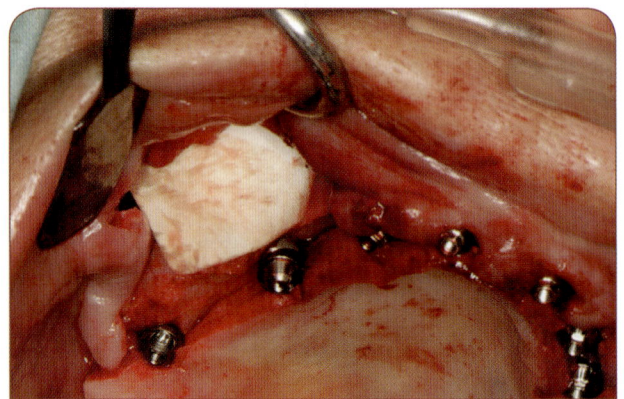

Fig. 18

Drilling and placing of 7 conventional bioner top DM implants. The sinus was filled with PRP and calcium sulfate and covered by Collagene AT membrane **(Fig. 18)**.

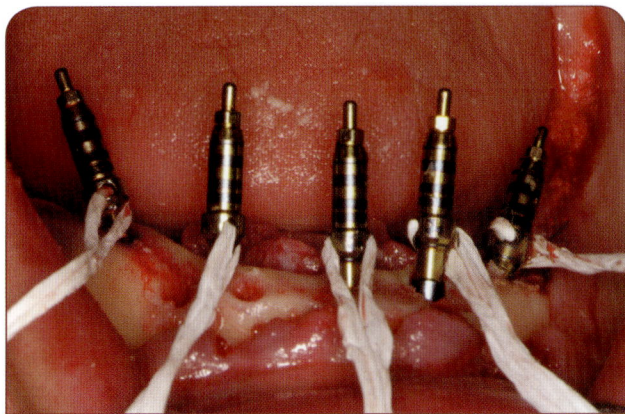

Fig. 19

Five mandibular bioner top DM 4 × 13 implants were drilled following the standard protocol of bioner **(Fig. 19)**.

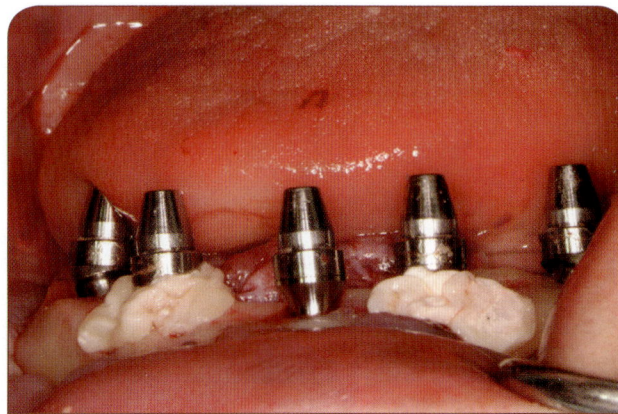

Fig. 20

Implants seated. Extraction socket filled with PRP and calcium sulfate **(Fig. 20)**.

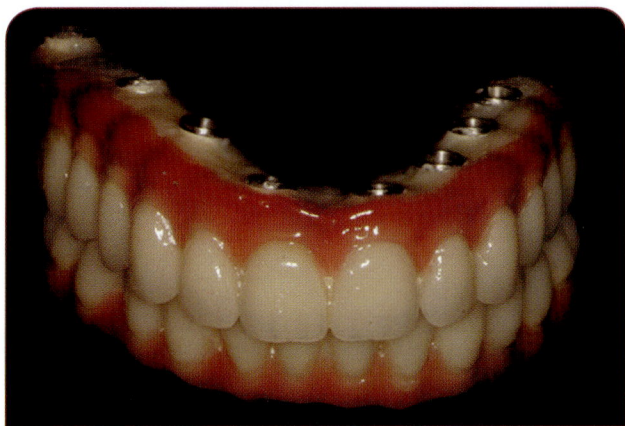

Fig. 21

Composite prosthesis made after surgery **(Fig. 21)**.

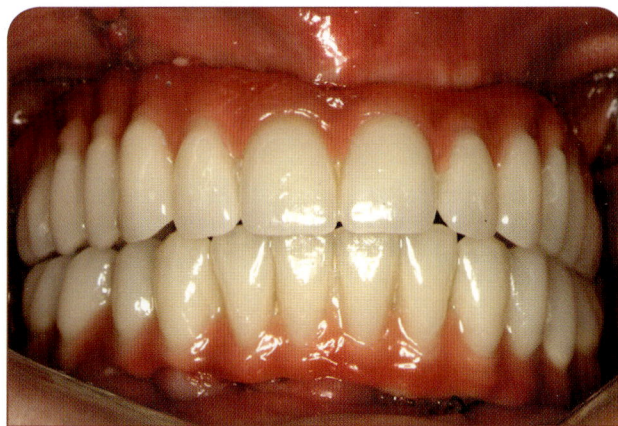

Fig. 22

Prosthesis fixed on the day of surgery **(Fig. 22)**.

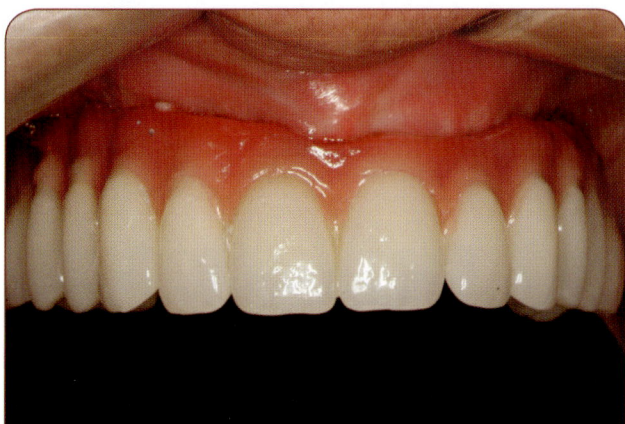

Fig. 23

Maxillary aesthetic prosthesis in place **(Fig. 23)**.

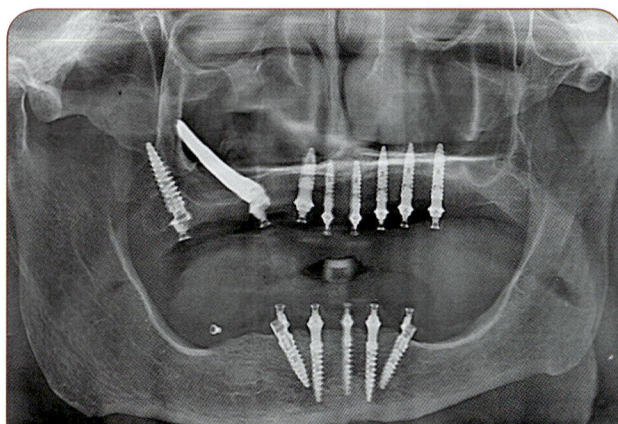

Fig. 24

Orthopantomogram (OPG) showing implants in position **(Fig. 24)**.

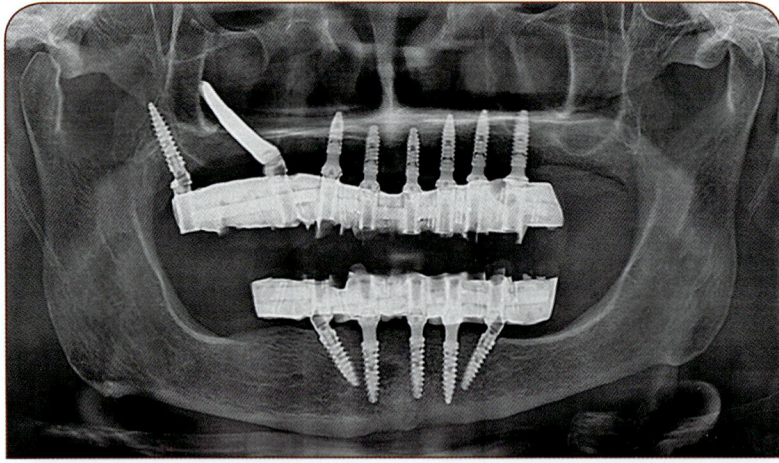

Fig. 25

Orthopantomogram (OPG) prosthesis in month **(Fig. 25)**.

Jin Y Kim

FULL MAXILLARY IMPLANT RECONSTRUCTION WITH ORTHODONTICS-PERIODONTICS TREATMENT IN THE MANDIBULAR ARCH

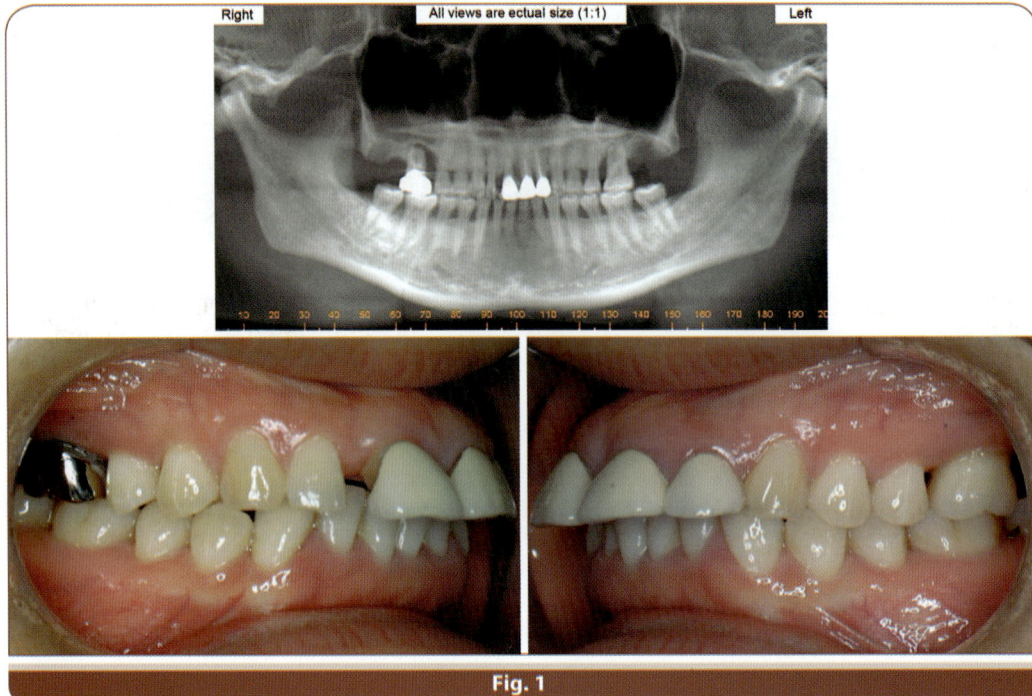

Fig. 1

Patient presented with generalized moderate periodontitis of teeth in the mandibular arch, and advanced periodontitis in the maxillary arch. Etiology in this case included poor dental care, malocclusion and trauma from occlusion/parafunction **(Fig. 1)**.

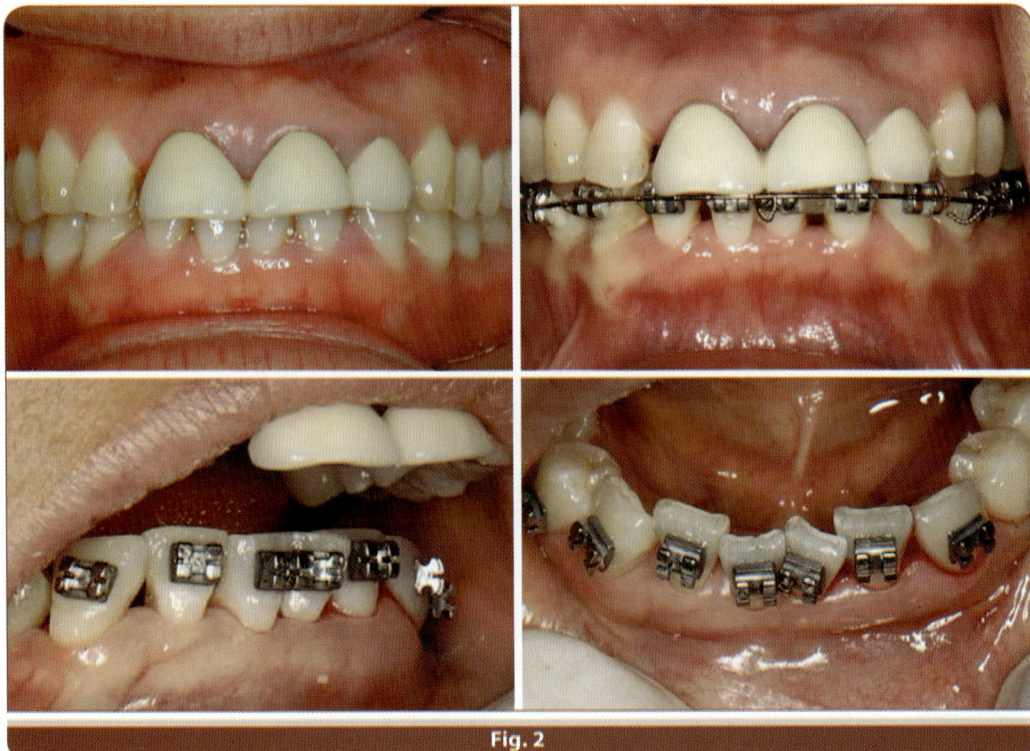

Fig. 2

Treatment included non-surgical and surgical periodontal therapy of the mandibular arch, followed by orthodontic therapy, and full arch implant therapy in the maxillary arch. Full clearance of natural teeth and comprehensive implant therapy was chosen as this approach allowed for correction the occlusion, and significant cosmetic improvement **(Fig. 2)**.

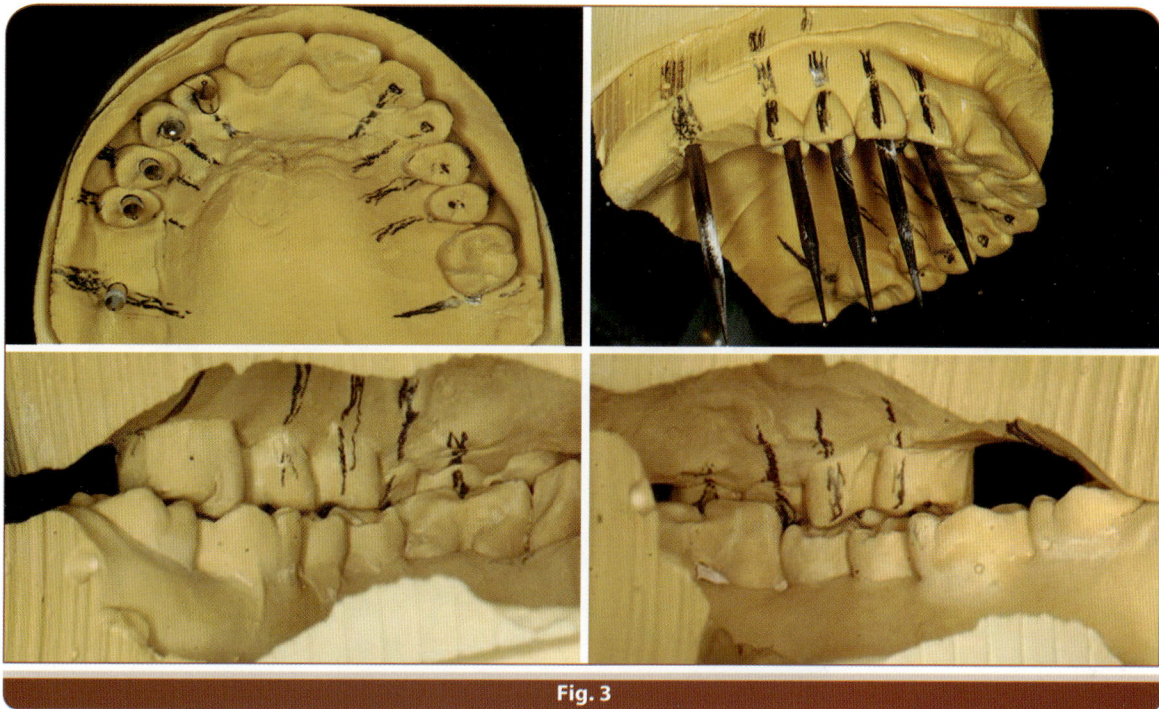

Fig. 3

Immediate implant placement on the day of maxillary teeth extraction, and functional immediate loading/immediate was planned **(Fig. 3)**.

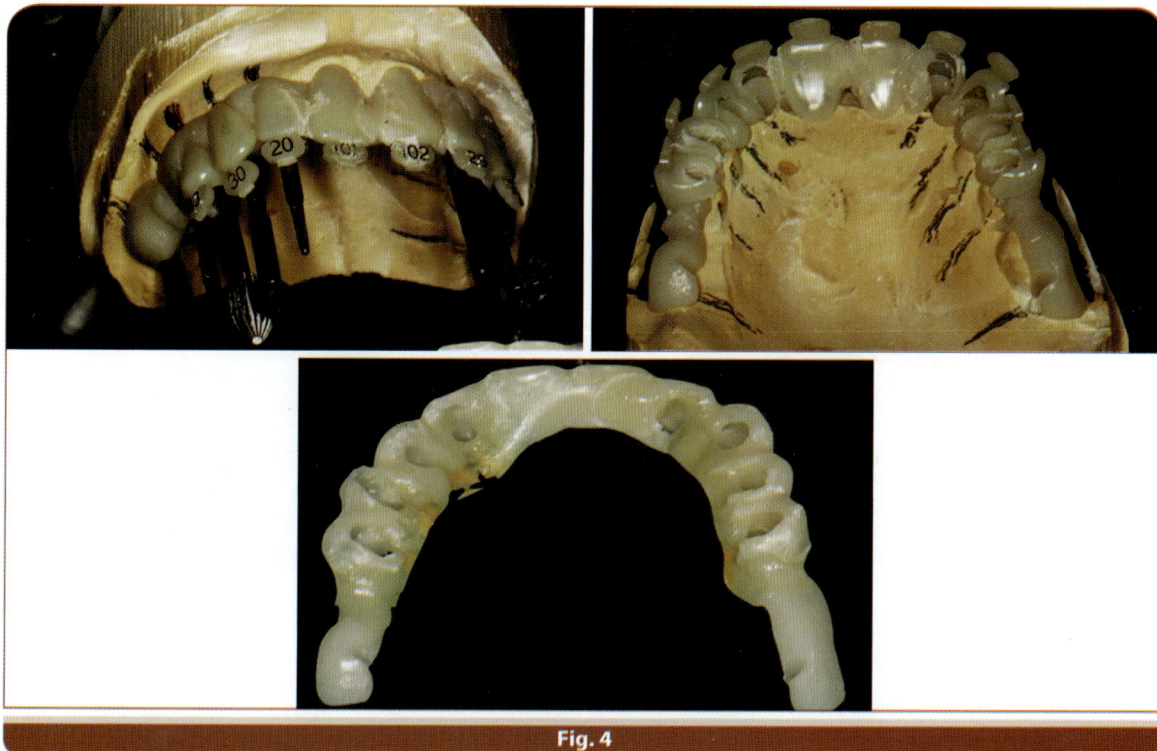

Fig. 4

Immediate functional prosthesis was fabricated for loading. This appliance was also used for precise placement of the implants in predetermined positions. Although this is analog approach, many times careful traditional planning yields better outcomes than the newer digital approaches **(Fig. 4)**.

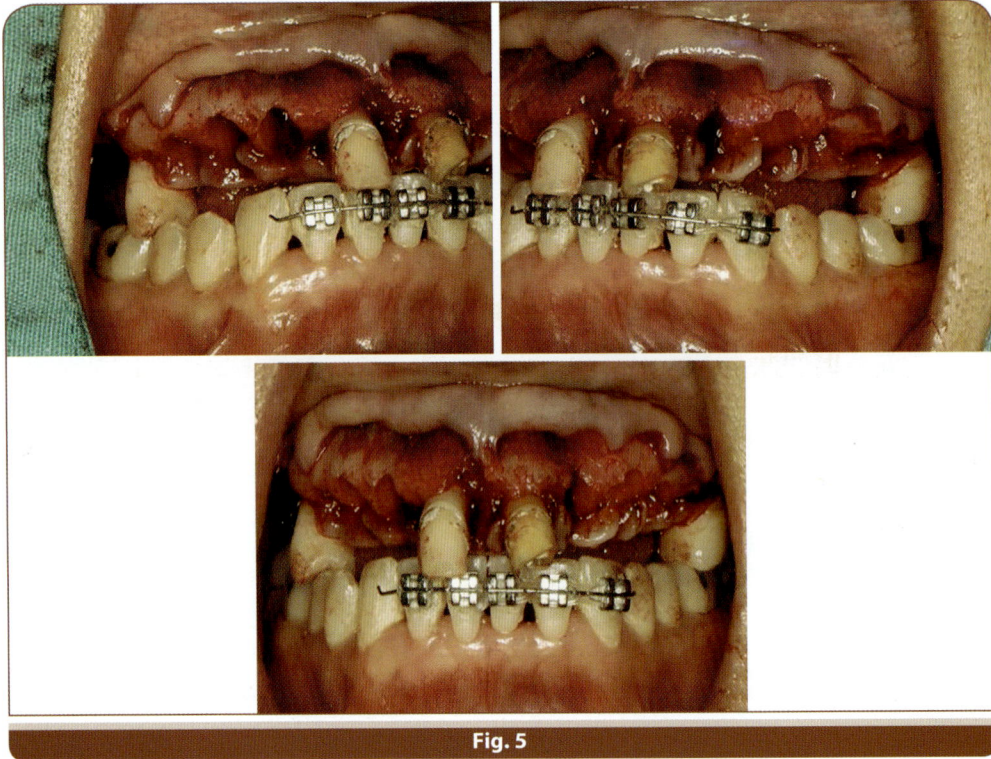

Fig. 5

A full thickness flap raised and extraction done keeping tripod contact with lower teeth **(Fig. 5)**.

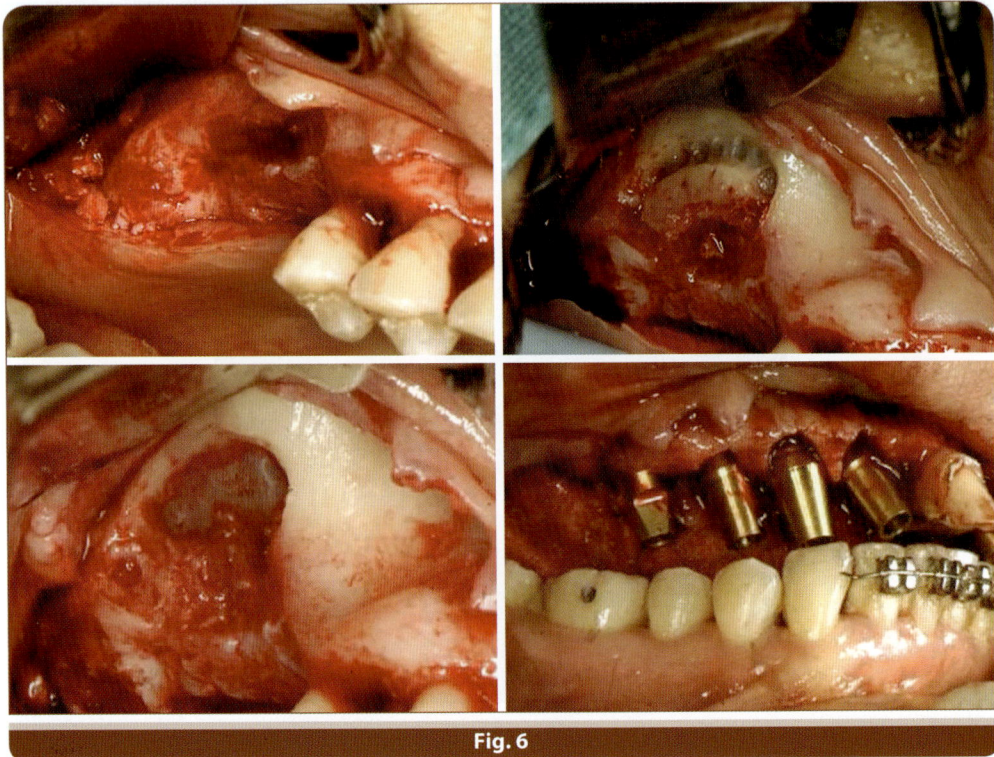

Fig. 6

Bilateral sinus grafts were performed, via the classic window access approach. Some implants placed in the sinus region were not included in the immediate load protocol **(Fig. 6)**.

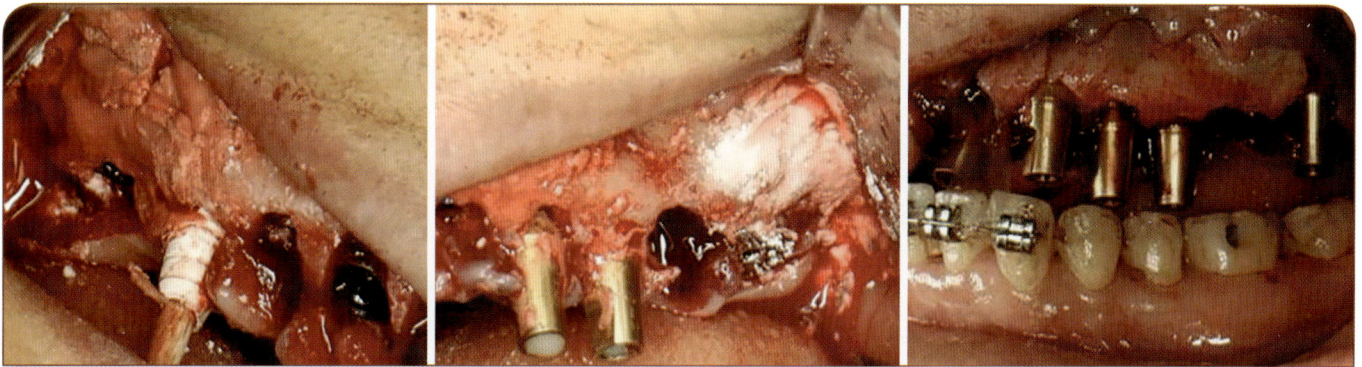

Fig. 7

Permanant abutments torqued to the implants **(Fig. 7)**.

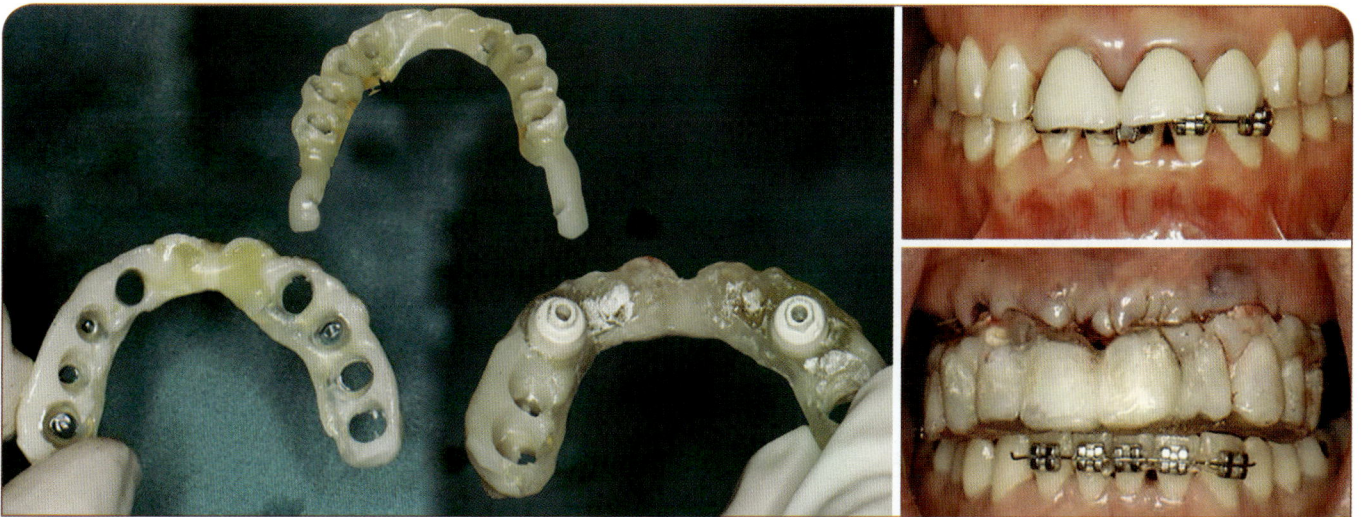

Fig. 8

The prosthesis used as a surgical template was converted to screw retained immediate functional prosthesis **(Fig. 8)**.

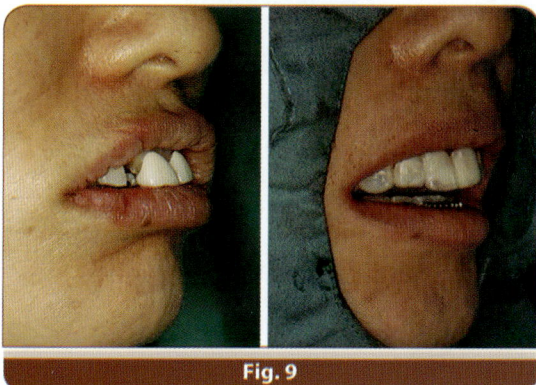

Fig. 9

The facial appearance immediately before, and after implant surgery **(Fig. 9)**.

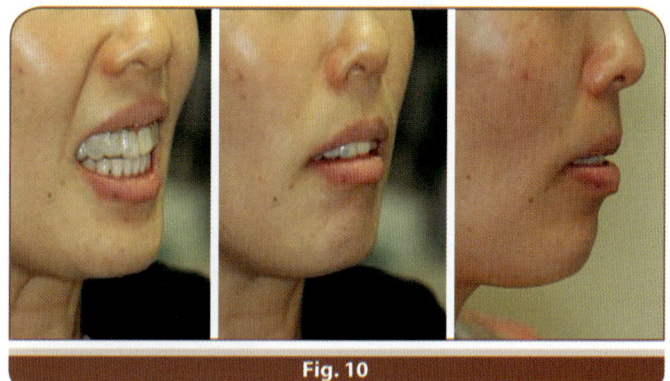

Fig. 10

Patient functioned in the prosthesis for 8 months **(Fig. 10)**.

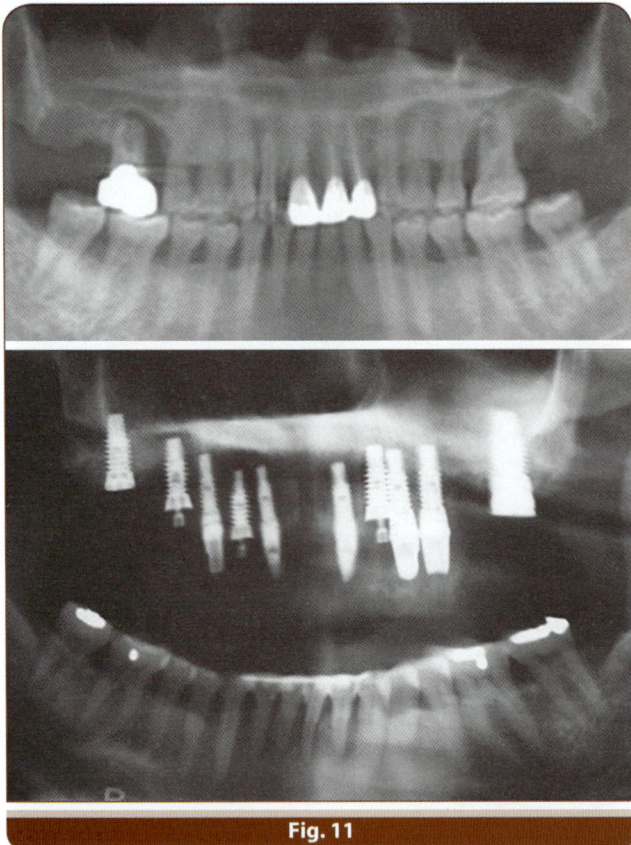

Fig. 11

Panoramic film images, presurgery, and immediate post-implant surgery **(Fig. 11)**.

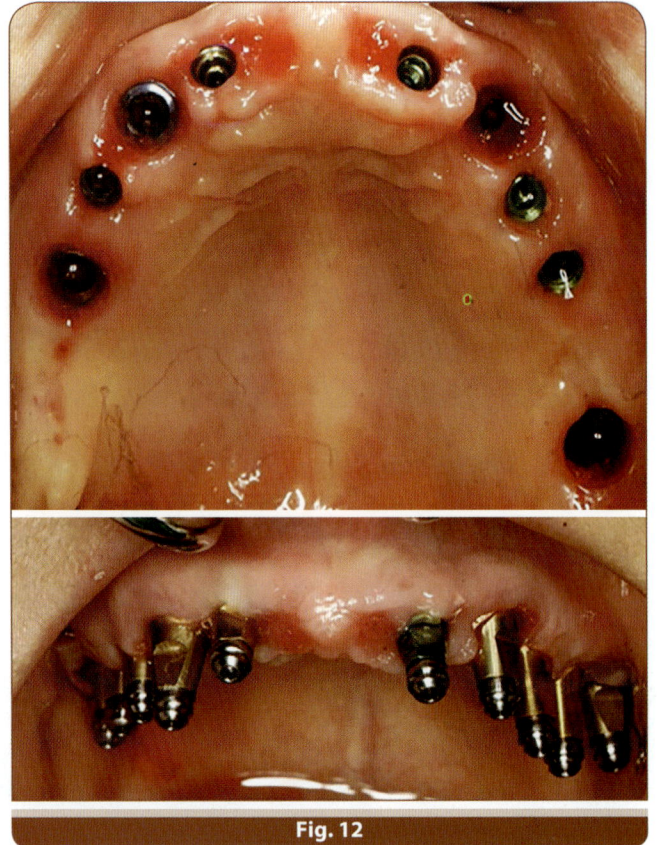

Fig. 12

At 8 months, all implants have fully osseointegrated **(Fig. 12)**.

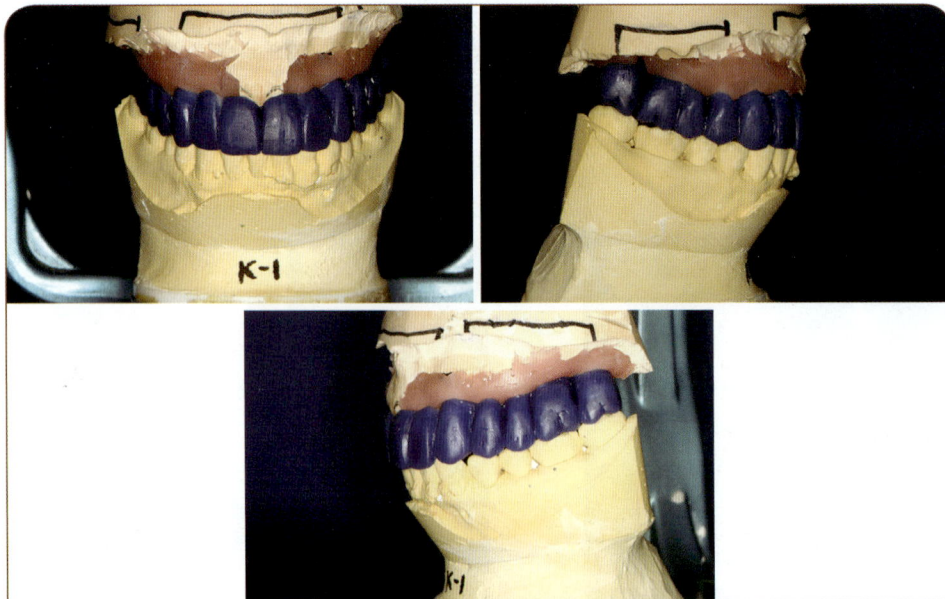

Fig. 13

Custom UCLA abutments were individually waxed up and cast **(Fig. 13)**.

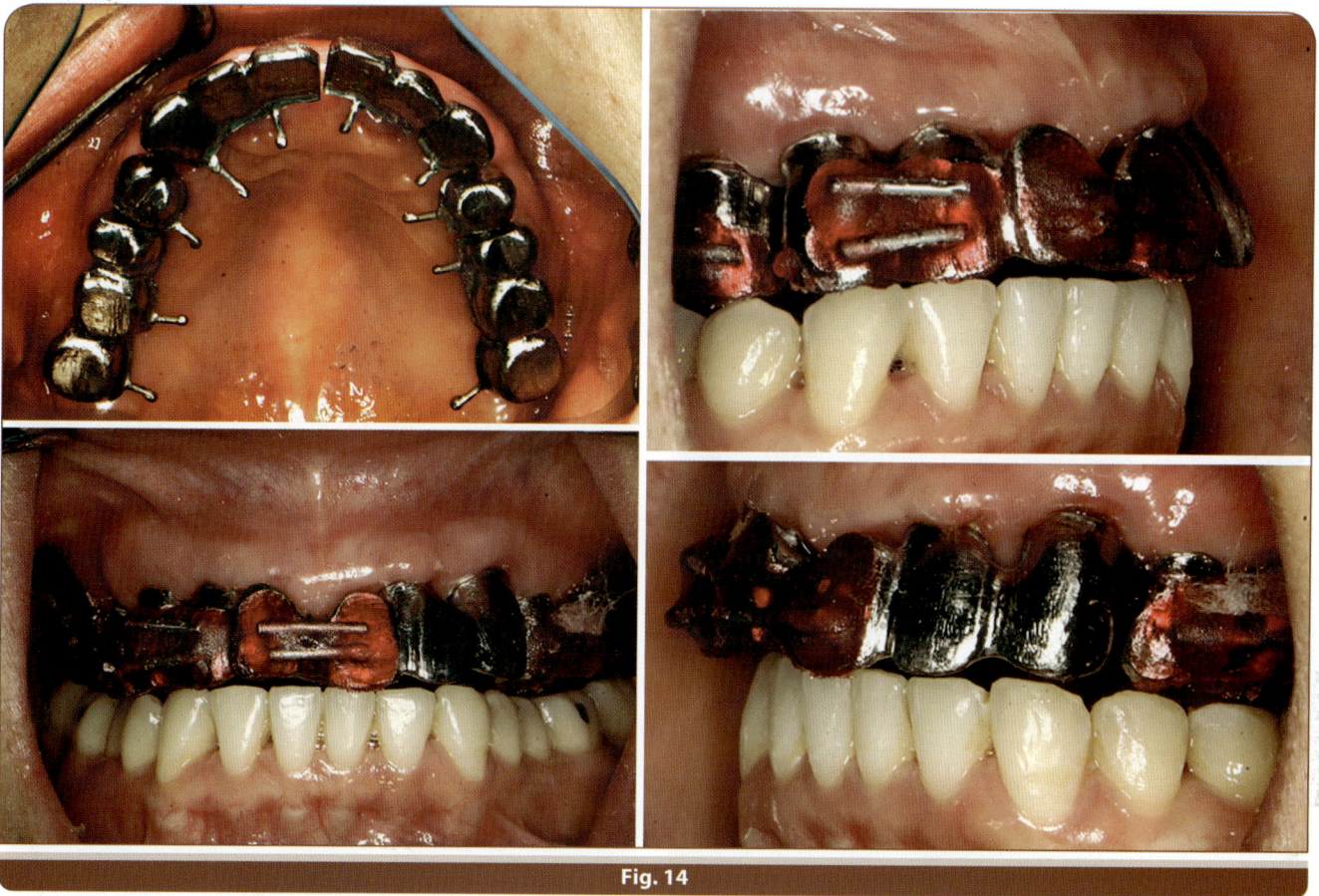

Fig. 14

Metal copings for the definitive restorations were individually waxed up and cast, tried in over custom UCLA abutments and luted, indexed, luted and soldered **(Fig. 14)**.

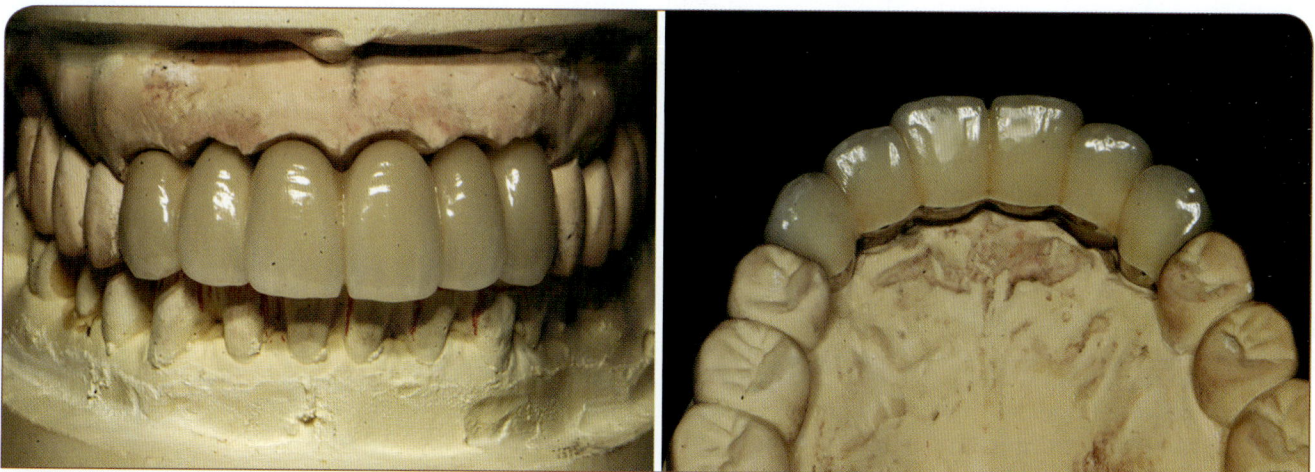

Fig. 15

Ceramic layering on the frame works **(Fig. 15)**.

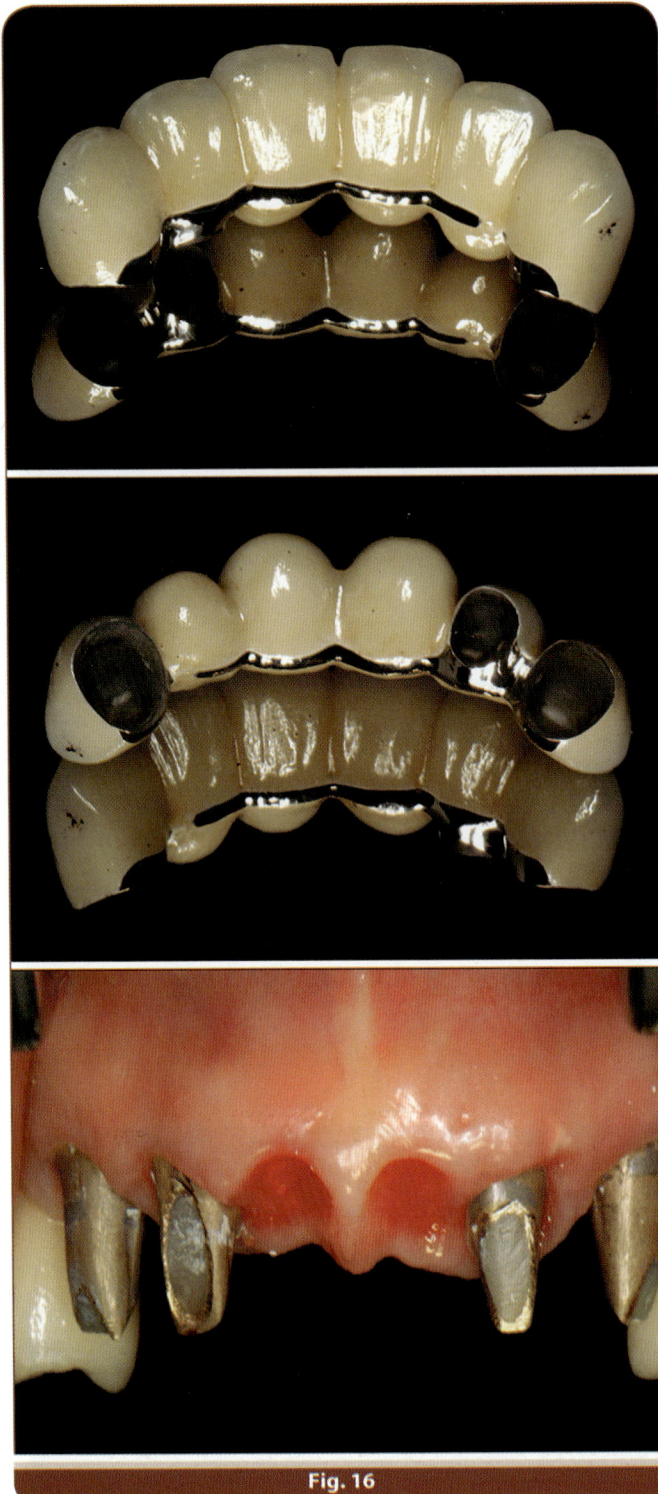

Fig. 16

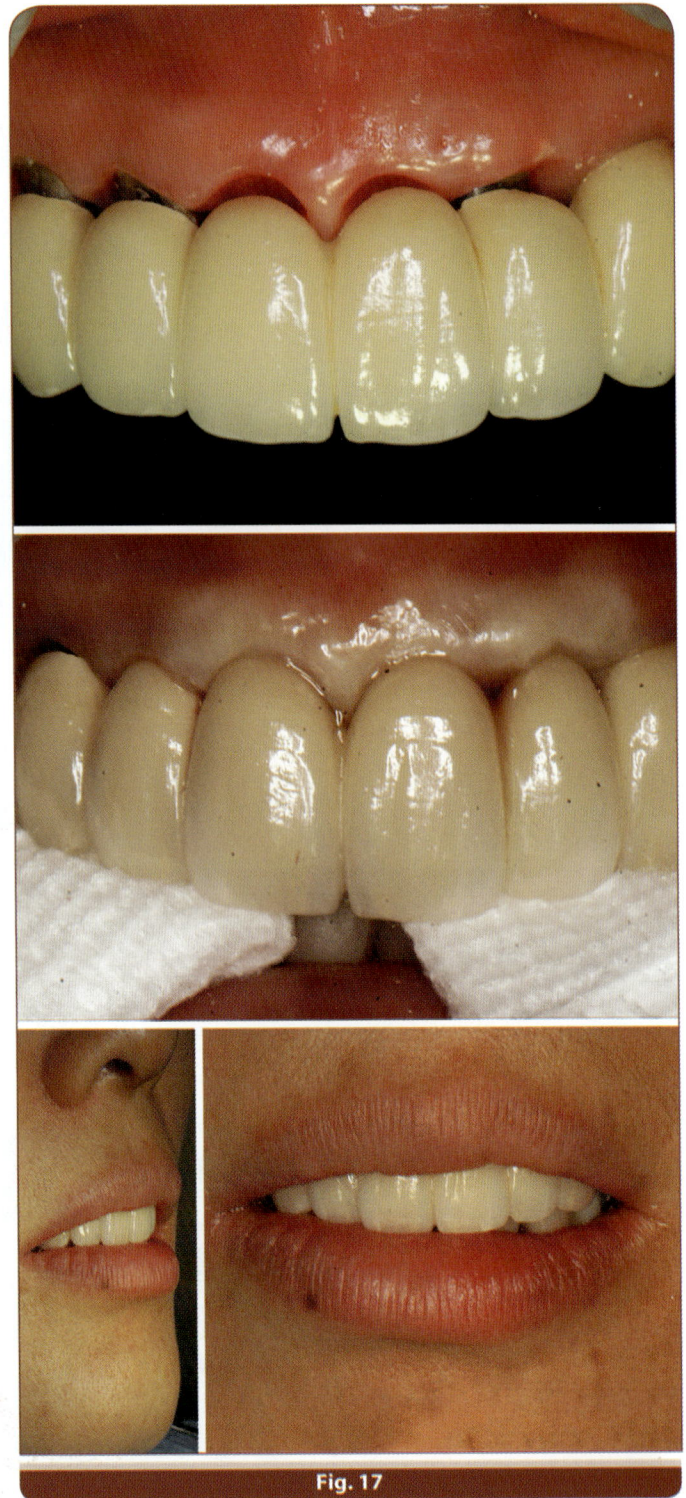

Fig. 17

Definitive cementable ceramo-metal restoration was fabricated with ovate pontics in the central incisor region **(Fig. 16)**.

Day of delivery of definitive prosthesis (2008) **(Fig. 17)**.

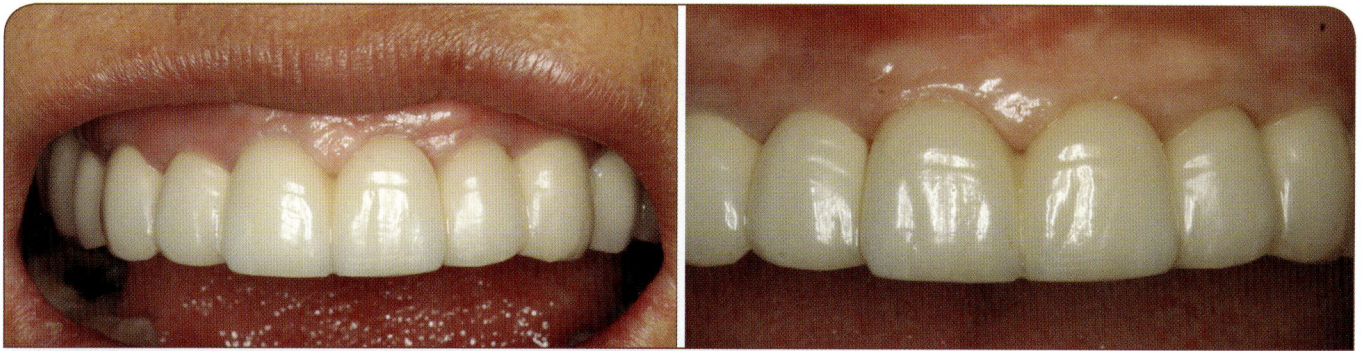

Fig. 18

6 years follow-up **(Fig. 18)**.

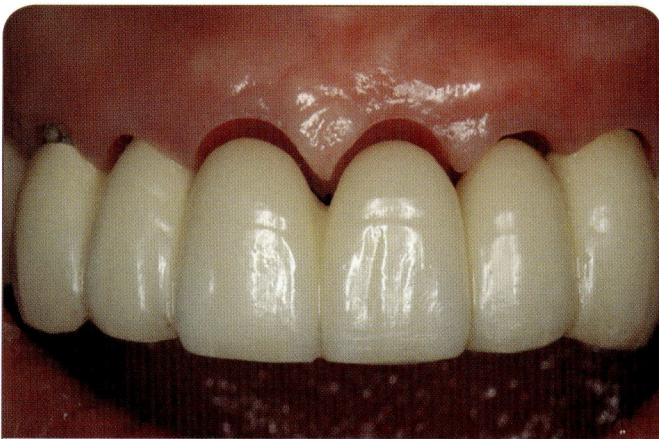

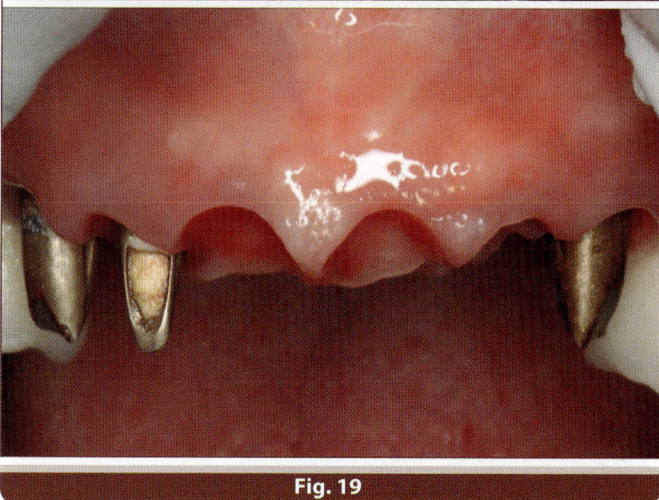

Fig. 19

The anterior prosthesis was decemented at year 8. Minor occlusal adjustment was carried out, and the bridge was recemented. The ovate form seems to have remained unchanged for 8 years **(Fig. 19)**.

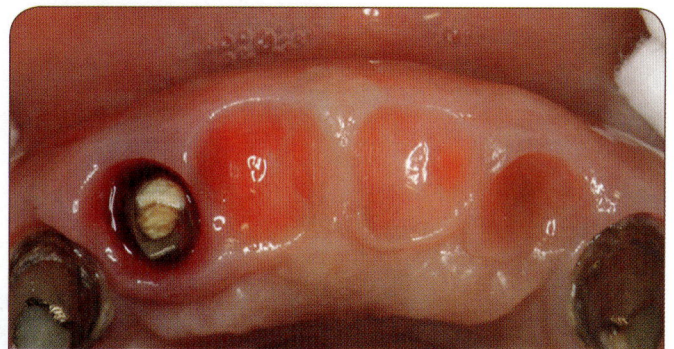

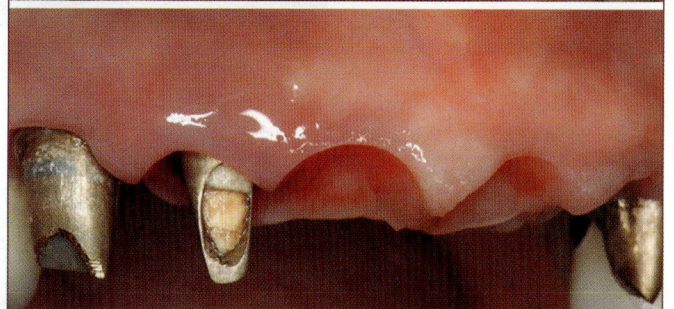

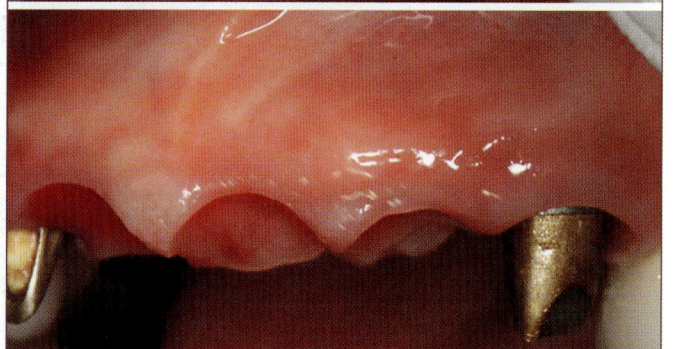

Fig. 20

Very nice gingival architecture achieved with ovate ponties **(Fig. 20)**.

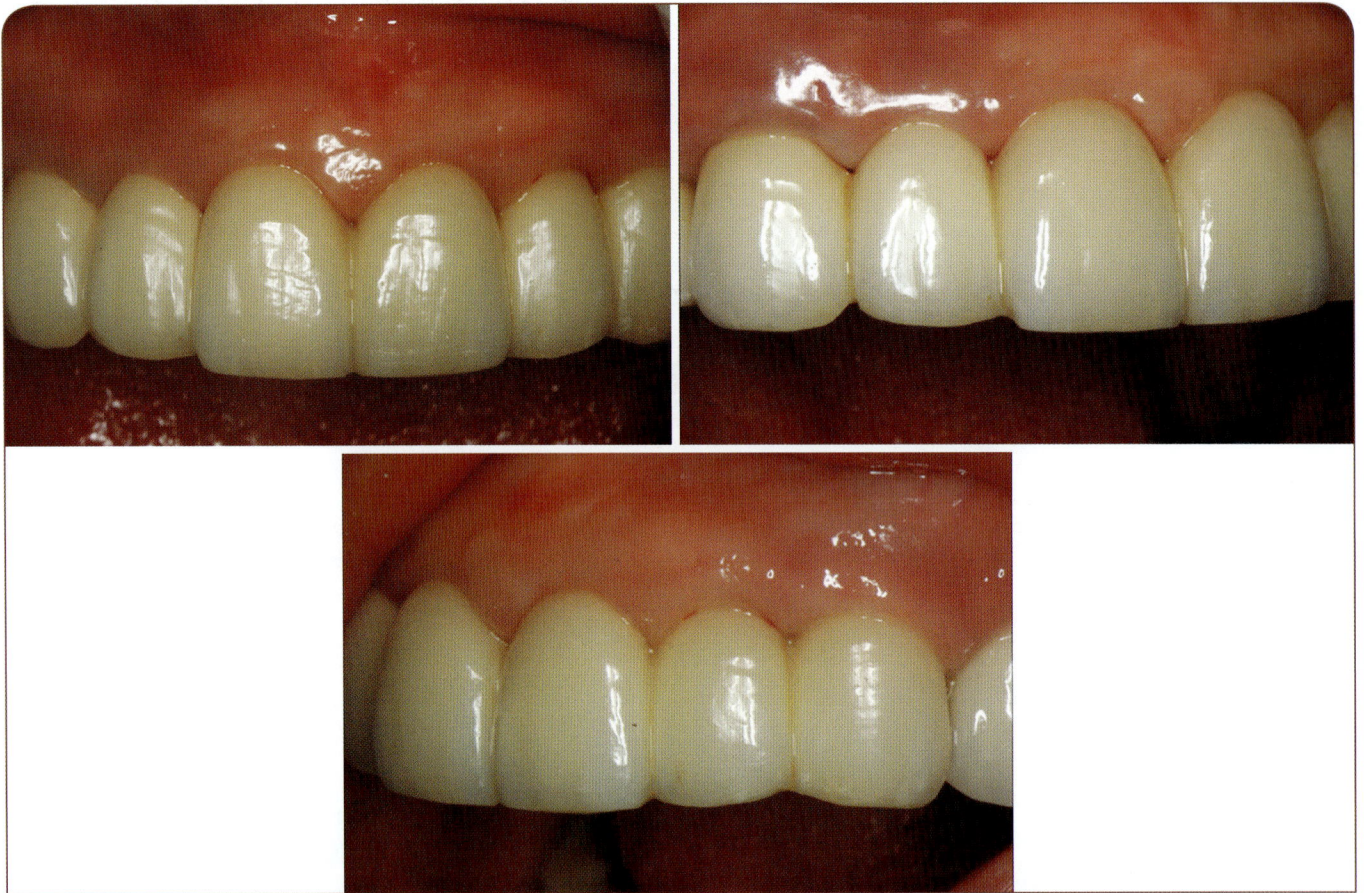

Fig. 21

Restorations and panoramic film after 9 years (9 year follow-up) **(Fig. 21)**.

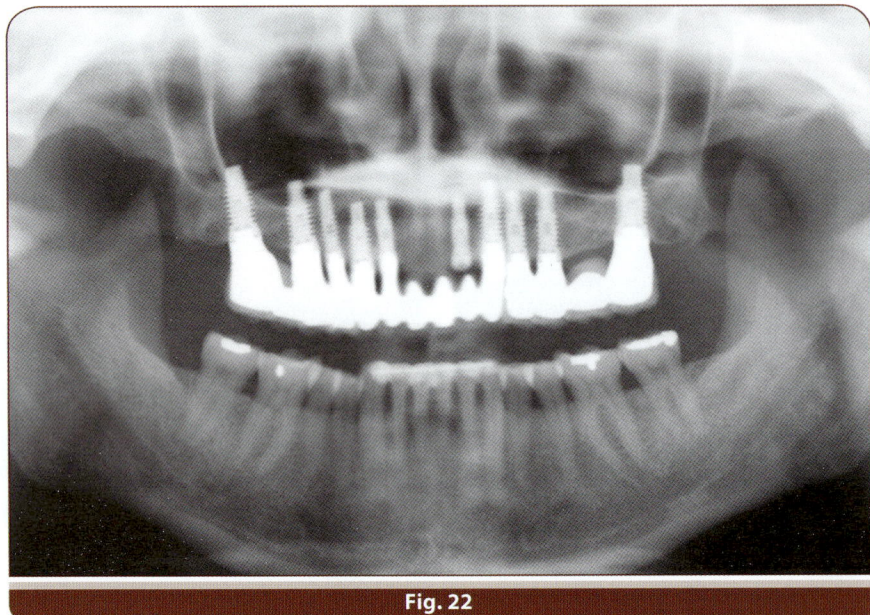

Fig. 22

9 years follow-up OPG **(Fig. 22)**.

CASE STUDY 107

Glenn Mascarenhas

PARTIAL ANODONTIA TREATED WITH ORTHODONTICS AND DENTAL IMPLANTS

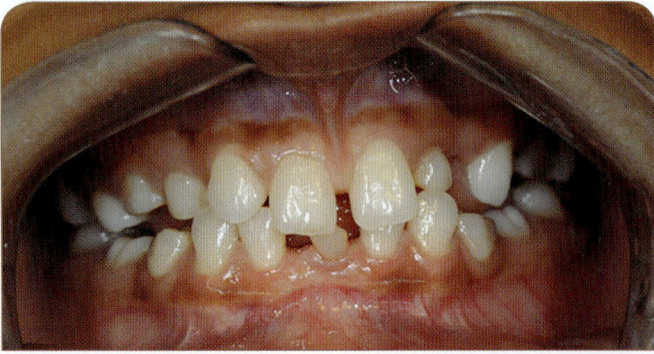

Fig. 1

A case of partial anodontia in a female patient aged 21 who was concerned about aesthetics and function (**Fig. 1**).

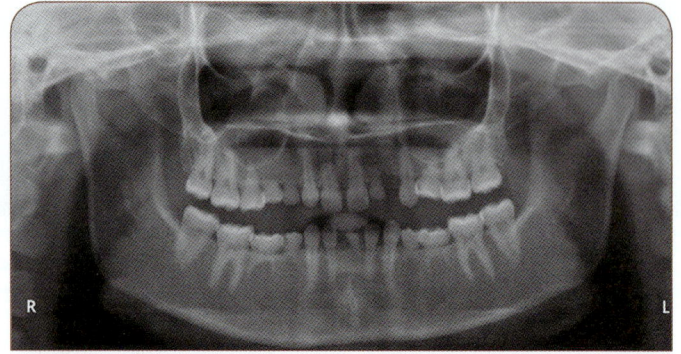

Fig. 2

Preoperative orthopantomogram (OPG). Missing some permanent incisors, premolars and third molars. Overretained deciduous teeth. (**Fig. 2**).

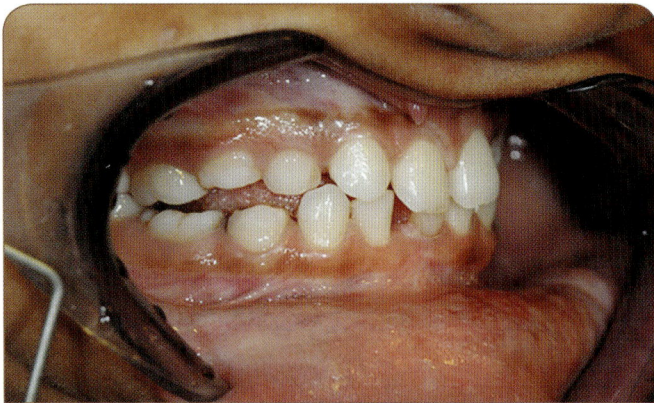

Fig. 3

Right lateral view (**Fig. 3**).

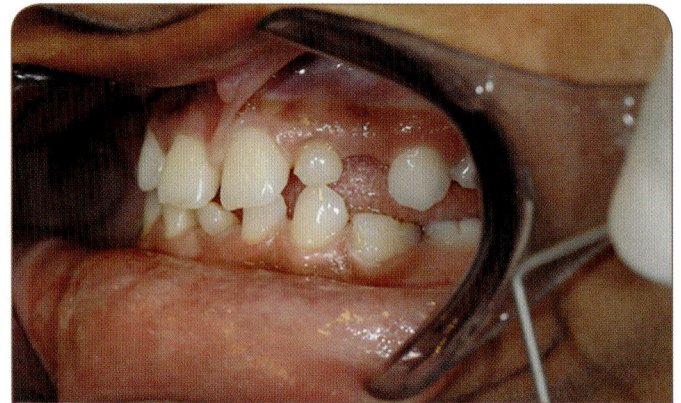

Fig. 4

Left lateral view (**Fig. 4**).

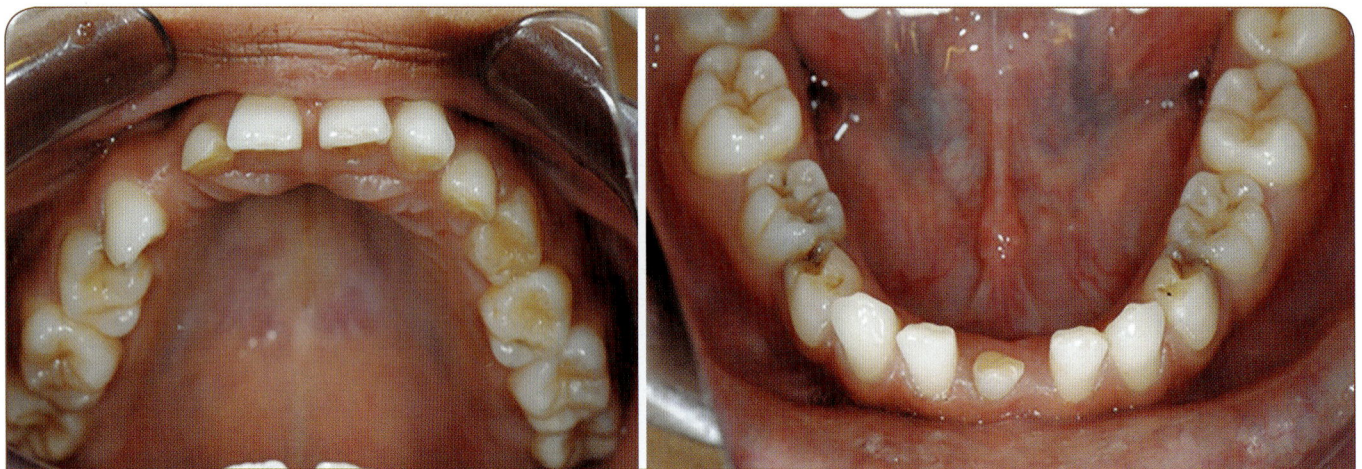

Fig. 5

Upper occlusal view. Lower occlusal view (**Fig. 5**).

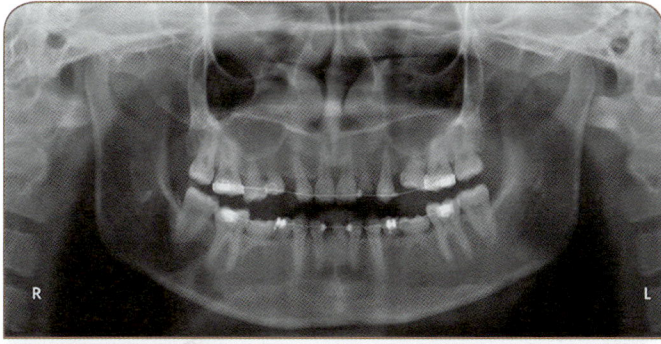

Fig. 6

Orthodontic treatment to bring about symmetry in spacing of residual dentition (**Fig. 6**).

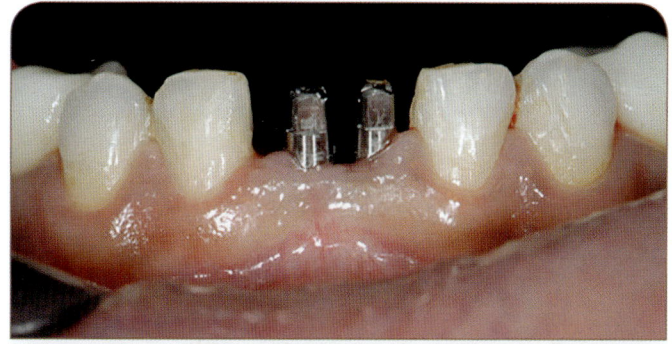

Fig. 7

Two single piece implants following orthodontic spacing for lower incisors (**Fig. 7**).

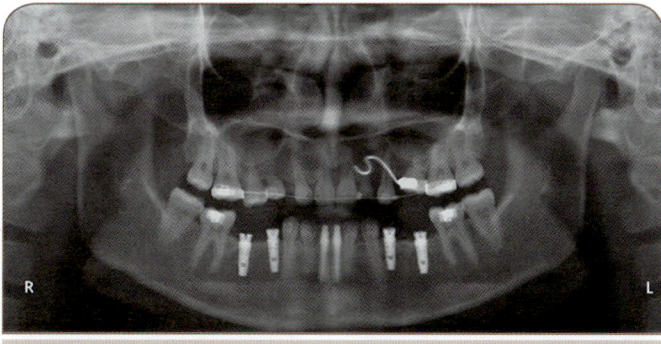

Fig. 8

Extraction of lower deciduous molars and implant placement for premolars (**Fig. 8**).

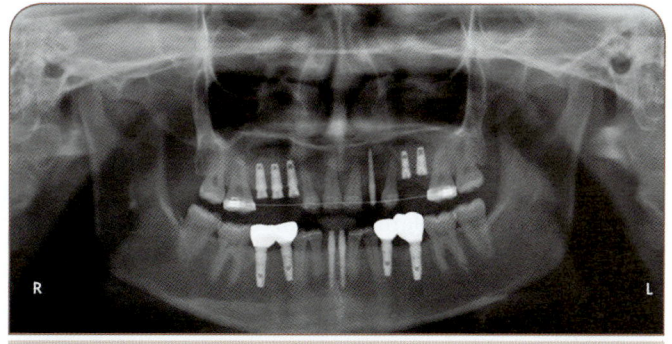

Fig. 9

Extraction of upper deciduous molars and implant placement with sinus grafting for permanent upper premolars and upper left lateral incisor (**Fig. 9**).

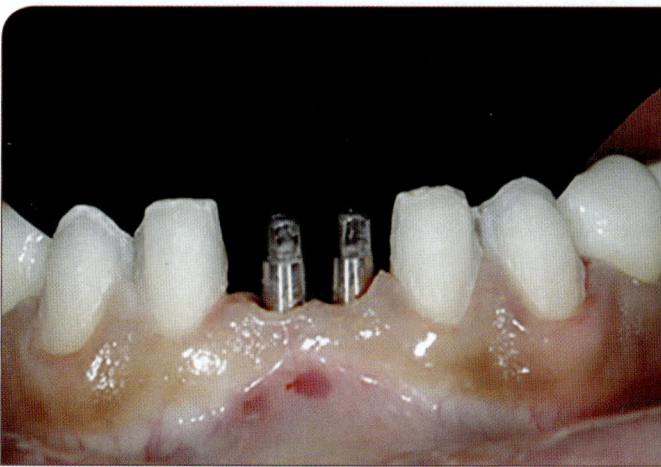

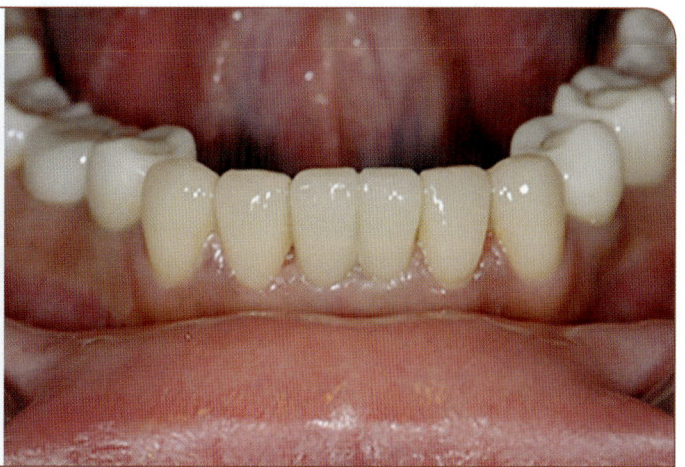

Fig. 10

Loading of lower implants with Zirconia crowns as well as veneers on adjacent incisors and canines (**Fig. 10**).

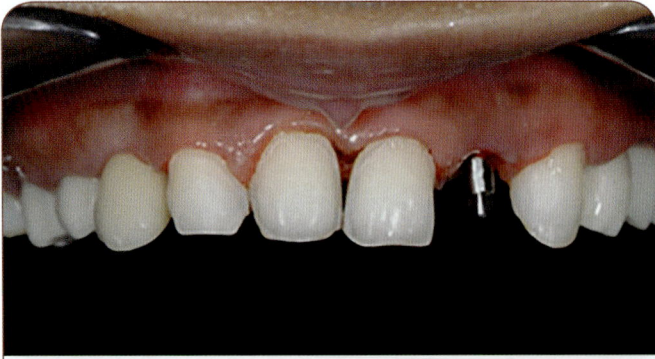

Fig. 11

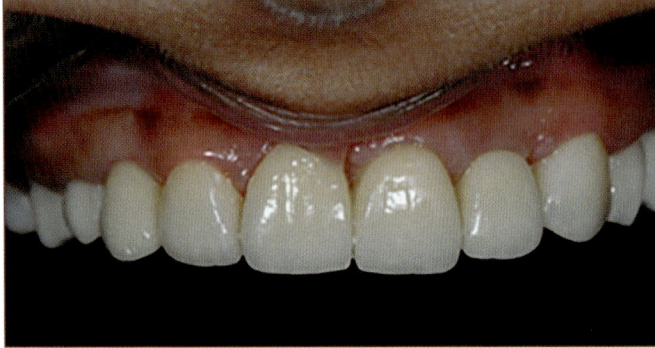

Loading of upper implants with Zirconia crowns as well as veneers on adjacent incisors & canines (**Fig. 11**).

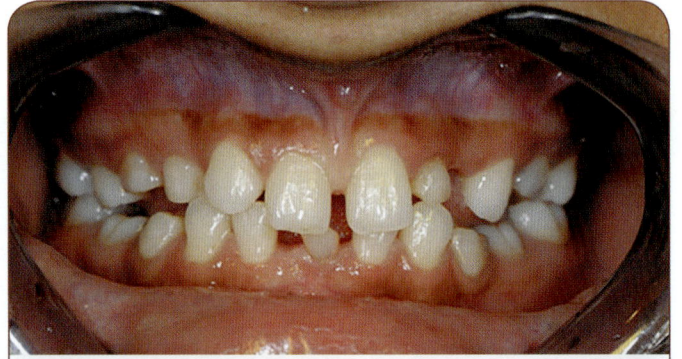

Fig. 12

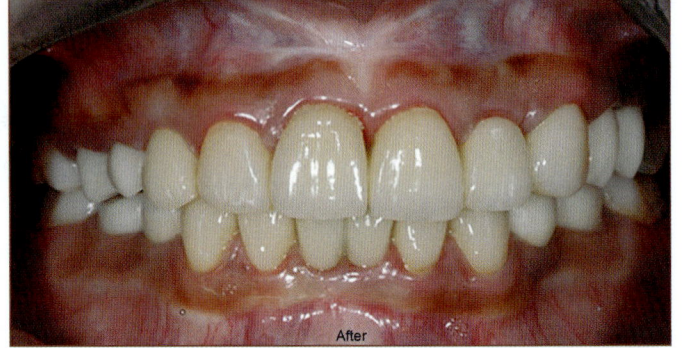

Before and after treatment (**Fig. 12**).

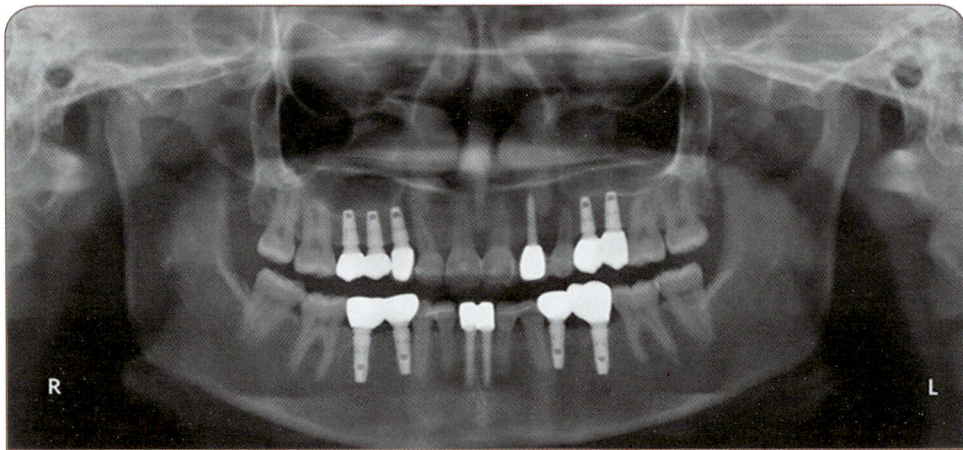

Fig. 13

Orthopantomogram post orthodontic and loading of implants (**Fig. 13**).

CASE STUDY 108

Praful Bali, Vani Kalra, Priyank Jayna

FULL MOUTH VISIO.LIGN PROSTHESIS FOR ENHANCED ESTHETICS AND FUNCTION

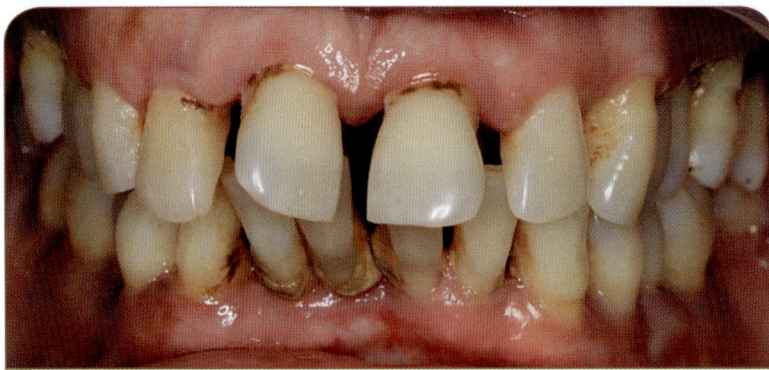

Fig. 1

A 56-year-old female patient presents with failing dentition—grade II and grade III mobility with most of the teeth and severe malocclusion **(Fig. 1)**.

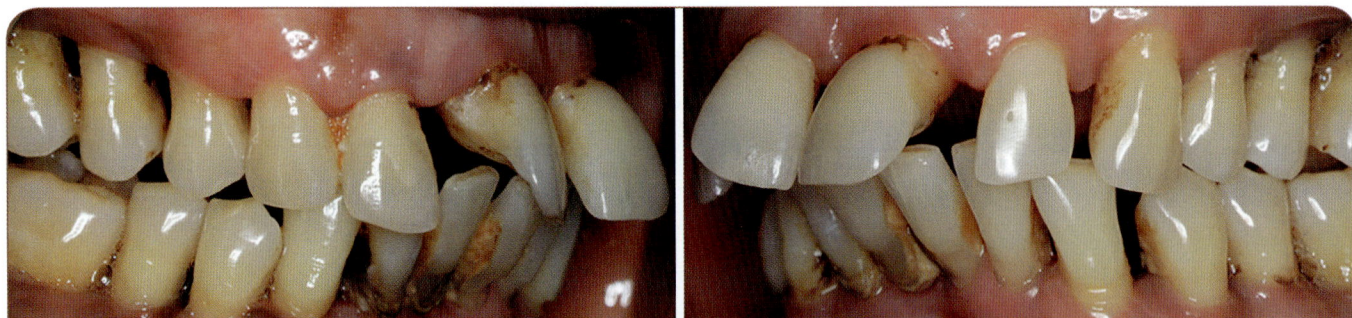

Fig. 2

Right and left lateral views of the failed dentition **(Fig. 2)**.

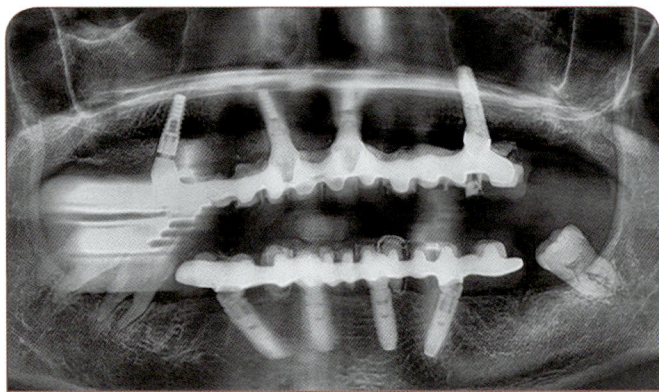

Fig. 3

Total extraction done. The upper and lower jaws are leveled and 4 blue sky implants (Bredent) are placed and 4 fast and fixed abutments screwed to the implants. The patient is given acrylic temporary immediate prosthesis for 3 months **(Fig. 3)**.

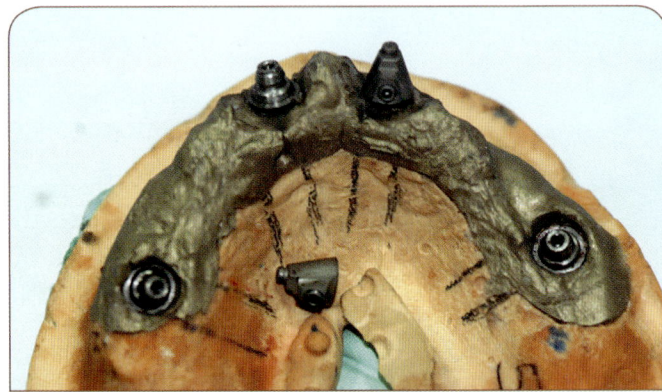

Fig. 4

For the definitive prosthesis transverse screws are planned for the upper anterior implants so that the screw holes are palatally oriented and the esthetics is not hampered. The view of the transverse screw abutments on the maxillary model **(Fig. 4)**.

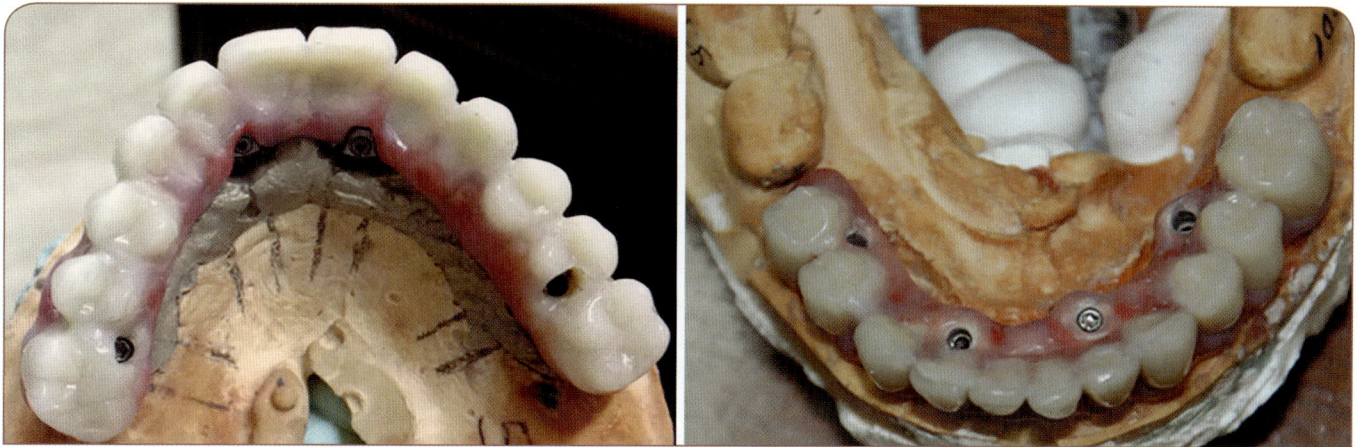

Fig. 5

The upper and lower models with the definitive visio.lign art work **(Fig. 5)**.

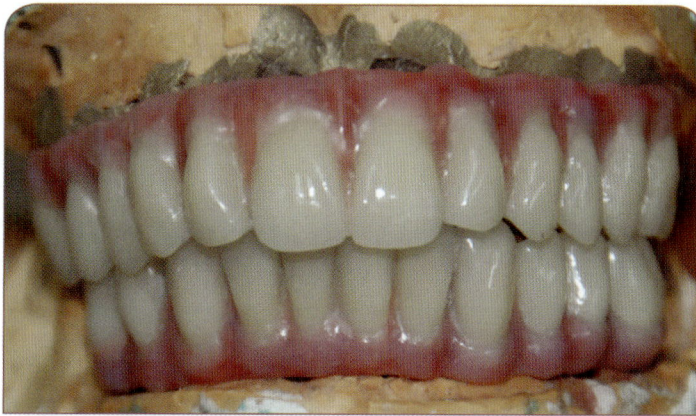

Fig. 6

Upper and lower models mounted on the articulator after face bow transfer. Visio.lign art work done **(Fig. 6)**.

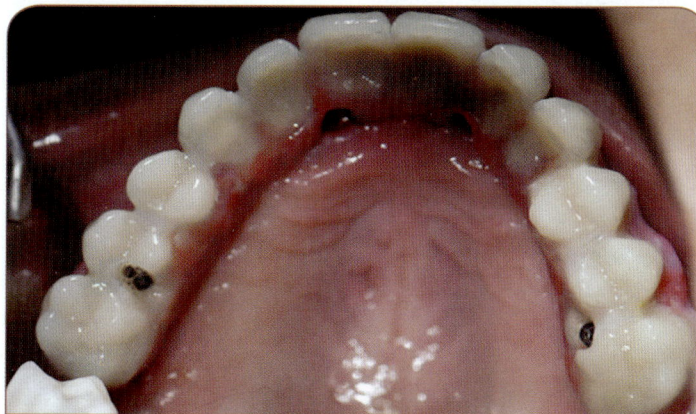

Fig. 7

The transverse screws are tightened palatally **(Fig. 7)**.

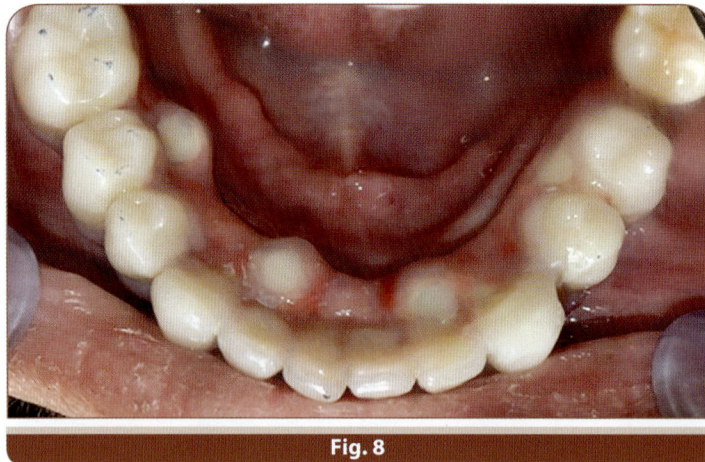

Occlusal view of the lower jaw **(Fig. 8)**.

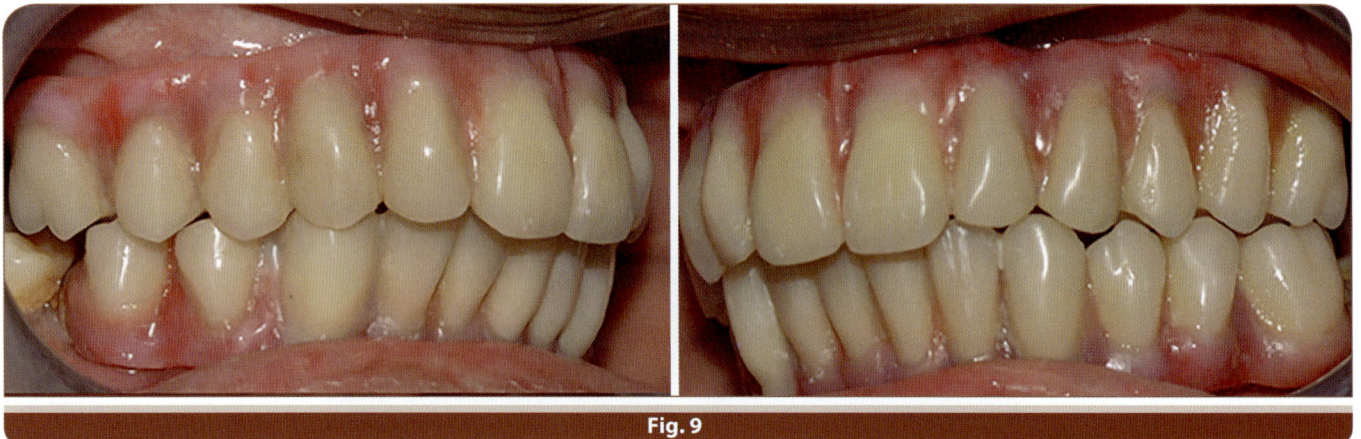

Right and left lateral view of the finished prosthesis **(Fig. 9)**.

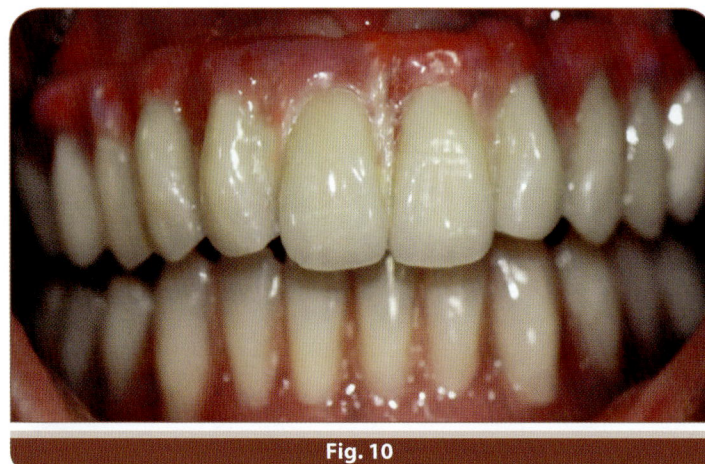

Facial view of the final visio.lign prosthesis **(Fig. 10)**.

Glenn Mascarenhas

Full Mouth Rehabilitation with Dental Implants 3D Printed Laser Sintered Frameworks in Segments with Porcelain Fused to the Metal

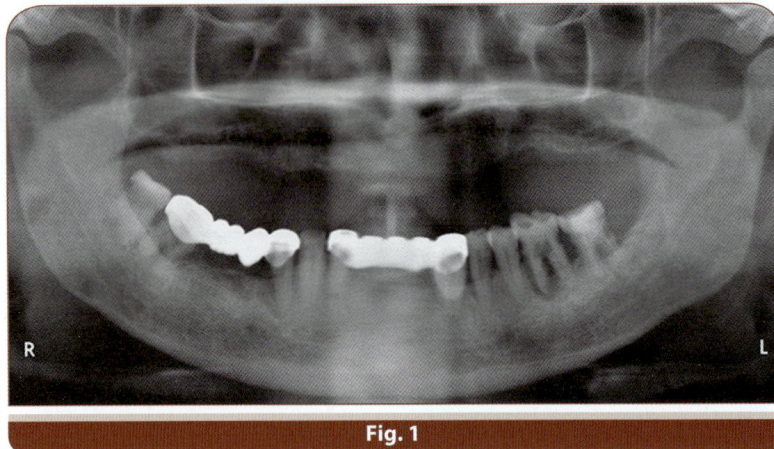

Fig. 1

Preoperative orthopantomogram (OPG) with edentulous maxilla and failing dentition in the mandible **(Fig. 1)**.

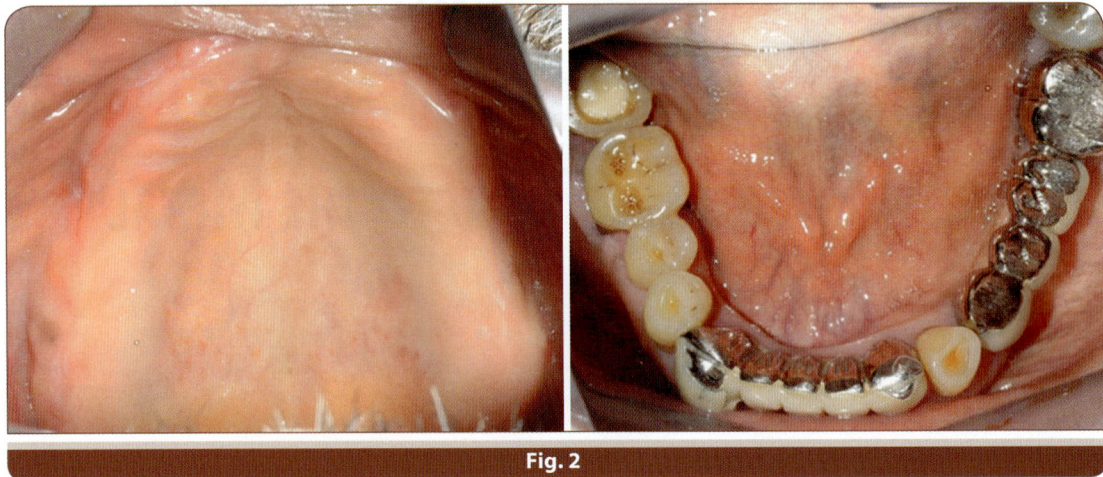

Fig. 2

Occlusal views of maxilla and mandible **(Fig. 2)**.

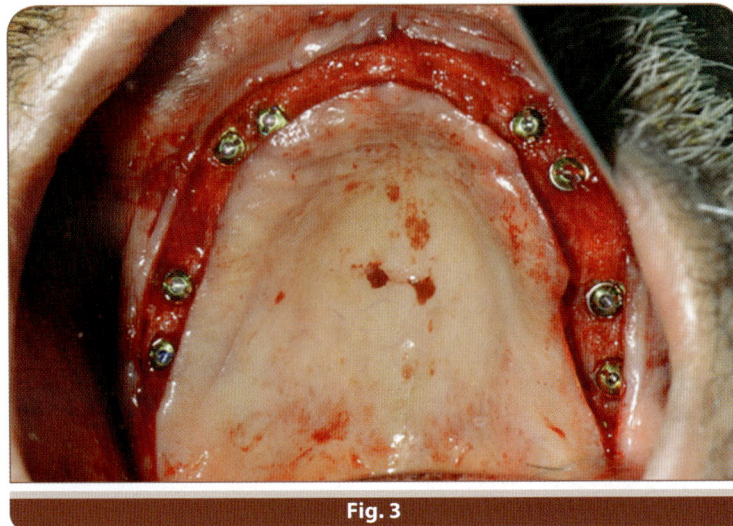

Fig. 3

Eight Dentium Superline implants inserted in the maxilla—all 4 posterior implants inserted after indirect sinus floor elevation with Platelet-rich fibrin (PRF) **(Fig. 3)**.

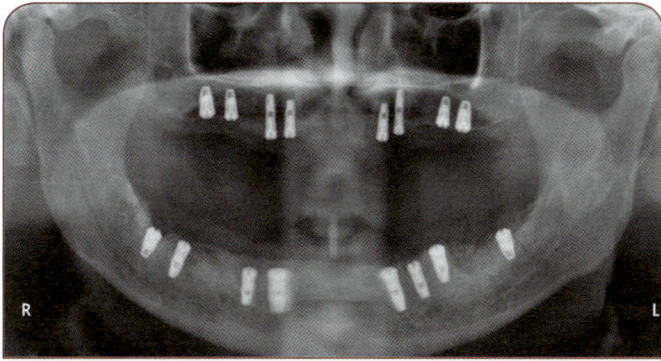

Fig. 4

Postoperative OPG with 8 Dentium Superline implants in the maxilla and 8 implants in the mandible **(Fig. 4)**.

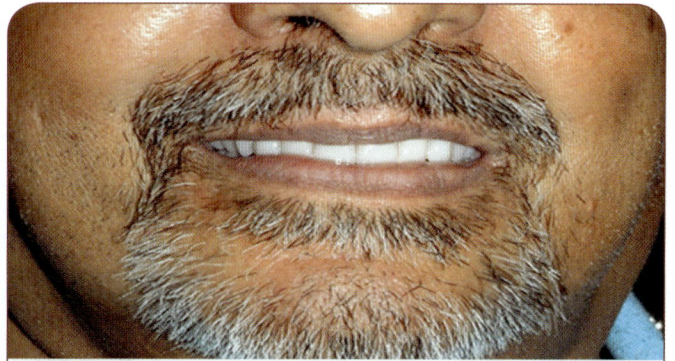

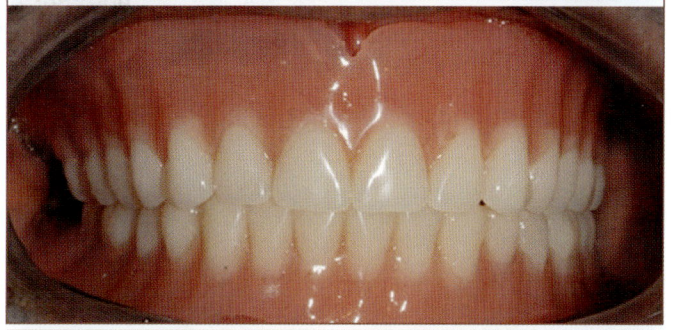

Fig. 5

Complete dentures fabricated as interim prosthesis **(Fig. 5)**.

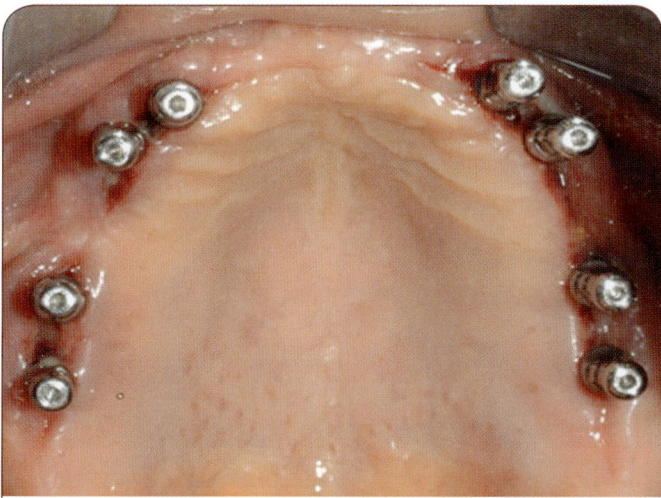

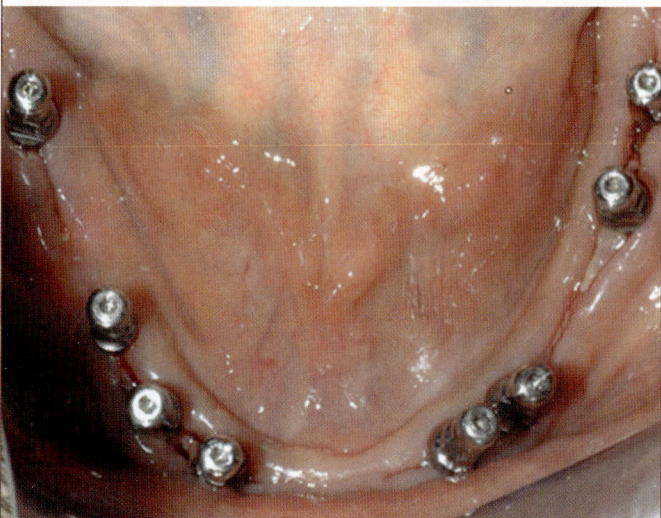

Fig. 6

3 months post operative, impression posts in place for closed tray impression technique **(Fig. 6)**.

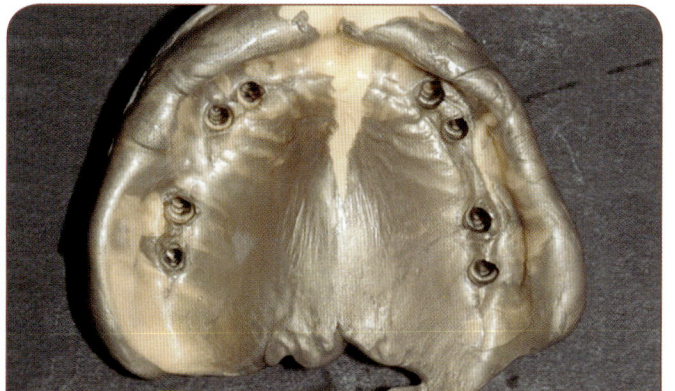

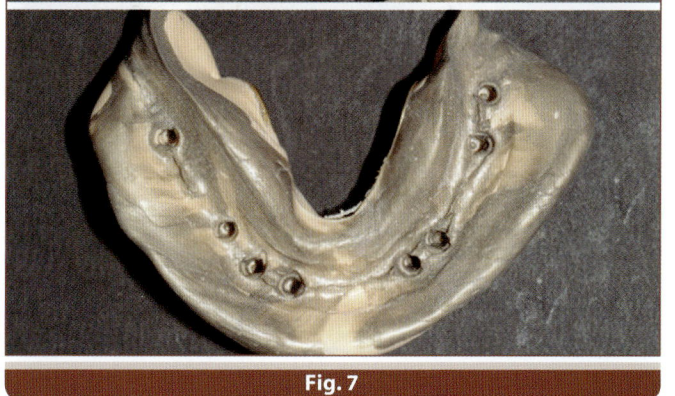

Fig. 7

Putty/wash polyvinyl siloxane impressions **(Fig. 7)**.

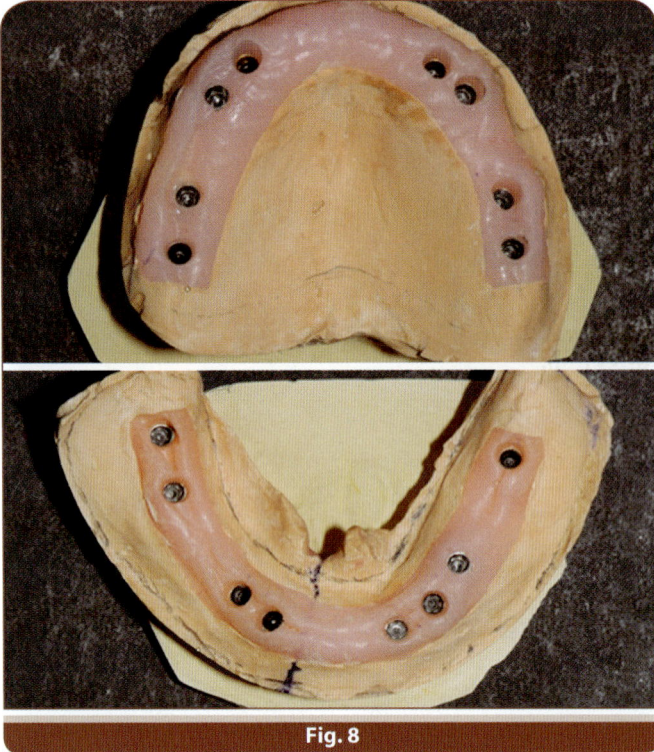

Fig. 8

Upper and lower working models **(Fig. 8)**.

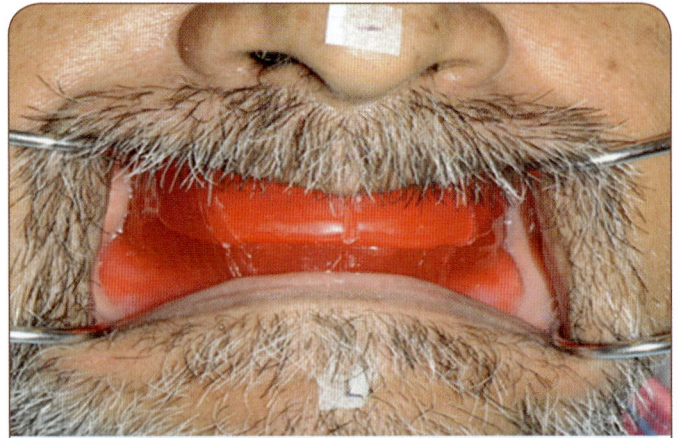

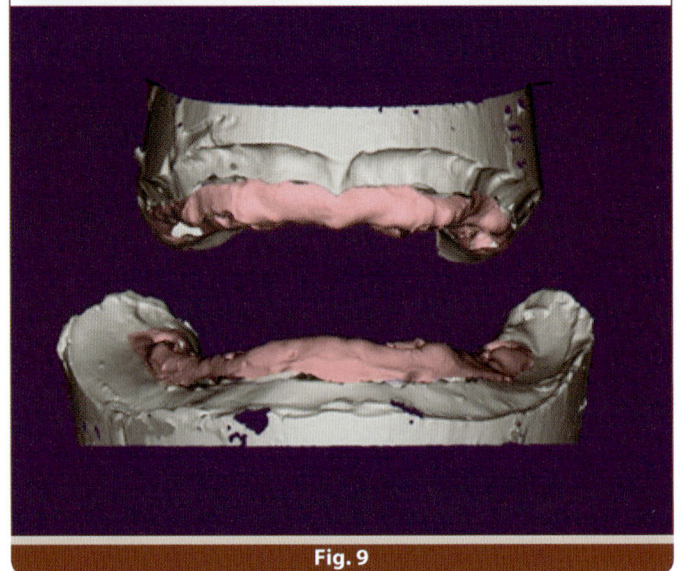

Fig. 9

Jaw relation recorded. Virtually articulated casts **(Fig. 9)**.

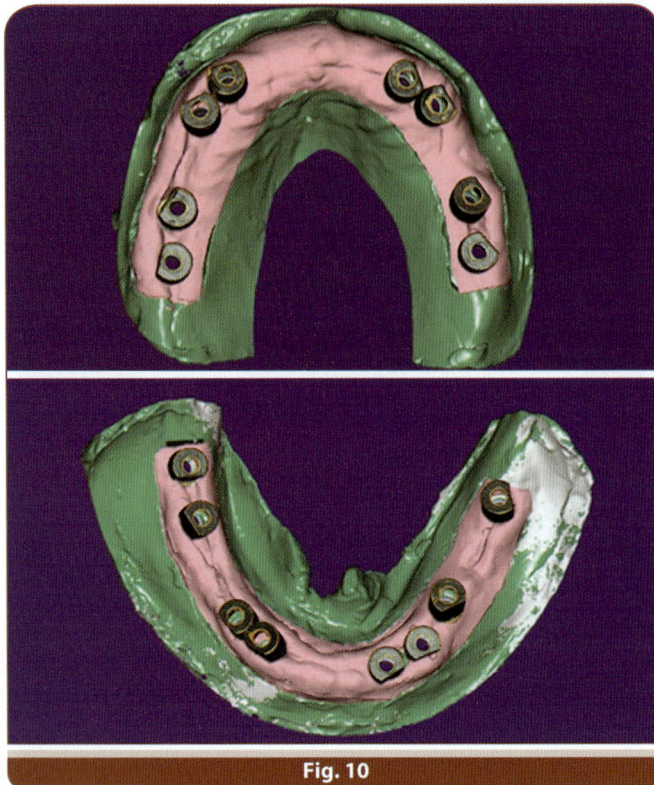

Fig. 10

Models with scan bodies **(Fig. 10)**.

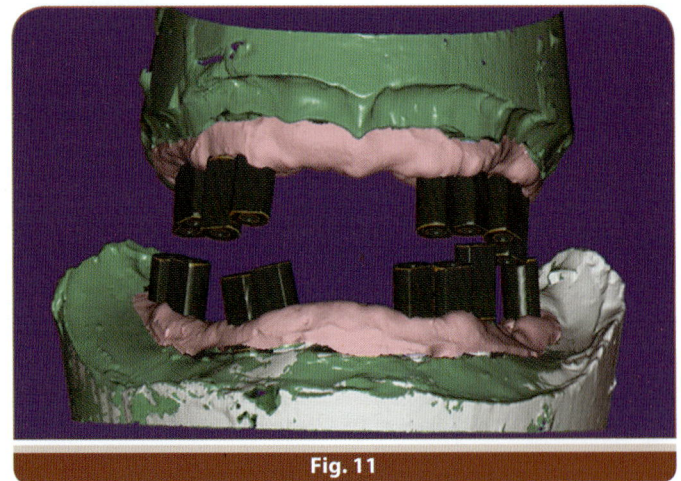

Fig. 11

Scan bodies with articulation **(Fig. 11)**.

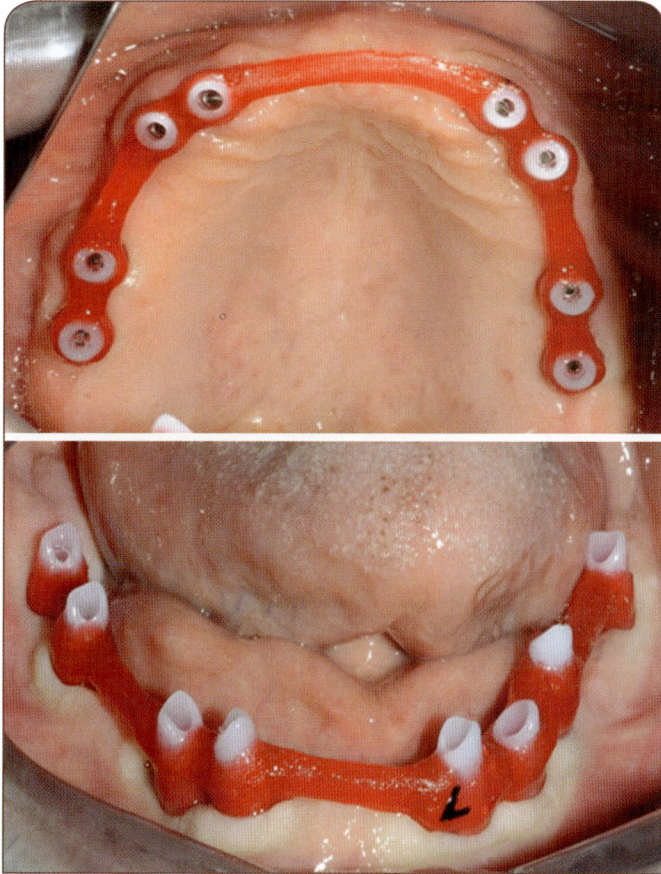

Fig. 12

Jig trial Duralay frameworks to verify accuracy of fit (Fig. 12).

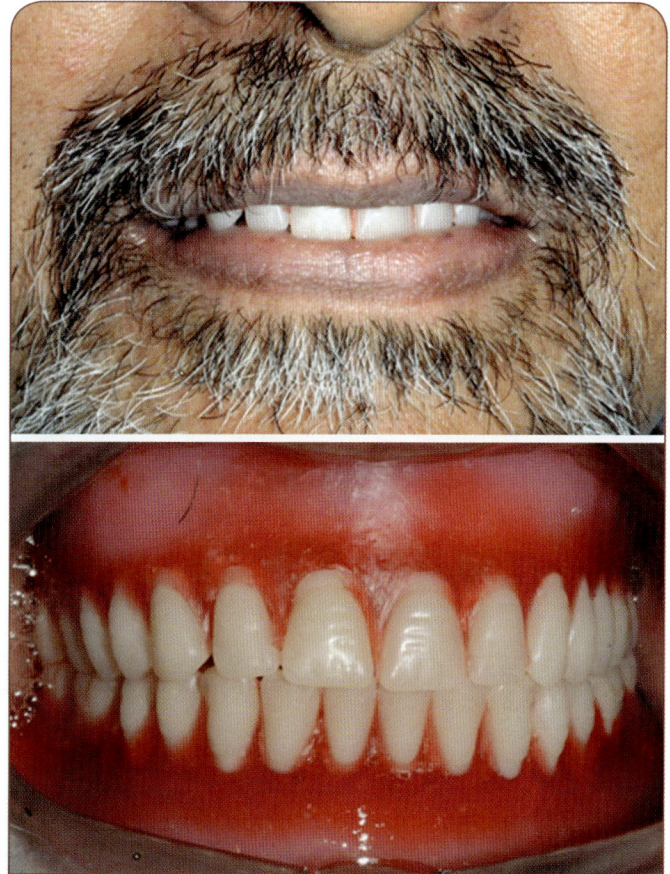

Fig. 13

Set-up trial (Fig. 13).

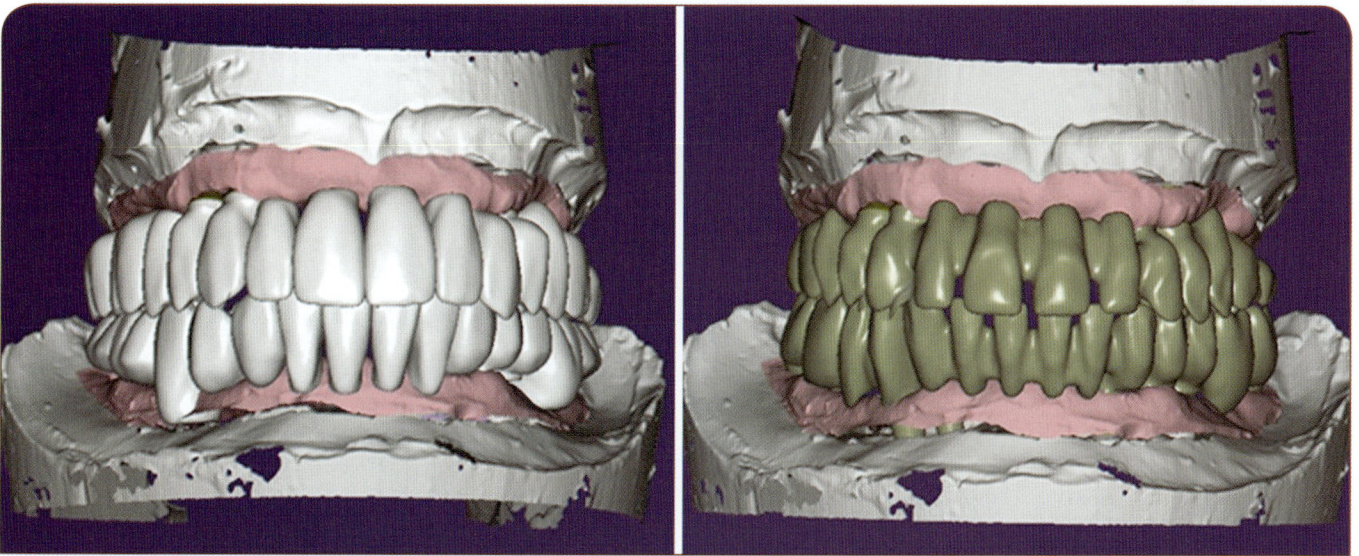

Fig. 14

Virtual prosthesis planned. Cut back for metal printing (Fig. 14).

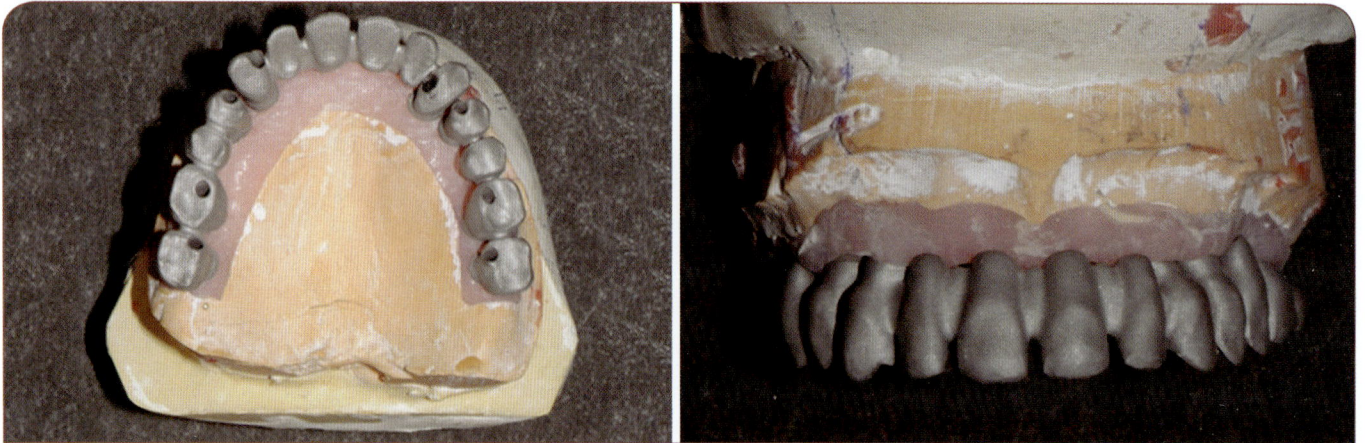

Fig. 15

3D printed - Laser sintered maxillary framework in 3 segments **(Fig. 15)**.

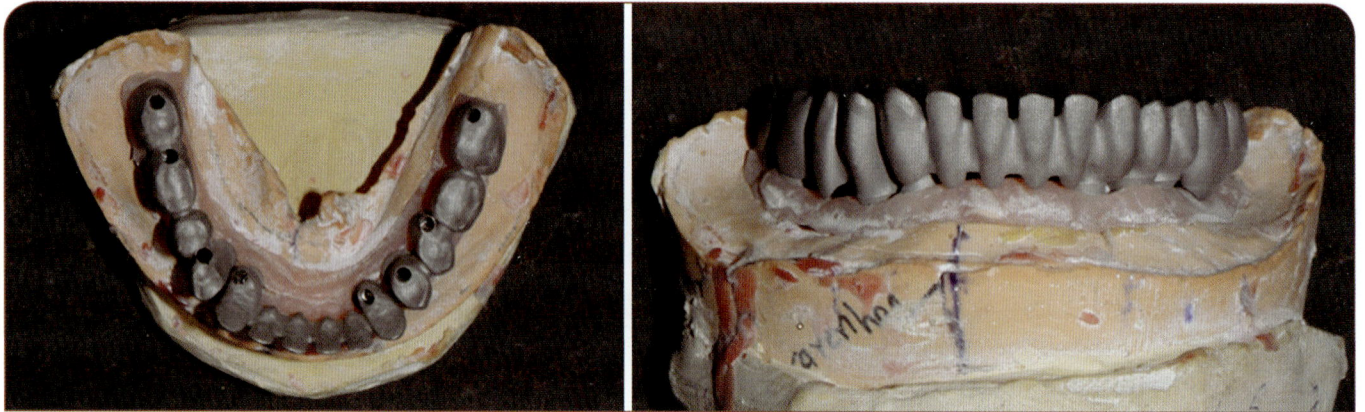

Fig. 16

3D printed—Laser sintered mandibular framework in 3 segments **(Fig. 16)**.

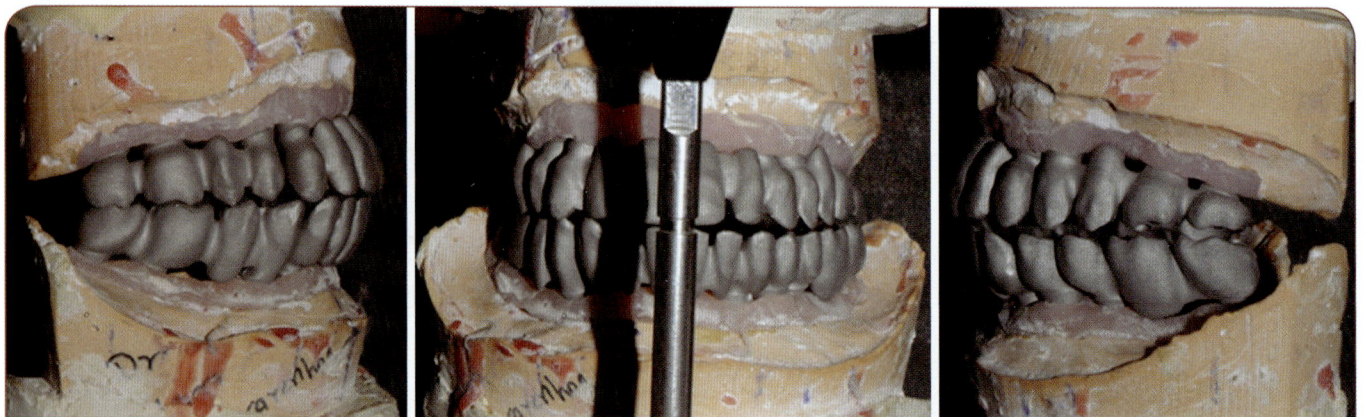

Fig. 17

3D printed frameworks on working models **(Fig. 17)**.

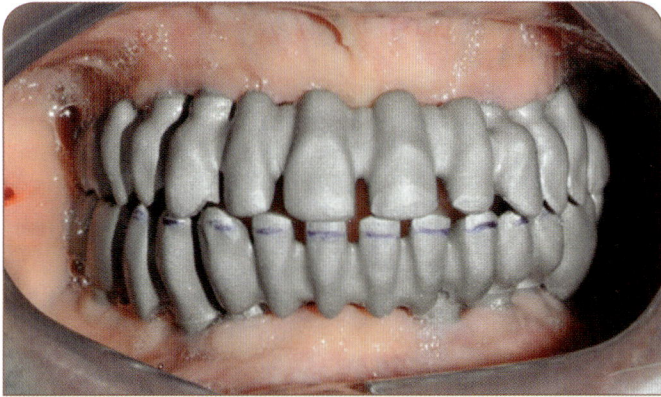

Fig. 18

Trial of 3D printed frameworks **(Fig. 18)**.

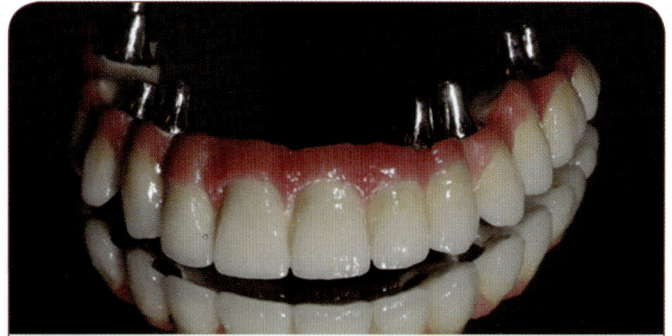

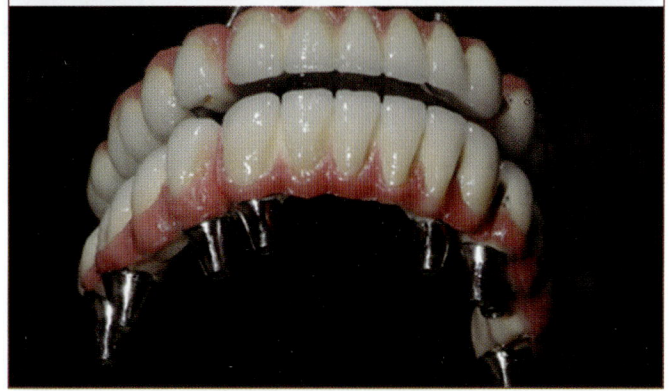

Fig. 19

3D printed upper and lower framework with porcelain fused to the metal **(Fig. 19)**.

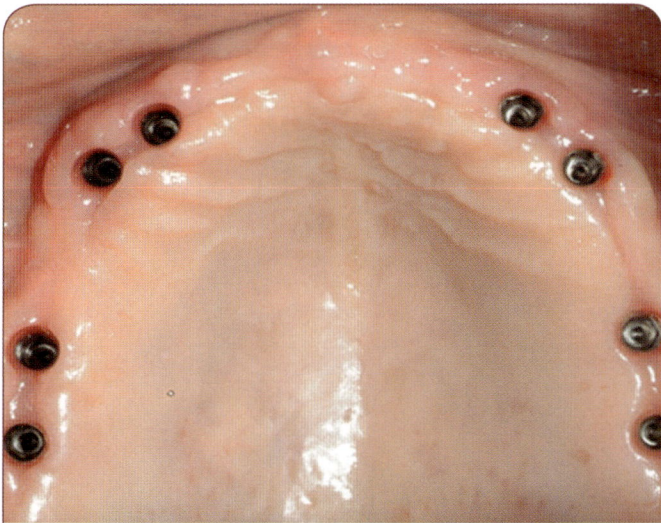

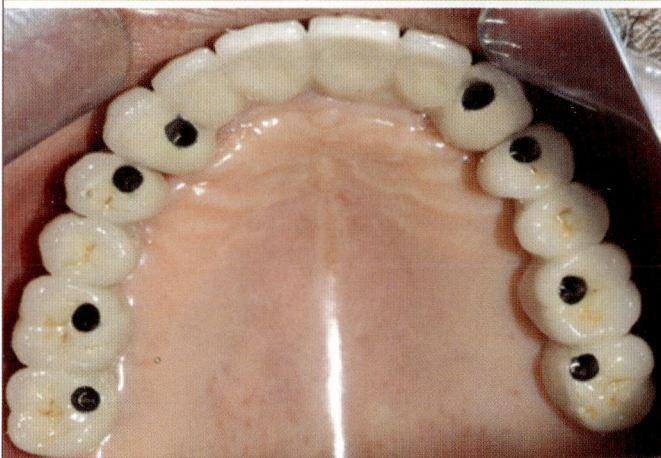

Fig. 20

Maxillary implants without healing abutments. Upper screw-retained prosthesis in situ **(Fig. 20)**.

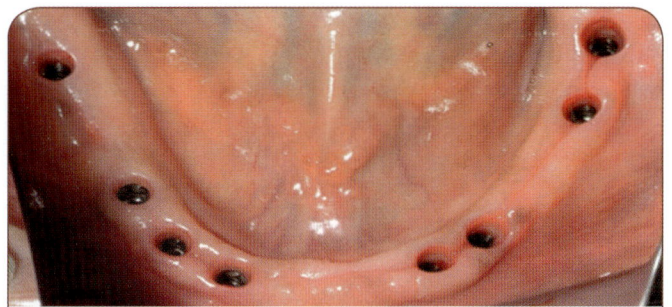

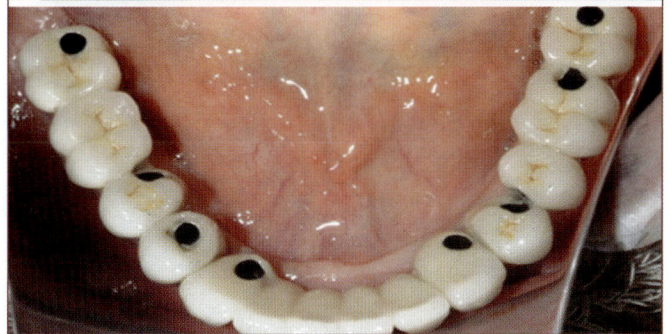

Fig. 21

Mandibular implants without healing abutments. Lower screw-retained prosthesis in situ **(Fig. 21)**.

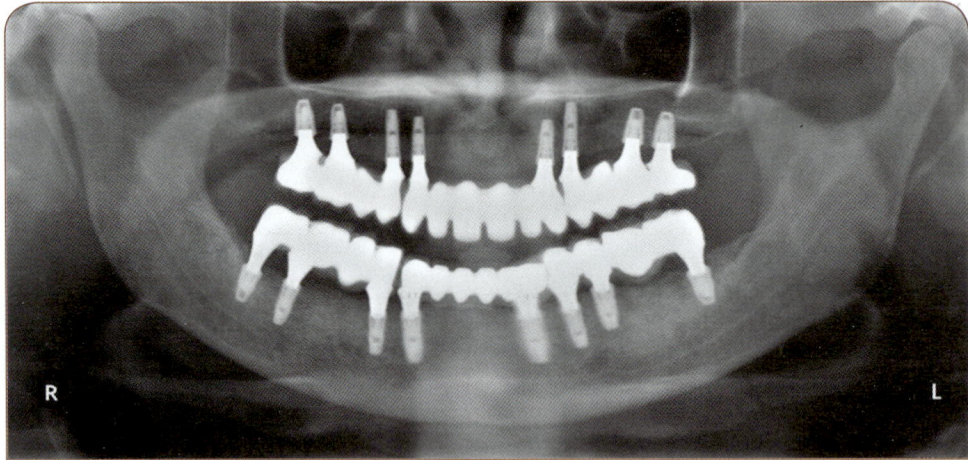

Fig. 22

Post-loading orthopantomogram (OPG) **(Fig. 22)**.

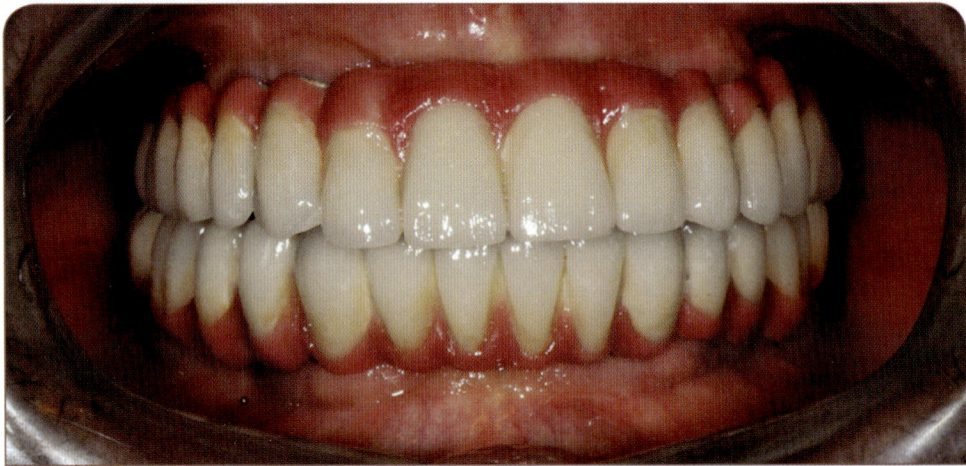

Fig. 23

Retracted view of prosthesis **(Fig. 23)**.

Lanka Mahesh

Extra Oral Cementation of an Implant Prosthesis Replacing a Single Posterior Tooth

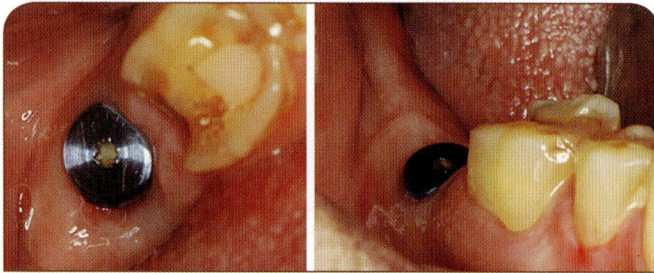

Fig. 1

A 45 year old male patient. A 5.11.5 Nobel replace select (Nobel Biocare) implant was placed immediately post extraction with a healing collar at the time of implant placement. Clinical view 3 months postoperative **(Fig. 1)**.

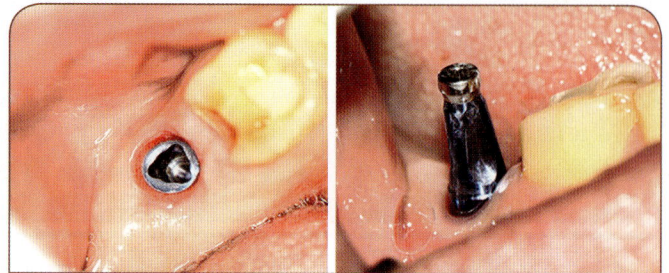

Fig. 2

Removal of the healing collar exhibits nice tissue around the implant. An impression post is screwed into place and verified with an IOPA X-ray to ensure correct seating **(Fig. 2)**.

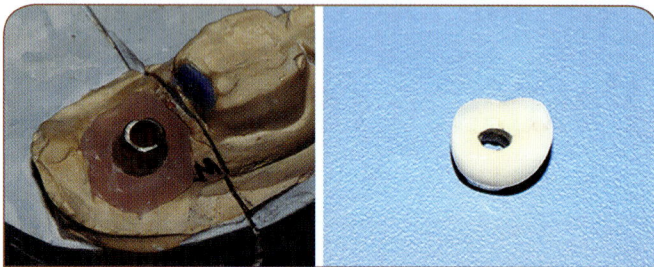

Fig. 3

The master cast with cotton and modelling wax placed into the abutment. The PFM prosthesis with an occlusal vent **(Fig. 3)**.

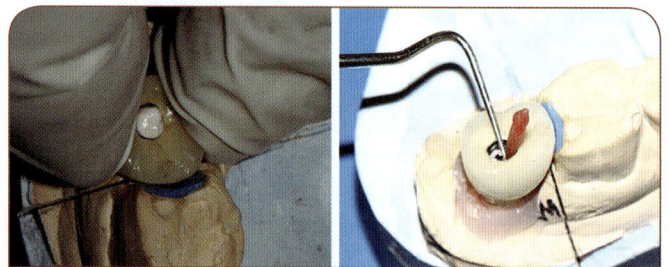

Fig. 4

The crown is cemented on the abutment with Rely X™ U200 with positive finger pressure. After the cement has set the occlusal cement and the wax and cotton pellet are removed with an explorer **(Fig. 4)**.

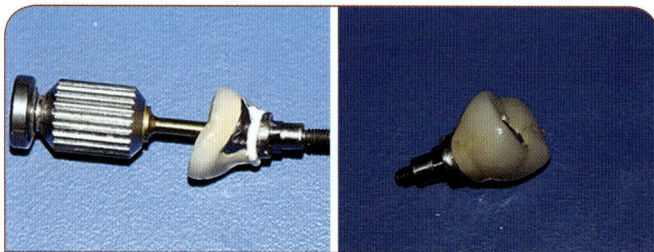

Fig. 5

A large quantity of cement is clearly visible on the abutment implant interface, after removal of the crown from the model. View after the excess cement is removed **(Fig. 5)**.

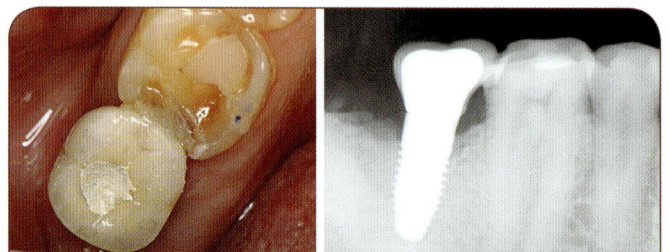

Fig. 6

The implant was torqued onto the abutment. The access hole was blocked with teflon tape and a temporary filling material, Cavit (3M). 4 years postoperative clinical and radiographic images show a stable peri-implant tissue response and stable crestal bone levels **(Fig. 6)**.

Glenn Mascarenhas

Full Arch Rehabilitation
Titanium Milled Framework with Individual
Zirconia Crowns

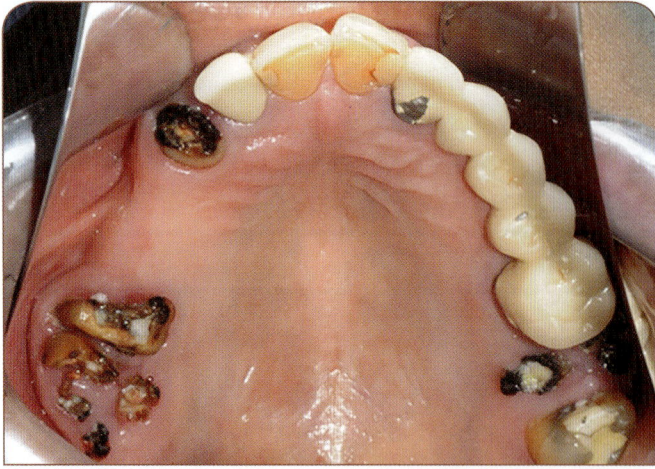

Fig. 1

Failing upper dentition in a female patient aged 58 years (**Fig. 1**).

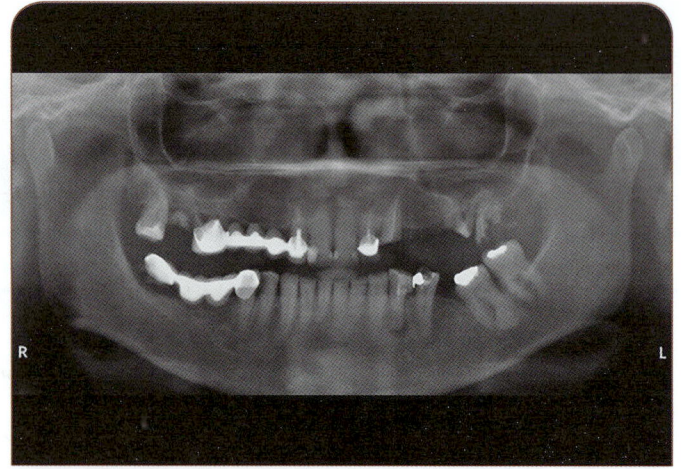

Fig. 2

Failing upper and lower right dentition. Chronic periapical infections in lower left premolars (**Fig. 2**).

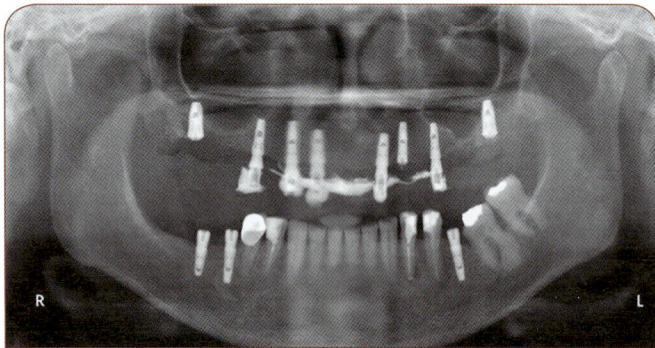

Fig. 3

Total upper extractions. Eight Dentium Superline implants placed in the maxilla and 3 implants in the mandible (**Fig. 3**).

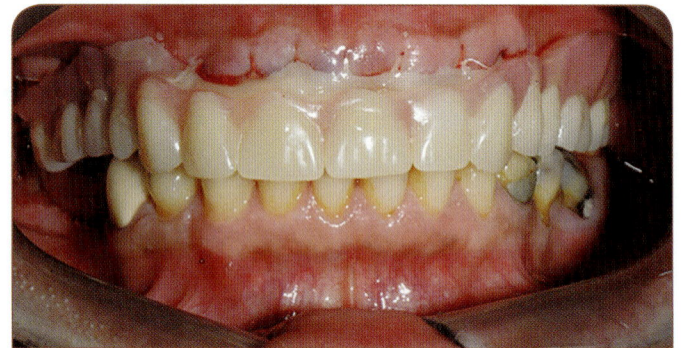

Fig. 4

Immediate temporary acrylic prosthesis placed on 5 implants (**Fig. 4**).

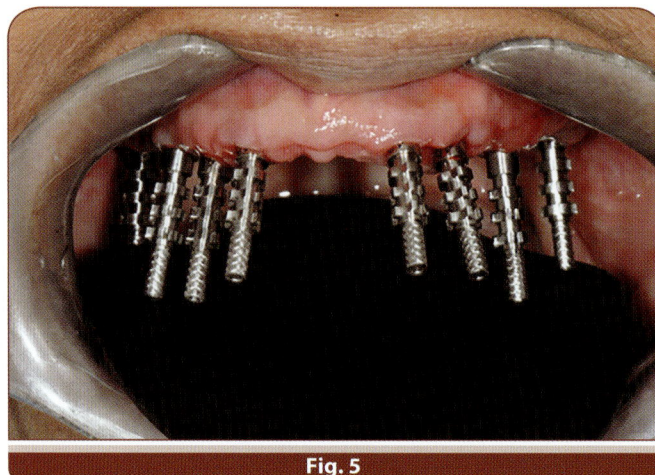

Fig. 5

Open tray impression made after 3 months of healing (**Fig. 5**).

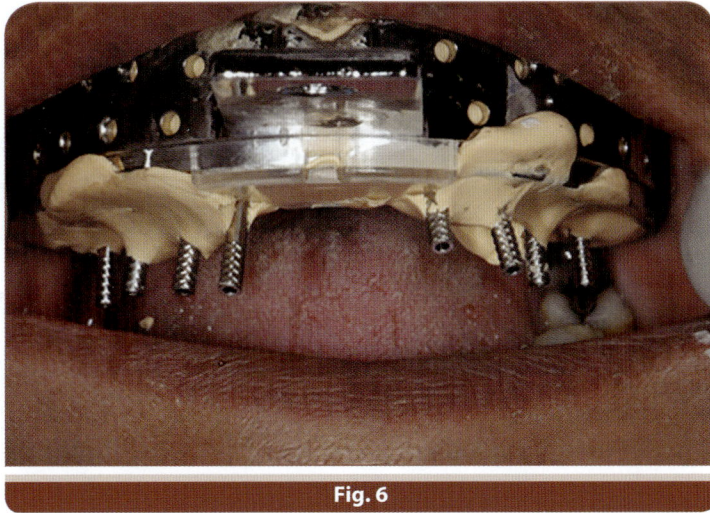

Fig. 6

Impression tray with polyvinyl siloxane (PVS) impression material for open tray impression technique **(Fig. 6)**.

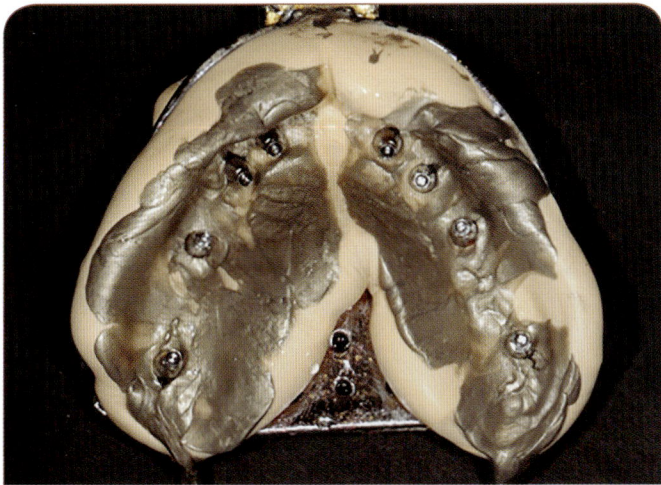

Fig. 8

Jaw relation recorded **(Fig. 8)**.

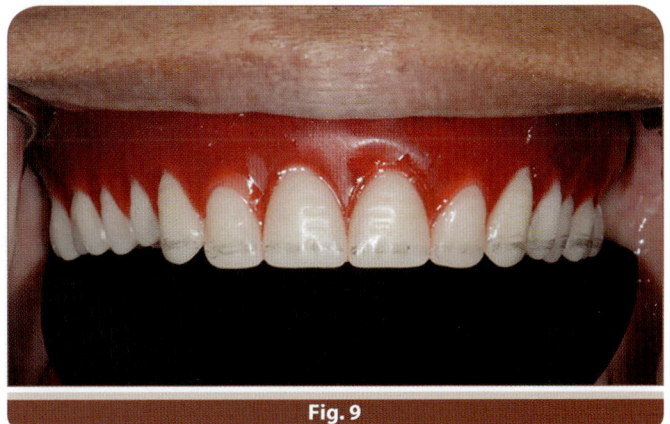

Fig. 7

Open tray impression with impression posts in place **(Fig. 7)**.

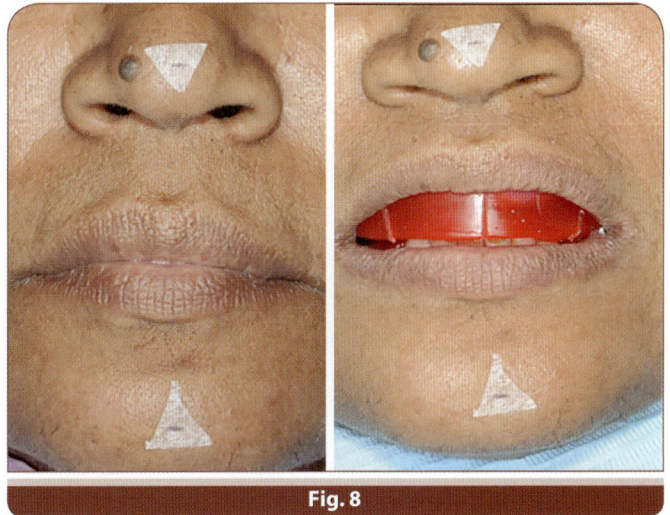

Fig. 9

Corrections being recorded during a set-up trial **(Fig. 9)**.

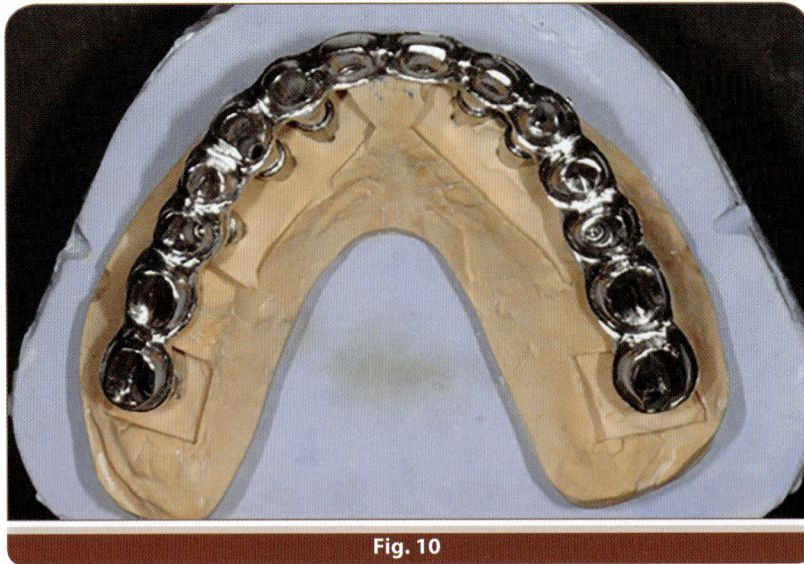

Fig. 10

Milled titanium framework for individual zirconia crowns (Malo bridge) **(Fig. 10)**.

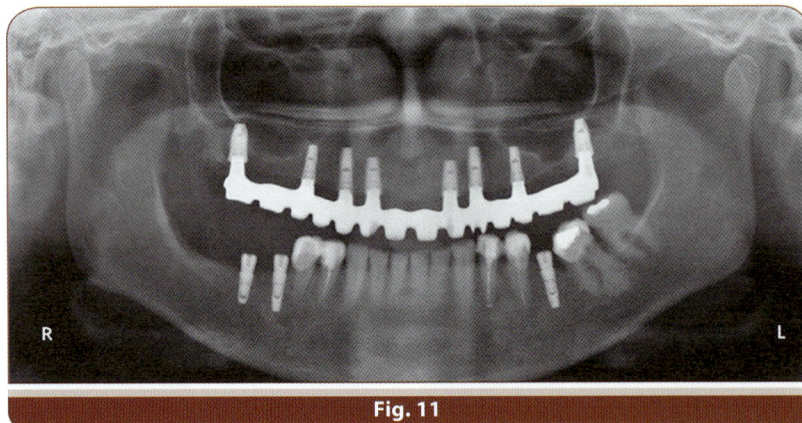

Fig. 11

Orthopantomogram (OPG) showing trial of milled titanium framework **(Fig. 11)**.

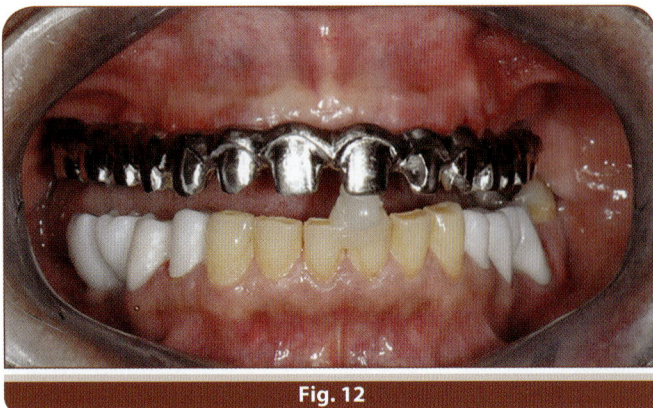

Fig. 12

Trial of milled framework and lower Zirconia copings **(Fig. 12)**.

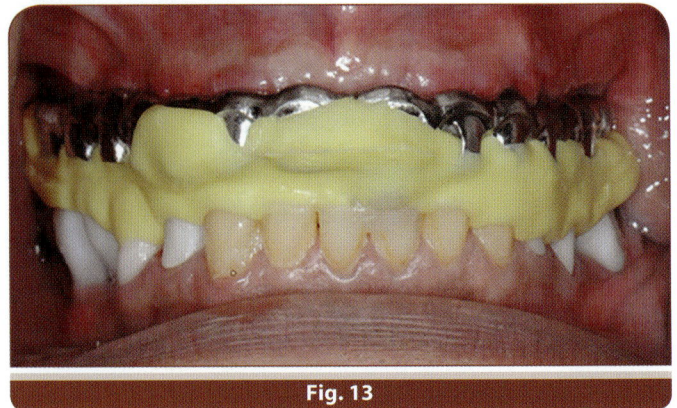

Fig. 13

Bite registration in Polyether **(Fig. 13)**.

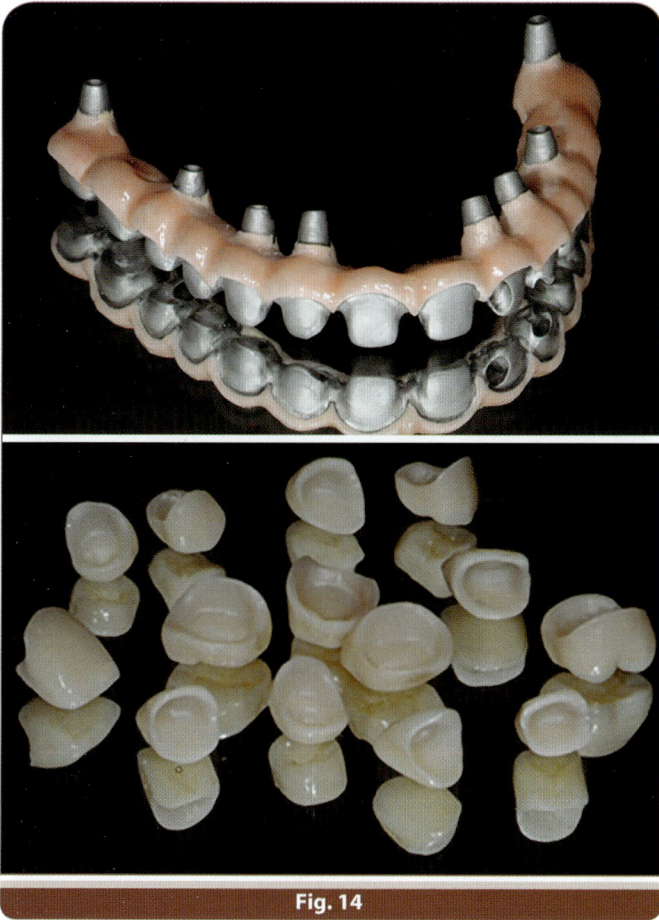
Fig. 14

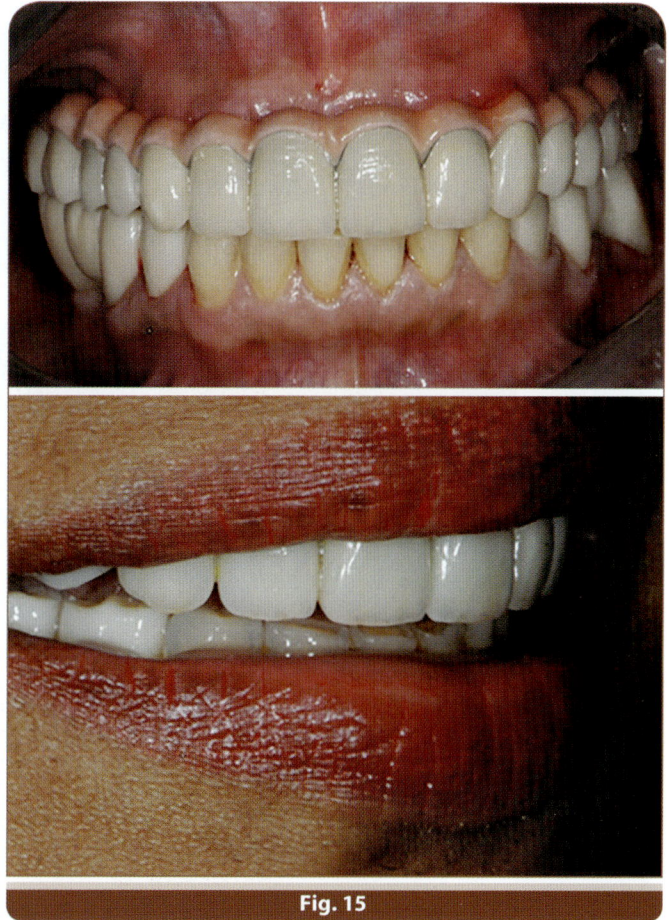
Fig. 15

Gingival Porcelain on framework. Layered Zirconia crowns for the anteriors and monolithic crowns for the posteriors (**Fig. 14**).

In centric occlusion. Natural aesthetics with individual crowns (**Fig. 15**).

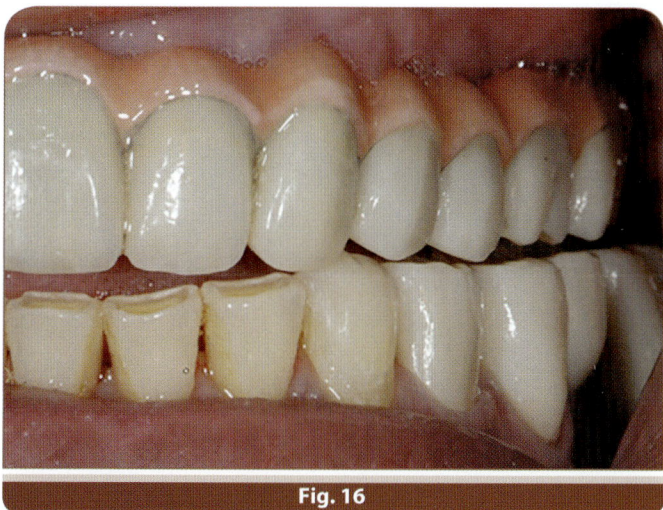
Fig. 16

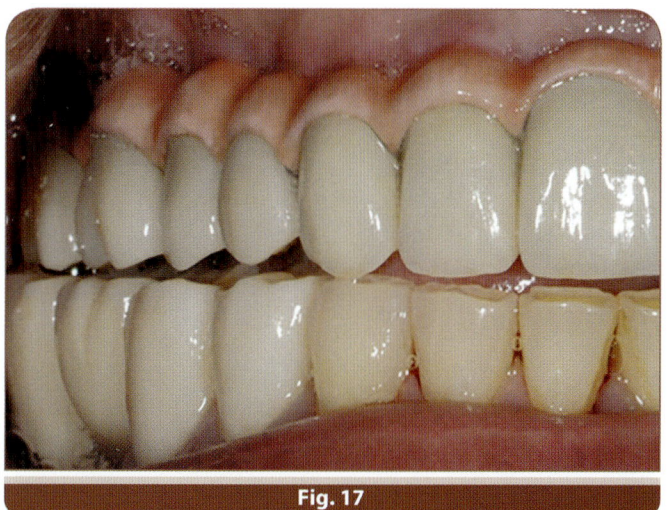
Fig. 17

Checking the left lateral excursion for canine guided occlusion (**Fig. 16**).

Checking the right lateral excursion for canine guided occlusion (**Fig. 17**).

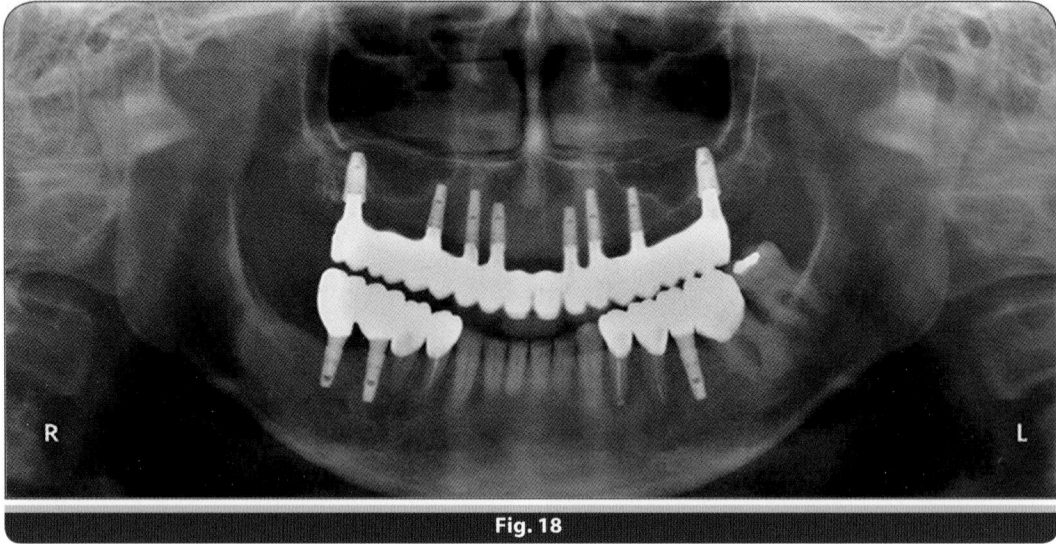

Orthopantomogram (OPG) of prosthesis (**Fig. 18**).

Praful Bali, Ashish Chowdhary

LOWER COMPLETE CERAMIC BRIDGE WORK ON "ALL ON 4"

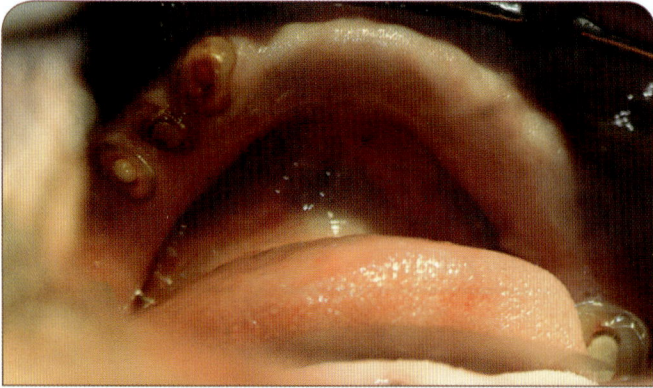

Fig. 1

Patient presents wearing an ill-fitting lower denture on some remaining lower teeth with the aim to fix the lower jaw with implants **(Fig. 1)**.

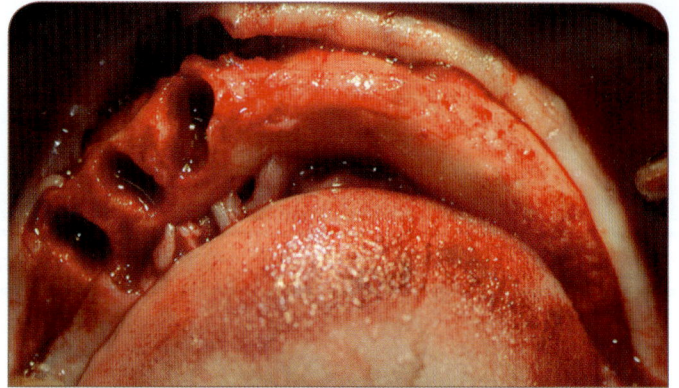

Fig. 2

Flap reflection done **(Fig. 2)**.

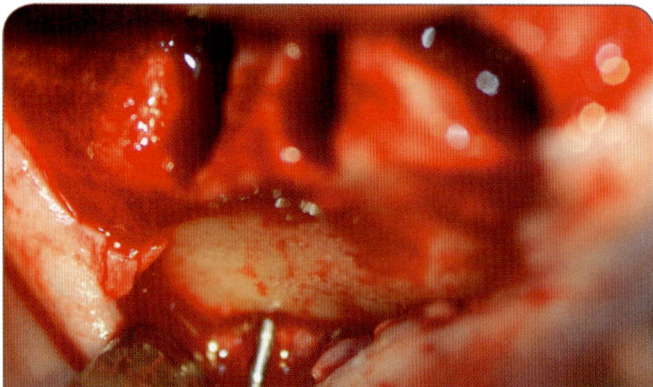

Fig. 3

Identification of the Mental canal exposing the nerve to evade possible injury to this vital structure **(Fig. 3)**.

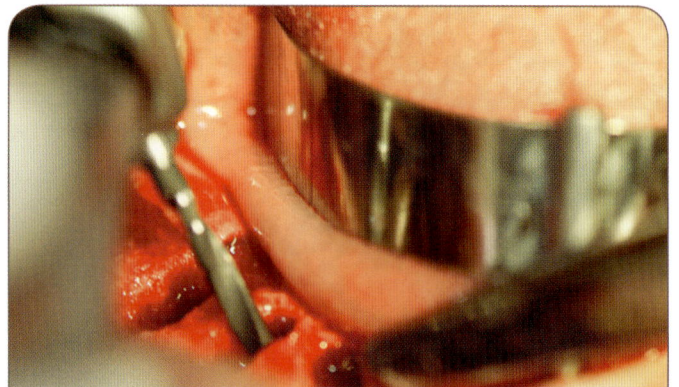

Fig. 4

2 mm drill to prepare site for tilted implant at 45 degrees **(Fig. 4)**.

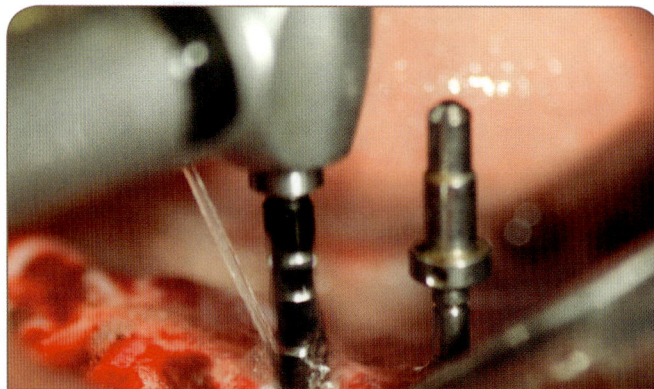

Fig. 5

Osteotomy site preparation for anterior straight implants **(Fig. 5)**.

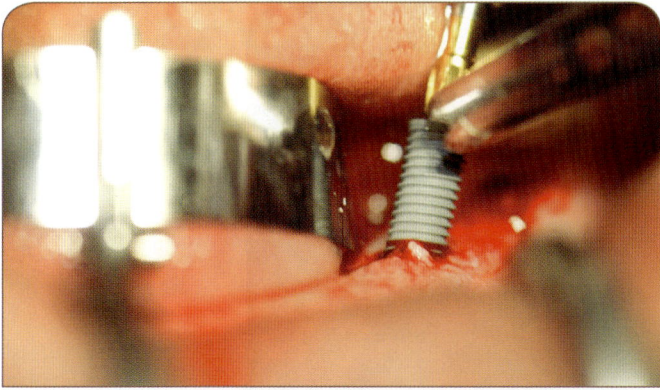

Fig. 6

Tilted implant placement in the posterior region (**Fig. 6**).

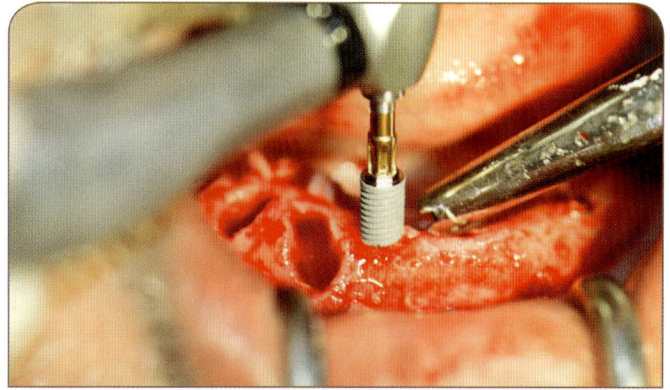

Fig. 7

Implant placement at 0 degrees in the anterior region (**Fig. 7**).

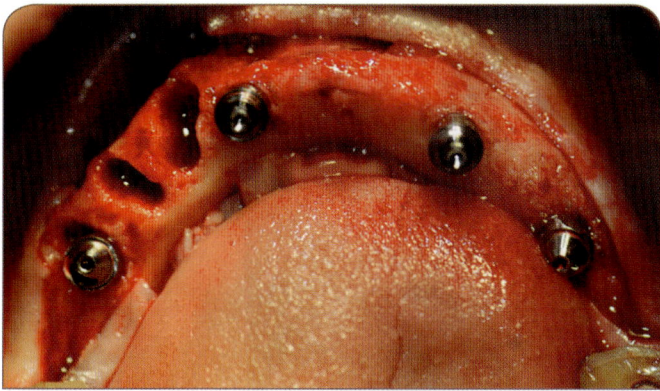

Fig. 8

Multiunit abutments torqued to the 4 implants (**Fig. 8**).

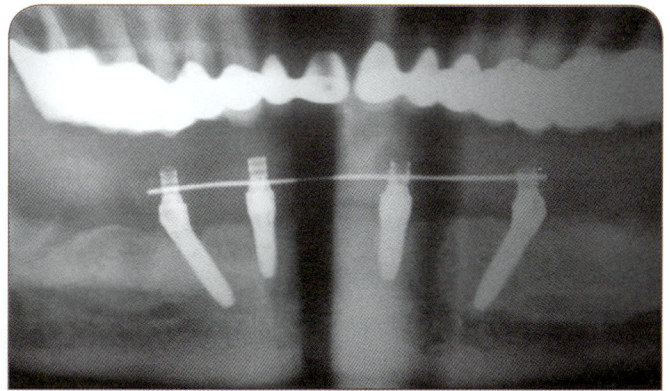

Fig. 9

Immediate postoperative OPG (**Fig. 9**).

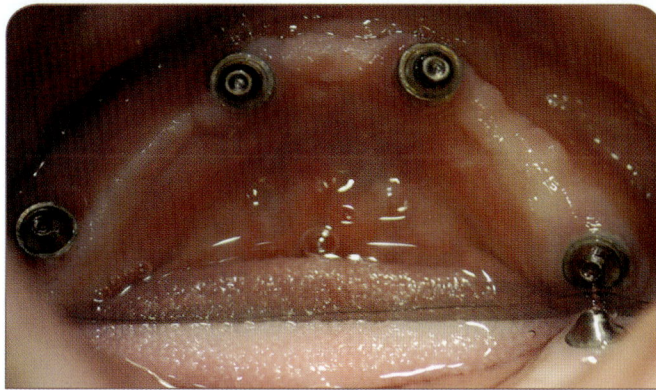

Fig. 10

3 months postoperative view of the lower arch (**Fig. 10**).

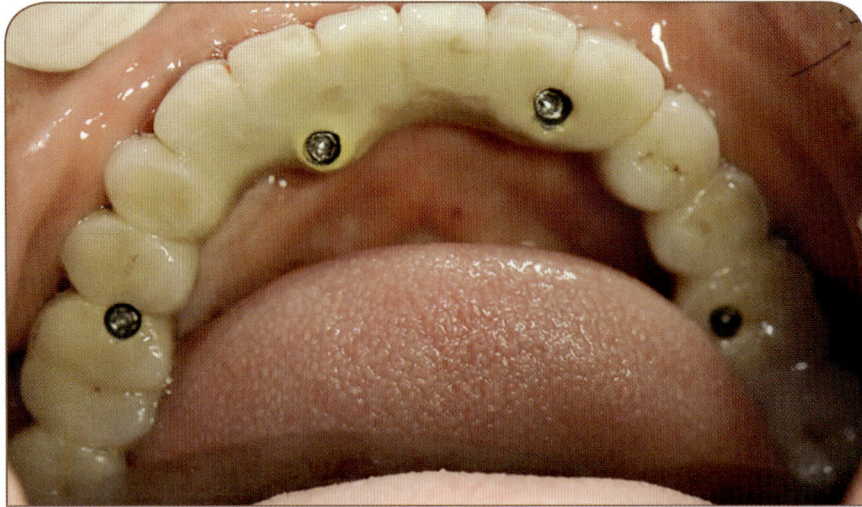

Fig. 11

A full arch ceramic final prosthesis made **(Fig. 11)**.

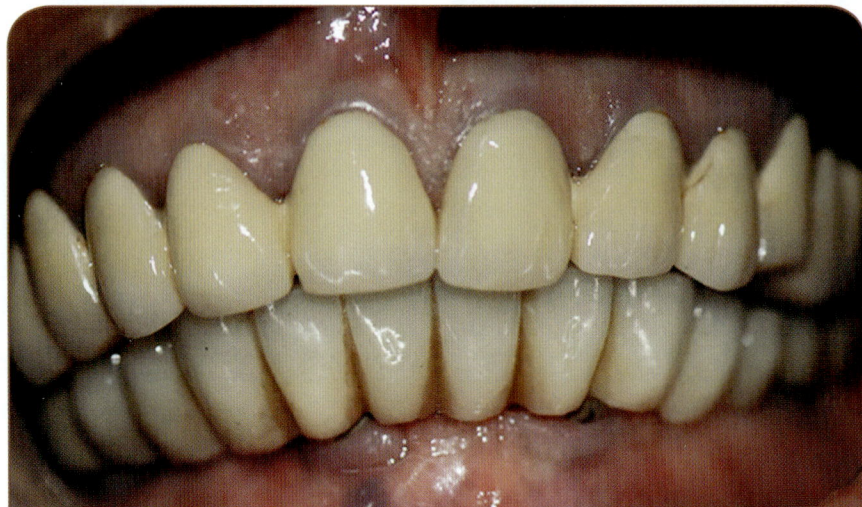

Fig. 12

Final facial view of the full arch ceramic prosthesis. Care taken to keep the pontic areas self cleansing **(Fig. 12)**.

CASE STUDY 113

Praful Bali, Shweta Gupta

Bio-HPP Framework for a Lower "Fast & Fixed" Prosthesis

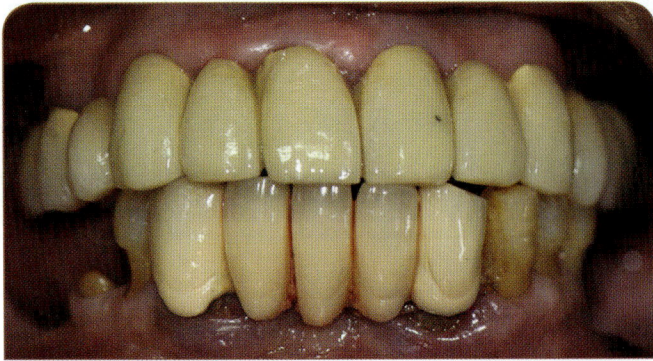

Fig. 1

Patient presents with a moving mandibular prosthesis and also grade 2 mobility with the remaining teeth. Patient is advised total extraction and rehabilitation with implants **(Fig. 1)**.

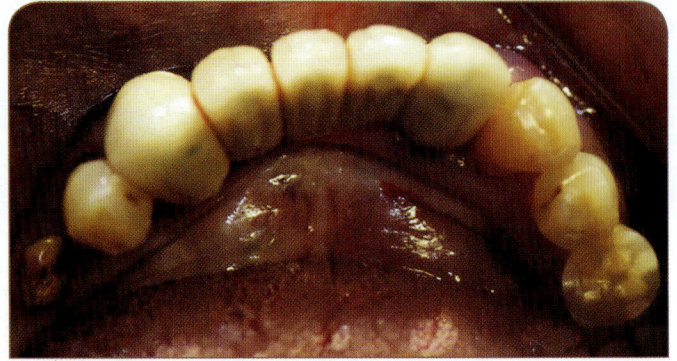

Fig. 2

Preoperative occlusal view of the failed dentition **(Fig. 2)**.

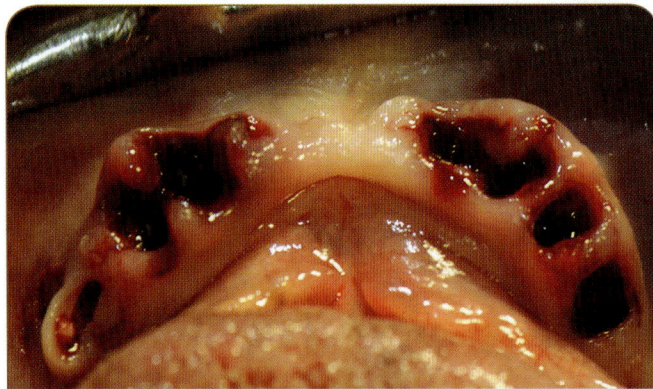

Fig. 3

All teeth are extracted and planned for a "Fast & Fixed" procedure **(Fig. 3)**.

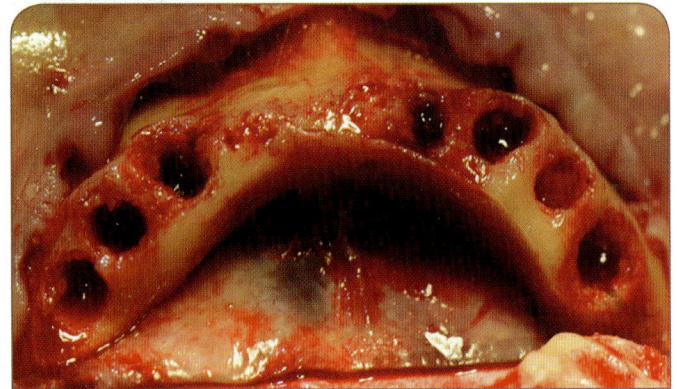

Fig. 4

Flap reflection is done with curettage of extraction sockets. The ridge is flattened where required **(Fig. 4)**.

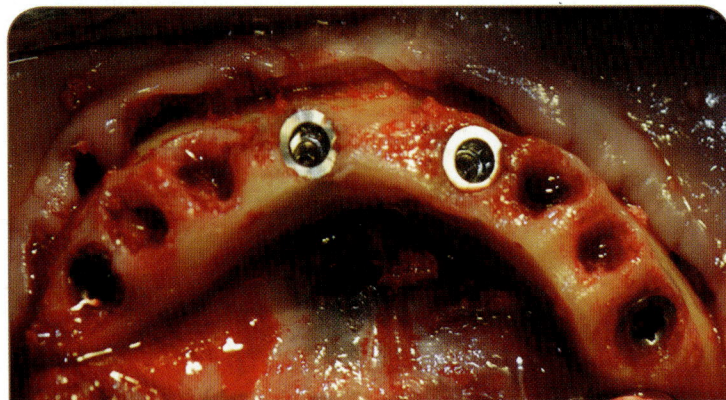

Fig. 5

4 Blue SKY Bredent implants placed: Posteriors at 45 degree and anteriors at 0 degree **(Fig. 5)**.

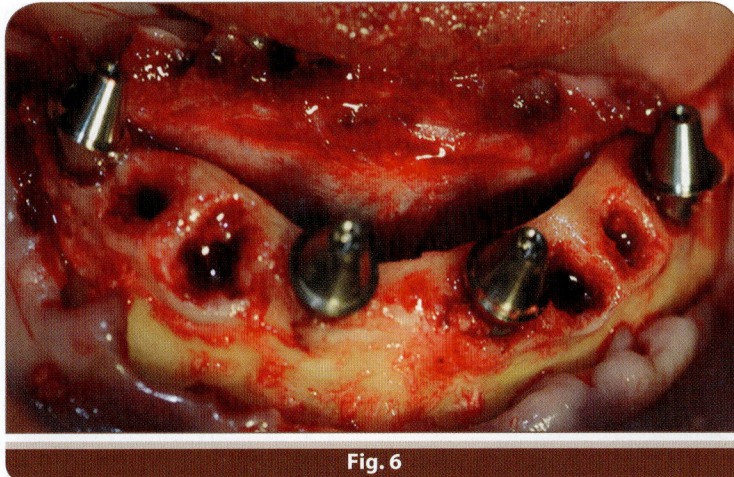

Fig. 6

"Fast & Fixed" abutments are torqued at 30 N/cm onto the 4 implants **(Fig. 6)**.

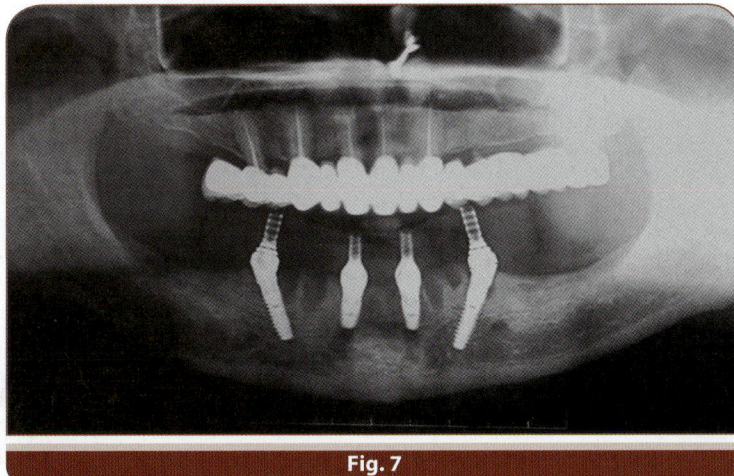

Fig. 7

Immediate postoperative OPG **(Fig. 7)**.

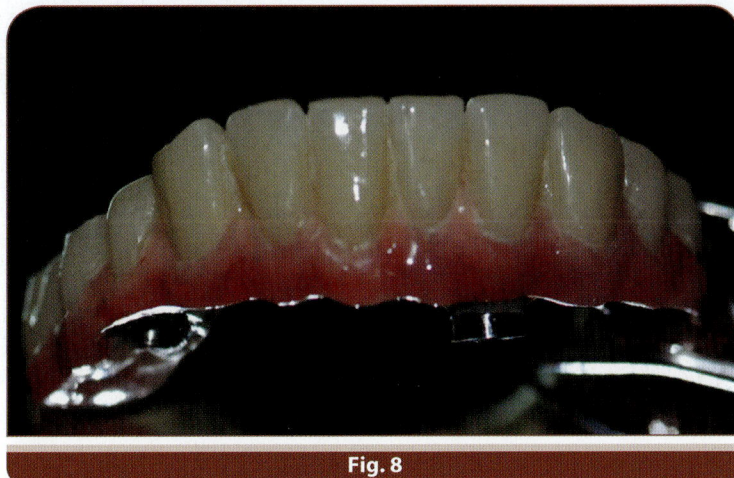

Fig. 8

The definitive prosthesis is made with Visio.lign over a Bio-HPP framework **(Fig. 8)**.

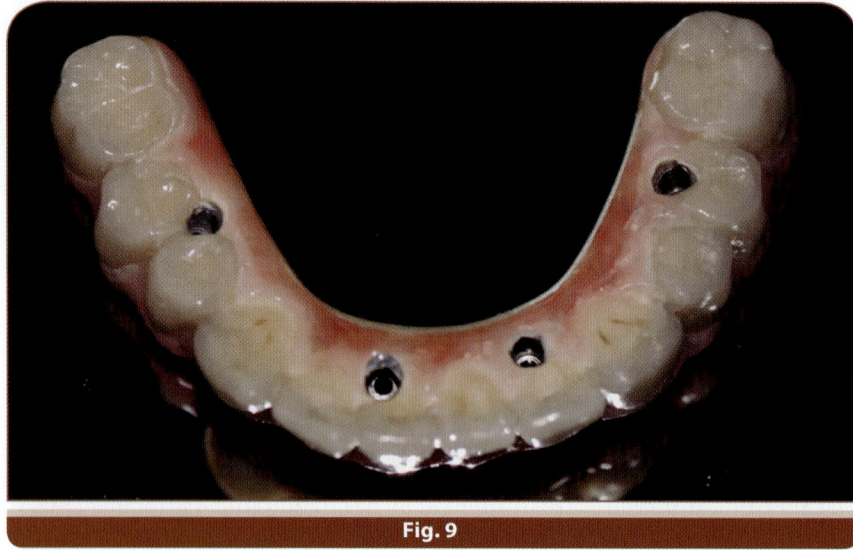

Fig. 9

Occlusal view of prosthesis with screw positions. One tooth each side is added as cantilever according to the prescribed AP spread **(Fig. 9)**.

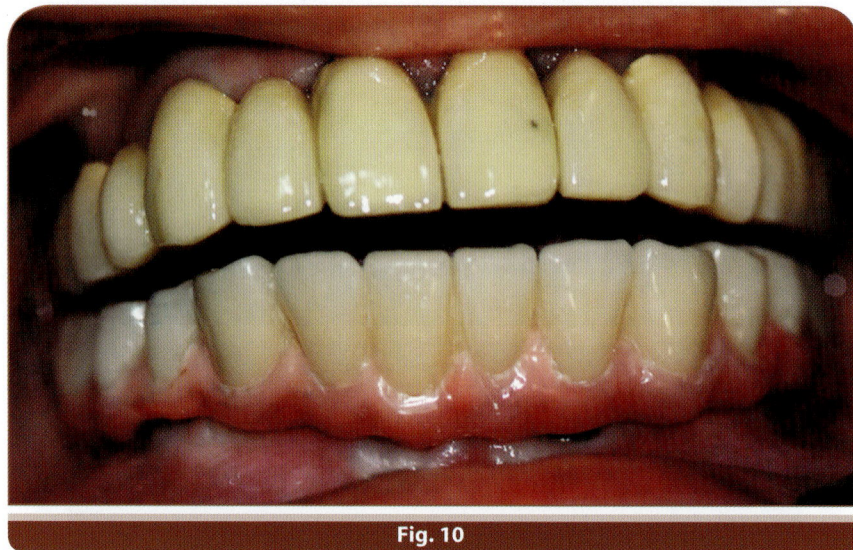

Fig. 10

Clinical view of the final prosthesis: The final Visio.lign- Bio HPP prosthesis is torqued at 15 N/cm **(Fig. 10)**.

Lanka Mahesh, Nitika Poonia

FULL MOUTH REHABILITATION WITH FIXED MAXILLARY HYBRID PROSTHESIS AND REMOVABLE IMPLANT SUPPORTED MANDIBULAR PROSTHESIS

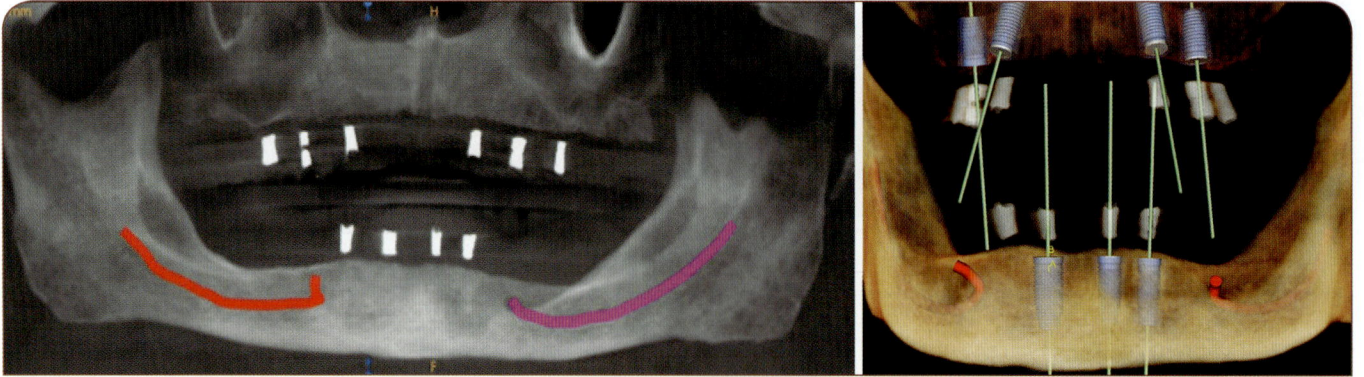

Fig. 1

Preoperative scan views showing enlarged sinuses and a high IAN bilaterally **(Fig. 1)**.

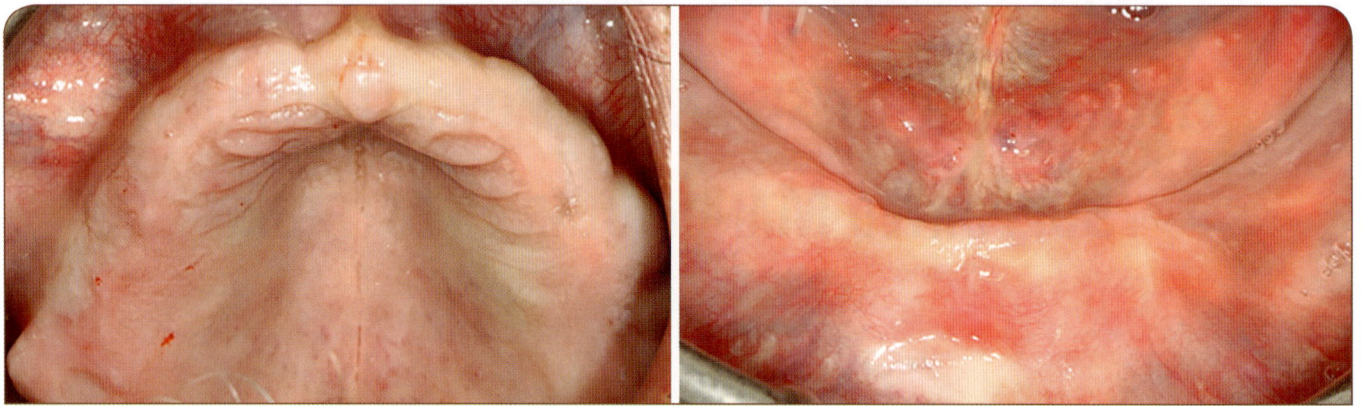

Fig. 2

Maxillary and mandibular preoperative view showing adequate soft tissue volume in both arches. The mandibular arch appears knife edge at the crest. Treatment plan included 6 intrasinus implants in the maxilla for a fixed hybrid prosthesis and 4 intraforamen implants in the mandible for a removable denture **(Fig. 2)**.

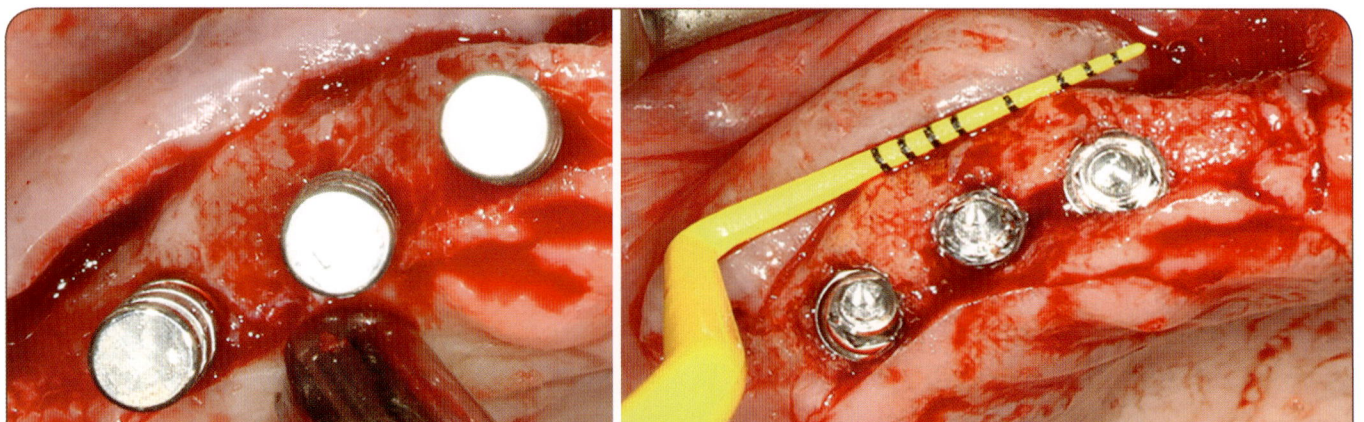

Fig. 3

Paralleling pins in the prepared osteotomies showing correct interimplant distance. 3 implants are inserted with a good volume of facial bone present (A.B. Dent). A periodontal probe is being used to highlight the same **(Fig. 3)**.

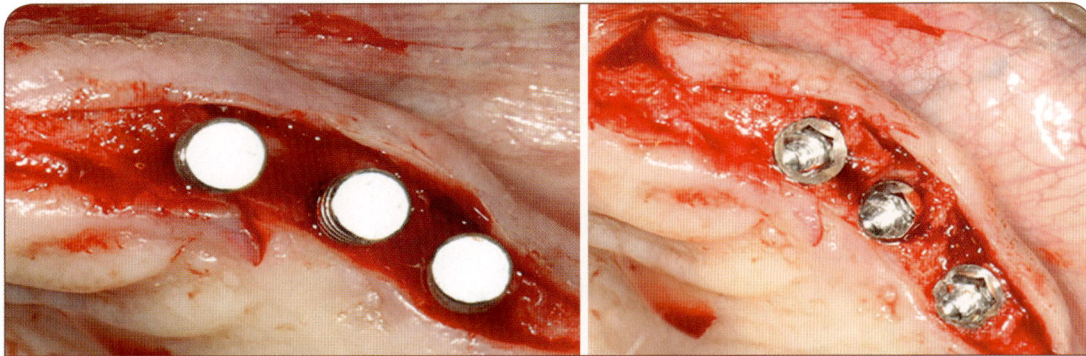

Fig. 4

The same protocol is followed on the left side. Implants are placed at the most distal aspects of available bone (mesial to the sinus) **(Fig. 4)**.

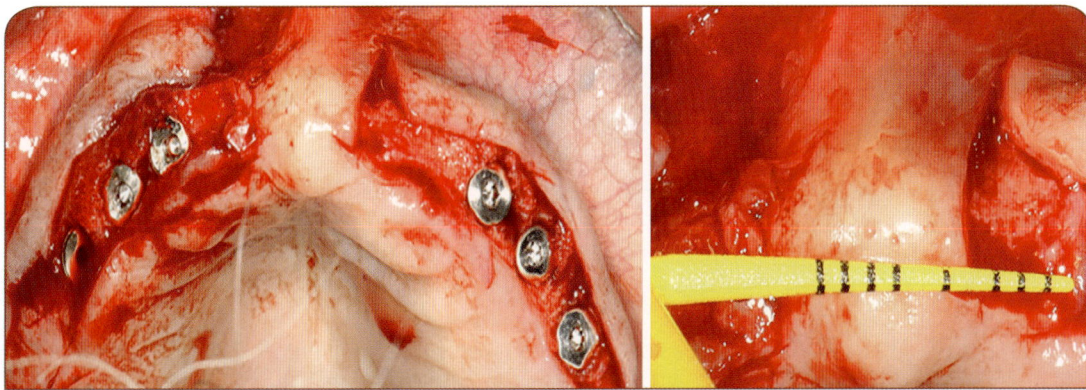

Fig. 5

A good A-P spread is achieved with correct implant placement, in such cases it is prudent not to place implants in the central incisor positions and to leave a band of 5 to 6 mm of tissue undisturbed which itself allows for proper spacing of implants and correct flap closure **(Fig. 5)**.

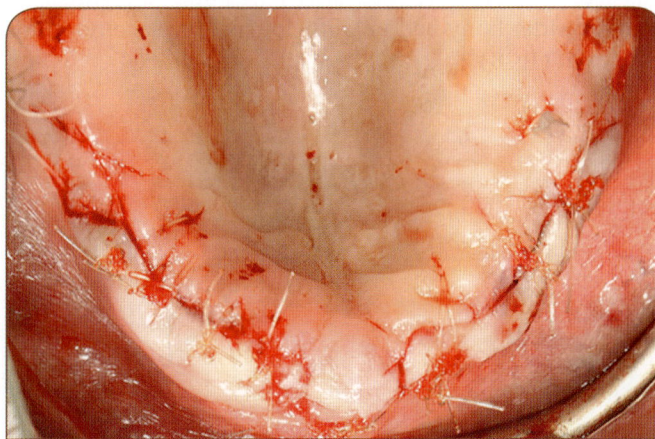

Fig. 6

Wound closure with 4–0 nylon. No interim prosthesis is given during the healing period to prevent inadvertent forces that may be transmitted to the underlying healing wound. Mini implants can be used as an alternative, should the patient be very desirous of a denture in the healing period **(Fig. 6)**.

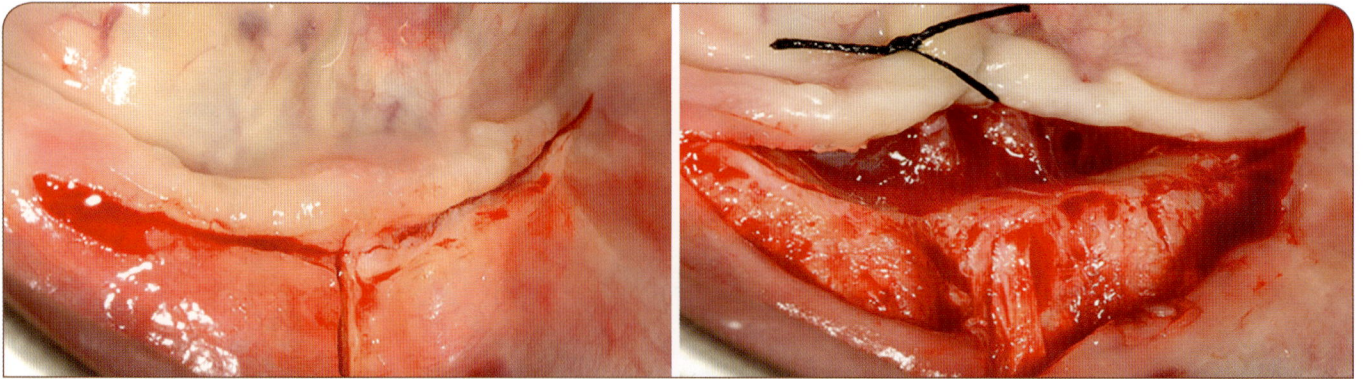

Fig. 7

The classic overdenture surgery incision with a crestal incision from tooth # 34–44 and a midfacial releasing incision is given to expose underlying bone, a lingual "tie back" suture is of immense help to aid in visibility. A sharp crest of the alveolus is clearly evident **(Fig. 7)**.

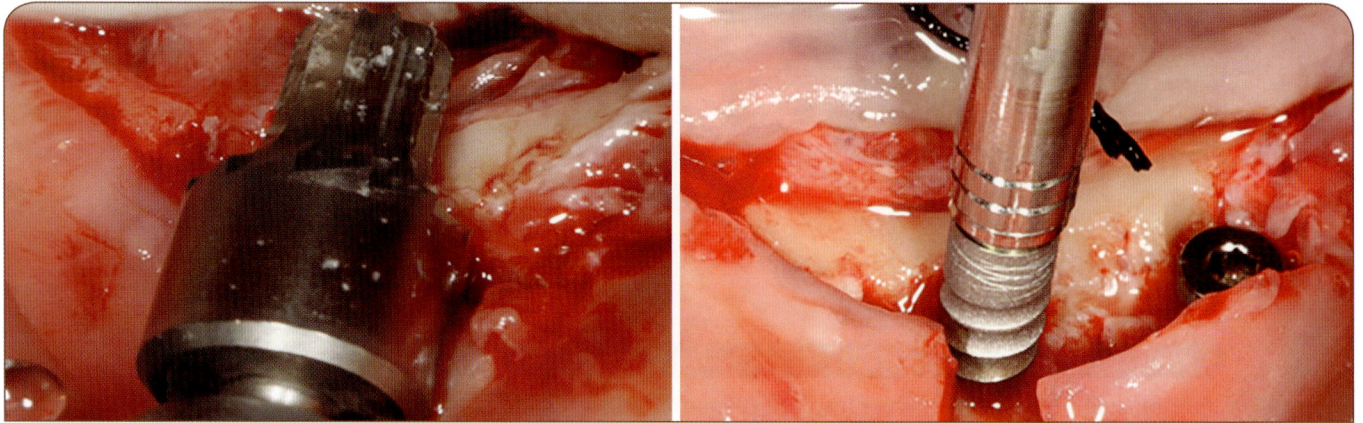

Fig. 8

A crestotome bur at 2500 rpm is used on a reverse mode to flatten the knife edge ridge. This procedure causes a decrease in available bone height but creates a wider bony bed to allow for fixture placement. After osteotomies are completed implants are placed in ABDE positions **(Fig. 8)**.

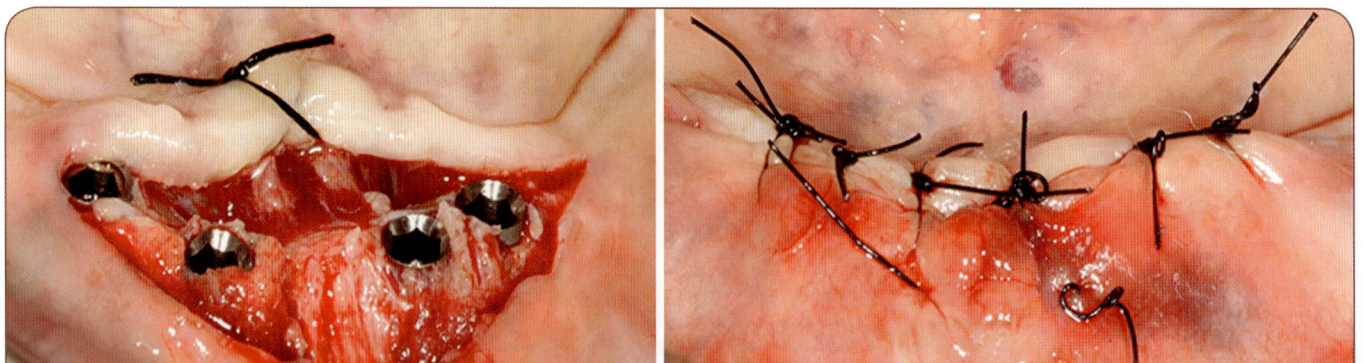

Fig. 9

Four implants (A.B Dent) are placed in equidistant positions and the wound closed with 3–0 polyamide sutures **(Fig. 9)**.

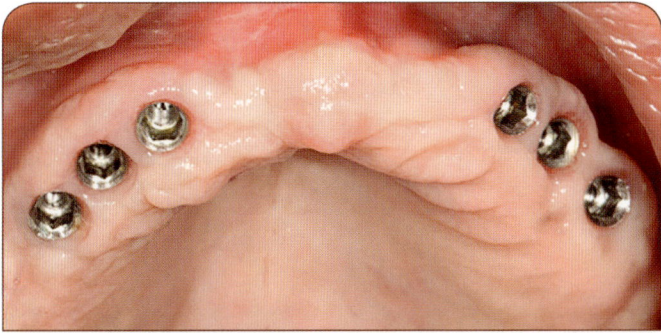

Fig. 10

The A-P spread of the implants is adequate to have the prosthesis accommodate a single molar on each side as a cantilever extension **(Fig. 10)**.

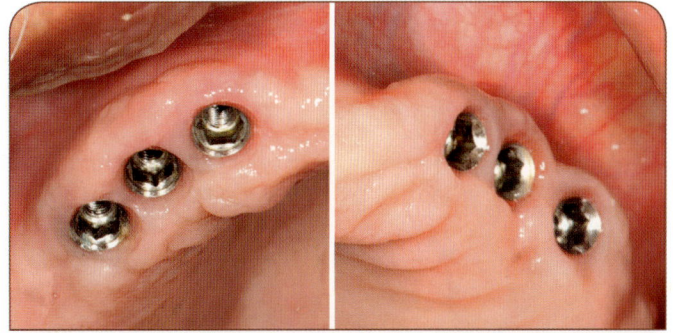

Fig. 11

An adequate band of keratinized tissue is evident around the implants **(Fig. 11)**.

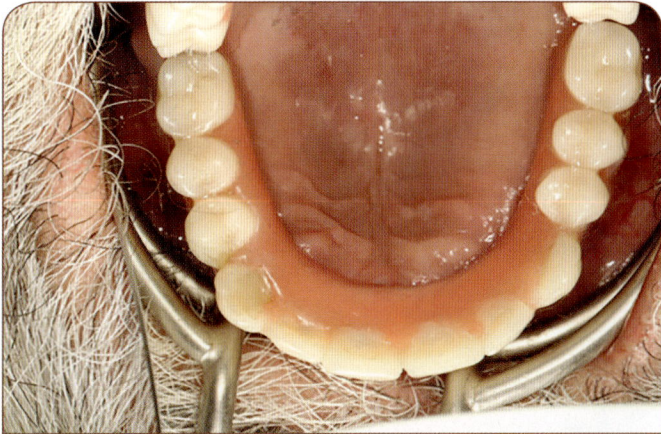

Fig. 12

The upper prosthesis at insertion **(Fig. 12)**.

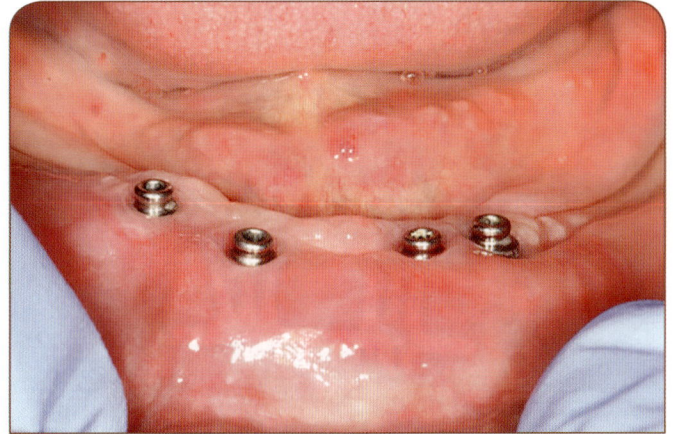

Fig. 13

Low attachments for the mandibular prosthesis. The implant positions are ideal to resist force from the opposite fixed dention, without getting dislodged **(Fig. 13)**.

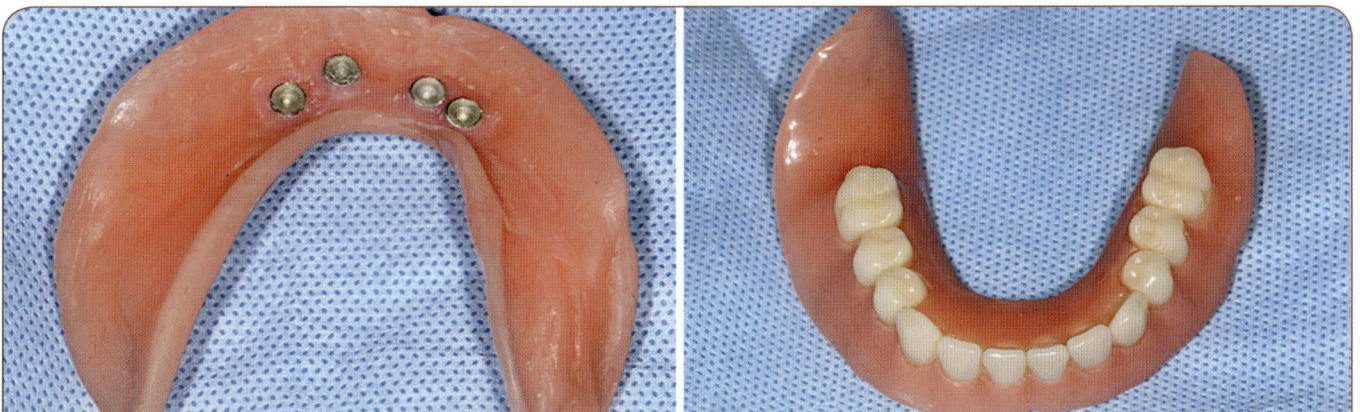

Fig. 14

Mandibular prosthesis: tissue surface and occlusal view **(Fig. 14)**.

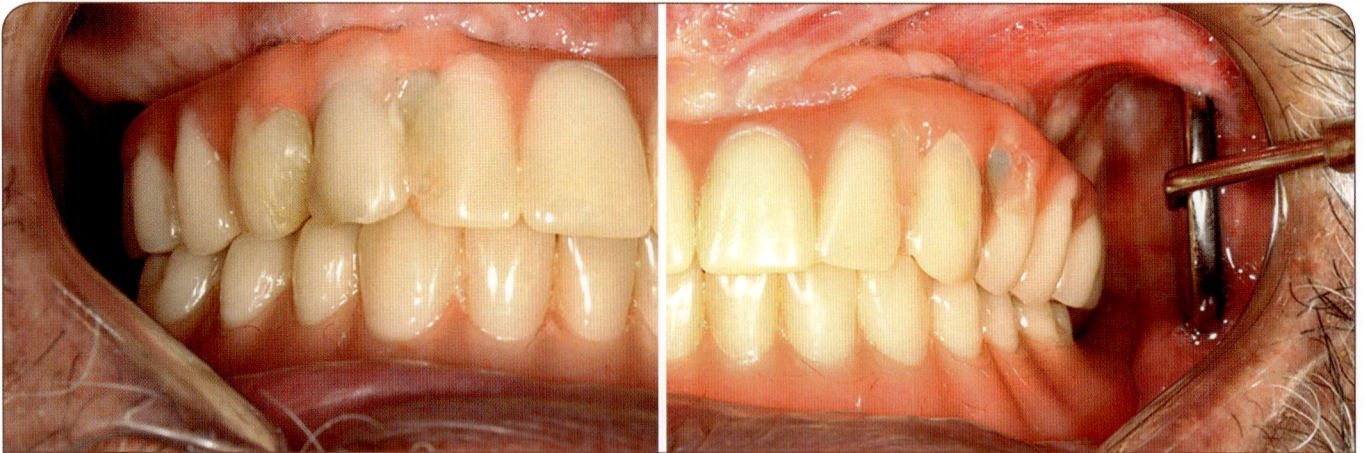

Fig. 15

The prosthesis in occlusion: left and right side views **(Fig. 15)**.

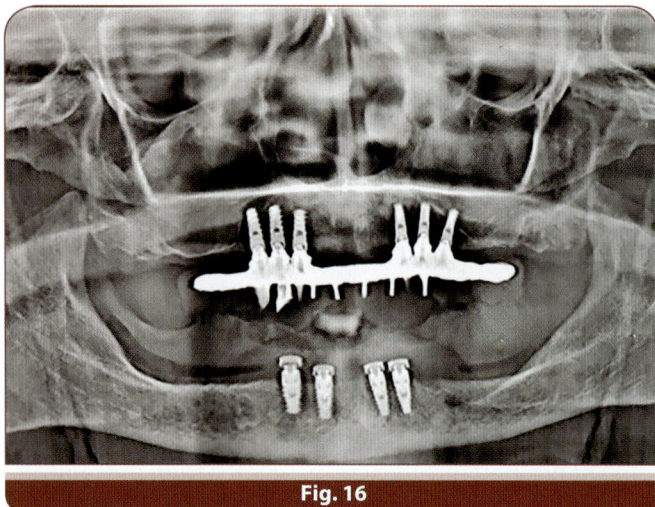

Fig. 16

Frontal view of the prosthesis **(Fig. 16)**.

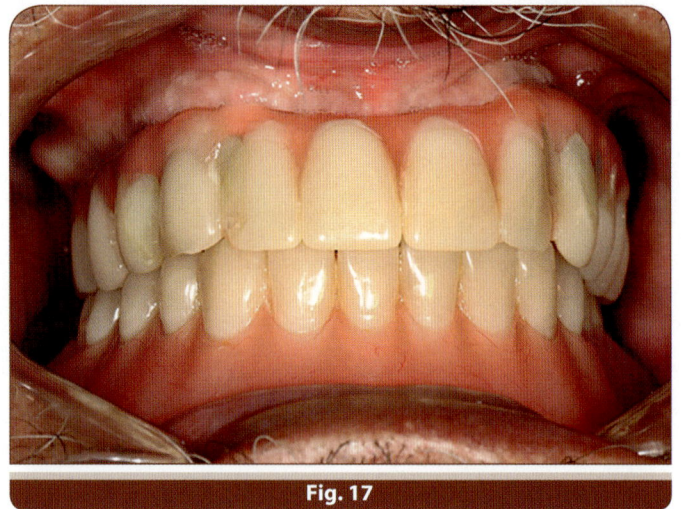

Fig. 17

Two years follow-up panorex showing a stable prosthesis and bone levels **(Fig. 17)**.

SECTION 8

Complications and Failures

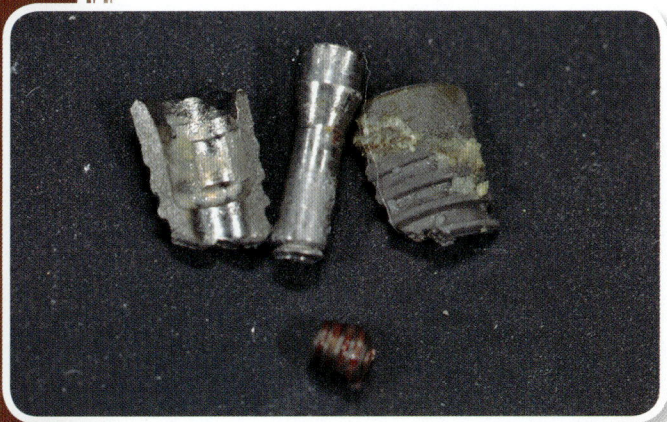

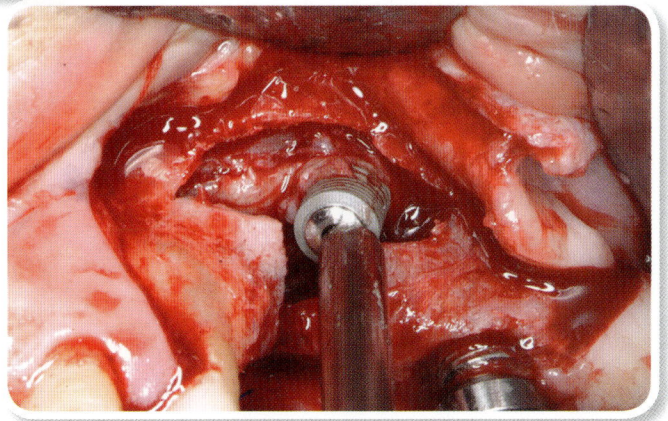

CASE STUDY 115

Lanka Mahesh, Vishal Gupta

Management of a Failed Implant Site with Simultaneous Implant Placement and GBR

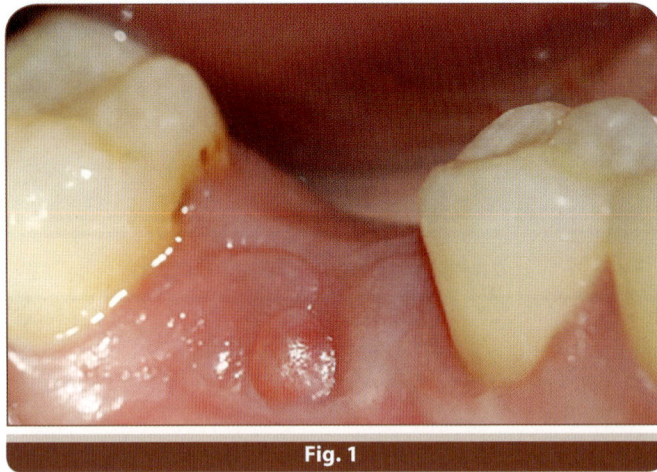

Fig. 1

A 33-year of female, history of implant placement 8 weeks prior. Complains of swelling and pain. Sinus tract visible **(Fig. 1)**.

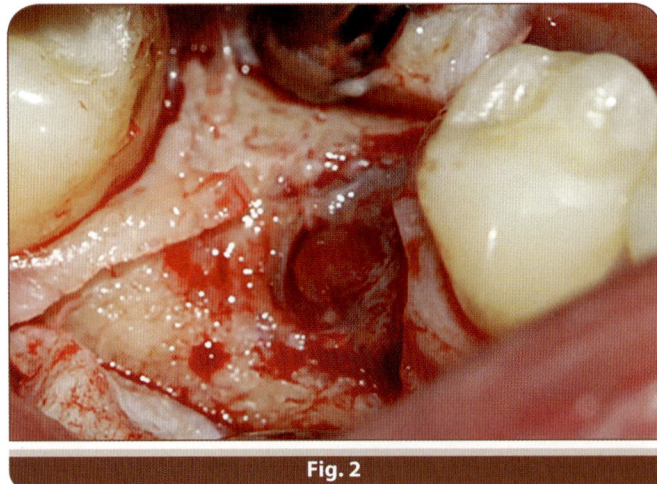

Fig. 2

After flap reflection fibrous encapsulation around implant visible **(Fig. 2)**.

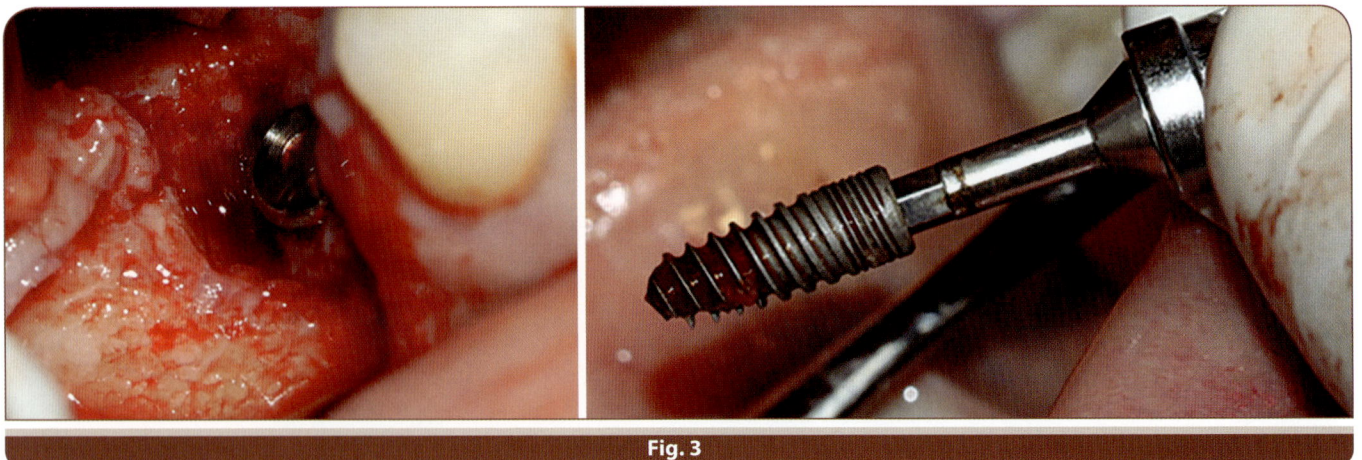

Fig. 3

Bony defect present. Implant reverse torqued removed and all granulation tissue removed from the site **(Fig. 3)**.

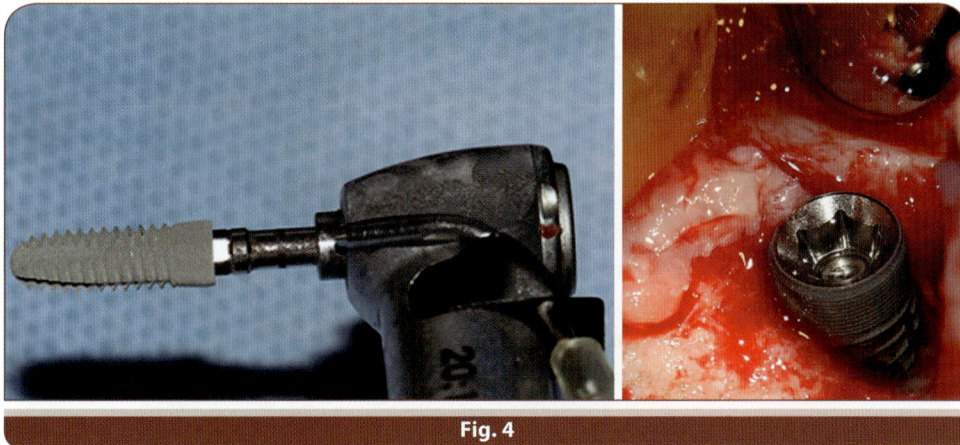

Fig. 4

Kelt 4.7/11.5 (Bioner implants) placed and torqued to 35 N.cm. Bony defect clearly visible on the mesial aspect of implant **(Fig. 4)**.

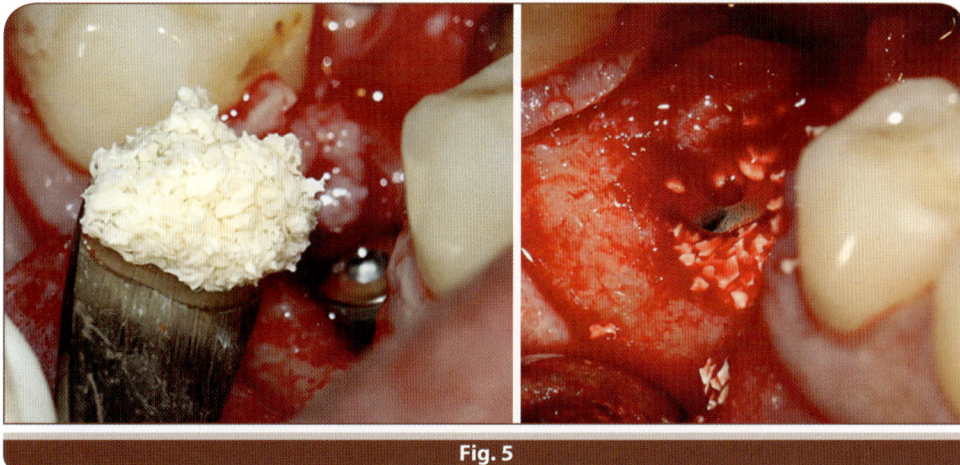

Fig. 5

Defect grafted with Cerabone (Botiss, GMBS). Graft material packed to completely fill the defect **(Fig. 5)**.

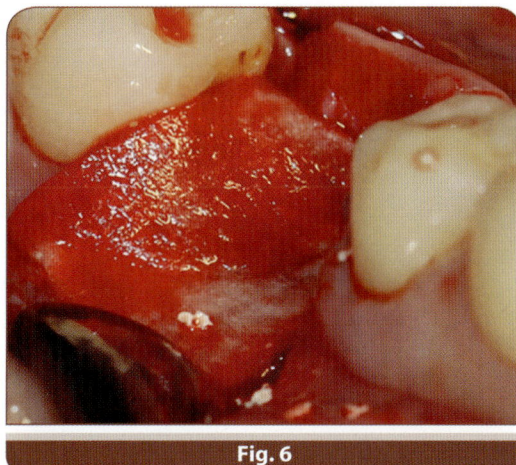

Fig. 6

Collagen membrane placement (RCM6) **(Fig. 6)**.

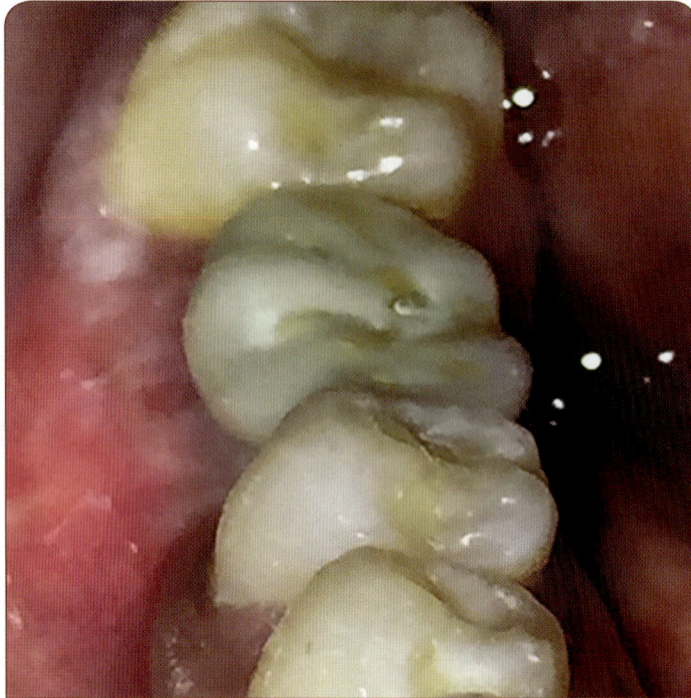

Fig. 7

Final prosthesis at insertion **(Fig. 7)**.

CASE STUDY 116

Lanka Mahesh, Nitika Poonia

MANAGEMENT OF A FAILED CASE WITH GBR REIMPLANTATION AND RST

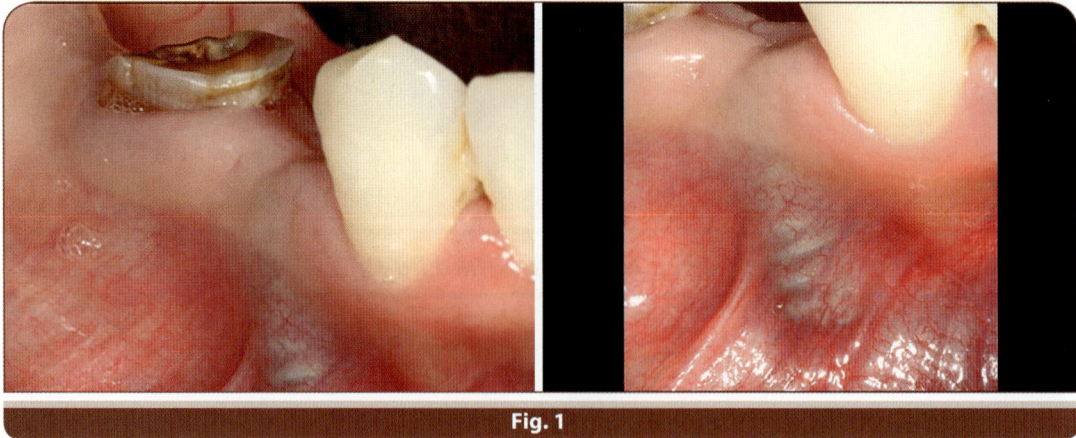

Fig. 1

A 47-year female patient with history of implant placement approximately 2 months prior. Complained of pain and discomfort **(Fig. 1).**

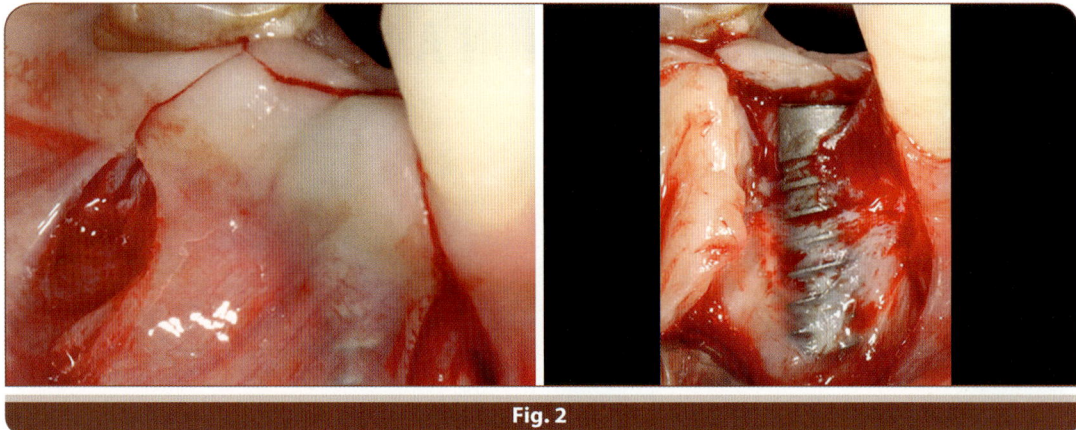

Fig. 2

After flap reflection implant threads visible. Buccal bone totally absent **(Fig. 2)**.

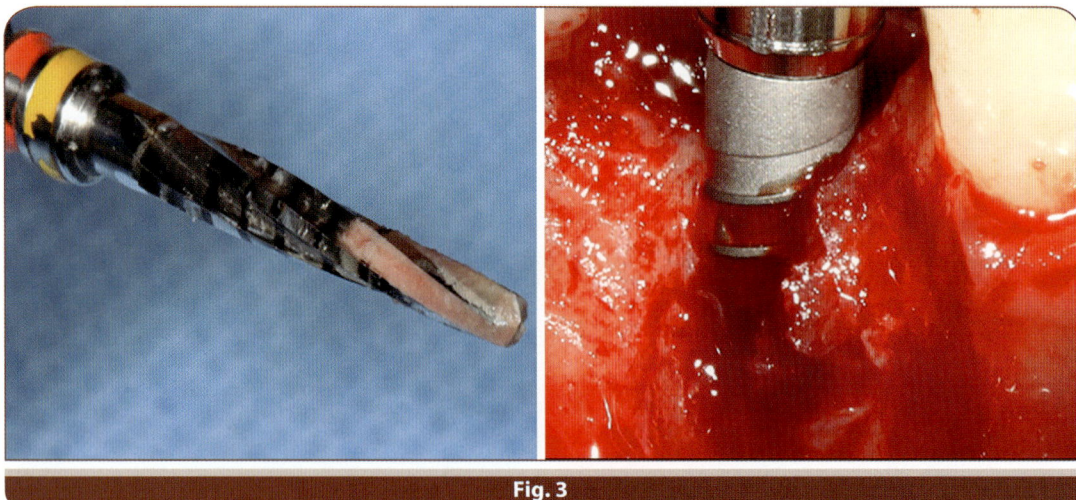

Fig. 3

New implant placed with minimal drilling protocol **(Fig. 3)**.

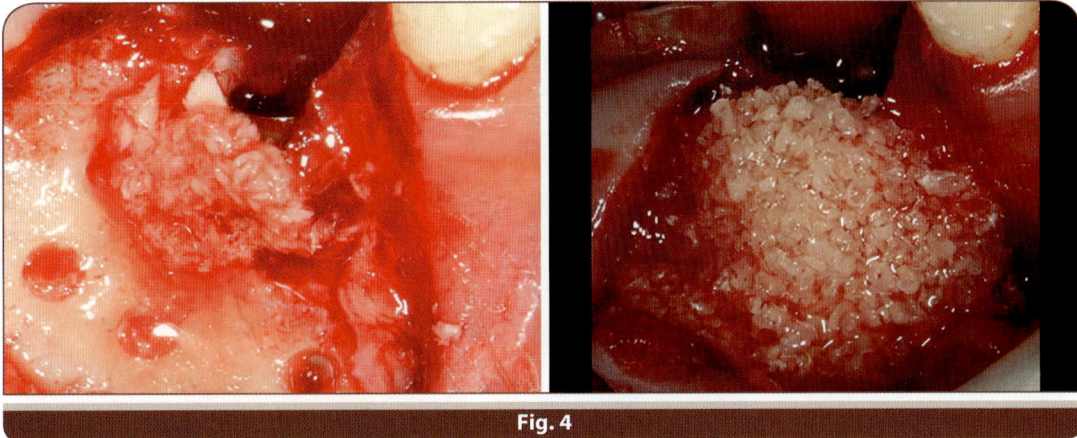

Fig. 4

Host bed prepared to initiate bleading and GBR with cerabone (bone graft) material done **(Fig. 4)**.

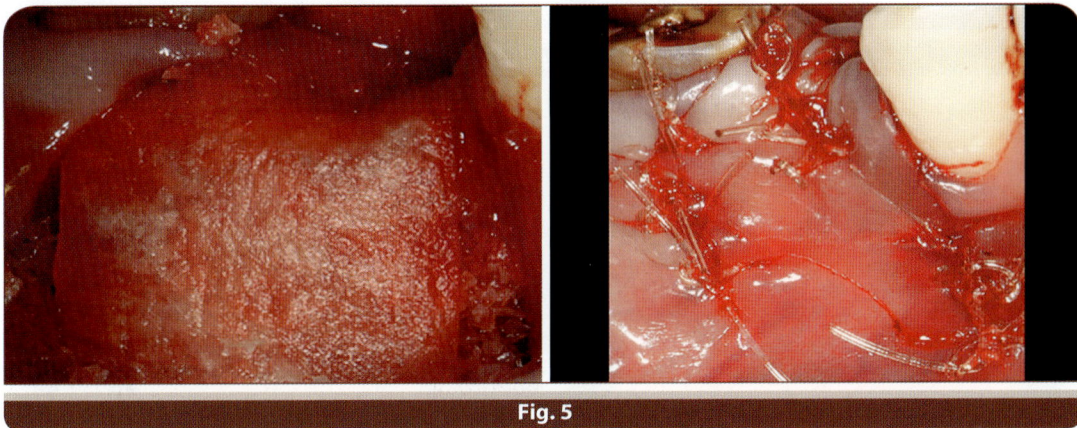

Fig. 5

Resorbable collagen membrane placed suture done **(Fig. 5)**.

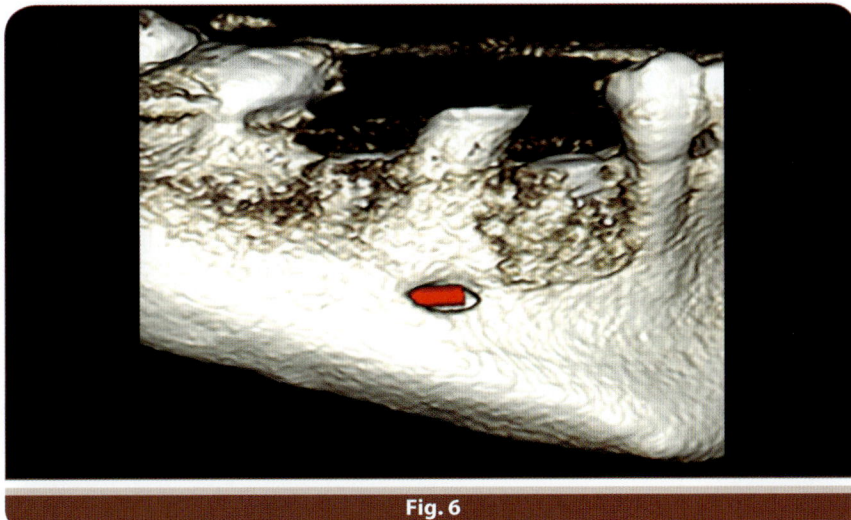

Fig. 6

CT scan showing new bone formation **(Fig. 6)**.

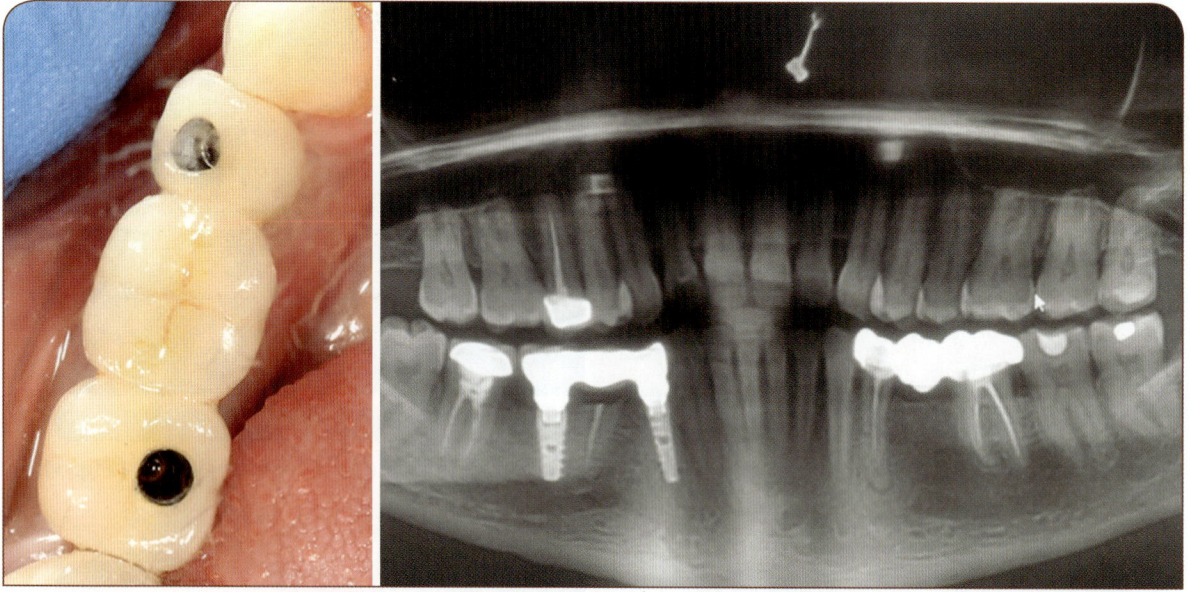

Fig. 7

Prosthesis at delivery and final panorex at 16 months **(Fig. 7)**.

José Luis Calvo Guirado

MANAGEMENT OF A MAXILLARY ARCH WITH FAILING IMPLANTS AND FRACTURED SCREWS

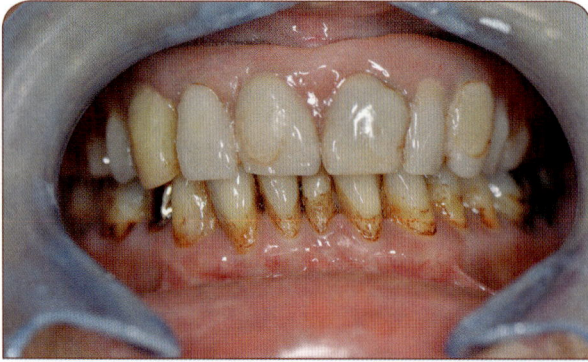

Fig. 1

A 61-year-old singer female patient complains about the upper implant retained denture. Bar retained a resin prostheses with composite on buccal part of the denture **(Fig. 1)**.

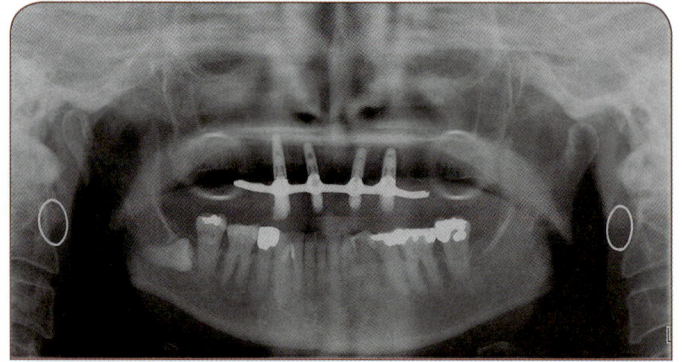

Fig. 2

Bar retained a resin prostheses placed on top of 4 implants, with immediate loading three years ago. All implants are moving **(Fig. 2)**.

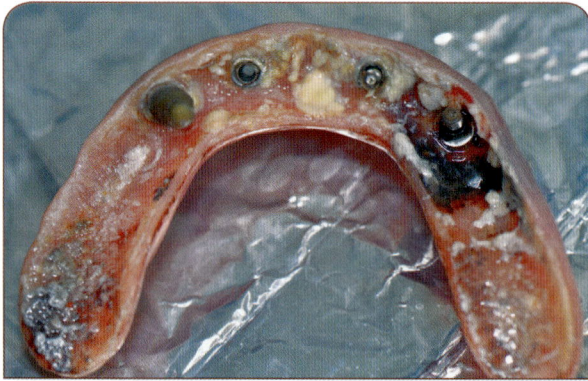

Fig. 3

One implant was lost, three screws are fractured. A lot of food retention **(Fig. 3)**.

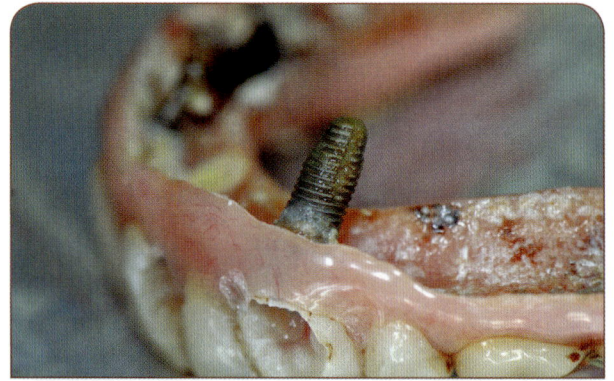

Fig. 4

Implant lost of osseointegration **(Fig. 4)**.

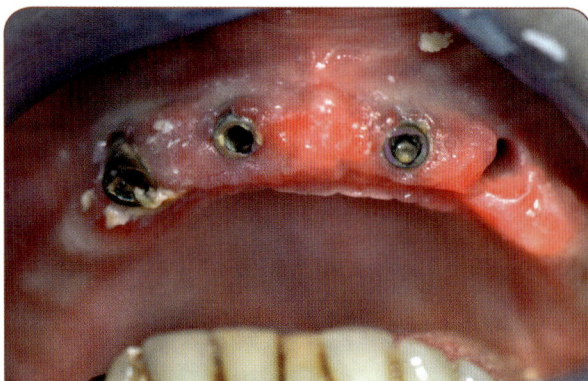

Fig. 5

Intraoral photo shows food retention, fractured passing screws, implant lost **(Fig. 5)**.

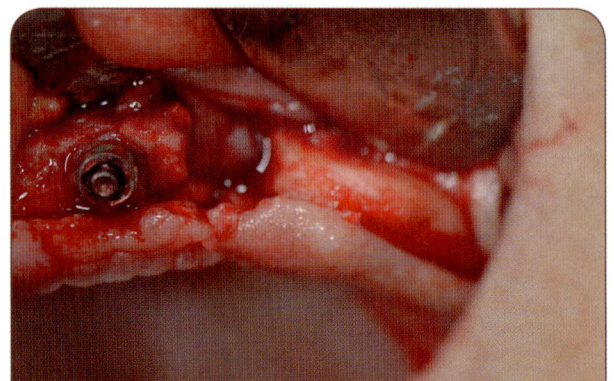

Fig. 6

Bone crater of implant lost **(Fig. 6)**.

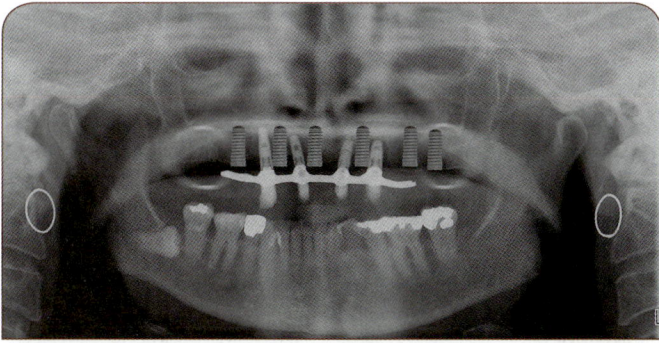

Fig. 7

Treatment plan was to place 6 implants in the upper jaw and keep at least 2 older implants for provisional denture retention **(Fig. 7)**.

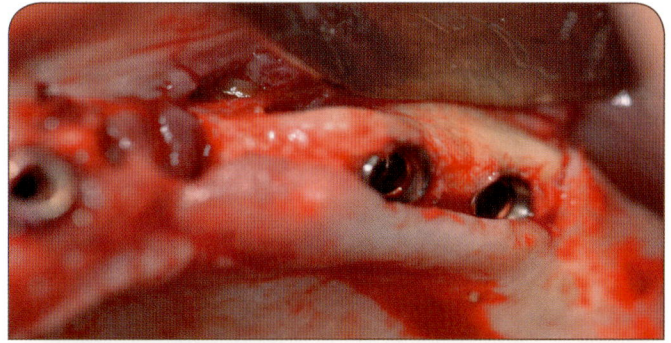

Fig. 8

Two bone level Straumann implants were placed on the upper left side **(Fig. 8)**.

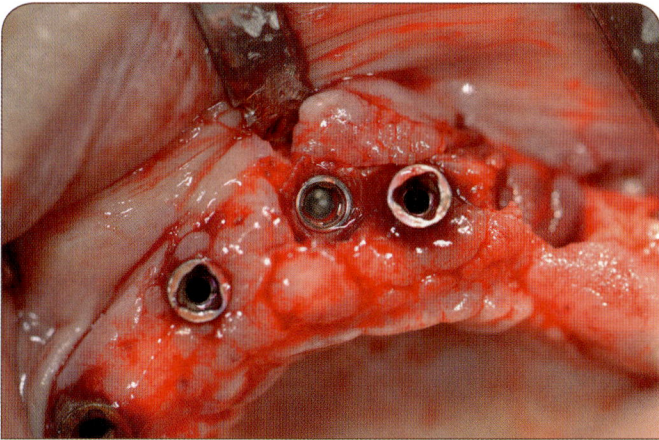

Fig. 9

Two bone level Straumann implants were placed in the center of the maxilla **(Fig. 9)**.

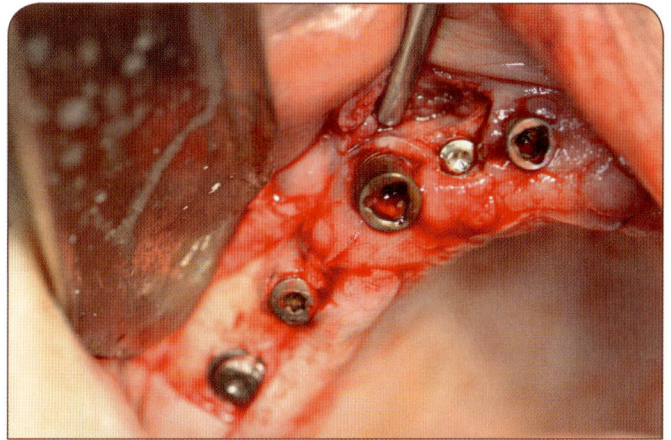

Fig. 10

Two bone level Straumann implants were placed on the upper right side **(Fig. 10)**.

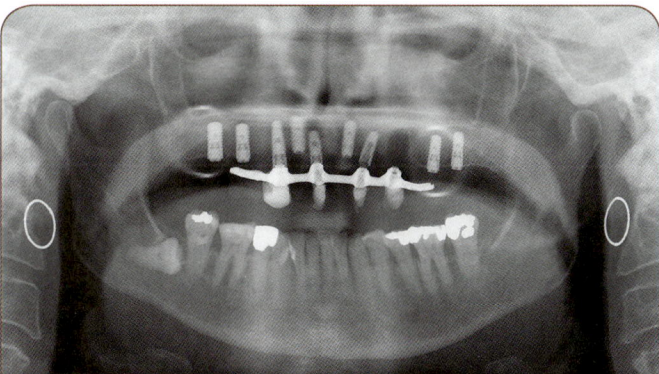

Fig. 11

Six bone level Straumann implants were placed in the hole maxilla **(Fig. 11)**.

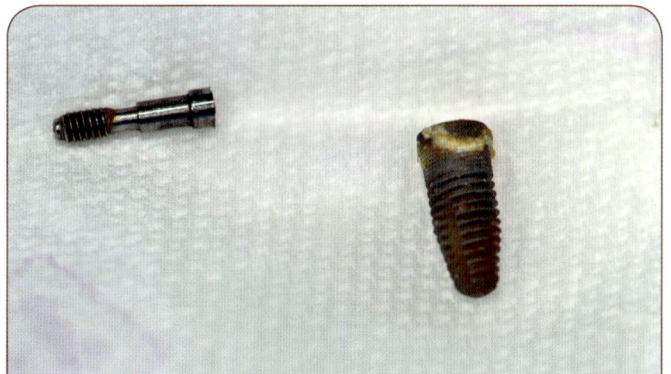

Fig. 12

Implant lost **(Fig. 12)**.

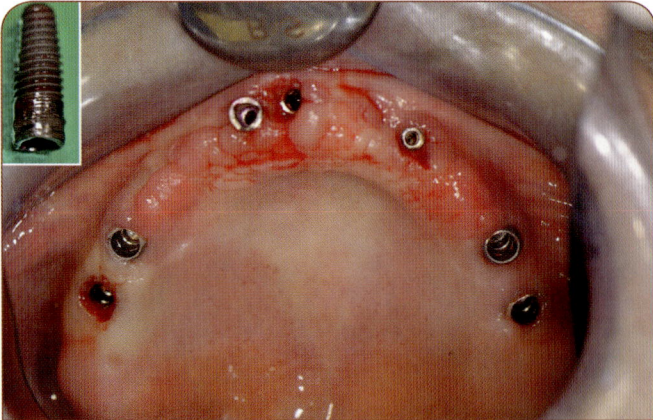
Fig. 13

Six bone level Straumann implants after 3 months of healing **(Fig. 13)**.

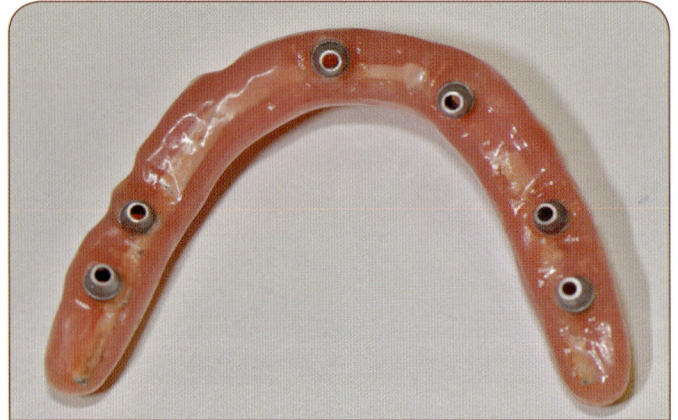
Fig. 14

The new screw retained resin denture **(Fig. 14)**.

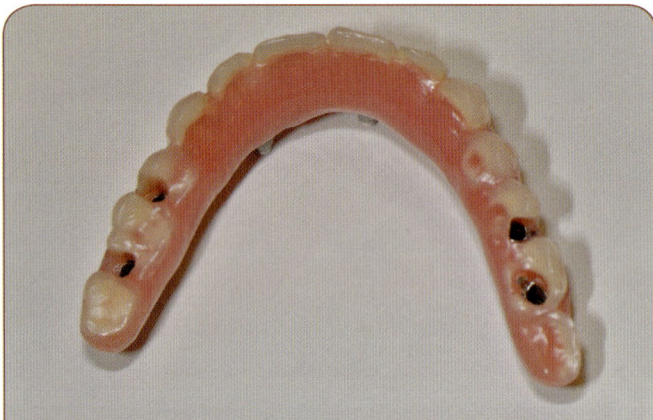
Fig. 15

The new screw retained resin denture **(Fig. 15)**.

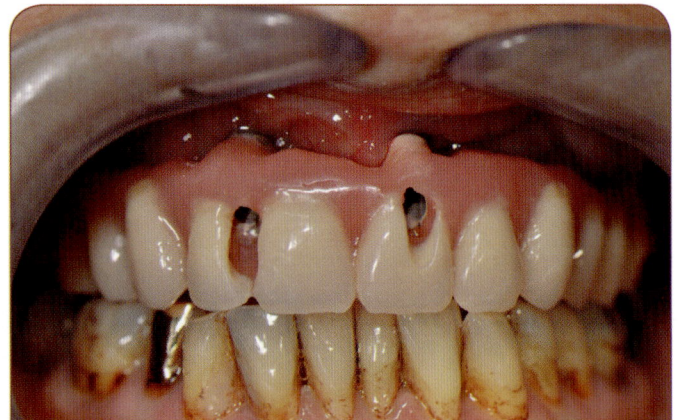
Fig. 16

The new screw retained resin denture **(Fig. 16)**.

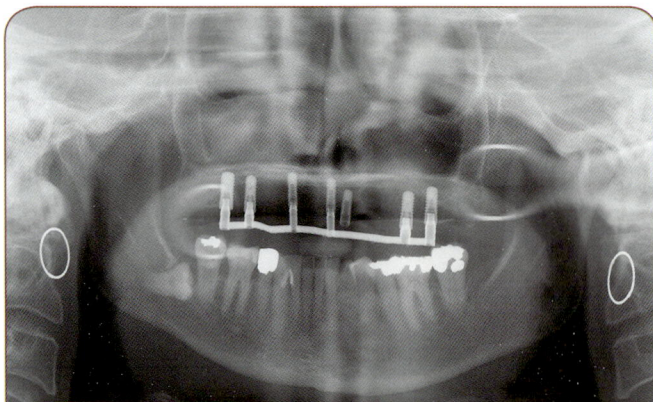
Fig. 17

The new screw retained resin denture bar checking **(Fig. 17)**.

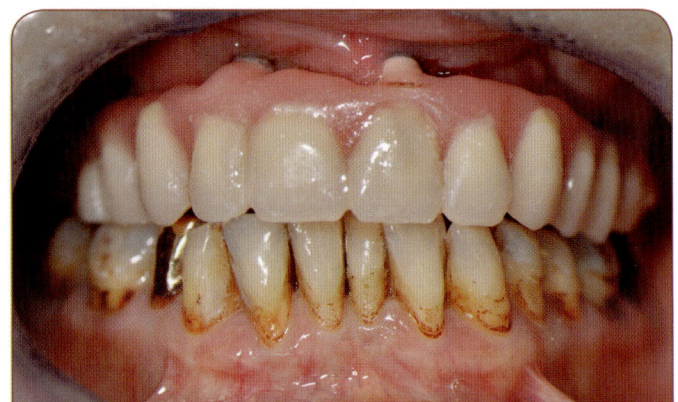
Fig. 18

The new screw retained resin denture in place **(Fig. 18)**.

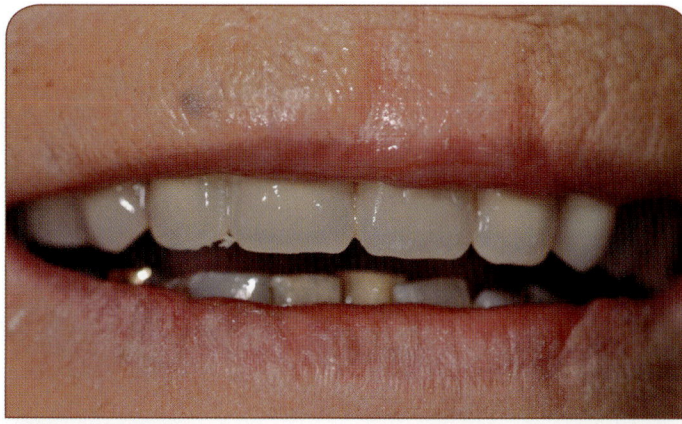

Fig. 19

The new screw retained resin denture with low smile **(Fig. 19)**.

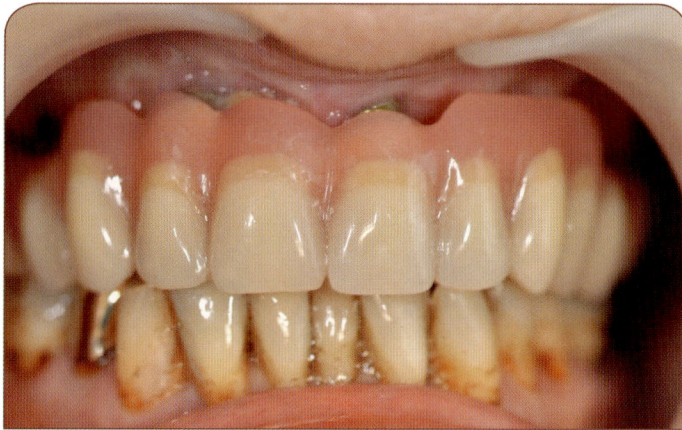

Fig. 20

The new screw retained resin denture in place after 2 years follow-up **(Fig. 20)**.

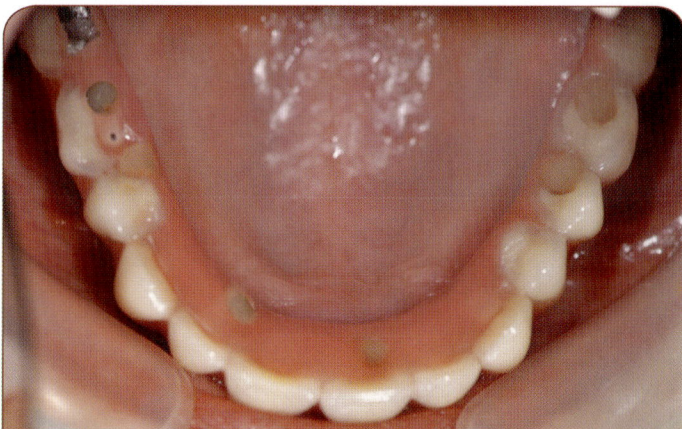

Fig. 21

The new screw retained resin denture in place after 2 years follow-up **(Fig. 21)**.

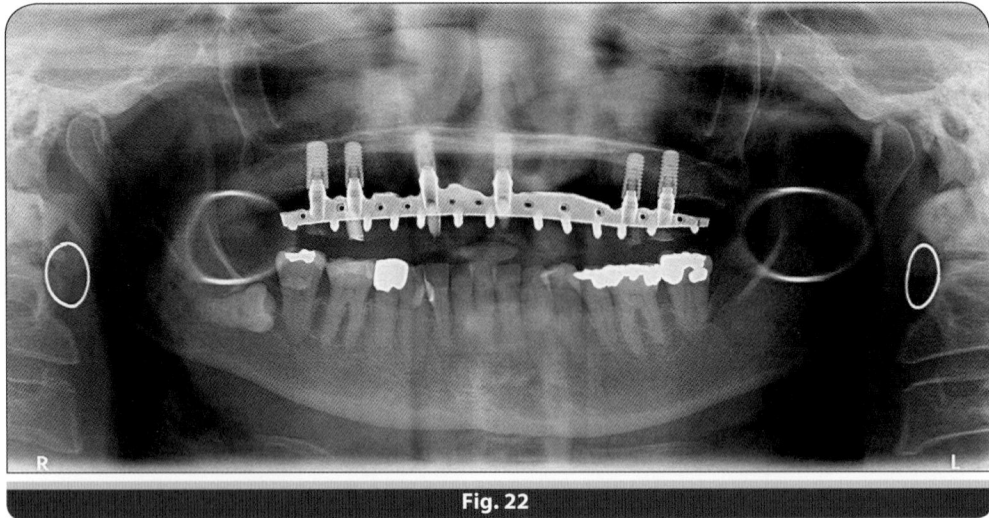

Fig. 22

The new screw retained resin denture in place after 2 years follow-up **(Fig. 22)**.

Lanka Mahesh

MALALIGNED IMPLANT FIXTURE REMOVAL AND REPLACEMENT WITH AN IMPLANT AND GBR IN CORRECT POSITION IN THE ESTHETIC ZONE

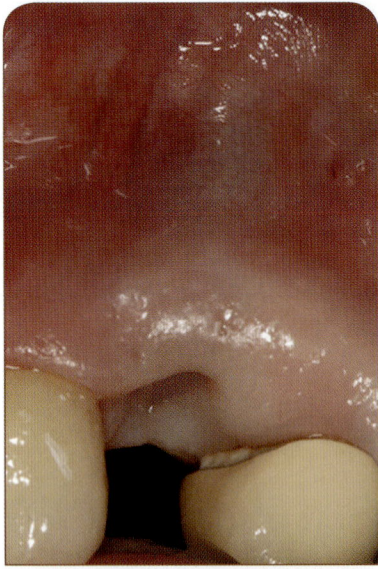

Fig. 1

Preoperative clinical view clearly showing the implant fixture below the mucosal tissue **(Fig. 1)**.

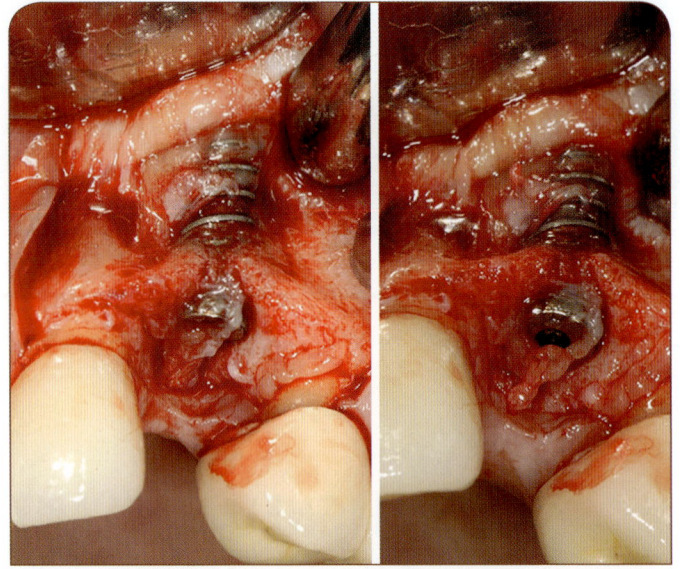

Fig. 2

After flap elevation the situation is evident. During implant placement in an immediate extraction site the operator misjudged the angulation and perforated the facial wall completely **(Fig. 2)**.

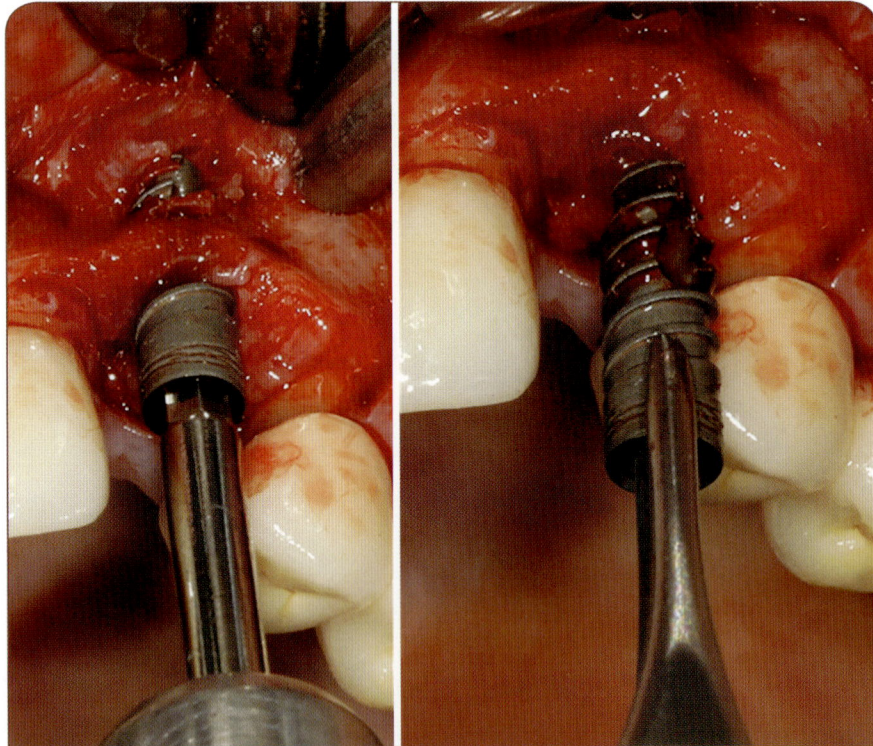

Fig. 3

The faulty implant is reverse torqued out (in this case due to lack of bony housing support it becomes a simple procedure) **(Fig. 3)**.

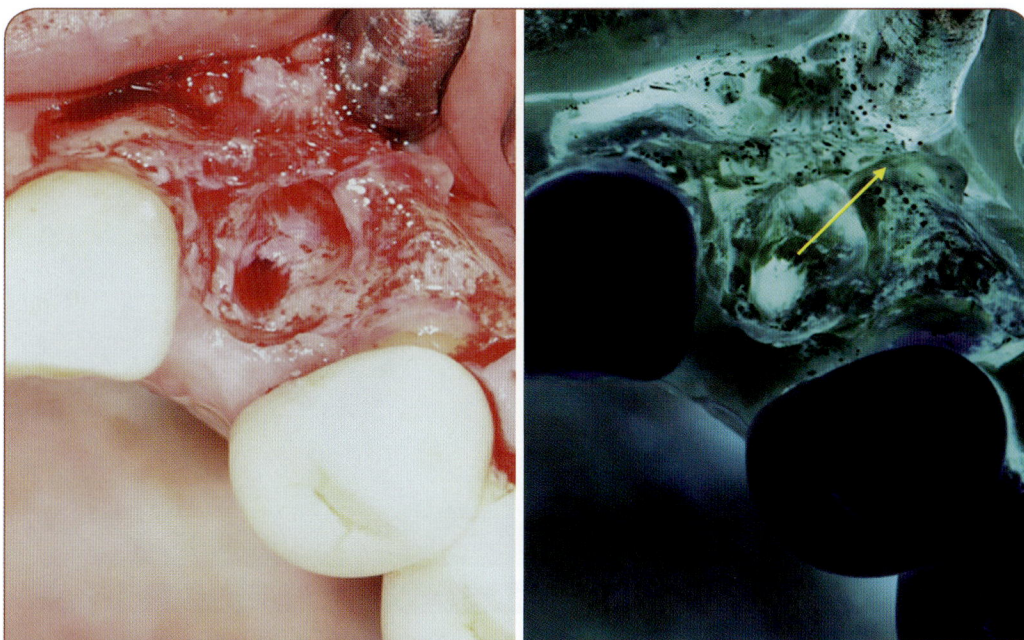

Fig. 4

The pilot drill osteotomy in correct position in a palatal orientation. The yellow arrow shows the new osteotomy site in relation to the previous facially directed implant position (Fig. 4).

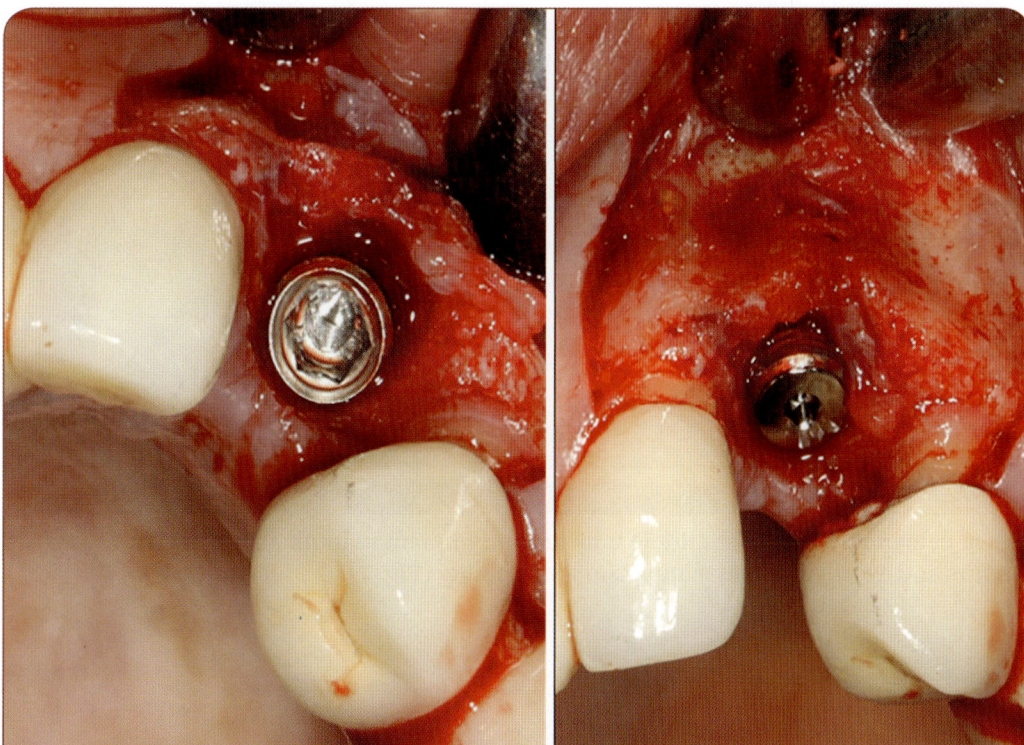

Fig. 5

A fresh fixture of 3.75/13 mm AB Dent is placed in correct position. The defect on the facial wall is evident (Fig. 5).

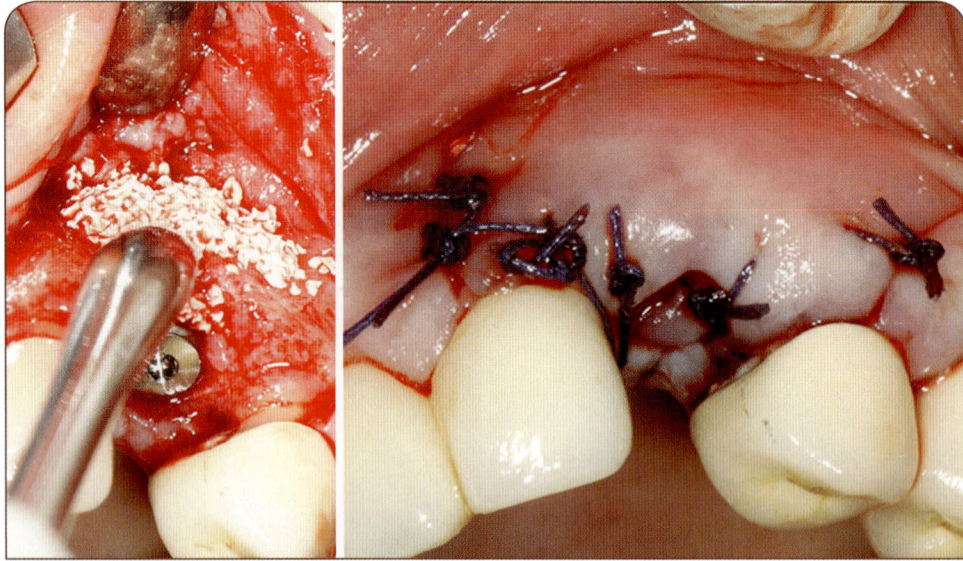

Fig. 6

A slow resorbing xenograft, Ti oss is placed on the defect site and closed with a resorbable collagen membrane, ossix plus (Datum dental). The surgical site is closed with 3-0 vicryl sutures the bulk of graft is evident immediately **(Fig. 6)**.

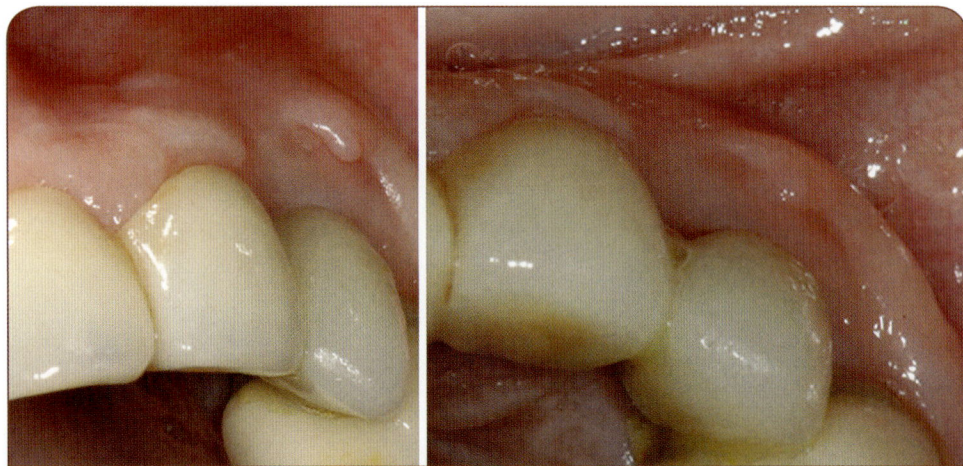

Fig. 7

At the time of crown cementation excellent tissue bulk around implant in tooth # 23 position. One year recall with soft stable tissue contours and excellent tissue maturation and stability **(Fig. 7)**.

José Luis Calvo Guirado

MANAGEMENT OF A FRACTURED IMPLANT IN THE MANDIBULAR POSTERIOR SEGMENT WITH GBR AND REIMPLANTATION

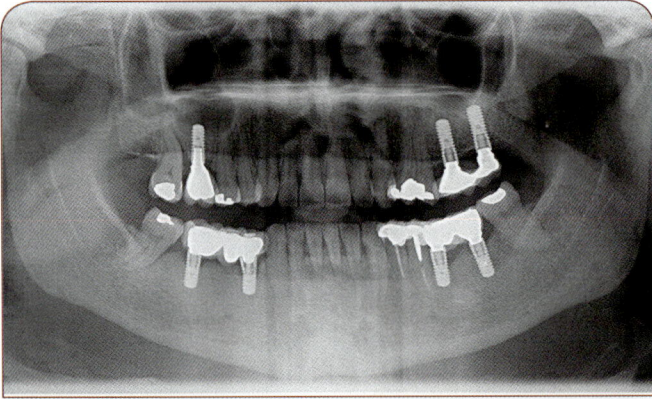

Fig. 1

A female patient 47 years old reports with pain in the right mandibular implanted area, she complains of moving bridge **(Fig. 1)**.

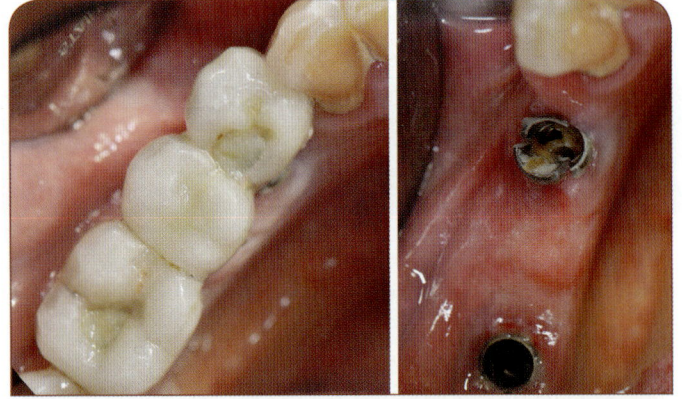

Fig. 2

Moving ceramic bridge, pain in the right mandibular implanted area **(Fig. 2)**.

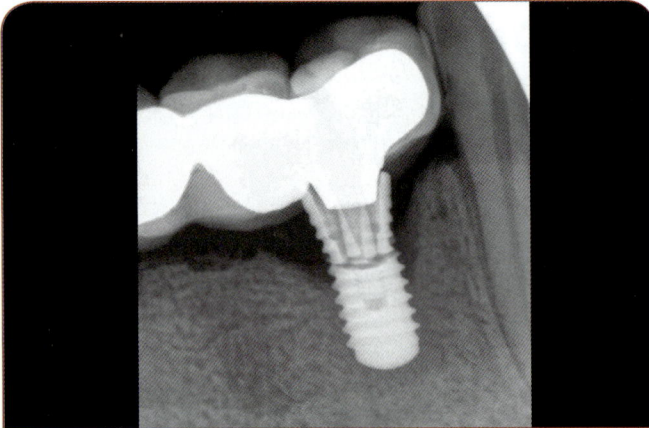

Fig. 3

Straumann bone level Roxolid 4.1 by 10 mm implant fractured, after rachtet is used in the wrong way **(Fig. 3)**.

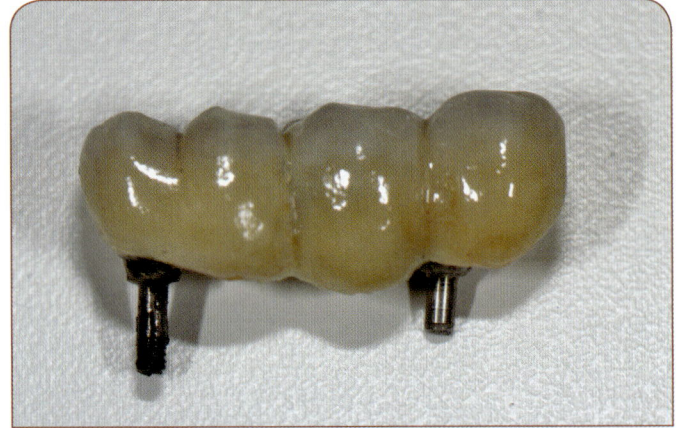

Fig. 4

Fractured anterior screw, after rachtet is used in the wrong way **(Fig. 4)**.

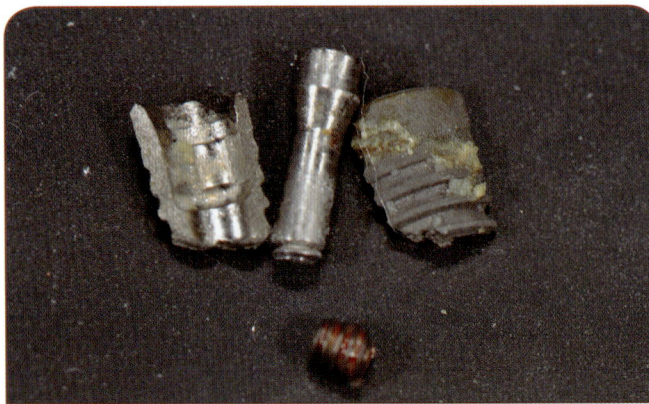

Fig. 5

Fractured implant portion taken out **(Fig. 5)**.

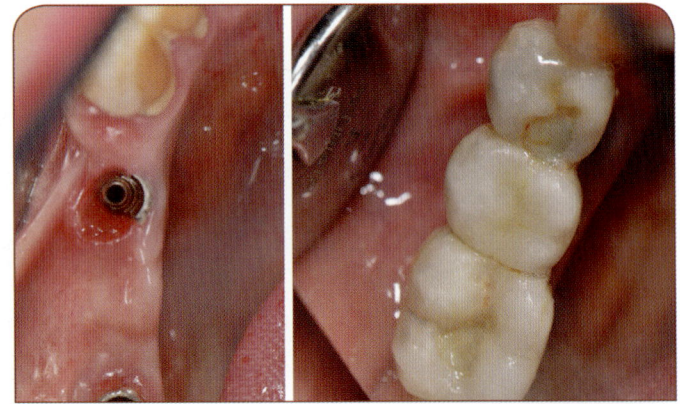

Fig. 6

Fractured anterior screw is visible **(Fig. 6)**.

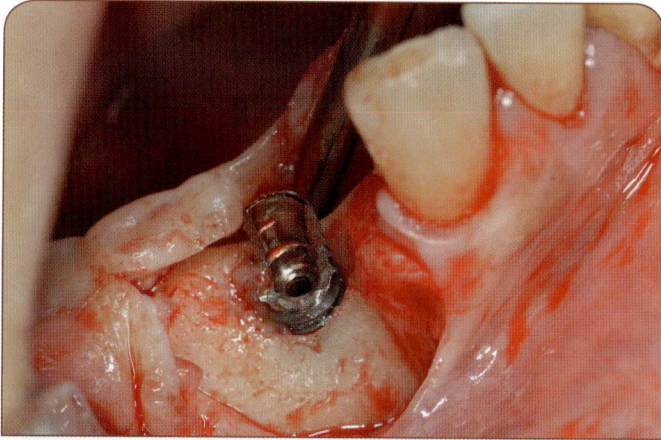
Fig. 7

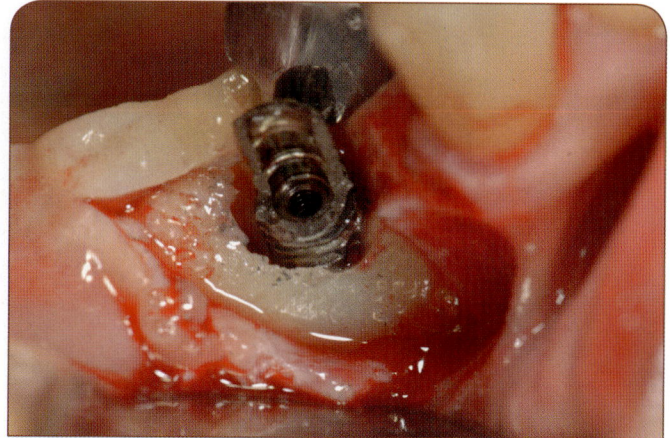
Fig. 8

Flap elevation done to expose the fractured implant **(Fig. 7)**.

Fractured implant in the extraction process **(Fig. 8)**.

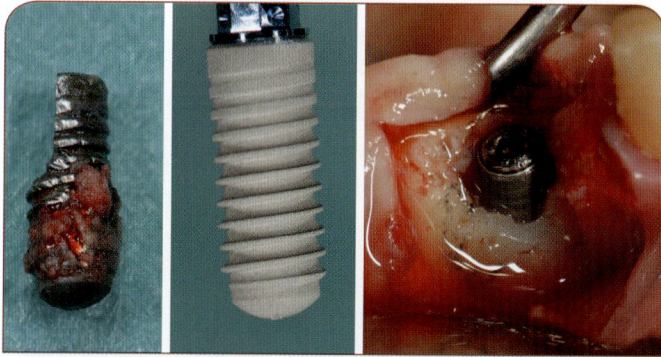
Fig. 9

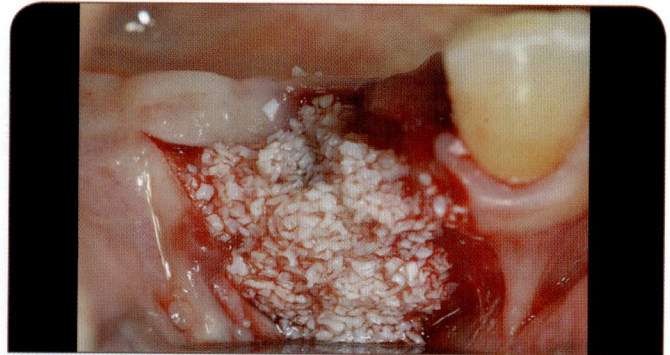
Fig. 10

After removal of the failed implant a 4.8 mm implant is placed in the same bone defect **(Fig. 9)**.

Xenograft Biomaterial is used to fill the dehiscence **(Fig. 10)**.

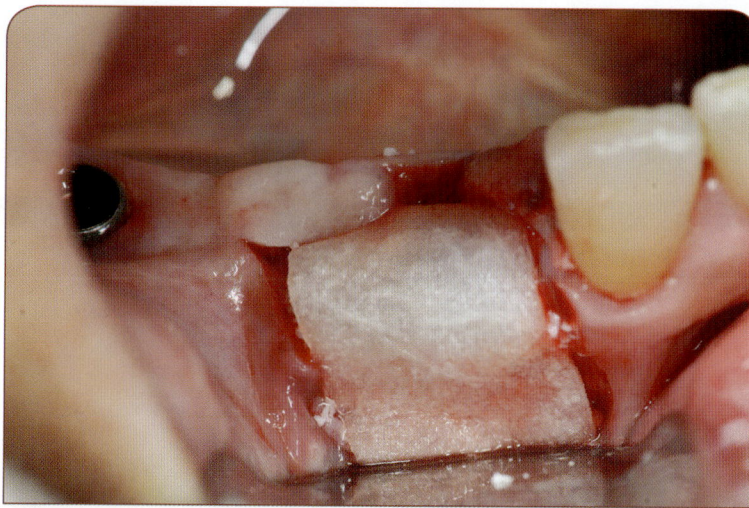
Fig. 11

A collagen membrane is placed **(Fig. 11)**.

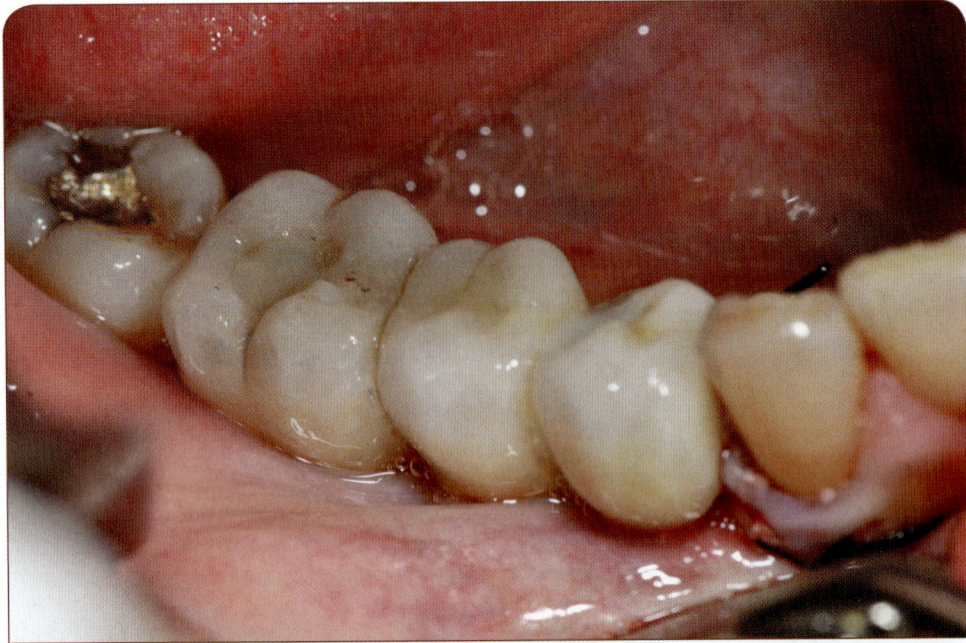

Fig. 12

Old bridge rachtet using the last implants and the anterior implant let to heal alone **(Fig. 12)**.

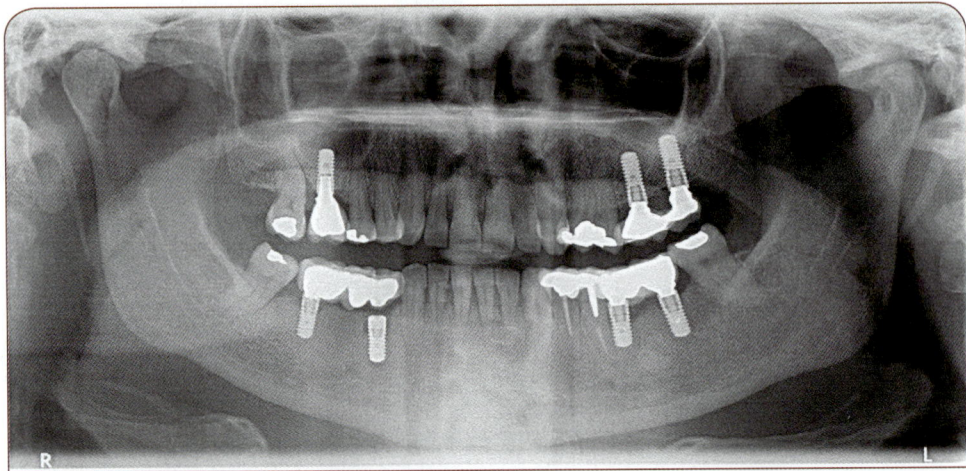

Fig. 13

Final X-ray with new implant in place **(Fig. 13)**.

Dong Seok Sohn

REMOVAL OF INTRUDED IMPLANT FROM MAXILLARY SINUS, FOLLOWED BY IMMEDIATE SINUS AUGMENTATION AND IMPLANT PLACEMENT

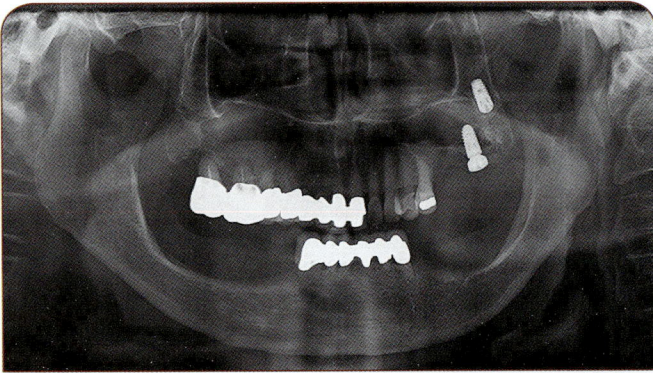

Fig. 1

A 76-year-old female patient referred due to intruded implant into sinus cavity. OPG showing implant in left maxillary sinus **(Fig. 1)**.

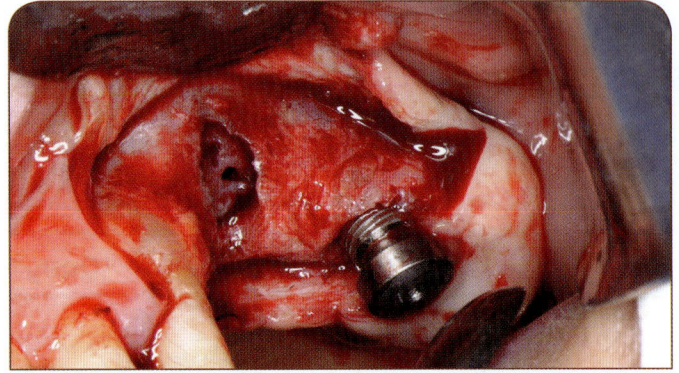

Fig. 2

Full thickness flap raised **(Fig. 2)**.

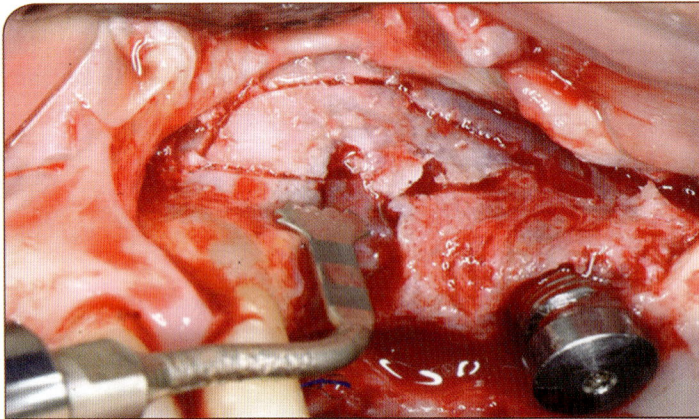

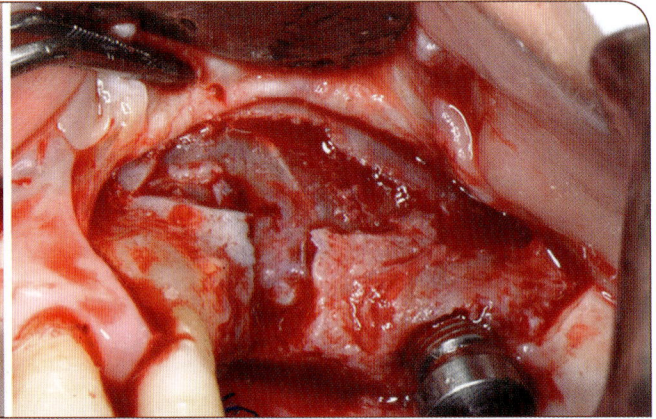

Fig. 3

Bony window prepared using a piezoelectric screw insert **(Fig. 3)**.

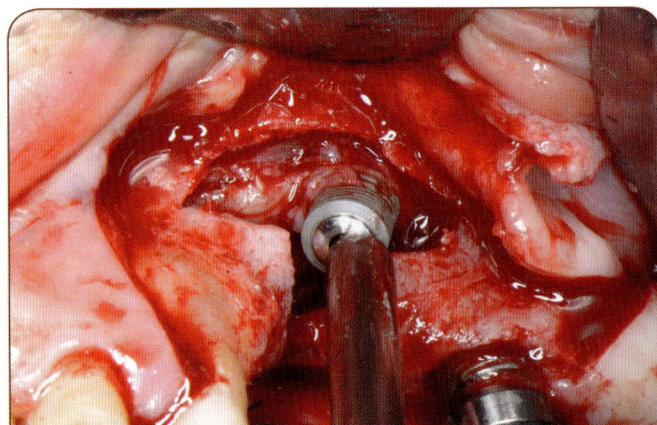

Fig. 4

Implant was suctioned with a saline flow by an aspirator **(Fig. 4)**.

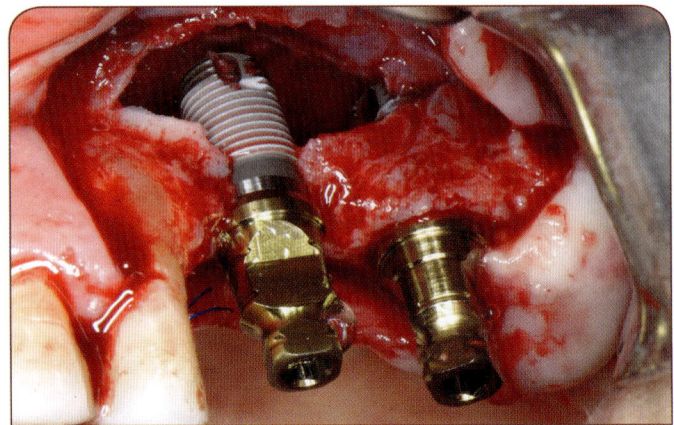

Fig. 5

Note the placement of a new implant at the site after elevator of sinus membrane **(Fig. 5)**.

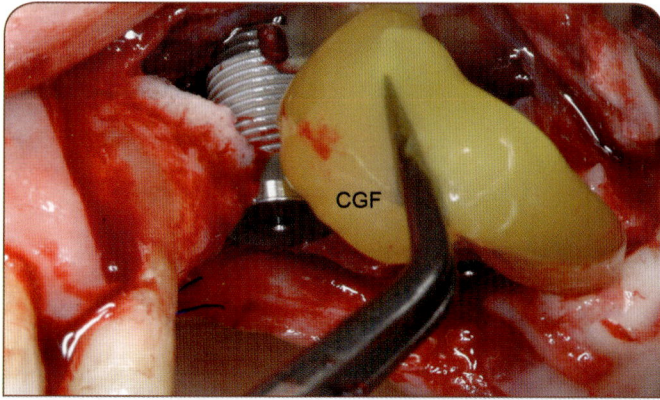

Fig. 6

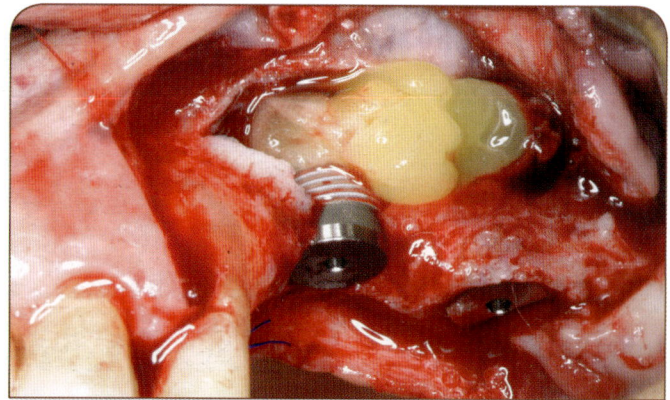

Fig. 7

A platelet rich fibrin block with concentrated growth factor (CGF) was grafted under the elevated sinus membrane to accelerate new bone formation in the sinus (Figs. 6 and 7).

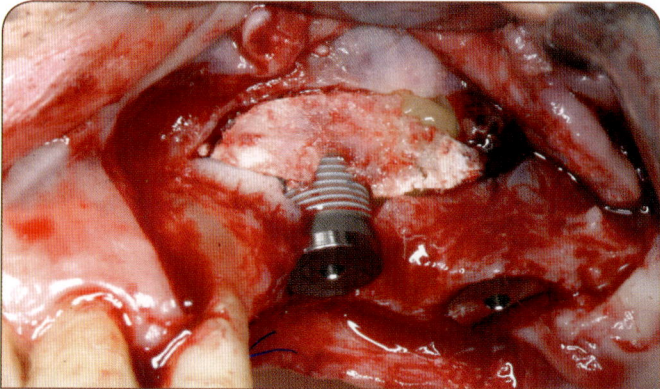

Fig. 8

The bony window was repositioned precisely into the excess window (Fig. 8).

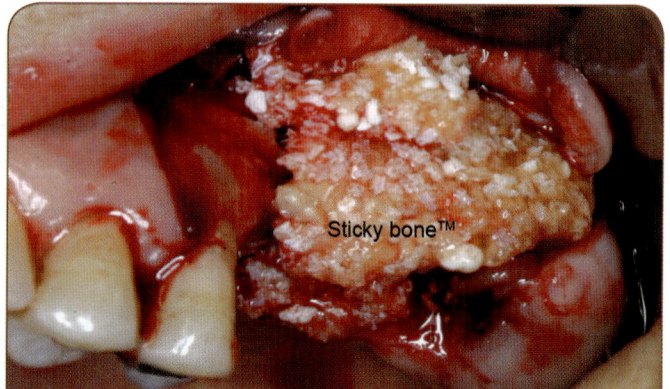

Fig. 9

Sticky bone placed (Fig. 9).

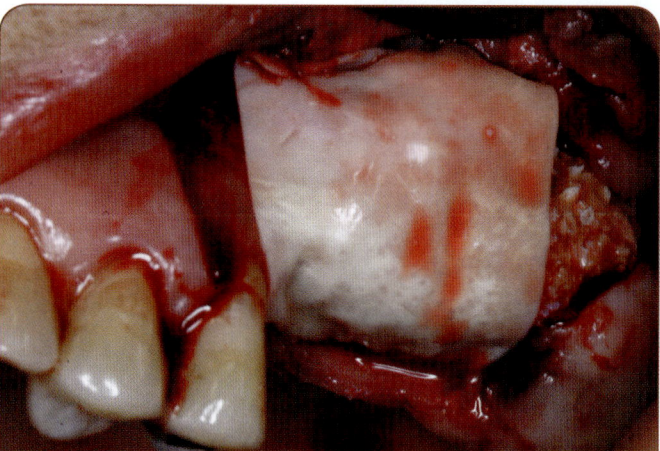

Fig. 10

Membrane placed over the entire assembly (Fig. 10).

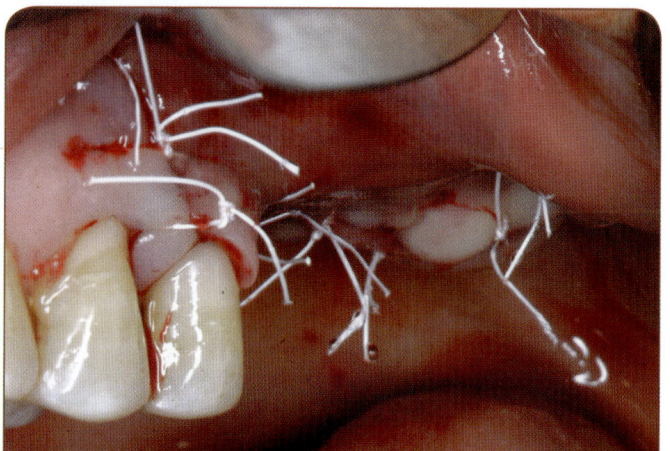

Fig. 11

Suture placement done (Fig. 11).

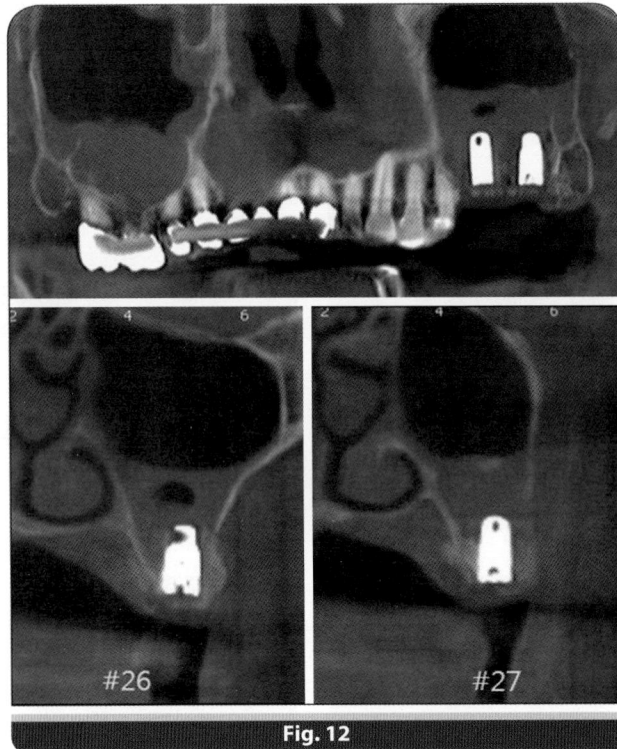

Fig. 12

Cone beam CT view showing bone formation at sites after 8 months of healing **(Fig. 12)**.

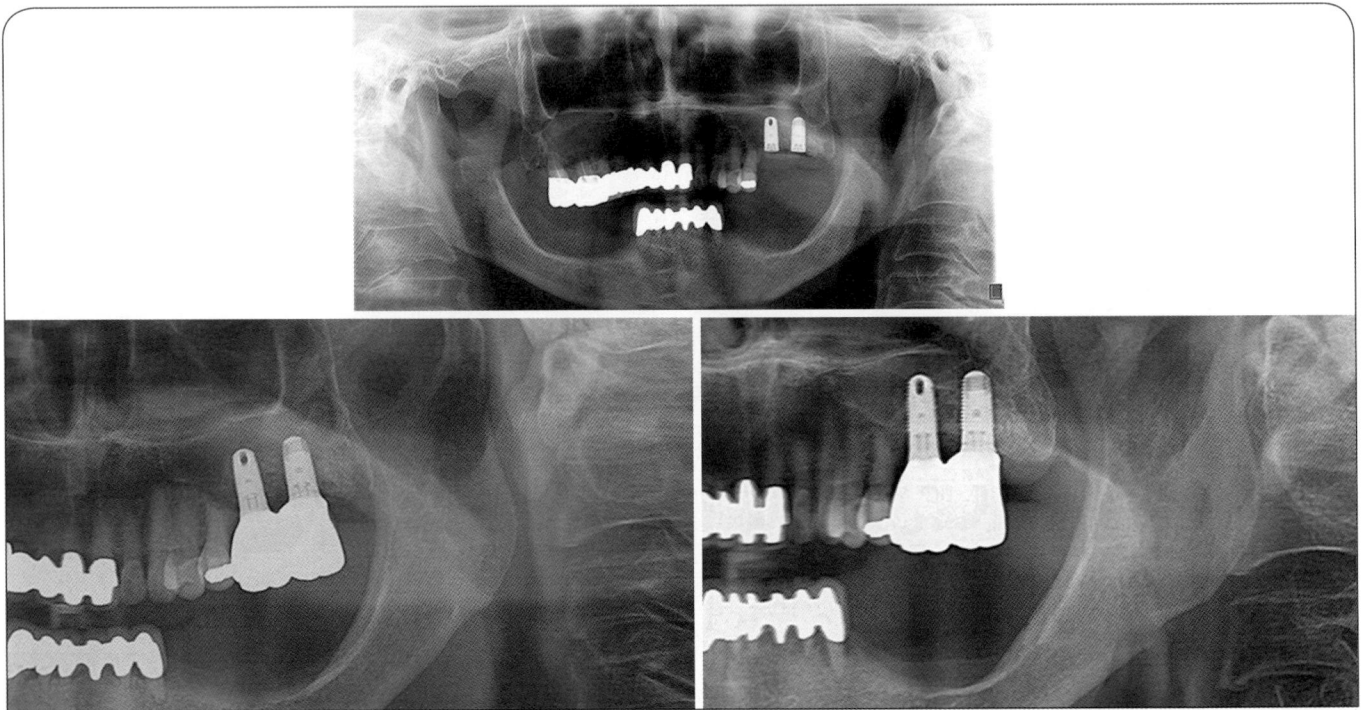

Fig. 13

OPG with final prosthesis. Perfect healing around the implant can be seen **(Fig. 13)**.

Tarun Kumar

MANAGEMENT OF AN IMPLANT THREAD EXPOSURE

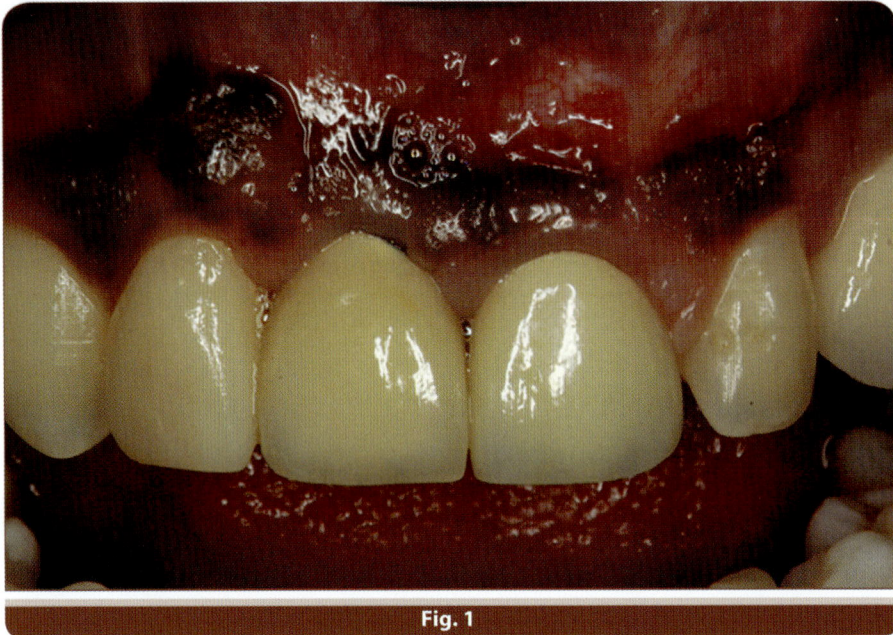

Fig. 1

A 24-year-old male patient came with a chief complaint of metal exposure in the implant retained prosthesis placed 2 years back. On examination, there was an exposure of implant thread in relation to tooth # 11 **(Fig. 1)**.

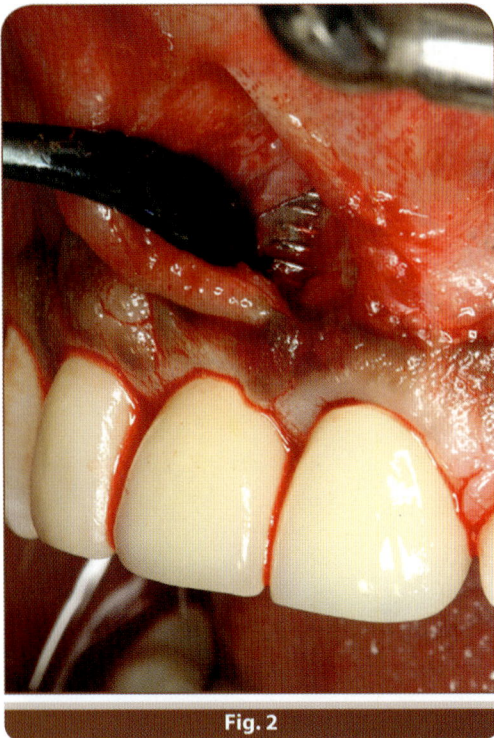

Fig. 2

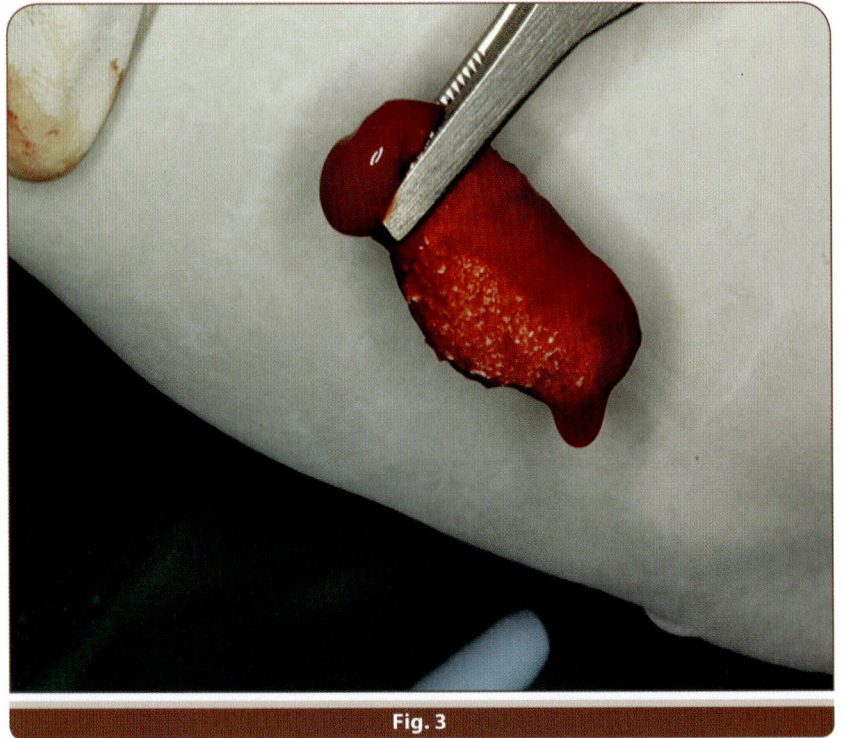

Fig. 3

Vertical releasing incision was given and subperiosteal tunnel was created keeping the marginal and papillary gingiva intact, exposing the implant surface followed by debridement of the implant surface **(Fig. 2)**.

A sticky bone was prepared using Xenograft and injectable platelet rich fibrin (i-PRF) **(Fig. 3)**.

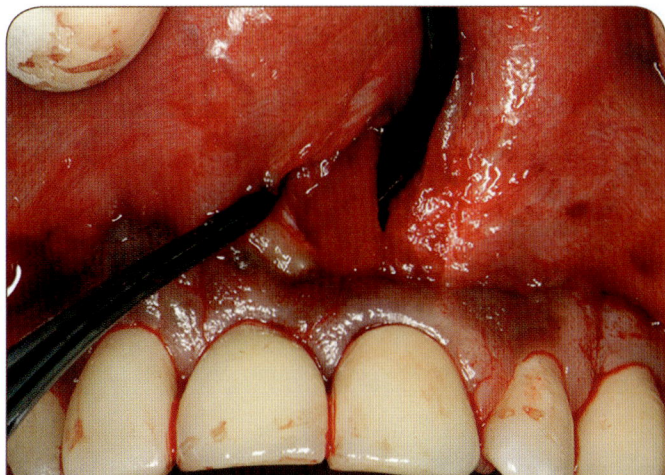

Fig. 4

Once coronal advancement of the gingival margin was established, collagen membrane was trimmed and adjusted to cover the sticky bone graft placed in the subperiosteal tunnel with a fine tipped curved forceps **(Fig. 4)**.

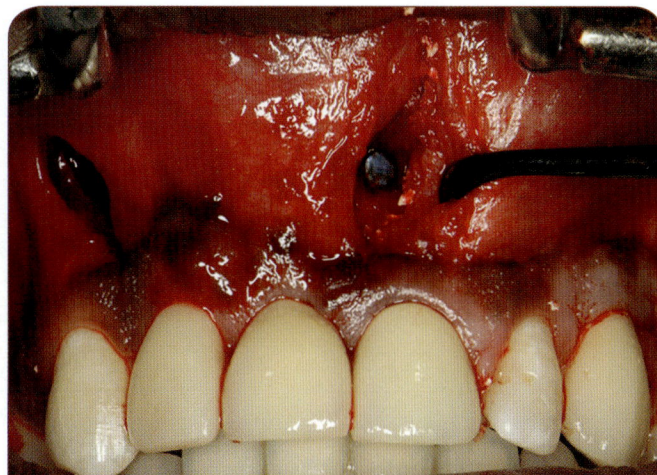

Fig. 5

The collagen membrane placed was secured using titanium screws **(Fig. 5)**.

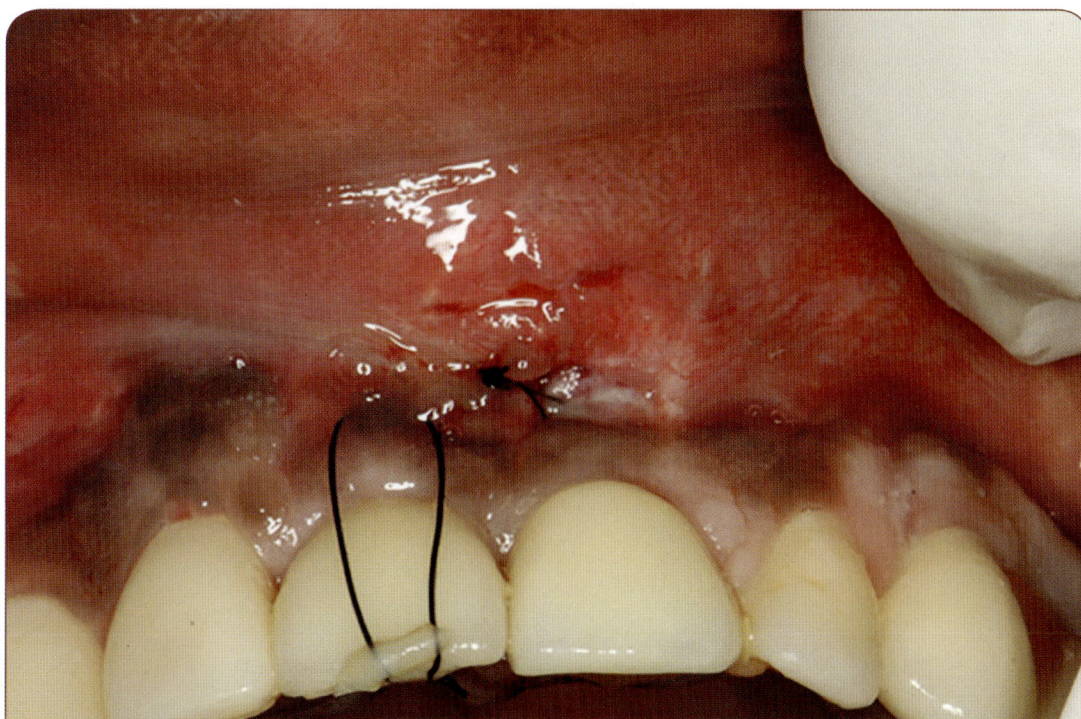

Fig. 6

The collagen membrane and mucogingival complex were then advanced coronally and stabilized in the new position with a coronally anchored suturing, by placing a horizontal mattress suture at approximately 2 to 3 mm apical to the gingival margin of the tooth (or within the band of keratinized gingiva). The suture was then tied to position the knot at the mid coronal point of the facial aspect of the tooth, which was secured with help of composite resin to prevent apical relapse of the gingival margin during initial stages of healing **(Fig. 6)**.

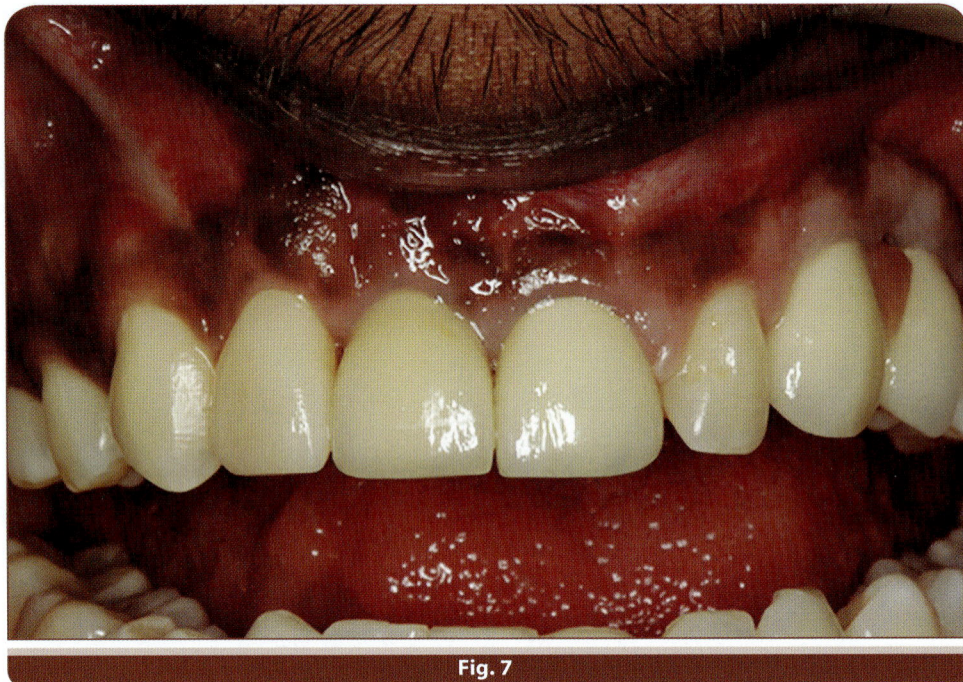

Fig. 7

There was adequate coverage of the exposed implant thread after 2 years of follow-up **(Fig. 7)**.

David Morales Schwarz , Hilde Morales

MANAGEMENT OF BUCCAL FENESTRATION DURING IMPLANT PLACEMENT IN ANTERIOR ZONE

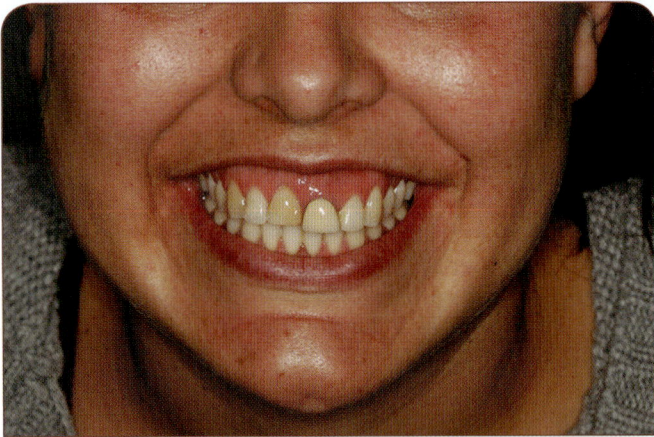

Fig. 1

A 31-year-old with no relevant medical history. We plan to remove tooth #21 and to place a top DM bioner implant **(Fig. 1)**.

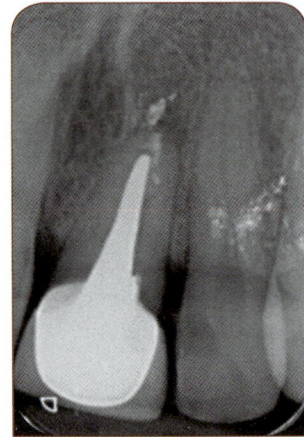

Fig. 2

Radiographic examination of teeth revealed poor prognosis **(Fig. 2)**.

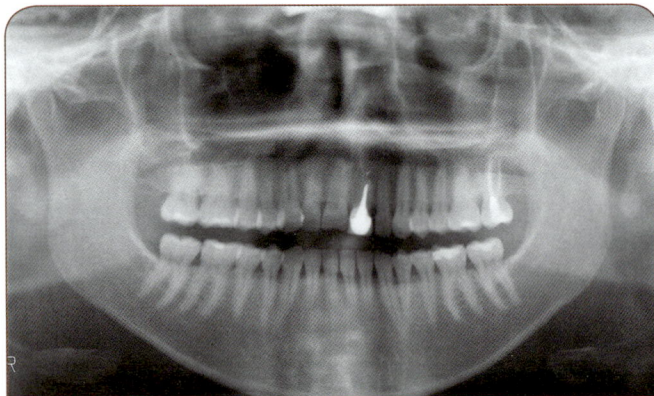

Fig. 3

Preoperative Orthopantomogram.

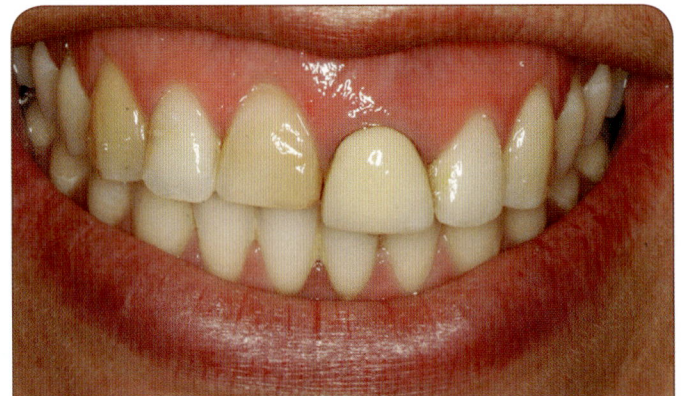

Fig. 4

We could see the difference between tooth #21 and tooth #11 gingival contour **(Fig. 4)**.

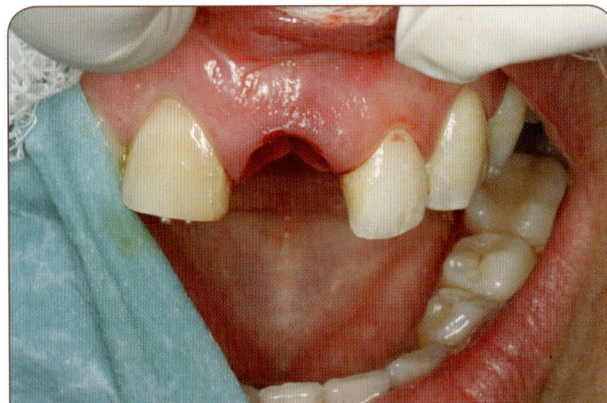

Fig. 5

Atraumatic extraction of #21 **(Fig. 5)**.

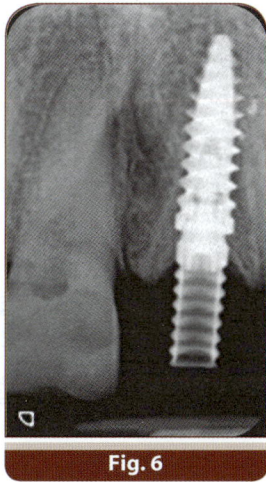

Fig. 6

Drilling 1200 RPM and placing 4 × 13 mm bioner top DM **(Fig. 6)**.

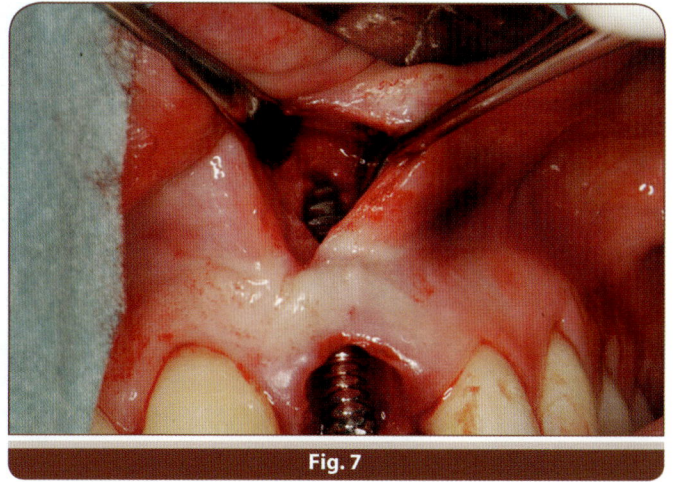

Fig. 7

An oval incision was made at the implant apex to see the fenestration **(Fig. 7)**.

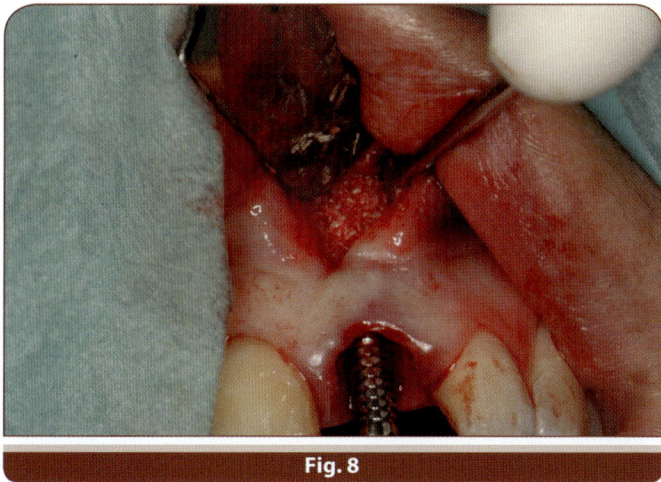

Fig. 8

We filled fenestration with Bio-Oss **(Fig. 8)**.

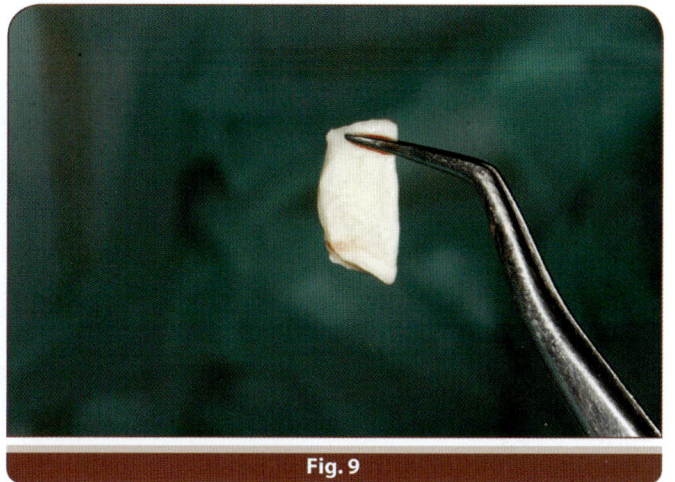

Fig. 9

Platelet rich plasma with calcium sulfate membrane **(Fig. 9)**.

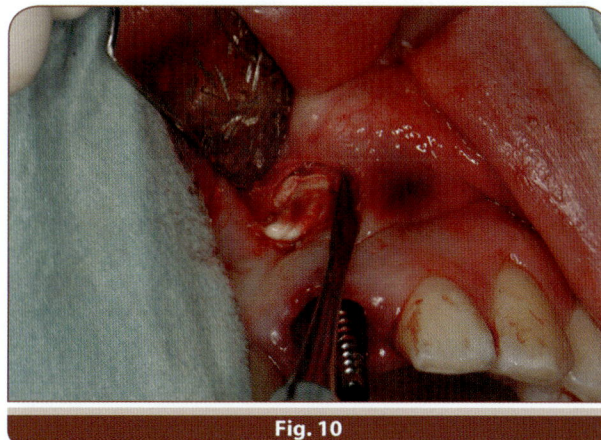

Fig. 10

Platelet rich plasma with calcium sulfate membrane was placed at the socket **(Fig. 10)**.

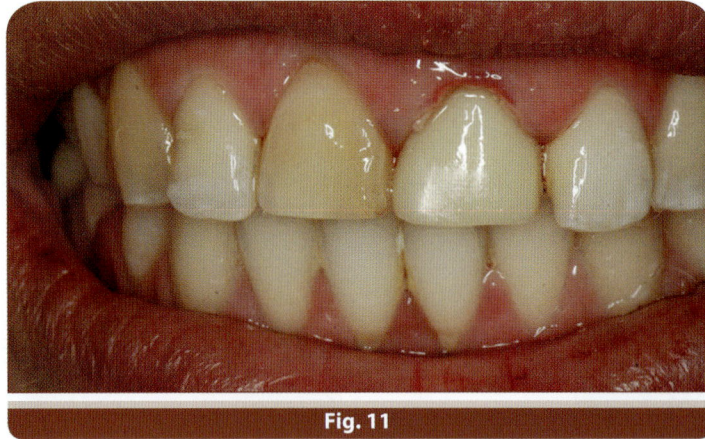

Fig. 11

Immediate loading of implant by provisional restoration **(Fig. 11)**.

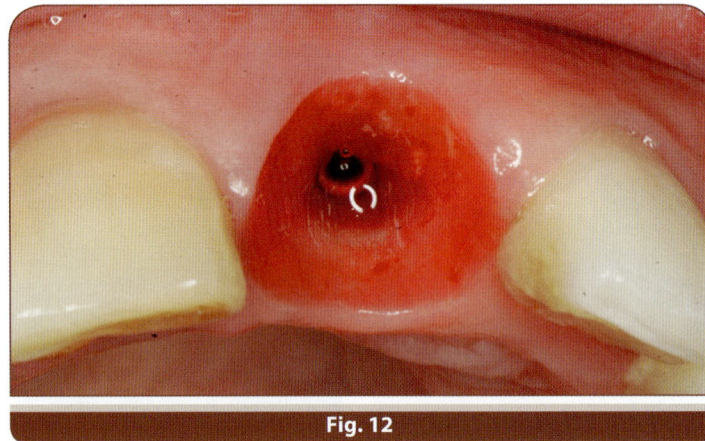

Fig. 12

The peri-implant soft tissue had been shaped and matured according to the contours of the provisional restoration. The emergence profile was used to duplicate the definitive restoration **(Fig. 12)**.

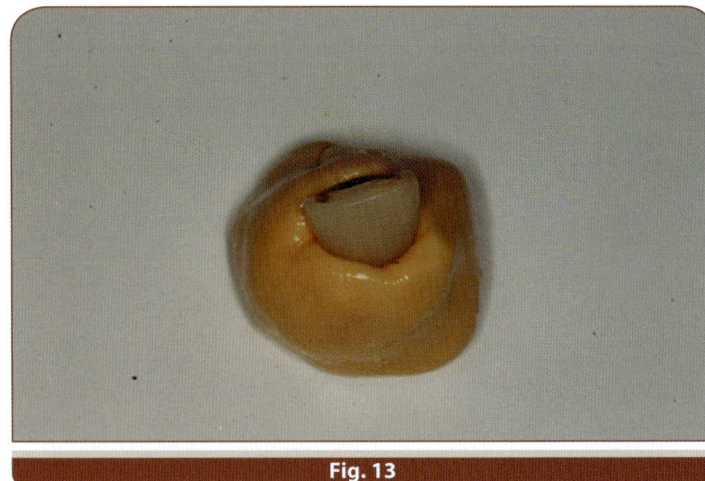

Fig. 13

The emergence profile was used to duplicate the definitive restoration **(Fig. 13)**.

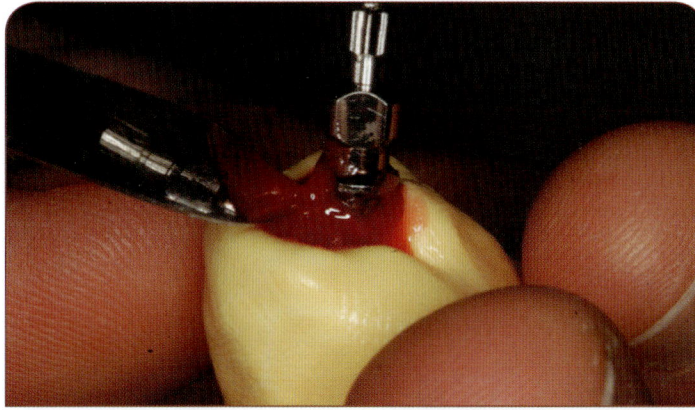

Fig. 14

Resin was added to fill the space between the provisional crown base and trimmed gingiva **(Fig. 14)**.

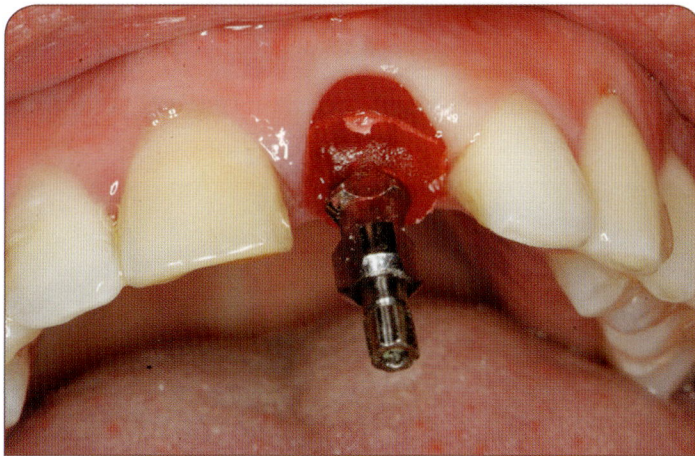

Fig. 15

The final impression was taken to make a definitive implant restoration **(Fig. 15)**.

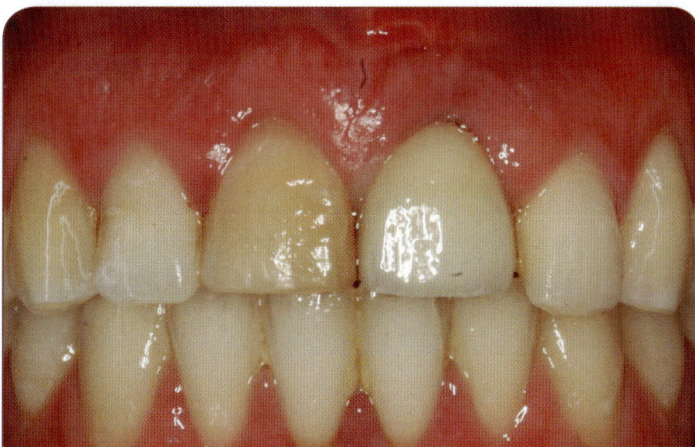

Fig. 16

Definitive implant restoration with an optimal emergence profile **(Fig. 16)**.

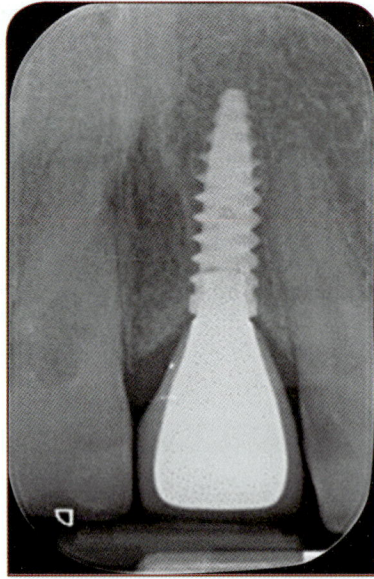

Fig. 17

Definitive implant restoration **(Fig. 17)**.

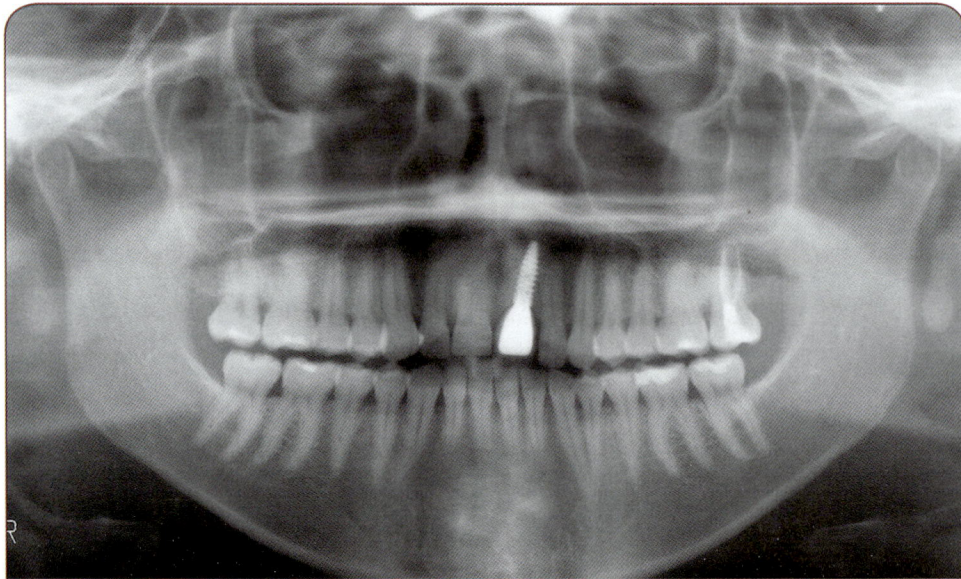

Fig. 18

Radiographic illustration showing properly healed implant site **(Fig. 18)**.

Lanka Mahesh, Vishal Gupta

REMOVAL OF IMPLANT DISPLACED INTO THE ANTRUM AND ITS MANAGEMENT

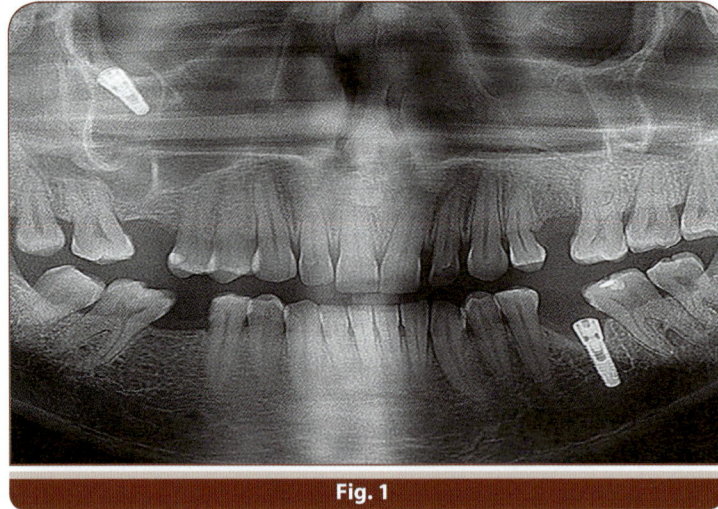

Fig. 1

Preoperative panorex of a 30-year-old male patient having undergone sinus grafting elsewhere and the implant displaced into the antrum and located at the inferior orbital floor **(Fig. 1)**.

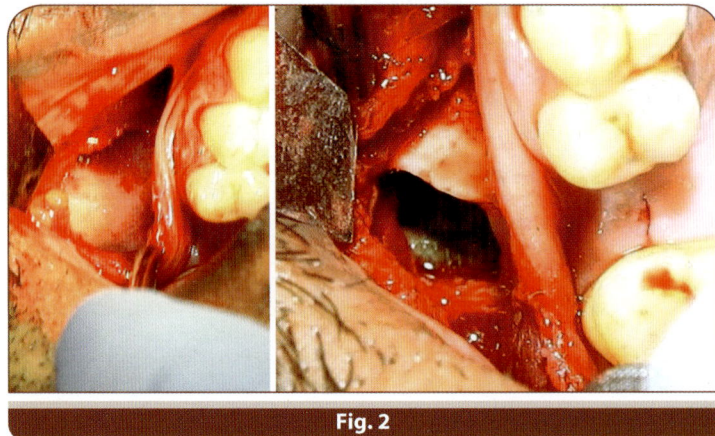

Fig. 2

Caldwell-Luc incision. The implant is dislodged with saline rinses at pressure and a fine long nosed narrow tweezer **(Fig. 2)**.

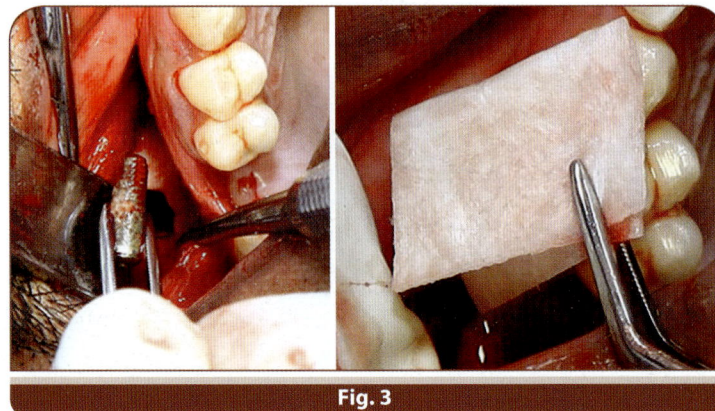

Fig. 3

The offending implant is removed and an antral wash is performed. NovaBone butty (NovaBone) is placed into the antrum. Double layer RCM membrane (ACE Surgical) is placed over the antrostomy site **(Fig. 3)**.

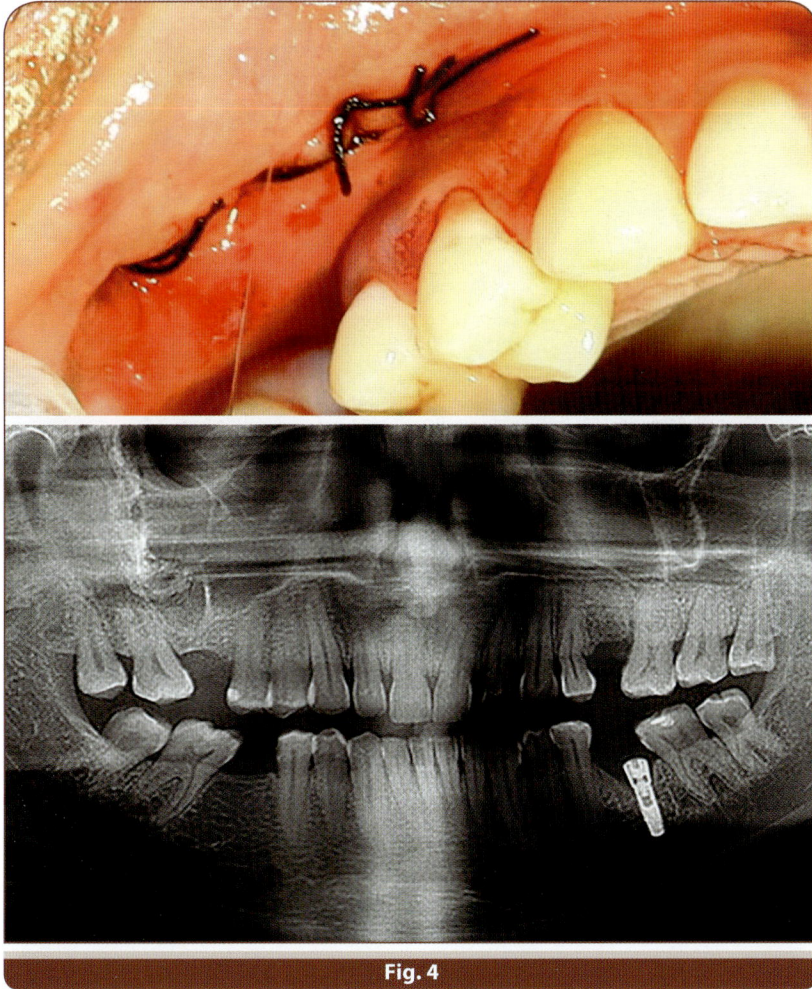

Fig. 4

Wound closure is achieved with simple interrupted 3-0 silk sutures. Immediate postoperative panorex demonstrates bone fill **(Fig. 4)**.

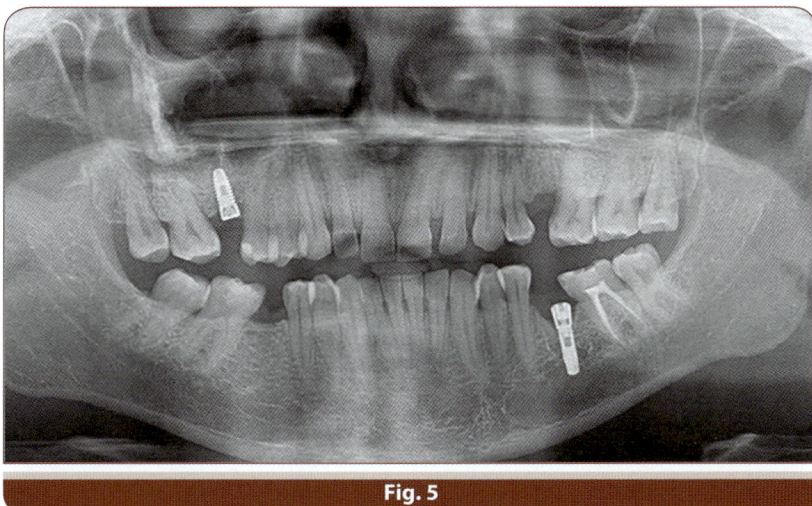

Fig. 5

Six months following the grafting procedure. A 3.8/11.5 kelt implant (Bioner) is placed in the region of 16 **(Fig. 5)**.

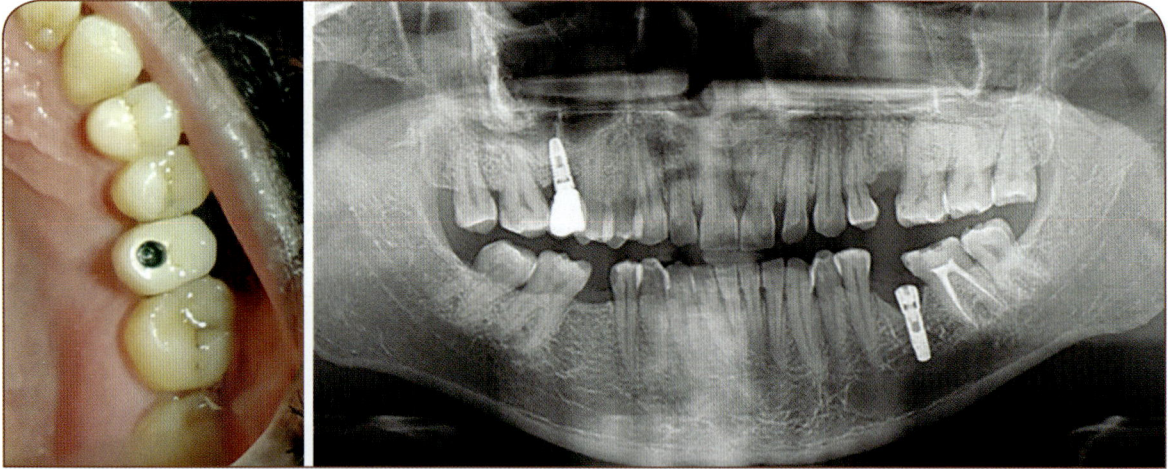

Fig. 6

The final SCR (screw cemented restoration) in place. Postoperative panorex demostrating good bone fill in the antrum and a stable prosthesis. The mandibular implant was restored subsequently **(Fig. 6)**.

CASE STUDY 124

Bassam F Rabie

MANAGING SOFT TISSUE COMPLICATION IN IMMEDIATE POST EXTRACTION IMPLANTS

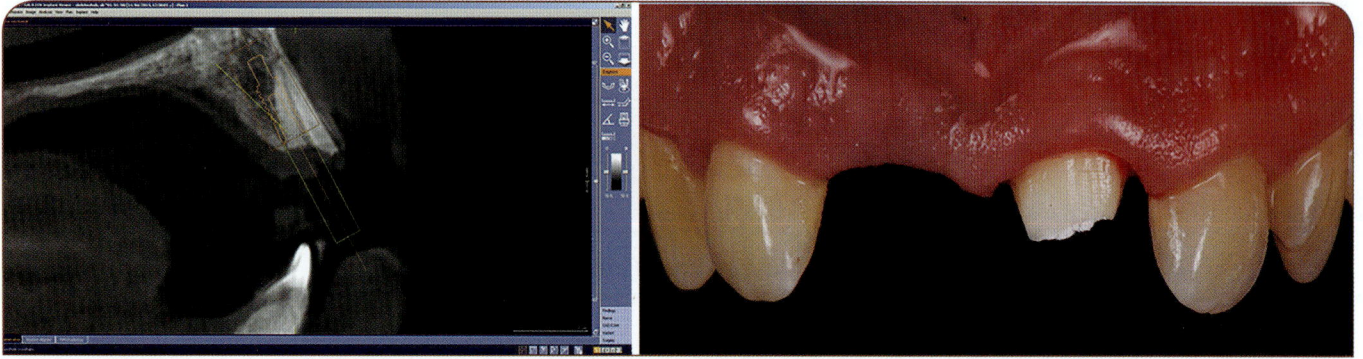

Fig. 1

Fractured upper centrals 3D planning on CBCT shows good amount of triangle bone housing palatal to the root **(Fig. 1)**.

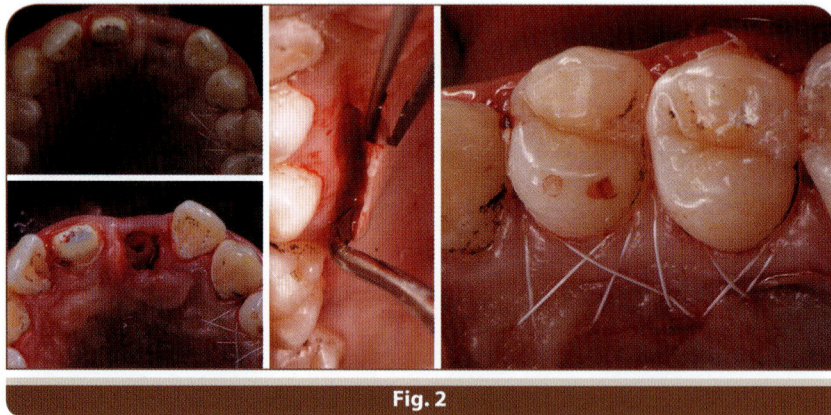

Fig. 2

Connective tissue harvested Small opening on top of the 3-week-old fractured central **(Fig. 2)**.

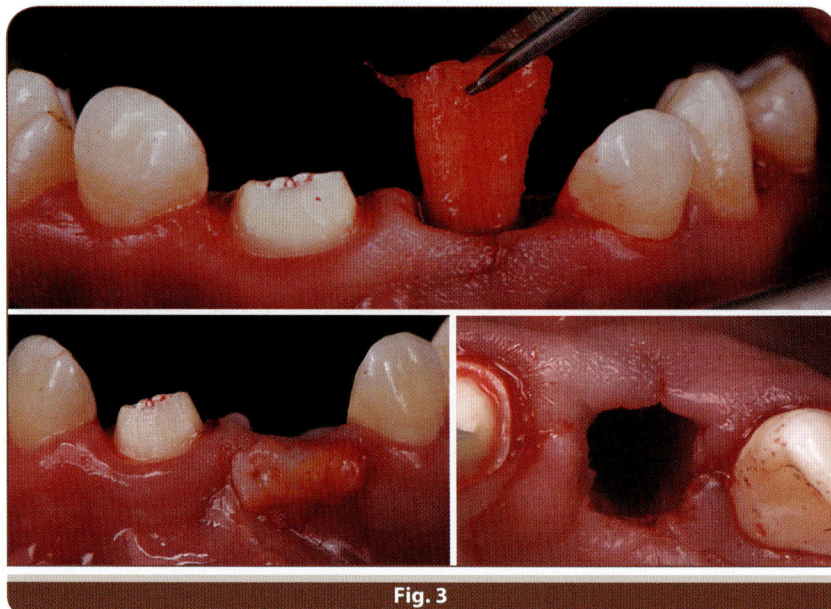

Fig. 3

Atraumatic extraction socket intact. Connective tissue in place ready to be inserted after tunneling in front of the socket **(Fig. 3)**.

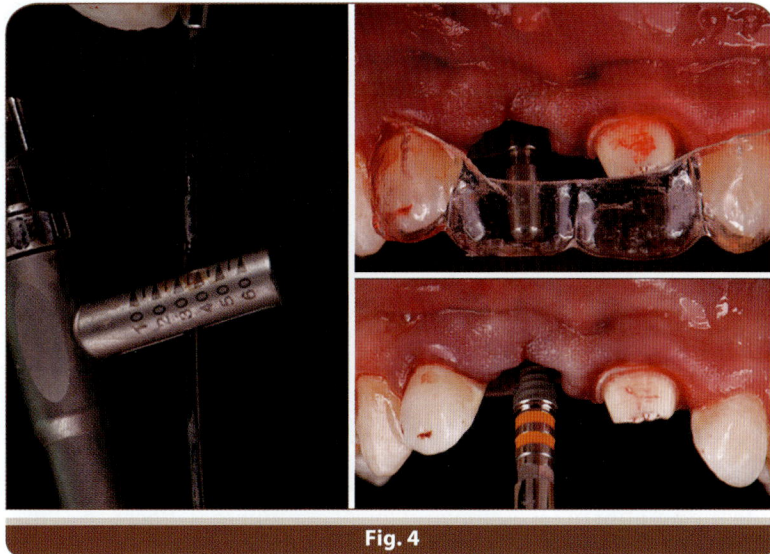

Fig. 4

Placement of the implant in the palatal bony housing with very good initial stability of around 40 Ncm guided by the conventional surgical stent **(Fig. 4)**.

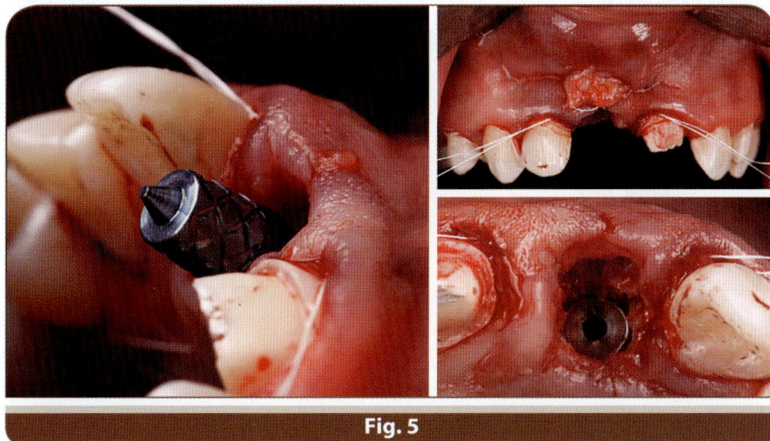

Fig. 5

Abutment body replica showing position of the implant with enough gap in front of it. CT placed in tunnel and allograft bone in the gap. All this to compensate for the remodelling **(Fig. 5)**.

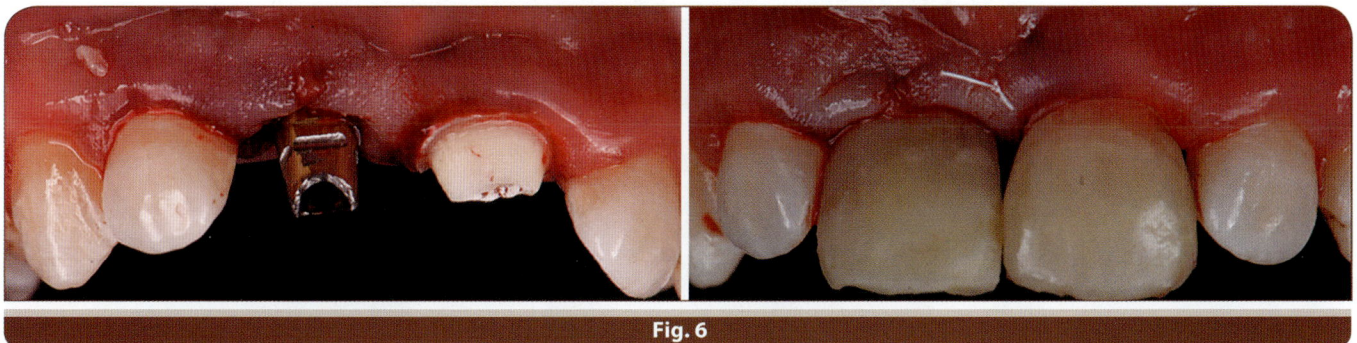

Fig. 6

Temporary abutment in place and conventional fabrication of a temporary crown, but the connective tissue unfortunately was lost during the surgery being sucked in the suction due to human assistant error. Notice the soft tissue around the implant temporary crown **(Fig. 6)**.

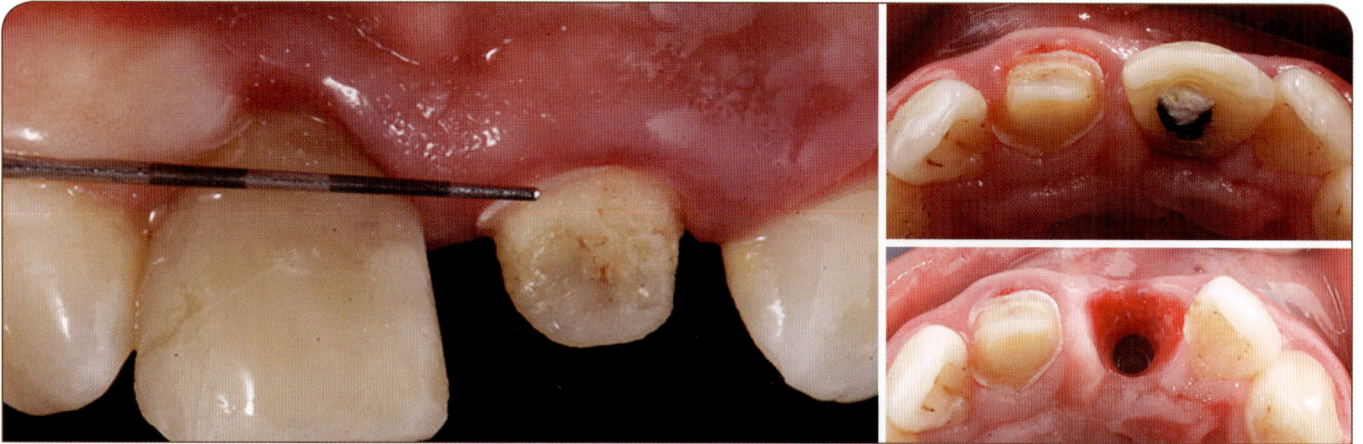

Fig. 7

After 3 weeks of healing, note the amount of recession and facial contour loss, because of the loss of the soft tissue graft **(Fig. 7)**.

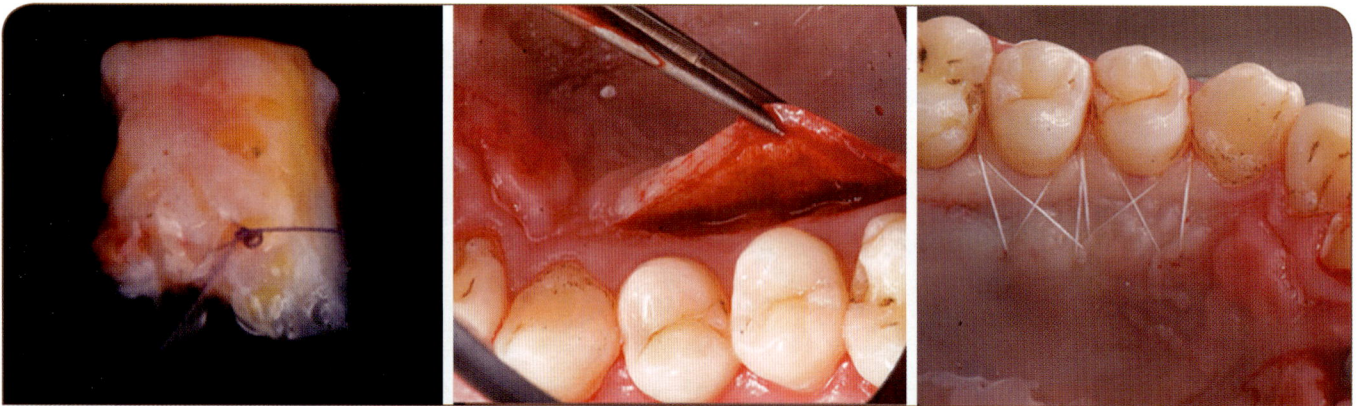

Fig. 8

So, to solve the complication, another tunneling around the integrated implant after 2 months is done and a new CT is harvested and folded and sutured with a 7/0 resorbable PGA suture to further thicken the graft **(Fig. 8)**.

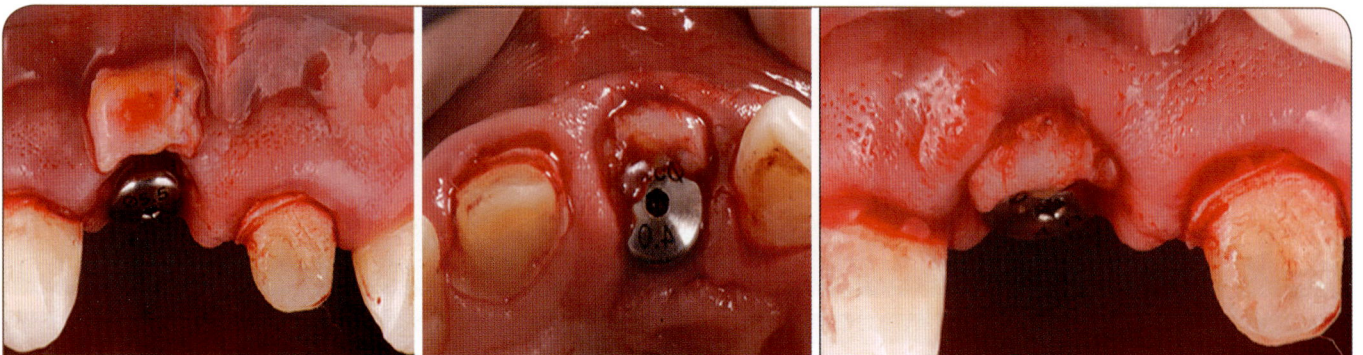

Fig. 9

CT graft in place and immediately the facial contour is gained. The left central incisor was root canaled **(Fig. 9)**.

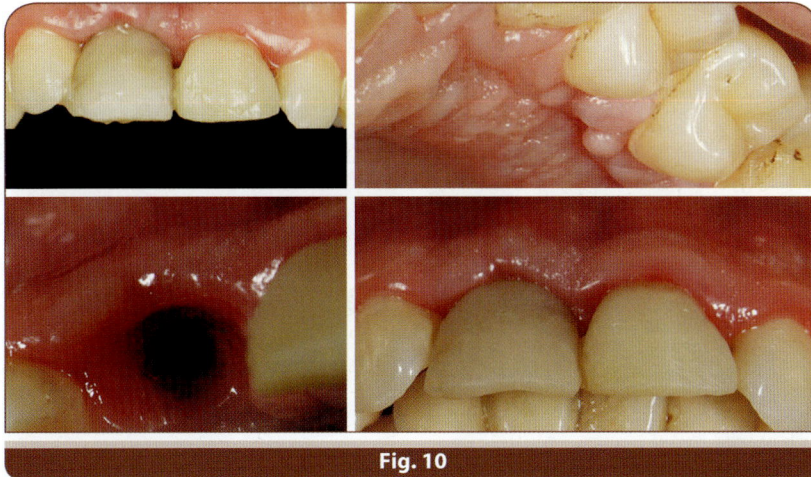

Fig. 10

Immediated temporization of implant. After another 3 weeks, the level of the soft tissue margins has been gained by the coronal advancement with the tunneling and graft **(Fig. 10)**.

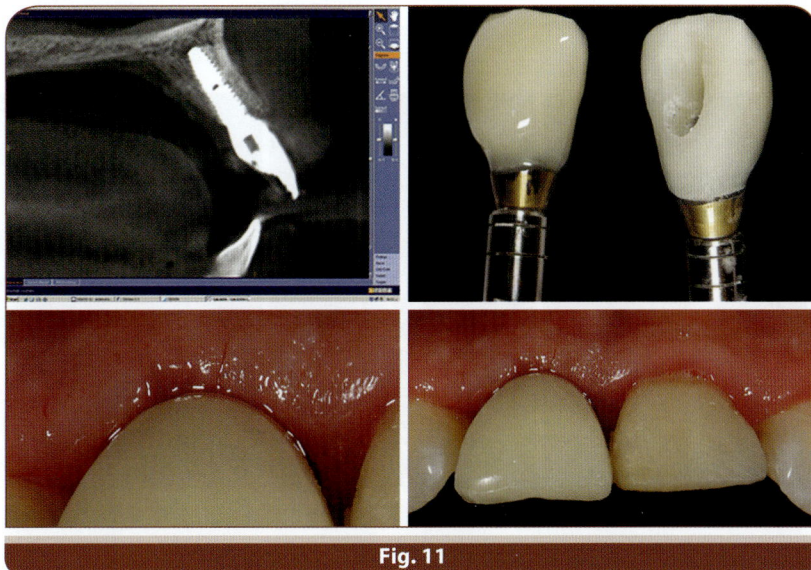

Fig. 11

A new CAD CAM temporary was fabricated and screw retained on the implant to further give time for the soft tissue to mature **(Fig. 11)**.

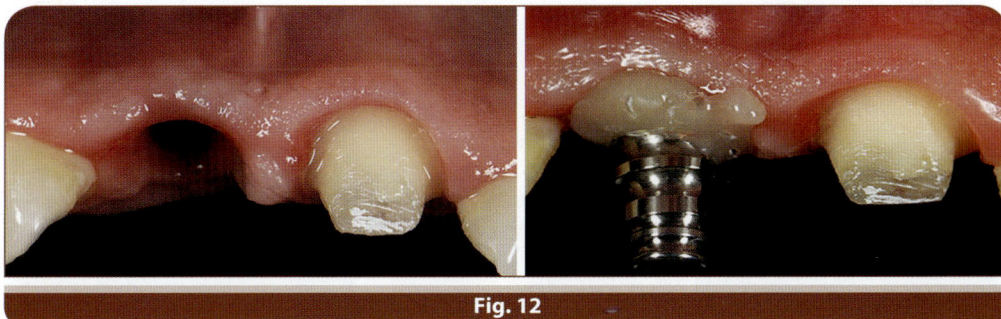

Fig. 12

After 6 weeks the temporary is removed. A tissue level impression is taken. Focus on the quality and shape and emergence of the soft tissue and Papilla around the implant **(Fig. 12)**.

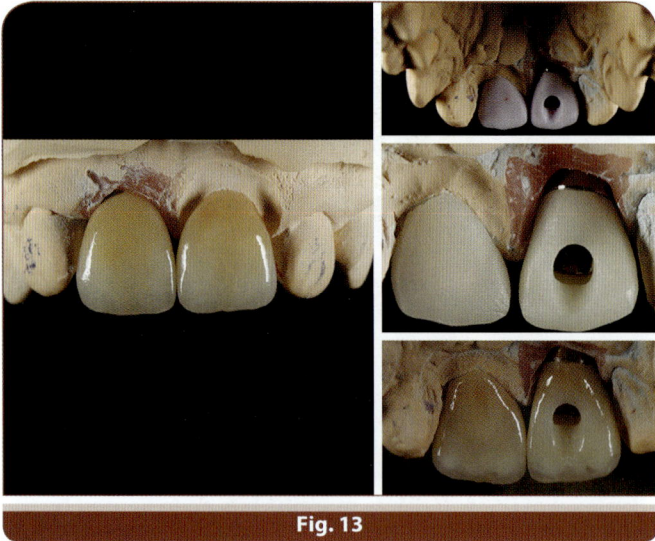

Fig. 13

CAD CAM E.max crowns where milled and cut back and porcelain added and characterized **(Fig. 13)**.

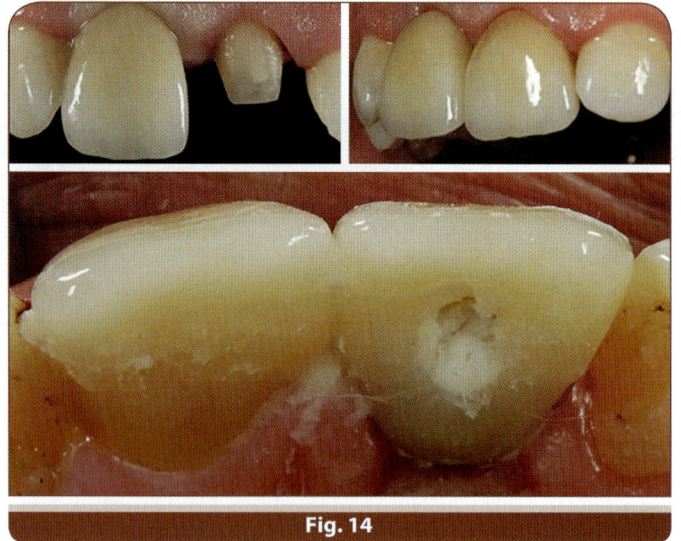

Fig. 14

Crow on natural-root canaled tooth was resin-bonded while the implant crown was finally cemented and left to set **(Fig. 14)**.

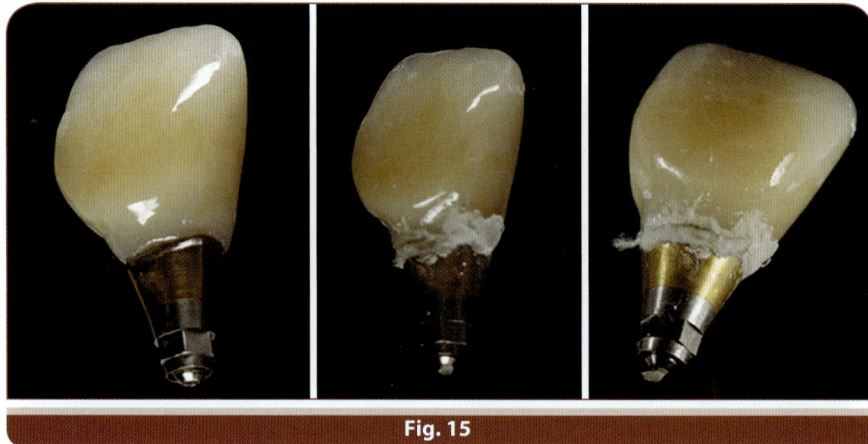

Fig. 15

After complete setting of the final cement, the excess was removed from the access hole and the crown abutment assembly was unscrewed. Now the excess cement is removed from the abutment crown interface, which is usually left under the tissue when cemented **(Fig. 15)**.

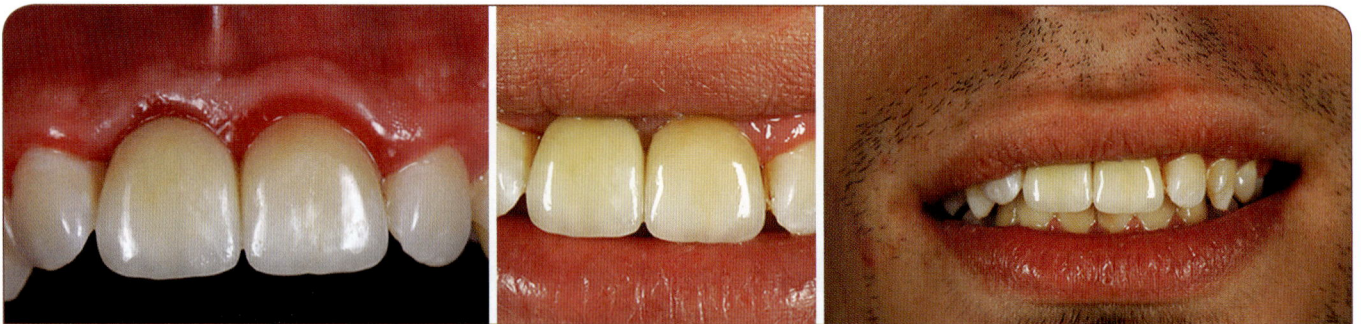

Fig. 16

After 3 years of loading **(Fig. 16)**.

CASE STUDY 125

Lanka Mahesh, Nitika Poonia

Removal of a Fractured Implant, Socket Grafting and Delayed Implant Placement

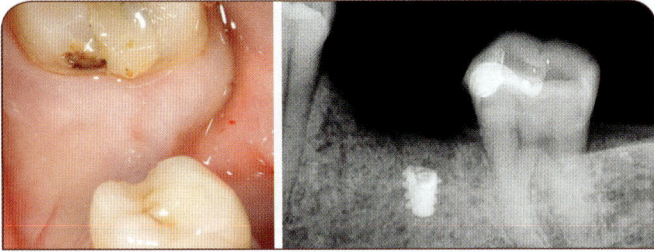

Fig. 1

Preoperative view of a referred case with soft tissue collapse in the operated site evident. The radiograph reveals a fractured xive (Dentsply) narrow diameter implant. Implant fractured after 2 months of loading due to a narrow diameter implant in a site which demanded a wider implant **(Fig. 1)**.

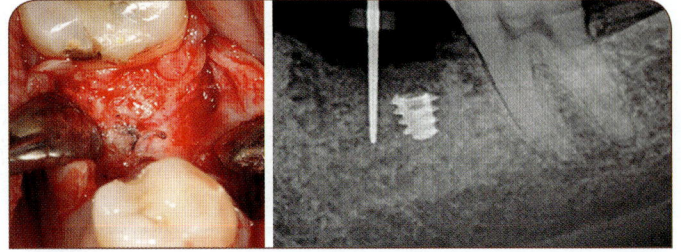

Fig. 2

A full thickness mucoperiosteal flap is raised to get adequate visibility of the site. A lancet drill is used at high speed and an endodontic file with a stopper is placed to determine exact position of the implant **(Fig. 2)**.

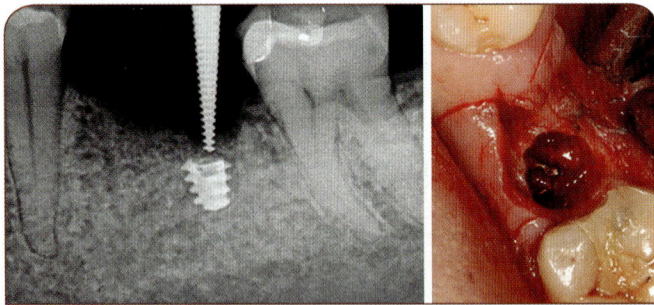

Fig. 3

After removal of coronal position a buck file is placed and another X-ray taken. The fractured implant is visible, with narrow fissure carbide burs on a high speed turbine airotor bone around the fractured segment is gently removed **(Fig. 3)**.

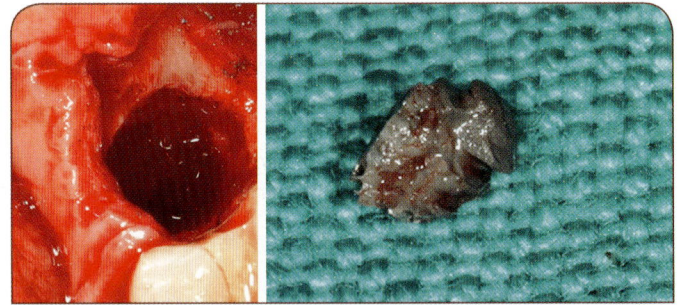

Fig. 4

The fractured implant is gently luxated out with the help of luxators. The fractured implant after explantation **(Fig. 4)**.

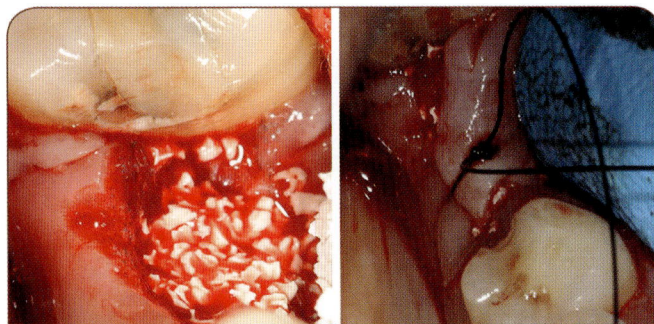

Fig. 5

An intraoperative decision was taken to graft the implant site and re-enter after 5 months for fresh implant placement. Bio-Oss (Geistlisch) was packed into the site closed with a collaplug (Zimmer Dental). The flap was released and approximated with 4-0 polyamide sutures **(Fig. 5)**.

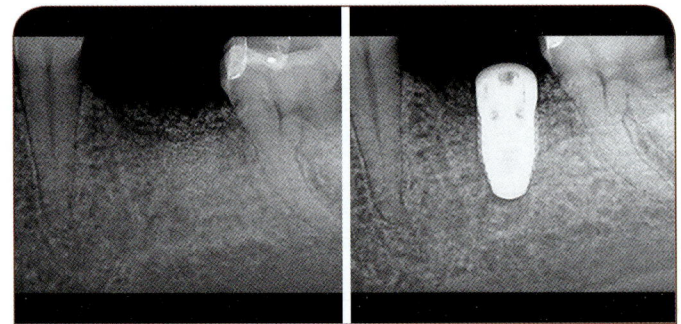

Fig. 6

Intraoral radiograph of the healed site 5 months postoperative shows a well healed site. A 5/10 mm implant fixture is inserted at 40 Ncm (Nobel groovy, Nobel Biocare) **(Fig. 6)**.

Bach Le

Retreatment of a Failing Dental Implant Site in the Esthetic Zone using the Screw Tent-Pole Technique with Mineralized Allograft

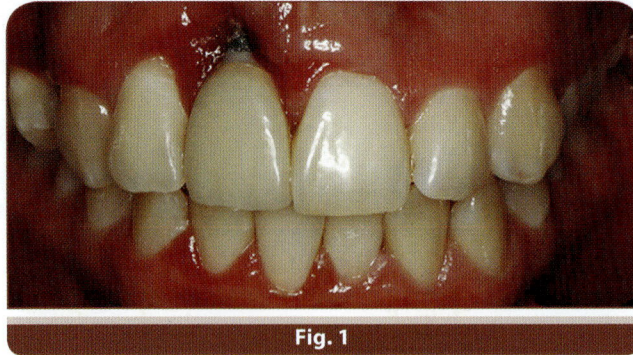

Fig. 1

Severe labial soft tissue defect with exposure of the implant collar at the right maxillary central incisor. There is also gingival recession on the right lateral incisor due to multiple previous surgical intervention causing gingival disharmony. Despite the appearance, there is no evidence of purulence or infection **(Fig. 1)**.

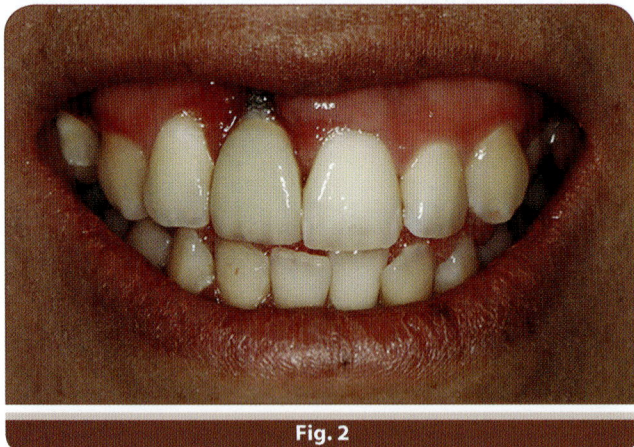

Fig. 2

High smile line revealing the unesthetic soft tissue defect **(Fig. 2)**.

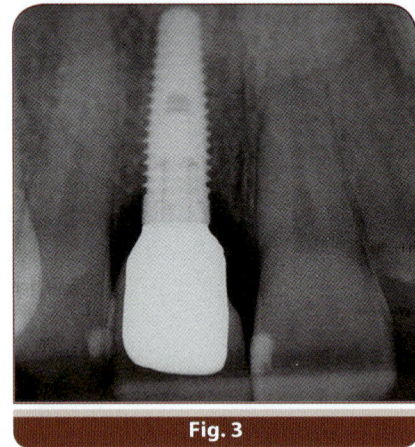

Fig. 3

Radiograph showing circumferential bone loss around the implant **(Fig. 3)**.

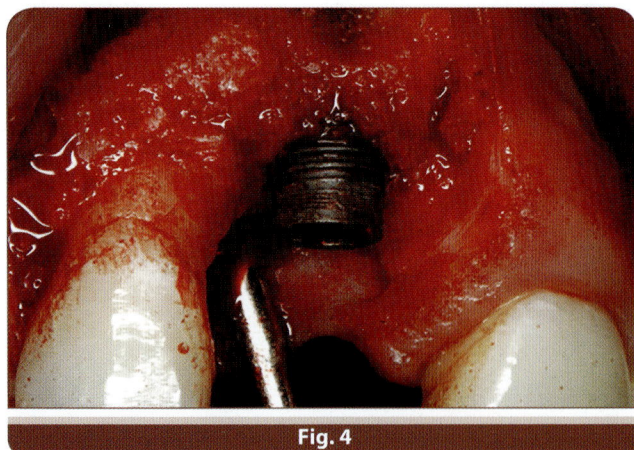

Fig. 4

Moderate circumferential crestal bone loss around the implant with poor prognosis for salvage. The decision was made to remove the implant with GBR repair of the defect **(Fig. 4)**.

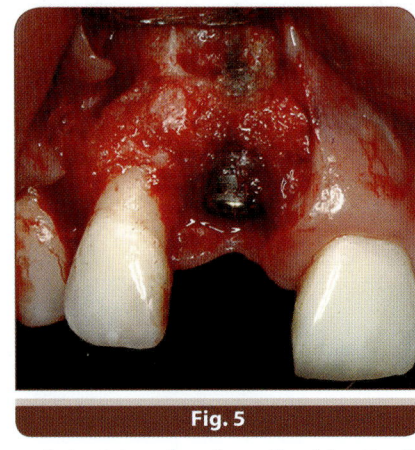

Fig. 5

An Open Book incision (as described by Bach Le) design was made with the vertical arm on the mesial to allow for flap rotation and coronal advancement of the gingival margin level on the distal to simultaneously correct the recession defect on the right lateral incisor **(Fig. 5)**.

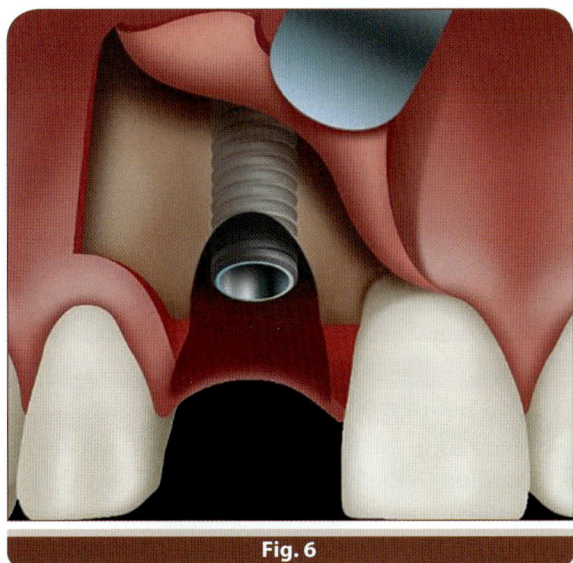

Fig. 6

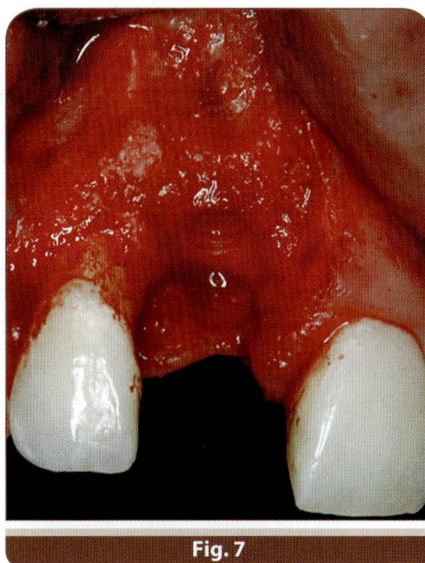

Fig. 7

Incision design: The "open book flap" design is utilized for better graft containment and allow for coronal advancement of the gingival margin. The flap is usually developed with a distal, curvilinear, vertical incision that follows the gingival margin of the distal tooth. A wide subperiosteal reflection is made up to the level of the nasal spine to expose 2 to 3 times the treatment area, and then the papilla is reflected on the mesial side of the edentulous site **(Fig. 6)**.

Removing the implant resulted in a 6 mm vertical bone defect with missing palatal and labial walls. Interproximal bone height of adjacent teeth were not compromised **(Fig. 7)**.

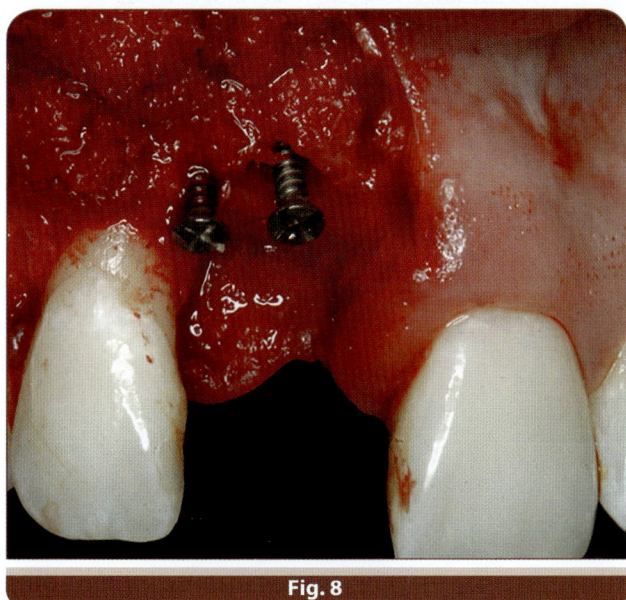

Fig. 8

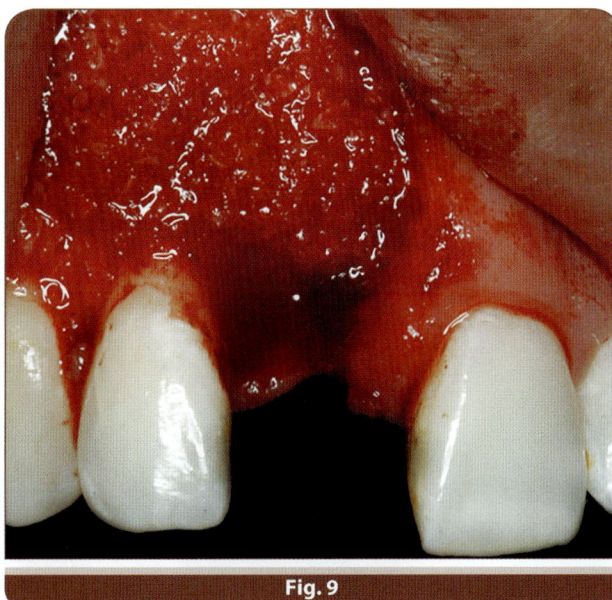

Fig. 9

Screw tent-pole technique used to tent the soft tissue matrix to support an bone graft material to promote vertical osseous regeneration **(Fig. 8)**.

A mineralized human allograft (MinerOss Cancellous) is placed into the defect and packed onto the labial bone surface of the adjacent tooth. Overcorrection of at least 30% of the normal alveolar ridge is done in anticipation of future bone graft remodeling and resorption **(Fig. 9)**.

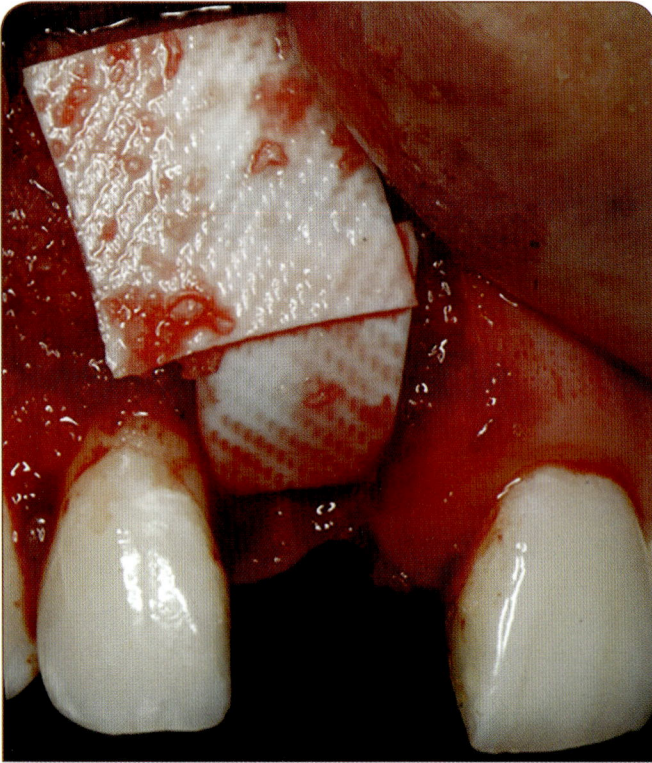

Fig. 10

Multiple cross-link resorbable collagen membranes (Ossix Plus) are placed over the graft **(Fig. 10)**.

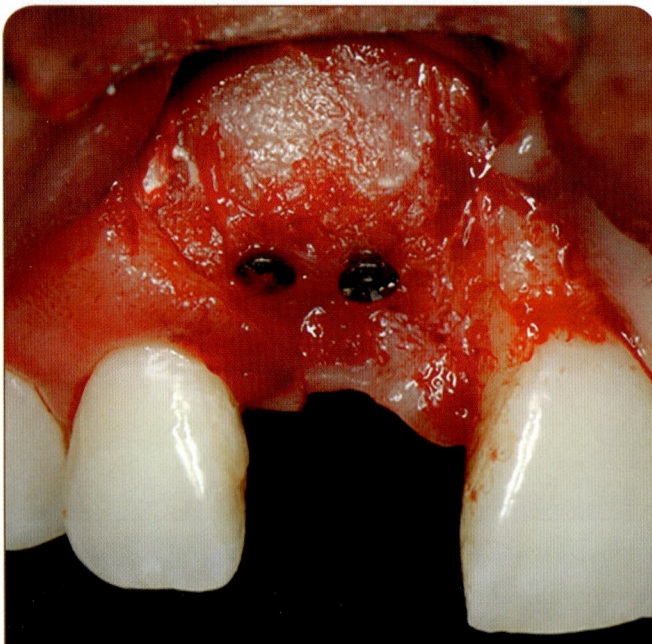

Fig. 11

Postoperative CT scan taken 1 year after GBR procedure shows restoration of hard tissue dimensions with new bone formation to the head of the screw **(Fig. 11)**.

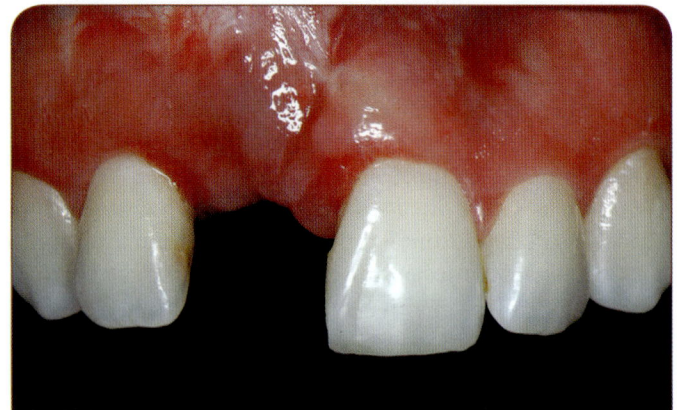

Fig. 12

One year after implant removal and GBR **(Fig. 12)**.

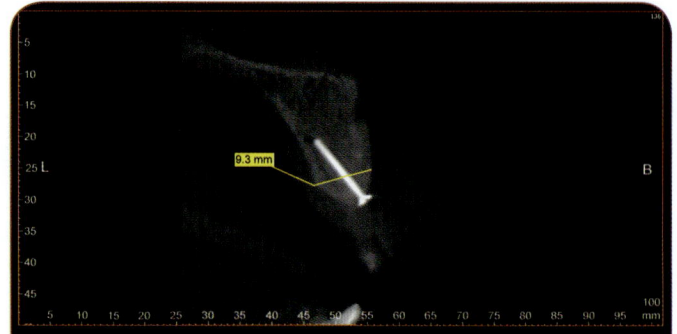

Fig. 13

One year after implant removal and GBR **(Fig. 13)**.

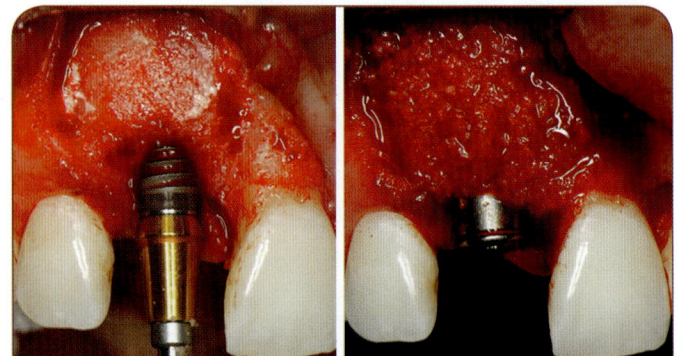

Fig. 14

Placement of a tapered implant (Biohorizons). Even though there is adequate labial bone thickness, an additional layer of mineralized human allograft is placed over the existing bone to increase soft tissue profile and improve alveolar ridge contour **(Fig. 14)**.

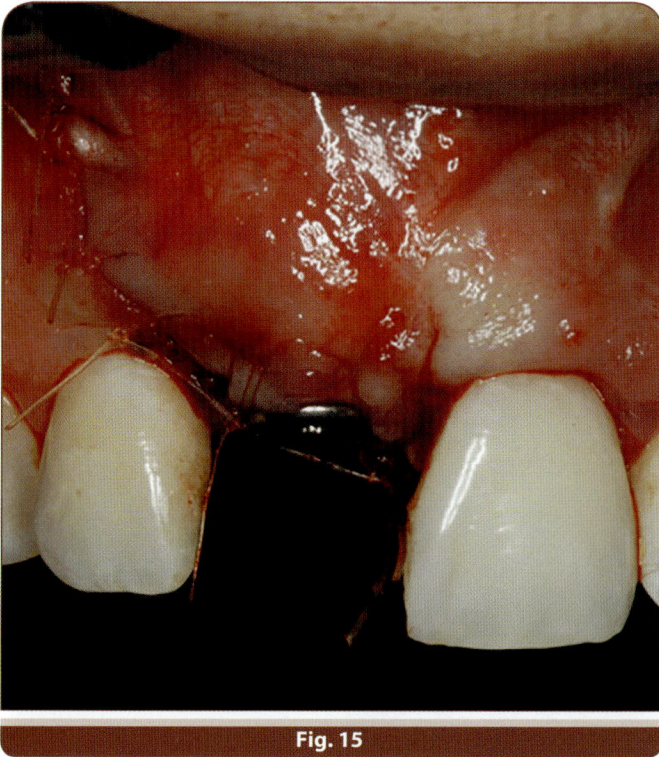

Fig. 15

A wide healing abutment was connected to the implant to create an additional tenting effect over the graft site and help to contour the overlying soft tissue. The simultaneous bone grafting is done with non-submerged implant placement **(Fig. 15)**.

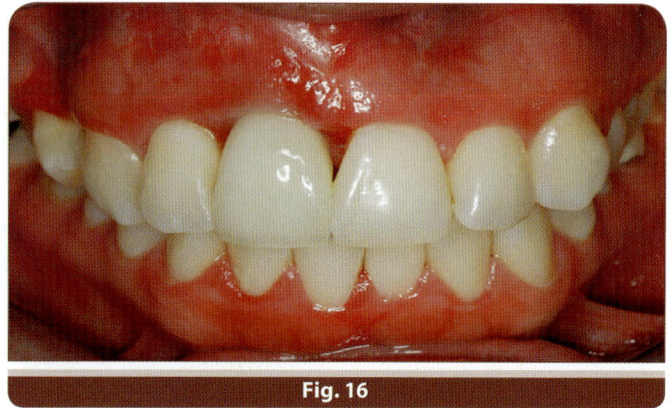

Fig. 16

Delivery of a screw-retained provisional restoration 3 months after implant placement **(Fig. 16)**.

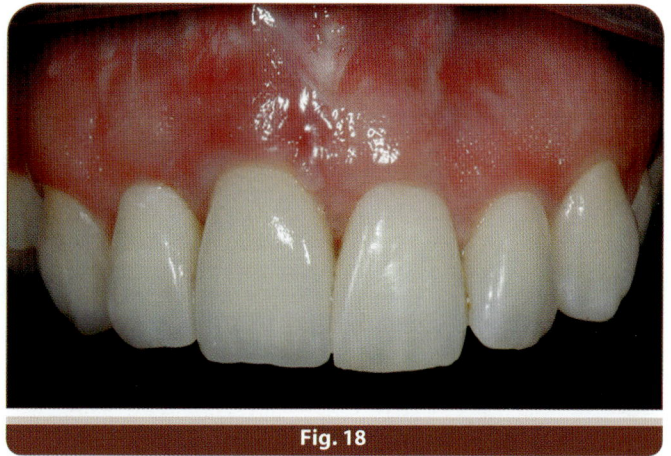

Fig. 18

Delivery of final restoration **(Fig. 18)**.

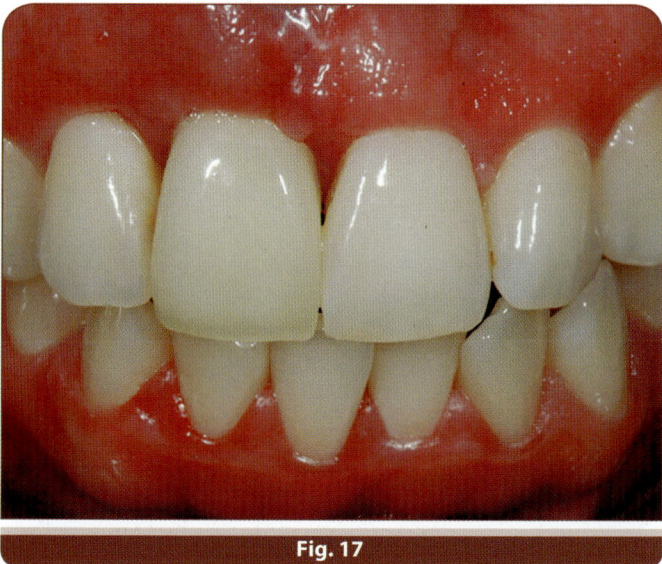

Fig. 17

Four months after delivery of provisional restoration. Note improvement in soft tissue architecture with increase in midline papilla fill **(Fig. 17)**.

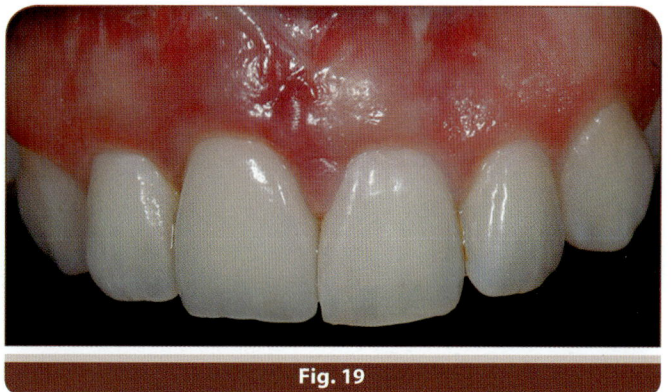

Fig. 19

Six years follow-up. Note continued improvement in soft tissue architecture and papilla fill. Note improvement in gingival margin level of the right lateral incisor with more symmetrical teeth size compared to pretreatment photo **(Fig. 19)**.

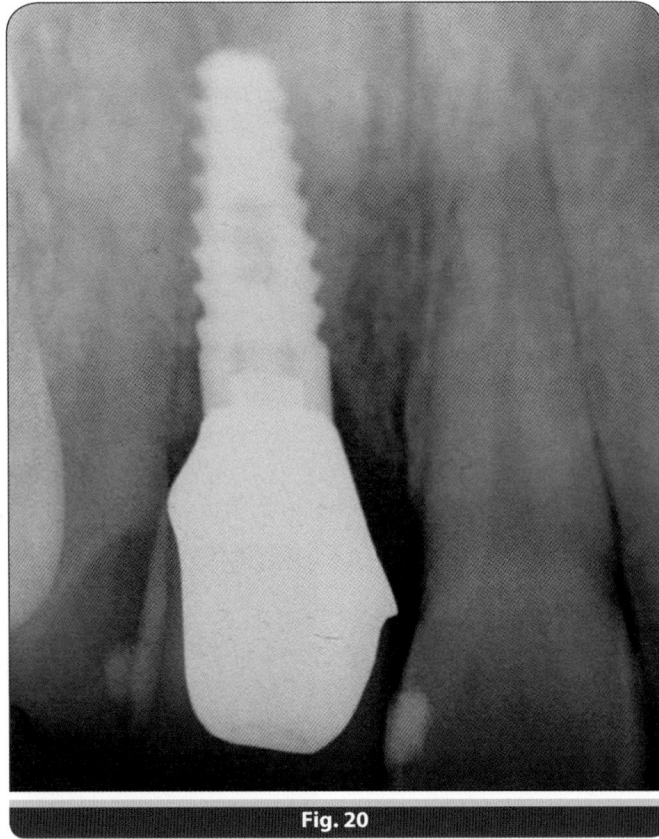

Fig. 20

Postoperative radiograph taken 6 years after delivery of definitive restoration shows stable peri-implant bone level **(Fig. 20)**.

Saj Jivraj

RESTORATION OF MALPOSITIONED IMPLANTS

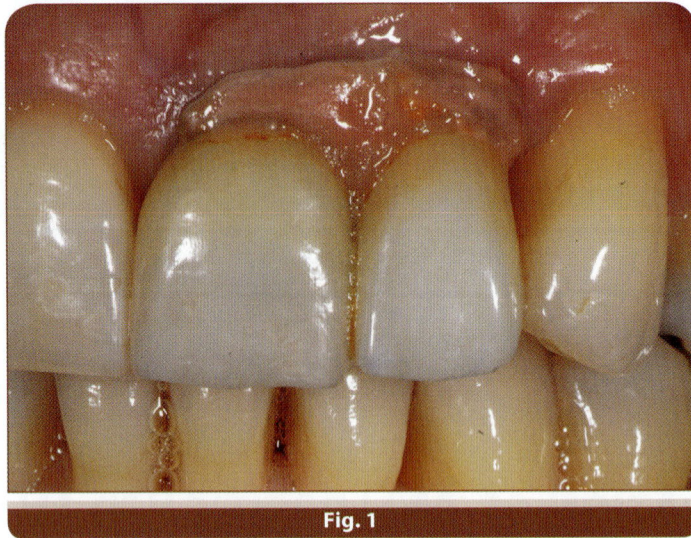

Fig. 1

Current restoration is a cemented implant supported restoration with pink composite. Implants placed, WP and NP, Cemented, Composite added, Asymmetrical **(Fig. 1)**.

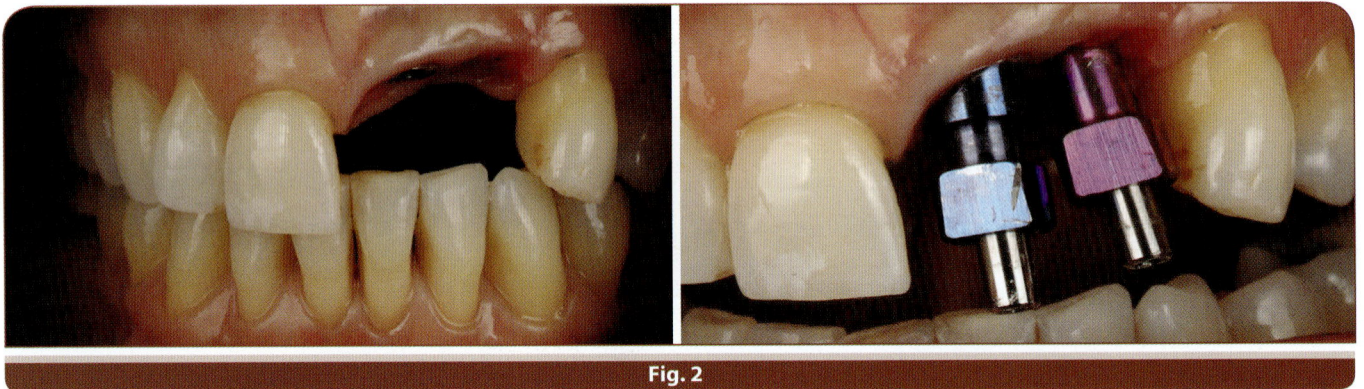

Fig. 2

Massive tissue loss, high smile line, Implants shallow **(Fig. 2)**.

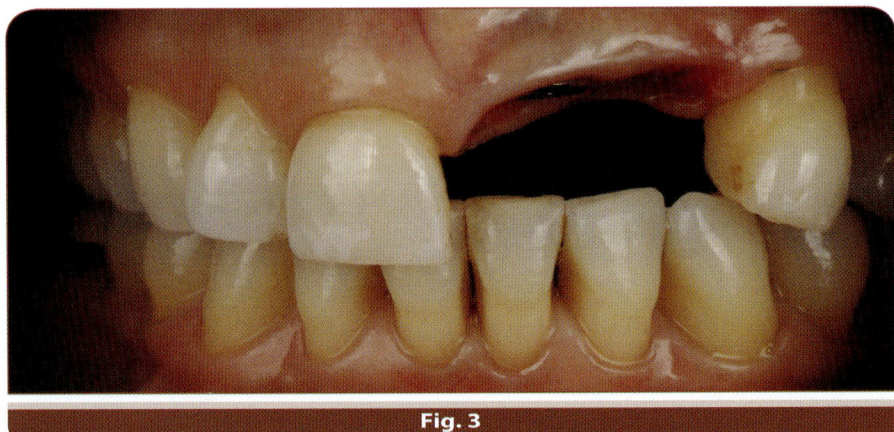

Fig. 3

Patient wants no surgery. We want to screw retain cleansable and esthetically pleasing **(Fig. 3)**.

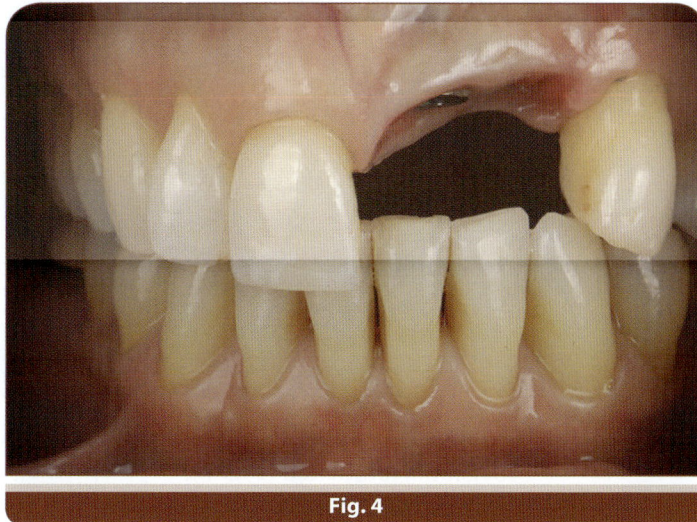

Fig. 4

Keep existing implants, test in provisional, definitive restoration and nightguard **(Fig. 4)**.

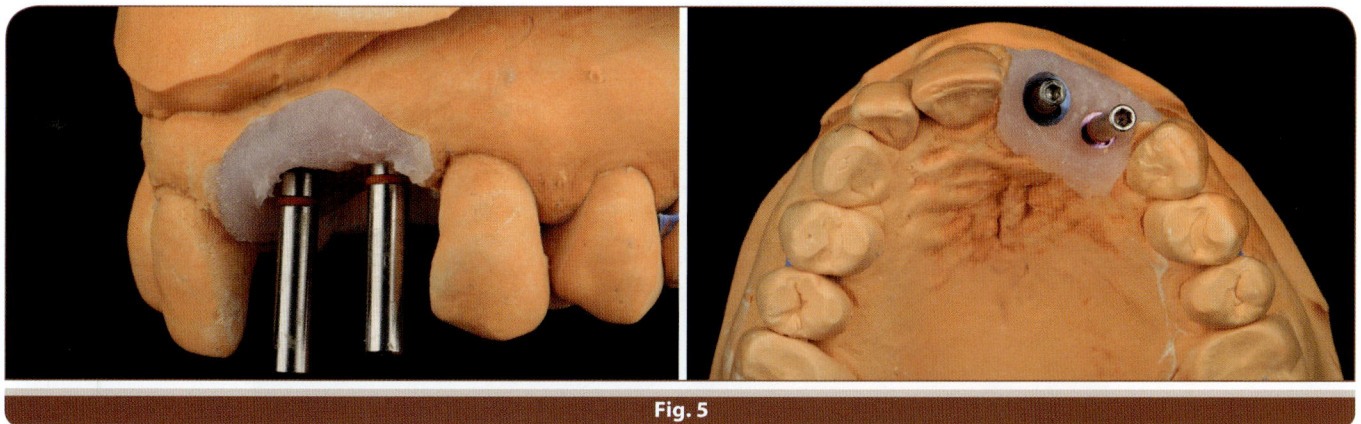

Fig. 5

Implant trajectory **(Fig. 5)**.

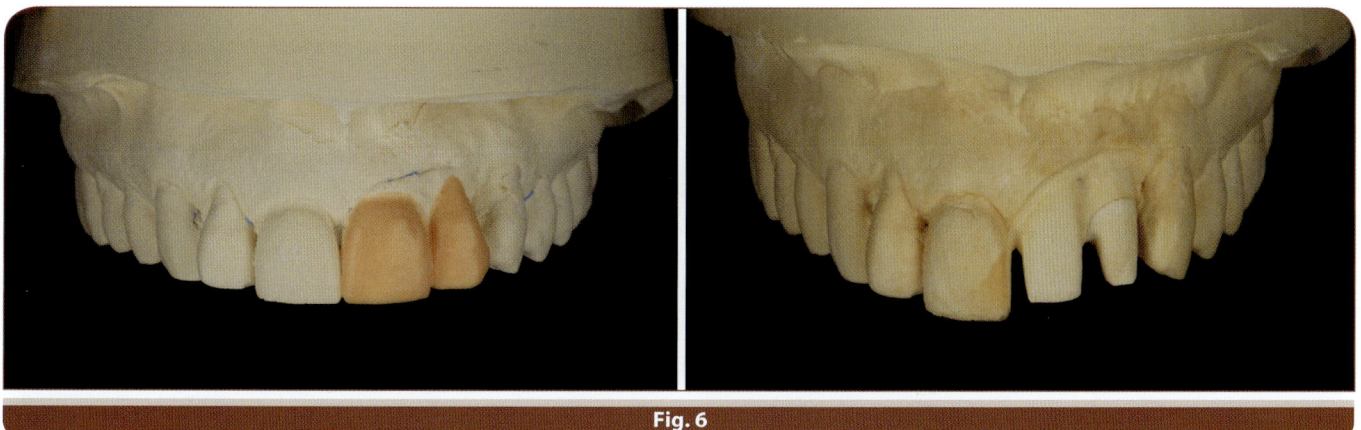

Fig. 6

Diagnostic wax-up for provisional restoration **(Fig. 6)**.

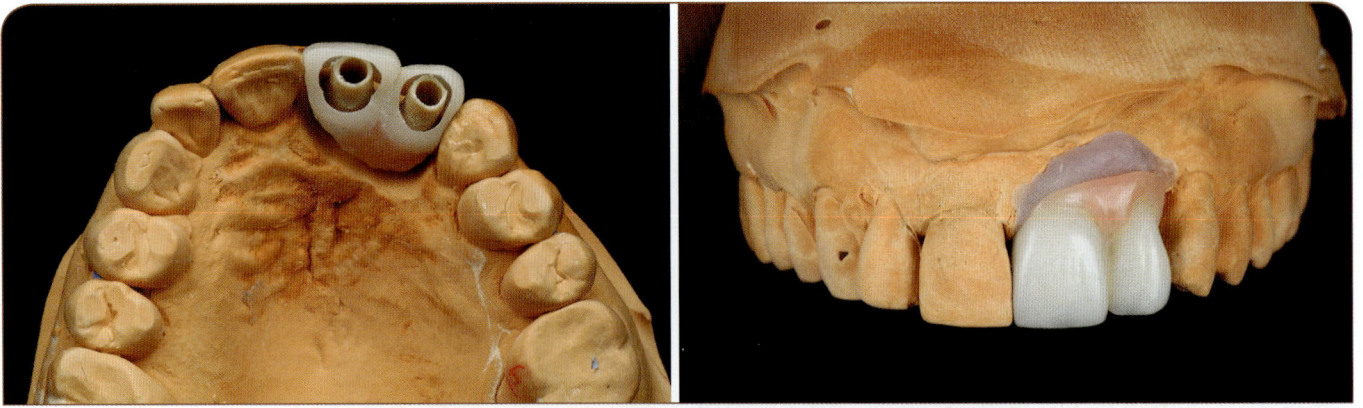

Fig. 7

Provisional fabricated **(Fig. 7)**.

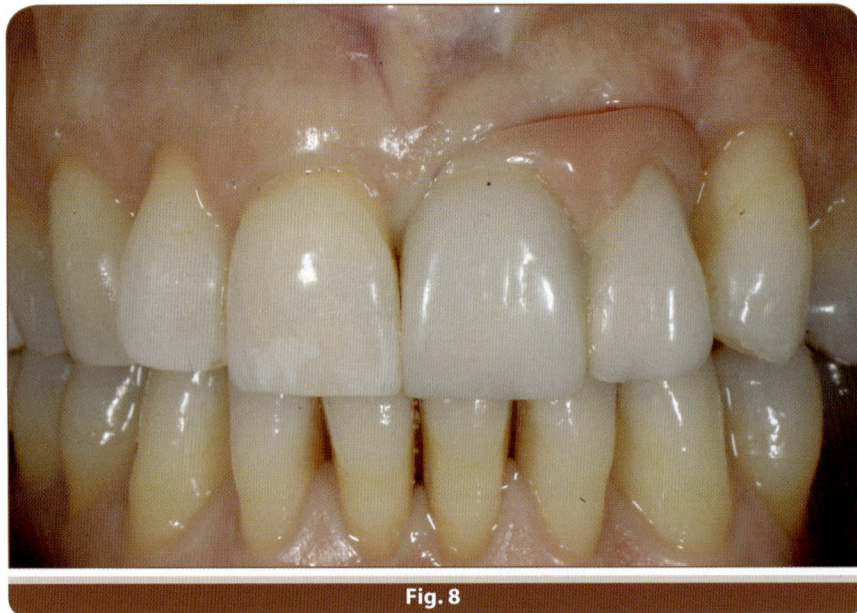

Fig. 8

Provisional intraorally **(Fig. 8)**.

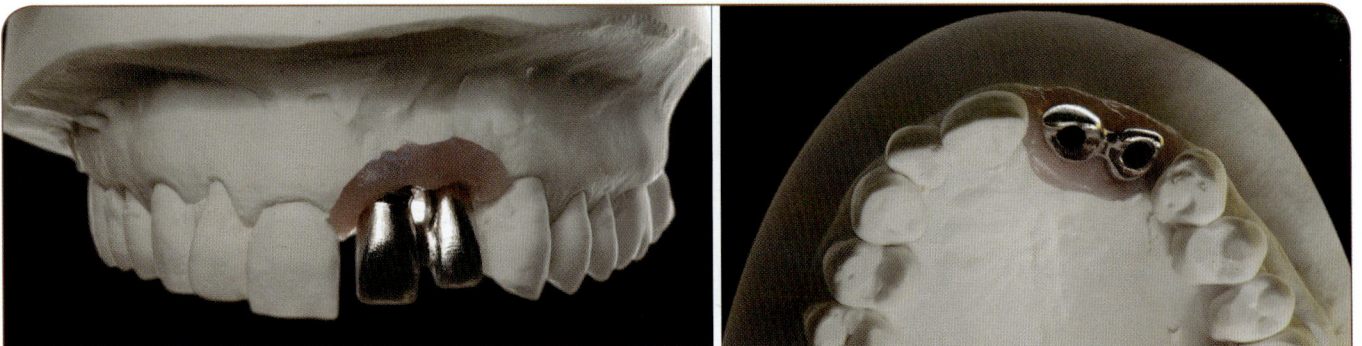

Fig. 9

Screw access channel bent, noble alloy used **(Fig. 9)**.

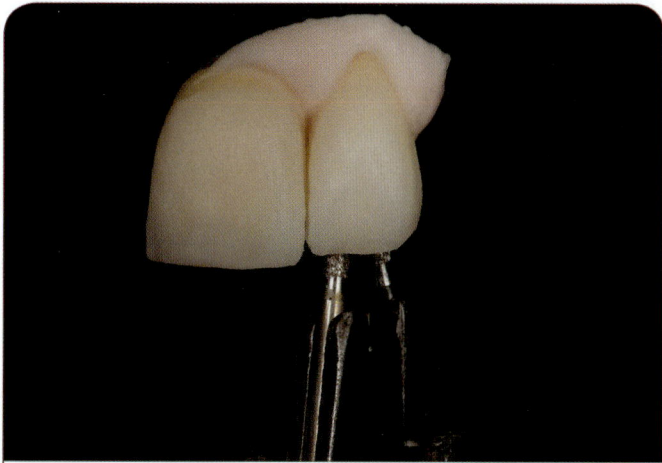

Fig. 10

Contours made cleansable (Fig. 10).

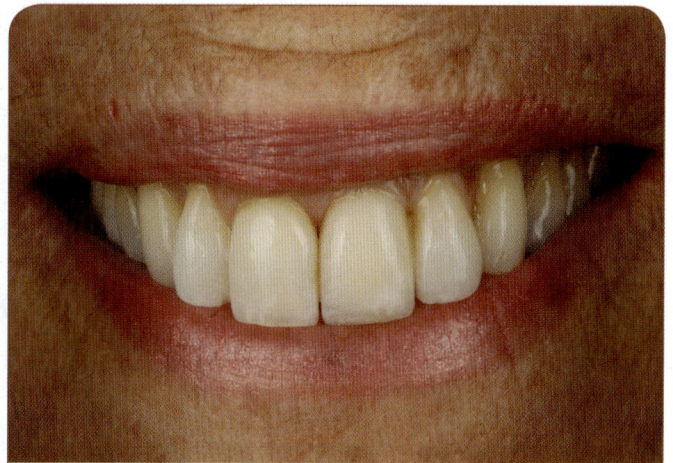

Fig. 11

Final restoration (Fig. 11).

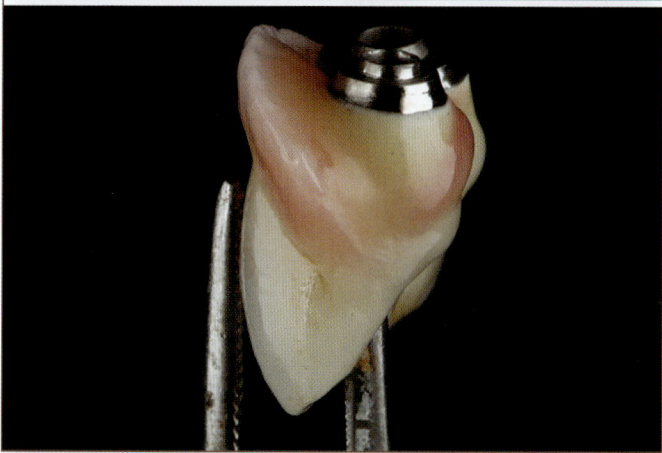

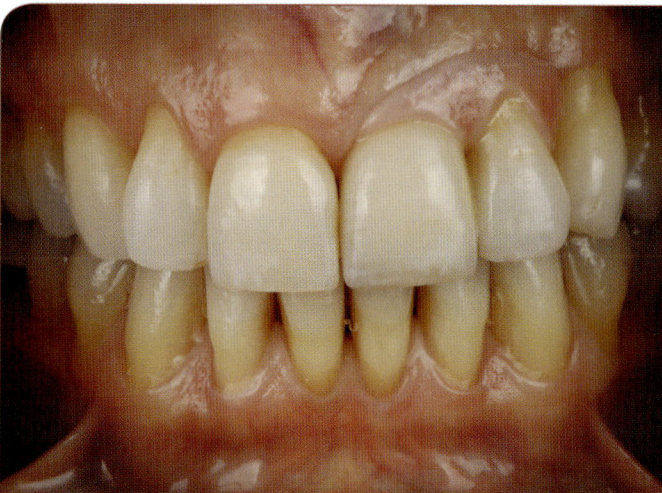

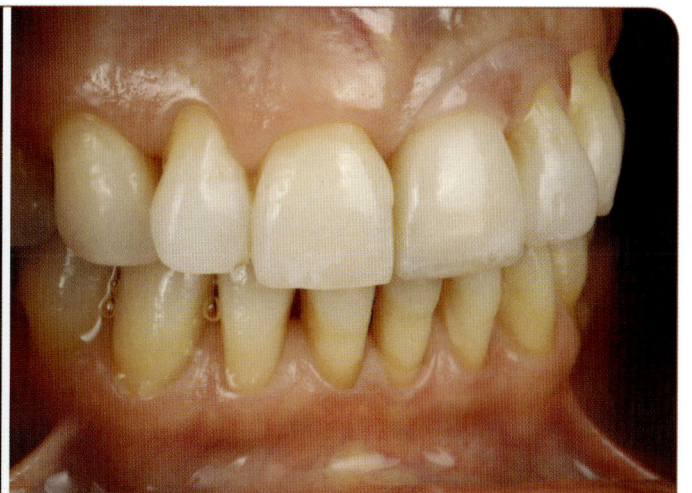

Fig. 12

Final restoration with pink ceramic (Fig. 12).

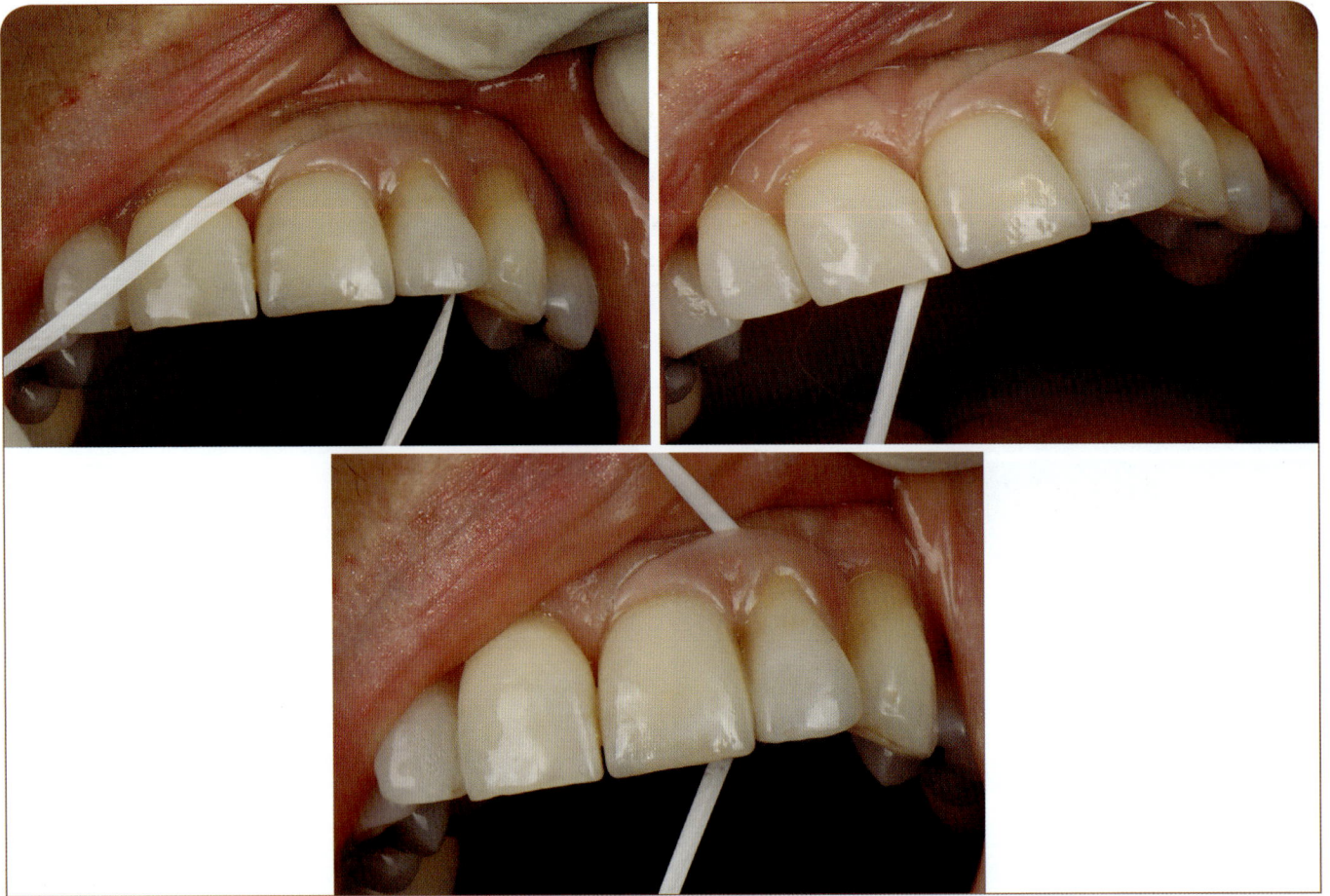

Fig. 13

Patient able to floss **(Fig. 13)**.

Tarun Kumar

MANAGEMENT OF TITANIUM MESH EXPOSURE

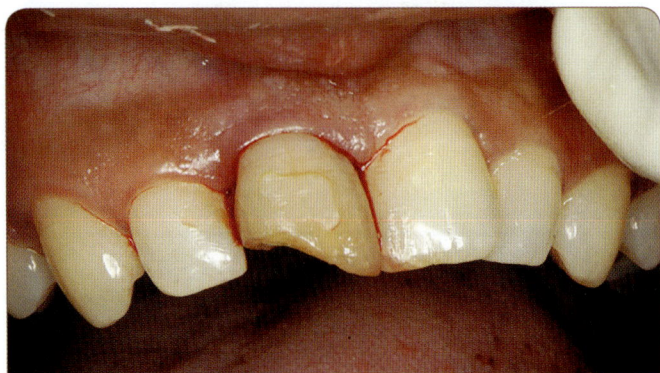

Fig. 1

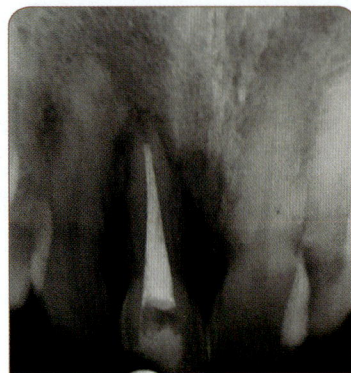

Fig. 2

A 24-year-old male patient came with a chief complaint of broken tooth in the upper right front tooth region of jaw and mobility with the same tooth.

His medical history was non-contributory. His past dental history revealed that he had got a Root Canal Treatment done in the same tooth 2 years back **(Fig. 1)**.

Owing to the poor prognosis of the endodontically failed tooth, it was extracted atraumatically after taking patient's consent **(Fig. 2)**.

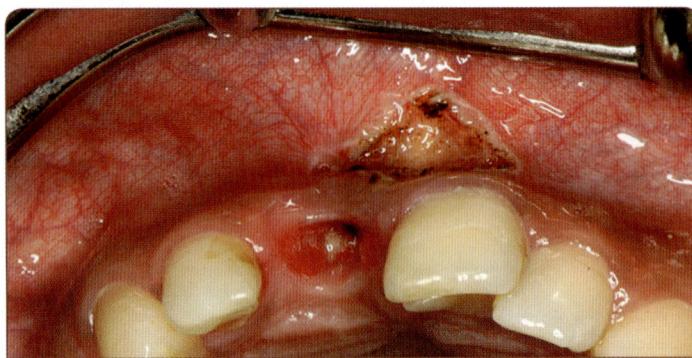

Fig. 3

After 8 weeks of healing of the extraction socket, laser assisted frenotomy was done with respect to the labial frenum in relation to tooth #11 and tooth #21 **(Fig. 3)**.

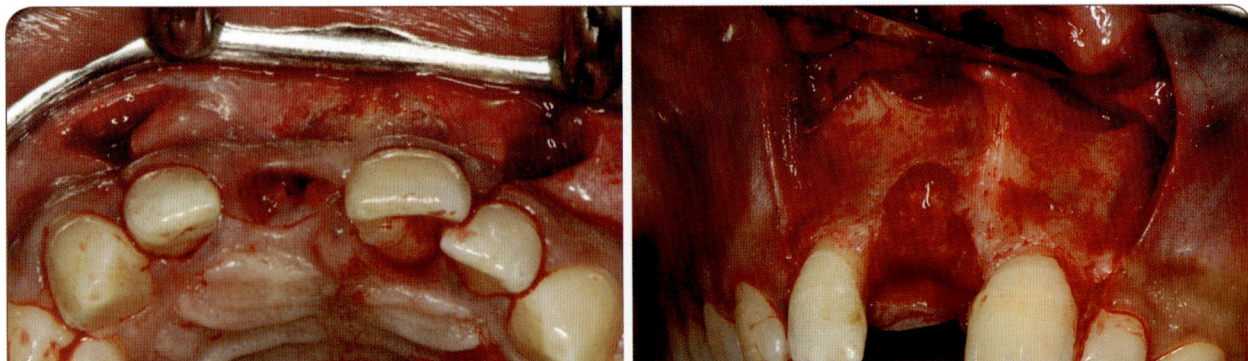

Fig. 4

Midcrestal, crevicular and 2 vertical releasing incisions not involving the interdental papillae were given. A full thickness mucoperiosteal flap was raised which revealed a bony defect in the edentulous site **(Fig. 4)**.

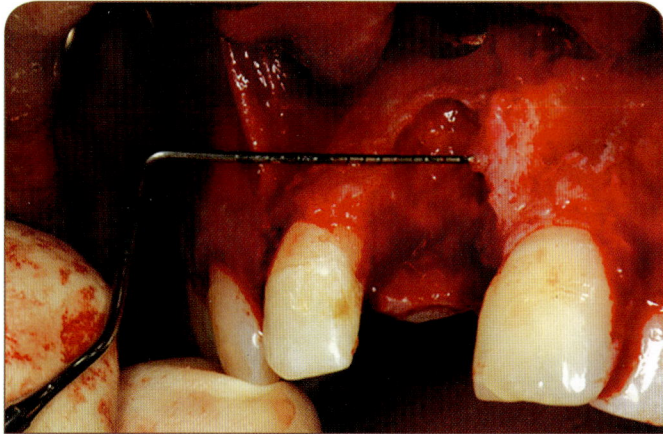
Fig. 5

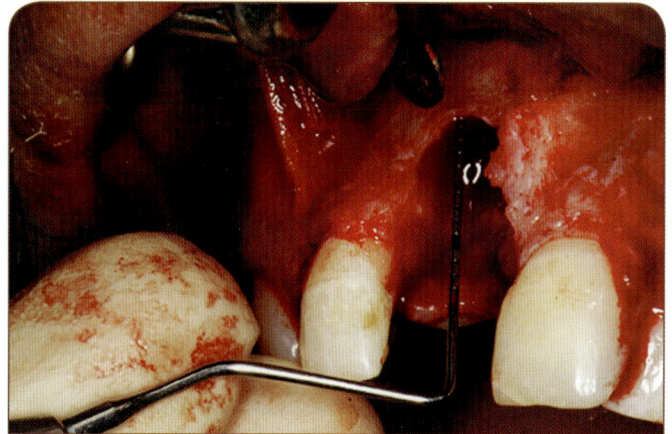
Fig. 6

After reflection of a full thickness mucoperiosteal flap, the length and the width of the bony defect was measured **(Figs. 5 and 6)**.

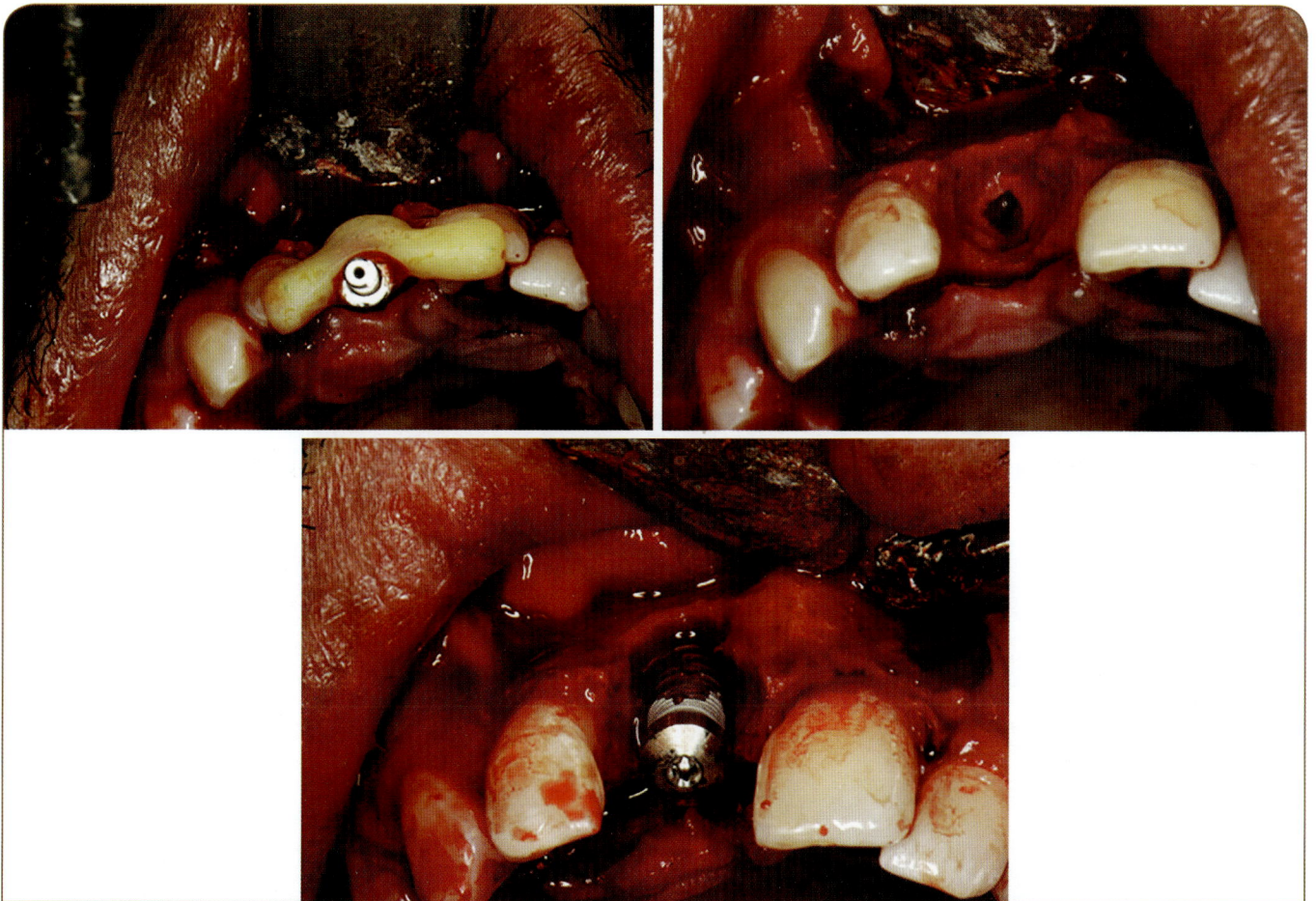
Fig. 7

Using the surgical stent which acts a guide for implant placement, osteotomy site was prepared followed by placement of 4.3 × 11 mm implant **(Fig. 7)**.

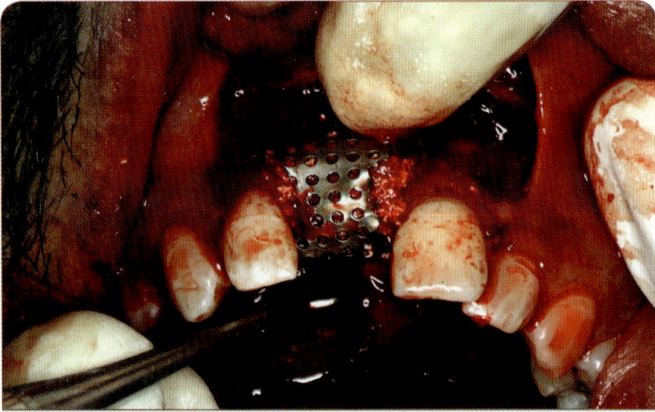

Fig. 8

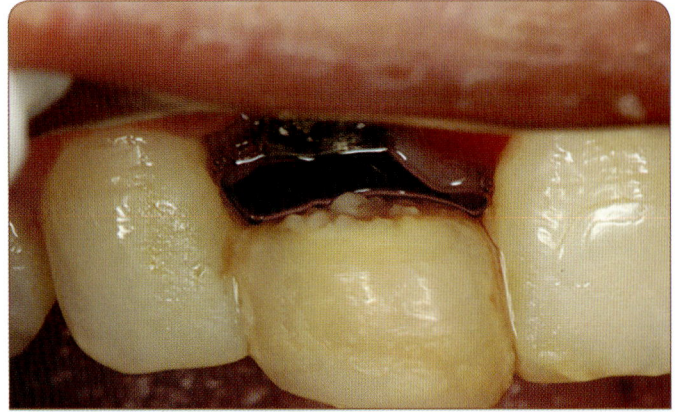

Fig. 9

Placement of titanium mesh over the osteotomy site that was grafted with a mixture of Xenograft and Autograft **(Fig. 8)**.

After implant placement patient was given a temporary crown in relation to tooth #11 which was fabricated to avoid any contact with the grafted osteotomy site **(Fig. 9)**.

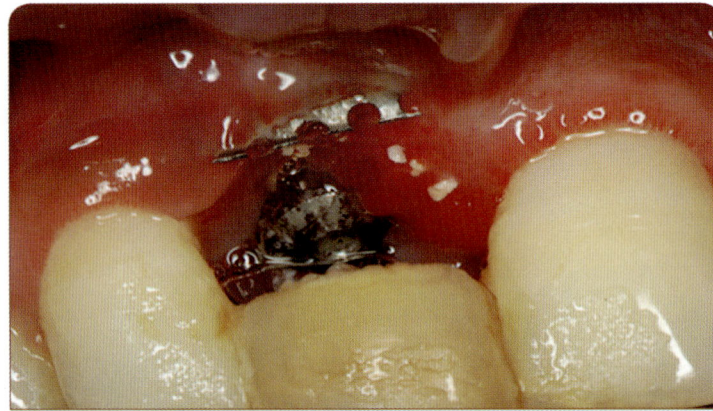

Fig. 10

20 days after the procedure, titanium mesh exposure was encountered **(Fig. 10)**.

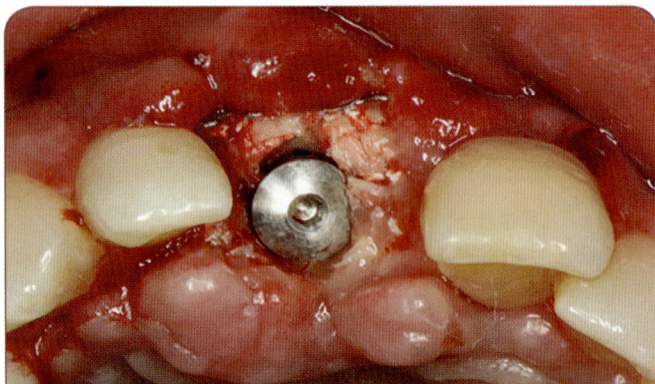

Fig. 11

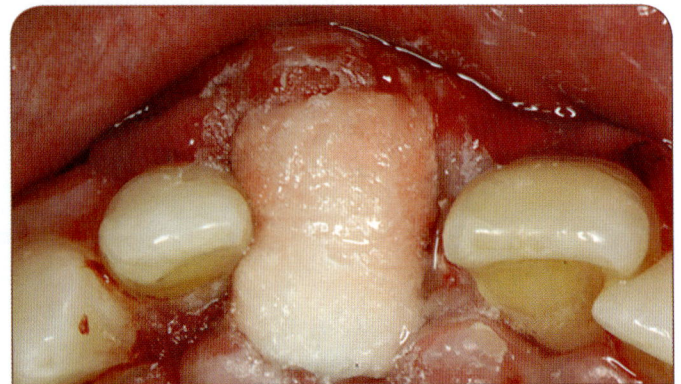

Fig. 12

The temporary crown was removed, exposed titanium mesh was trimmed and CollaTape was placed over it followed by placement of fibrin glue over it **(Figs. 11 and 12)**.

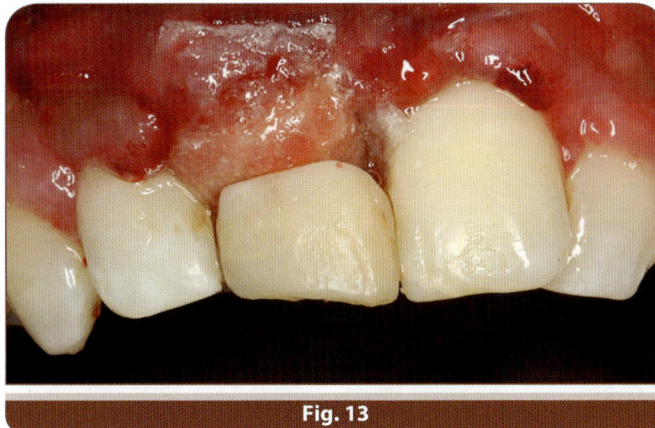

Fig. 13

Uneventful healing with the treated mesh exposure site was observed **(Fig. 13)**.

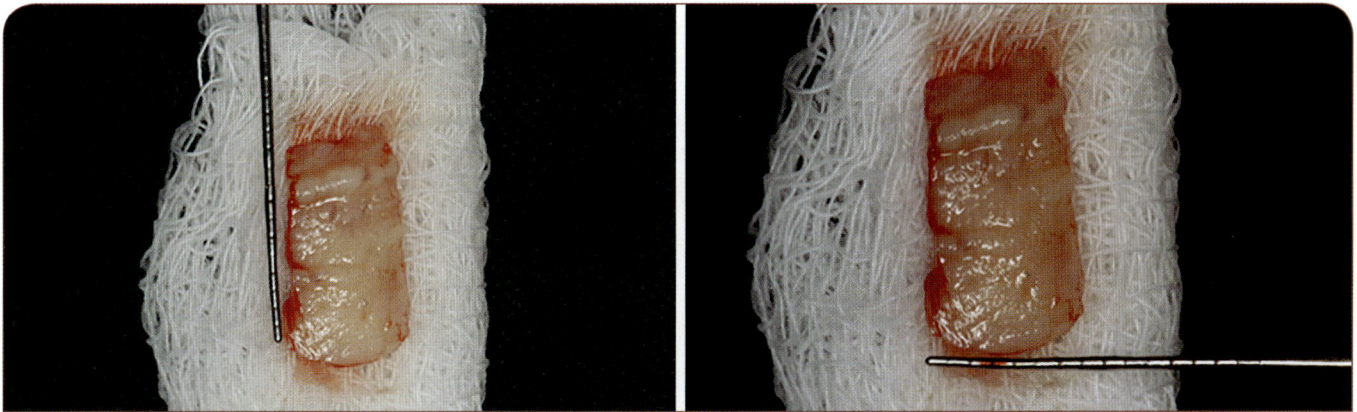

Fig. 14

A 6 × 10 mm free gingival graft was harvested from the palate, 1 mm apical to the gingival margin of adjacent teeth with a no. 15 scalpel blade. Followed which all the adipose and glandular tissues on the graft were removed using a scraping motion with a no. 15 scalpel blade **(Fig. 14)**.

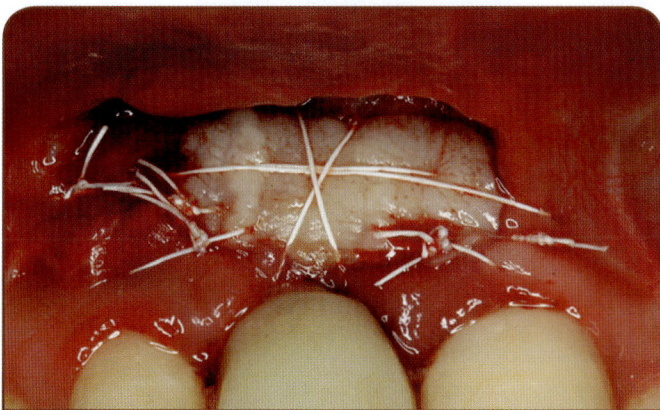

Fig. 15

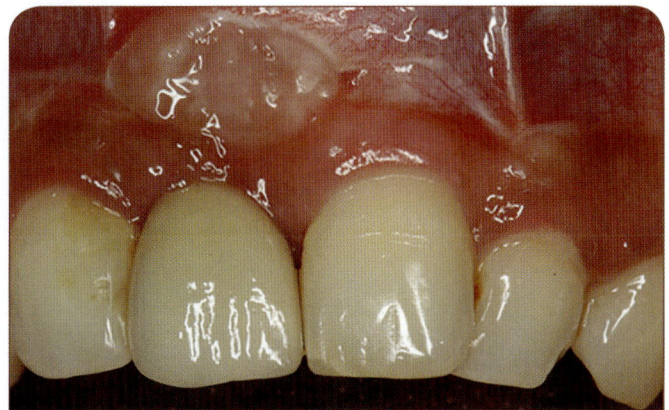

Fig. 16

After the donor tissue had been shaped appropriately, it was placed on the recipient bed and fixed with periosteal sutures **(Fig. 15)**.

The insufficient width of the keratinized gingiva was sufficiently augmented by the soft tissue grafting and the final prosthesis was delivered to the patient **(Fig. 16)**.

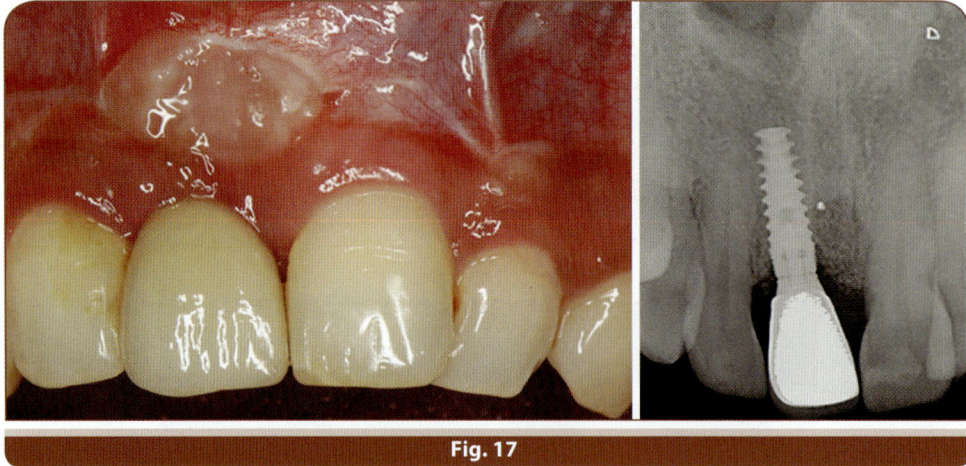

Fig. 17

There was uneventful healing and no complications were further encountered on 2 years of follow-up. Intraoral peri-apical radiograph revealing minimal amount of crestal bone loss after 2 years **(Fig. 17)**.

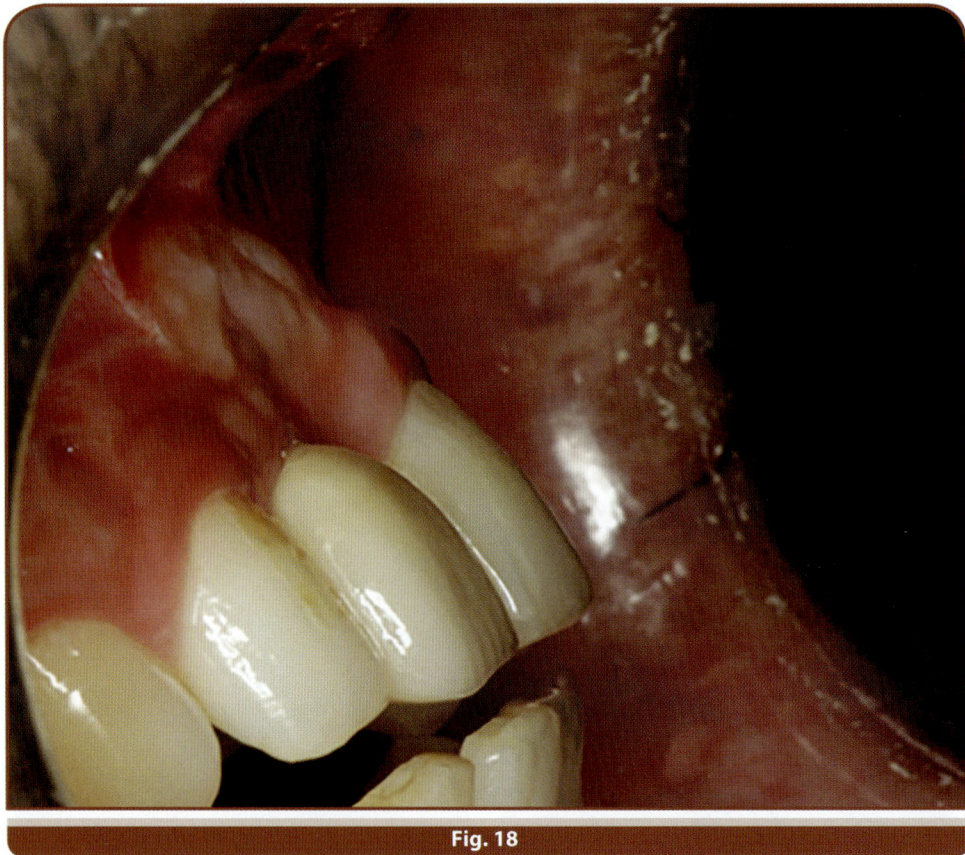

Fig. 18

Lateral view of the beautiful hard and soft tissue augmentation **(Fig. 18)**.

CASE STUDY 129

Praful Bali

Esthetic Management of Complication after 12 years of Implant Placement

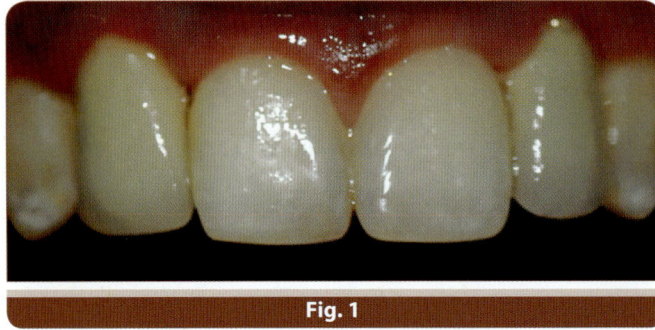

Fig. 1

Tooth #12,22 were implanted in 2002. The position and placement was not good but due to the low lip line of the patient the metal ceramic crowns were accepted by the patient **(Fig. 1)**.

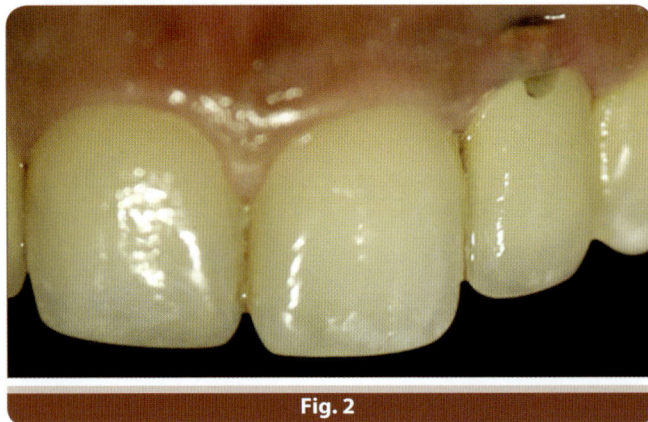

Fig. 2

After 12 years, in 2014 the patient returned with pain in the left implant restoration. She wanted to change the crown and requested if better esthetic work could be done **(Fig. 2)**.

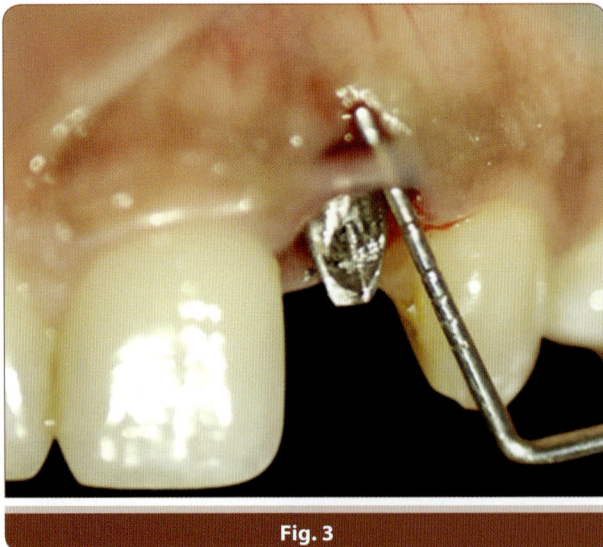

Fig. 3

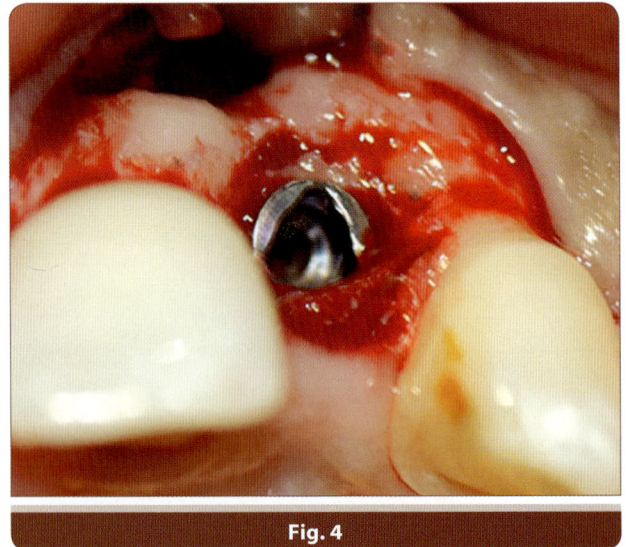

Fig. 4

The impinching crown was removed and all possibilities including implant removal, GBR and re-implantation explained to the patient. The patient chose the more conservative treatment of a soft tissue graft to boost the thin biotype **(Fig. 3)**

The abutment was removed and a full thickness flap was raised to expose the implant. Note the implant was placed without any esthetic considerations and hence the buccal position and vertically high implant. But the implant is well osseointegrated **(Fig. 4)**.

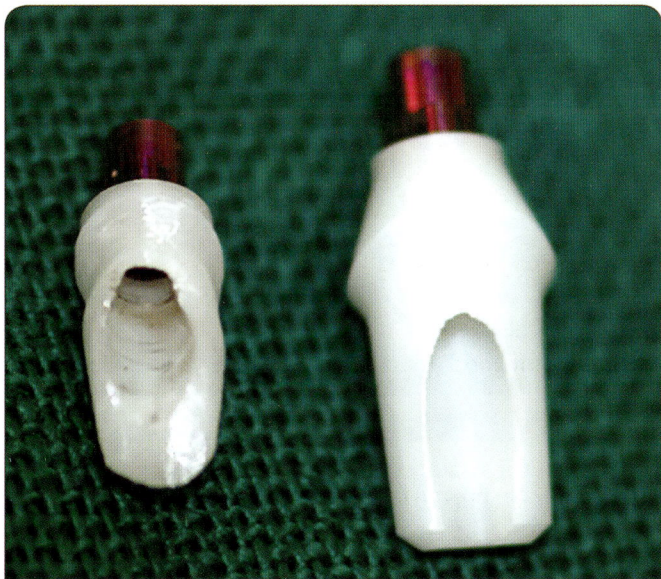

Fig. 5

A stock Zirconia abutment is reshaped. A concavity is created to accommodate the soft tissue and create a seal **(Fig. 5)**.

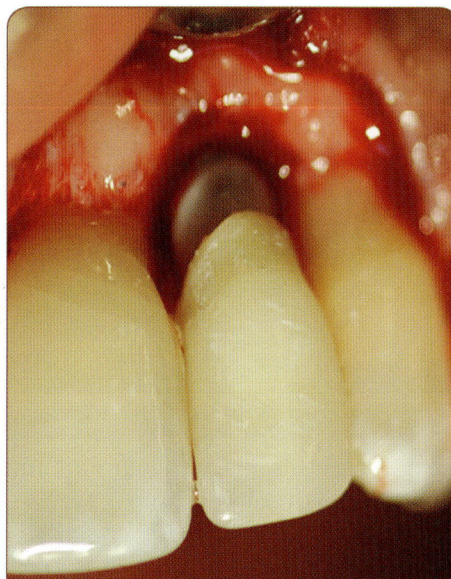

Fig. 6

A Procera Zirconia abutment is reshaped and torqued to the implant. An acrylic temporary is cemented to the abutment. Note the concavity purposely made to create a soft tissue seal around the neck of the implant **(Fig. 6)**.

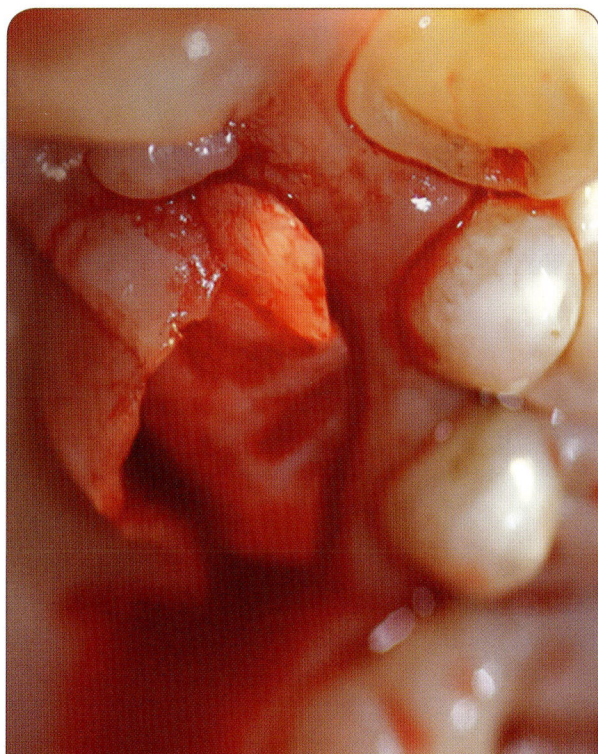

Fig. 7

A Pedicle Connective tissue graft is taken from the palate **(Fig. 7)**.

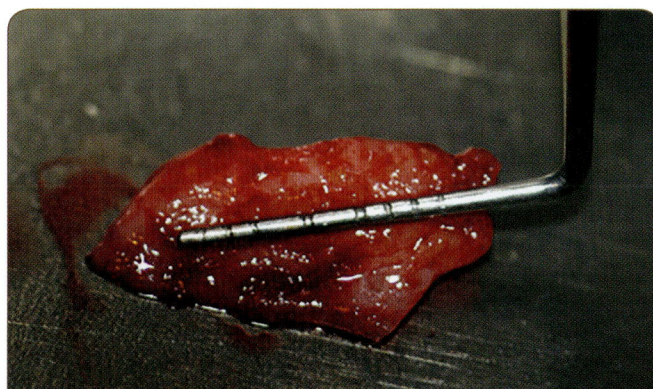

Fig. 8

A thick connective tissue is incised **(Fig. 8)**.

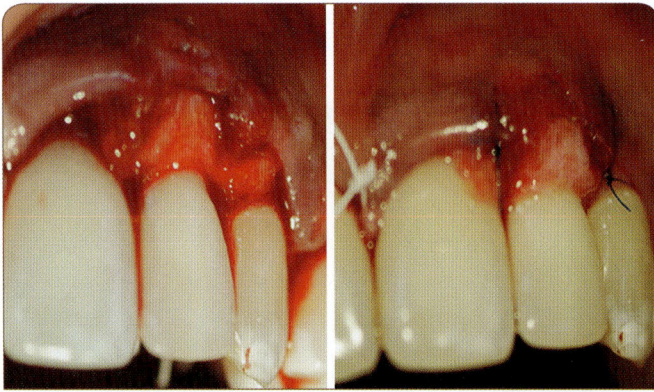

Fig. 9

The connective tissue is placed at the abutment bone interface and sutured over it **(Fig. 9)**.

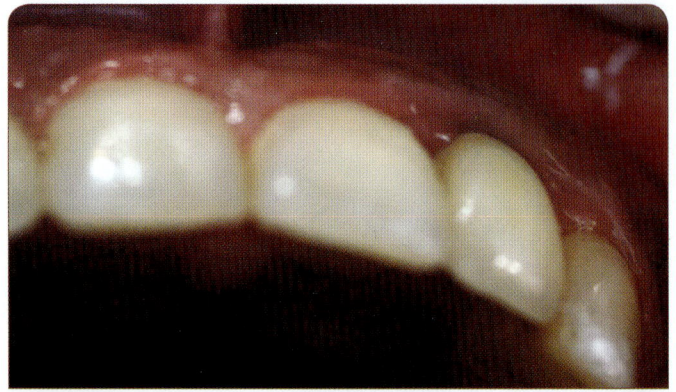

Fig. 10

The bulk of the tissue seen post healing of 2 months. Nice papilla fill too **(Fig. 10)**.

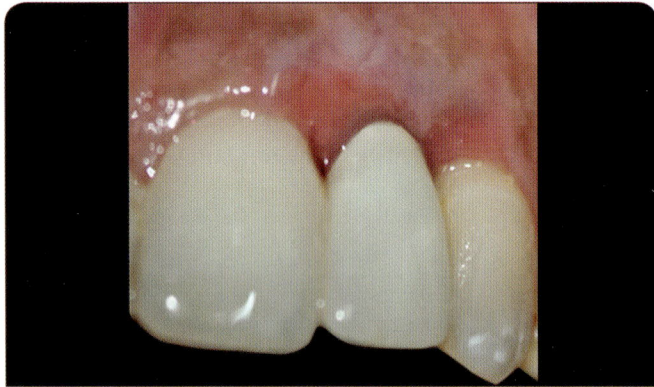

Fig. 11

A permanent Zirconia crown is cemented 2 months after the procedure. The level of the issue has certainly become much more positive. Patient is instructed to keep very good oral hygiene around the new restoration **(Fig. 11)**.

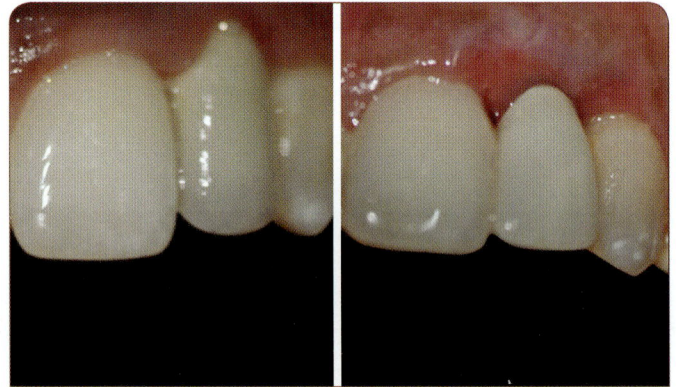

Fig. 12

Pre- and Post-comparison: A reasonably good overall result achieved in a compromised case by CT graft **(Fig. 12)**.

SECTION 9

Implant Overdentures

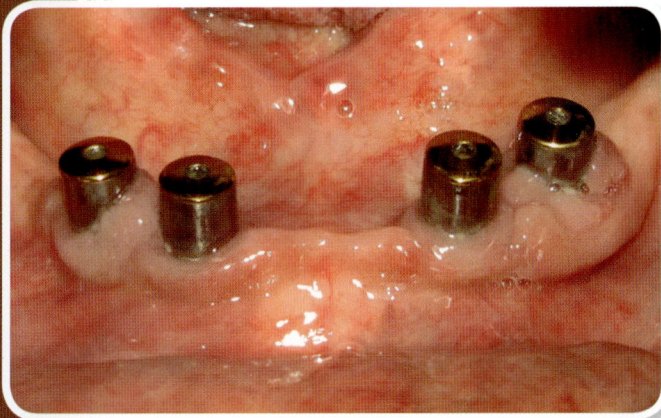

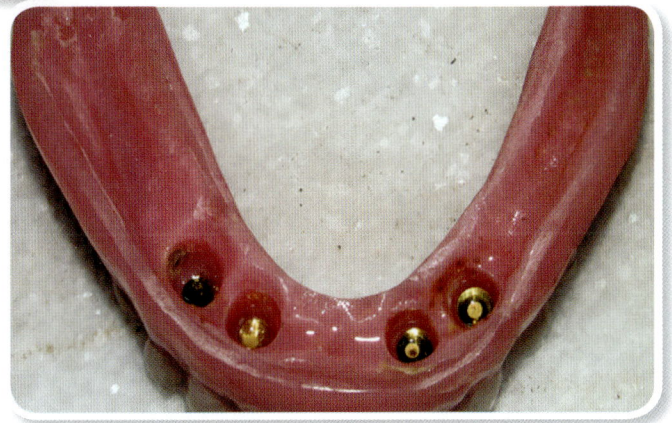

Praful Bali, Vani Kalra

MAGNETS FOR RETENTION AND STABILITY OF LOWER IMPLANT SUPPORTED DENTURE

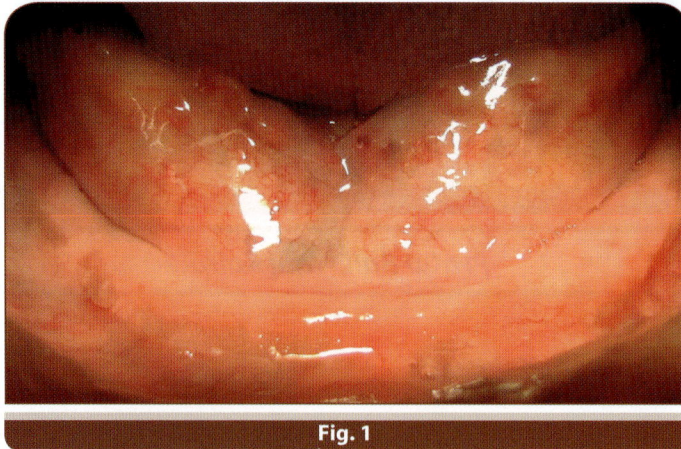

Fig. 1

A male patient 77 years of age wants to get implants done to stabilize the loose lower denture. Patient already has a denture and wants an option to use the same **(Fig. 1)**.

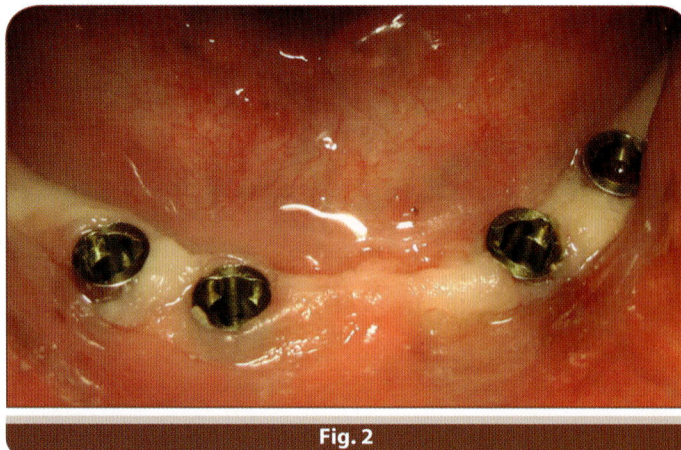

Fig. 2

4 Nobel Biocare 4.3/13 implants are placed parallel doing a flap less surgery. This is two week post operative view **(Fig. 2)**.

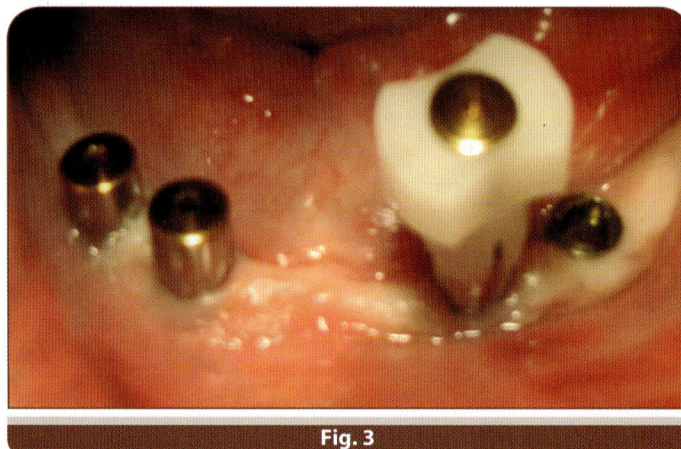

Fig. 3

The male and female parts of the attachments are put one by one to the implants **(Fig. 3)**.

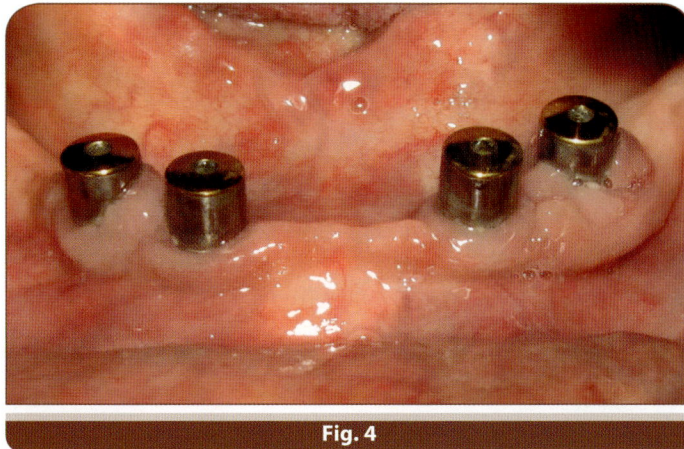

Fig. 4

3 mm height male part are placed on to the implants and torqued to 15 Ncm **(Fig. 4)**.

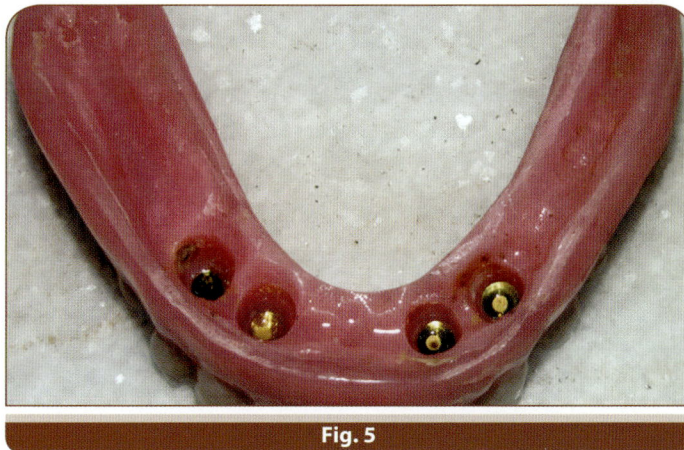

Fig. 5

The patient's denture is relieved in the area of the male part to allow space for the magnets (female part). Magnetic attachments are transferred of the inner surface of the existing denture using self curing acrylic **(Fig. 5)**.

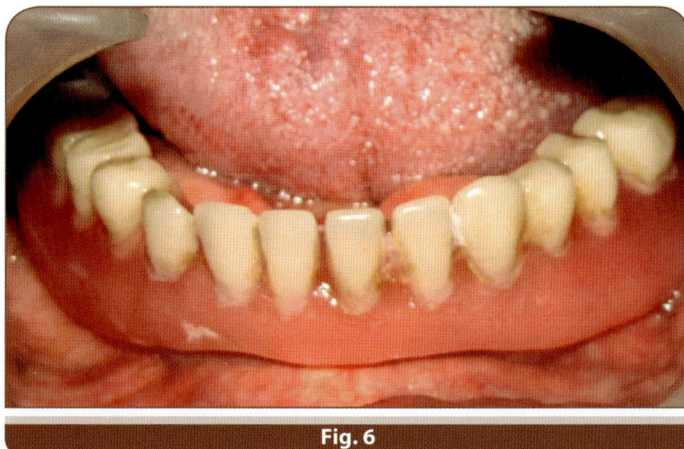

Fig. 6

Patient's existing denture is not stable with magnetic attachments and the patient is restored to function **(Fig. 6)**.

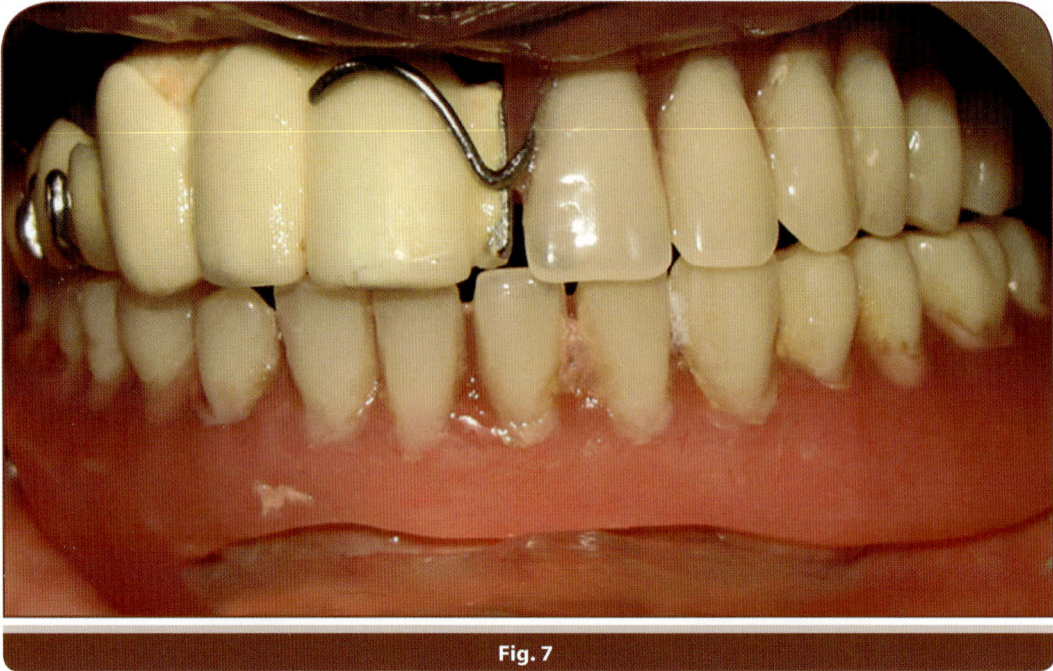

Fig. 7

Final facial view **(Fig. 7)**.

CASE STUDY 131

Gregori M Kurtzman

Lower Hader Clip Eclipse Overdenture

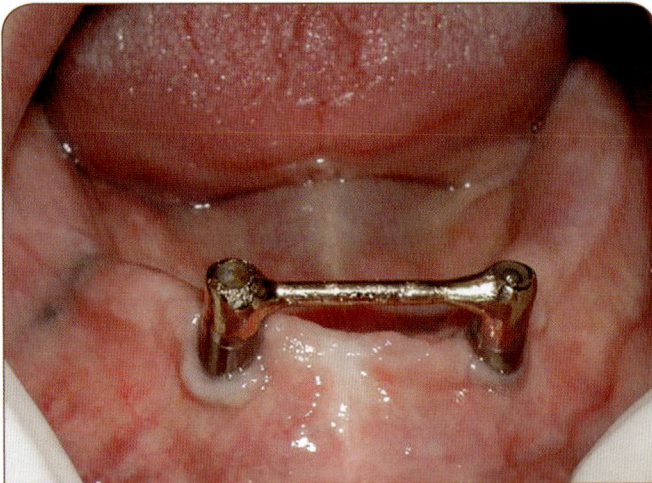

Fig. 1

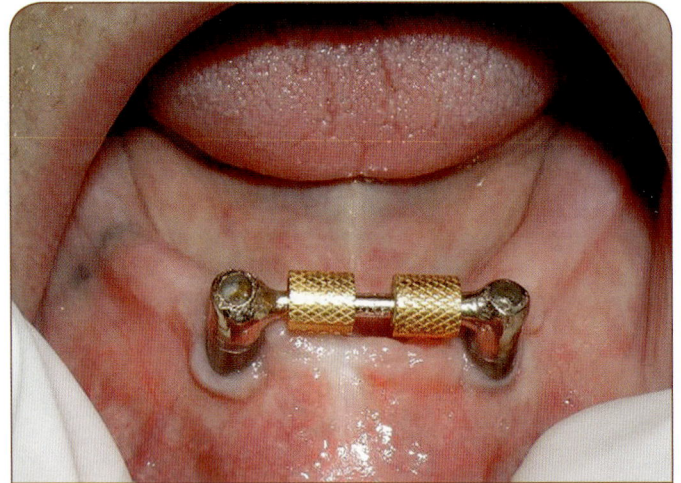

Fig. 2

Patient is a 68-year-old male who had two implants placed two years ago in the mandible cuspid positions. These had been restored with a cast bar and the prosthetics secured to the overdenture superstructure with a single Hader clip. A full denture was worn on the maxillary arch. The patient presented requesting a new set of dentures and indicated that his lower denture had insufficient retention.

Examination indicated that the overdenture bar was of sufficient length to accommodate two Hader clips, which would increase retention in the new denture **(Fig. 1)**.

Two Hader clips with metal housings were placed on the bar at maximum spread **(Fig. 2)**.

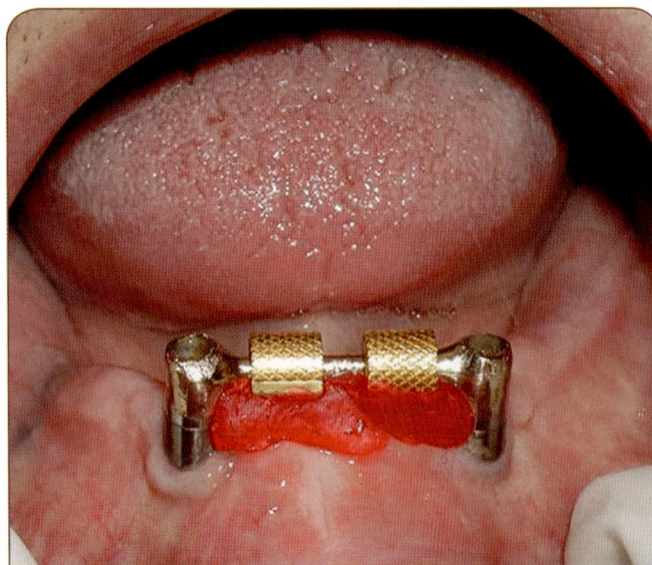

Fig. 3

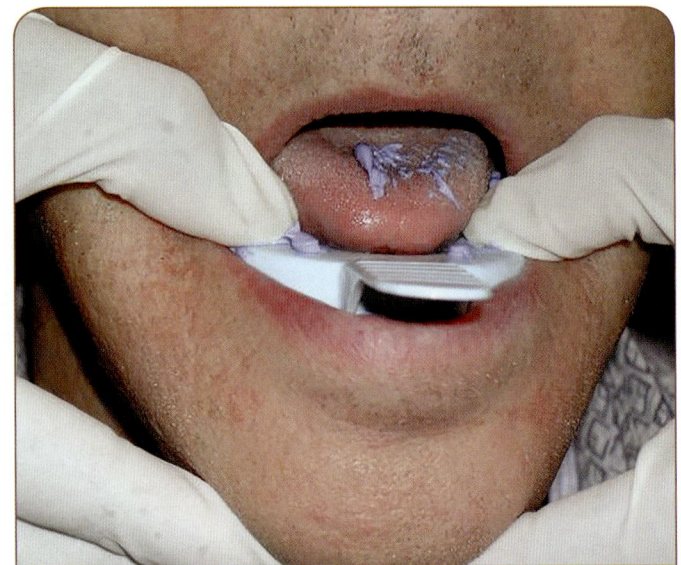

Fig. 4

Beading wax was placed under the bar to prevent impression material from locking under the superstructure **(Fig. 3)**.

A full arch polyvinyl siloxane (PVS) impression was made **(Fig. 4)**.

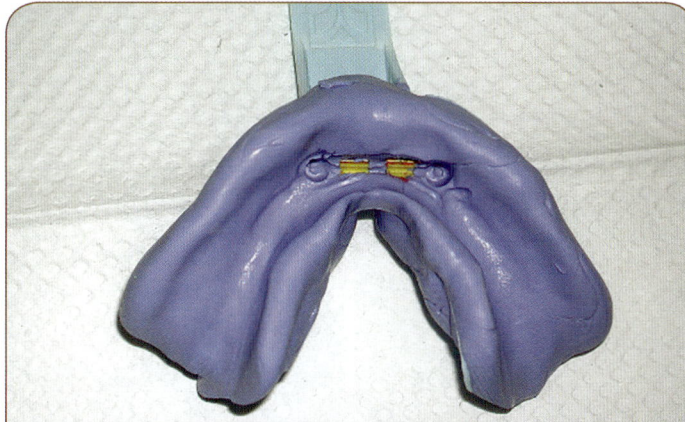

Fig. 5

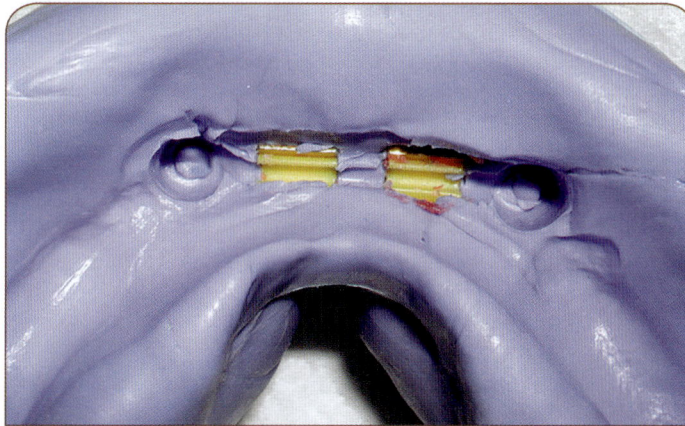

Fig. 6

Hader attachments in their metal housings were picked up in the impression **(Figs. 5 and 6)**.

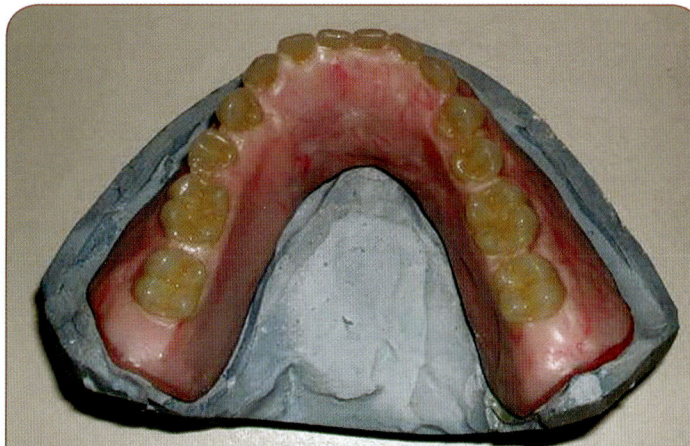

Fig. 7

The setup of teeth utilizing Eclipse setup and contour material on the previously cured base is returned for try-in in a light proof bag. Mandibular try-in showing the "bubble gum" colored Eclipse setup and contour material **(Fig. 7)**.

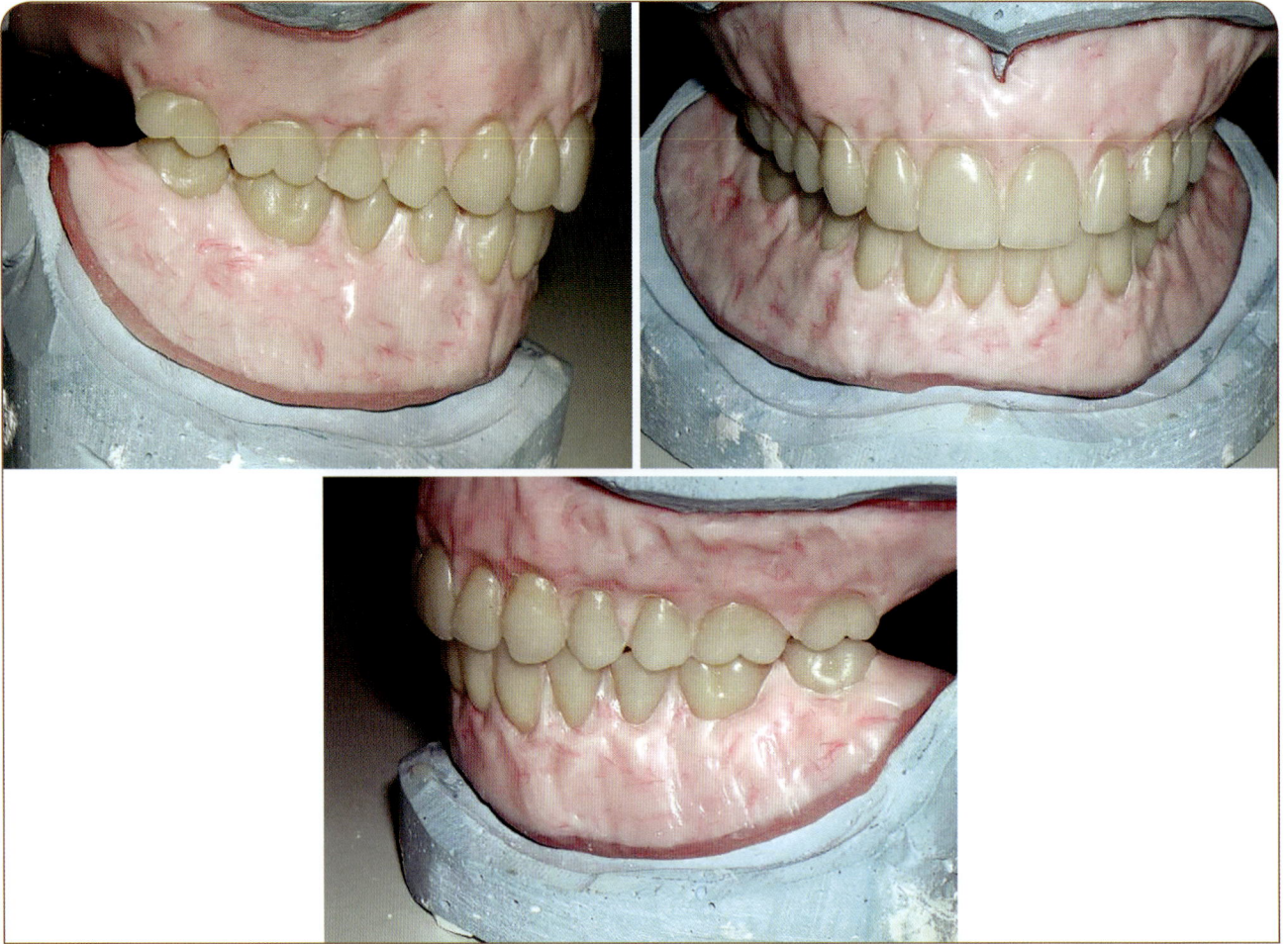

Fig. 8

Articulated try-in showing the "bubble gum" colored Eclipse setup and contour material on the master casts **(Fig. 8)**.

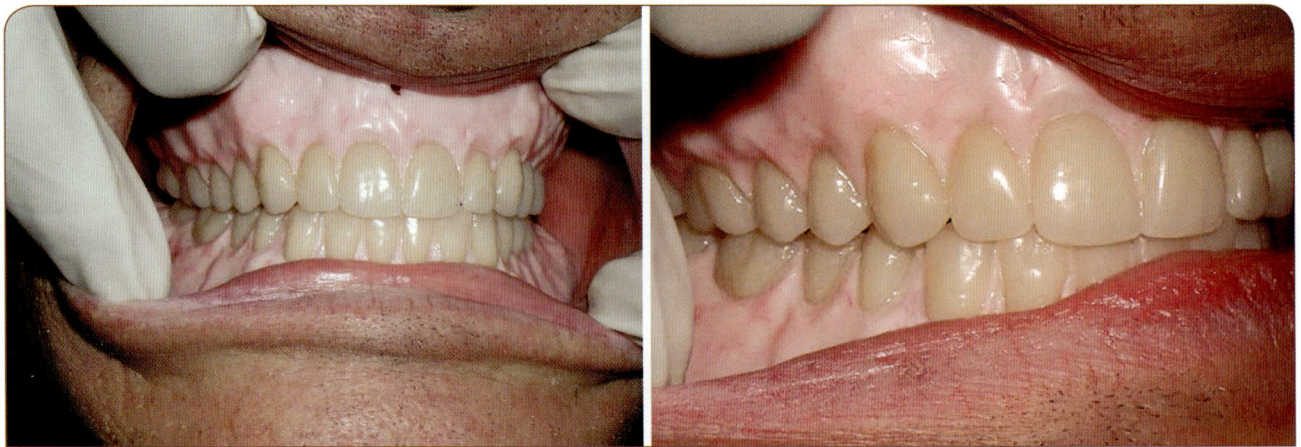

Fig. 9

Try-in showing the "bubble gum" colored Eclipse setup and contour material intraorally **(Fig. 9)**.

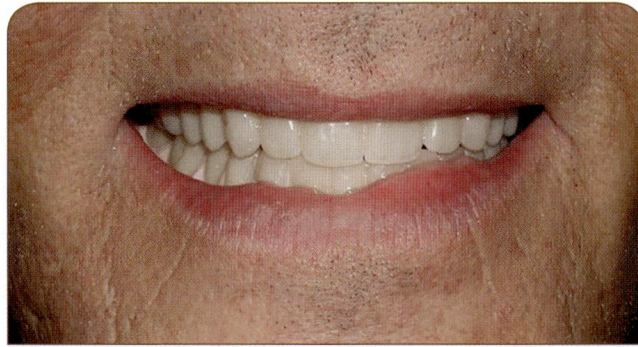

Fig. 10

Natural smile showing the teeth at try-in **(Fig. 10)**.

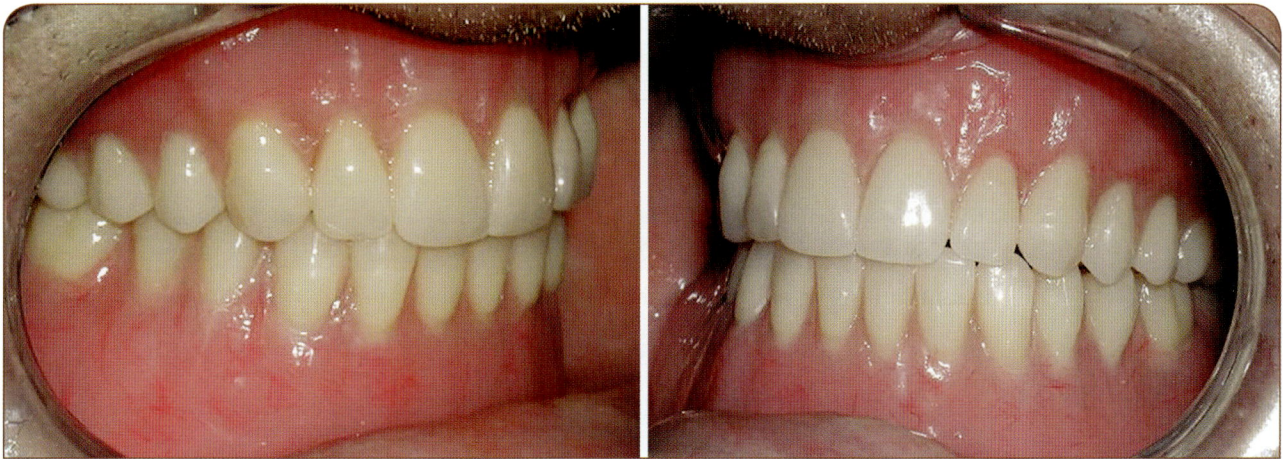

Fig. 11

Finished and cured Eclipse dentures intraorally. Note "bubble gum" color of the material has changed to a natural appearance after curing **(Fig. 11)**.

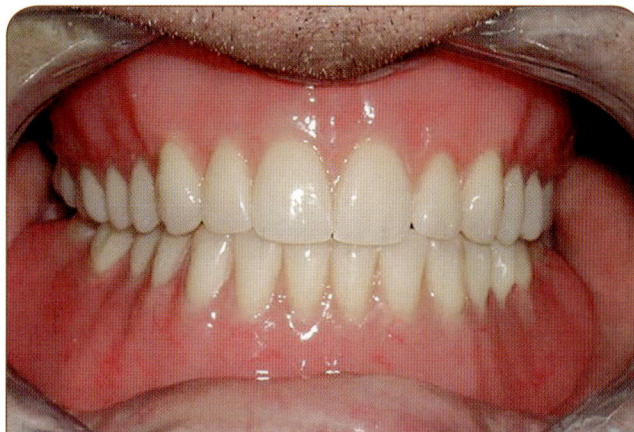

Fig. 12

Lab work by Joel Cash and Beehive Lab **(Fig. 12)**.

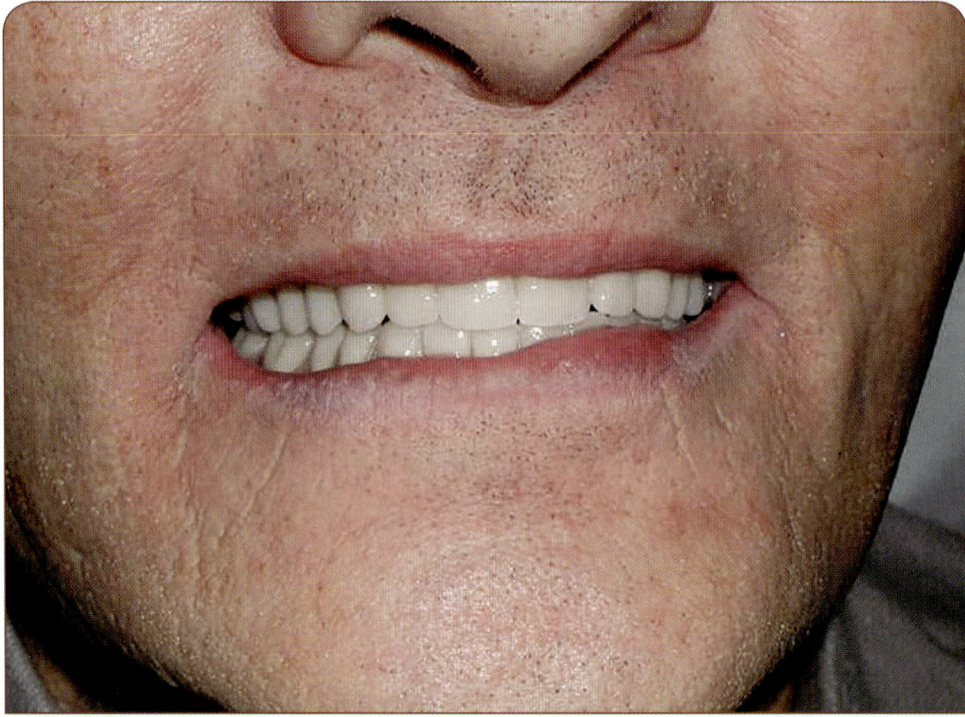

Fig. 13

Patient smiling showing the finished Eclipse dentures **(Fig. 13)**.

Gregori M Kurtzman

Fully Edentulous Arch
CAD/CAM Bar-Overdenture

A 92-year-old white male. Full maxillary denture opposing a failing natural tooth bar-overdenture. Patient has minimal vestibule which would make use of a conventional denture difficult. Implants used: Southern Implants

- LL 2nd premolar—Co-Axis 24 degree 4 × 15 mm
- LL canine—Taper 4 × 13 mm
- LR right lateral incisor—Taper 4 × 13 mm
- LR 1st premolar—Co-Axis 24 degree 4 × 15 mm

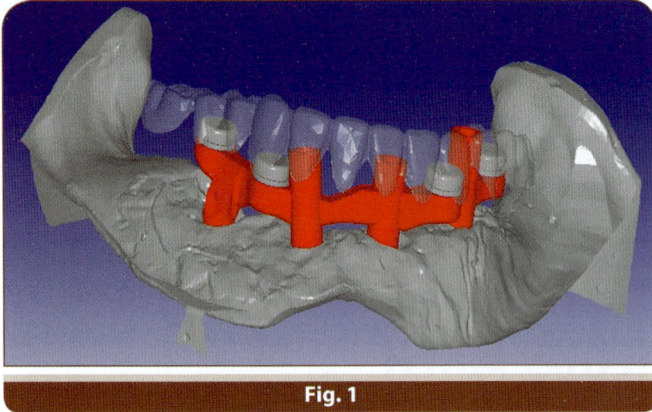

Fig. 1

Virtual designed overdenture bar (red) on the virtual model with Locator attachments shown on the bar and overlay of where the wax setup teeth would be in relation to the bar **(Fig. 1)**.

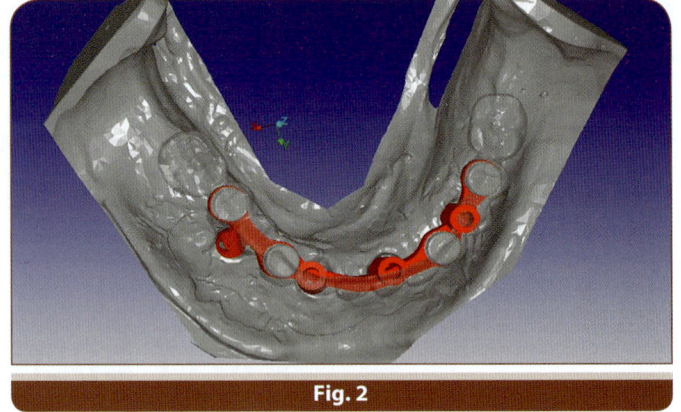

Fig. 2

Occlusal view of the virtual designed. Overdenture bar (red) on the virtual model with Locator attachments shown on the bar and overlay of where the wax setup teeth would be in relation to the bar **(Fig. 2)**.

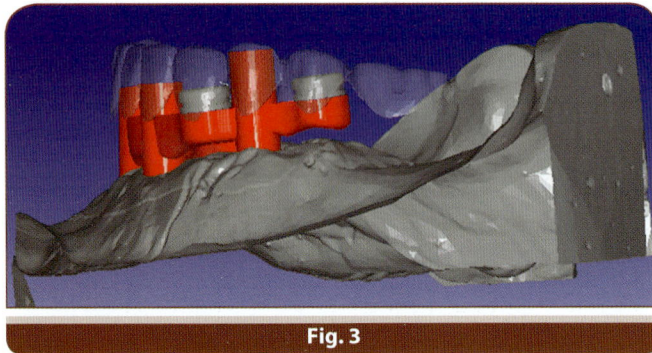

Fig. 3

Left side view of the virtual designed Overdenture bar (red) on the virtual model with Locator attachments shown on the bar and overlay of where the wax setup teeth would be in relation to the bar **(Fig. 3)**.

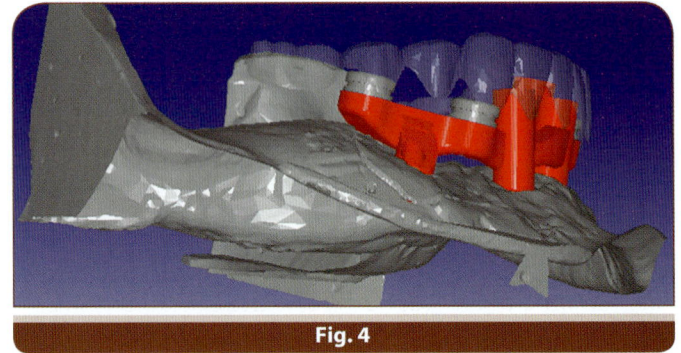

Fig. 4

Right side view of the virtual designed. Overdenture bar (red) on the virtual model with Locator attachments shown on the bar and overlay of where the wax setup teeth would be in relation to the bar **(Fig. 4)**.

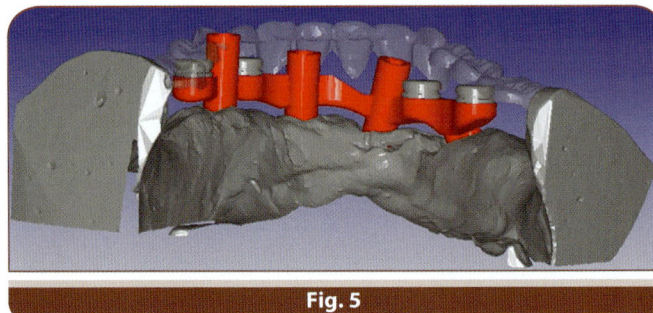

Fig. 5

Lingual view of the virtual designed. Overdenture bar (red) on the virtual model with Locator attachments shown on the bar and overlay of where the wax setup teeth would be in relation to the bar **(Fig. 5)**.

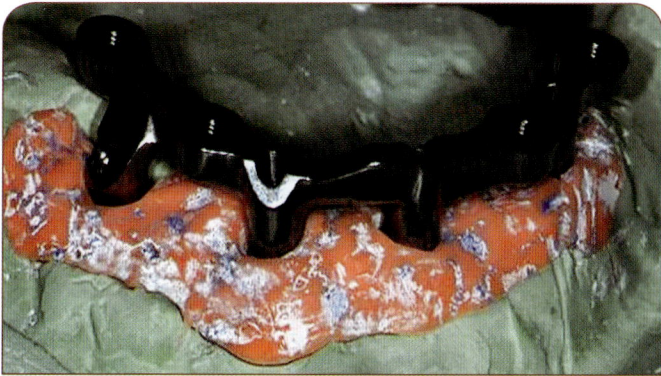

Fig. 6

Titanium CAD/CAM milled overdenture bar on the soft tissue model with threaded receptor sites for the Locator attachments to be placed on the bar **(Fig. 6)**.

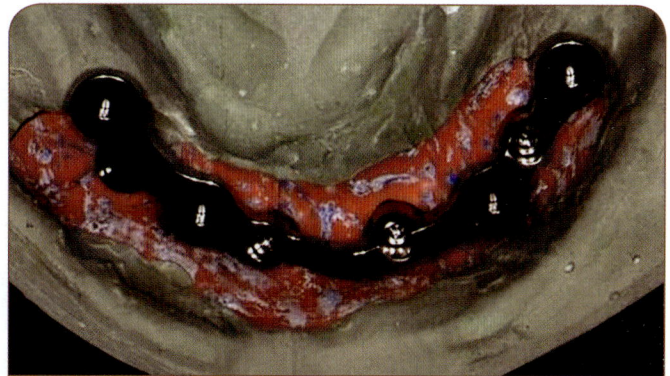

Fig. 7

Occlusal view of the titanium CAD/CAM milled overdenture bar on the soft tissue model with threaded receptor sites for the Locator attachments to be placed on the bar **(Fig. 7)**.

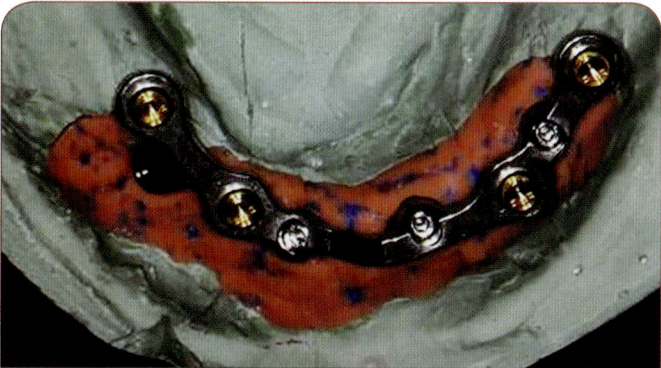

Fig. 8

Occlusal view of the titanium CAD/CAM milled overdenture bar on the soft tissue model with Locator female portion of the attachments threaded into the bar **(Fig. 8)**.

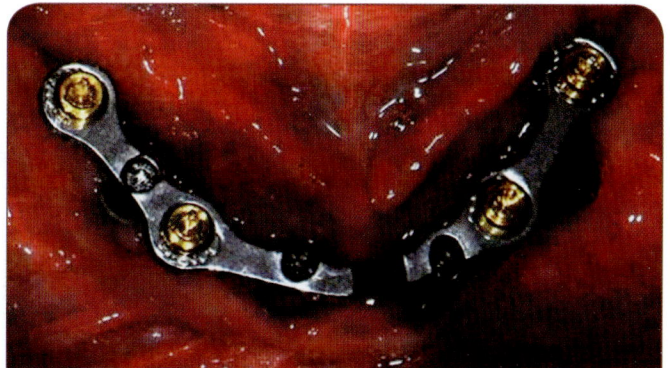

Fig. 9

Occlusal view of the titanium CAD/CAM milled overdenture bar intraorally with the Locator female portion of the attachments on the bar **(Fig. 9)**.

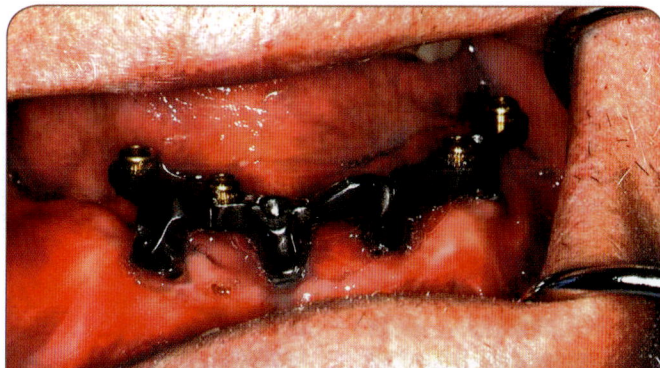

Fig. 10

Lateral view of the titanium CAD/CAM milled overdenture bar intraorally with the Locator female portion of the attachments on the bar **(Fig. 10)**.

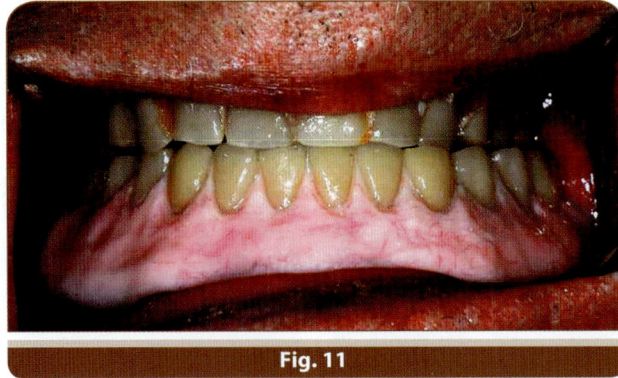

Fig. 11

Eclipse (uncured) denture setup seated on the overdenture bar intraorally to verify occlusion with the old maxillary full denture **(Fig. 11)**.

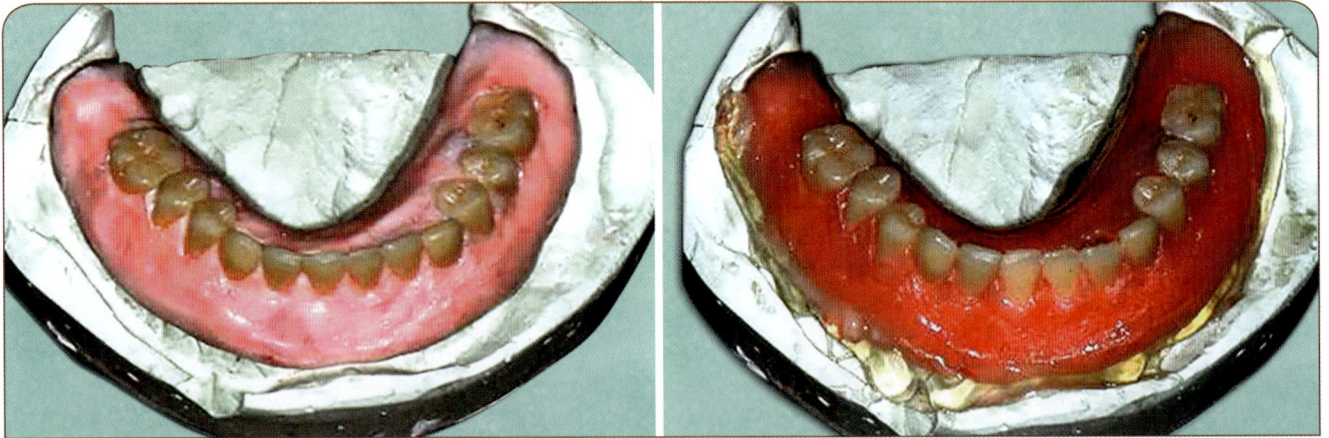

Fig. 12

Eclipse denture setup uncured on left on the master cast and following light-curing in the Eclipse curing unit **(Fig. 12)**.

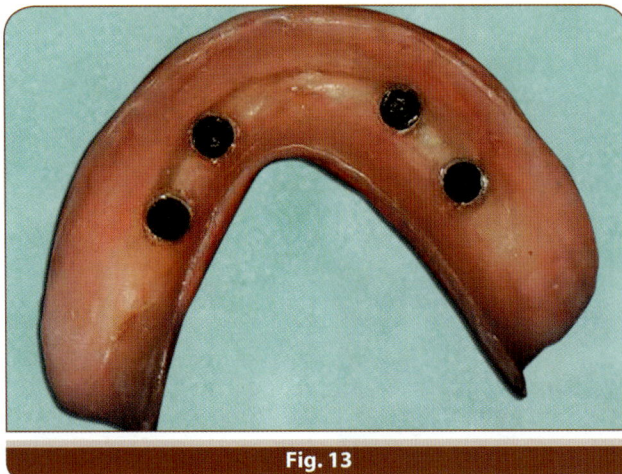

Fig. 13

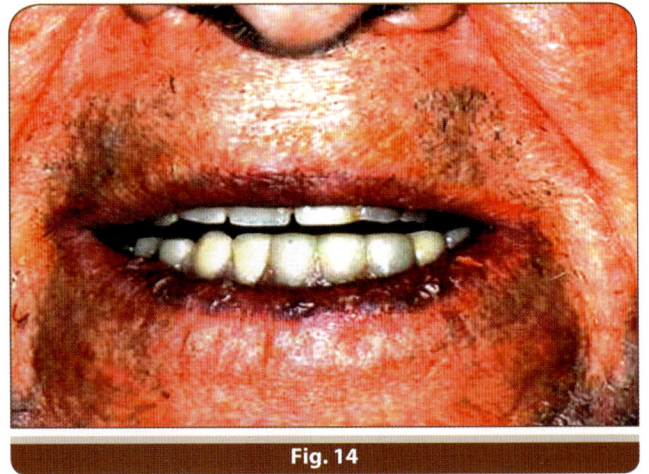

Fig. 14

Tissue side view of the processed Eclipse overdenture with Locator males in metal housings luted to the denture **(Fig. 13)**.

Finished overdenture on the overdenture bar intraorally **(Fig. 14)**.

Gregori M Kurtzman

FULLY EDENTULOUS ARCH HYBRID PROSTHESIS CAD/CAM MILLING RESIN OVERLAY TO TITANIUM FRAME

A 61-year-old white female. Periodontally involved maxillary teeth with poor prognosis. Patient wished a fixed approach. Special considerations: bilateral sinus augmentation was required to placed the posterior fixtures.

Implants used: Southern Implants
- 1st molars bilaterally = 6 × 13 mm
- 1st premolars bilaterally = 5 × 15 mm
- Canines bilaterally = 4 × 15 mm

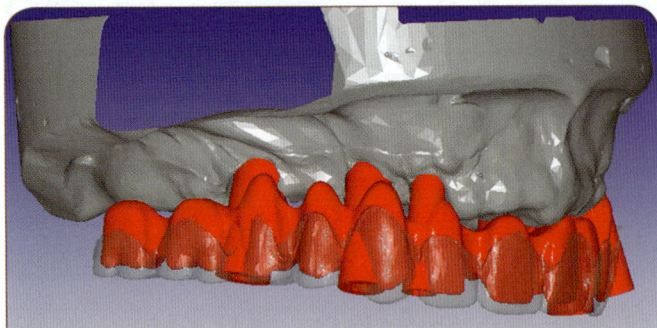
Fig. 1

Virtual model with frame in red and overlay by the teeth (semi transparent). Right lateral view **(Fig. 1)**.

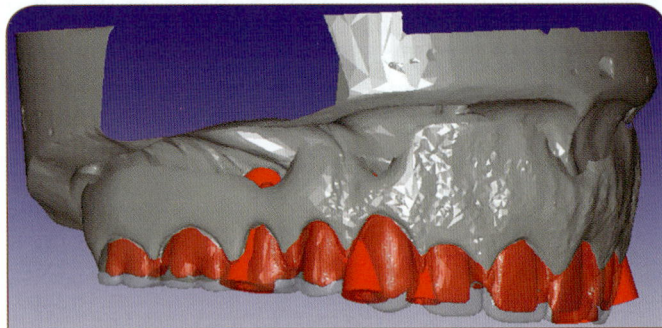
Fig. 2

Virtual model with frame in red and overlay by the teeth (semi transparent) and gingiva. Right lateral view **(Fig. 2)**.

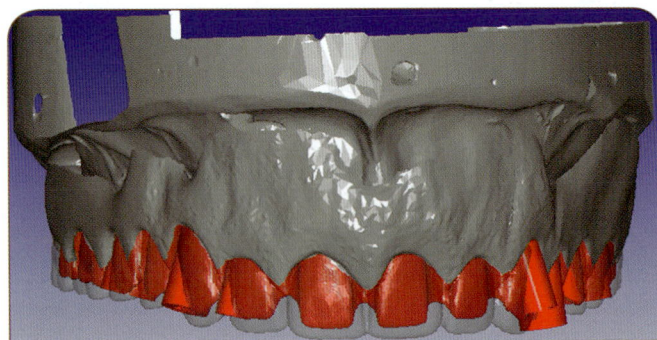
Fig. 3

Virtual model with frame in red and overlay by the teeth (semi transparent) and gingiva. Buccal view **(Fig. 3)**.

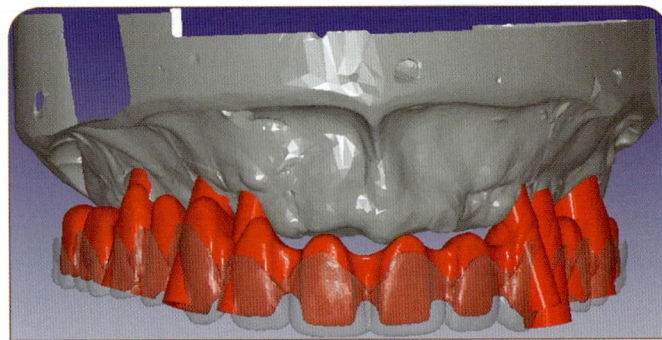
Fig. 4

Virtual model with frame in red and overlay by the teeth (semi transparent). Buccal view **(Fig. 4)**.

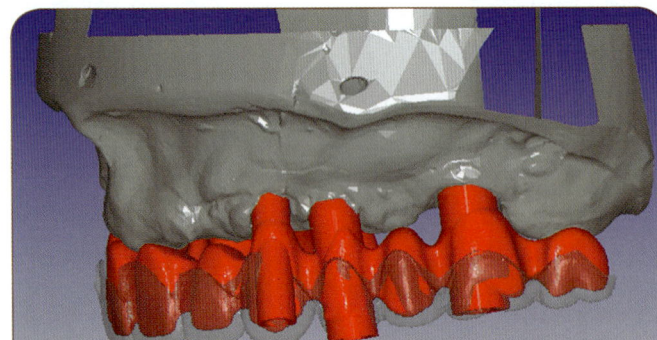
Fig. 5

Virtual model with frame in red and overlay by the teeth (semi transparent). Left lateral view **(Fig. 5)**.

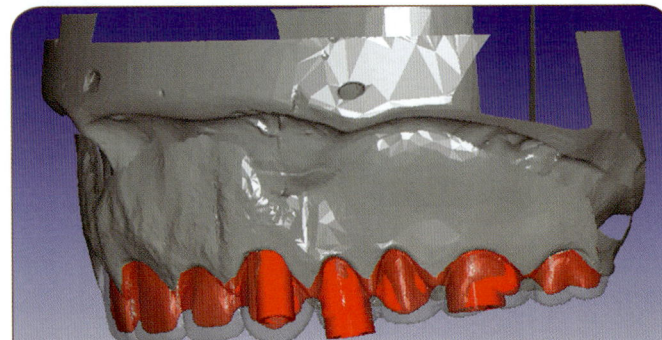
Fig. 6

Virtual model with frame in red and overlay by the teeth (semi transparent) and gingiva. Left lateral view **(Fig. 6)**.

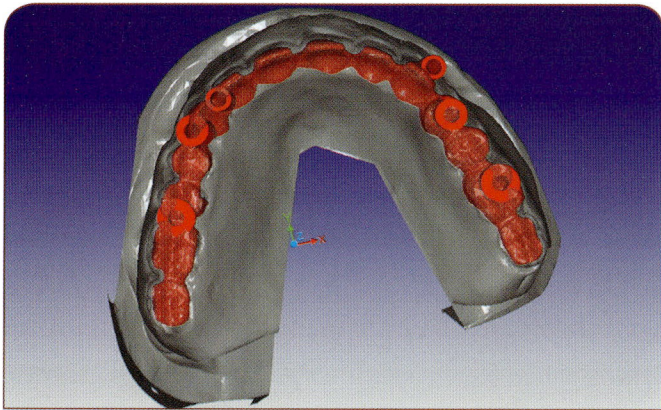

Fig. 7

Virtual model with frame in red and overlay by the teeth (semi transparent) with gingiva. Occlusal view **(Fig. 7)**.

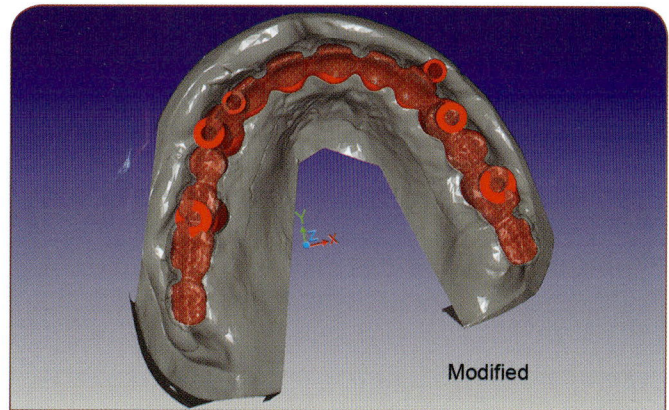

Modified

Fig. 8

Virtual model with frame in red and overlay by the teeth (semi transparent). Occlusal view **(Fig. 8)**.

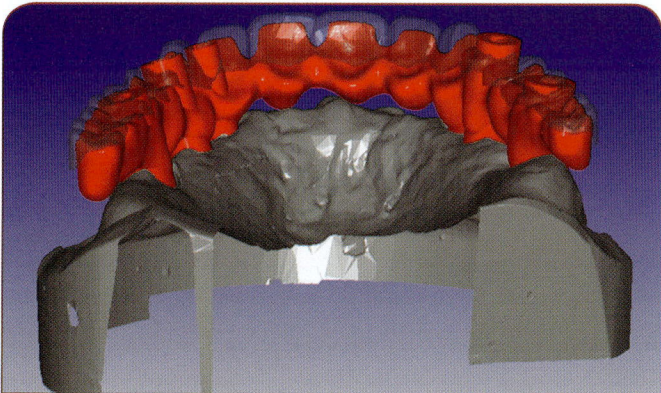

Fig. 9

Virtual model with frame in red and overlay by the teeth (semi transparent). Lingual view **(Fig. 9)**.

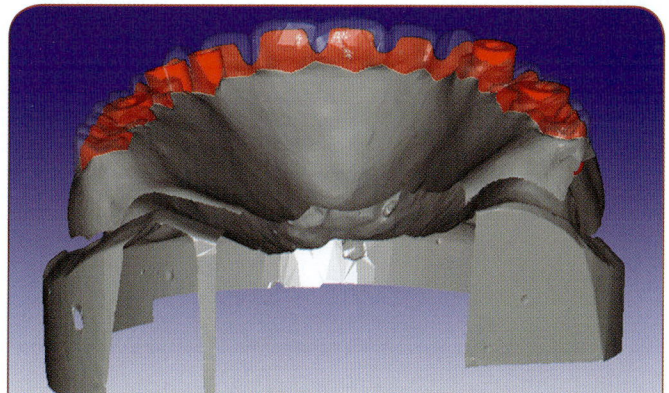

Fig. 10

Virtual model with frame in red and overlay by the teeth (semi transparent) with gingiva. Lingual view **(Fig. 10)**.

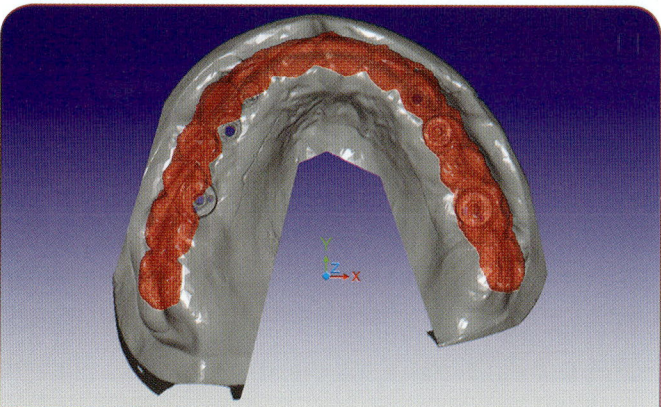

Fig. 11

Virtual model with frame in red and overlay by the teeth (semi transparent) with gingiva. Occlusal view **(Fig. 11)**.

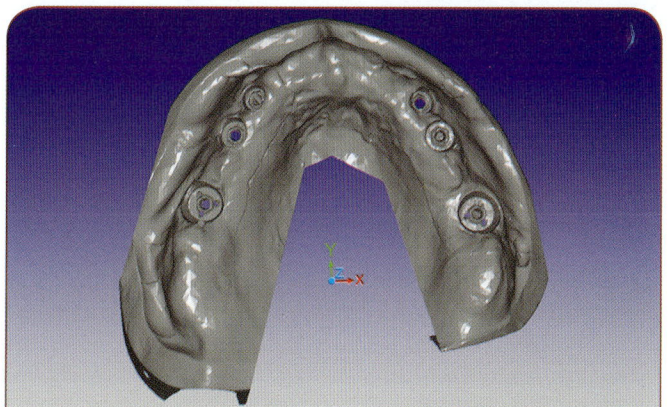

Fig. 12

Virtual model with implant connectors. Occlusal view **(Fig. 12)**.

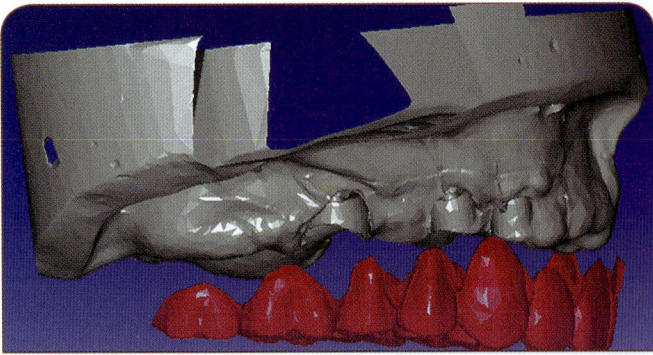

Fig. 13

Virtual model with teeth in red. Right lateral view **(Fig. 13)**.

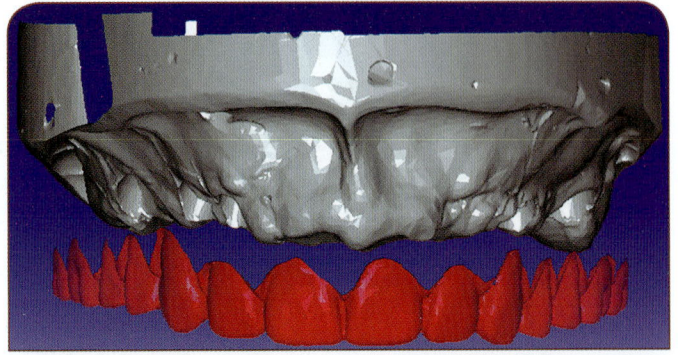

Fig. 14

Virtual model with teeth in red. Facial view **(Fig. 14)**.

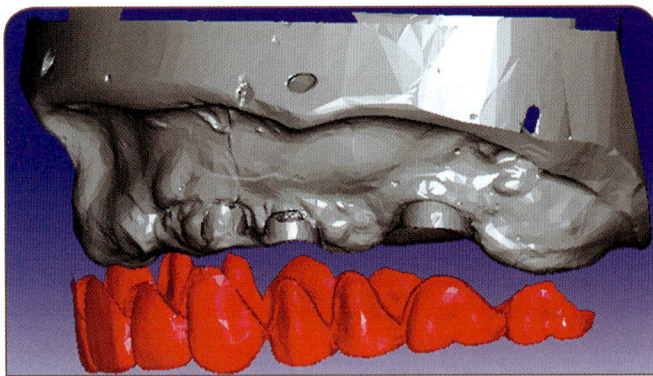

Fig. 15

Virtual model with teeth in red. Left lateral view **(Fig. 15)**.

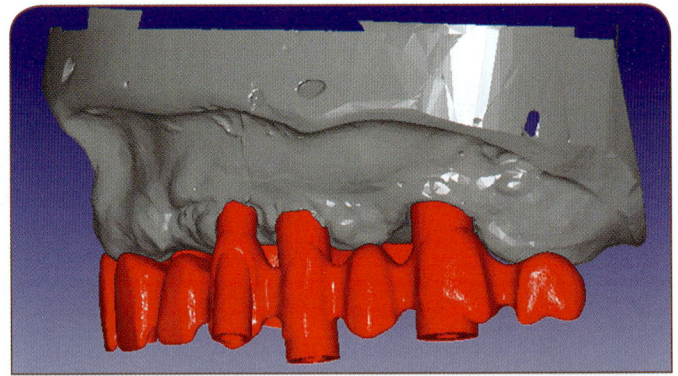

Fig. 16

Virtual model with frame in red. Left lateral view, demonstrating implant emergence on the facial of the canine **(Fig. 16)**.

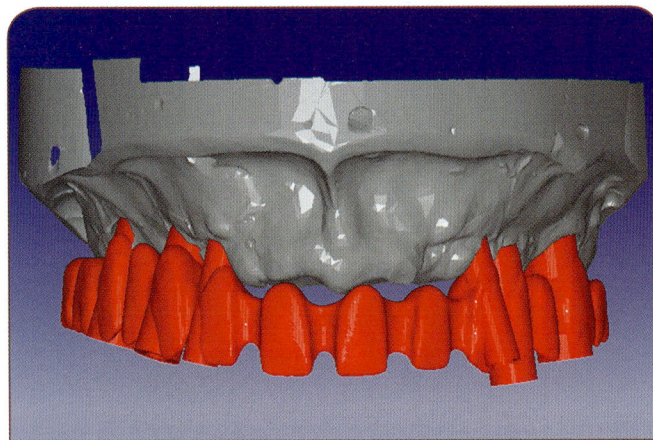

Fig. 17

Virtual model with frame in red. Buccal view, demonstrating implant emergence on the facial of the canine **(Fig. 17)**.

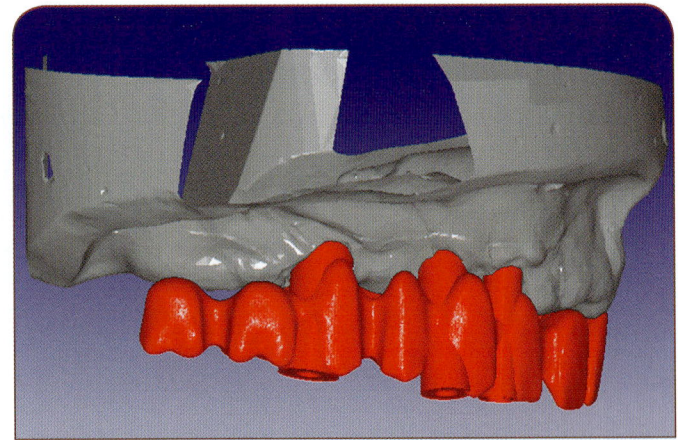

Fig. 18

Virtual model with frame in red. Right lateral view **(Fig. 18)**.

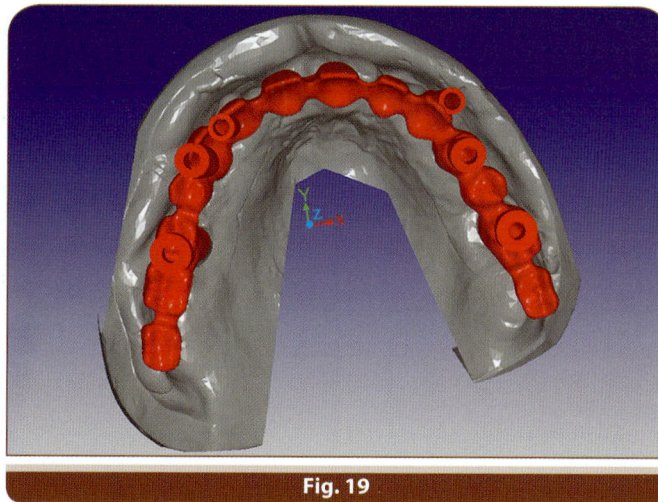

Fig. 19

Virtual model with frame in red. Occlusal view, demonstrating implant emergence on the facial of the left canine **(Fig. 19)**.

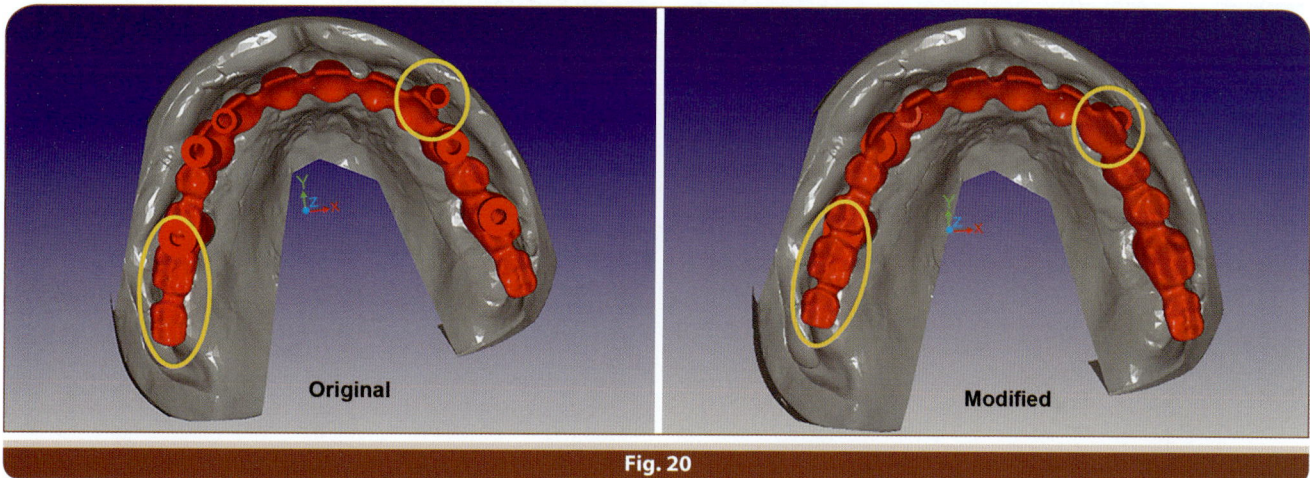

Fig. 20

Virtual model with frame in red. Occlusal view, showing modification of the virtual frame **(Fig. 20)**.

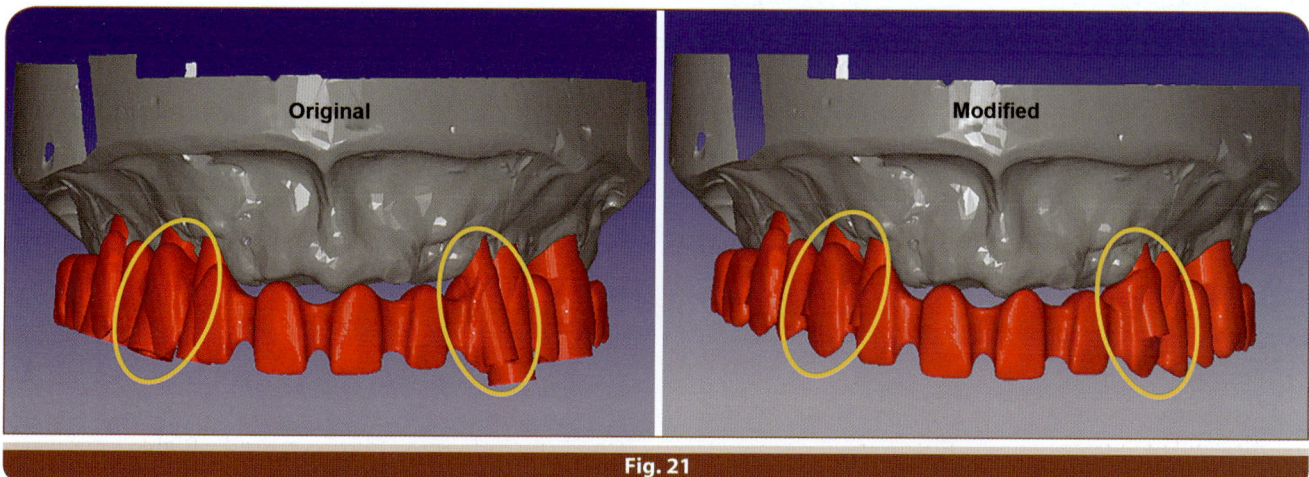

Fig. 21

Modifications of the virtual frame—facial view **(Fig. 21)**.

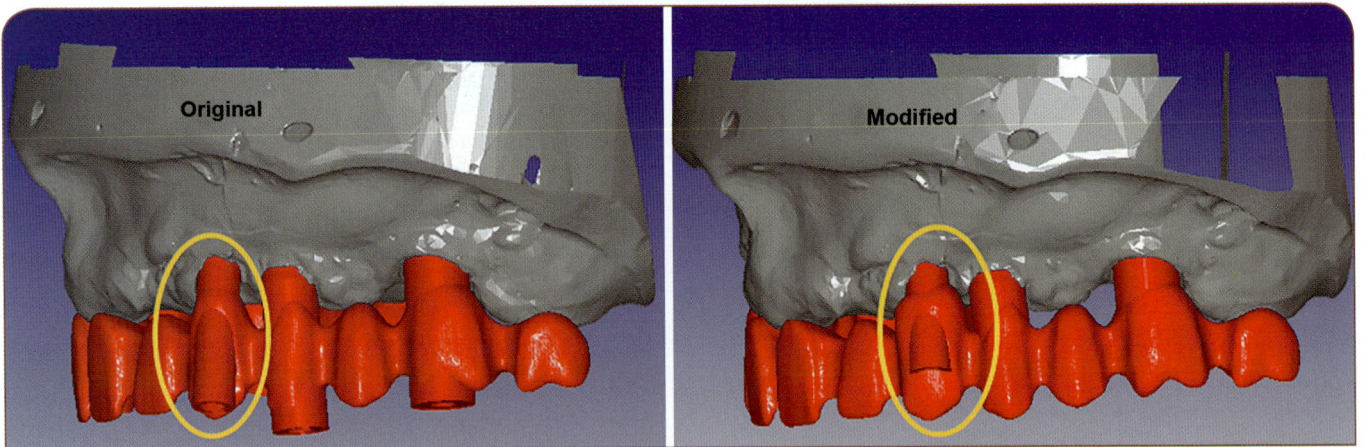

Fig. 22

Modifications of the virtual frame—left buccal view **(Fig. 22)**.

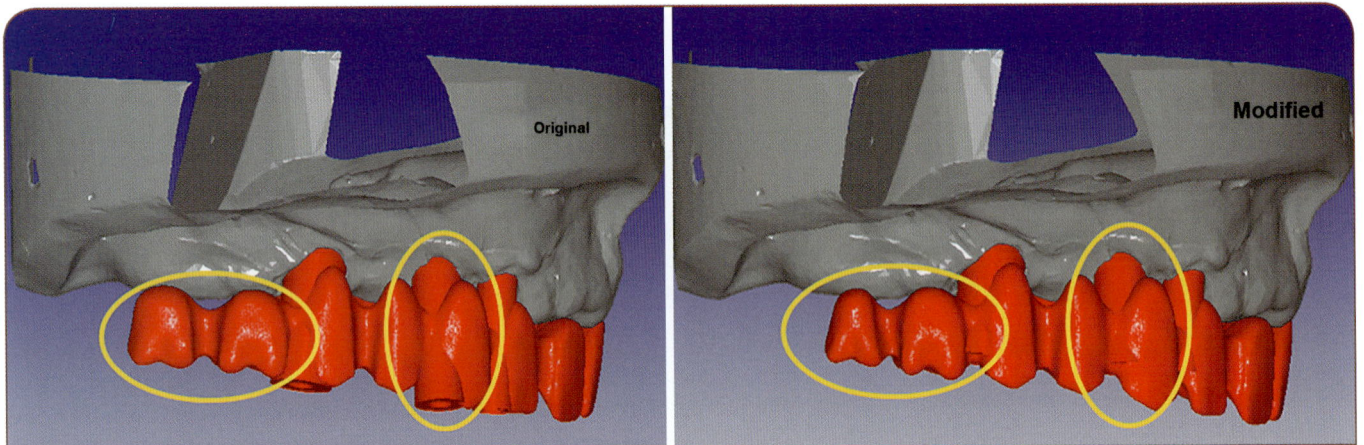

Fig. 23

Modifications of the virtual frame—right buccal view **(Fig. 23)**.

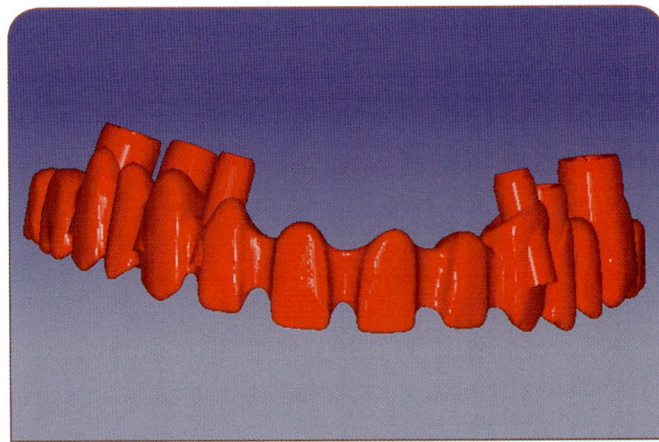

Fig. 24

Virtual frame. Facial view **(Fig. 24)**.

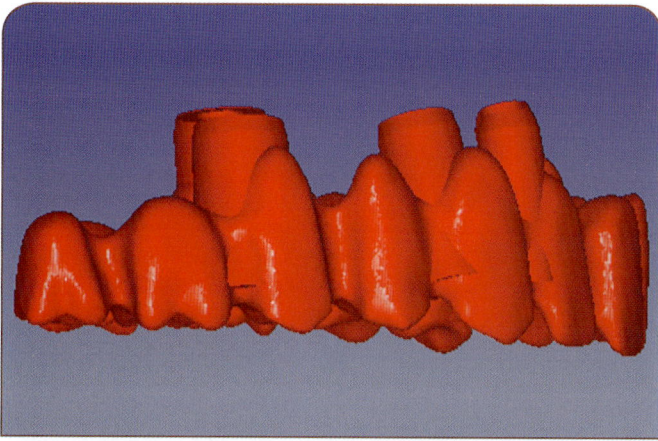

Fig. 25

Virtual frame. Right lateral view (**Fig. 25**).

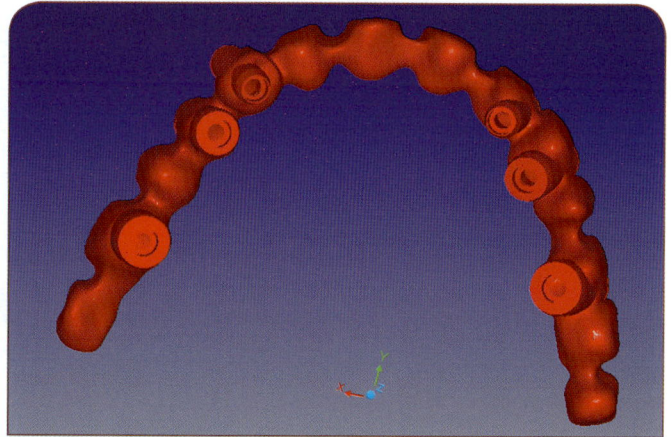

Fig. 26

Virtual frame. Gingival view (**Fig. 26**).

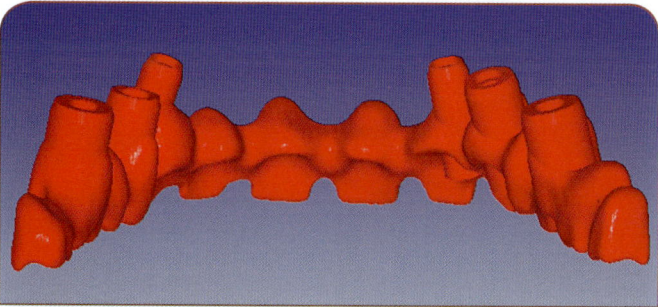

Fig. 27

Virtual frame. Lingual view (**Fig. 27**).

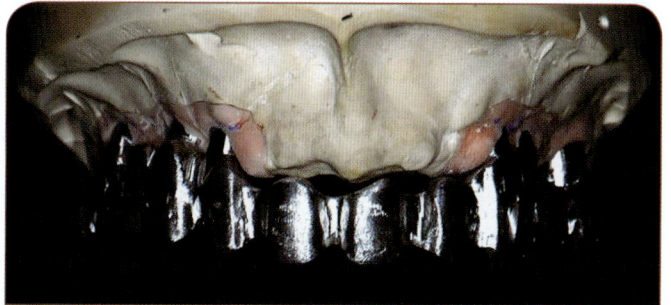

Fig. 28

CAD/CAM milled frame for a fixed hybrid full arch prosthetic. Note emergence of the screw access hole on the left canine on the facial surface (**Fig. 28**).

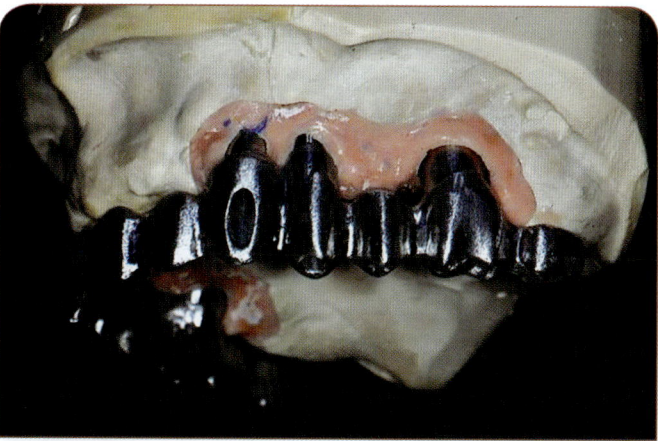

Fig. 29

CAD/CAM milled frame for a fixed hybrid full arch prosthetic. Note emergence of the screw access hole on the left canine on the facial surface (**Fig. 29**).

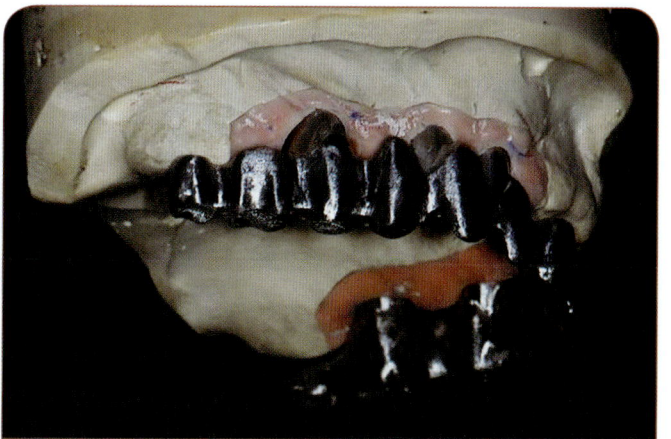

Fig. 30

CAD/CAM milled frame for a fixed hybrid full arch prosthetic. Note emergence of the screw access hole on the left canine on the facial surface (**Fig. 30**).

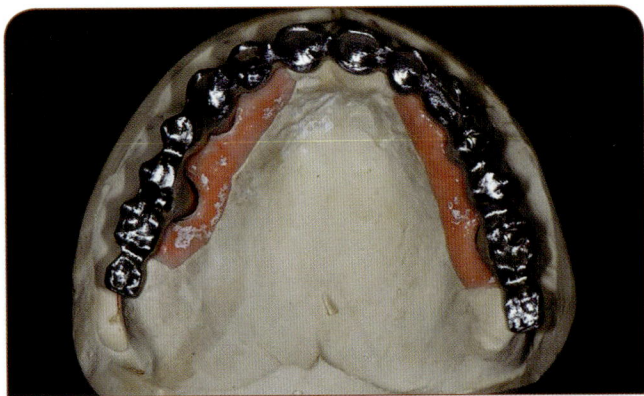

Fig. 31

CAD/CAM milled frame for a fixed hybrid full arch prosthetic **(Fig. 31)**.

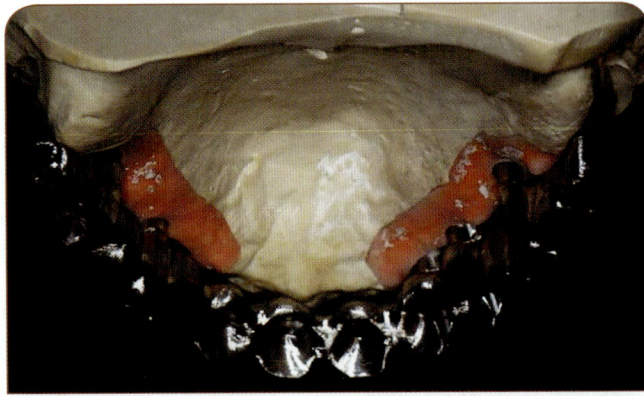

Fig. 32

CAD/CAM milled frame for a fixed hybrid full arch prosthetic **(Fig. 32)**.

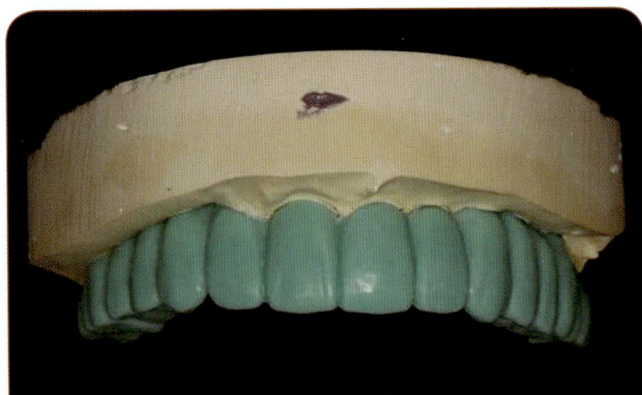

Fig. 33

Waxup on the CAD/CAM milled hybrid frame to full contour **(Fig. 33)**.

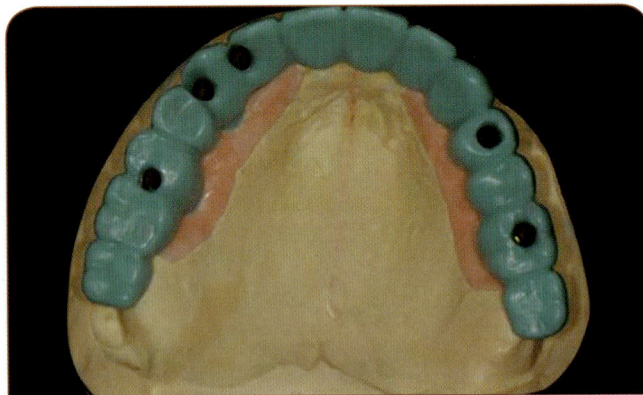

Fig. 34

Waxup on the CAD/CAM milled hybrid frame to full contour. Screw access holes on all but the left canine can be seen **(Fig. 34)**.

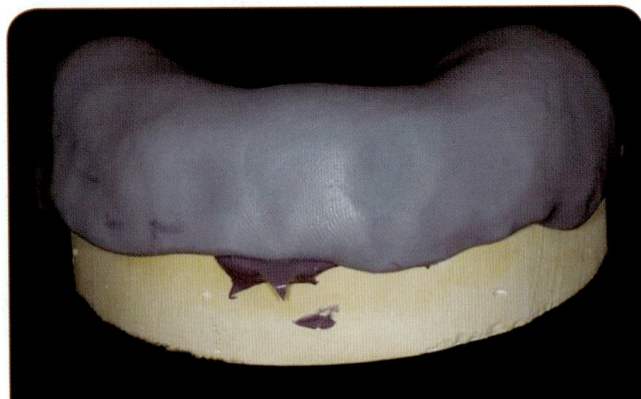

Fig. 35

Silicone stent fabricated over the waxup on the CAD/CAM milled hybrid frame **(Fig. 35)**.

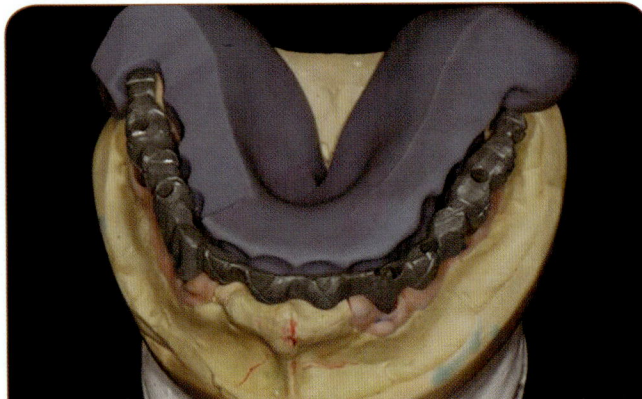

Fig. 36

Waxup has been removed from the CAD/CAM milled hybrid frame after a silicone stent was fabricated **(Fig. 36)**.

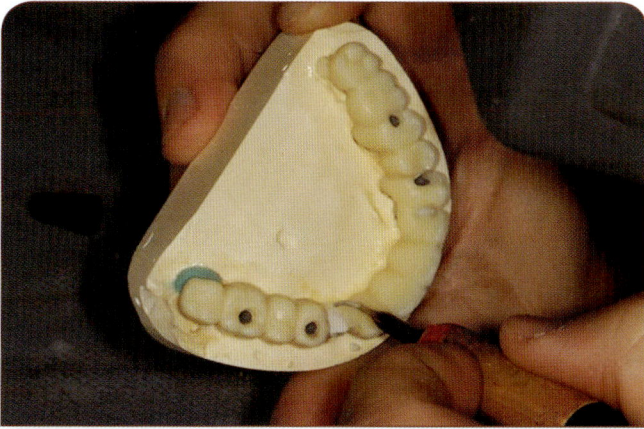

Fig. 37

Fig. 38

Radica (Dentsply) a light-curable resin that has thermoplastic properties prior to light-curing is injected into the silicone mold to get the basic shape of the desired teeth. A electric spatula is used to refine and add material to layer enamel shade on the dentin shade previously placed **(Fig. 37)**.

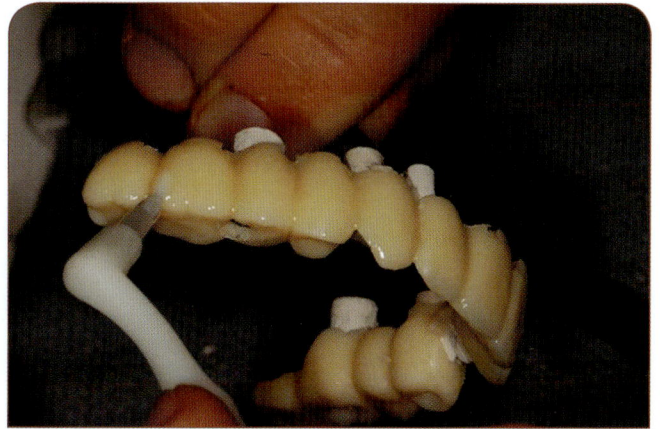

Following shaping of the Radica resin, before light-curing to prevent an air inhibited layer from forming on the exterior surface of the resin, Eclipse Air Barrier Sealer (ABS) (Dentsply) is brushed on all surfaces **(Fig. 38)**.

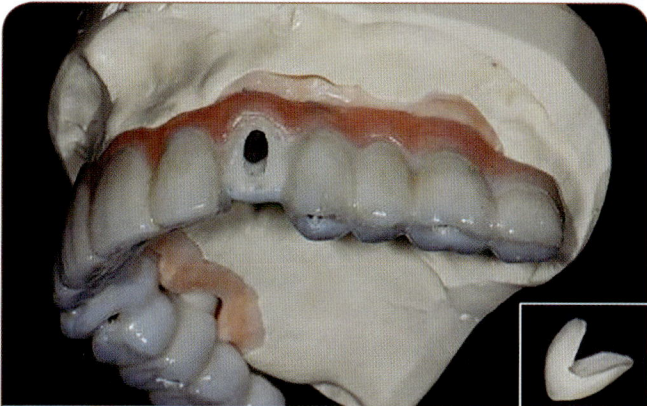

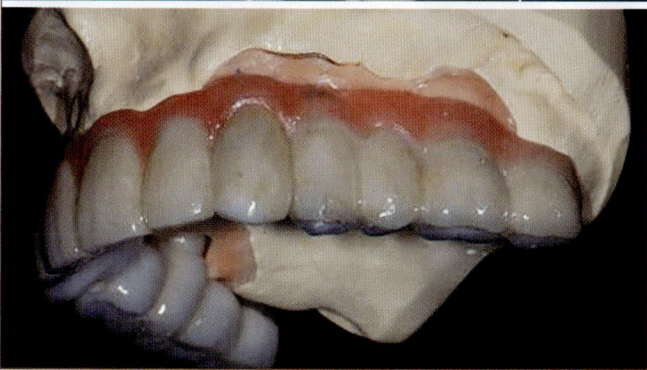

Fig. 39

Fig. 40

Finished Radica resin to CAD/CAM milled metal hybrid frame with overlay off on left and seated on right to cover the screw access hole emerging on the facial of the left canine **(Fig. 39)**.

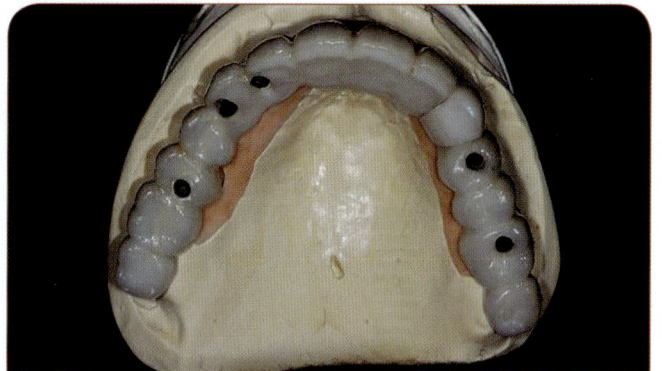

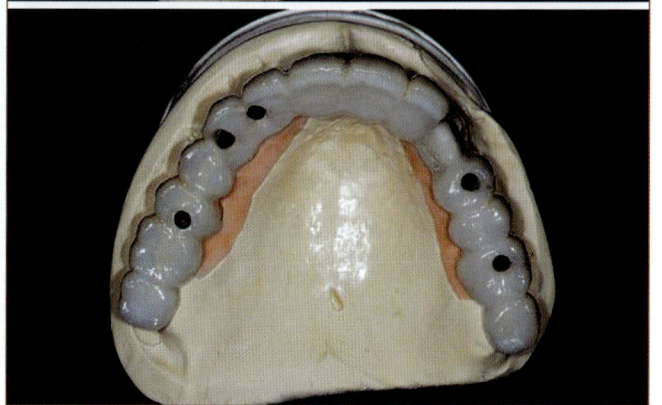

Finished Radica resin to CAD/CAM milled metal hybrid frame with overlay off on left and seated on right to cover the screw access hole emerging on the facial of the left canine **(Fig. 40)**.

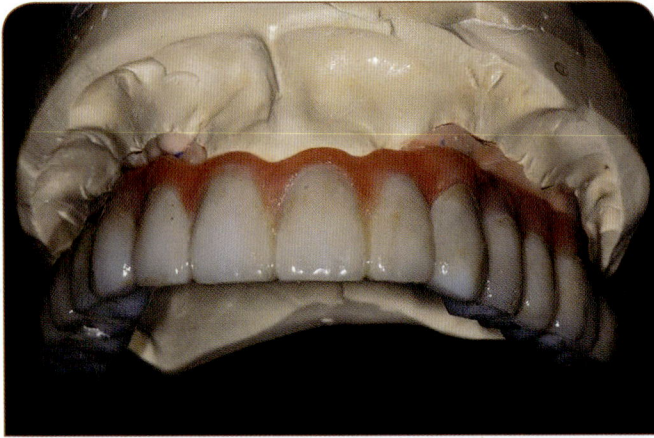

Fig. 41

Finished Radica resin to CAD/CAM milled metal hybrid frame with overlay seated to cover the screw access hole emerging on the facial of the left canine **(Fig. 41)**.

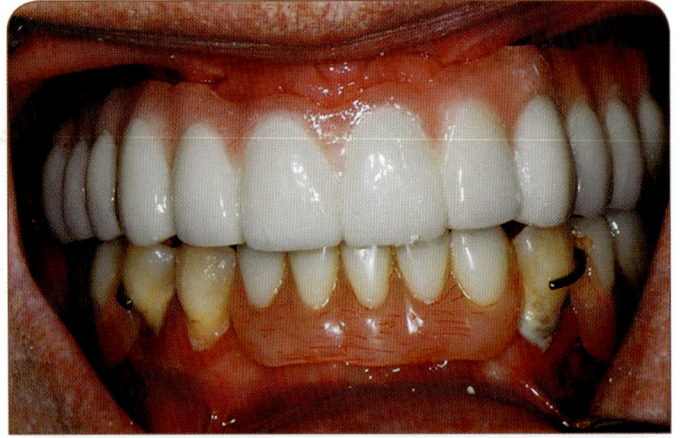

Fig. 42

Finished Radica resin to CAD/CAM milled metal hybrid frame with overlay off on the left canine showing the screw access hole emerging on the facial of the left canine seated intraorally **(Fig. 42)**.

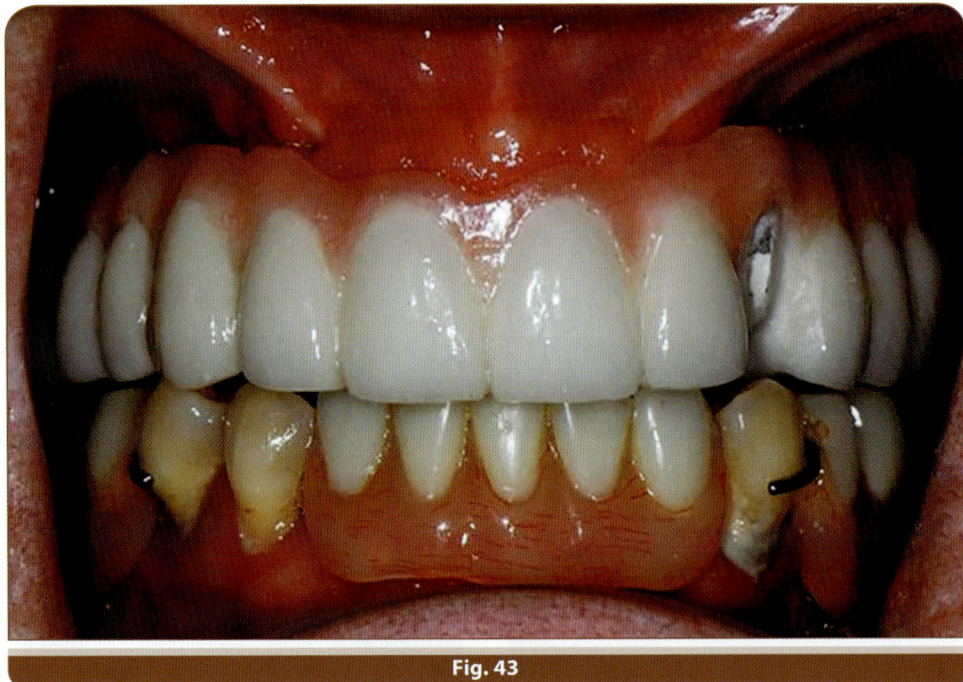

Fig. 43

Finished Radica resin to CAD/CAM milled metal hybrid frame with overlay seated to cover the screw access hole emerging on the facial of the left canine seated intraorally **(Fig. 43)**.

Gregori M Kurtzman, Douglas F Dompkowski

Fully Edentulous Arch Hybrid Prosthesis CAD/CAM Milling Denture Teeth to Metal Frame

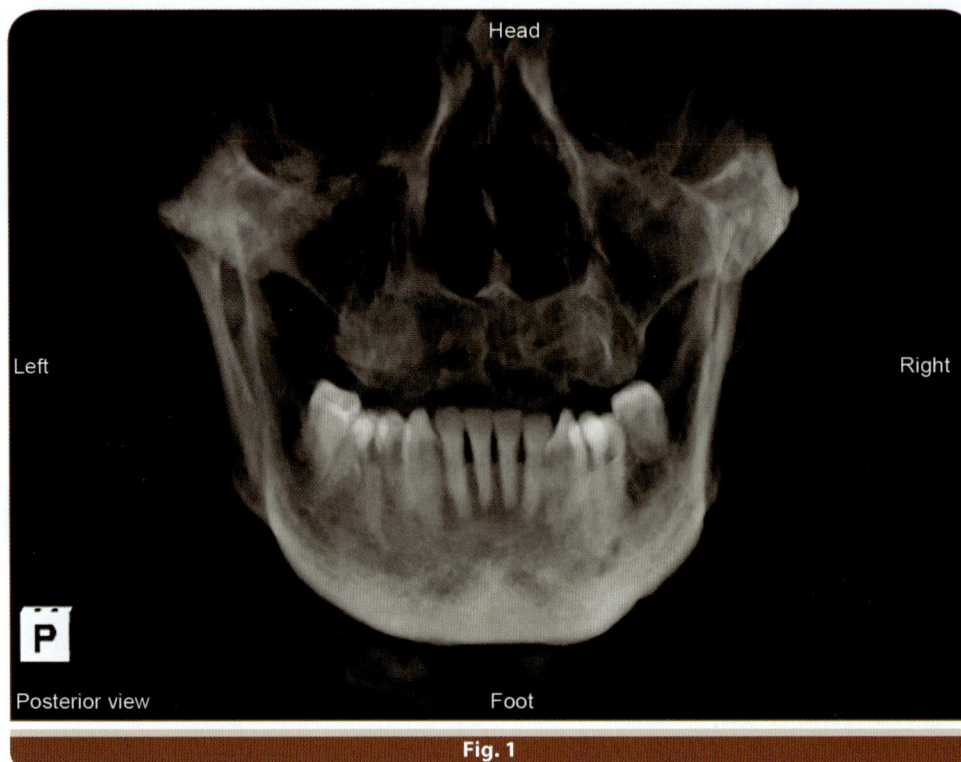

Fig. 1

A 48-year-old female presented requesting consultation for an implant retained fixed prosthesis in the maxillary arch. Patient indicated she had been wearing a full upper denture for over 20 years and was unhappy with both the esthetics and stability of the prosthesis. Cone beam computed tomography (CBCT) was made and was noted adequate bone in the maxilla to place implants for a fixed prosthesis **(Fig. 1)**.

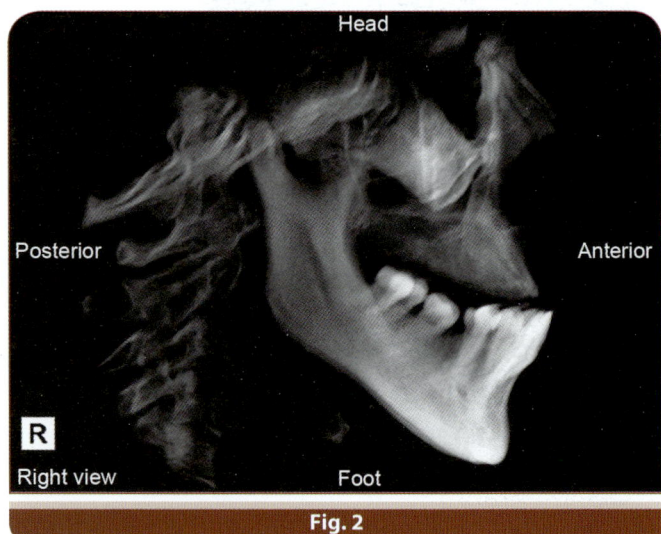

Fig. 2

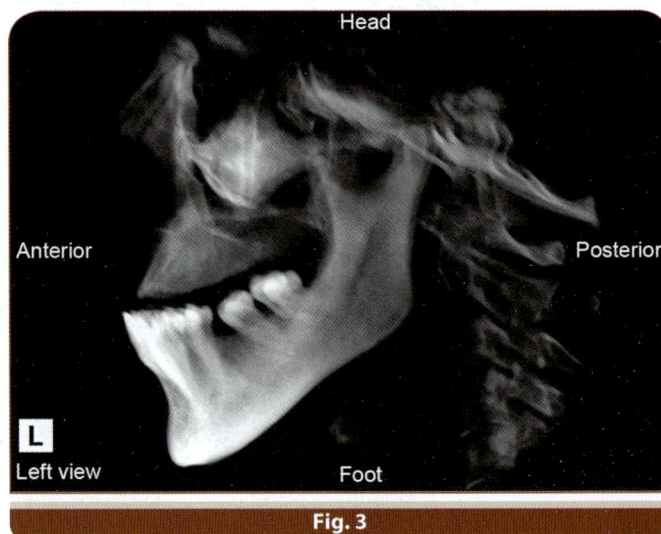

Fig. 3

Right side cephalometric view of the CBCT scan demonstrates a steep angle to the premaxilla that could hamper implant placement in a prosthetic guided implant positioning in the incisor area **(Fig. 2)**.

Left side cephalometric view of the CBCT scan demonstrates a steep angle to the premaxilla that could hamper implant placement in a prosthetic guided implant positioning in the incisor area **(Fig. 3)**.

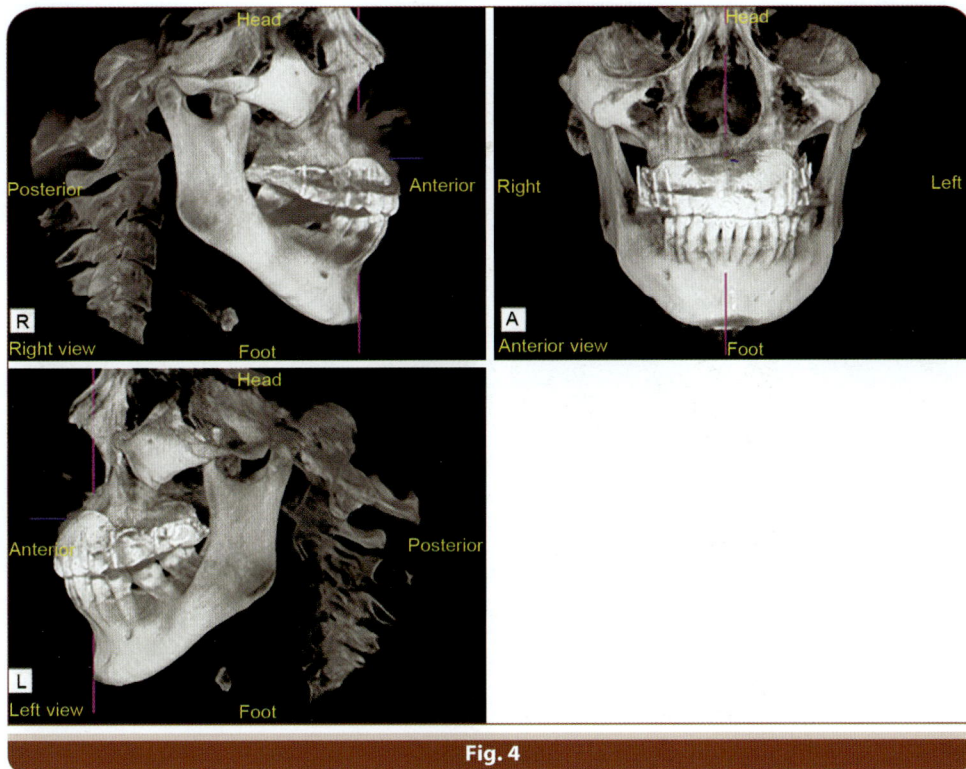

Fig. 4

Secondary CBCT scan with replica of the existing full maxillary denture fabricated from radiopaque acrylic (Jet XR) to check implant possible positions based on the tooth positions dictated by the prosthetics **(Fig. 4)**.

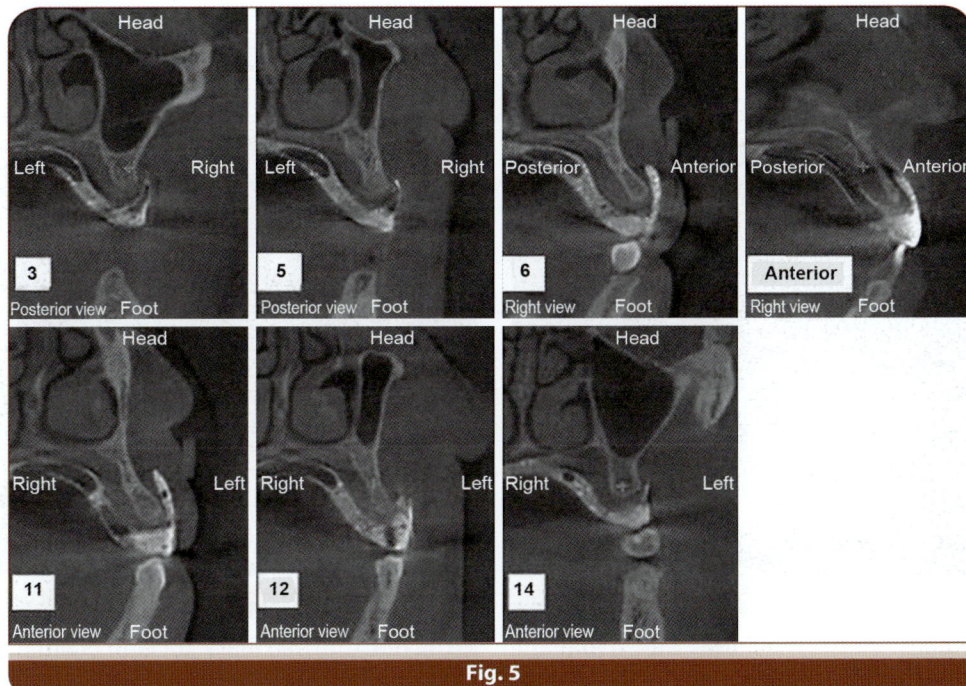

Fig. 5

Serial sections of the maxilla with the radiopaque denture in place demonstrating very narrow bone available for implant placement in the incisor area and adequate height in the posterior molar area for implant placement **(Fig. 5)**.

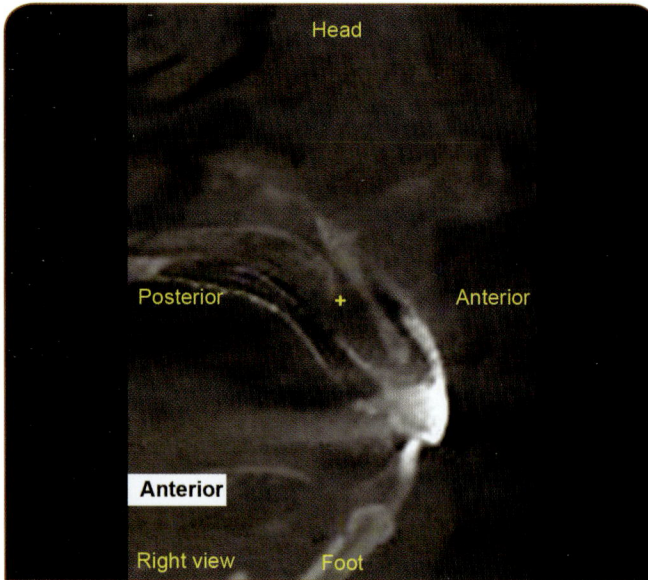

Fig. 6

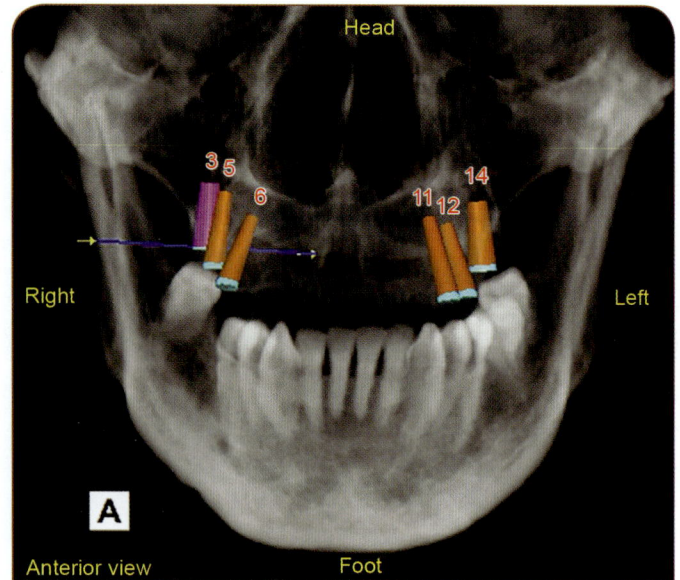

Fig. 7

Although, there is adequate height, the severe resorption in the central incisor area had left only the denser palatal plate with no width to place implants in this area **(Fig. 6)**.

To avoid the maxillary incisor positions and avoid the steep angle of the premaxilla which would complicate the prosthetics, implants were planned for the canine, 1st premolar and 1st molar sites bilaterally **(Fig. 7)**.

Implants planned are:

- 1st molars: 5 × 13 mm taper implants (Southern Implants)
- 1st premolars: 4 × 15 mm 12 degree Co-Axis implants (Southern Implants)
- Canines: 4 × 15 mm 12 degree Co-Axis implants (Southern Implants).

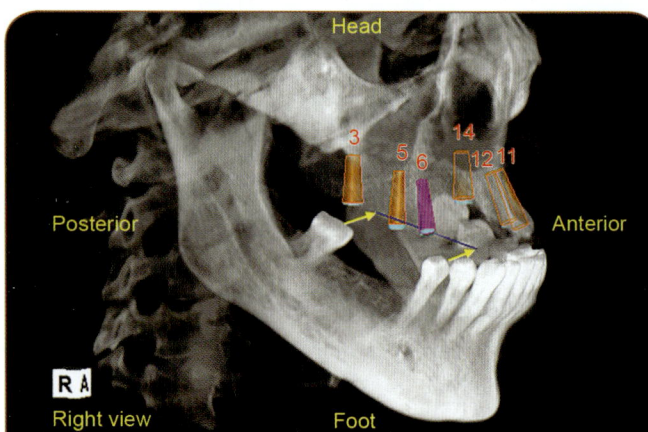

Fig. 8

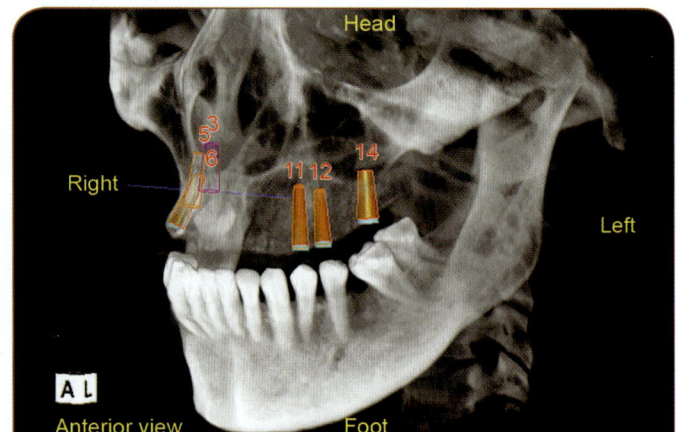

Fig. 9

To avoid the maxillary incisor positions and avoid the steep angle of the premaxilla which would complicate the prosthetics, implants were planned for the canine, 1st premolar and 1st molar sites bilaterally **(Fig. 8)**.

To avoid the maxillary incisor positions and avoid the steep angle of the premaxilla which would complicate the prosthetics, implants were planned for the canine, 1st premolar and 1st molar sites bilaterally **(Fig. 9)**.

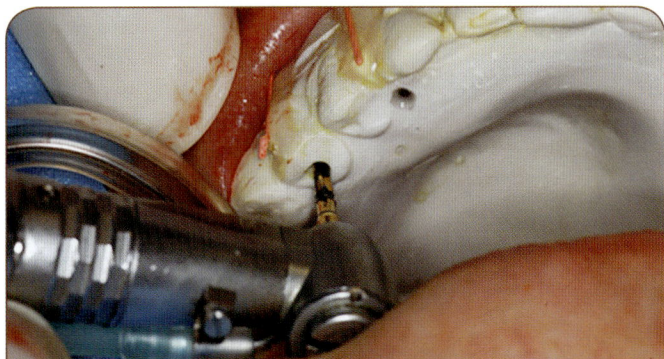

Fig. 10

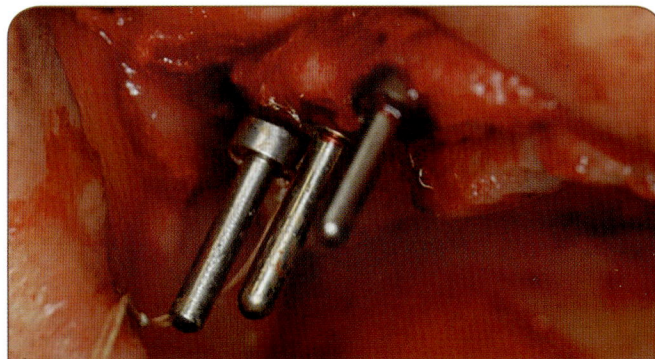

Fig. 11

The radiopaque denture is used as a surgical stent with pilot holes placed at the desired locations based on the CBCT scan taken. A pilot drill is used to engage the bone through the soft tissue without flapping initially **(Fig. 10)**.

A full thickness flap is created and the pilot holes deepened and guide pins placed to verify parallelism between the implants on the right side **(Fig. 11)**.

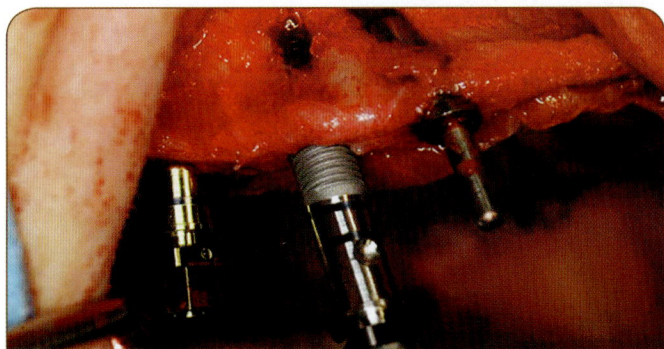

Fig. 12

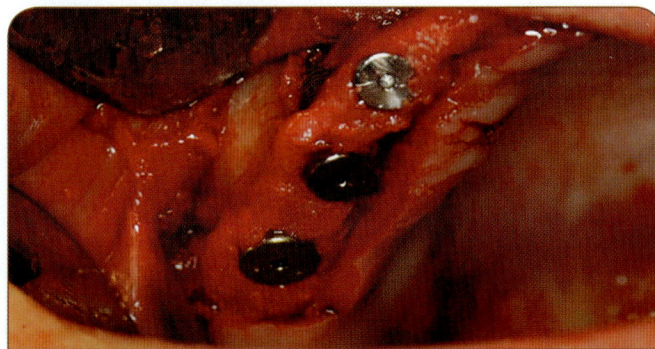

Fig. 13

Osteotomies were continued to accommodate the implants selected. Note perforations in the buccal plate that will be grafted **(Fig. 12)**.

Implants have been placed on the right side and cover screws affixed to the implants. Perforation can be seen on the buccal plate at the implant at the 1st premolar site **(Fig. 13)**.

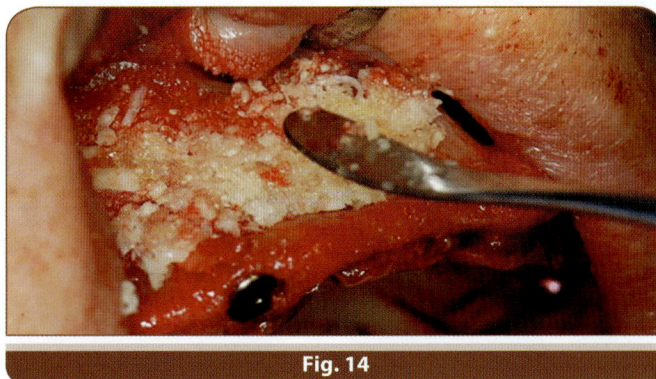

Fig. 14

DynaBlast® (Keystone Dental), a demineralized bone matrix with cancellous bone chips was placed on the buccal to fill the perforations in the buccal plate and help eliminate the undercut present on the buccal. The process of guided positioning, implant placement and grafting was repeated on the left side. Flaps were closed with 3-0 silk sutured in an interrupted patter **(Fig. 14)**.

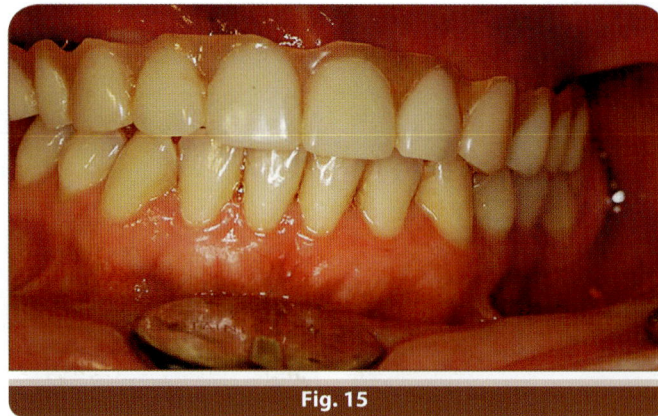

Fig. 15

The existing denture was modified with removal of the buccal flanges to accommodate the grafting of the buccal across the entire arch. Patient was instructed to use denture adhesive and stick to a soft diet till ready to be restored in 6 months **(Fig. 15)**.

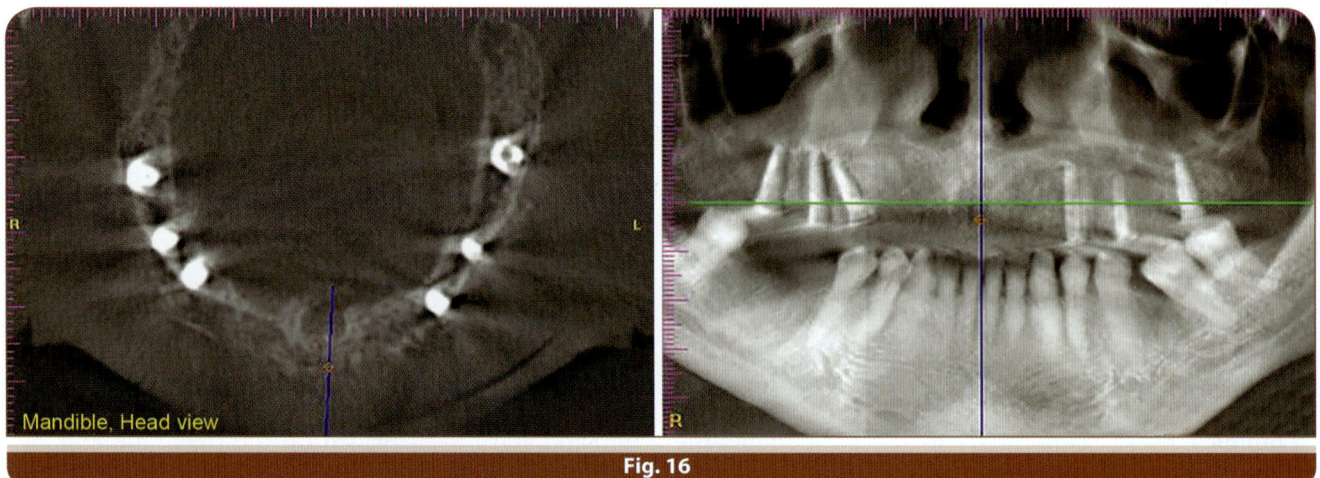

Fig. 16

CBCT scan taken at 6 months post-implant placement. Note in horizontal view all implants are surrounded by bone **(Fig. 16)**.

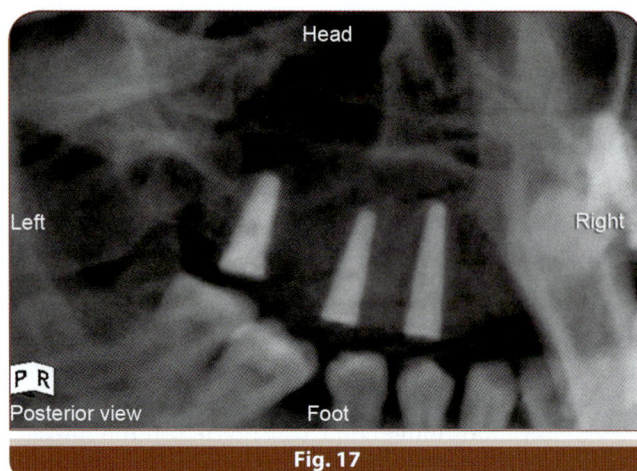

Fig. 17

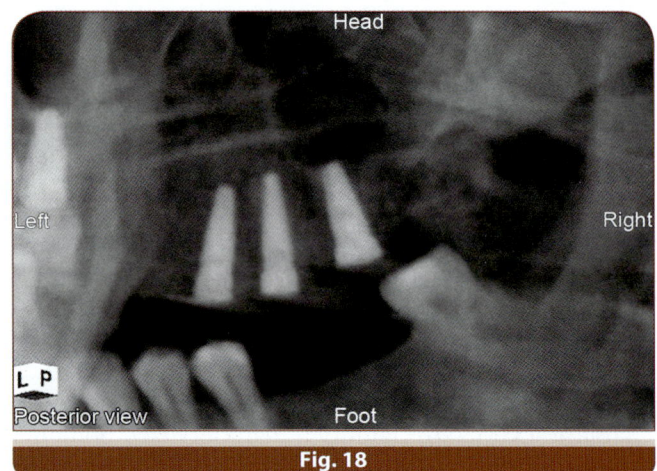

Fig. 18

Right side cephalometric view of the CBCT demonstrating integrated implants **(Fig. 17)**.

Left side cephalometric view of the CBCT demonstrating integrated implants **(Fig. 18)**.

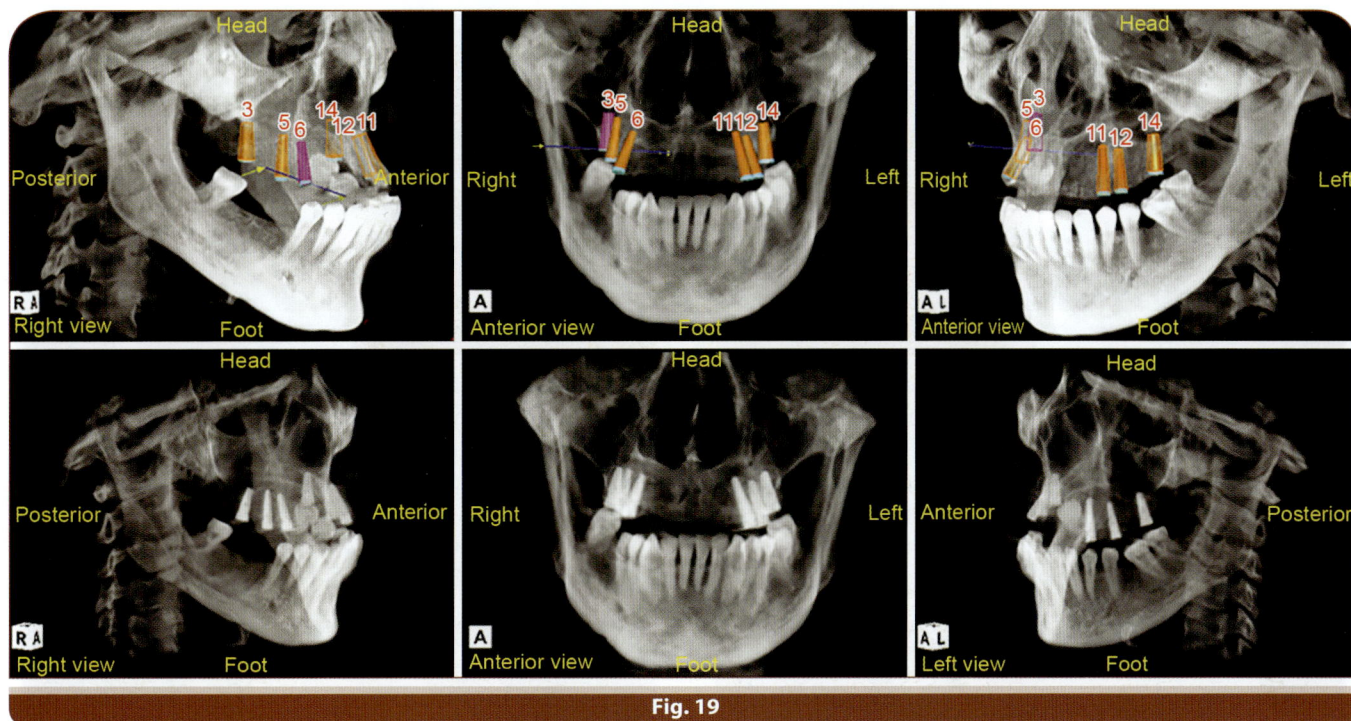

Fig. 19

CBCT comparison of the planned implant positions and implant positioned achieved demonstrating good surgical guidance **(Fig. 19)**.

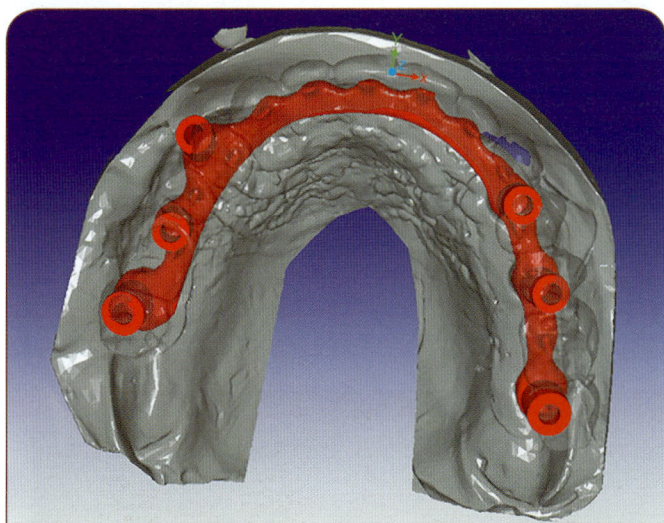

Fig. 20

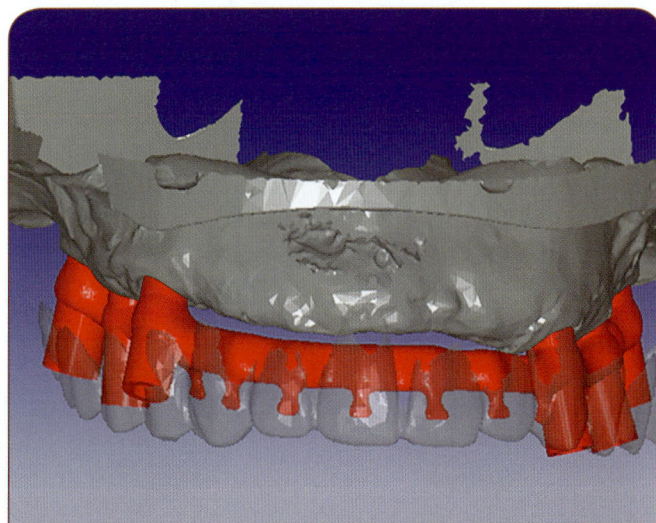

Fig. 21

Occlusal view of a virtual scan of the soft tissue model fabricated from an open tray impression of the implants. The planned prosthesis is shown in red to support a fixed hybrid full arch bridge with denture teeth on the frame. Teeth can be seen from a scan of the wax setup to ensure that the hybrid frame lays within the prosthetically driven restoration **(Fig. 20)**.

Buccal view of a virtual scan of the soft tissue model fabricated from an open tray impression of the implants. The planned prosthesis is shown in red to support a fixed hybrid full arch bridge with denture teeth on the frame. Teeth can be seen from a scan of the wax setup to ensure that the hybrid frame lays within the prosthetically driven restoration **(Fig. 21)**.

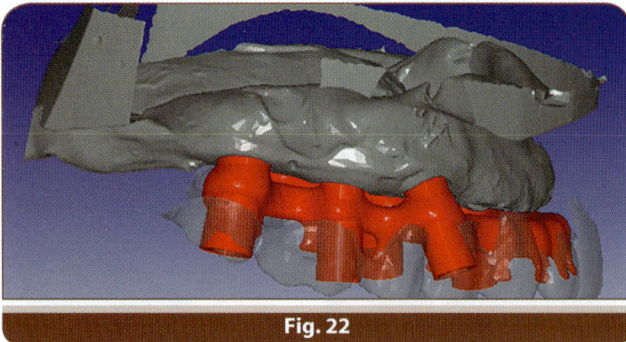

Fig. 22

Right lateral view of a virtual scan of the soft tissue model fabricated from an open tray impression of the implants. The planned prosthesis is shown in red to support a fixed hybrid full arch bridge with denture teeth on the frame. Teeth can be seen from a scan of the wax setup to ensure that the hybrid frame lays within the prosthetically driven restoration **(Fig. 22)**.

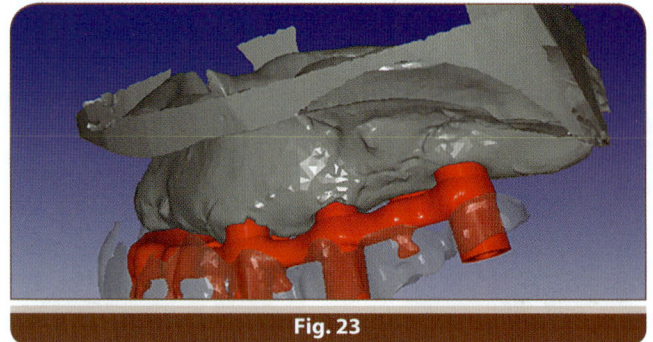

Fig. 23

Left lateral view of a virtual scan of the soft tissue model fabricated from an open tray impression of the implants. The planned prosthesis is shown in red to support a fixed hybrid full arch bridge with denture teeth on the frame. Teeth can be seen from a scan of the wax setup to ensure that the hybrid frame lays within the prosthetically driven restoration **(Fig. 23)**.

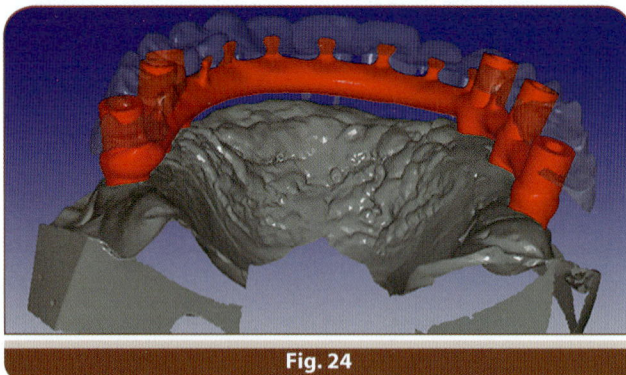

Fig. 24

Lingual view of a virtual scan of the soft tissue model fabricated from an open tray impression of the implants. The planned prosthesis is shown in red to support a fixed hybrid full arch bridge with denture teeth on the frame. Teeth can be seen from a scan of the wax setup to ensure that the hybrid frame lays within the prosthetically driven restoration **(Fig. 24)**.

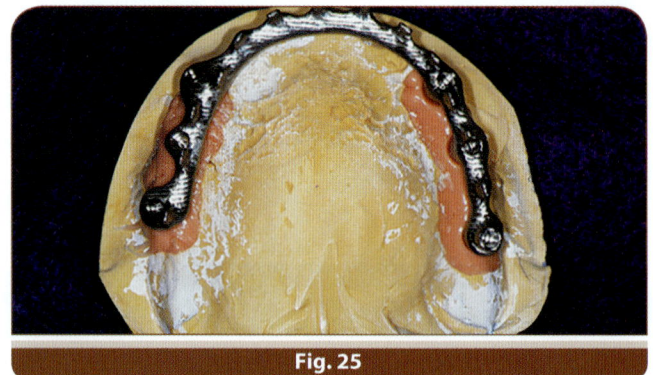

Fig. 25

Occlusal view of the CAD/CAM milled Chrome Cobalt hybrid framework (Dentsply) on the soft tissue model. The frame has been designed to retain denture teeth on the frame with complete wrap of the frame **(Fig. 25)**.

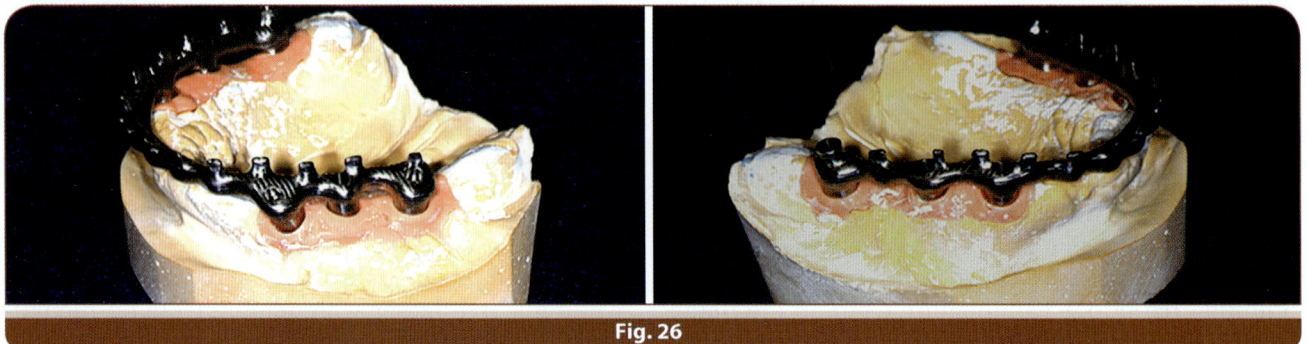

Fig. 26

Lateral view of the CAD/CAM milled Chrome Cobalt hybrid framework (Dentsply) on the soft tissue model. The frame has been designed to retain denture teeth on the frame with complete wrap of the frame **(Fig. 26)**.

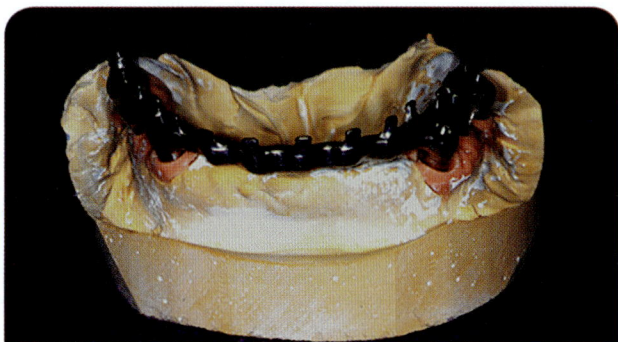

Fig. 27

Buccal view of the CAD/CAM milled Chrome Cobalt hybrid framework (Dentsply) on the soft tissue model. The frame has been designed to retain denture teeth on the frame with complete wrap of the frame **(Fig. 27)**.

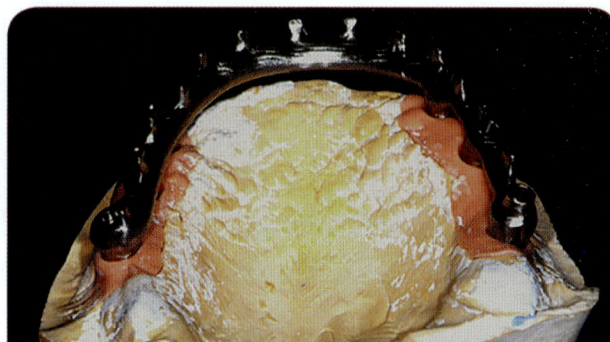

Fig. 28

Lingual view of the CAD/CAM milled Chrome Cobalt hybrid framework (Dentsply) on the soft tissue model **(Fig. 28)**.

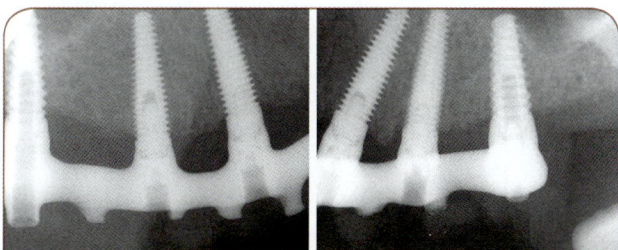

Fig. 29

Radiographic verification of passive intraoral fit of the CAD/CAM milled hybrid framework **(Fig. 29)**.

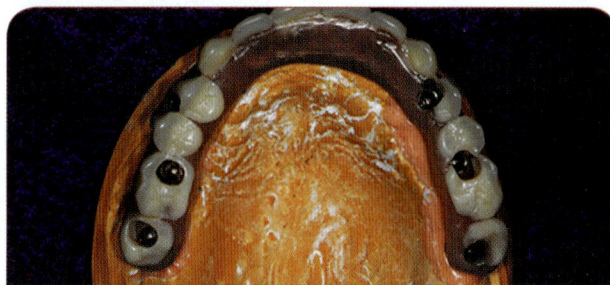

Fig. 30

Occlusal view of the CAD/CAM milled Chrome Cobalt hybrid framework (Dentsply) on the soft tissue model. Denture teeth have been processed to the CAD/CAM milled frame with Eclipse light-curable denture resin (Dentsply). Screw access holes for the hybrid prosthesis can be noted **(Fig. 30)**.

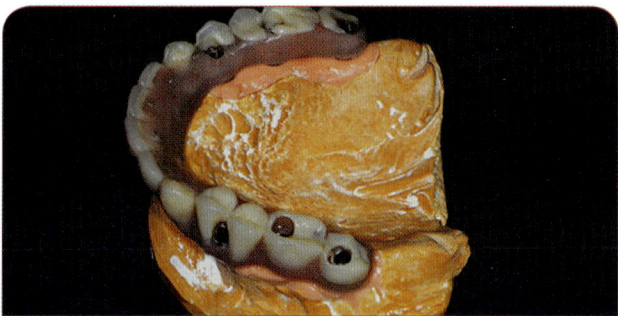

Fig. 31

Right side view of the CAD/CAM milled Chrome Cobalt hybrid framework (Dentsply) on the soft tissue model. Denture teeth have been processed to the CAD/CAM milled frame with Eclipse light-curable denture resin (Dentsply). Screw access holes for the hybrid prosthesis can be noted **(Fig. 31)**.

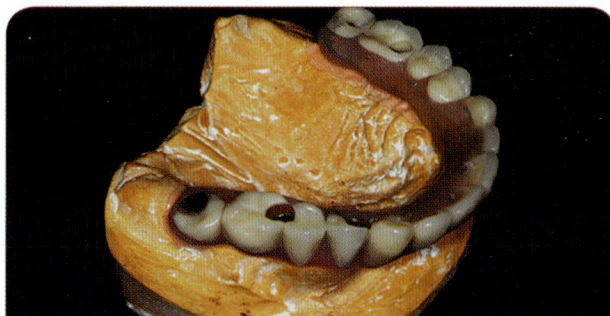

Fig. 32

Left lateral view of the CAD/CAM milled Chrome Cobalt hybrid framework (Dentsply) on the soft tissue model. Denture teeth have been processed to the CAD/CAM milled frame with Eclipse light-curable denture resin (Dentsply). Screw access holes for the hybrid prosthesis can be noted **(Fig. 32)**.

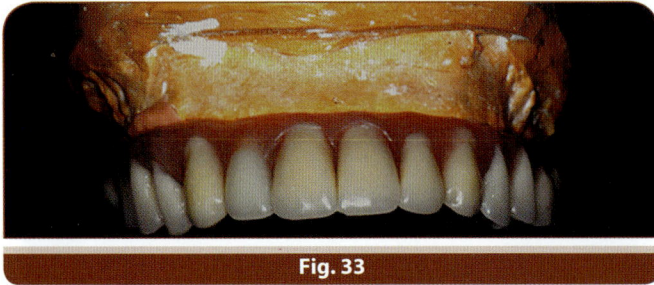

Fig. 33

Buccal view of the CAD/CAM milled Chrome Cobalt hybrid framework (Dentsply) on the soft tissue model. Denture teeth have been processed to the CAD/CAM milled frame with Eclipse light-curable denture resin (Dentsply). Screw access holes for the hybrid prosthesis can be noted **(Fig. 33)**.

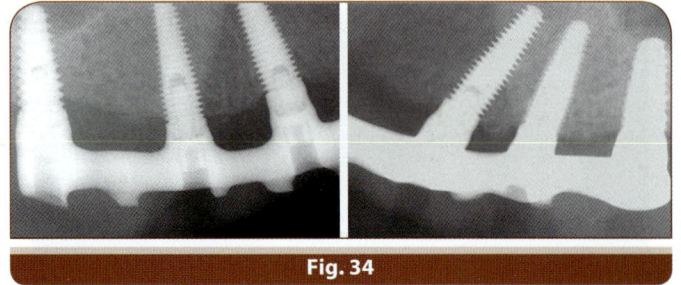

Fig. 34

Radiographs of the finished hybrid prosthesis intraorally verifying fit of the prosthesis to the implants **(Fig. 34)**.

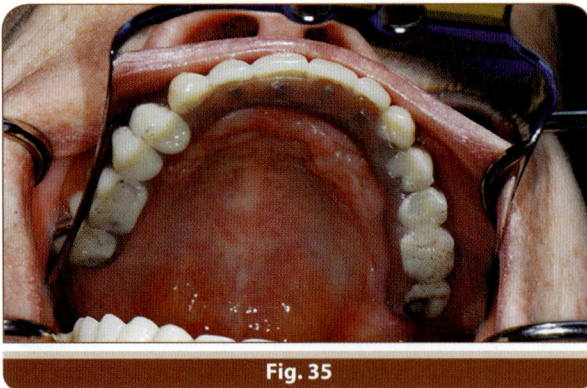

Fig. 35

Occlusal view of the CAD/CAM milled Chrome Cobalt hybrid framework (Dentsply) on the soft tissue model. Denture teeth have been processed to the CAD/CAM milled frame with Eclipse light-curable denture resin (Dentsply). Screw access holes for the hybrid prosthesis have been sealed with PTFE tape and flowable composite (VersaFlo, Centrix Dental, Shelton, CT, USA) **(Fig. 35)**.

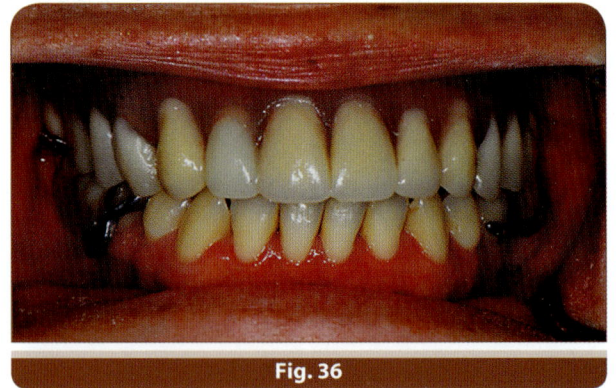

Fig. 36

Buccal view of the CAD/CAM milled Chrome Cobalt hybrid framework (Dentsply) on the soft tissue model. Denture teeth have been processed to the CAD/CAM milled frame with Eclipse light-curable denture resin (Dentsply) **(Fig. 36)**.

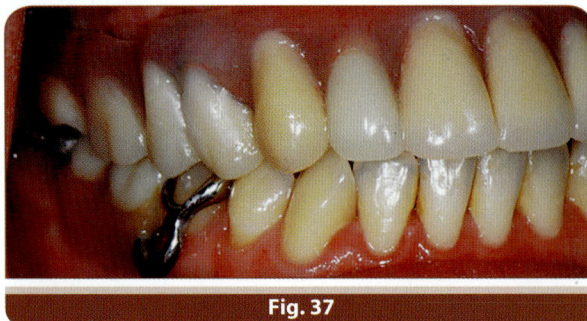

Fig. 37

Right lateral view of the CAD/CAM milled Chrome Cobalt hybrid framework (Dentsply) on the soft tissue model. Denture teeth have been processed to the CAD/CAM milled frame with Eclipse light-curable denture resin (Dentsply) **(Fig. 37)**.

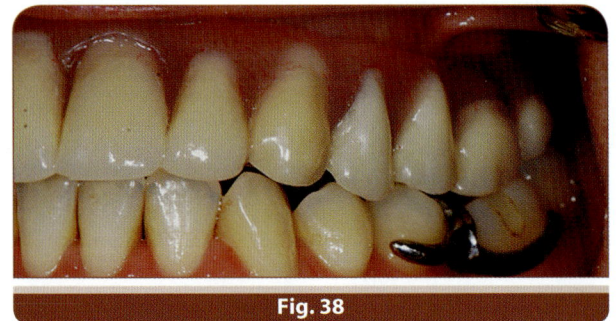

Fig. 38

Left lateral view of the CAD/CAM milled Chrome Cobalt hybrid framework (Dentsply) on the soft tissue model. Denture teeth have been processed to the CAD/CAM milled frame with Eclipse light-curable denture resin (Dentsply) **(Fig. 38)**.

Gregori M Kurtzman

PARTIALLY EDENTULOUS ARCH HYBRID PROSTHESIS

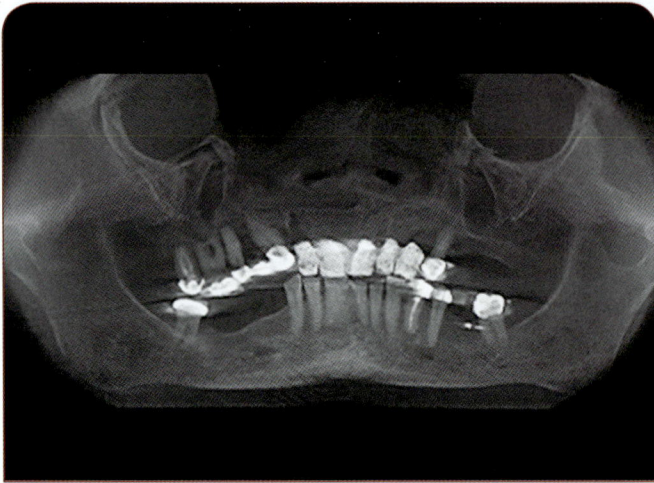

Fig. 1

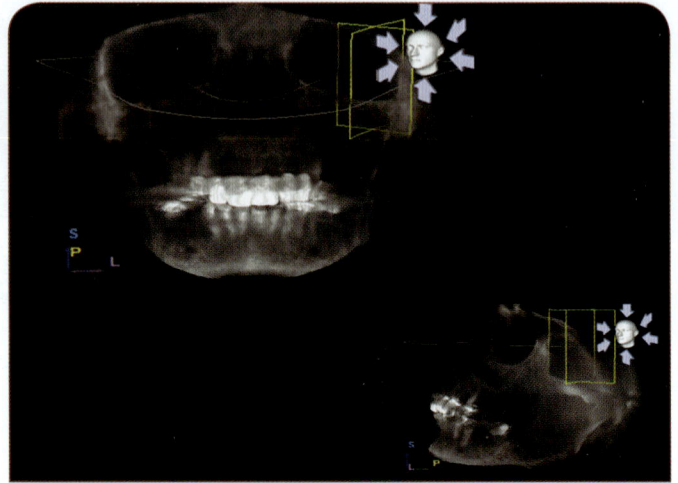

Fig. 2

An 86-year-old white female failing fixed prosthesis from the right lateral incisor to the left cuspid. Grade 2 (moderate) mobility was noted of the bridge. Patient stated she did not want a removable prosthetic in either arch as she had tried these in past and was unable to wear them due to gagging issues. Lower anterior's have moderate wear. Occlusal stops on natural 2-31, 6-27, 12-21 **(Fig. 1)**.

An impression was taken of the maxillary arch and a vacuform stent was fabricated on the cast. The teeth to be replaced were removed from the cast to the level of the gingiva. The vacuform stent was filled with a radiopaque acrylic resin (Jet XR, Lang Dental) and inserted on the cast and allowed to set. Upon setting acrylic flash was removed. Teeth were extracted and the radiopaque stent was inserted and a CBCT scan was taken to determine osseous anatomy in relation to where the teeth needed to be positioned prosthetically **(Fig. 2)**.

Due to the angulation of the available bone (Triangle of bone) Co-Axis implants (Southern Implants) with a 12 degree angle correction in the implant platform were immediately placed into osteotomies at the three extraction sites. A flat healing screw was placed on each implant and a full arch removable Essix provisional inserted to be utilized during the healing and osseointegration period. The Essix was relieved over each of the implants, so that during function no pressure would be placed on the implants that might hamper integration.

After 6 months of healing and integration the implants were exposed utilizing a tissue punch and healing abutments placed to replace the healing screws. The Essix provisional was modified to avoid contact with the healing abutments.

The soft tissue was allowed to heal for two weeks and then the restorative phase of treatment was begun.

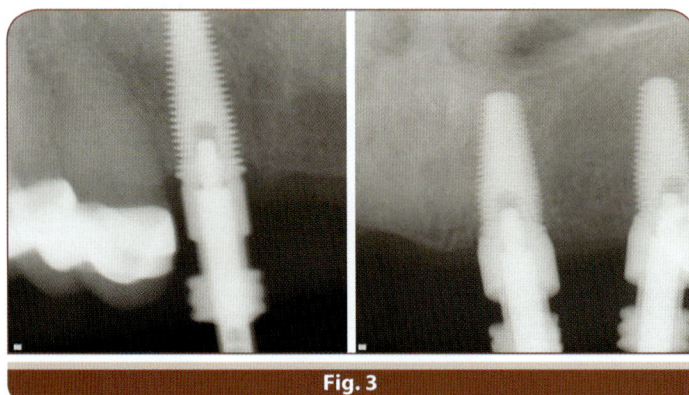

Fig. 3

Radiographs of open tray impression heads in the Southern implants fixtures to verify seating of the parts. Implants at the left central and cuspid are Co-Axis fixtures with 12 degree angle correction in implant **(Fig. 3)**.

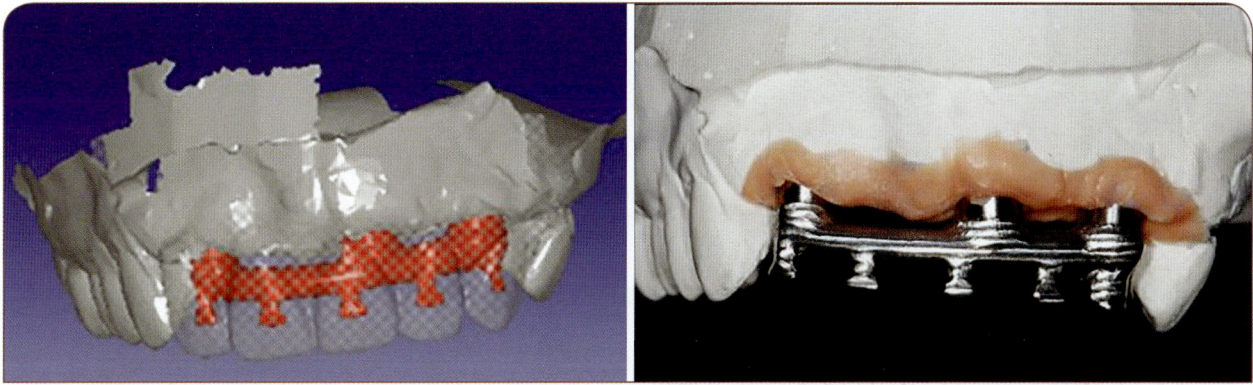

Fig. 4

Virtual frame (left) prior to milling and the finished milled titanium CAD/CAM Dentsply Compartis ISUS frame (Labial View) **(Fig. 4).**

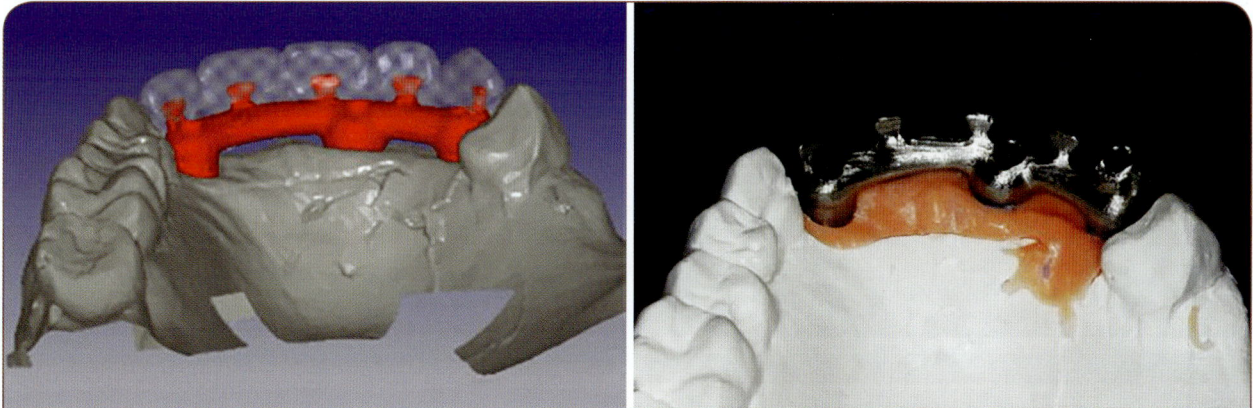

Fig. 5

Virtual frame (left) prior to milling and the finished milled titanium CAD/CAM Dentsply Compartis ISUS frame (Palatal View) **(Fig. 5).**

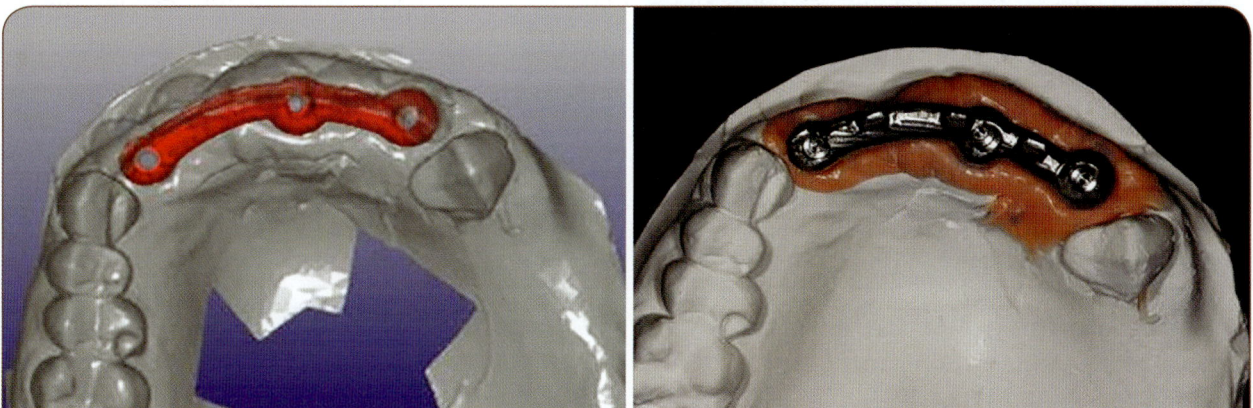

Fig. 6

Virtual frame (left) prior to milling and the finished milled titanium CAD/CAM Dentsply Compartis ISUS frame (Occlusal View) **(Fig. 6).**

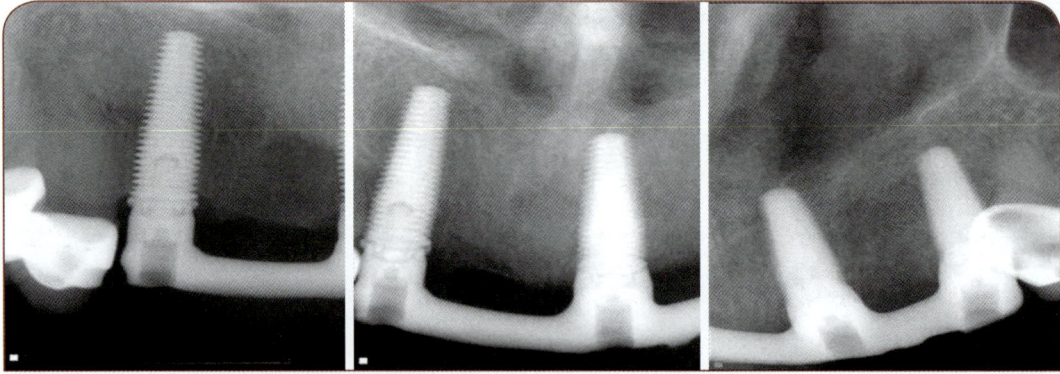

Fig. 7

Radiographs of the final finished prosthesis demonstrating fit of the Dentsply Compartis ISUS CAD/CAM milled frame **(Fig. 7)**.

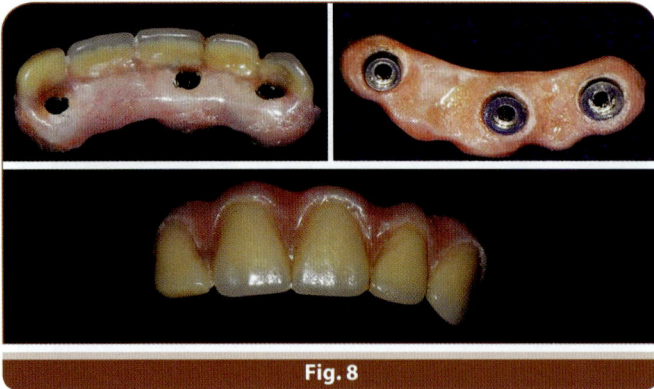

Fig. 8

Finished milled titanium CAD/CAM Dentsply Compartis ISUS frame **(Fig. 8)**.

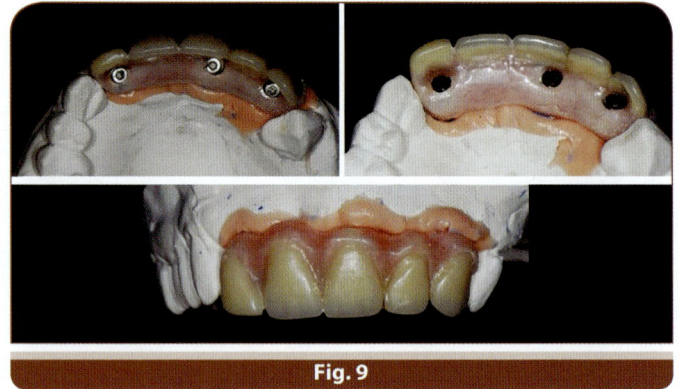

Fig. 9

Finished milled titanium CAD/CAM Dentsply Compartis ISUS frame on the working cast **(Fig. 9)**.

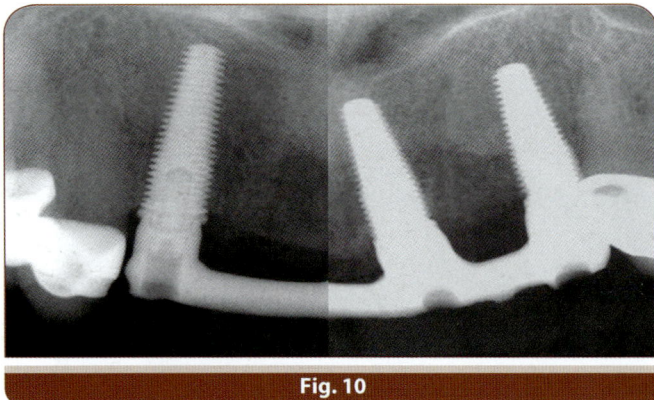

Fig. 10

Radiographs of the Dentsply Compartis ISUS CAD/CAM milled for demonstrating fit **(Fig. 10)**.

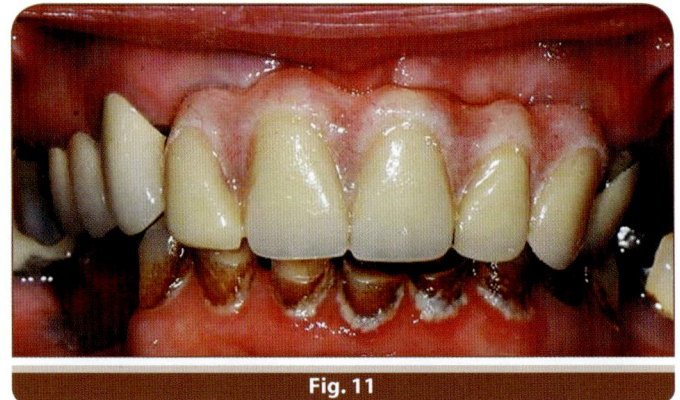

Fig. 11

Finished milled titanium CAD/CAM Dentsply Compartis ISUS frame intraorally on this 89-year-old patient. Many other problems to address here, next step a good cleaning **(Fig. 11)**.

Gregori M Kurtzman

Partially Edentulous Arch Hybrid Prosthesis CAD/CAM Milling-Posterior

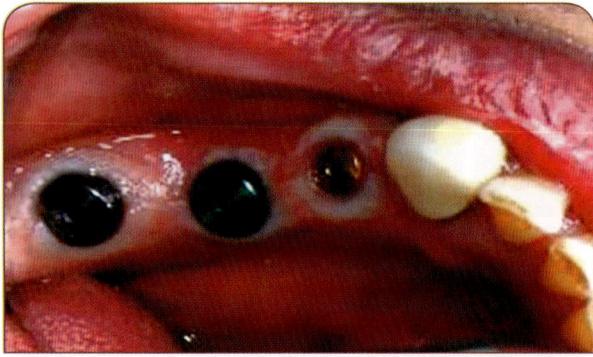

Fig. 1

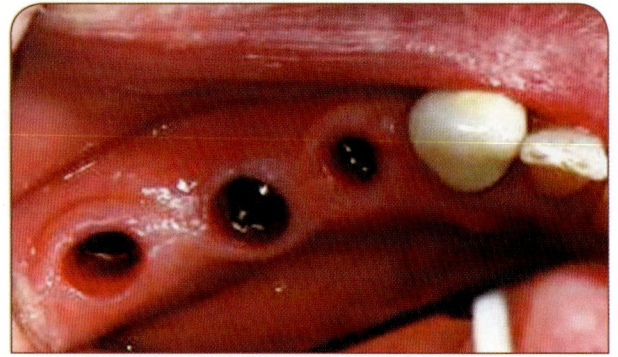

Fig. 2

A 63-year-old white male with failure of natural abutments Left lower quadrant necessitating implant placement after extraction. Implants used: Southern Implants. Lower left posterior following implant healing, ready for restorative phase to begin **(Fig. 1)**.

Healing abutments have been removed demonstrating tissue tunnels through the gingiva to the implant platforms with no inflammation and good keratinization **(Fig. 2)**.

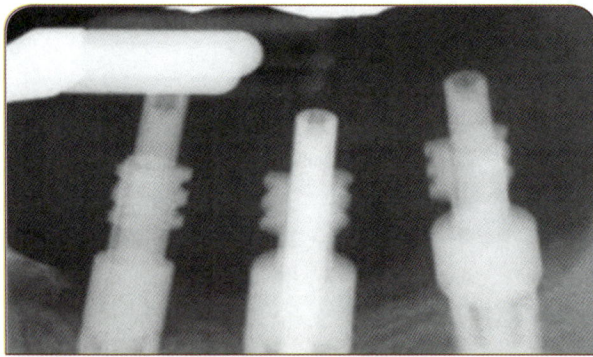

Fig. 3

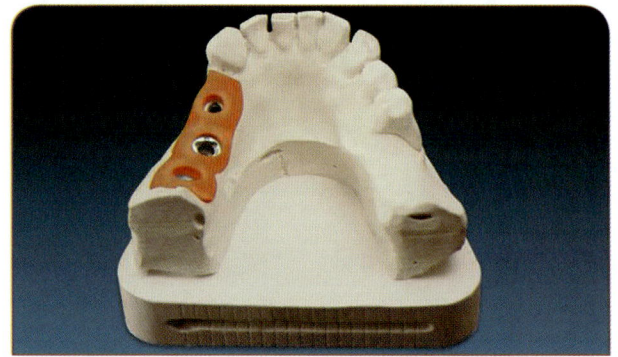

Fig. 4

Open tray impression abutments have been placed and an intraoral radiograph taken to verify mating of the parts to the implant with no gaps **(Fig. 3)**.

Soft tissue model fabricated of the arch containing the implants from the open tray implant impression **(Fig. 4)**.

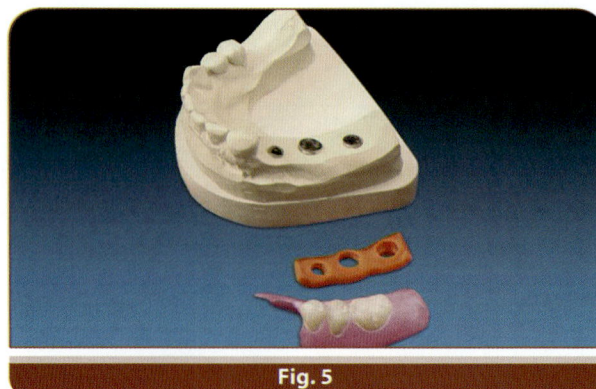

Fig. 5

Soft tissue moulage removed from the implant cast for access to the implant analogs and a wax setup of the teeth to be replaced **(Fig. 5)**.

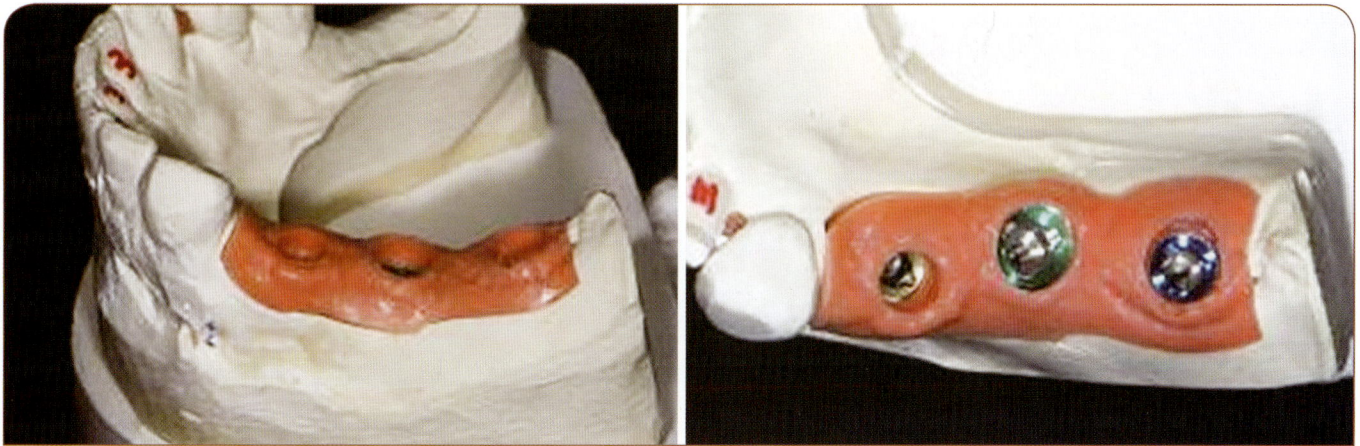

Fig. 6

Soft tissue implant model demonstrating the implant platforms **(Fig. 6)**.

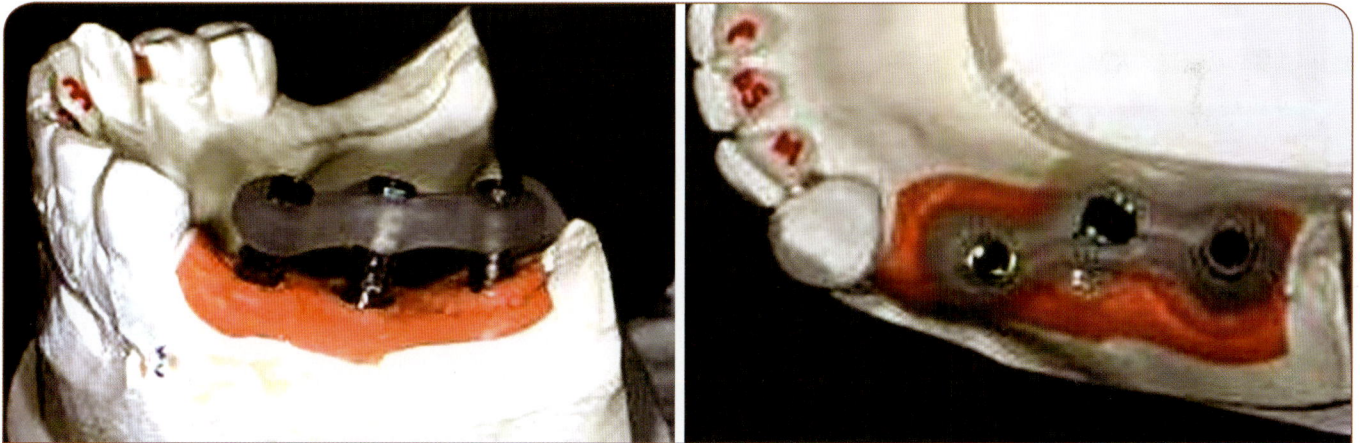

Fig. 7

A verification stent was fabricated using titanium temporary cylinders and acrylic on the soft tissue model to be used to verify accuracy of the impression prior to fabrication of the CAD/CAM milled prosthetic framework **(Fig. 7)**.

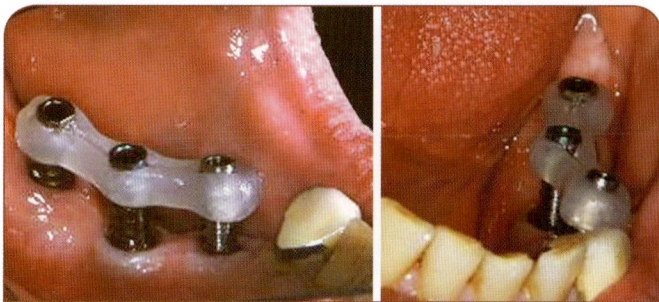

Fig. 8

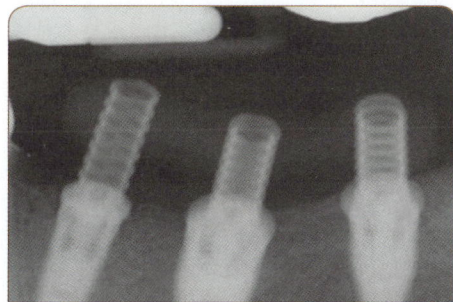

Fig. 9

Verification stent tried intraorally to check accuracy of the soft tissue model that was fabrciated from the open tray implant impression **(Fig. 8)**.

Intraoral radiograph of the verification stent to verify passive and full seating of the verification stent on the implants **(Fig. 9)**.

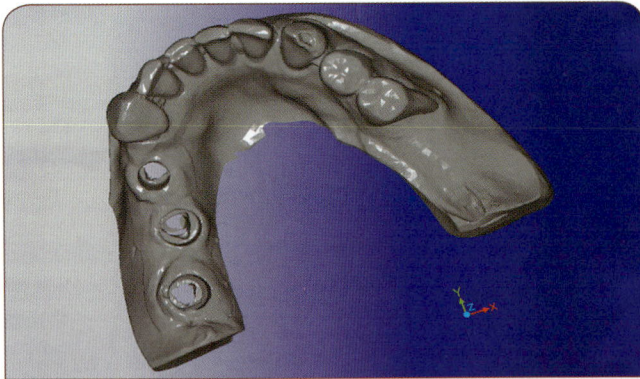

Fig. 10

Virtual model showing implant connectors and positions. Occlusal view **(Fig. 10)**.

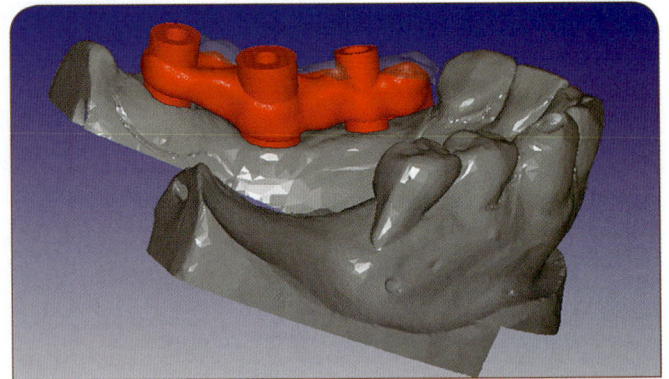

Fig. 11

Virtual model with frame in red and overlay of the teeth (semi transparent). Lingual view. As can be noted the implant positions do not correspond well with the virtual teeth from the waxup and will require modification of the planned prosthesis design prior to milling **(Fig. 11)**.

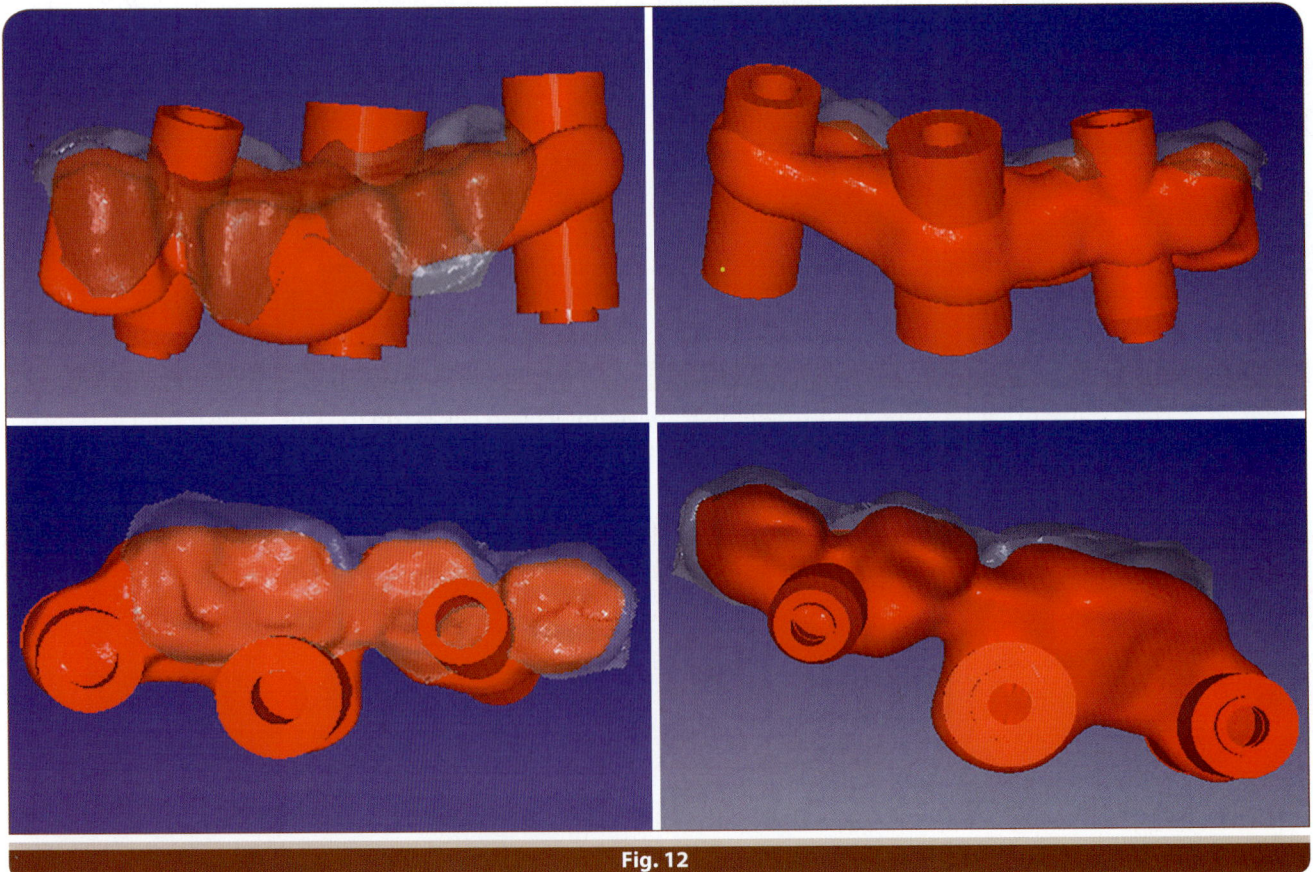

Fig. 12

Virtual frame in red and overlay of the teeth (semi transparent). Buccal, Lingual, Occlusal and Gingival view
As can be noted the implant positions do not correspond well with the virtual teeth from the waxup and will require modification of the planned prosthesis design prior to milling **(Fig. 12)**.

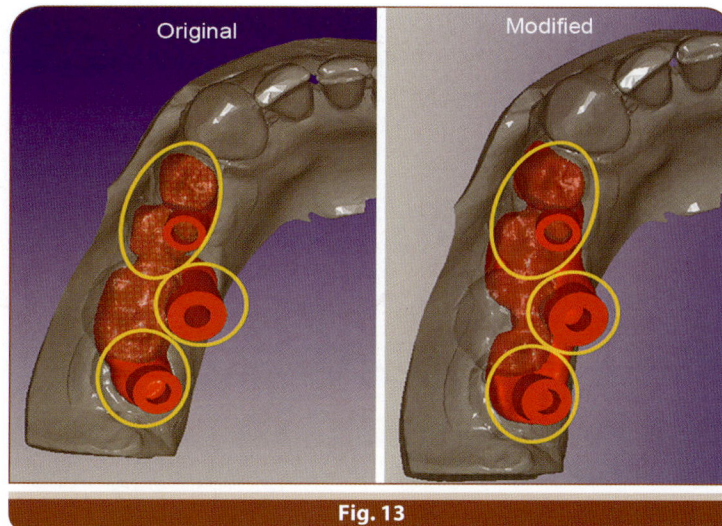

Fig. 13

Virtual model with frame in red and overlay of the teeth (semi transparent). Occlusal view **(Fig. 13)**.

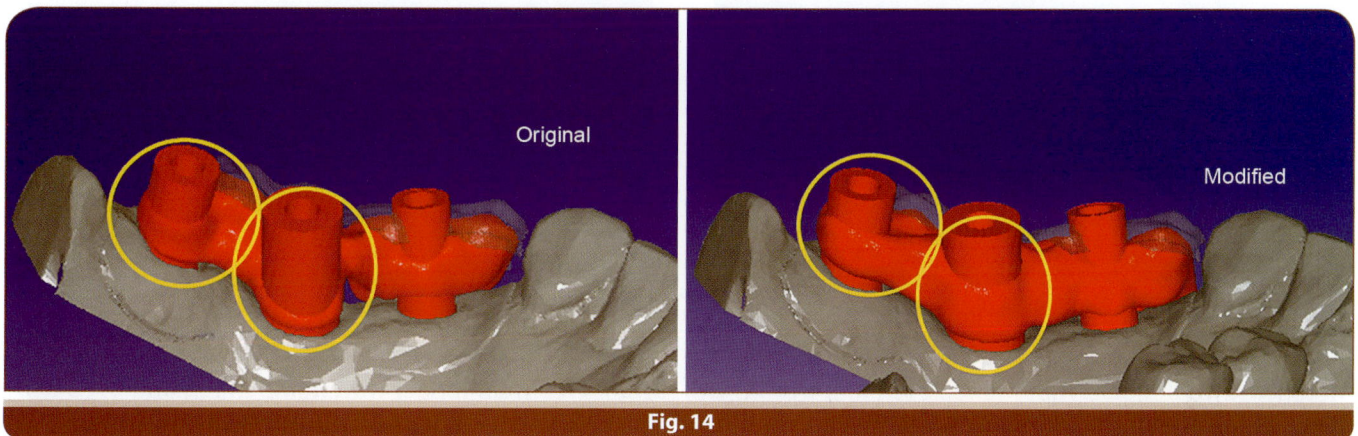

Fig. 14

Virtual model with frame in red and overlay by the teeth (semi transparent). Lingual view **(Fig. 14)**.

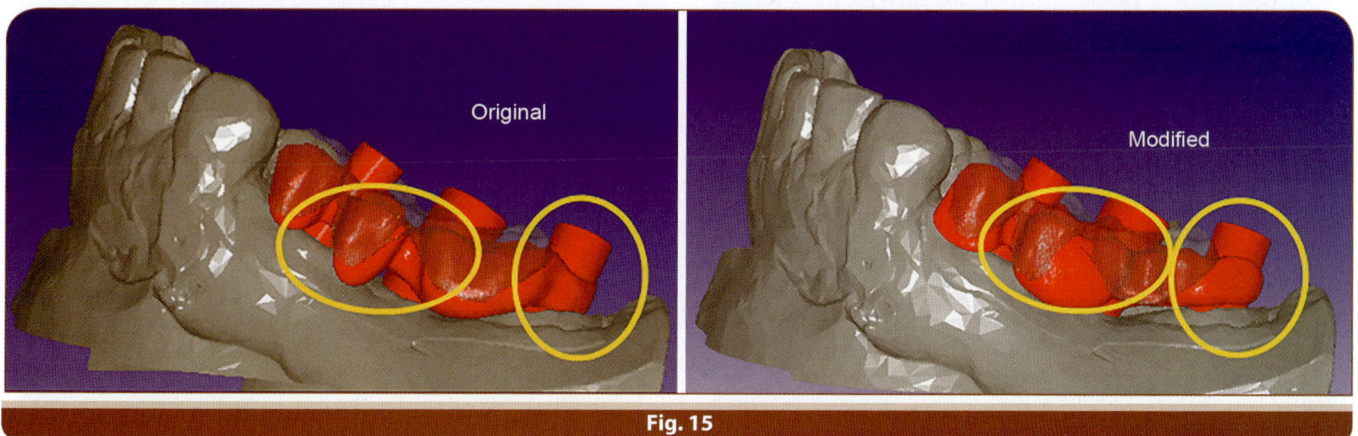

Fig. 15

Virtual model with frame in red and overlay by the teeth (semi transparent). Buccal view **(Fig. 15)**.

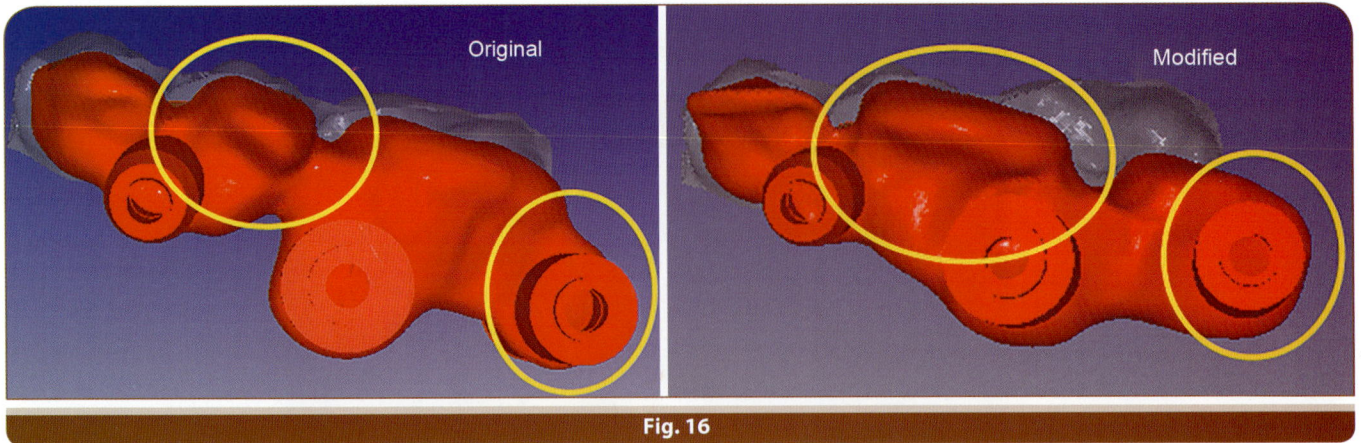

Virtual frame in red and overlay by the teeth (semi transparent). Gingival view **(Fig. 16)**.

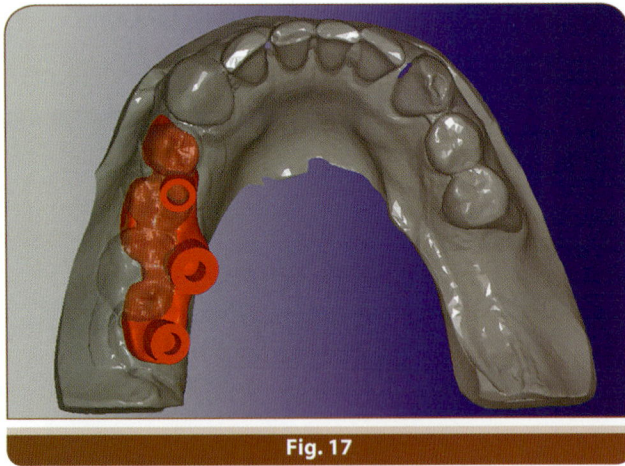

Modified virtual model with frame in red and overlay by the teeth (semi transparent). Occlusal view **(Fig. 17)**.

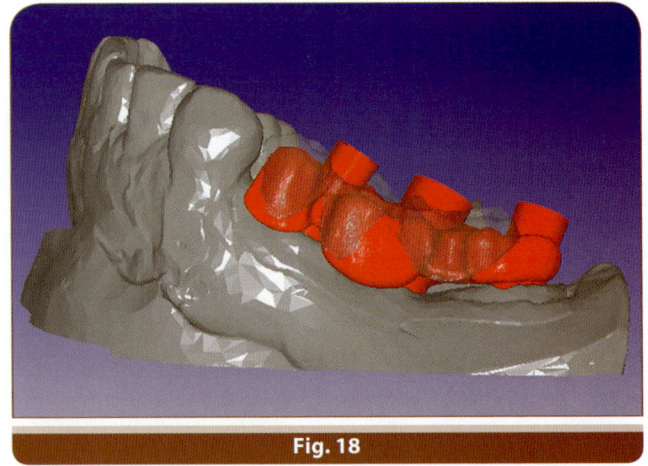

Modified virtual model with frame in red and overlay by the teeth (semi transparent). Buccal view **(Fig. 18)**.

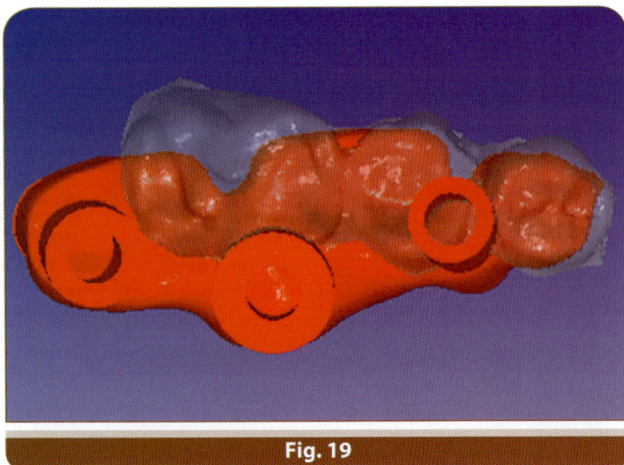

Modified virtual frame in red and overlay by the teeth (semi transparent). Occlusal view **(Fig. 19)**.

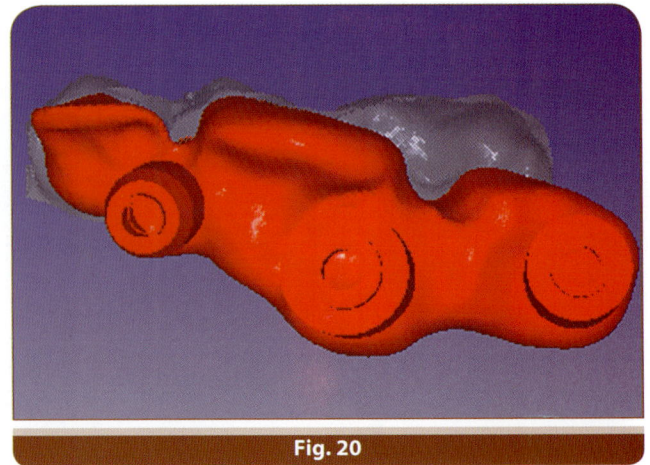

Modified virtual frame in red and overlay by the teeth (semi transparent). Gingival view **(Fig. 20)**.

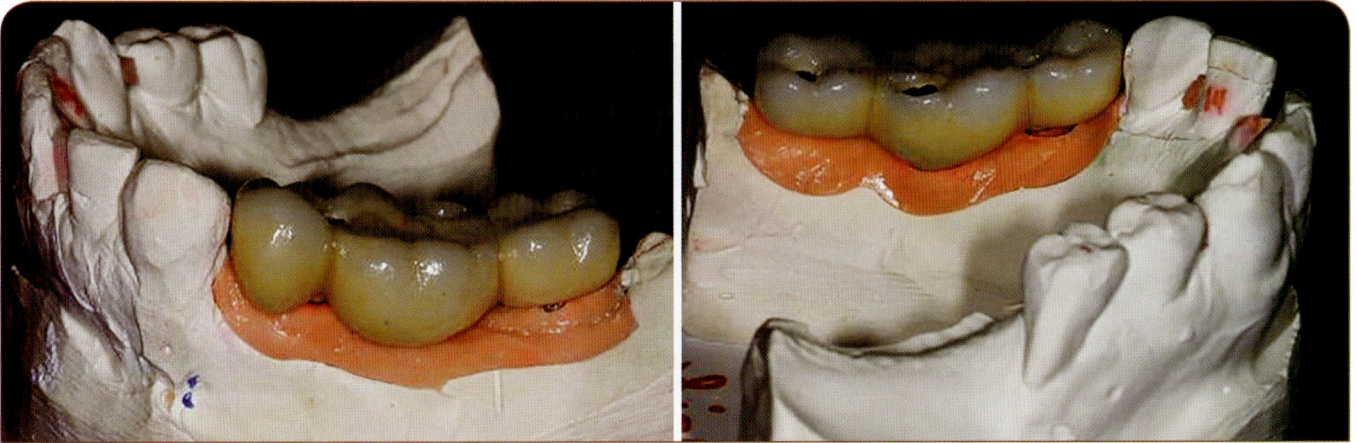

Fig. 21

CAD/CAM milled titanium prosthetic frame for the splinted 3 unit implant prosthesis with porcelain fused to the frame on the soft tissue model. Bridge is a screw retained prosthesis **(Fig. 21)**.

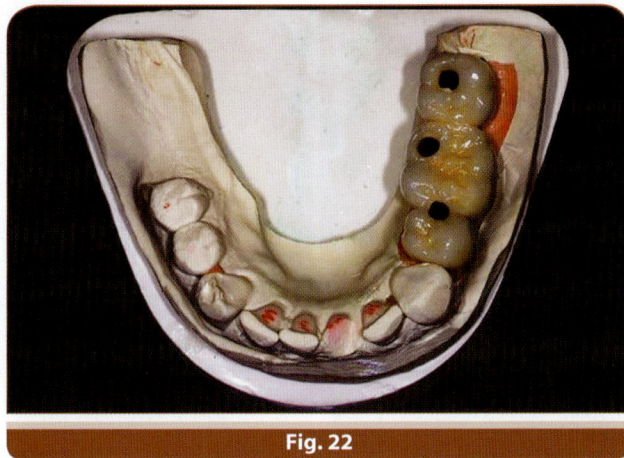

Fig. 22

CAD/CAM milled titanium prosthetic frame for the splinted 3 unit implant prosthesis with porcelain fused to the frame on the soft tissue model. Bridge is a screw retained prosthesis **(Fig. 22)**.

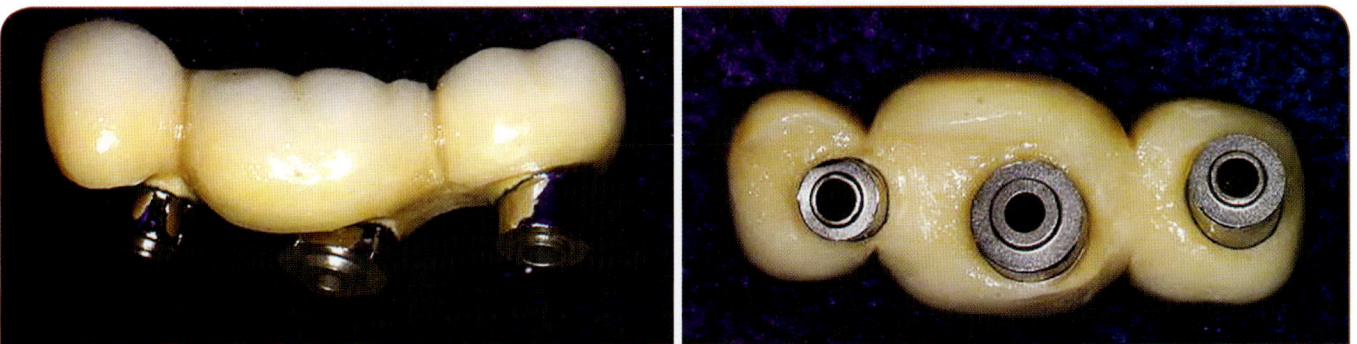

Fig. 23

CAD/CAM milled titanium prosthetic frame for the splinted 3 unit implant prosthesis with porcelain fused to the frame. Bridge is a screw retained prosthesis **(Fig. 23)**.

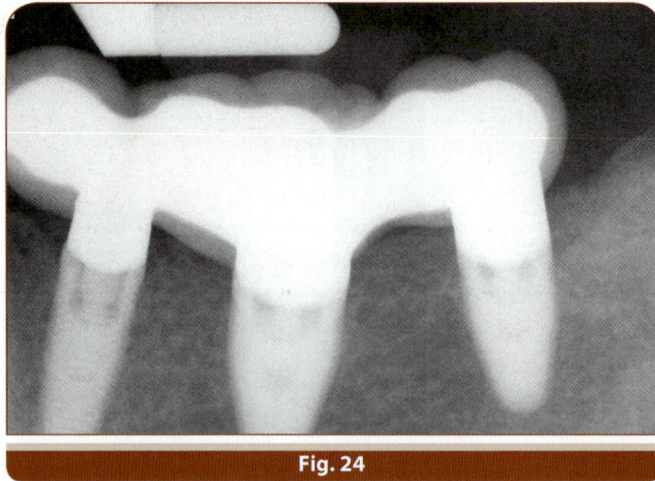

Fig. 24

Radiograph intraorally to verify full seating of the CAD/CAM milled titanium prosthetic frame for the splinted 3 unit implant prosthesis with porcelain fused to the frame **(Fig. 24)**.

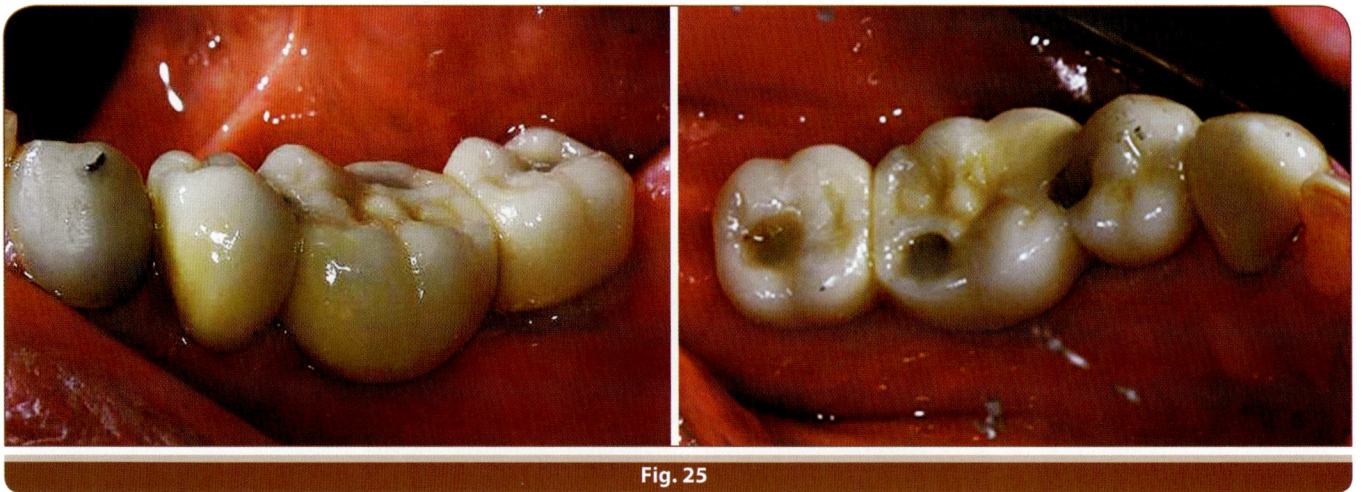

Fig. 25

Inserted CAD/CAM milled titanium prosthetic frame for the splinted 3 unit implant prosthesis with porcelain fused to the frame intraorally. Bridge is a screw retained prosthesis and the screw access holes have been sealed with PTFE tape and a flowable composite resin **(Fig. 25)**.

Gregori M Kurtzman

REPLACEMENT OF A FRACTURED OVERDENTURE BAR WITH A CAD/CAM MILLED LOCATOR BAR OVERDENTURE

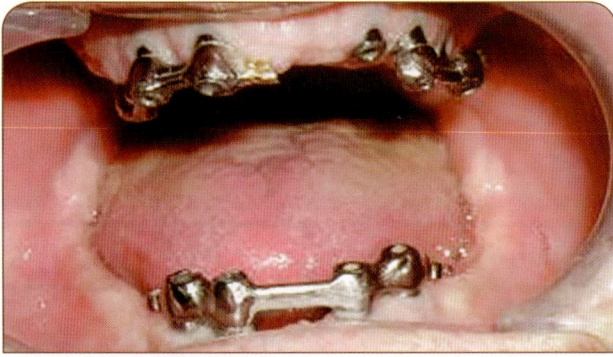

Fig. 1

Patient presented with the chief complaint of broken upper prosthesis. The implants were placed and restored at NYU in 1993. Lower left posterior following implant healing, ready for restorative phase to begin **(Fig. 1)**.

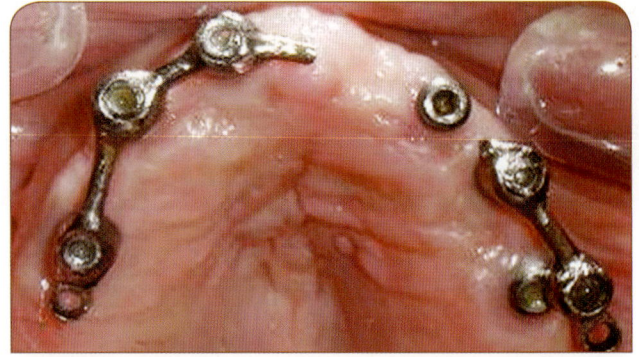

Fig. 2

Appears that the upper was fabricated from stock abutments with stock bars soldered between them. A section of the bar was missing as well as an abutment head and another fixation screw **(Fig. 2)**.

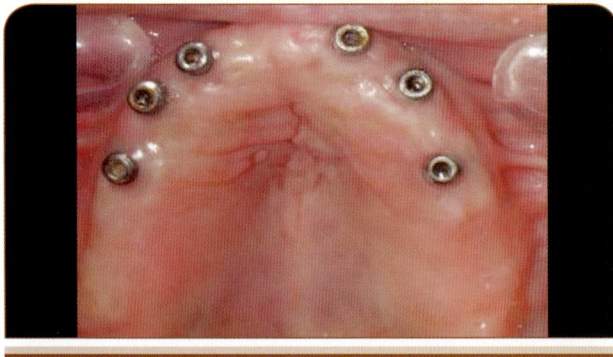

Fig. 3

Implants identified as Corevent's with TSI cemented heads. Old bar was removed and implants checked for mobility. There was no mobility and the soft tissue was healthy **(Fig. 3)**.

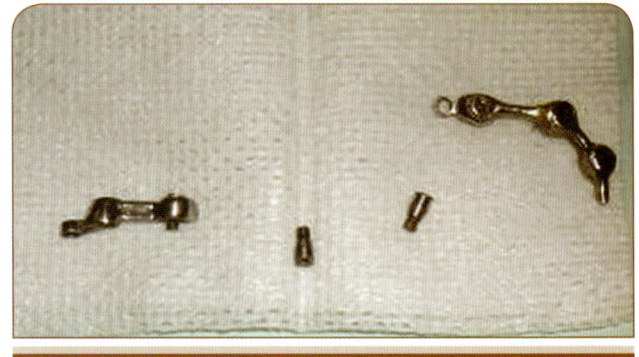

Fig. 4

Portions of the old bar and fixation screws **(Fig. 4)**.

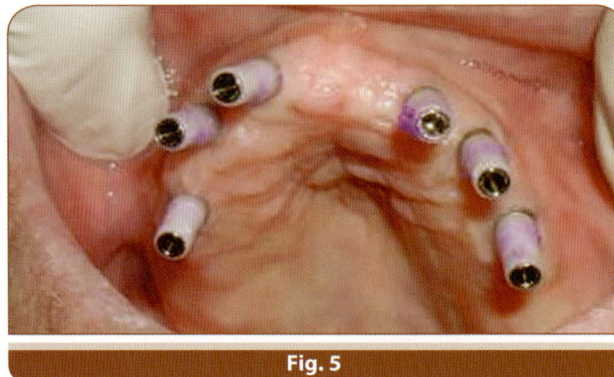

Fig. 5

Since the TSI was only available until 1995 took some effort but was able to locate 6 UCLA sleeves and long pins to use as impression heads. The sleeves were coated with (PVS) adhesive **(Fig. 5)**.

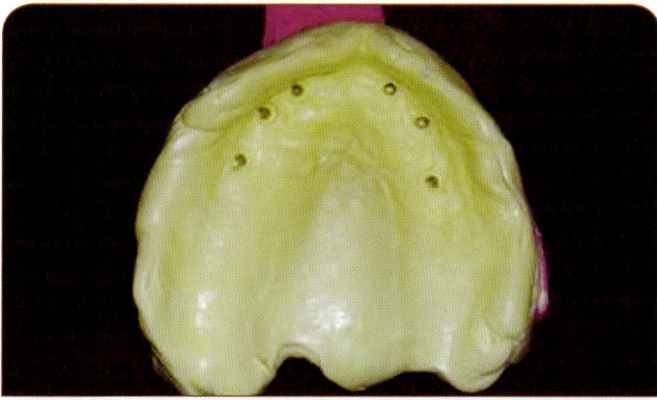

Fig. 6

An open tray impression was taken with a heavy body polyvinyl siloxane (PVS) **(Fig. 6)**.

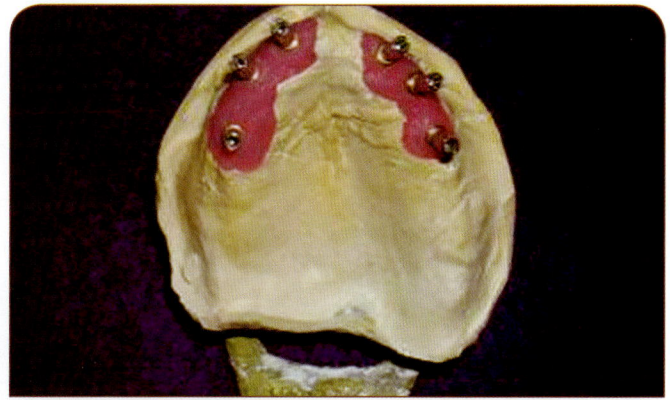

Fig. 7

Soft tissue master model fabricated and long pins shown in place **(Fig. 7)**.

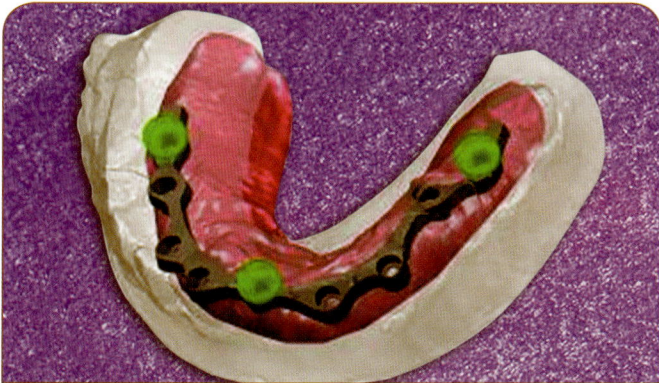

Fig. 8

A virtual scan of the soft tissue model and overlay of a scan of the wax try in previously developed and tried intraorally. The overdenture bar was designed in the PC. The green circles signify Locator attachments **(Fig. 8)**.

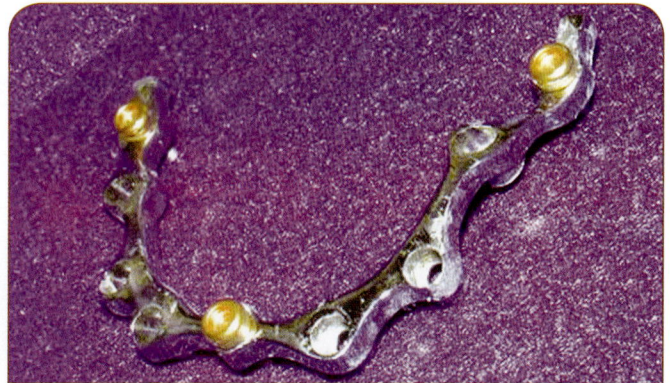

Fig. 9

The final CAD/CAM milled Camstructure bar (Sinlab bar) fabricated from a solid block of titanium. Holes tapped through the bar to accept threaded Locator attachments **(Fig. 9)**.

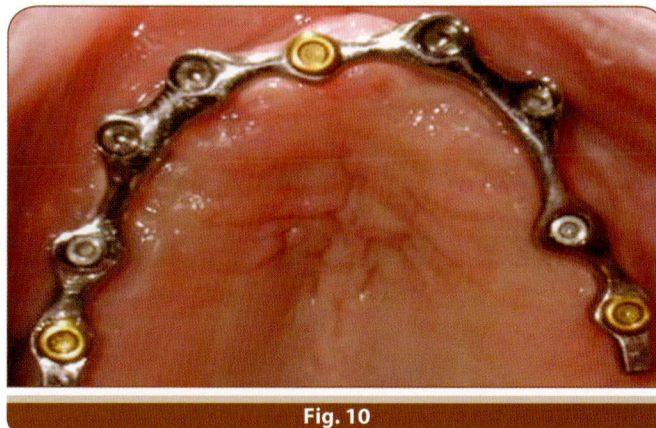

Fig. 10

The finished CAM structure bar intraorally **(Fig. 10)**.

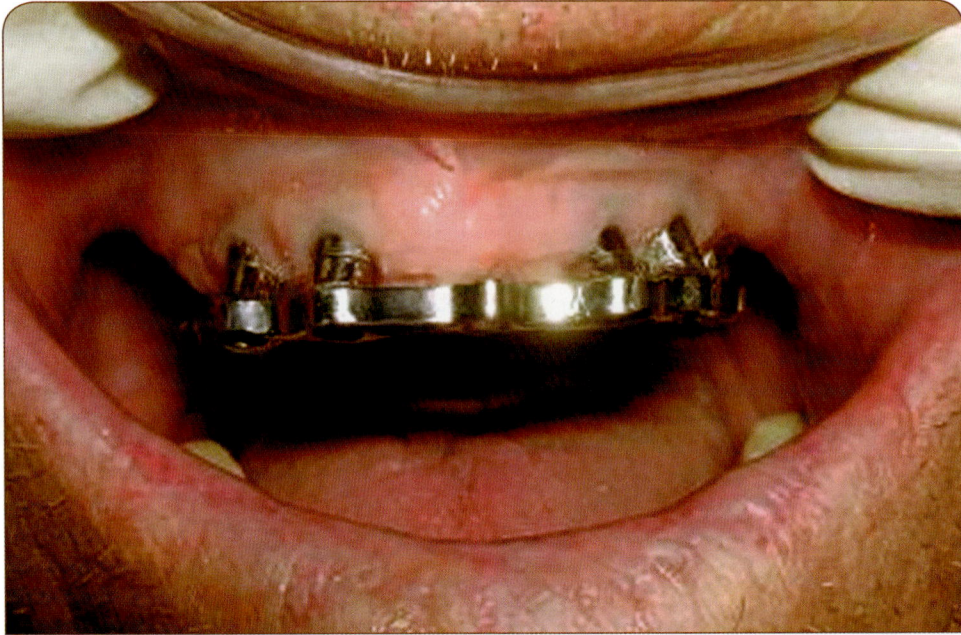

Fig. 11

Buccal view of the inserted CAM structure bar (locators not present in the bar in this view) **(Fig. 11)**.

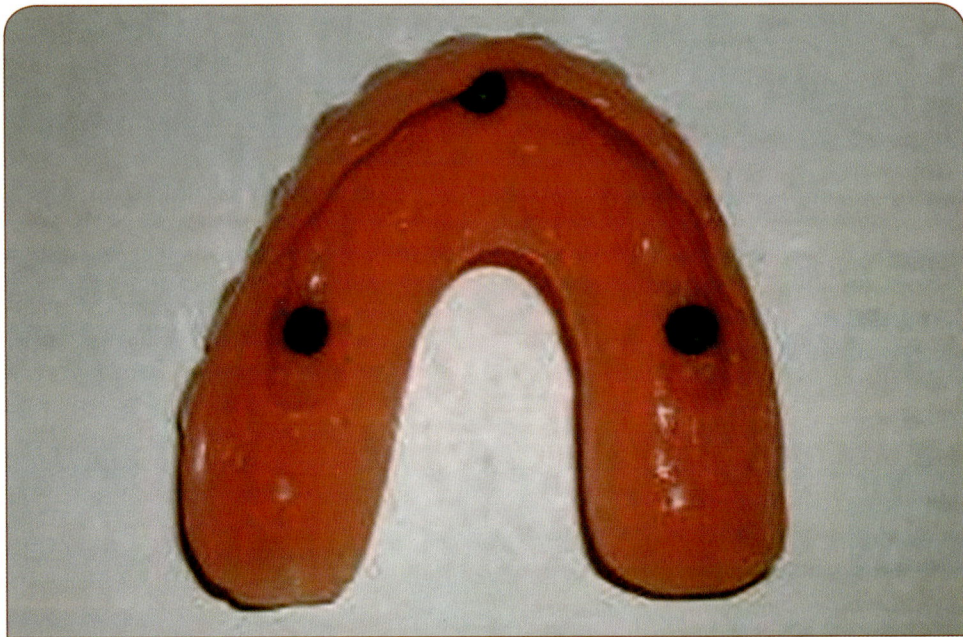

Fig. 12

Internal of the new denture with black processor male locators in their metal housings **(Fig. 12)**.

INDEX